Aging and the Heart

Aging and the Heart

A Post-Genomic View

José Marín-García
Director
The Molecular Cardiology and Neuromuscular Institute
Highland Park, New Jersey

With the collaboration of

Michael J. Goldenthal
Senior Research Scientist
The Molecular Cardiology and Neuromuscular Institute
Highland Park, New Jersey

Gordon W. Moe
Associate Professor
University of Toronto
St. Michael Hospital
Toronto, Canada

Springer

José Marín-García, M.D.
Director, The Molecular Cardiology
and Neuromuscular Institute
Highland Park, New Jersey

ISBN: 978-0-387-74071-3 e-ISBN: 978-0-387-74072-0

Library of Congress Control Number: 2007931956

Printed on acid-free paper.

9 8 7 6 5 4 3 2 1

springer.com

To my wife, Danièle, and daughter Mèlanie, with love

Preface

Cardiac aging, like aging in general, is a complex process involving numerous cellular and molecular changes, which along the way contribute to the expression of the multiple phenotypes of aging, "the different faces" of cardiac aging. Several plausible theories have been considered to explain aging, e.g., evolutionary, free radical, and somatic mutation. However, at this time it is most likely that these different theories are intertwined with each other without a definitive "winner", reflecting a mixture of genetic and epigenetic elements found in most aged individuals with cardiovascular defects. The demonstration in numerous animals models of the dramatic alterations in life span achieved by gene engineering or lifestyle modifications, such as caloric restriction and exercise, further underscores the interplay of both genetic and environmental factors in aging, as well their acting through molecular and signaling pathways operative in the heart and the vasculature.

That aging and decreasing heart function occurred together has been amply documented, and our current knowledge of age-associated cardiac pathologies has outpaced our understanding of the basic mechanisms underlying these processes. At present, Genomic, Proteomic, Recombinant DNA and other techniques are increasingly being applied to study cardiac cells structural and functional changes in diverse pathologies, as well as in aging in general, and in the aging heart in particular. An ever increasing number of animal models have contributed greatly to our understanding of the multiple pathways and molecules participating in the development of cardiovascular aging dysfunction and aging-associated diseases. With the availability of the Human Genome Project and novel and exciting molecular technologies, the unraveling of the underlying basic mechanisms of cardiac aging have already begun.

In preparing this book it has been our major objective to present each chapter as clearly and as comprehensively as possible providing current information available on theories and developmental mechanisms of aging, including biochemical, cellular, molecular, genetic and epigenetic data. The genetic and molecular basis of cardiovascular aging will be thoroughly discussed together with a comprehensive assessment of the bioenergetic changes occurring in human and animal models of cardiac aging, diagnostic progress and future therapeutic modalities.

Besides presenting a detailed review of the most pertinent investigative works from multiple sources, we have also tried to add as much explanatory ideas and concepts generated from our own work on cardiovascular aging. Furthermore, we have discussed what in our opinion is the future of this important field, mainly from the standpoint of basic research. Notwithstanding, we have also acknowledged the great contributions from the past, and are certain they will continue in the future

The chapters in this book have been arranged in a way that the readers can to some degree recognize and appreciate the current thoughts and ideas on the particular field/subject. Furthermore, we have tried to include as much as possible original and creative scientific works, but aware of our limitations we must accept that this is a work still in progress.

We are hopeful that this book will be a valuable guide to aging and the heart from a post-genomic perspective, and also an important introduction to new ideas and future progress. Although we do not expect that this book will make anyone an expert in the field, certainly it will provide a overall-grasp of-theories and perspectives that may shape the present and future understanding of Cardiovascular Aging.

Finally, I want to thank Drs. Goldenthal and Moe for their contribution, for their enthusiasm and for their dedication to make this endeavor all worthy.

"........... Time will pass, inevitably
Death will follow, consequently
After a healthy and productive aging, hopefully"

José Marín-García

Highland Park, NJ

Contents

Part I Introduction to a Post-Genomic View of Aging and the Aging Heart

1 Post-Genomic View of Aging: Definitions, Theories and Observations 3
Overview 3
Definitions 4
Longevity 4
Gene-Longevity Association Studies 4
Longevity Genes from Model Systems 8
Theories of Aging 12
Evolutionary Theories 12
Molecular/Genome Mutations/Deletions Theory 14
Wear-and Tear- Theories 16
(a) FRTA 16
(b) Cross-Linkage Theory 19
(c) DNA-Repair Theory 19
(d) Cellular Garbage Theory 19
(e) The Membrane Theory of Aging 19
(f) The Hayflick Theory 19
Reliability Theory 19
Neuro-Endocrine/Immunological Theory 20
Hormesis and Aging 21
Gender Issues in Aging 21
Advances on Aging and the Genome 22
Epidemiology/Human Populations 24
Population Aging 24
Modifying/ Delaying Aging 25
Is Aging Reversible? 26
References 26

2 Overview of Cardiovascular Aging 33
Overview 33
Introduction 33
Biophysiology of CV Aging 34
Mechanisms/Signaling Pathways in the Aging Heart 35
Telomeres and CV Aging 35
Cellular Damage/Cell Loss, Mitochondria and CV Aging 37
ROS Generation and CV Aging 41
Inflammation and CV Aging 45

Neuroendocrine Mechanisms in CV Aging ... 45
Adrenergic (and Muscarinic) Receptors in the Aging Heart ... 46
Cardiac G Protein-Coupled Receptors ... 47
Thyroid Hormone/SERCA in the Aging Heart ... 48
Growth hormone (GH) and IGF-1 ... 49
Autophagy and CV Aging ... 51
Cardiac Function in Aging ... 52
Genetic Make-up in Cardiac Aging ... 52
Epigenetic and Environmental Factors in Cardiac Aging ... 53
Epidemiology of CV Aging and Population Differences ... 55
Aging is Not a Disease, Rather a Risk Factor ... 56
Modifying/Delaying CV Aging ... 57
Stem Cells and CV Aging ... 58
Dietary and Lifestyle Change ... 58
Conclusion ... 58
Summary ... 59
References ... 60

Part II Methodologies, Cardiac Phenotypes and Adaptation

3 Molecular and Cellular Methodologies: A Primer ... 71
Overview ... 71
Introduction ... 71
Cell Culture: Studying Isolated Cardiomyocytes and Vascular Cells in Aging ... 72
Observations in Endothelial and Smooth Muscle Cells ... 73
Cell and Tissue Transfection and Gene Transfer in Cardiovascular Studies ... 74
Knock-out Transgenic Animal Models ... 77
Gene Profiling: Transcriptome and Proteomic Analysis ... 78
Proteomic Analysis ... 81
DNA Damage and Mutations in Aging ... 83
Types of DNA Damage ... 83
Microsatellite Instability ... 83
Single-Strand versus Double-Strand Damage ... 83
Comet Assay ... 84
DNA Repair Enzymes in Aging ... 85
Mutation Analysis ... 87
Telomere Analysis ... 88
Cell-Engineering and Transplantation ... 89
Tissue Engineering ... 91
Conclusion ... 92
Summary ... 93
References ... 94

4 Molecular and Cellular Phenotypes of Cardiovascular Aging ... 103
Overview ... 103
Introduction: Morphological Changes in the Aging Heart ... 103
Fibrosis ... 105
Apoptosis (Programmed Cell Death), Necrosis and Myocardial Remodeling ... 106
Mitochondria, ETC and ROS ... 110
Autophagy and Cardiac Aging ... 113

Post-translational Changes Associated with Aging 115
Glycation 117
DNA Damage 117
Types of Damage 117
Role of DNA Repair 123
Mitochondrial DNA Repair 128
DNA Repair and Human Diseases of Aging 129
Telomeres and Telomere-related Proteins 131
Conclusion 134
Summary 135
References 135

Part III Aging of the Cardiovasculature and Related Systems

5 Aging of the Vasculature and Related Systems 149
Overview 149
Introduction 149
Arterial Remodeling and Aging 149
Endothelial Cell Function and Remodeling 155
Role of Cell Senescence 155
Mechanisms of Cell Senescence 157
Functional Effects of Endothelial Cell Senescence 158
Endothelial Aging and Oxidative Stress 160
Endothelial Dysfunction is Central to the Vascular Aging Phenotype 162
Aging and Vascular Smooth Muscle Cells (SMCs) 162
Mechanisms and Significance of Vascular SMC Senescence 164
Markers of SMC in Aging and Aging-Related Diseases 165
Thrombosis, Fibrinolysis and Inflammation in Aging 166
Angiogenesis/Neovascularization in Aging 168
Conclusion 169
Summary 169
References 170

6 Aging and the Cardiovascular-Related Systems 181
Overview 181
Introduction 181
The Aging Immune System 182
Aging and Neurohormonal Regulation 191
Aging and Skeletal Muscle 194
Aging and the Blood-Brain Barrier 196
Conclusion 198
Summary 199
References 200

Part IV Cardiovascular Diseases in Aging

7 Cardiomyopathy and Heart Failure in Aging 209
Overview 209
Introduction 209

Clinical Considerations 209
Etiology and Precipitating Factors 209
Clinical Presentation and Diagnostic Challenges 210
Pharmacotherapy of Heart Failure in the Elderly 211
Disease Management Programs for Heart Failure in the Elderly 212
Device and Replacement Therapy in the Elderly 212
Pathophysiologic Considerations 213
Basic Mechanisms Mediating Aging-Related Cardiac Dysfunction and Heart Failure 213
Myocardial Remodeling and Aging 213
Genomics 216
HCM 216
DCM and RCM 218
Animal Models of Cardiomyopathy and HF 222
Conclusion 230
Summary 230
References 231

8 Atherosclerosis, Hypertension and Aging 239
Overview 239
Introduction 239
Lipoprotein Oxidation and Modification 244
Inflammation and Atherosclerosis 246
The Cap of the Atherosclerotic Lesion and its Rupture 250
Biomarkers 250
Gene Expression Profiling and Atherosclerosis 251
Therapeutic Approaches 254
The Role of Altered Immunity in Atherosclerosis in Aging 255
Acute Coronary Syndrome in the Elderly 256
Myocarditis in the Elderly Population 258
Hypertension in the Elderly 259
Genetics and Environmental Factors in Essential or Primary Hypertension 261
Identification of Primary Risk Genes and Candidate Genes in Essential Hypertension 262
Conclusion 264
Summary 264
References 265

9 Metabolic Syndrome, Diabetes and Cardiometabolic Risks in Aging 277
Overview 277
Introduction 277
The Metabolic Syndrome and the Concept of Cardiometabolic Risks 278
The Effects of CB1 Blockade on Cardiometabolic Risk 280
Clinical Management and Trials with Metabolic Syndrome 281
Cardiometabolic Risk Factor in the Elderly 282
Endogenous Sex Hormones and Metabolic Syndrome in the Elderly 283
Leptin and Metabolic Syndrome in the Elderly 284
Metabolic Syndrome and Oxidative Stress in the Elderly 284
Cardiac Remodeling and Insulin Resistance in the Elderly 285
Cardiometabolic Risk Factors and Cardiovascular Disease in the Elderly 286

Metabolic Syndrome, Diabetes and Cognitive Decline in the Elderly 286
Genes Involved in Metabolic Syndrome 289
Diabetes in the Elderly 291
Genes Associated with Diabetes 291
Relationship Between Metabolic Syndrome and Diabetes 294
Conclusion 295
Summary 295
References 296

10 Gender and Cardiovascular Diseases in Aging 307
Overview 307
Introduction 307
Gender Effect/Mechanisms on Specific CVDs 308
Cell Death 309
Age-Associated CVDs and Gender 309
Heart Failure (HF) 309
Dysrhythmias 313
Cardiac Hypertrophy 316
Hypertension 318
Coronary Artery Disease (CAD) 320
Gender and Specific CV Markers 324
Cardiac Troponin (cTn) 324
C-reactive Protein 324
Phospholipase A(2) 325
E-selectin/Atherosclerosis 325
Lipid Peroxides (LPO) 326
Mitochondria 326
Resistin 327
Adiponectin 327
Gender-Specific Gene Profiling 327
Gene Polymorphisms in Gender-Specific Age-Related CVDs 327
Pharmacogenomics and Gender 328
Conclusions 329
Summary 330
References 331

11 Cardiac Dysrhythmias and Channelopathies in Aging 339
Overview 339
Introduction 339
Sympathetic Nerve System in Aging 340
Electrophysiological Studies in Animal Models of Aging 341
Atrial Dysrhythmias 342
Sinoatrial Node Dysfunction (SND) 342
Atrioventricular Nodal Reentrant Tachycardia (AVNRT) 343
Atrial Fibrillation 344
AV Conduction in Aging 345
LQT and Sudden Death 346
Syncope/Tilt Test 350
Pacer Therapy in the Elderly 351
Advanced Heart Failure 351

Pacemaker Implantation as an Adjunct Therapy for Atrial Fibrillation 352
Ventricular Dysrhythmias 352
Premature Ventricular Beats 352
Ventricular Tachycardia (VT) 353
Ventricular Fibrillation (VF) 354
Dysrhythmogenic Right Ventricular Dysplasia in the Elderly (DRVD) 354
Antidysrhythmic Therapy in Aging 355
Channelopathies 355
Introduction to Channelopathies 355
Calcium and Potassium Currents 355
Sarcolemmal K_{ATP} Channels in Aging 356
Calcium Channels 357
Connexins 358
KCNQ Potassium Channel 359
Mitochondrial Channels 359
Ion Channels/Transporters in Mitochondria 360
Mitochondrial Ca^{2+}-Channels/Transporter 360
Mitochondrial Ca^{2+} Cycling 361
Ca^{2+} Transporter in Aging 361
Mitochondrial K^+ Channels 364
K^+ Uniporter/$K_{\mathbf{ATP}}$ Channel 364
Mitochondrial K_{ATP} Channel in Aging 365
Mitochondrial PTP 367
Mitochondrial PTP in Aging 367
Pharmacogenetics/Pharmacogenomics in Dysrhythmias/Channelopathies of Aging ... 370
Pharmacogenetics and Pharmacogenomics 370
Conclusions 371
Summary 372
References 375

Part V Genetics

12 Genetics of Life Span: Lessons from Model Organisms 387
Overview 387
Introduction 387
Insulin/IGF-1 Pathway in *C. elegans* 388
Insulin/IGF Signaling in Other Eucaryotes 390
Tissue-Specific Roles of Insulin/IGF-Signaling 392
Metabolic Pathways Involved in Longevity in *C. elegans* 392
SIR/Sirtuins 395
TOR 397
Other Genetic Factors in Aging Drosophila 398
Mouse Models of Aging 401
Models for Premature Aging Syndromes and Progeria 404
Conclusion 406
Summary 406
References 407

13 Profiling the Aging Cardiovascular System: Transcriptional, Proteomic, SNPs, Gene Mapping and Epigenetics Analysis 417
Overview 417
Introduction 417
Transcriptional Gene Profiling 418
Normal Aging Studies 418
Age-associated Myocardial Transcription Responses to Oxidative and Ischemic Stress 420
CR in Heart and Skeletal Muscle 422
Transcriptome Profiling in Age-associated Cardiac Diseases 424
Proteomic Analysis 425
Cell Proteomics in Aging 427
Genetics of Aging 429
Mapping of Genes Involved in Aging 429
Genome Wide Scans 429
SNP Analysis in Aging and Aging Associated Disease Susceptibility 430
Lipoproteins (APOE) 430
ACE 431
KLOTHO 431
Epigenetics 432
DNA Methylation 432
Chromatin Modifications 432
Conclusion 433
Summary 434
References 435

Part VI Therapies

14 Translational Research: Gene, Pharmacogenomics and Cell-Based Therapy in the Aging Heart 443
Overview 443
Introduction 443
Primary Targets in Reversing Cardiovascular and Cardiac Aging Damage 444
Attenuating Cell Death and Remodeling 444
Initiating Pro-Survival Pathways 446
Modulation of Cardioprotection Pathways as a Potential Strategy 447
Attenuating the Generation of OS and Reducing ROS 450
Directly Targeting Mitochondrial Dysfunction and Structural Defects 452
Removing "Biological Garbage" (Targeting Lysosomes, Proteasomes and Other Approaches for Enhancing Catabolic Remediation) 455
Targeting the Nucleus 457
Genomic Instability 459
Attack at the Level of Transcription 460
Targeting the Sarcomere and SR 461
Conclusion and New Horizons 461
Summary 462
References 463

15 Nutrition and Exercise in Cardiovascular Aging: Metabolic and Pharmacological Interventions ... 471
Overview ... 471
Introduction ... 471
Caloric Restriction (CR) ... 472
Overview of CR in Comparative Models ... 472
Tissue-Specific and Cardiovascular-Specific Transcriptional and Proteomic Profiling of CR ... 472
CR in Heart and Skeletal Muscle ... 472
Specific Pathways Affected ... 473
Oxidative Stress and ROS ... 473
Mitochondria Function and Biogenesis ... 474
MtDNA Damage and Repair ... 476
Genomic Instability ... 477
IGF/Growth Hormone/SIR Involvement ... 477
Vascular Inflammation ... 480
Dissection of the CR Process: Which Aspect of the Diet Does the Signaling ... 481
Development of CR Mimetics ... 482
Resveratrol Studies ... 482
Conclusions ... 484
New Directions ... 484
Pharmacological Reversal of Aging ... 484
Role of Exercise ... 485
Gene Profiling ... 485
Specific Pathways Affected ... 486
Ischemia/Reperfusion/Apoptosis/Remodeling ... 486
Mitochondrial Function and Stress Responses ... 487
Myocardial Signaling ... 487
Vasodilatation/Endothelial-Dependent Effects ... 488
Clinical Applications of Exercise ... 488
Summary ... 489
References ... 490

Part VII The Future of Aging Research

16 Aging and the Frontier Ahead ... 499
Overview ... 499
Introduction ... 499
New Focus on Genetic Analysis in Aging Research ... 500
Animal Models: Can Simpler Models Suffice? ... 500
Advances in Human Genotyping and Gene Analysis ... 501
Longevity and Frailty Genes ... 501
Methods of Genetic Analysis ... 502
Mitochondrial DNA and Aging ... 504
Cellular Models ... 505
Search for Biomarkers of Human Aging ... 506
Systems Biology: Improved Networking-Enlarging the Perspective ... 513
Reversing Aging and/or Dysfunction of Age-Associated Diseases ... 516
Targeting Cellular Atrophy and Depletion in Aging ... 517

Stem Cells as both Primary Targets of Aging and a Potential Treatment Plan 518
Targeting Specific Organelles in Aging: Mitochondria/Lysosome 521
Pharmacogenomics and Nutrigenomics 523
Conclusion 524
Summary 525
References 526

Glossary 539

Index 559

Part I
Introduction to a Post-Genomic View of Aging and the Aging Heart

Chapter 1
Post-Genomic View of Aging: Definitions, Theories and Observations

Overview

From birth to death, aging is a continuous and extremely complex multifactorial process that involves the interaction of genetic, epigenetic and environmental factors, and in which the incidence of diseases increases as well as the possibility of dying. The variability of the aging phenotype among individuals of the same species as well as the variability in longevity among species strongly suggests the mediating influence of both genetic and environmental factors in dictating the life span. For example, several genetic polymorphisms are known to confer extreme longevity in animal models, and a number of observations suggest that similar polymorphisms may operate in humans. The spectrum of the aging phenotype may vary from disease and disability to absence of pathology and preservation of function. At present, humans over age 65 are more likely to be active and productive than at any other time in history and life expectancy, disability rates, and health and wealth indicators have all shown significant improvement in the last 25 years. The US census bureau reported that average life expectancy in 2004 was 77.9 years, up from about 47.3 in 1900 with a projection of 79.2 years for 2015. This increase appears to be largely due to improvements in health care, nutrition, and overall standard of living for most people. Furthermore, recent observations have shown that good health, with a balanced emotional state in early life may be associated with greater longevity, although further research is needed to understand this connection. On the other hand, healthy, comfortable older age continues to elude many individuals, particularly members of certain racial, ethnic, and socio-economic groups.

Rather than individual chronological age, aging may be more closely related to epigenetic and environmental factors, including stress and the absence of disease. The aging human populations may develop different physiological or anatomical defects and may die from different age-dependent diseases. Diseases such as Alzheimer disease, cardiovascular disease, osteoporosis, cancer, diabetes, and arthritis, affect too many older men and women, and seriously compromises the quality of their lives.

At present, in spite of intensive interest and significant progress in aging research, there is not yet a universal agreement on one specific theory of aging. On the contrary, the number of theories is large, some more favored by investigators than others, although in the final analysis many if not all of these theories may work together. In this chapter, an outline of common but important definitions of age and aging, together with an analysis of the better-known theories, gender differences, and epidemiological information on aging will be presented.

J. Marín-García, *Aging and the Heart*,

Definitions

Life Span, the length of time lived by the individual.

Life span can mean:

Life expectancy, the average life span expected of a group.
Maximum life span, the maximum life span observed in a group under ideal conditions.
Mean or average life span, statistical description of the expected life span.
Longevity, the length of the individual life span with survival beyond the average life span for that particular species/race.
Chronological life span, the number of years since birth/Life span in units of time.

Organismal Senescence, the gathering of the processes of deterioration, which follow the period of development.
Cellular senescence, the phenomenon where cells lose the ability to divide (involving DNA damage, including shortening of telomeres, and cells either senesce, or self-destruct [via apoptosis] if the damage cannot be repaired).
Biological age, age assessed by biological markers (e.g., telomere length).
Gerontology, the study of aging.
Geriatrics, the study of the diseases of the aging.

Longevity

Longevity is a multifactorial quantitative trait that refers to the life span expected of an individual or species, extending from birth to death. According to Luciani et al. [1] longevity contains a chance or probability component resulting from the interaction between chances of survival and unpredictable events that occur throughout life. Environmental changes that reduce mortality, e.g., advances in medicine, have a profound impact on the individual life span [2]. In developed countries advances in the treatment of severe diseases, including cardiovascular diseases (CVD), and improvements in nutrition and living conditions (environmental hygiene, social welfare and healthcare systems) have led to a dramatic reduction in the death rate at young ages before 1950, and at old ages after 1950 [3]. As a result, the mean life span has experienced a remarkable increase in the developed world where more and more people are celebrating their 100th birthday; however, there is not yet a clear explanation for the heterogeneity of the life span. Why do some people reach advanced ages while others do not? To answer this question one must look at individual factors such as lifestyle, behavior, socio-economic background and the individual genetic make-up [2].

Gene-Longevity Association Studies

In the study of longevity, late-death ($\geq$ than 90 years old) is of great interest since it might be the result of successful aging. Furthermore, families with long-living individuals may offer an important contribution toward understanding the inherited/familial component of longevity. Using twin data several investigators have observed a correlation between genetics and life span, and evidence that longevity tends to aggregate in families have been reported [4–7]. In 1998, Perls et al. found that the chances for survival until 80–94 years old by siblings of centenarian was four times as high as those for siblings of individuals at 73 years of age [4]. More recently, these investigators reported that compared with 1900 birth cohort survival data from the US, male siblings of centenarians were at least 17 times as likely to attain age 100 themselves, while female siblings were at least 8 times as likely [8]. Nevertheless, and in spite of these interesting observations, the basis for the genetic component to confer human longevity still remains largely undefined.

Elegant genetic studies from simpler organisms (e.g., yeast, *C. elegans*) have identified a number of highly-conserved factors, which not only have been shown to modulate life span in a large number of animal models, but also have functional homologues in humans; these include specific growth factors (GH, IGF-1), receptors, signaling mediators, transcriptional factors and players in chromatin remodeling. Of particular interest, is that nearly all the factors identified thus far have demonstrable effect on cardiac and cardiovascular function, and can modulate the cell's responsiveness to Oxidative Stress (OS). The conservation of these elements in evolution has allowed these simpler models of cellular aging to be surrogate models for further identification of genes and factors involved in the aging pathways, as well as the elucidation of a number of environmental factors, which can either retard or accelerate aging, including nutrients and stress stimuli. On the other hand, these observations have also showed species-specific variations, which caution against the wholesale translation of findings from other systems to human. Benedictis et al [2]. in their review article on human gene-longevity association studies suggested that in the assessment of the genetics of longevity two major arguments should to be taken into account. The first involves the definition of the phenotype. Longevity is, in fact, the net outcome of cumulative mortality over all age-classes, and cumulative mortality is historically controlled. Second, classical approaches to the study of human genetics, which are aimed at detecting co-segregation of genetic markers in pedigrees, are not easy to implement since this requires the sampling of pedigrees that include two or more very old individuals, possibly in more than one generation, which is a rare occurrence. According to these investigators, this difficulty applies equally to parametric (lod score) and non-parametric (sib-pair) methods of assessing linkage. Moreover, the continuous changes in environmental and life style conditions render a direct comparison between the age of death of parents and that of their offspring virtually meaningless. Gene-longevity association studies of unrelated individuals, which search for non-random associations between polymorphisms at candidate loci and aging, are the most frequent type reported in the literature. Although we must recognize that different studies may display dissimilar results, negative findings for genes whose variants are well-known risk factors in age-related diseases have been found. Since 1990, several studies have been published, in which a number of gene polymorphisms showed a significant correlation with longevity, and reduced incidence of CVD as depicted in Table 1.1. For example, the TLR4 ASP299GLY polymorphism has a significantly lower frequency in patients affected by myocardial infarction compared to controls, whereas centenarians show a higher frequency for this allele [9]. These data are suggestive that people genetically predisposed to developing weak inflammatory activity, seem to have fewer chances of developing CVD and subsequently live longer if they do not become affected by serious infectious diseases. These findings are also in agreement with increasing data showing how the genetic background may exert the opposite effect with respect to inflammatory components in CVD and longevity, as discussed in a later chapter.

Santoro et al. [27] have recently evaluated the involvement of mitochondrial DNA (mtDNA) in human longevity since aging and longevity, as complex traits that have a significant genetic component, likely depend on a number of nuclear gene variants interacting with mtDNA variability, both inherited and somatic. This analysis revealed that the genetics for complex traits, including aging and longevity, is more complicated than previously thought. For instance, suppression of specific gene effects on phenotype by nonallelic genes (epistasis) has been documented between nuclear gene polymorphisms and mtDNA variability (both somatic and inherited), as well as between mtDNA somatic mutations (tissue specific) and mtDNA inherited variants (haplogroups and sub-haplogroups); therefore, these multiple interactions must be considered as additional players capable of explaining in part the aging and the longevity phenotype. We agree with these investigators that testing this hypothesis is one of the main challenges in the genetics of aging and longevity. It is well established that mitochondria are major producers of reactive oxygen species (ROS) in cells, and that

Table 1.1 Human genes whose polymorphisms is associated with longevity

Gene	Function	Disease associated	References
ApoE	Lipoprotein metabolism	AD, CVD	10–14
ApoB	Cholesterol homeostasis (LDL)	CAD	11, 15–16
ACE	Angiotensin converting enzyme	MI, AD, EH	13, 17
Fibrinogen	Plasma coagulation factor	CAD	18
Prothrombin	Blood coagulation	MI	18
ND2 (nt5178) of mtDNA	NADH dehydrogenase subunit 2, OXPHOS	MI, atherogenesis in diabetes	19–21
J haplotype of mtDNA	Not determined	Mitochondrial diseases (LHON), AD	22, 23
C150T of mtDNA	MtDNA replication	None	24, 25
TLR4 ASP299GLY	Toll-R receptor involved in innate immunity	MI	9
GH1	Growth hormone/ Insulin/IGF-1 signaling	Not determined	26

AD: Alzheimer disease; CAD: Coronary artery disease; CVD: Cardiovascular disease; EH: Essential hypertension; MI: Myocardial infarction; MtDNA: Mitochondrial DNA; GH, growth hormone

organelle dysfunction may lead to metabolic defects in both vascular and smooth muscle cells with resulting vascular dysfunction. What is less well known is that mtDNA polymorphisms may play a significant role in aging and senescence. Takagi et al. [20] have found that a C to A transversion in mtDNA at nucleotide 5178 of the NADH dehydrogenase subunit 2 (ND2) gene, resulting in a Leu/Met substitution at amino acid 237, was more frequently present in Japanese centenarians than in controls, and in subsequent studies demonstrated that the C5178A polymorphism was associated with anti-atherosclerotic effects in diabetic subjects [21]. To determine whether the C5178A (Leu237Met) polymorphism in the mitochondrial ND2 gene is associated with a low prevalence of myocardial infarction (MI) in a case-control study, the genotype of ND2 gene was assessed either with a polymerase chain reaction-restriction fragment length polymorphism (PCR-RFLP) or by a colorimetry-based allele-specific DNA probe assay.

Multivariate logistic regression analysis with adjustment for age, gender, body mass index, smoking status, hypertension, diabetes mellitus, hypercholesterolemia, and hyperuricemia demonstrated that the frequency of the 5178A genotype was significantly higher in controls than in subjects with MI. Taken together, these findings suggest that the 5178A genotype of mitochondrial ND2 gene polymorphism is protective against MI and it may also explain, at least in part, its contribution to longevity.

In contrast, polymorphisms at PAI-1 loci, encoding the plasminogen activator inhibitor type 1 are associated with an increased risk of ischemic heart disease in elderly men [28], consistent with findings of high PAI-1 activity in populations with angina pectoris [29] and in post–MI patients [30]. However, the impact of moderately increased PAI-1 activities associated with the PAI-1 4G/4G have failed to show any significant effect on mortality in the general population [28]. It is well-established that the 4G/5G polymorphism affects PAI-1 gene transcription with lower levels of plasma PAI-1 in the presence of the 5G allele, while the 4G/4G genotype is associated with higher PAI-1 levels. Moreover, in a population-based study of Dutch elderly (with a follow-up of 7.8 years) assessing the relative risks for cardiovascular events and all-cause mortality with respect to PAI-1 activity and 4G/5G genotype, the 4G/4G genotype was unexpectedly associated with a decreased risk of stroke, transient ischemic attack and cardiovascular mortality [31]. In addition, subjects with high plasma PAI-1 activity were at increased risk of stroke, CV mortality and all cause mortality. Thus, these findings suggest that the 4G allele appeared to provide protective effect against stroke, perhaps as a result of the associated inhibition of fibrinolysis leading to atherosclerotic plaque stabilization and increased neutralization of potentially neurotoxic tPA. Gene/longevity association studies for those genes whose variability contributes significantly to general mortality, may be better assessed by cross-sectional analysis [2].

As indicated in Table 1.1, a consistent positive association has been reported between both apolipoprotein B (apoB) and apolipoprotein E allele polymorphisms and longevity implicating a significant role for cholesterol homeostasis in longevity. To examine whether the prevalence of genetic risk factors for coronary artery disease (CAD) is lower in individuals who have reached an extremely old age, Kervinen et al [11]. analyzed the allele frequencies of apolipoprotein E (apo E) and B (apo B) polymorphisms, and plasma lipoprotein(a) levels in nonagenarians and in younger control groups and found that the frequency of the ε4 allele of apo E was significantly lower in the nonagenarians than in middle-aged and young adults. In addition, the frequency of *Eco*RI allele R- of apo B was low in the nonagenarians, whereas the allele frequency for the *Xba*I polymorphism of apo B and plasma lipoprotein(a) concentrations did not differ between the nonagenarians and the younger groups. The presence of these potential genetic risk factors for CAD, namely the ε4 allele of apo E and the R-allele of apo B, decreases the probability of an individual reaching an extremely old age, and therefore these alleles are less likely to be present in the very old population. The apo E genotype/allele distributions have been shown to significantly vary between centenarians and young people in a variety of populations [10], and the e4 allele has been proposed to be a frailty gene, (i.e., the apo E ε4 carrier has an increased rate of mortality compared to the rest of the population) rather than a longevity gene. However, data from a study of 253 individuals of Italian ancestry matched for origin, including 100 free-living healthy octo- and nonagenarians, 62 disabled octo- and nonagenarians, and 91 healthy adult controls do not support the potential association between apo E polymorphism and longevity or disability in this population [32] likely due to population-specific interactions between gene pools and environment.

In addition to the control of gene and phenotypic expression by both environmental and epigenetic influences, the control of gene action by epistatic interactions as well as global regulators likely play a critical role in aging.

Interestingly, a kindred with familial hypercholesterolemia in which one-third of the relatives with a mutant LDL receptor gene have normal plasma cholesterol concentrations was reported by Hobbs et al. [33] The proband, a 9-yr-old boy with a plasma cholesterol value greater than 500 mg/dl, was homozygous for a point mutation that changes Ser156 to Leu in the LDL receptor. The mutant gene was identified in heterozygous form in 17 of the mother's relatives, five of whom had normal LDL-cholesterol values. The pedigree was consistent with dominant transmission of a single gene that ameliorates or suppresses the hypercholesterolemic effect of the LDL receptor mutation.

As pointed out by Benedictis et al. [2] a decline or increase in specific gene variants in the genetic pool of the oldest-old (as compared to those of younger individuals) may reflect the capability of these variants to compensate time-related damages in crucial cell pathways. Studies with centenarians have stressed that this subgroup through a combination of environmental circumstance, lifestyle and genetic background have escaped most of the major age-related diseases including neoplasms [34], exhibit a complex remodeling of immune responses and feature in particular a largely conserved or even up-regulated innate immunity, with an associated elevation of moderate inflammation [35]. Interestingly, gene polymorphisms, which may be risk factors for severe diseases, have failed to reveal any association with longevity or they yielded completely unexpected results, such as the high incidence in centenarians of the D/D ACE genotype or no longevity association with the 4G/4G PAI-1 genotype [13, 17]. The positive association between mtDNA inheritance and longevity on the other hand, may reflect both the essential role and need that mtDNA plays in cell metabolism (OXPHOS) as well as a potential role as a sensor/trigger of apoptotic cell death, autophagy and oxidative stress as discussed in Chapter 4.

Aging and longevity are related in a rather complex way with the ability to cope with a variety of stressors including OS [2]. Observations from both model organisms and healthy centenarians have highlighted the importance of the capacity to cope with stress for attaining longevity. Accordingly, common genetic risk factors defined primarily or solely on the basis of their involvement in specific diseases, such as CVD are probably not the key to longevity albeit playing a contributory role. Their effect on mortality appears to be smaller as compared to the effects of "master" genes located at the cluster of the aging network such as genes in the GH/IGF1/insulin signaling pathway, which we will describe in several chapters of this book. Consequently, a current focus of human longevity research includes the search for stress-response genes that have been conserved by evolution. Furthermore, multidisciplinary approaches integrating demographic, molecular genetic, biochemical, and clinical methods are increasingly needed to decipher the complex network of factors that controls aging and longevity in higher organisms.

Longevity Genes from Model Systems

Findings from model systems have shown that individual genes may have significant effect on life span, a number of which are listed in Table 1.2. The major genetic model organisms used in aging research are the bakers' yeast (*Saccharomyces cerevisiae*), filamentous fungus (*Podospora anserina*), soil roundworm (*Caenorhabditis elegans*), fruit fly (*Drosophila melanogaster*), and mouse (*Mus musculus*).

Study of the aging process in *Podospora anserina* is relatively easy, and is currently under intense observation in several laboratories to identify genes involved in life span definition. In this model organism, cellular senescence is accompanied by a drastic reorganization of the internal membrane network (mitochondria, endoplasmic reticulum, nuclear membrane). At the molecular level, it is correlated with extensive mtDNA defects. Early studies suggested that this senescence can be triggered by the accumulation of a cytoplasmic and infectious element, whose nature is still unknown [37]. Recent evidence suggests that longevity in this model, measured in centimeters of growth, is in part under the control of numerous nuclear genes encoding and regulating mitochondrial respiratory metabolism, a key determinant of *Podospora* life span, as well as other less defined genetic elements and environmental conditions. Moreover, loss of function of the mitochondrial cytochrome pathway

Table 1.2 Model systems used for genes-longevity association (modified after Jazwinski) [36]

Saccharomyces	Caenorhabditis	Drosophila	Mouse
LAG1	daf-2	sod1	Prop-1
LAC1	daf-12	cat1	p66shc
RAS1	age-1/daf-23	mth	mclk1
RAS2	daf-18	IIS	
PHB1	akt-1/akt-2		
PHB2	daf-16		
CDC7	daf-12		
BUD1	ctl-1		
RTG2	old-1		
RPD3	spe-26		
HDA1	clk-1		
SIR2	mev-1		
SIR4-42	IIS		
UTH4	aak-2		
YGL023			
SGS1			
RAD52			
FOB1			

IIS: Insulin/IGF-1 signaling

leads to the compensatory induction of an alternative oxidase, to decreased ROS production, mtDNA stabilization and to a striking increase in life span [38]. This model illustrates several aspects of aging/senescence unique to this fungus as well as conserved features shared by many models including the primary role of mitochondrial bioenergy, ROS production and mtDNA defects.

Reports on the increased in mRNA level of heat shock proteins (Hsp) genes in aged *Drosophila* suggest that expression of Hsp might be beneficial in preventing the damage induced by aging, and that overexpression of the small mitochondrial Hsp22 extends *Drosophila* life span and increases resistance to OS [39]. Morrow et al. have demonstrated that targeted expression of Hsp22 within motorneurons increases *Drosophila* mean life span by more than 30 %. Hsp22 shows beneficial effects on early-aging events since the premortality phase displays the same increase as the mean life span, and flies expressing Hsp22 in their motorneurons maintain their locomotor activity longer as assessed by a negative geotaxis assay. The motorneurons-targeted expression of Hsp22 also significantly increased fly resistance to both OS induced by paraquat (up to 35 %) and thermal stress. Also, these investigators have shown that *Drosophila* not expressing the mitochondrial small Hsp22 have a 40 % decrease in life span, dying faster than matched controls and display a decrease of 30 % in locomotor activity compared with controls [40]. Moreover, the absence of Hsp22 also sensitizes flies to mild stress. Taken together, these findings suggest that Hsp22 is a key player in cell-protection mechanisms against oxidative injuries and aging in *Drosophila*, and further confirm the essential role that mitochondria play in aging.

There is increasing evidence that aging is hormonally regulated by an evolutionarily conserved insulin/IGF-1 signaling (IIS) pathway, and mutations in IIS components affect life span in *C. elegans, Drosophila melanogaster* and mice. According to Hwangbo et al. [41] aging in *Drosophila* is slowed when insulin-like signaling is reduced; life expectancy is extended by more than 50 % when the insulin-like receptor (InR) or its receptor substrate (chico) are mutated, or when insulin-producing cells are ablated. However, when insulin affects aging, or whether insulin signals regulate aging directly or indirectly through secondary hormones are not yet known. In addition, *C. elegans* life span is also extended when insulin signaling is inhibited in certain tissues, or when repressed in adult worms, mediated by the forkhead transcription factor (FOXO) encoded by daf-16. Previously, Kenyon et al. reported that mutations in the gene daf-2 can cause fertile, active, adult *C. elegans* hermaphrodites to live more than twice as long as wild type [42]. This life span extension, the largest yet reported in any organism, requires the activity of a second gene, daf-16. Both genes also regulate formation of the dauer larva, a developmentally arrested larval form that is induced by crowding and starvation and is very long-lived. These findings raise the possibility that the longevity of the dauer is not simply a consequence of its arrested growth, but rather results from a regulated life span extension mechanism that can be uncoupled from other aspects of dauer formation. Taken together daf-2 and daf-16 provide intriguing information on how life span can be extended. Moreover, the conserved nature of these genes actions on aging has been demonstrated. The *D. melanogaster* insulin-like receptor mediates phosphorylation of dFOXO, the fly equivalent of nematode daf-16 and mammalian FOXO3a. Likewise, dFOXO regulates *D. melanogaster* aging when activated in the adult pericerebral fat body [43]. In addition, this limited activation of dFOXO reduces expression of the *Drosophila* insulin-like peptide dilp-2 synthesized in neurons, and represses endogenous insulin-dependent signaling in peripheral fat body. These findings suggest that autonomous and non-autonomous roles of insulin signaling combine to control aging. A diagram showing the involvement of conserved elements in the insulin/IGF-1 signaling pathway is shown in Figure 1.1.

In yeast mother cells, *SIR* genes are determinants of life span since null mutations in *SIR2* shorten life span and an extra copy of *SIR2* can extend life span [44]. These effects appear to primarily derive from the silencing of chromatin in the ribosomal DNA (rDNA) repeats by Sir2p, mediated through its histone deacetylase activity. This silencing reduces rDNA gene expression and suppresses recombination that would generate toxic extrachromosomal rDNA circles (ERCs) [45]. In yeast mother cells, aging results from an asymmetry of cell division, leading to the accumulation of ERCs and

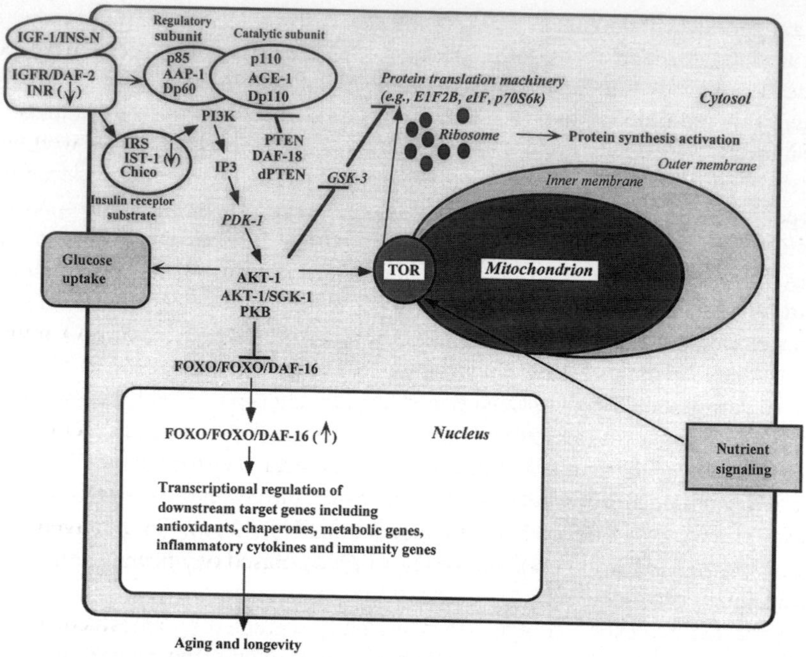

Fig. 1.1 Elements in insulin and IGF-1 signal transduction pathway are linked with aging and longevity
Shown are highly conserved homologues involved in this pathway in *C. elegans* (INS-N, DAF-2, ISI, AAP-1, AGE-1, DAF-18, IST-1, AKT-1/SGK-1, DAF-16), Drosophila (INR, Dp60, Dp110, Chico, dPTEN, PKB, dFOXO) and human (IGF, IGFR, p85, p110, PTEN, IRS, AKT-1, FOXO), which involves a cascade of phosphorylation events that converge on the FOXO/DAF-16 modulating its entry to the nucleus to set in motion a concerted transcriptional regulation of downstream target genes. A role of TOR, and GSK-3 in controlling protein synthesis and ribosomal biogenesis is also involved in aging and longevity with some interfacing with the insulin/IGF-1 signaling pathway. As indicated by the arrows, DAF-2/ insulin receptor and insulin receptor substrate signaling leads to reduced longevity, whereas FOXO/DAF-16 signaling increased longevity.

perhaps other deleterious molecules. In *C. elegans*, although aging appears different that in yeast (the soma of adults has only post-mitotic cells), a *SIR2* homolog, *Sir-2.1*, can regulate their life span since transgenic worms with extra copies of *Sir-2.1* live longer as well as display enhanced stress resistance [46]. Interestingly, this effect however is not mediated by silencing rDNA or modulating ERC formation, a process unique to yeast. Furthermore, *Sir-2.1* and its regulation of *C. elegans* life span are dependent on the expression of daf-16 and *Sir-2.1* is thought to be an upstream element in the insulin signaling pathway regulating life span [46]. Recent studies have demonstrated that SIR-2.1 interacts with 14-3-3 proteins to transcriptionally activate DAF-16 and extend life span and impact stress resistance [47].

Mutations in other downstream elements of this pathway have been shown to reduce signaling and provide longevity in *C. elegans*, [48–51] and other downstream elements including ER stress proteins have been implicated using gene profiling analysis [52].

Sir2 proteins by their biochemical activity as NAD-protein deacetylases might keep track of the metabolic rate by the amount of available NAD, and couple this status to regulatory events, such as the silencing of chromatin. Moreover, homologues of SIR2 have been identified and implicated in cellular senescence in flies as well as in a variety of mouse and human cells (including mammalian cardiac myocytes) [53–56]. SIR2 genes appear to be operative in regulating aging in many different organisms, albeit as pointed out by Guarente [57], some of the molecular events that it controls may be species-specific (i.e., rDNA silencing in yeast and insulin signaling/dauer formation in worms).

More roles for the SIR2 homologues (there are seven SIR-related proteins [sirtuins] with distinct subcellular localizations and functions in human cells) in mammalian cells have been revealed including the deacetylation and activation of mammalian acetyl-CoA synthetases [58], a role in DNA base-excision repair [59], roles in metabolic regulation [60], fat mobilization [61], and insulin secretion [62, 63]. These multiple roles SIR2 play in aging and physiology as well with respect to caloric restriction are more extensively discussed in a later section and are currently viewed as a potential target for pharmacological modulation to treat both disease of aging and may be eventually be applicable to expanding human longevity.

Giannakou et al. have studied the timing of the effect of reduced IIS on life span and the role of a potential target tissue, the fat body of adult *Drosophila*, containing an overexpressed allele of dFOXO, a downstream effector of IIS [64]. This study found that FOXO transcription factors and the adipose tissue are evolutionarily conserved in the regulation of aging, and that the reduction of IIS in the adult was sufficient to mediate its effects on both life span and fecundity. Furthermore, most long-lived IIS mutants also show increased resistance to OS. Interestingly, in *Drosophila* and in mice, the long-lived phenotype of several IIS mutants is restricted to females. Recently, van Heemst et al. prospectively evaluated in human subjects the incidence of selected polymorphic variants in genes encoding elements in the IIS pathway and gauged their impact on body height and longevity using multivariate analysis [26]. Based on the expected effects (increased or decreased signaling) of the selected variants components (e.g., GHRHR, GH1, IGF-1, INS, IRS1), composite IIS scores to estimate IIS pathway activity were determined. In women, lower IIS scores were significantly associated with lower body height and improved old age survival. Moreover, multivariate analyses showed that these results were most pronounced for specific variants including the *GH1* SNP, *IGF1 CA* repeat and IRS1 SNP. In females, for variant allele carriers of the GH1 SNP, body height was 2 cm lower and mortality 0.80-fold reduced when compared with wild-type allele carriers. The conclusion was that in females, genetic variation causing reduced IIS activation is beneficial for old age survival and this effect was stronger for the GH1 SNP than for variation in other conserved IIS genes previously found to affect longevity in model organisms.

Aging of eukaryotic organisms is affected by their nutritional state and by their ability to prevent or repair oxidative damage. Furthermore, the signaling pathways that control metabolism and OS responses also influence the life span. When nutrients are abundant, the IIS pathway promotes growth and energy storage but shortens life span. On the other hand, the transcription factor FOXO, which is inhibited by IIS, extends life span in conditions of low IIS activity. In addition, activation of the stress-responsive Jun-N-terminal kinase (JNK) pathway may also increase life span. Wang el al. demonstrated that JNK requires FOXO to extend life span in *Drosophila* and that JNK antagonizes IIS, causing nuclear localization of FOXO and inducing its targets, including growth control and stress defense genes [65]. JNK and FOXO also restrict IIS activity systemically by repressing IIS ligand expression in neuroendocrine cells. Therefore, the convergence of JNK signaling and FOXO on IIS signaling provides a model to explain the effects of stress and nutrition on longevity. A conserved MST-FOXO signaling pathway has been recently reported to mediate OS responses and extend mammalian life span. Lehtinen et al. [66] have shown that the protein kinase MST1 mediates OS-induced cell death in primary mammalian neurons by directly activating the FOXO transcription factors. MST1 phosphorylates FOXO proteins at a conserved site within the forkhead domain that disrupts their interaction with 14-3-3 proteins, promotes FOXO nuclear translocation and induces cell death in neurons. This study extended the MST-FOXO signaling link to nematodes by demonstrating that knockdown of the *C. elegans* MST1 ortholog CST-1 resulted in a shortened life span and accelerated tissue aging, while CST-1 overexpression enhanced life span and delayed aging, and that the CST-1-induced life span extension occurs in a daf-16-dependent manner. Identification of the FOXO transcription factors, as major and evolutionarily conserved targets of MST1, suggested that MST kinases play important roles in diverse biological processes, including cellular responses to OS and longevity. Taken together, these studies provide another important mechanism by which metabolic and stress responses are integrated via phosphorylation of FOXO proteins.

Theories of Aging

Nobody really knows why we get older. It is possible that after an organism passes reproductive age its use to future generations is limited and it just slowly fades away. It is possible that the organism changes as it gets older, but why the organism's cells behave this way is not completely understood. The theories of aging are many, and the most popular may be that as cells age they become less efficient and less able to rid themselves of waste and toxic products, and eventually they are no longer able to work at all – and die.

At the outset it should be mentioned that to establish a new, fundamental theory or view on a subject that has been so extensively handled by investigators is extremely difficult. Moreover, it is important to realize that there is not yet a common, universal theory of aging; but rather many diverse perspectives, which significantly are not necessarily mutually exclusive. Instead, they may better be held together, at least at the molecular and cellular levels, where they address the questions of "is aging programmed?" or "is aging accidental?" In this section we will describe the better-known general theories of aging. Later in Chapter 2 we will further discuss these theories more specifically in reference to cardiovascular (CV) aging.

Evolutionary Theories

The search for a general biology of aging has utilized terms of evolutionary biology, which correlate the developmental processes of plants and organisms in an effort to resolve their inherited relationship and developmental evolution. However, attempts to explain "late-life mortality plateaus" by using evolution theory have largely failed since they required highly specialized, elaborate and unrealistic assumptions. It is our view that evolutionary theory is likely to be more applicable to explaining early reproductive success, rather than later failures such as aging and death. According to these theories, aging is the result of investing resources in reproduction, rather than the maintenance of the body (the Disposable Soma Theory or DST), in light of the fact that accidents, predation and disease will eventually kill the organism no matter how much energy is devoted to repair the body. According to Weinert and Timiras, the concept of an evolutionary tradeoff is a central premise in both the DST and the Antagonistic Pleiotropy Theory (APT) [67]. The DST explains why we live for a certain period of time but does not attempt to delineate the specific cause of aging. On the other hand, the APT suggests that some genes may be selected for their beneficial effects early in life, but these can have unselected deleterious effects with age contributing to senescence. More specific evolutionary theories have been postulated and they are not necessary mutually exclusive, i.e., late-acting deleterious mutations could accumulate in populations over evolutionary time. Haldane invoked *population genetics*, the study of the allele frequency distribution and change under the influence of the four evolutionary forces: natural selection, genetic drift, mutation, and gene flow. This also takes account of population subdivision and population structure in space, and as such, attempts to explain such phenomena as adaptation and speciation. Population genetics was an essential component in the modern evolutionary synthesis (MES). Also, MES may be explained in terms of a new synthesis, the modern synthesis, the evolutionary synthesis, neo-Darwinian synthesis or neo-Darwinism, which integrates Charles Darwin's theory of the evolution of species by natural selection, Mendel's theory of genetics as the basis for biological inheritance, random genetic mutation as the source of variation, and mathematical population genetics. The primary founders of MES were Sewall Wright, JBS Haldane and RA Fisher, who also laid the foundations for the related discipline of *quantitative genetics* or the study of continuous traits (such as height or weight) and their underlying mechanisms. Using these constructs, late-acting deleterious mutations could accumulate in populations over evolutionary time through genetic drift. And it is these later-acting deleterious mutations, which are believed to cause, or perhaps more correctly allow, age-related mortality. Peter Medawar formalized this perspective in his mutation accumulation theory of aging [69]. "The force of natural selection weakens with increasing age – even in a theoretically immortal population, provided only that it is exposed to real hazards of mortality. If a genetic disaster happens late enough in individual life, its consequences may be completely unimportant". The 'real hazards of mortality' are typically predation, disease and accidents. So, even an immortal population, whose fertility does not decline with time, will have fewer individuals alive in older age groups. This is called 'extrinsic mortality'. Young cohorts, not depleted in numbers yet by extrinsic mortality, contribute far more to the next generation than the few remaining older cohorts, so the force of selection against late-acting deleterious mutations, which only affect these few older individuals, is very weak. The mutations may not be selected against, and therefore may spread over evolutionary time into the population.

In his excellent review reflecting on the evolution of senescence and death, WR Clark [70], noted that Medawar was among the first to recognize what has become a foundation stone of contemporary evolutionary theories of aging: the declining force of natural selection with age of the individual. Harmful genetic events that are expressed prior to the reproductive period in an animal's life history will be strongly selected against, whereas the expression of such genes at later stages will not be subject to negative selection. In addition, Medawar speculated that spontaneously arising variants of genes that display a harmful effect only later in life termed – senescence effector alleles – would simply accumulate in a species over evolutionary time; the allelic variants of the genes responsible for Huntington's chorea and Alzheimer disease are often cited as examples. Moreover, harmful genetic alterations could arise in senescence regulator genes, as well as in the senescence effector genes themselves. We concur with Clark that this concept of senescence regulator genes, which was not followed up for several decades after Medawar proposed it, may be his most important contribution to thinking about the evolution of senescence. According, to Charlesworth [71], the idea that a senescent decline in the performance of biological systems must have an evolutionary basis traces back almost to the beginnings of evolutionary biology. At first sight, the almost universal existence of senescence in species of multicellular organisms appears paradoxical, since natural selection may cause the evolution of increased, not decreased, fitness [72]. Many biologists have the opinion that senescence reflects an inevitable process of damage accumulation with age [73], and that similarly senescence can be seen in complex machines such as cars [74]. Charlesworth pointed out [71], that unicellular organisms, such as bacteria, and the germ lines of multicellular organisms have been able to propagate themselves without senescence over billions of years, implying that biological systems are capable of continuous repair and maintenance to avoid senescence at the cellular level, and therefore senescence cannot just be an unavoidable cumulative result of damage. The significant amount of variation among different species in their rates of senescence also clearly indicates that aging is subject to variation and selection that is suggested by the presence of both quantitative genetic variation and major gene mutations affecting the rate of aging [72, 75, 76].

The major testable prediction made by the evolutionary theory is that species, which have high extrinsic mortality in nature, will age more quickly and have shorter intrinsic life span. This is because there is too little time before death occurs by extrinsic causes for the effects of deleterious mutations to be expressed and, therefore, selected against. This is borne out among mammals, the best studied in terms of life history. There is a correlation among mammals between body size and life span, such that larger species live longer than smaller species in controlled/optimum conditions, but there are notable exceptions. For instance, many bats and rodents are similarly sized, yet bats live much, much longer. For instance, the little brown bat, half the size of a mouse, can live 30 years in the wild. A mouse will live 2–3 years even with optimum conditions. The explanation is that bats have fewer predators, therefore low extrinsic mortality. Thus more individuals survive to later ages so the force of selection against late-acting deleterious mutations is stronger. Fewer late-acting deleterious mutations = slower aging = longer life span. Birds are also warm-blooded and similarly sized to many small mammals, yet live often 5–10 times as long. They clearly have fewer predation pressures compared with ground-dwelling mammals. And seabirds, which generally have the fewest predators of all birds, live longest.

Also, when examining the body-size vs. life span relationship, predator mammals tend to have longer life span than prey animals in a controlled environment such as a zoo or nature reserve. The explanation for the long life span of primates (such as humans, monkeys and apes) relative to body size is that their intelligence and often sociality helps them avoid becoming prey. Being a predator, being smart and working together all reduce extrinsic mortality.

Another evolutionary theory of aging was proposed by GC Williams and involves antagonistic pleiotropy [77]. A single gene may affect multiple traits (pleiotropy). Some traits that increase fitness early in life may also have negative effects later in life. But because many more individuals are alive at young ages than at old ages, even small positive effects early can be strongly selected for, and large negative effects later may be very weakly selected against. Williams suggested the following example: perhaps a gene codes for calcium deposition in bones which promotes juvenile survival and will therefore be favored by natural selection; however this same gene promotes calcium deposition in the arteries, causing negative effects in old age. Therefore negative effects in old age may reflect the result of natural selection for pleiotropic genes, which are beneficial early in life. In this case, fitness is relatively high when Fisher's reproductive value is high and relatively low when Fisher's reproductive value is low. We agree with Gavrilov and Gavrilova [78] that evolutionary theories of aging are useful when they open new opportunities for further research by suggesting testable predictions, although they may have been harmful when they are used to impose limitations on aging studies. As pointed out by Gavrilov and Gavrilova [79], manifold difficulties occur in incorporating evolutionay theory to explain late-life mortality plateaus in aging whereas it may be more proficient to explain reproduction rather than aging and death. Finally, it is apparent that the evolutionary theories of aging are not ultimate completed theories; they are rather a set of ideas that require further research and validation.

Molecular/Genome Mutations/Deletions Theory

The genetics of aging is an extremely exciting research area that can be used to test the theories of aging. According to Hekimi [80], each animal species displays a specific life span, rate of aging and characteristic pattern of development of age-dependent diseases. Significantly, the genetic basis of these related features are being studied experimentally in invertebrate and vertebrate model systems as well as in humans through medical records. At present, three types of mutants are being analyzed: (1) short-lived mutants that are prone to age-dependent diseases and might be models of accelerated aging; (2) mutants that show overt molecular defects but that do not live shorter lives than controls, and can be used to test specific theories about the molecular causes of aging and age-dependent diseases; and (3) long-lived mutants that might advance the understanding of the molecular physiology of slow-aging animals and may help in the discovery of molecular targets that could be used to manipulate rates of aging to benefit human health. Accumulation of mutations occur in the mitochondrial genome (together with respiratory chain defects forming the basis for "the mitochondrial theory of aging") and nuclear DNA (often termed genomic instability) that will lead to damage/dysfunction of proteins, membranes, organelles and cells, and finally to cell death and aging. The DNA damage may be secondary to a number of insults, including oxygen free radicals, toxins, chemicals or radiation, together with an ineffectual DNA repair machinery with aging ("DNA repair theory") and errors in DNA replication.

Analysis of genome-wide transcription by DNA microarrays and serial analysis of gene expression (SAGE) are increasingly used to detect changes with age in several model systems. These techniques allow the compilation of a blueprint or molecular signature of normal aging, and its comparison with slowing or acceleration of aging by specific interventions in *Drosophila melanogaster*, mice and *C. elegans* [81–84].

Studies of human centenarians and their relatives have identified a significant genetic aspect underlying the ability to survive to exceptional ages. In one study, the mortality rate of centenarian siblings was shown to be, on average, half the mortality rate of the US year 1900 cohort [8, 85]. This sustained life-long reduction in mortality rate suggests that the effect is due to genetic rather than environmental or socio-economic factors. Another study supported the idea that exceptional longevity has a genetic component by using a genome-wide scan of 308 individuals belonging to 137 sibships demonstrating exceptional longevity to identify a locus on chromosome 4 that exhibited significant linkage with exceptional longevity and therefore is likely to contain gene(s) that promote longevity [86]. Moreover, as we have previously noted, an increasing number of polymorphic gene variants (listed in Table 1.1) have been identified with differential distribution in the very old and in centenarians. Genetic analysis of human longevity is particularly important since most of the genetic aspects of aging are mainly studied in short-lived model organisms.

An outgrowth of the DNA/Genetic theory is the *Cell senescence/Telomere/Telomerase Theory of Aging*. Telomeres are specialized DNA-protein structures located at the end of chromosomes, which shorten with each replication, unless they are preserved by the action of the enzyme telomerase reverse transcriptase (TERT). During aging their length is progressively reduced in most somatic cells, with incomplete synthesis of the lagging strand resulting in telomere shortening every time the cells divide. After a number of cell cycles, telomere length reaches a critical size, cellular replication stops and the cell becomes senescent. This phenomenon is called telomere-driven senescence versus the stress-induced premature senescence (which can occur independently of telomere shortening). Telomerization, the expression of TERT in a number of cultured cell-types, including endothelial cells and cardiomyocytes, leads to recovery of telomerase activity stopping the initiation of senescence [87–90]. Significantly, telomere shortening and the cell's replicative life span is not only achieved by incomplete lagging strand synthesis, but is in great part based on telomeric DNA damage. In telomerase-negative cells, during DNA replication *in vitro*, telomeres shorten due to multiple causes including the inability of DNA polymerases to fully copy the lagging strand, DNA end processing and random DNA damage, often caused by OS and the short telomeres activate replicative senescence and irreversible cell cycle arrest. According to von Zglinicki and Martin-Ruiz, telomere length acts as an indicator of replicative history, of the probability of cell senescence, and of accumulated OS [91]. In addition, in most human cells telomeres shorten during aging *in vivo*, suggesting that telomere length could be a biomarker of aging and age-related morbidity. These investigators noted that there are two different possibilities: (1) In a tissue-specific fashion, short telomeres might indicate senescence of stem cells, and this might contribute to age-related functional attenuation in this tissue. (2) Short telomeres in one tissue might act as risk markers for age-related disease residing in a completely different tissue. Although recent observations appear to support both approaches, the impact of cell senescence on tissue aging *in vivo* is still questionable. In another study, the same group of investigators measured white blood cell telomere length at baseline in 598 participants of the Leiden 85-plus Study (mean age at baseline 89.8 years), and obtained second telomere measurements from 81 participants after an average time span of between 4 and 13 years [92]. At baseline, telomere length was not predictive for mortality involving cardiovascular causes, cancer or infectious diseases, and longitudinal measurements of telomere length were highly unstable in a large fraction of subjects. Thus the conclusion was that blood monocyte telomere length is not a predictive indicator for age-related morbidity and mortality at ages over 85 years, possibly because of a high degree of telomere length instability in this group. On the other hand, these investigators have reported more recently a potential correlation between telomere length in peripheral blood mononuclear cells and ventricular function, as assessed by echocardiographic determination of ejection fraction (EF) in a group of 85-year old subjects recruited from the community as part of the Newcastle 85+ Study [93]. In this study, sex and telomere length were significant predictors of EF while current smoking, blood pressure, plasma high sensitivity C-reactive protein (CRP), and use of cardiovascular medications were not. Thus aging may affect myocardial function in the oldest old, and this may be independent of other specific disease processes. In the future it may be possible to introduce telomerase in cells *in vivo*, keeping in mind that free radicals damage the DNA (*Free Radical Theory of Aging*).

Wear-and Tear- Theories

This set of theories refer to a progressive, accumulative damage that the body can not repair by itself, including:

(a) The Free Radical Theory of Aging (FRTA).
(b) Cross-linkage theories (a result of metabolism, cross-links form between molecules and lead to rigidity, leading the molecules to no longer function properly).
(c) DNA-repair theory (DNA cannot keep up with the damage caused by factors like pollution, environment, and the slow repair mechanism associated with aging).
(d) Garbage accumulation theory.

(a) FRTA

The groundbreaking original paper on FRTA [94] was published in 1956. This is one of the better-known theories, and has generated a massive amount of research designed to support or refute the theory; however, it is still somewhat debatable. Parenthetically, FRTA is the most widely accepted theory. Not only scientists, but also lay people, have taken a particularly strong interest in this theory, as evidenced by the sales of supplemental antioxidants.

Free radicals (FRs) are molecules carrying an unpaired electron. They are extremely reactive compounds that will come to have a new electron in any way possible. In this process, the free radical will attach itself to another molecule modifying it biochemically. As FRs steal an electron from other molecules, they may convert these molecules into *de novo* FRs, or break down or alter their chemical structure. These aggressive compounds induce damage to cellular macromolecules such as DNA, lipids and proteins. The main FRs and non-FRs mimics are called reactive oxygen species" or ROS, including superoxide radical (SOR), hydroxyl radical (OHR), hydroperoxyl radical (HPR), alkoxyl radical (AR), peroxyl radical (PR) and nitric oxide radical (NOR). Other molecules that are technically not FRs, but act much like them, are singlet oxygen and hydrogen peroxide (H_2O_2). As a measure of the significant potency of FR, they also play predominant roles in other theories, including the Mitochondrial, Membrane and Cross-link theories, as well as being central elements in FRTA. Furthermore, recent observations suggest that only some of these damaged macromolecules can be removed and their accumulation in the aging cell might exceed the cell ability to get rid off of this "garbage" (The Garbage theory). Moreover, the "garbage" limits the function of the cellular repair systems creating a positive feedback loop causing cellular aging. Notwithstanding their role in cell damage, ROS are also important housekeeping signaling molecules, for example in the p53 and NF-κB pathways.

Some of the strongest indications in support of FRTA have come from life span extension in *Drosophila* and *C. elegans* transgenic studies [95, 96]. Compared to normal controls transgenic flies equipped with enhanced antioxidant defenses (overexpressed superoxide dismutase [CuSOD] or catalase) had up to 30 % longer average and maximum life spans; a reduction of age-related accumulation of oxidative damage to protein and DNA; reduced DNA damage when exposed to radiation, and many other improved indices of oxidant damage [97]. Increased expression of Cu-SOD (which neutralizes SOR) and catalase (which neutralizes H_2O_2) in *Drosophila* was associated with increased longevity and increased resistance to OS. Long-lived mutant *C. elegans* are also OS resistant and have significant age-dependent increase in SOD and catalase activities [98]. Moreover, antioxidant compounds (synthetic mimetics of catalase and SOD) can delay aging in *C. elegans.* [99]

Further support for FRTA comes from interspecies comparison of FR production, oxidative damage, and antioxidant levels. For instance, the white-footed mouse (*Peromyscus leucopus*) lives about twice as long as the house mouse (*Mus musculus*) although their metabolic rates are similar. At age 3.5 years, the rates of mitochondrial SOR and H_2O_2 generation was 40 % less in heart and 80 % less in brain in *Peromyscus*, while catalase and glutathione peroxidase (GPx) activities were about twice as high in *Peromyscus*, and the level of damaged proteins was 80 % higher in *Mus* mice [100]. The lower rate of mitochondrial superoxide and H_2O_2 generation, higher activities of catalase and GPx and low levels of protein oxidative damage in the longer-lived *Peromyscus* species supports FTRA and the role of OS in aging. Pigeons and rats have similar body mass and metabolic rates, yet rates of heart, liver and brain mitochondrial SOR and H_2O_2 generation are 10 times less in pigeons, while their levels of catalase and GPx are higher. As noted by Beckman and Ames [95], interspecies comparisons of oxidative damage, antioxidant defenses, and oxidant generation provide some important corroborating evidence that oxidants are significant determinants of life span.

On the other hand, initial studies found that ubiquitous overexpression of CuSOD does not extend life span in transgenic mouse strains as it does in flies [101]. Similarly, dietary antioxidants may decrease the accumulation of ROS in mice, but they fail to extend their life span [102]. Interestingly, several studies have suggested that modulation of catalase levels may be more related than SOD levels to longevity in mice [103–104]. In studies of long-lived dwarf mice, Brown-Borg and Rakoczy reported significantly elevated *catalase* in livers and kidneys from dwarf mice compared to age-matched control mice; conversely, marked reduction was found in liver catalase levels in short-lived growth hormone (GH) transgenic mice with accelerated aging [103].

These studies have been extended by a recent study, which found that transgenic mice that over-express human catalase localized to the mitochondria (MCAT) exhibited significant increases (over 20 %) in both their median and maximum life span [104]. These transgenic mouse strains with over a 50-fold increase in catalase expression in cardiac and skeletal muscle mitochondria also displayed reduced severity in age-dependent arteriosclerosis, reduced OS (e.g., H_2O_2 production and oxidative damage) and increased genomic stability as indicated by reduced levels of mtDNA deletions in both heart and skeletal muscle. The observation that a relatively large increase in life span results from the up-regulation of a single gene involved in boosting antioxidant defenses, and its targeting to the mitochondria, buttresses the notion that mitochondrial ROS and OS play a critical role in determining life span, and are to date the most compelling support for FRTA. It will be critical to see if these findings are applicable to other species including larger mammals and humans. A role of mitochondrial-generated ROS and OS in leading to cellular senescence and aging is illustrated in Figure 1.2.

It is also noteworthy that stress conditioning can lead to a positive compensatory response (*hormesis*), that protects against oxidative damage in part by both activating antioxidant defenses and reducing ROS generation and extends life span, a critical concept which we will revisit frequently throughout this book [105]. For example, rodents exposed to chronic radiation exhibit reproducible

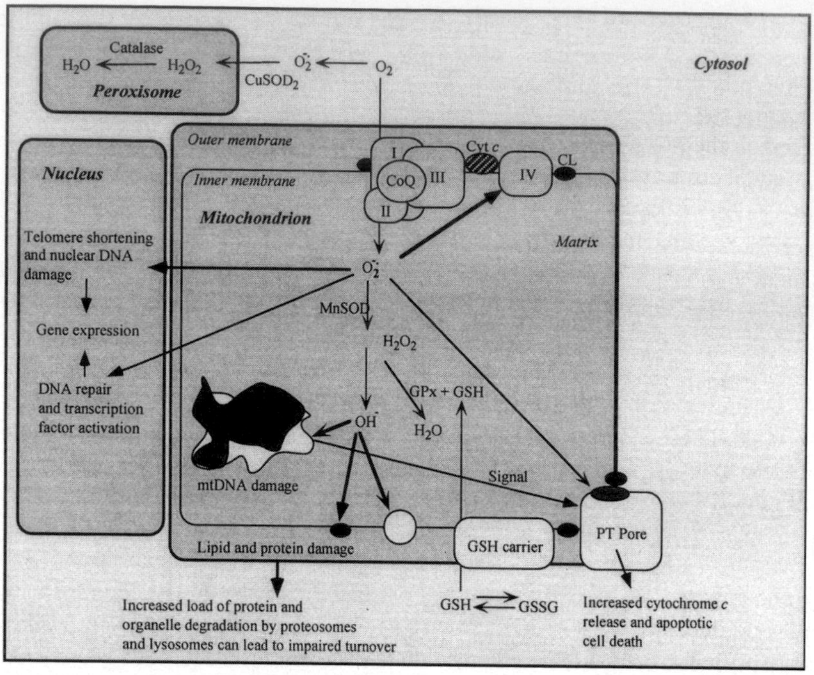

Fig. 1.2 Molecular and subcellular events leading to oxidative stress-induced senescence and aging Aging-accumulated damage to proteins, lipids and mtDNA caused by mitochondrial-generated ROS including H_2O_2, superoxide (O_2^-) and hydroxyl radicals (OH^-), leads to PT pore opening and apoptotic cell death, telomere shortening and nuclear DNA damage as well as modulated DNA repair and gene expression in the nucleus and increased load for protein/organelle turnover triggering cell senescence. Also shown are antioxidant factors in peroxisomes (catalase), mitochondria (GPx, GSH and MnSOD) and in the cytosol (CuSOD), which function to scavenge ROS and reduce their impact.

increased life span [106]. This can be explained if radiation exposure produces a stable activation of cellular defenses [67]. Similarly caloric restriction (CR), which can be viewed as another form of moderate stress conditioning, can prolong the life span of almost every organism in which it has been used. Considerable evidence has shown that dietary restriction including reduction in caloric intake impacts cellular metabolism including redox remodeling, reducing ROS production and upregulating antioxidant defenses [107]. In isolated mitochondrial preparations from rodents, CR both reduced ROS generation and attenuated the accumulation of oxidative damage [108]. Although the increased-longevity effects of CR is an attractive methodology; it is important to keep in mind that CR may affect the function of many other molecular, cellular, and organ systems. The potential correlation of CV function and CR as well as whether this approach is applicable to humans are addressed in depth in Chapter 15.

A relationship between free radical-mediated oxidative damage and aging has also been demonstrated in humans [95]. Mecocci et al. have examined markers of oxidative damage to DNA, lipids, and proteins in muscle biopsy specimens from humans aged 25–93 years, and found an age-dependent increase in 8-hydroxy-2-deoxyguanosine (a marker of oxidative damage to DNA), in malondialdehyde (MDA), a marker of lipid peroxidation, and to a lesser extent in protein carbonyl groups, a marker of protein oxidation [109]. Therefore these findings provide further correlative support for a contributory role of oxidative damage in human aging. Nevertheless, a direct cause-and-effect relationship between the accumulation of oxidatively mediated damage and aging remains to be established [110].

(b) Cross-Linkage Theory

This theory suggests that as a result of metabolism, cross-links form between molecules that lead to rigidity, leading the molecules to no longer function properly. This theory is also referred to as the "Glycosylation theory of aging". Glucose and other simple sugars in the presence of O_2 result in the production of advanced glycation end-products (AGE), which bind to proteins causing further cross-linking. While increasing evidence supports a prominent role for increased AGE in aging particularly in the vascular system (discussed in Chapter 4) and in aging-associated diseases such as atherosclerosis and diabetes, by most accounts this cross-linking is secondary to the development of oxidative stress and free radicals and metabolic dysfunction.

(c) DNA-Repair Theory

DNA cannot keep up with the damage caused by factors like pollution, environment, and the slow repair mechanism associated with aging.

(d) Cellular Garbage Theory

This theory encompasses both the membrane and the Hayflick limit theories involves the accumulation of by-products of normal cellular metabolism that are found in the aging cells ("cellular senescence" theory). These by-products may be inert (e.g., lipofuscins) or reactive (e.g., ROS), and together with other molecules are in a cross-linked state (e.g., DNA, lipids, proteins), and cannot be broken down by lysosomes. This "garbage" is particularly abundant in post-mitotic cells (cardiomyocytes and neurons) where it interferes with normal cell functioning by the loss of proteins, organelles, (e.g., mitochondria) and the overall reduction of cellular mass.

(e) The Membrane Theory of Aging

This theory refers to the age-related changes affecting the cells ability to transfer molecules, heat and electrical processes that impair their function. With aging membranes lipids decrease and become more rigid, dysfunctional and unable to block the accumulation of toxic products. These cellular toxins/lipofuscin will deposit in growing amount with aging in the brain, heart and other organs. Similarly there will be changes in ion transfer (Na^+ and K^+) that will affect heat and electron transfer.

(f) The Hayflick Theory

The central premise of this theory relates to findings that human somatic cells are limited in the number of times that they can divide, and suggests that to live longer there is a need to slow down the rate of cell division. Changes in cell proliferation could be accomplished by a number of changes, including dietary (see Chapter 15 on CR) and lifestyle as well as well as by invoking signaling elements of senescence pathways. Interestingly, both growth factors and OS can modulate cell proliferation.

Reliability Theory

Reliability theory suggests that biological systems start their adult life with a high load of initial damage. This theory predicts that even those systems that are entirely composed of non-aging elements will nevertheless deteriorate with age, if these systems contain a high level of redundancy in irreplaceable elements. From this systemic perspective, aging, therefore, is predicted to be a direct consequence of system redundancy. While intuitively system redundancy has clear positive benefits including overall damage tolerance, which decreases mortality and increases life span, damage tolerance permits defects to be accumulated over time resulting in aging.

According to Gavrilov and Gavrilova [79], this theory also predicts the late-life mortality deceleration with subsequent leveling-off, as well as the late-life mortality plateaus, as an inevitable consequence of redundancy exhaustion at extreme old ages. More simply put, at very high ages (e.g., achieved by centenarians), some aging phenomena disappear as redundancy in the number of elements declines.

This theory explains why mortality rates increase exponentially with age (the Gompertz law) in many species, by taking into account the initial defects in newly formed systems. The law states that death rate is a sum of an age-independent component (Makeham term) and an age-dependent component (Gompertz function), which increases exponentially with age, (i.e., the larger the quantity of death with age, the faster it will grow). When external causes of death are rare (e.g., living conditions, low mortality countries, etc.) the age-independent mortality component is often negligible, and the formula is simplified to a Gompertz law of mortality [111]. The reliability theory also suggests a rationale for mortality convergence at higher ages.

The Gompertz-Makeham law in the age window of about 30–80 years rather accurately predicts the age dynamics of human mortality. Beyond 80 years the death rates do not increase as fast as predicted by this law (this is called the late-life mortality deceleration). Fundamentally, this theory may be helpful in developing a comprehensive theory of aging and longevity integrating mathematical methods with specific biological findings. Other investigators have suggested (primarily based on studies of *Drosophila* aging) that the features of the components assumed by this theory are most likely under the control of natural selection, which ultimately leaves us with mortality patterns that are shaped by evolution [112].

Neuro-Endocrine/Immunological Theory

This theory deals mainly with the wear and tear that overwhelms the repair mechanisms of the organism and focuses on the interaction and integration of the neuroendocrine and immune systems. The nervous system is linked to the endocrine system by the hypothalamus via the pituitary gland. By synthesizing and secreting neurohormones, often called *releasing hormones*, the hypothalamus controls the secretion of hormones from the anterior pituitary gland – among them, gonadotropin-releasing hormone (GnRH). The hypothalamus sets off various chain reactions whereby an organ releases a hormone which in turn stimulates the release of another hormone, which in turn stimulates yet another bodily response.

In the young, the body's hormone levels tend to be high, accounting for among other things, menstruation in women and high libido in both sexes. The growth hormones (GH) that help us to form muscle mass, hGH, testosterone and thyroid, drop dramatically with age so elderly individuals even if they have not gained weight, will have increased fat-to-muscle ratio. Furthermore, aging causes a drop in hormone production, produces a decline in the body's ability to repair and regulate itself as well. Since the production of different hormones is highly interrelated, decline in the production of any one hormone is likely to have a feedback signaling effect on other organs and levels of other hormones as well. As noted by Weinert and Timiras [67], the integration of the neuro-endocrine-immune systems play an essential role throughout the sequential stages of life and changes in these systems functions are paramount for aging and in aging-related diseases as discussed in Chapter 6.

Hormesis and Aging

Hormesis refers to a biological adaptive response to stimuli that may have a detrimental effect but when applied at low level/dosage may be beneficial to the survival of an organism [113]. The biological response deploys an impressive array of adaptations that may be turned on in response to various stresses, including physiological stress, as well as exposure to radiation, toxic chemicals, and dietary alterations. For instance, Hart and colleagues have shown that DNA repair efficiency and fidelity are markedly enhanced in caloric restricted diets although the implications of these findings for human populations remains to be further investigated and established [114]. The reasons for the hormesis phenomenon are not completely understood. It is possible that a low dose challenge with a toxin may jumpstart certain repair mechanisms in the body, and these mechanisms are efficient enough that they not only neutralize the toxin's effect, but even repair other defects not caused by the toxin. Another explanation is that an insult present at low doses interacts with genetic signaling systems that upregulate gene expression, whereas high doses cause overt toxicity.

Hormesis in aging is characterized by a beneficial response to stress through physiological adaptations, as exemplified in life span extension by irradiation and calorie restriction. The initial observation that reduced food intake has a beneficial effect on rat life span was made over 70 years ago. In the decades that followed, researchers have successfully applied this method to increase the life span of a very wide range of model systems, including mice, hamsters, dogs, fish, invertebrate animals, and yeast. CR extends life by slowing and/or delaying the aging processes. Recent experiments with *C. elegans* suggest that the TOR (target of rapamycin) pathway, rather than insulin-like signaling, might be involved in mediating the life-extending effect of dietary restriction [115, 116]. Recent evidence has also suggested a contributory role of translational inhibition in the longevity response to dietary restriction in *C. elegans*; [117] TOR is a highly-conserved, established component of the nutrient response pathway regulating levels of ribosomal proteins (e.g., ribosomal-protein p70 S6 kinase (p70 S6K) and impacting translational initiation factor activities and has been found to effect ribosome biogenesis as well as the process of translation itself. Reducing levels of p70 S6K or specific translation-initiation factors (e.g., eIF4E, eIF2b and eIF4G) increases the *C. elegans* life span, presumably by shifting cells to physiological states that favor maintenance and repair [117]. Interestingly, recent studies have confirmed similar findings of extended life span by decreased TOR signaling in yeast [118] and overexpression of dominant-negative alleles of TOR or S6K in *Drosophila* [119].

Using rodent as a model system, Masoro has reported that the level of food restriction that results in life extension and retarded aging also enhances their ability to cope with intense stressors [113]. Moreover, this level of dietary restriction (DR) leads to a modest increase in the daily peak concentration of plasma free corticosterone, which strongly points to DR as a low-intensity stressor. Furthermore, in an effort to integrate DR, Hormone-IGF-1 Axis Hypothesis and Oxidative Damage Attenuation Hypothesis under a single theory Masoro suggests that hormesis may be the umbrella encompassing those hypothesis, each playing a similar role in life-extending and anti-aging action [120]. For a more comprehensive discussion on caloric restriction and aging, the reader is directed to Chapter 15.

Gender Issues in Aging

In a variety of organisms, including human, females live longer and sex-dependent genes influence life span [121–123]. The effect of a gene on a multifactorial trait is contingent on the physiological background in which the gene is expressed. If the age-related physiological scenario changes in males and females differently, the effects of a certain gene on disease or survival could vary between the sexes, which indicates that males and females may follow different pathways toward extreme longevity [124].

It is apparent that females live longer than males, and estrogen may be the cause. It is worth noting that the direct genomic effect of estrogen is mediated by the interaction of its receptor (ER) with specific target sequences of DNA termed estrogen response elements, (ERE) and this interaction of ERs with ERE can be affected by differences in the ERE sequence, the ER subtype and/or dimerization of ERs [125]. On the other hand, there are also "non-genomic" effects of estrogen, which are independent of gene transcription or protein synthesis and involve steroid-induced modulation of cytoplasmic or cell membrane-bound regulatory proteins. Relevant biological actions of steroids have been associated with this signaling in different tissues [126]. Furthermore, signaling regulatory cascades such MAPK, PI3K and tyrosine kinases are modulated through non-transcriptional mechanisms by steroid hormones. Moreover, steroid hormone receptor modulation of cell membrane-associated molecules such as ion channels and G-protein-coupled receptors has been detected in a number of tissues. Binding of estrogens to receptors increases the expression of longevity-associated genes. By activation of the MAPK and NFκB signaling pathways, this binding can result in an upregulation of antioxidant enzymes including SOD and GPx, suggesting a mechanism by which mitochondria from females produce fewer ROS than those from males [127].

Baba et al. have examined the interaction of insulin signaling pathway, estrogen and OS [128]. Using a targeted knock-in strategy; they generated a homologous murine model replacing Pro-1195 with Leu in the gene encoding the insulin receptor. Mice homozygous for this mutant allele died in the neonatal stage from diabetic ketoacidosis, while heterozygous mice exhibited the suppressed kinase activity of the insulin receptor (InsR) but grew normally without spontaneously developing diabetes during adulthood. When heterozygous mice were evaluated for longevity phenotypes under conditions of OS (i.e., 80 % oxygen), mutant female mice survived 33.3 % longer than wild-type female mice, whereas mutant male mice survived 18.2 % longer than wild-type male mice. These results suggested that mutant mice acquired more resistance to OS, but the benefit of the longevity mutation was more pronounced in females than males. Moreover, MnSOD activity in mutant mice was significantly upregulated, suggesting that the suppressed insulin signaling leads to an enhanced antioxidant defense. Estrogen treatment of mutant mice resulted in elevated survival of mice with OS. Conversely both mutant and wild-type female mice had reduced survival response to OS when ovarectomized. Compared with wild-type mice, estrogen exhibited a significant influence in InsR mutants, suggesting that estrogen modulates insulin signaling in mutant mice. In addition, it was found that survival under OS conditions was further augmented when their diet was restricted. Taken together, these data suggest that distinct insulin, estrogen, and dietary signals can act in a cooperative way to enhance the resistance to OS in mice.

Advances on Aging and the Genome

Currently, there is a growing body of literature focusing on the identification of genes involved in multifactorial diseases of the old and in longevity. Nevertheless, important issues remains unanswered, including the definition of phenotype, if earlier and later onset phenotypes have loci in common, and how to rank or reject the many candidate disease loci found in different studies [129]. As pointed out by Vijg and Suh [130], future investigations are likely to involve large-scale case-control studies, in which large numbers of genes, corresponding to entire gene functional modules, will be assessed for all possible sequence variation and associated with detailed phenotypic information on each individual over extended periods of time. This should eventually unravel the genetic factors that contribute to each particular aging phenotype

We concur with these authors that aging, which affects all organ systems, is clearly one of the most complex phenotype that we know, and that insight into the genetic components of longevity and aging would offer the unprecedented opportunity to postpone and prevent some, if not all, late-life illnesses. Currently, the causes of aging still remain in great part unknown, probably because our limitations in studying aging systems; on the other hand, ample information has been gathered about individual cellular components at various ages, but without achieving a clear understanding of the integrated genomic circuits that control mechanisms of aging, survival, and stress responses. These authors further noted that with the emergence of functional genomics, we finally have the opportunity to study aging in a comprehensive manner, through a systems approach, and the opportunity to understand the dynamic network of genes that determines the physiology of an individual organism over time [131].

We have dealt earlier with the theories of aging and comment on the interactions of the genome and aging, outlining the paramount role played by mitochondria and telomeres. Point mutations and deletions of mtDNA have been found to increase with aging in several tissues in human, rodents and monkeys. Recently, the impact of mtDNA mutation has been more directly addressed experimentally by creating homozygous knock-in mice that express a proof-reading-deficient version of Polγ, the nuclear-encoded catalytic subunit of mtDNA polymerase γ [132]. The knock-in mice developed a three to five-fold increase in the levels of point mutations, as well as an increased amount of deleted mtDNA. The increase in somatic mtDNA mutations was associated with reduced life span and premature onset of aging-related phenotypes, including heart enlargement, thus providing a causative link between mtDNA mutations and aging. Furthermore, the accumulation of age-dependent mtDNA point mutations and deletions in post-mitotic tissues has been found significantly elevated in individuals with either mutations in the mitochondrial helicase Twinkle or in Polγ suggesting that the activity of proteins involved in mtDNA replication may be targeted in aging [133].

Experimental evidence indicates that short telomeres accumulate prior to senescence and that replicative senescence is not triggered by the first telomere to reach a critical minimal threshold length. These observations are compatible with limited repair of short telomeres by telomerase-dependent or telomerase-independent DNA repair pathways. Deficiencies in telomere repair may result in accelerated senescence and aging as well as genetic instability that facilitates malignant transformation as shown in Figure 1.3 [134]. Molecules that may have a significant role in the repair of telomeric DNA prior to replicative senescence include ATM, p53, PARP, DNA-PK, Ku70/80, the human hRad50-hMre11-p95 complex, BRCA 1 and 2 and the helicases that are implicated in Bloom's and Werner's syndrome.

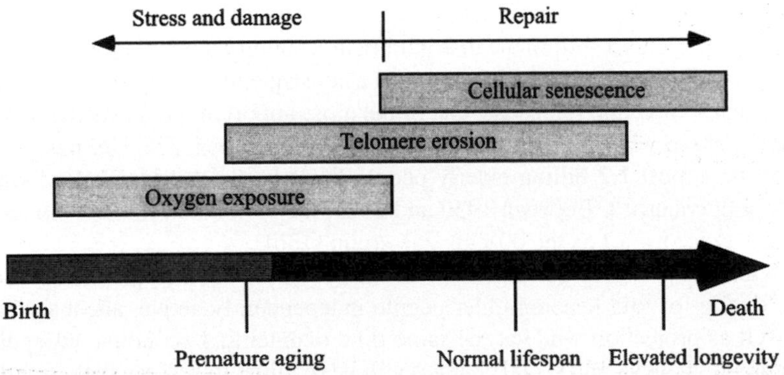

Fig. 1.3 The correlation of oxidative stress, telomeric damage and cell senescence with premature aging, normal aging and increased longevity.

As observed by Stewart and Weinberg [135], the cell phenotype of senescence operates to circumscribe the proliferative potential of mammalian cells, and the key regulators of these phenotypes are the telomeres whose erosion below a certain length can trigger crisis. The relationship between senescence and telomere function is rather complex; a number of physiological stresses as well as dysfunction of the complex molecular structures at the ends of telomeric DNA can trigger senescence. On the other hand, cells can escape senescence by inactivating the Rb and p53 tumor suppressor proteins and can surmount crisis by activating a telomere maintenance mechanism. Interestingly, the loss of a functional telomere influences biological functions as diverse as aging and carcinogenesis.

Notwithstanding, our current knowledge of aging and senescence has outpaced our understanding of the basic mechanisms underlying these processes. At present with the availability of the Human Genome Project (HGP) and an ever increasing number of animals models, as well as new and exciting molecular technologies, the unraveling of the underlying basic mechanisms of aging have already begun. We concur with Vijg and Suh that progress in functional genomics has brought us to the threshold of identifying genetic components of longevity and aging, and that no longer should attempts to identify genes be restricted to pedigree analysis. High-throughput genotyping of single nucleotide polymorphisms (SNPs) in the regulatory and coding regions of candidate human genes can be used directly to assess genetic variants in association with age and age-associated diseases in case-control studies in different geographical regions. We also need to evaluate adequate, well-defined population samples, in which people are monitored for various health parameters and biological samples are taken [132]. Large population surveys have now begun or are in the planning stage. In the UK the Biobank initiative, is a project that will follow the health of half a million volunteers, aged 45–69, for many years, collecting information on environmental and lifestyle factors and linking these to medical records and biological samples. While the genetic component of longevity by itself is important, it may be of much greater interest to elucidate the genetics of the various individual phenotypes that together comprise the aging phenome, and in the aging phenotype in populations monitored from middle age to old age. These longitudinal studies will provide an assessment of all stages in the progression of a disease, rather than at a single time. Furthermore, with the availability of large populations of individuals under such study it will be possible to find the genes that control human longevity and aging.

Epidemiology/Human Populations

Population Aging

Population aging represents a shift in the distribution of a country's population towards greater ages. This shift is in part related to increased longevity, as a consequence of improvements in human living conditions and health care, and represents one of the most important human achievements occurring not only in the western world, but also in less advanced countries. The UN has projected that by 2025 there will be almost 1.2 billion elderly people living in the world, 71 % of which are likely to be in developing countries. Between 1950 and 2025, the "Old" Old (those who are 80 years and above) will grow twice as fast as the 60-plus-age group [136].

However, with aging we are confronted with important issues, i.e., providing and maintaining an acceptable quality of life, keeping older people independently active, adequate health and productivity, as well as protection while at the same time maintaining economic prosperity in society. Multiple economic, financial and social changes will be required to achieve these goals. Importantly, the quality of life with active aging, depends on a number factors including, social, economic, personal and behavioral factors, as well as health and social services, environment, gender and culture.

In promoting active aging healthy and active life styles, including healthy nutrition policies, and prevention of chronic illnesses have to be encouraged.

Notwithstanding the above progress, population aging is not only the result of increased life expectancy, but is also related to a decline in fertility. An increase in longevity raises the average age of the population by raising the number of years that each person is old relative to number of years in which he is young, and decline in fertility increases the average age of the population by changing the ratio of people born recently to people born further in the past (the old). Of these two forces, it is declining fertility that is the dominant contributor to population aging in the world today [137]. While the large decline in total fertility rate is primarily responsible for the population aging that is taking place in the world's most developed countries, in developing countries where the fertility is, at least comparatively, high they may experience even faster population aging than the currently developed countries in the future. Parenthetically, the majority of the developed countries (with the exception of the United States) have fertility rates below their replacement levels, and their population growth is largely based on immigration together with an increased aging population, which arises from previous large generations now enjoying longer life expectancy.

Modifying/ Delaying Aging

The positive effect of CR on aging and longevity in rodents, as well as the activation of a genetic pathway in response to starvation in nematodes and mice has been reported. This genetic pathway may be conserved across phyla and might help delay aging, particularly human aging. On the other hand, Le Bourg [138] posed the question if delaying aging by hormesis may be more helpful than studying the effect of the genetic pathway used to survive starvation since these studies have largely been directed more to analysis of a rescue program used to resist starvation rather than to active in ad libitum-fed animals; therefore, it is not clear if aging can be delayed under the usual living conditions of animals and humans. Hormesis has been proposed as a way of studying aging under normal living conditions, because ad libitum-fed animals subjected to mild stresses can live slightly longer than control animals and display increased resistance to strong stresses. We agree with Le Bourg that it would be of interest to study the response to non-lethal stresses rather than lethal ones in animals subjected to a mild stress inducing hormesis, because elderly people are more often confronted by such non-lethal stresses (e.g., temperature drop in winter) than by lethal ones. Similarly, following the principles of hormesis, others scientists have suggested that the stress response may also counteract the negative effects of aging, and several mild stresses have been reported to increase longevity (irradiation, heat and cold shock, hypergravity, exercise, etc.). In particular one of them, hypergravity decreases the rate of behavioral aging. At this time the mechanisms whereby these stresses increase longevity are not clear, although they may involve metabolic regulation and induction of stress protein such as heat shock proteins (HSPs). It is worth noting than in response to increased level of ROS in the senescent heart, genes encoding mitochondrial stress proteins including both heat shock and antioxidant response proteins, such as HSP60, HO-1 and GPx are up-regulated [139]. Levels of HSP60 protein have been found increased in association with increased level of protein import into mitochondria indicating that defective mitochondrial protein import is not the primary cause of mitochondrial dysfunction [140]. A slight longevity increase have been reported in young adult flies of both sexes submitted to heat shock (37°C) for 1–3 weeks, although it was only observed with the lowest heat shock; longer shocks had neutral or negative effects [141]. Interestingly, the experimental flies with increased longevity did not show a delayed behavioral aging in contrast to hypergravity, but survived longer at 37°C than control flies. This higher thermotolerance was not associated with an increased HSP70 induction, suggesting that these stresses in comparison with hypergravity and other mild stresses may have dissimilar effects on aging and longevity.

Is Aging Reversible?

Our current understanding of aging is that it cannot be prevented nor reversed. Aging in general, is a complex process, of many causes, which involves numerous cellular and molecular changes and that along the way contribute to the expression of the multiple phenotypes of aging. Aging is universal in the animal kingdom where a tradeoff is being paid by most species between the energy that is expended in reproduction and what is used in the organismal body maintenance. Nevertheless, the changes of aging that gradually occurs in cells, tissues, organ and systems can be modulated, reduced or delayed by preventative means, like dietary restriction, and in human by following a healthy lifestyle. From the lower to the higher species in the animal kingdom similar basic changes occur with aging, although each organism ages in a unique way with its own timetable. Although the aging process brings a progressive decline in endurance/power and the risk of disease increases, healthy aging with adequate maintenance of body functions is still within the individual reach. Moreover, the emphasis should be not on the loss that occurs with aging, but rather on the gains that aging may bring to humans, and others species in the animal kingdom (e.g., elephants), such as increasing knowledge, leadership, well being, relationships and creativity.

References

1. Luciani F, Valensin S, Vescovini R, Sansoni P, Fagnoni F, Franceschi C, Bonafe M, Turchetti G. A stochastic model for CD8(+)T cell dynamics in human immunosenescence: implications for survival and longevity. J Theor Biol 2001;213:587–597
2. De Benedictis G, Tan Q, Jeune B, Christensen K, Ukraintseva SV, Bonafe M, Franceschi C, Vaupel JW, Yashin AI. Recent advances in human gene-longevity association studies. Mech Ageing Dev 2001;122:909–920
3. Vaupel JW, Carey JR, Christensen K, Johnson TE, Yashin AI, Holm NV, Iachine IA, Kannisto V, Khazaeli AA, Liedo P, Longo VD, Zeng Y, Manton KG, Curtsinger JW. Biodemographic trajectories of longevity. Science 1998;280:855–860
4. Perls TT, Bubrick E, Wager CG, Vijg J, Kruglyak L. Siblings of centenarians live longer. Lancet 1998;351:1560
5. Gudmundsson H, Gudbjartsson DF, Frigge M, Gulcher JR, Stefansson K. Inheritance of human longevity in Iceland. Eur J Hum Genet 2000;8:743–749
6. Carmelli, D. Intrapair comparisons of total life span in twins and pairs of sibs. Hum Biol 1982;54:525–537
7. Yashin AI, Iachine IA, Harris JR. Half of the variation in susceptibility to mortality is genetic: findings from Swedish twin survival data. Behav Genet 1999;29:11–19
8. Perls TT, Wilmoth J, Levenson R, Drinkwater M, Cohen M, Bogan H, Joyce E, Brewster S, Kunkel L, Puca A. Life-long sustained mortality advantage of siblings of centenarians. Proc Natl Acad Sci USA 2002;99: 8442–8447
9. Candore G, Aquino A, Balistreri CR, Bulati M, Di Carlo D, Grimaldi MP, Listi F, Orlando V, Vasto S, Caruso M, Colonna-Romano G, Lio D, Caruso C. Inflammation, longevity, and cardiovascular diseases: role of polymorphisms of TLR4. Ann N Y Acad Sci 2006;1067:282–287
10. Gerdes LU, Jeune B, Ranberg KA, Nybo H, Vaupel JW. Estimation of apolipoprotein E genotype-specific relative mortality risks from the distribution of genotypes in centenarians and middle-aged men: apolipoprotein E gene is a "frailty gene," not a "longevity gene". Genet Epidemiol 2000;19:202–210
11. Kervinen K, Savolainen MJ, Salokannel J, Hynninen A, Heikkinen J, Ehnholm C, Koistinen MJ, Kesaniemi YA. Apolipoprotein E and B polymorphisms – longevity factors assessed in nonagenarians. Atherosclerosis 1994;105:89–95
12. Louhija J, Miettinen HE, Kontula K, Tikkanen MJ, Miettinen TA, Tilvis RS. Aging and genetic variation of plasma apolipoproteins: Relative loss of the apolipoprotein E4 phenotype in centenarians. Arterioscler Thromb. 1994;14:1084–1089
13. Schachter F, Faure-Delanef L, Guenot F, Rouger H, Froguel P, Lesueur-Ginot L, Cohen D.Genetic associations with human longevity at the APOE and ACE loci. Nat Genet 1994;6:29–32
14. Jian-Gang Z, Yong-Xing M, Chuan-Fu W, Pei-Fang L, Song-Bai Z, Nui-Fan G, Guo-Yin F, Lin H. Apolipoprotein E and longevity among Han Chinese population. Mech Ageing Dev 1998;104:159–167
15. De Benedictis G, Falcone E, Rose G, Ruffolo R, Spadafora P, Baggio G, Bertolini S, Mari D, Mattace R, Monti D, Morellini M, Sansoni P, Franceschi C. DNA multiallelic systems reveal gene/longevity associations not detected by diallelic systems. The APOB locus. Hum Genet 1997;99:312–318

16. De Benedictis G, Carotenuto L, Carrieri G, De Luca M, Falcone E, Rose G, Yashin AI, Bonafe M, Franceschi C. Age-related changes of the 3'APOB-VNTR genotype pool in ageing cohorts. Ann Hum Genet 1998; 62: 115–122
17. Faure-Delanef L, Baudin B, Beneteau-Burnat B, Beaudoin JC, Giboudeau J, Cohen D.Plasma concentration, kinetic constants, and gene polymorphism of angiotensin I-converting enzyme in centenarians. Clin Chem 1998;44:2083–2087
18. Mari D, Mannucci PM, Duca F, Bertolini S, Franceschi C. Mutant factor V (Arg506Gln) in healthy centenarians. Lancet 1996;347:1044
19. Tanaka M, Gong JS, Zhang J, Yoneda M, Yagi K. Mitochondrial genotype associated with longevity. Lancet 1998;351:185–186
20. Takagi K, Yamada Y, Gong JS, Sone T, Yokota M, Tanaka M. Association of a 5178C→A (Leu237Met) polymorphism in the mitochondrial DNA with a low prevalence of myocardial infarction in Japanese individuals. Atherosclerosis 2004;175:281–286
21. Matsunaga H, Tanaka Y, Tanaka M, Gong JS, Zhang J, Nomiyama T, Ogawa O, Ogihara T, Yamada Y, Yagi K, Kawamori R. Antiatherogenic mitochondrial genotype in patients with type 2 diabetes. Diabetes Care 2001;24:500–503
22. De Benedictis G, Rose G, Carrieri G, De Luca M, Falcone E, Passarino G, Bonafe M, Monti D, Baggio G, Bertolini S, Mari D, Mattace R, Franceschi C. Mitochondrial DNA inherited variants are associated with successful aging and longevity in humans. FASEB J 1999;13:1532–1536
23. Rose G, Passarino G, Carrieri G, Altomare K, Greco V, Bertolini S, Bonafe M, Franceschi C, De Benedictis G. Paradoxes in longevity: sequence analysis of mtDNA haplogroup J in centenarians. Eur J Hum Genet 2001;9:701–707
24. Zhang J, Asin-Cayuela J, Fish J, Michikawa Y, Bonafe M, Olivieri F, Passarino G, De Benedictis G, Franceschi C, Attardi G. Strikingly higher frequency in centenarians and twins of mtDNA mutation causing remodeling of replication origin in leukocytes. Proc Natl Acad Sci USA 2003;100:1116–1121
25. Niemi AK, Moilanen JS, Tanaka M, Hervonen A, Hurme M, Lehtimaki T, Arai Y, Hirose N, Majamaa K. A combination of three common inherited mitochondrial DNA polymorphisms promotes longevity in Finnish and Japanese subjects. Eur J Hum Genet 2005;13:166–170
26. van Heemst D, Beekman M, Mooijaart SP, Heijmans BT, Brandt BW, Zwaan BJ, Slagboom PE, Westendorp RG. Reduced insulin/IGF-1 signalling and human longevity. Aging Cell 2005;4:79–85
27. Santoro A, Salvioli S, Raule N, Capri M, Sevini F, Valensin S, Monti D, Bellizzi D, Passarino G, Rose G, De Benedictis G, Franceschi C. Mitochondrial DNA involvement in human longevity. Biochim Biophys Acta 2006;1757:1388–1399
28. Heijmans BT, Westendorp RG, Knook DL, Kluft C, Slagboom PE. Angiotensin I-converting enzyme and plasminogen activator inhibitor-1 gene variants: risk of mortality and fatal cardiovascular disease in an elderly population-based cohort. J Am Coll Cardiol 1999;34:1176–1183
29. Juhan-Vague I, Pyke SM, Alessi MC, Jespersen J, Haverkate F, Thompson SG. Fibrinolytic factors and the risk of myocardial infarction or sudden death in patients with angina pectoris. Circulation 1996; 94:2057–2063
30. Hamsten A, Wiman B, de Faire U, Blomback M. Increased plasma levels of a rapid inhibitor of tissue plasminogen activator in young survivors of myocardial infarction. N Engl J Med 1985; 313:1557–1563
31. Hoekstra T, Geleijnse JM, Kluft C, Giltay EJ, Kok FJ, Schouten EG. 4G/4G genotype of PAI-1 gene is associated with reduced risk of stroke in elderly. Stroke 2003;34:2822–2828
32. Bader G, Zuliani G, Kostner GM, Fellin R. Apolipoprotein E polymorphism is not associated with longevity or disability in a sample of Italian octo- and nonagenarians. Gerontology 1998;44:293–299
33. Hobbs HH, Leitersdorf E, Leffert CC, Cryer DR, Brown MS, Goldstein JL Evidence for a dominant gene that suppresses hypercholesterolemia in a family with defective low density lipoprotein receptors.J Clin Invest 1989;84:656–664
34. Bonafe M, Valensin S, Gianni W, Marigliano V, Franceschi C. The unexpected contribution of immunosenescence to the leveling off of cancer incidence and mortality in the oldest old. Crit Rev Oncol Hematol 2001;39: 227–233
35. Franceschi C, Olivieri F, Marchegiani F, Cardelli M, Cavallone L, Capri M, Salvioli S, Valensin S, De Benedictis G, Di Iorio A, Caruso C, Paolisso G, Monti D. Genes involved in immune response/inflammation, IGF1/insulin pathway and response to oxidative stress play a major role in the genetics of human longevity: the lesson of centenarians. Mech Ageing Dev 2005;126:351–361
36. Jazwinski SM. Aging and longevity. Acta Biochim Pol. 2000;47:269–279
37. Jamet-Vierny C, Rossignol M, Haedens V, Silar P. What triggers senescence in Podospora anserina? Fungal Genet Biol 1999;27:26–35
38. Lorin S, Dufour A, Sainsard A. Mitochondrial metabolism and aging in the filamentous fungus *Podospora anserina*. Biochim Biophys Acta 2006:1757:604–610

39. Morrow G, Samson M, Michaud S, Tanguay RM. Overexpression of the small mitochondrial Hsp22 extends Drosophila life span and increases resistance to oxidative stress. FASEB J 2004;18:598–599
40. Morrow G, Battistini S, Zhang P, Tanguay RM. Decreased life span in the absence of expression of the mitochondrial small heat shock protein Hsp22 in Drosophila. J Biol Chem 2004;279:43382–43385
41. Hwangbo DS, Gershman B, Tu MP, Palmer M, Tatar M. Drosophila dFOXO controls life span and regulates insulin signalling in brain and fat body. Nature 2004;429:562–566
42. Kenyon C, Chang J, Gensch E, Rudner A, Tabtiang R. A C. elegans mutant that lives twice as long as wild type. Nature. 1993;366:461–464
43. Hwangbo DS, Gershman B, Tu MP, Palmer M, Tatar M. Drosophila dFOXO controls life span and regulates insulin signalling in brain and fat body. Nature 2004;429:562–566
44. Kaeberlein M, McVey M, Guarente L. The SIR2/3/4 complex and SIR2 alone promote longevity in Saccharomyces cerevisiae by two different mechanisms. Genes Dev 1999;13:2570–2580
45. Sinclair D, Guarente L. Extrachromosomal rDNA circles – a cause of aging in yeast. Cell 1997;91:1033–1042
46. Tissenbaum HA, Guarente L. Increased dosage of a sir-2 gene extends life span in C. elegans. Nature 2001;410:227–230
47. Berdichevsky A, Viswanathan M, Horvitz HR, Guarente L. C. elegans SIR-2.1 interacts with 14-3-3 proteins to activate DAF-16 and extend life span. Cell 2006;125:1165–1177
48. Morris JZ, Tissenbaum HA, Ruvkun G. A phosphatidylinositol-3-OH kinase family member regulating longevity and diapauses in Caenorhabditis elegans. Nature 1996;382:536–539
49. Koutarou D, Kimura KD, Tissenbaum HA, Liu Y, Ruvkun G. daf-2, an insulin receptor-like gene that regulates longevity and diapause in Caenorhabditis elegans. Science 1997;277:942–946
50. Ogg S, Paradis S, Gottlieb S, Patterson GI, Lee L, Tissenbaum HA, Ruvkun G. The Fork head transcription factor DAF-16 transduces insulin-like metabolic and longevity signals in C. elegans. Nature 1997;389: 994–999
51. Lin K, Dorman JB, Rodan A, Kenyon C. daf-16: an HNF-3/forkhead family member that can function to double the life-span of Caenorhabditis elegans. Science 1997;278:1319–1322
52. Viswanathan M, Kim SK, Berdichevsky A, Guarente L. A role for SIR-2.1 regulation of ER stress response genes in determining C. elegans life span. Dev Cell 2005;9:605–615
53. Haigis MC, Guarente LP. Mammalian sirtuins – emerging roles in physiology, aging, and calorie restriction. Genes Dev 2006;20:2913–2921
54. Lemieux ME, Yang X, Jardine K, He X, Jacobsen KX, Staines WA, Harper ME, McBurney MW. The Sirt1 deacetylase modulates the insulin-like growth factor signaling pathway in mammals. Mech Ageing Dev 2005;126:1097–1105
55. Langley E, Pearson M, Faretta M, Bauer UM, Frye RA, Minucci S, Pelicci PG, Kouzarides T. Human SIR2 deacetylates p53 and antagonizes PML/p53-induced cellular senescence. EMBO J 2002;21:2383–2396
56. Alcendor RR, Kirshenbaum LA, Imai S, Vatner SF, Sadoshima J. Silent information regulator 2alpha, a longevity factor and class III histone deacetylase, is an essential endogenous apoptosis inhibitor in cardiac myocytes. Circ Res 2004;95:971–980
57. Guarente L. SIR2 and aging – the exception that proves the rule. Trends Genet 2001;17:391–392
58. Hallows WC, Lee S, Denu JM. Sirtuins deacetylate and activate mammalian acetyl-CoA synthetases. Proc Natl Acad Sci USA 2006;103:10230–10235
59. Mostoslavsky R, Chua KF, Lombard DB, Pang WW, Fischer MR, Gellon L, Liu P, Mostoslavsky G, Franco S, Murphy MM, Mills KD, Patel P, Hsu JT, Hong AL, Ford E, Cheng HL, Kennedy C, Nunez N, Bronson R, Frendewey D, Auerbach W, Valenzuela D, Karow M, Hottiger MO, Hursting S, Barrett JC, Guarente L, Mulligan R, Demple B, Yancopoulos GD, Alt FW. Genomic instability and aging-like phenotype in the absence of mammalian SIRT6. Cell 2006;124:315–329
60. Rodgers JT, Lerin C, Haas W, Gygi SP, Spiegelman BM, Puigserver P. Nutrient control of glucose homeostasis through a complex of PGC-1alpha and SIRT1. Nature 2005;434:113–118
61. Picard F, Kurtev M, Chung N, Topark-Ngarm A, Senawong T, Machado De Oliveira R, Leid M, McBurney MW, Guarente L. Sirt1 promotes fat mobilization in white adipocytes by repressing PPAR-gamma. Nature 2004;429:771–776
62. Moynihan KA, Grimm AA, Plueger MM, Bernal-Mizrachi E, Ford E, Cras-Meneur C, Permutt MA, Imai S. Increased dosage of mammalian Sir2 in pancreatic beta cells enhances glucose-stimulated insulin secretion in mice. Cell Metab 2005;2:105–117
63. Bordone L, Motta MC, Picard F, Robinson A, Jhala US, Apfeld J, McDonagh T, Lemieux M, McBurney M, Szilvasi A, Easlon EJ, Lin SJ, Guarente L. Sirt1 regulates insulin secretion by repressing UCP2 in pancreatic beta cells. PLoS Biol 2006;4:e31
64. Giannakou ME, Goss M, Junger MA, Hafen E, Leevers SJ, Partridge L. Long-lived Drosophila with overexpressed dFOXO in adult fat body. Science 2004;305:361

65. Wang MC, Bohmann D, Jasper H. JNK extends life span and limits growth by antagonizing cellular and organism-wide responses to insulin signaling. Cell 2005;121:115–125
66. Lehtinen MK, Yuan Z, Boag PR, Yang Y, Villen J, Becker EB, DiBacco S, de la Iglesia N, Gygi S, Blackwell TK, Bonni A. A conserved MST-FOXO signaling pathway mediates oxidative-stress responses and extends life span. Cell 2006;125:987–1001
67. Weinert BT, Timiras PS. Theories of aging. J Appl Physiol 2003;95:1706–1716
68. Haldane JBS New paths in genetics. London: Allen & Unwin; 1941
69. Medawar, PB. An unsolved problem of biology. London: H. K. Lewis; 1952
70. Clark WR. Reflections on an unsolved problem of biology: the evolution of senescence and death. Adv Gerontol 2004;14:7–20
71. Charlesworth B. Fisher, Medawar, Hamilton and the evolution of aging. Genetics 2000;156:927–931
72. Rose MR. The evolutionary biology of aging. Oxford: Oxford University Press; 1991, Chapter 1
73. Comfort A. The biology of senescence. Edinburgh, UK: Churchill Livingstone; 1979
74. Gavrilov LA, Gavrilova NS. The biology of life-span: a quantitative approach. Switzerland: Harwood, Chur; 1991
75. Wachter KW, Finch CE. Between Zeus and the Salmon: the biodemography of longevity. Washington, DC: National Academy Press; 1997
76. Finch CE. Longevity, senescence, and the genome. Chicago, IL: University of Chicago Press; 1990
77. Williams, GC. Adaptation and natural selection. Princeton, NJ: Princeton University Press; 1966
78. Gavrilov LA, Gavrilova NS. Evolutionary theories of aging and longevity. Scientific World Journal 2002;2:339–356
79. Gavrilov LA, Gavrilova NS. The reliability theory of aging and longevity. Journal of Theoretical Biology 2001;213:527–545
80. Hekimi S. How genetic analysis tests theories of animal aging. Nat Genet 2006;38:985–991
81. Pletcher SD, Macdonald SJ, Marguerie R, Certa U, Stearns SC, Goldstein DB, Partridge L. Genome-wide transcript profiles in aging and calorically restricted Drosophila melanogaster. Curr Biol 2002;12:712–23
82. Weindruch R, Kayo T, Lee CK, Prolla TA. Microarray profiling of gene expression in aging and its alteration by caloric restriction in mice. J Nutr 2001;131:918S–923S
83. Zou S, Meadows S, Sharp L, Jan LY, Jan YN. Genome-wide study of aging and oxidative stress response in Drosophila melanogaster. Proc Natl Acad Sci USA 2000;97:13726–13731
84. Halaschek-Wiener J, Khattra JS, McKay S, Pouzyrev A, Stott JM, Yang GS, Holt RA, Jones SJ, Marra MA, Brooks-Wilson AR, Riddle DL. Analysis of long-lived C. elegans daf-2 mutants using serial analysis of gene expression. Genome Res 2005;15:603–615
85. Perls T, Kunkel L, Puca A. The genetics of aging. Curr Opin Genet Dev 2002;12:362–369
86. Puca AA, Daly MJ, Brewster SJ, Matise TC, Barrett J, Shea-Drinkwater M, Kang S, Joyce E, Nicoli J, Benson E, Kunkel LM, Perls T. A genome-wide scan for linkage to human exceptional longevity identifies a locus on chromosome 4. Proc Natl Acad Sci USA 2001;98:10505–10508
87. Oh H, Taffet GE, Youker KA, Entman ML, Overbeek PA, Michael LH, Schneider MD. Telomerase reverse transcriptase promotes cardiac muscle cell proliferation, hypertrophy, and survival. Proc Natl Acad Sci USA 2001;98:10308–10313
88. Young AT, Lakey JR, Murray AG, Mullen JC, Moore RB. In vitro senescence occurring in normal human endothelial cells can be rescued by ectopic telomerase activity. Transplant Proc 2003;35:2483–2485
89. Steinert S, Shay JW, Wright WE. Transient expression of human telomerase extends the life span of normal human fibroblasts. Biochem Biophys Res Commun 2000;273:1095–1098
90. Yang J, Chang E, Cherry AM, Bangs CD, Oei Y, Bodnar A, Bronstein A, Chiu CP, Herron GS. Human endothelial cell life extension by telomerase expression. J Biol Chem 1999;274:26141–26148
91. von Zglinicki T, Martin-Ruiz CM. Telomeres as biomarkers for ageing and age-related diseases. Curr Mol Med 2005;5:197–203
92. Martin-Ruiz CM, Gussekloo J, van Heemst D, von Zglinicki T, Westendorp RG. Telomere length in white blood cells is not associated with morbidity or mortality in the oldest old: a population-based study. Aging Cell 2005;4:287–289
93. Collerton J, Martin-Ruiz C, Kenny A, Barrass K, von Zglinicki T, Kirkwood T, Keavney B. Telomere length is associated with left ventricular function in the oldest old: the Newcastle 85+ study. Eur Heart J 2007;28:172–176
94. Harman, D. Aging: a theory based on free radical and radiation chemistry. J Gerontal 1956; 11:298–300
95. Beckman K, Ames, B. The free radical theory of aging matures. Physiol Rev 1998; 78:548–581
96. Sohal, R., Weindruch R. Oxidative stress, caloric restriction, and aging. Science 1996;273:59–63
97. Orr WC, Sohal RS. Extension of life-span by overexpression of superoxide dismutase and catalase in Drosophila melanogaster. Science 1994;263:1128–1130

98. Larsen PL. Aging and resistance to oxidative damage in Caenorhabditis elegans. Proc Natl Acad Sci USA 1993;90:8905–8909
99. Melov S, Ravenscroft J, Malik S, Gill MS, Walker DW, Clayton PE, Wallace DC, Malfroy B, Doctrow SR, Lithgow GJ. Extension of life-span with superoxide dismutase/catalase mimetics. Science 2000;289:1567–1569
100. Sohal RS, Ku HH, Agarwal S. Biochemical correlates of longevity in two closely related rodent species. Biochem Biophys Res Commun 1993;196:7–11
101. Huang TT, Carlson EJ, Gillespie AM, Shi Y, Epstein CJ. Ubiquitous overexpression of CuZn superoxide dismutase does not extend life span in mice. J Gerontol A Biol Sci Med Sci 2000;55:B5–B9
102. Mehlhorn RJ. Oxidants and antioxidants in aging. In: Timiras PS, editor. Physiological basis of aging and geriatrics. 3rd ed. Boca Raton, FL: CRC, 2003. p. 61–83
103. Brown-Borg HM, Rakoczy SG. Catalase expression in delayed and premature aging mouse models. Exp Gerontol 2000;35:199–212
104. Schriner SE, Linford NJ, Martin GM, Treuting P, Ogburn CE, Emond M, Coskun PE, Ladiges W, Wolf N, Van Remmen H, Wallace DC, Rabinovitch PS. Extension of murine life span by overexpression of catalase targeted to mitochondria. Science 2005;308:1909–1911
105. Finkel T, Holbrook NJ. Oxidants, oxidative stress and the biology of ageing. Nature 2000;408:239–247
106. Caratero A, Courtade M, Bonnet L, Planel H, Caratero C. Effect of a continuous gamma irradiation at a very low dose on the life span of mice. Gerontology 1998;44:272–276
107. Hyun DH, Emerson SS, Jo DG, Mattson MP, de Cabo R. Calorie restriction up-regulates the plasma membrane redox system in brain cells and suppresses oxidative stress during aging. Proc Natl Acad Sci U S A 2006;103:19908–19912
108. Merry BJ. Molecular mechanisms linking calorie restriction and longevity. Int J Biochem Cell Biol 2002;34:1340–1354
109. Mecocci P, Fano G, Fulle S, MacGarvey U, Shinobu L, Polidori MC, Cherubini A, Vecchiet J, Senin U, Beal MF. Age-dependent increases in oxidative damage to DNA, lipids, and proteins in human skeletal muscle. Free Radic Biol Med 1999;26:303–308
110. Kregel KC, Zhang HJ. An integrated view of oxidative stress in aging: basic mechanisms, functional effects, and pathological considerations. Am J Physiol Regul Integr Comp Physiol 2007;292:R18–R36
111. Gompertz B. On the nature of the function expressive of the law of human mortality and on a new mode of determining life contingencies. Philos. Trans Roy Soc Lond A 1825;115:513–585
112. Rose MR, Rauser CL, Mueller LD, Benford G. A revolution for aging research. Biogerontology 2006;7:269–277
113. Masoro EJ. Overview of caloric restriction and ageing. Mech Ageing Dev 2005;126:913–922
114. Duffy PH, Feuers RJ, Hart RW. Effect of chronic caloric restriction on the circadian regulation of physiological and behavioral variables in old male B6C3F1 mice. Chronobiol Int 1990;7:291–303
115. Houthoofd K, Braeckman BP, Johnson TE, Vanfleteren JR. Life extension via dietary restriction is independent of the Ins/IGF-1 signalling pathway in Caenorhabditis elegans. Exp Gerontol 2003;38:947–954
116. Houthoofd K, Vanfleteren JR. The longevity effect of dietary restriction in Caenorhabditis elegans. Exp Gerontol 2006;41:1026–1031
117. Hansen M, Taubert S, Crawford D, Libina N, Lee SJ, Kenyon C. Life span extension by conditions that inhibit translation in Caenorhabditis elegans. Aging Cell 2007;6:95–110
118. Powers RW III, Kaeberlein M, Caldwell SD, Kennedy BK, Fields S. Extension of chronological life span in yeast by decreased TOR pathway signaling. Genes Dev 2006;20:174–184
119. Kapahi P, Zid BM, Harper T, Koslover D, Sapin V, Benzer S. Regulation of life span in Drosophila by modulation of genes in the TOR signaling pathway. Curr Biol 2004;14:885–890
120. Masoro EJ. The role of hormesis in life extension by dietary restriction. Interdiscip Top Gerontol 2007;35:1–17
121. Proust J, Moulias R, Fumeron F, Bekkhoucha F, Busson M, Schmid M, Hors J. HLA and longevity. Tissue Antigens 1982;19:168–173
122. Dorak; Ivanova R, Henon N, Lepage V, Charron D, Vicaut E, Schachter F. HLA-DR alleles display sex-dependent effects on survival and discriminate between individual and familial longevity. Hum Mol Genet 1998;7: 187–194
123. De Benedictis G, Carotenuto L, Carrieri G, De Luca M, Falcone E, Rose G, Cavalcanti S, Corsonello F, Feraco E, Baggio G, Bertolini S, Mari D, Mattace R, Yashin AI, Bonafe M, Franceschi C. Gene/longevity association studies at four autosomal loci (REN, THO, PARP, SOD2). Eur J Hum Genet 1998;6:534–541
124. Franceschi C, Motta L, Valensin S, Rapisarda R, Franzone A, Berardelli M, Motta M, Monti D, Bonafe M, Ferrucci L, Deiana L, Pes GM, Carru C, Desole MS, Barbi C, Sartoni G, Gemelli C, Lescai F, Olivieri F, Marchegiani F, Cardelli M, Cavallone L, Gueresi P, Cossarizza A, Troiano L, Pini G, Sansoni P, Passeri G, Lisa R, Spazzafumo L, Amadio L, Giunta S, Stecconi R, Morresi R, Viticchi C, Mattace R, De Benedictis G, Baggio G. Do men and women follow different trajectories to reach extreme longevity? Italian Multicenter Study on Centenarians (IMUSCE). Aging (Milano) 2000;12:77–84

125. Gruber CJ, Gruber DM, Gruber IM, Wieser F, Huber JC. Anatomy of the estrogen response element. Trends Endocrinol Metab 2004;15:73–78
126. Simoncini T, Mannella P, Fornari L, Caruso A, Varone G, Genazzani AR. Genomic and non-genomic effects of estrogens on endothelial cells. Steroids 2004;69:537–542
127. Vina J, Sastre J, Pallardo FV, Gambini J, Borras C. Role of mitochondrial oxidative stress to explain the different longevity between genders: protective effect of estrogens. Free Radic Res 2006;40:1359–1365
128. Baba T, Shimizu T, Suzuki Y, Ogawara M, Isono K, Koseki H, Kurosawa H, Shirasawa T. Estrogen, insulin, and dietary signals cooperatively regulate longevity signals to enhance resistance to oxidative stress in mice. J Biol Chem 2005;280:16417–16426
129. Slagboom PE, Heijmans BT, Beekman M, Westendorp RG, Meulenbelt I. Genetics of human aging. The search for genes contributing to human longevity and diseases of the old. Ann N Y Acad Sci 2000;908:50–63
130. Vijg J, Suh Y. Genetics of longevity and aging. Annu Rev Med 2005;56:193–212
131. Vijg J, Suh Y. Functional genomics of ageing. Mech Ageing Dev 2003;124:3–8
132. Trifunovic A, Wredenberg A, Falkenberg M, Spelbrink JN, Rovio AT, Bruder CE, Bohlooly-YM, Gidlof S, Oldfors A, Wibom R, Tornell J, Jacobs HT, Larsson NG. Premature ageing in mice expressing defective mitochondrial DNA polymerase. Nature 2004;27:417–423
133. Wanrooij S, Luoma P, van Goethem G, van Broeckhoven C, Suomalainen A, Spelbrink JN. Twinkle and POLγ defects enhance age-dependent accumulation of mutations in the control region of mtDNA. Nucleic Acids Res 2004;32:3053–3064
134. Lansdorp PM. Repair of telomeric DNA prior to replicative senescence. Mech Ageing Dev 2000;118:23–34
135. Stewart SA, Weinberg RA. Telomeres: cancer to human aging. Annu Rev Cell Dev Biol 2006;22:531–557
136. Iliescu ML, Zanoschi G. Population aging and public health. The active aging concep Rev Med Chir Soc Med Nat Iasi 2005;109:120–123
137. Weil, DN. The economics of population aging. In: Rosenzweig MR, Stark O, editors. Handbook of population and family economics. New York: Elsevier; 1997, p. 967–1014
138. Le Bourg E. Delaying aging: could the study of hormesis be more helpful than that of the genetic pathway used to survive starvation? Biogerontology 2003;4:319–324
139. Marin-Garcia J, Goldenthal MJ, Pi Y. Mitochondrial and nuclear gene expression in the senescent heart. Unpublished data.
140. Craig EE, Hood DA. Influence of aging on protein import into cardiac mitochondria. Am J Physiol 1997;272:H2983–H2988
141. Le Bourg E, Valenti P, Lucchetta P, Payre F. Effects of mild heat shocks at young age on aging and longevity in Drosophila melanogaster. Biogerontology 2001;2:155–164

Chapter 2
Overview of Cardiovascular Aging

Overview

Cardiovascular (CV) aging can be defined as a phenomenon of progressive and cumulative decline in the heart's physiological functions, which inevitably occurs over time in all living organisms, and eventually will terminate in death. While normal chronological aging cannot be prevented there are certain things we can do to slow down "pathological aging." Because aging results from the combined acceleration of inflammation, depletion, and wear and tear, individualized interventions in the aging patient might help to reduce morbidity by decreasing those periods of functional decline common in old individuals. In this way, the health span will come closer to matching the life span. It is not clear whether aging in general, and CV aging in particular occur fundamentally thru genetic processes (intrinsic factors) or from an accumulation of abnormal macromolecules or extrinsic factors, such as DNA, proteins and lipids (mostly damaged by environmental factors, including reactive oxidative species [ROS]) or from a combination of both intrinsic and extrinsic elements; nevertheless, because the continuous marked increase in life expectancy and life span, researchers and clinicians must be aware of the effects of aging and the available treatment modalitics.

Introduction

Cardiac aging is a rather complex multifactorial process unlikely to be dependent on a unique, singular, pathway or determined gene(s) or gene products. On the contrary, a number of specific and non-specific pathways and genes appear to play a role in the general regulation/modulation of life span, and cardiac aging in particular. At the molecular level, multiple mechanisms interplay in cardiac aging either in parallel or in series, including the involvement of somatic mutations, telomere loss, defects in protein turnover, protein functional decline with accumulation of defective proteins, (i.e., impaired induction of heat shock proteins and decline in chaperone function) and mitochondrial defects. Most of these mechanisms produce significant damage to cardiac macromolecules.

From a cardiovascular standpoint, some mechanisms appear to be more at work than others, in particular the molecular stresses that defective mitochondrial bioenergetics and biogenesis may bring to cardiomyocytes, as well as alterations in hormonal and inflammatory signaling and telomere shortening. Identification of the totality of the mechanisms/pathways contributing to cardiac aging is probably an unattainable goal, although important work in this regard is currently in progress. A promising development is the availability of high output genetic screening applied to both new animal model systems as well as human subjects. Furthermore, approaches such as integrative physiology could be used to assess/monitor the function of the heart non-invasively and without

J. Marín-García, *Aging and the Heart*,

perturbing cardiovascular hemodynamics. For instance, using optical coherent tomography (OCT) the contractility of the heart of adult *Drosophila* was evaluated by Wolf et al. [1]. They were able to accurately distinguish between normal and abnormal cardiac function based on measurements of internal cardiac chamber dimensions *in vivo*. Decreased contractility with cardiomegaly was found in association with mutations in cardiomyocyte sarcomeric or cytoskeletal proteins, including troponin I, tropomyosin 2 or δ-sarcoglycan, recapitulating in this animal model the cardiac phenotypes associated with specific mutations that cause human dilated cardiomyopathy (DCM.) This approach could be employed to screening genes that could also be involved in the cardiomyopathy of aging. Later on in this chapter, further discussion will be presented about the feasibility and practicality of using animal models in the study of CV aging, together with the mechanisms that may bring about CV aging.

Biophysiology of CV Aging

The processes of biological CV aging are mechanistically connected to reduced physiological reserve, abnormal drug handling, and pharmacodynamic responses. Thus, an intrinsic, continuous and irreversible process of progressive decline in its molecular and physiological function characterizes the aging heart, and this cardiac deterioration is the most common cause of death in elderly people. When cardiac disease is added to this normal process it may be called extrinsic cardiac aging. The aging human heart displays alterations in the histology of the vasculature and hemodynamics, including the development of large resistance vessels with intima-media-thickening and increasing deposition of matrix substance, which ultimately will lead to reduced compliance and increased vessel stiffness and endothelial dysfunction [2, 3]. Furthermore, with aging, there is increased left ventricular mass relative to chamber volume, decreased diastolic function [4–6] and decreased β-adrenergic sympathetic responsiveness [7]. While interactions between advanced age, disease and physical inactivity need to be considered when interpreting age-associated changes in cardiovascular function, the "aging process" in itself occurs independently of changes on cardiac structure and performance, such as cardiac hypertrophy and prolonged myocardial contractility. Cellular mechanisms thought to be involved in cardiac aging, include prolonged action potential (AP) duration, altered myosin heavy chain (MHC) isoform expression and sarcoplasmic reticulum (SR) function, all of which may lead to changes in cardiac excitation–contraction (E-C) coupling. Cardiac E-C coupling cycle or cardiac cycle has been shown to be prolonged with increased age, probably due to cytosolic Ca^{2+} overload-induced dysregulation [7]. The cytosolic Ca^{2+} load is dependent on multiple factors, including membrane structure and permeability, regulatory proteins within the membrane, and ROS levels, which affect both membrane structure and function. However, the link between advanced age and altered cardiac E-C coupling is not yet fully understood.

At present, significant progress is being made in our understanding of the molecular and cellular changes that underlie the aging processes. Rapidly evolving technologies continue to unravel how genes control cell and tissue function. For example, the technique of DNA microarray gene profiling permits a comparison of expression of tens of thousands of genes at one time to determine which genes are turned on or off in a particular cell or condition. The USA's National Institute of Aging (NIA) has at present a collection of 15,000 mouse genes, including genes active in early development, and this repository is available to research institutions worldwide. Verified sequences of each gene in the set are also available, and by comparing the sequence information with genes that have already been well studied, scientists may be able to determine the function of these genes in mice and eventually in humans.

Mechanisms/Signaling Pathways in the Aging Heart

Telomeres and CV Aging

Most of the current theories on CV aging stand by the principle that accumulation of nuclear and mtDNA damage, of variable severity, will result in senescence of cardiomyocytes since DNA can be easily oxidized and damaged by a number of insults, including diet, toxins, pollution, environment, as well as other epigenetic influences and lifestyle. Despite a variety of DNA repair systems, DNA damage including base modification, large-scale rearrangements, single-strand and double-strand breaks produced over a lifetime accumulate in aging. Evidence of this aging-associated DNA damage is most evident in mtDNA, presumably because of its proximity to the formation of ROS as well as to the less extensive protection provided by mitochondrial-based DNA repair systems. However, as previously noted in Chapter 1, telomeres are particular aging-sensitive areas of nuclear chromosomes.

Located at the end of chromosomes, telomeres are DNA-protein structures which have been shown to be indispensable in maintaining not only the stability and integrity of the genome but are integral to the regulation of life span of both cultured cardiomyocytes and the entire organism [8]. The telomeric complex is composed of noncoding double-stranded repeats of G-rich tandem DNA sequences (TTAGGG in humans) that are extended several kilobase pairs, the enzyme telomerase, (consisting of a catalytic telomerase reverse transcriptase [TERT] and a telomerase RNA component [Terc] serving as a template for the synthesis of new telomere DNA repeats) and numerous associated proteins with structural and regulatory roles that participate in the control of telomere length and capping. In most somatic cells, including vascular endothelial cells (ECs), smooth muscle cells (SMCs), and cardiomyocytes, telomerase activity is insufficient, and telomere shortening occurs with increasing cell division, resulting in irreversible cell growth arrest and cellular senescence. For instance, ECs from human abdominal aorta display age-dependent telomere shortening and increased frequency of aneuploidy [9]. Moreover, a greater rate of age-associated telomere loss has been found in ECs from intimal regions of human iliac arteries [10] and abdominal arteries [11]. Age-dependent telomere shortening may trigger defective cellular function, vascular dysfunction and compromised viability of the aged organism (as illustrated in Fig. 2.1). Moreover, increasing evidence suggests an association between telomere length and cardiovascular disease (CVD). For instance several studies have documented telomere attrition and evidence of cellular senescence in vascular cells in coronary artery disease (CAD) and human atherosclerosis [12–14]. Vascular SMCs from atherosclerotic fibrous caps expressed markers of senescence (e.g., senescence-associated β-galactosidase) not seen in normal vessels, and markedly shorter telomeres than normal vessels compared with normal medial vascular SMC; telomere shortening was closely associated with increasing severity of atherosclerosis [12]. Average telomere length in leukocytes of 10 patients with severe CAD was significantly shorter than in 20 controls with normal coronary angiograms after adjustment for age and sex [13]. Telomere length was shorter in white blood cells from hypertensive men with carotid artery plaques compared to hypertensive men without plaques and multivariate analysis indicated that telomere length was a significant predictor of the presence of carotid artery plaques [14].

Interestingly, in the Newcastle 85+ study telomere length was found to be a predictor of LV ejection fraction (EF) in the oldest old subjects (85+ years of age) [15], in which longer telomeres were associated with a significant increase in EF as measured by echocardiography. Nevertheless, whether telomere shortening is a direct cause of the cardiovascular pathology of aging or a consequence is not known.

Since telomere dysfunction and telomere shortening have been observed with aging in SMCs, endothelial, and white blood cells, they may be the primary factors in predisposing vascular tissues to atherosclerosis, and to a decreasing capacity for neovascularization [8]. Interestingly, attrition of

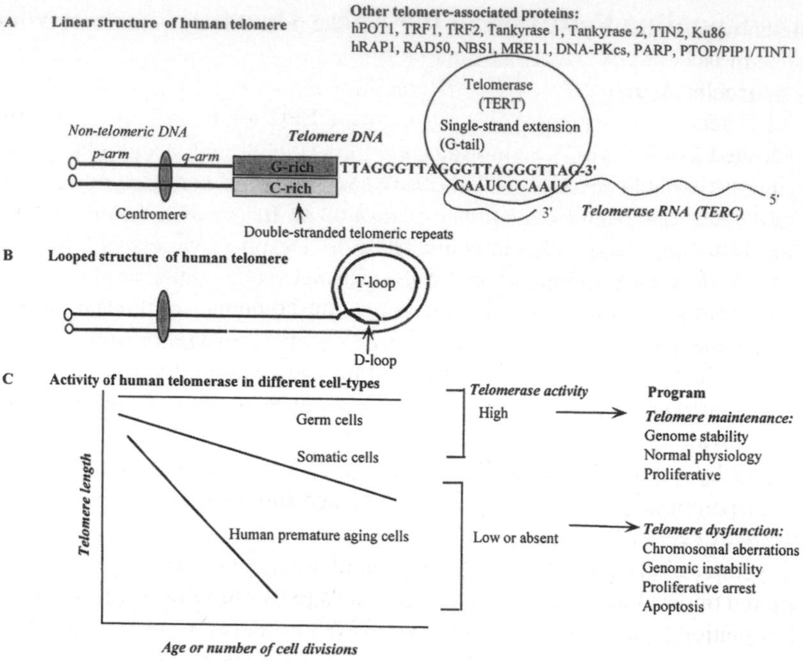

Fig. 2.1 Telomeres, telomerase and cell proliferation
A) Linear structure of telomeres present at the ends of the chromosomes (one end at the Q arm is shown here) are composed of a tandem repeated sequence in telomeric DNA, a telomerase ribonucleoprotein complex including a catalytic telomerase reverse transcriptase holoenzyme (TERT), a RNA component and additional telomeric proteins (listed on top) B) Looped structure of telomere shows formation of T-loop and D-loop region. C) Telomere length decreases in aging in somatic cells but not in germ cells. As telomerase activity is low or absent in most somatic cells, progressive telomere erosion occurs with each mitotic division during normal aging. In germ cells (and tumor cells) containing high telomerase activity- no change in telomere length is seen with aging or progressive divisions. Accelerated telomere attrition is associated with human premature aging. Some of the phenotypic changes associated with telomere length are shown on the bottom right.

telomere length is most prominent under conditions of high oxidative stress (OS), whose prevalence is likely linked in hypertensive and diabetic individuals, and in individuals with CAD. As we discuss further in Chapter 4, under conditions of mild chronic OS, the loss of telomere integrity is a major trigger for the onset of premature senescence [16]. Kurz et al. recently demonstrated that glutathione-dependent redox homeostasis plays a key role in the preservation of telomere function in endothelial cells [17]. Increasing intracellular OS in human umbilical vein ECs (HUVECs) by treating cells with inhibitors of glutathione synthesis caused premature EC senescence with diminished telomere integrity. Incubation of ECs with H_2O_2 induced the nuclear export of TERT into the cytosol and loss of nuclear telomerase activity, and the onset of EC replicative senescence [18]. Similarly, cultivation of ECs resulted in an increased endogenous ROS formation starting after 29 population doublings concomitant with nuclear TERT export and senescence onset. Incubation of ECs with the antioxidant N-acetylcysteine, or with the statin atorvastatin, reduced the intracellular ROS formation and delayed nuclear export of TERT protein, loss in the overall TERT activity, and the onset of replicative senescence.

Recent observations have demonstrated that telomere biology also plays a significant role in the functional augmentation of endothelial progenitor cells (EPCs) by statins [19]. The *ex vivo* culturing of EPCs leads to premature replicative senescence brought about by uncapping of telomeres associated with loss of telomere repeat-binding factor (TRF2) and telomeric dysfunction rather than telomere shortening. Co-treatment of the cultured EPCs with statins delayed their premature senescence, in part by induction of TRF2 expression at the post-translational level. While the ability of EPCs to sustain ischemic tissue repair may be limited in the aging heart, estrogens which have been shown to accelerate recovery of the endothelium after vascular injury, were able to inhibit the onset of EPC senescence and significantly increase EPC telomerase activity [20]. Incubation of *ex vivo* cultivated EPCs with 17β-estradiol in a dose-dependent fashion significantly increased TERT transcript levels as gauged by RT-PCR. The finding that this anti-senescent effect of estrogen was significantly inhibited by pharmacological blockers of the phosphoinositide-3 kinase (PI3K) activity confirmed the role of PI3K/Akt pathway in mediating TERT induction by estrogen also suggested by elevated Akt phosphorylation in estrogen-treated EPCs. In addition, EPCs treated with 17β-estradiol exhibited significantly enhanced mitogenic potential and release of VEGF protein; moreover, EPCs treated with both 17β-estradiol and VEGF were more likely to integrate into the network formation than those treated with VEGF alone. Others have shown that estrogen also promotes cardiovascular protection via non-nuclear effects of estrogen receptor signaling leading to endothelial nitric oxide synthase (eNOS) activation also utilizing the P13K/Akt pathway [21]. The production of NO by cultured vascular ECs which could be induced by repeated exposure to the NO donor *S*-nitroso-penicillamine reduced EC senescence and delayed age-dependent inhibition of telomerase activity [22].

Telomerase inactivation during aging may also be related to the oxidized low-density lipoprotein (LDL)-accelerated onset of EPC senescence, which leads to the impairment of proliferative capacity and network formation [23]. Oxidized LDL-induced EPC senescence was accompanied by a 50% reduction in telomerase activity. The cardiovascular protective effects of estrogens promoted via indirect actions on lipoprotein metabolism, and through direct effects on vascular ECs and SMCs likely contribute to the lower incidence of CVD observed in premenopausal women compared with men. In this regard, it is noteworthy that women have a decelerated rate of age-dependent telomere attrition over men [24].

Several observations primarily in studies with human fibroblasts support the concept that the average telomere length is better maintained in conditions of low OS generated by either addition of antioxidants, low oxygen or overexpression of antioxidant enzymes [25–27]. Selective targeting of antioxidants directly to the mitochondria can counteract telomere shortening and increase life span in fibroblasts under mild OS [28]. These studies have led to the proposal that mitochondrial dysfunction may be a key mechanism underlying the loss of cellular proliferative capacity characterizing replicative senescence through enhanced telomere shortening (Fig. 2.2), and the generation of ROS may signal the nucleus to limit cell proliferation through telomere shortening and telomeres as sensors to damaged mitochondria [29].

Furthermore, there is increasing evidence that telomere dysfunction is an important factor in the pathogenesis of human and experimental CVDs associated with aging including hypertension, atherosclerosis, and heart failure (HF) (Fig. 2.3) and is increasingly viewed as an important potential therapeutic target in their treatment.

Cellular Damage/Cell Loss, Mitochondria and CV Aging

Cell damage occurs at random in any organ or tissue, including the heart, although the number of damaged cells required to affect cardiac function is unknown. When assessing cell damage in the heart (or any other similar organ) one should be mindful of the significant difference between using *in vitro* compared to *in vivo* approaches, with cells in culture reaching a limit in their potential for cell division/differentiation, which may not occur in *in vivo* [30]. Therefore caution should be exercised in the interpretation of data collected from different methodologies. Previous observations have shown that under physiological and pathological conditions, ROS are abundantly generated

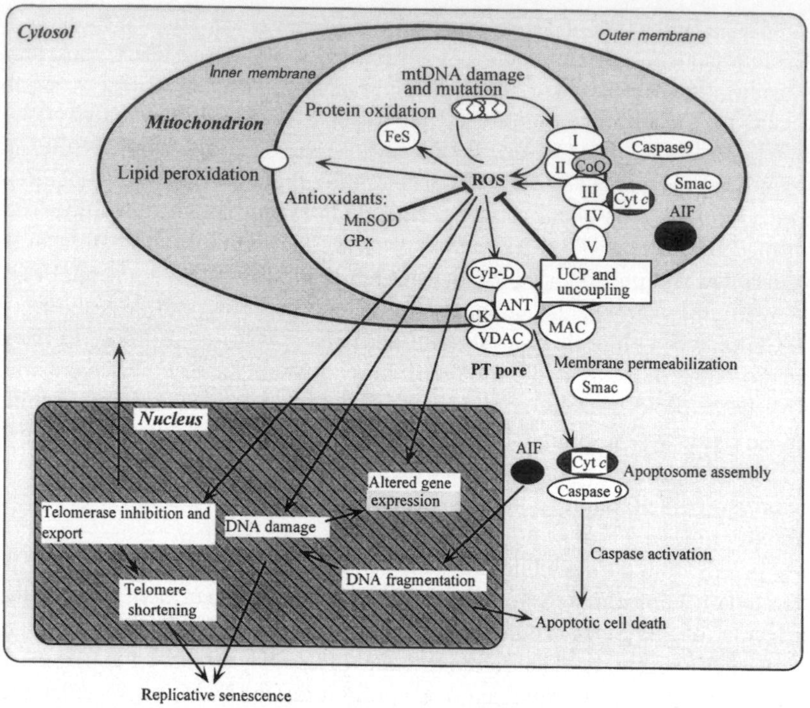

Fig. 2.2 Mitochondrial ROS production contributes to telomere-dependent replicative senescence
Production of ROS by aberrant mitochondrial respiratory complexes thought to occur in aging leads to mtDNA and protein damage and lipid peroxidation, PT pore and apoptotic progression (via cytochrome *c* release, membrane permeabilization, apoptosome formation and nuclear DNA fragmentation). ROS also affects the nucleus by reducing telomerase activity and increasing its export from the nucleus, causing direct DNA damage and activating specific gene expression – all of which contribute to the signaling of replicative senescence. Also depicted is the involvement of antioxidant response both in the mitochondria (e.g., MnSOD and GPx) and in the cytosol, which can remove ROS by scavenging free radicals.

in mitochondria, mainly during aging and in ischemia-reperfusion of the heart. Moreover, mitochondrial dysfunction and ROS generation may play a significant part in the loss of postmitotic cells, such as cardiomyocytes. Confirming this, *in vitro* studies of H_2O_2-treated cardiomyocytes in our laboratory and others have shown that increased mitochondrial OS and declining mitochondrial energy production lead to the activation of apoptotic pathways [31, 32]. However, whether this also occurs in the aging heart *in vivo* is not known.

Although the role of apoptosis in normal myocardial aging is presently under considerable debate (as discussed further in Chapter 4), cardiomyocyte apoptosis has been confirmed by data demonstrating that the aging rat heart had significantly elevated levels of cytochrome *c* release from mitochondria, as well as decreased levels of the antiapoptotic protein Bcl-2, whereas levels of the proapoptotic protein Bax were unchanged [33]. Moreover, preliminary evidence from both animal models and human clinical studies suggests that apoptosis also plays a contributory role in aging-associated cardiovascular diseases including cardiomyopathy and HF, increased susceptibility to ischemia and myocardial infarction (MI), and atherosclerosis [34–37].

The mitochondrial-mediated intrinsic apoptotic pathway, which has been documented in the aging and failing heart, may play a significant role in the development of cardiac dysfunction and pathogenesis. This pathway also features an extensive dialogue between the mitochondria, the nucleus and other subcellular organelles (described in more detail in Chapter 4). Central to the early triggering events in the intrinsic apoptotic pathway, the release to the cytosol of a number of

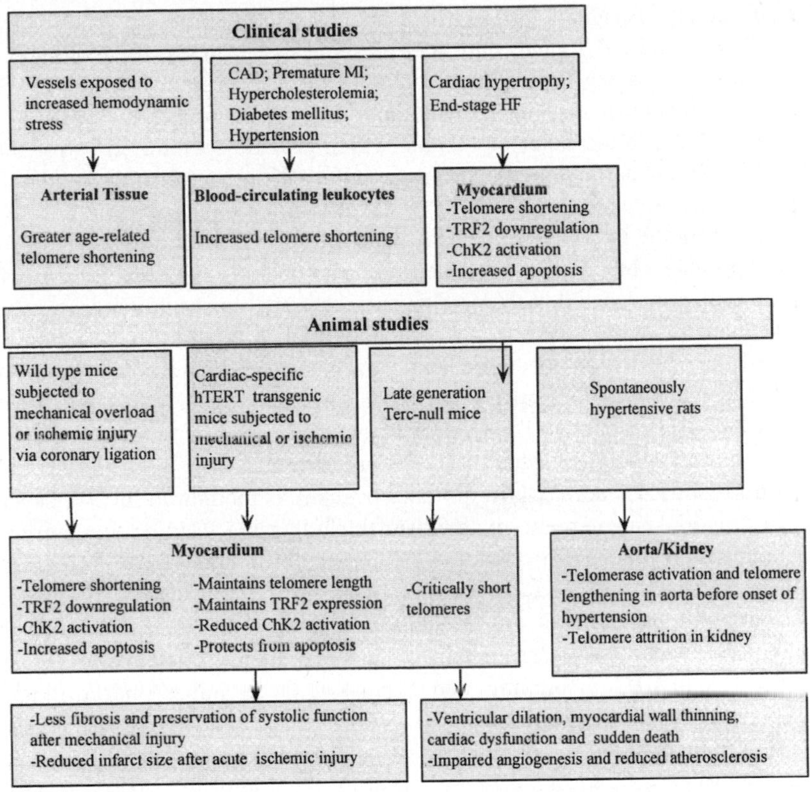

Fig. 2.3 Telomeres and telomerase in human and animal's models with cardiovascular disease (CVD) Telomere and telomerase phenotype in different tissues from patients with indicated CVD, and selected animal models of CVD.

mitochondrial-specific proteins from the mitochondrial intermembrane space including cytochrome *c*, Endonuclease G (EndoG), AIF (apoptosis inducing factor) and Smac/Diablo subsequently leads to downstream caspase activation, nuclear DNA fragmentation and cell death [38]. The release of EndoG and AIF, and their subsequent translocation to the nucleus, specifically affect degradation of nuclear DNA, even in the absence of caspase activation [39, 40]. In addition, AIF loss-of-function studies in transgenic mice have recently revealed that this mitochondrial flavoprotein also plays an essential function in mitochondrial respiration and aerobic energy and loss of this mitochondrial-based protein leads to impaired cardiac contractility and oxidative phosphorylation (OXPHOS) deficiency [41, 42]. Studies employing knockdown of EndoG using lentiviral-delivered RNAi have demonstrated that EndoG function is essential for ischemia-mediated nuclear DNA degradation in postnatal cardiomyocytes and was associated with an increase to caspase-independent pathways occurring during early cardiac differentiation [43].

Both Smac/Diablo and cytochrome *c* are released from the mitochondria and become subsequently involved in cytosolic caspase activation. Smac binds and inhibits cytosolic antiapoptotic signaling complexes (e.g., IAPs) that modulate apoptosis whereas cytosolic cytochrome *c* binds Apaf-1 along with dATP and promotes recruitment of procaspase-9 into the apoptosome, a multi-protein complex resulting in cytosolic caspase activation [44, 45]. The release of these mitochondrial peptides primarily involves an outer membrane permeabilization mediated by proapoptotic cytosolic factors Bax, Bak and tBID. In addition, a group of BH3-only proteins termed executioner proteins including Bnip3, PUMA, Bid, Bad, HGTD-P, and Noxa have been identified that also serve this function in response to ischemia-reperfusion in heart and/or brain [37]. In response to both external pro-death signals largely provided by the extrinsic apoptosis pathway (e.g., ischemia/hypoxia, cytotoxic cytokine TNF-α and Fas ligand) and nuclear signals (e.g., p53), these proapoptotic factors translocate to mitochondria where they bind outer membrane proteins (e.g., VDAC) leading to channel and pore formation in the outer membrane [38]. Activation of mitochondrial apoptosis-induced channels (MAC) in the outer membrane which provide specific pores for the passage of intermembrane proteins, in particular cytochrome *c*, to the cytosol are also regulated by Bcl-2 family proteins [46].

Protein release from the intermembrane space and cristae, where the majority of cytochrome *c* is located, also appears to be closely associated with the opening of the voltage-sensitive permeability transition (PT) pore located at the contact sites between inner and outer membranes, which is responsive to membrane potential changes, mitochondrial ROS and Ca^{2+} overload, pro-oxidant accumulation and NO [47]. Recent studies in the postischemic heart have noted that PT pore opening in reperfused hearts increased along with reperfusion time and concurs with cytochrome *c* release from mitochondria [48]. However unlike MAC, PT pore is not specific to apoptotic cell death and is a feature of necrotic cell death (as further discussed in Chapter 4).

The composition of the PT pore, while still controversial, is thought to involve several key components of mitochondrial bioenergetic metabolism, including the adenine nucleotide translocator (ANT), mitochondrial creatine kinase, the outer membrane porin molecule (VDAC) and inner membrane cyclophilin D (shown in Fig. 2.2). Opening of the PT pore promotes significant changes in mitochondrial structure and metabolism, including increased mitochondrial matrix volume leading to mitochondrial swelling, release of matrix calcium, altered cristae, and cessation of ATP production secondary to ETC uncoupling, and dissipation of the mitochondrial membrane potential [47, 49]. Scorrano et al. have proposed that cytochrome *c* efflux in apoptosis is coordinated with the activation of a mitochondrial remodeling pathway characterized by changes in inner mitochondrial membrane morphology and organization, ensuring the complete release of cytochrome *c* as well as the onset of mitochondrial dysfunction, which might further contribute to the aging and/or failing heart phenotype [50].

Opposing the progression of this pathway, antiapoptotic proteins (e.g., Bcl-2), localized to the outer mitochondrial membrane, either directly compete with or impede the proapoptotic factor activities, fortify, or remodel the mitochondrial membranes and their channels thereby preventing mitochondrial disruption and inhibiting PT pore opening. In addition, both the extrinsic and intrinsic pathways are regulated by a variety of endogenous inhibitors of apoptosis including FLICE, XIAP and ARC.

Studies with the multifaceted ARC which acts on targets in both the intrinsic and extrinsic pathway, have demonstrated that ARC is cardioprotective stemming the release of cytochrome *c* and hypoxia-induced injury in the heart, although its role in aging has not yet been assessed [51].

The endoplasmic reticulum (ER) has been recently recognized as an important organelle in the intrinsic pathway, mediating cell death elicited by a subset of stimuli such as OS [52]. Similar to their roles in transducing upstream signals to the mitochondria, proapoptotic proteins appear to relay upstream death signals to the ER triggering the release of Ca^{2+}, which in turn can rapidly accumulate in mitochondria promoting PT pore opening [53, 54]. Pro-survival factors from the growth factor signaling pathways (e.g., IGF-1) also can inhibit the progression of the apoptotic pathway.

Interestingly, p66Shc, a protein that is localized in the mitochondria, has recently been identified as an important component in the control of life span, regulation of the mitochondrial transmembrane potential and control of the OS response in mammals [55–57]. Despite its lacking a conventional mitochondrial targeting sequence, a fraction of cytoplasmic p66Shc protein localizes in the mitochondria remaining in an inactive form in a complex with mitochondrial heat shock protein HSP70 [56]. The activated monomeric form of p66Shc occurs upon its dissociation from HSP70 in response to stresses including OS and UV light, and can directly react with reduced cytochrome *c* to generate H_2O_2 which in turn induces mitochondrial permeability and apoptosis [58]. Mice containing a homozygous deletion of the p66shc gene have an extended life span (by 30 %), lower ROS levels and increased stress resistance [55]. In addition, acting downstream of tumor suppressor p53, p66Shc is required for p53-mediated stimulation of intracellular oxidant production, and induction of cytochrome *c* release and apoptosis [56, 57]. Interestingly, deletion of p66shc gene in mice decreased the tissue damage resulting from hindlimb ischemia, reduced overall systemic and tissue OS, and vascular cell apoptosis [59]. Wildtype mice showed a marked decrease in capillary density and exhibited muscle fiber necrosis in response to ischemic insult. In contrast, p66Shc $^{-/-}$ mice displayed decrease in minimal capillary density and myofiber death. Moreover, p66Shc deletion reduced early atherogenesis in animals fed a high-fat diet [60]. A more extensive discussion of the multi-faceted p66Shc is presented in Chapter 9.

As suggested by experimental models, mitochondria-related apoptosis is a contributory mechanism of aging. Compared to myocytes from younger animals, myocytes derived from the hearts of old mice displayed increased levels of markers of cell death and senescence [61]. It is possible that apoptosis in cardiac aging may be a protective mechanism to get rid of those damaged, potentially dangerous cells in a mechanistic effort to incline the balance toward healthy cells, although, we do not know where this balance is. On the other hand, the marked accumulation of mtDNA mutations in strains of transgenic mice overexpressing proofreading-deficient polymerase γ (discussed in Chapter 1) was unexpectedly not associated with increased markers of OS or defective cellular proliferation, but rather correlated with the induction of apoptotic markers, particularly in tissues characterized by rapid cellular turnover. The levels of apoptotic markers which are increased during aging in normal mice, increased further in these transgenic mouse strains and correlated with the accumulation of mtDNA mutations in the heart [62].

Recent studies examining senescence in cultured human fetal cardiomyocytes have noted growth arrest and morphological changes in association with senescence associated β-galactosidase activity [63]. Studies with glioma cells stained for senescence-associated β-galactosidase activity, a biomarker specific for senescent cells, showed that the enlarged cells gave a distinctive positive staining reaction [64]. This senescence phenotype appears to be dependent on the continuous expression of p16INK4A. It has been proposed that the induced expression of p16INK4A in these cells reverted their immortal phenotype, and caused immediate cellular senescence. Interestingly, increased expression of p16INK4A has also been detected in aging cardiomyocytes [61]. Proteins implicated in growth arrest and senescence, such as p27Kip1, p53, p16INK4a, and p19ARF, were also present in myocytes of young mice, and their expression increased with age. Furthermore, DNA damage and myocyte death have been found to exceed cell formation in older mice, leading to a decline in the number of myocytes, and HF. Interestingly, this effect did not occur in transgenic mice in which cardiac stem cell-mediated myocyte regeneration compensated for the extent of cell death, and prevented ventricular dysfunction.

Mice containing an IGF-1 transgene had attenuated levels of senescence-associated gene products (e.g., p27Kip1, p53, p16INK4a, and p19ARF) and Akt phosphorylation in myocytes, and compared to wild-type mice exhibited decreased levels of myocyte DNA damage and cell death. Unfortunately, neither myocyte mitochondrial structure nor function were evaluated [61].

ROS Generation and CV Aging

ROS, by-products of normal metabolic processes are highly reactive, small oxygen-containing molecules that play an essential role in OS levels and signaling of the aging heart. In the mitochondria, ROS are generated from electrons produced (or leaked) from the electron transport chain (ETC) at complexes I and III although non-mitochondrial sources of ROS generation are both active and physiologically relevant in the heart. The inefficiency of electron transfer through the mitochondrial

ETC and altered level of antioxidant defenses underlie the accumulation of ROS and oxidative stress in the aging heart [65]. As we noted in Chapter 1, a causative role for ROS in the aging process, known as the free radical theory of aging (FRTA) presupposes that in biological systems ROS attack molecules and cause a decline in the function of organ systems, eventually leading to failure and death. Moreover, the bioenergetic dysfunction that occurs with aging further increases the accumulation of ROS. Mitochondrial ROS generation is increased in cells with abnormal ETC function as well as under physiological and pathological conditions where oxygen consumption is increased with respiratory complex I in particular playing a major role in the formation of superoxide radicals [66]. A decline in complex I activity (in concert with increased state 4 respiration) elevates ROS production during aging. This promotes the generation of prooxidant compounds, leading to modulation of PT pore opening, abnormal mitochondrial membrane potential, and induction of cell death.

Among its many targets in the cardiomyocyte, ROS causes extensive damage in particular to mitochondrial macromolecules (e.g., carbohydrates, DNA, lipids and proteins) proximal to its source as well as reduced fluidity in the mitochondrial inner-membrane. Age-associated mitochondrial membrane changes include increased membrane rigidity, elevated levels of cholesterol, phosphatidylcholine, omega-6 polyunsaturated fatty acids (PUFA) and 4-hydroxy-2-nonenal with decreased levels and oxidative modifications in omega-3 PUFA and cardiolipin, a unique inner membrane phospholipid [67]. These changes are potentially responsible for the increased susceptibility of the aging heart to the damaging effects of ischemia/reperfusion (I/R), including mitochondrial Ca^{2+} overload, opening of the PT pore and cell death. Under the appropriate conditions, the aging myocardium may exhibit increased permeability of the inner mitochondrial membrane to solutes causing mitochondrial swelling, "proton leak", reduced ETC efficiency and uncoupling of OXPHOS from respiration which would limit net ATP production [68]. Unpublished studies from our laboratory have confirmed increased PT pore sensitivity to Ca^{2+} in senescent rat myocardial mitochondria, and these findings are consistent with previous observations of enhanced Ca^{2+} vulnerability and Ca^{2+}-induced damage in mitochondria from senescent animals hearts [69, 70].

Oxidative modification of proteins, such as carbonylation, nitration, and the formation of lipid peroxidation adducts such as 4-hydroxynonenal (HNE) and malondialdehyde (MDA), are by-products of oxidative damage secondary to ROS [71, 72]. Several studies support across-the-board or global increases in levels of some protein oxidative modifications [73]. For instance, protein carbonyls have been reported to increase exponentially with age, particularly in the last third of life span reaching a level such that on average one out of every three protein molecules carries the modification and the modified proteins are likely dysfunctional either as enzymes or structural proteins [74]. Other studies have focused on specific proteins (and specific residues within those proteins) that are modified with age. While modifications in membrane-localized ANT and in the protein subunits of respiratory complexes I to V secondary to ROS-mediated nitration, carbonylation, HNE and MDA adduct formation and an associated decline in enzymatic activity *in vitro* have been reported [75, 76], a recent study of bovine heart submitochondrial particles found that proteins sustaining oxidative damage generated from *in vivo* basal level of ROS were primarily localized in the mitochondrial matrix [77]. Superoxide is also especially damaging to the Fe-S centers of metabolic enzymes (e.g., complex I, aconitase, and succinate dehydrogenase). Inactivation of the Krebs cycle enzyme, mitochondrial aconitase by superoxide, which generates Fe (II) and H_2O_2, increases formation of the highly reactive hydroxyl radical [75, 78], and in aging mouse heart, this enzyme was also a prominent target of MDA-adduct formation resulting in significant age-related decline in its activity [75].

Another type of reactive free radical, peroxynitrite formed from NO reacting with superoxide radicals is a strong oxidant associated with age-related modification of specific proteins generally detected as tyrosine nitration of targeted subunits. Viner et al. have demonstrated significant age-dependent loss in the sarcoplasmic reticulum Ca^{2+}-ATPase (SERCA) activity in parallel with accumulation of significant amount of nitrotyrosine in skeletal muscle [79]. Significant increases in nitrotyrosine in SERCA were also found in aging rat heart [80], and in atherosclerotic plaques and vessels from rabbits and from human subjects [81]. While it has been demonstrated that peroxynitrite reacts *in vitro* with mitochondrial membranes from bovine heart to significantly inhibit the activities of respiratory complexes I and V as well as resulting in 3-nitrotyrosine accumulation in selective complex I and V subunits [82], this has not been demonstrated in aging. However, a recent analysis of the aging cardiac proteome in rats with regards to 3-nitrotyrosine has identified substantial modification in over 48 proteins, including many involved in bioenergetics such as cytosolic proteins of glycolysis (i.e., α-enolase, α-aldolase, GAPDH), mitochondrial proteins involved in electron transport, TCA cycle, fatty acid β-oxidation and OXPHOS (i.e., 3-ketoacyl-CoA thiolase, acetyl-CoA acetyltransferase, malate dehydrogenase, creatine kinase, electron-transfer flavoprotein, F1-ATPase (ATP synthase) and VDAC/porin), as well as proteins involved in cardiomyocyte structural integrity (i.e., desmin) [83].

Another central premise of the mitochondrial theory of aging suggests that somatic mutations in mtDNA, induced by oxygen free radicals, are a primary cause of energy decline. A large body of evidence has shown that oxidative damage affects nucleic acids, and in particular mtDNA, by the induction of single- and double-strand breaks, base damage, and modification (including 8-oxoguanosine formation) resulting in the generation of point mutations and deletions [84, 85]. Data collected from a number of animal studies demonstrated that with aging there is progressive accumulation of mtDNA damage, including large-scale mtDNA deletions in the heart. These findings are consistent with numerous studies with human subjects that have found specific large-scale mtDNA deletions (e.g., 4977 bp) to be significantly increased in individuals over 40 years of age and at highest levels in cardiac tissues.

While several types of myocardial mtDNA deletions increase with aging, their relative incidence in cardiac tissue is significantly lower in rats as compared to humans, with variable prevalence in different tissues [86, 87]. Significant accumulation of a 4.2 kb mtDNA deletion has been found in the myocardium of senescent mice compared to young or middle-aged animals [88]. Similarly, in Fischer 344 x Brown Norway F1 hybrid rats (5, 18 and 36 months of age), specific mtDNA deletions of 8–9 kb have been detected in the right and left ventricle and their abundance increased with age in parallel with reduced complex IV enzyme activity in individual cardiomyocytes (assessed by *in situ* histochemistry), marked tissue fibrosis and diminished myocyte contractility [89]. Furthermore, Pak et al. reported that over 40 % of cardiac mtDNA deletions in the aging rat heart contain unique point mutations located near the deletion breakpoints [90].

Increased levels of mtDNA point mutations have also been reported in aging humans. Several investigators have found increased levels of mutations at specific sites within the mtDNA D-loop control region in skin fibroblasts and skeletal muscle of aging individuals [91, 92], albeit not in cardiac tissues of elderly subjects [93]. No evidence for increased point mutations in the D-loop region were found in brain, skeletal muscle or heart of aged mice (25–26 month-old) [94].

The role of point mutations and deletions in mtDNA in aging has been tested experimentally by several independent groups using different transgenic mouse strains and constructs of the previously described proofreading-deficient version of Polγ, the nuclear-encoded catalytic subunit of mtDNA polymerase [62, 95]. These mutant mice developed between a three- and eight-fold increase in the levels of mtDNA point mutations, as well as increased amounts of deleted mtDNA associated with a reduced life span and premature onset of aging-related phenotypes, including cardiomegaly, providing a causative link between mtDNA mutations and aging. However, no significant accumulation of ROS or of ROS damage, changes of antioxidant enzymes nor markers of oxidative stress were found in tissues of the mice [96]. The finding of respiratory deficiency and increased evidence of apoptosis in these transgenic strains rather than ROS suggest their potential involvement as primary inducers of this aging phenotype. As a result, the overall relevance of these transgenic models to normal aging processes including human has been recently questioned [97].

Given the abundant evidence that ROS and ROS-mediated effects are increased in aging, ROS neutralization by mitochondrial antioxidants such as superoxide dismutase (SOD), glutathione peroxidase (GPx) and glutathione (GSH) becomes of increased significance in the aging heart. Studies in the aging rat heart suggest that interfibrillar (but not subsarcolemmal) mitochondria display a significantly higher rate of oxidant production, and marked reductions in selected antioxidants including mitochondrial ascorbate and reduced glutathione (GSH) levels [98]. Moreover, significant age-related increases in both cardiac MnSOD and GPx activities were also found in both subpopulations of mitochondria, possibly as an adaptive mechanism to cope with increased mitochondrial production of superoxide and H_2O_2 [99].

Currently, the use of a wide range of antioxidants are being considered as a method of reversing the accumulation of ROS, and therefore aging, a subject which we examine in greater detail in Chapter 15. A partial list of agents being used includes L-carnitine and α-lipoic acid (often used in combination), coenzyme Q_{10}, melatonin and mimetics of the antioxidant enzyme SOD. However, caution is required in their use since this therapeutic approach may also override the beneficial effects provided by ROS within the cytosol as signaling molecules. A more highly targeted approach employing synthetic peptide antioxidants containing dimethyltyrosine, which are cell-permeable and concentrate 1,000-fold in the mitochondria, has demonstrated the capacity to significantly reduce mitochondrial ROS and cell death in cultured cells, and when applied in an *ex vivo* heart model of ischemia effectively improved contractile force [100]. Similarly, other bioactive molecules with antioxidant activity have been selectively delivered to the mitochondria to decrease lipid peroxidation and oxidative protein damage. For instance, generation of a synthetic ubiquinone analog (termed *mitoQ*), incorporating a lipophilic triphenylphosphate cation results in positively charged lipophilic molecules which target negatively charged energized mitochondria, rapidly permeate the lipid bilayers and accumulate at high levels within mitochondria from heart and brain [101]. Another modified antioxidant, a synthetic analog of vitamin E (MitoVitE), can be incorporated into the heart mitochondrial matrix attenuating oxidative damage.

As we have previously noted, the most compelling support for the free radical theory of aging recently came from the work of Schriner et al. [102] with a transgenic mouse strain (MCAT) harboring a 50-fold increase in its expression of the antioxidant catalase in cardiac and skeletal muscle mitochondria. Although there have been occasional reports of mitochondrial-localized catalase, the great majority of this H_2O_2-degrading enzyme is normally found in the peroxisome in most cell-types. The MCAT strain with elevated catalase activity displayed reduced severity in age-dependent atherosclerosis, reduced OS (e.g., H_2O_2 levels and oxidative damage) and reduced levels of mtDNA deletions in heart and skeletal muscle resulting in both median and maximum life span increases of about 20 % compared to wild-type controls. Unfortunately, other laboratories have been unable to replicate this remarkable finding suggesting the possibility that the genetic background of the mouse strain employed may be a primary determinant in the anti-aging phenotype observed, rather than arising solely from the presence of the catalase transgene.

Recently, Ren et al. have provided further support for a role of catalase in interfering with cardiac aging. They evaluated contractility and intracellular Ca^{2+} indices in cardiomyocytes from young and old transgenic mice with and without cardiac overexpression of catalase [103]. Contractile indices analyzed included peak shortening (PS), time-to-90 % PS (TPS-90), time-to-90 % relengthening (TR-90), half-width duration (HWD), maximal velocity of shortening/relengthening (+/−dL/dt) and intracellular Ca^{2+} levels or decay rate. While aging depressed +/−dL/dt, prolonged HWD, TR-90 and intracellular Ca^{2+} decay, these aging-induced mechanical defects were nullified or significantly attenuated by catalase overexpression. Moreover, levels of advanced glycation endproduct (AGE), elevated by 5-fold in aged controls compared with young mice, were significantly reduced by catalase. The age-mediated decline of expression levels of myocardial Na^+/Ca^{2+} exchanger (NCX) and Kv(1.2) K^+ channels was also significantly attenuated in the transgenic aged strains although age-mediated decline of SERCA2a was not affected. These findings suggest that catalase protects cardiomyocytes from aging-induced contractile defect possibly via improved intracellular Ca^{2+} handling.

Inflammation and CV Aging

Current evidence indicates that major chronic aging-related diseases such as atherosclerosis, arthritis, dementia, osteoporosis, and CVDs, are inflammation-related, and inflammation is likely the underlying basis for the molecular alterations that link aging and age-related diseases (as further discussed in Chapter 6).

OS and redox dysfunction, which appear to be inextricably linked with aging, are critical risk factors for age-related inflammation [104]. Much of this is mediated by the activation of redox-sensitive transcription factors and dysregulated gene expression in the nucleus by age-related OS. Besides ROS and NO other molecules and signal transduction pathways such as inflammatory signaling are actively involved in aging. Key players involved in the inflammatory process are the age-related upregulation of NF-κB, IL-1β, IL-6, TNF-α, cyclooxygenase-2, adhesion molecules, and inducible NO synthase. Through this increased expression of inflammatory components, aging unleashes a series of profound subcellular changes outside the nucleus of the cardiovascular cells and in the membranes and membrane-bound organelles (e.g., mitochondria), which dictate the electrophysiological and metabolic functioning of cardiovascular cells, as well as relating to the further control and generation of OS.

Inflammatory markers have increasingly been identified as significant independent risk indicators for cardiovascular events. While adults over the age of 65 have experienced a high proportion of such events, the available epidemiological data comes mainly from middle-aged subjects. Kritchevsky et al. [105] have examined the role that inflammatory markers play in predicting the incidence of CVD specifically in older adults. Interestingly, IL-6, TNF-α and IL-10 levels appear to predict cardiovascular outcomes in adults <65 years. Data on C-reactive protein (CRP) was rather inconsistent and appeared to be less reliable in old age than in middle age. In addition, fibrinogen levels have some value in predicting mortality but in a non-specific manner. They concluded that in the elderly, inflammatory markers are non-specific measures of health and may predict both disability and mortality, even in the absence of clinical CVD. Interventions designed to prevent CVD through the modulation of inflammation may be helpful in reducing disability and mortality. The role of increased inflammatory markers such as IL-6 and IL-1β as risk factors in aging, and in the development of MI has also been reported [106]. Analysis of polymorphisms in *IL-6* gene promoter (−174 G>C) has indicated that elderly patients with acute coronary syndrome (ACS) carrying *IL-6* −174 GG genotypes exhibited a marked increase in one year follow-up mortality rate, suggesting that *IL-6* −174 G→C polymorphisms can be added to the other clinical markers such as CRP serum levels and a history of CAD, useful in identifying elderly male patients at higher risk of death after ACS [107].

Neuroendocrine Mechanisms in CV Aging

The neuroendocrine theory of aging elaborates mainly on the wear and tear occurring in the aging neuroendocrine system. This system is a complicated network governed by the release of hormones largely regulated by the hypothalamus, which controls a large assortment of chain-reactions in numerous target organs and which in turn regulates other glands to release their hormones. It also responds to the body hormone levels as a guide to modulate overall hormonal activity. For example, if cortisol damages the hypothalamus, then over time it becomes a vicious cycle of continued hypothalamic damage, leading to an ever-increasing degree of cortisol production and thus more hypothalamic damage. This damage could then lead to hormonal imbalance as the hypothalamus loses its ability to control the system. A more comprehensive appraisal of the hypothalamus/cortisol and the aging heart is presented in Chapter 6. In this sub-section, our discussion will be limited to the cause-effect relationship of specific elements of neuroendocrine regulation including cardiac adrenergic and G protein-coupled receptors, thyroid hormone, GH and IGF-1, and their role in the dysfunction of the aging heart.

Adrenergic (and Muscarinic) Receptors in the Aging Heart

Cardiac β-adrenergic receptor (β-AR) responsiveness in model systems and in humans *in vivo* decreases with aging, and the mechanisms by which this may occur include the down-regulation and decreased agonist binding of β1-receptors, uncoupling of β2-receptors, and abnormal G protein-mediated signal transduction [108]. While age-dependent changes in human adrenergic receptors are well established, little is known about possible age-dependent alterations in human cholinergic receptors [109]. In the human heart, there are muscarinic receptors that are predominantly of the M_2 subtype that couple to the inhibitory G protein G_i [110, 111]. Stimulation of these receptors also causes inhibition of adenylyl cyclase activity and a decrease in heart rate as well as in β-adrenoceptor-mediated increases in ventricular contractility [112–114].

In healthy humans, ganglionic blockade unmasks a clear age-related decrease in cardiac responses to isoproterenol but not to epinephrine. It has been hypothesized by Leenen et al. that an age-related decrease in neuronal uptake (which affects epinephrine but not isoproterenol) may offset a parallel decrease in β-receptor-mediated responses [115] These investigators found that healthy aging in human is associated with decreased cardiac responsiveness to the β-agonist epinephrine, and this decrease can be balanced by concomitant decreases in buffering of these responses by neuronal uptake and the arterial baroreflex. Wth aging, a decline in cardiac function, in part due to decreased α- and β-AR-mediated contractility occurs. While defects in β-AR signaling are known to occur in the aging heart, which components of the α1-AR signaling cascade are responsible for the aging-associated deficit in α1-AR contractile function, have just begun to be identified. These include protein kinase C (PKC) and associated anchoring proteins including receptors for activated C kinase (RACKs).

Age can significantly influence the cardiovascular responses to α-adrenergic stimulation, and phenylephrine, by acutely increasing afterload, has been shown to be effective in revealing the left ventricular systolic dysfunction occurring with aging. Moreover, it appears that the increase in systolic blood pressure in response to an α-adrenergic challenge is significantly influenced not only by age but also by gender [115]. Recently, Hees et al. have analyzed the effects of β-adrenergic stimulation on LV filling, and its major determinant, relaxation, in an aging population. They found that aging was accompanied by a blunted inotropic but preserved chronotropic response to steady-state dobutamine infusion and although LV filling reserve declines with age, relaxation reserve does not [116].

Using a Langendorff-perfused hearts isolated from 5-month adult and 24-month old aging Wistar rats, Korzick et al. [117] have measured cardiac contractility (dP/dt) following maximal α1-AR stimulation with phenylephrine. Evaluation of the subcellular distribution of PKCα and PKCε, and their respective anchoring proteins RACK1 and RACK2 by Western immunoblot analysis revealed that the subcellular translocation of PKCα and PKCε, in response to α1-AR stimulation, was disrupted in the aging myocardium. Moreover, age-related reductions in RACK1 and RACK2 levels were also observed, suggesting that alterations in PKC-anchoring proteins may contribute to impaired PKC translocation and defective α1-AR contraction in the aged rat heart. Interestingly, this group of investigators subsequently sought to determine whether age-related defects in α1-AR contraction could be reversed by chronic exercise training (treadmill) in 4-month adult and 24-month aged rats [118]. They found that the age-related decrease in α1-AR contractility in the rat heart can be partially reversed by exercise, suggesting that alterations in PKC levels underlie, at least in part, exercise training-induced improvements in α1-AR contraction. In addition, in the Fischer 344 rat both aging and gender mediate substantial alterations in various PKC isoforms interactions with other signaling factors such as ERK1/2 to form signaling modules (SMS) [119]. Senescence was associated with increased cytosolic and mitochondrial PKCα levels in both males and female, whereas increases in cytosolic PKCα-ERK1/2 SMS were only observed in aged females. Mitochondrial PKCδ and PKCδ-ERK1/2 SMS increased in both male and female with age however increases in cytosolic PKCδ were only observed in aged males. Nuclear and mitochondrial PKCδ-ERK1/2 SMS were 3.5- and 4.8-fold greater in males compared to females, respectively, and increases in mitochondrial-PKCε-ERK1/2 SMS were also specific to aged males. It is thought that these substantial age and gender-associated differences in the magnitude and distribution of cardiac PKC-ERK1/2 signaling modules may in part underlie the age-related reductions in ischemic stress reserves, particularly apparent in aged women as well as differences in cardioprotection with aging.

The cardiac effects of α1-adrenergic stimulation, both in cardiomyocyte Ca^{2+} -transient and cardiac PKC activity have been assessed by Montagne et al. in 3-month and 24-month old Wistar rats [120]. Their findings suggested that the negative effect of α1-adrenergic stimulation on cardiomyocyte Ca^{2+} transient observed in old rats could be related to the absence of α1-adrenergic-induced PKC translocation.

Notwithstanding these findings, the effect of aging on the human sympathetic nervous system remains a controversial issue. However, the interest in this subject is currently increasing, mainly because diverse cardiac pathologies, including essential hypertension, CAD, HF and dysrhythmias increase with age, and the sympathetic nervous system may be an important pathophysiological component [121]. Interestingly, in a study on the role of the sympathetic nervous system in aging and HF, Kaye and Esler [122] found no additive effect of aging in the activation of the sympathetic nervous system that occurs in HF, suggesting that other factors such as CAD and MI may impact the increased incidence of HF with aging.

Cardiac G Protein-Coupled Receptors

Cardiac G protein-coupled receptors (GPCRs) that function through stimulatory G protein Gαs, such as β_1- and β_2-ARs, play a key role in cardiac contractility. $G\alpha_{i2}$ levels increases with age in both human atria resulting in diminished levels of both basal and receptor-mediated adenylyl cyclase activity [123] Similarly, significant increases were found in $G\alpha_{i2}$ levels by immunoblot analysis in left ventricles of 24-month old Fischer 344 rats with reduced levels of both basal and receptor-mediated adenylyl cyclase activity [124]. These elevated levels of G_i may subsequently increase the receptor-mediated activation of G_i through multiple GPCRs. Increased G_i activity is likely to have an adverse effect on heart function since G_i-coupled signaling pathways in the heart reduce both the rate and force of contraction, which is in part mediated through cAMP-mediated phosphorylation of phospholamban [125]. Investigation of the effects of age on G protein-coupled receptor signaling in human atrial tissue also showed that the density of atrial muscarinic acetylcholine receptor (mAChR) increases with age but reaches statistical significance only in patients with diabetes [126]. Interestingly, in elderly subjects of similar ages, those with diabetes have 1.7-fold higher levels of $G\alpha_{i2}$ and twofold higher levels of $G\beta_1$. Other studies have reported that right atrial mAChR density significantly decreased in advanced age [127]. The disparity between these studies could be explained by differences in age between patients groups; one study examined only adults with an age range from 41–85 years [126], while the other study group's age ranged from 5 days to

76 years [127]. In this regard it is interesting to note that Oberhauser et al. found that acetylcholine release in human atria which is controlled by muscarinic M(2)-receptors is significantly reduced in atria of patients >70 years of age and patients with late diabetic complications suggesting that locally impaired parasympathetic activity may be a contributory risk factor in sudden cardiac death in the elderly and in diabetic patients [128].

Although structurally closely related to insulin, the relaxin family peptides act on a group of four G protein-coupled receptors now known as relaxin family peptide (RXFP) receptors [129]. Interestingly, relaxin and its receptor are often involved in pathologies that are considered to be age-related such as fibrosis, wound healing and in response to myocardial infarction. First identified as a substance influencing the reproductive tract [130], relaxin subsequently has been characterized as a peptide hormone with a two-chain structure similar to insulin with a wide array of cardiovascular and neuropeptide functions [131]. Relaxin affects collagen metabolism, inhibiting collagen synthesis and enhancing its breakdown by increasing matrix metalloproteinases. It also enhances angiogenesis and is a potent renal vasodilator. Activation of two of the leucine-rich receptors RXFP1 or RXFP2 causes increased cAMP accumulation and the initial response for both receptors is the result of Gs-mediated activation and GoB-mediated inhibition of adenylate cyclase; RXFP1 has a higher affinity for relaxin, while RXFP2 primarily binds to insulin-like peptide 3. Since drugs acting at RXFP1 may have clinical potential in treating diseases involving tissue fibrosis such as cardiac and renal failure, the relaxin systems may represent an important pharmacological target in clinical management of aging, and in particular age-related cardiac pathologies [132].

Thyroid Hormone/SERCA in the Aging Heart

The sarcoplasmic reticulum Ca^{2+} ATPase (SERCA) is a transmembrane protein that pumps cytoplasmic Ca^{2+} into the sarcoplasmic reticulum and in this context plays an important role in regulating the concentration of calcium around the contractile elements in cardiomyocytes. In the aging/senescent heart the expression of the SERCA gene is downregulated contributing to abnormal calcium homeostasis and impairment of cardiac function. However, the molecular mechanisms that regulate the SERCA gene expression in the heart during aging are still unclear. In our laboratory we have found new evidence that implicates a decrease in thyroid hormone (TH) responsiveness in the aging heart (unpublished data). This decrease in large part involves the binding of the TH receptor (TR) and retinoid X receptors (RXR) heterodimer to TH-responsive elements (TREs) located in the *SERCA* and cardiac myosin heavy chain (*MHC*) gene promoters.

Age-associated changes in the TR and RXRs could explain the age-associated changes in SERCA and MHC expression. Long et al. have reported that although no significant changes in RXRα or RXRβ mRNA levels occur in the aging rat heart, both α1 and α2 TR mRNA levels decreased significantly between 2 and 6 months of age [133]. During this time period, the mRNA levels for α-MHC declined by more than half, whereas β-MHC mRNA levels remained low and unchanged. On the other hand, between 6 and 24 months, when mRNA levels for β-MHC increased and α-MHC continued to decrease, there was a significant decline in TRβ1 and RXRγ mRNA levels accompanied by a reduction in the TRβ1 and RXRγ protein levels. These findings suggest that the decline in α-MHC gene expression may be biphasic and in part due to a decline in α1 (and possibly α2) TR levels between 2 and 6 months of age, and a decline in TRβ1 and RXRγ levels at later age.

The aging-mediated downregulation of MHC and SERCA mediated by myocardial TH/TR signaling-mediated transcriptional control can be reversed with exercise [134]. While the expression of myocardial TRα1 and TRβ1 proteins are significantly lower in sedentary aged rats than in sedentary young rats, their expression is significantly higher in exercise-trained aged rats than in sedentary aged rats. Furthermore, the activity of TR binding to the TRE transcriptional regulatory elements in the α-MHC and SERCA promoters and the myocardial expression of α-MHC and SERCA (both mRNA and protein) were upregulated with exercise training in the aging heart, in association with changes in the myocardial TR protein levels. In addition, plasma 3,3′-triiodothyronine (T3) and thyroid hormone levels which decrease in aging [135, 136], are increased with exercise training. The reversal of aging-induced downregulation of myocardial TR signaling-mediated transcription of MHC and SERCA genes by exercise training, appears to be related to the cardiac functional improvement observed in trained aged hearts

The identification of the specific mechanisms contributing to decreased TH signaling in the aging heart may provide significant insights into possible therapeutic keeping in mind that in the aging heart decreased TH activity may be a physiological adaptation. It is possible that therapies which increase SERCA activity might improve cardiac function in the senescent heart. On the other hand, it has been shown that a decrease in SERCA activity contributes to the functional abnormalities observed in senescent hearts, and that Ca^{2+} cycling proteins can be targeted to improve cardiac function in senescence [137]. The well-established decline in myocardial SERCA content with age may also contribute to the increased development of impaired function after I/R in aging subjects. Furthermore, the ratio of SERCA to either phospholamban or calsequestrin decreased in the senescent human myocardium [138]. Decreased rates of Ca^{2+} transport mediated by the SERCA isoform are responsible for the slower sequestration of cytosolic Ca^{2+} and consequent prolonged muscle relaxation times in the aging heart.

SERCA is a prominent target of oxidative/nitrative damage in aging as we have noted in the previous section. Knyushko et al. [80] have found that senescent Fischer 344 rat heart showed a 60 % decrease in SERCA activity relative to that of young adult hearts, and this functional reduction in activity could be attributed, in part, to both a lower abundance of SERCA protein, and increased 3-nitrotyrosine modifications of multiple tyrosines within the cardiac SERCA protein. Nitration in the senescent heart was found to increase by more than two nitrotyrosines per Ca^{2+}-ATPase molecule, coinciding with the appearance of partial nitrated Tyr(294), Tyr(295) and Tyr(753) residues. In contrast, skeletal muscle SERCA exhibited a homogeneous pattern of nitration, with full site nitration of Tyr(753) in the young, with additional nitration of Tyr(294) and Tyr(295) in the senescent muscle. The nitration of these latter sites correlates with diminished transport function in both types of muscle, suggesting that these sites have a potential role in the downregulation of ATP utilization by the Ca^{2+}-ATPase under conditions of nitrative stress.

Growth hormone (GH) and IGF-1

Reduced signaling of insulin and highly conserved insulin-like peptides can profoundly affect organismal life span as we have discussed in Chapter 1. Mutations in genes involved in the insulin/insulin-like growth factor 1 IGF-1 signal response pathway have been reported to significantly extend life span in diverse species, including yeast, nematodes, fruit flies, and rodents. Intriguingly, the long-lived mutants, share important phenotypic characteristics, including reduced insulin signaling, enhanced sensitivity to insulin, and reduced IGF-1 plasma levels. In the nematode and the fly, secondary hormones downstream of insulin-like signaling also appear to regulate aging. However, the relative order and significance in which the hormones act in mammals has been difficult to resolve since there is a complex network of interacting and interdependent signaling molecules including insulin, IGF-1, growth hormone (GH), and TH, affecting multiple inter-acting cellular pathways [139]. For instance, while endocrine manipulations in animal models can slow aging without concurrent costs in reproduction, these bring inevitable increases in stress resistance [140].

Several mutant mouse strains have been instrumental in providing models of life span and aging modulation. These include GH-deficient/resistant animals which have a prolonged life span compared with their normal siblings. Studies have indicated that the Ames and Snell dwarf mouse strain and GH receptor/GH binding protein knockout (GHR-KO) do not experience aging at the same rate as their normal siblings but are subject to delayed aging. The Snell and Ames Dwarf mice are homozygous for recessive mutations at the pituitary-1 (pit1) *Pit-1,* or *Prop-1 locus*, respectively, which encode transcription factors controlling pituitary development [141]. Both Snell and Ames Dwarf mice demonstrate increased longevity (50 % in males and 64 % in females) compared to their wild-type controls, which has been generally attributed to GH/IGF-1 deficiency [142]. Mice homozygous for such a mutation are deficient in serum GH, thyroid-stimulating hormone (TSH), and prolactin as well as IGF-1.

While the mechanism of increased life span has not been fully delineated, there is increased support for the centrality of insulin signaling in the control of mammalian aging and for the involvement of this pathway in extending the life span of IGF-1-deficient mice. In the Snell dwarf mouse, GH deficiency leads to reduced insulin release and alterations in insulin signaling, including a decreased IRS-2 pool level, a reduction in PI3K activity and its association with IRS-2, decreased docking of p85 to IRS-2, and preferential docking of IRS-2 to p85–p110 leading to reduced insulin levels, enhanced insulin sensitivity, alterations in carbohydrate and lipid metabolism, reduced generation of ROS, enhanced resistance to stress, reduced oxidative damage, and delayed onset of age-related disease [141, 143, 144]. These alterations would establish a physiological homeostasis that favors longevity. Mouse longevity is also increased by fat-specific disruption of the insulin receptor gene *FIRKO* [145].

While a lower level of circulating growth hormone and an enhanced life span was found in transgenic mice expressing bovine growth hormone (bGH) [146], mouse mutant models containing high plasma GH but a 90 % lower IGF-1 also live longer than wild-type mice. This suggests that reduction in plasma IGF-1 levels may be primarily responsible for a major portion of the life span increase in dwarf, GH-deficient, and GHRBP-null mice [144, 147]. Further evidence for the direct role of IGF-1 signaling in the control of mammalian aging has also been provided by mouse strains in which the loss of a single copy of the *igf1r* gene (encoding the IGF receptor) results in a 26 % increase in mouse life span [148].

Moreover, GH/IGF-1 receptor system not only plays an important role in determining organism development and life span and but is in itself affected by age. IGF-1 decreased linearly with age in both sexes, with significantly higher levels in men than women [149]. The decrease in GH-induced IGF-1 secretion in the elderly suggests that resistance to the action of GH may be a secondary contributing factor in the low plasma IGF-1 concentrations [150].

It has also been argued that decreased IGF-1 level with age may contribute to the increase in cardiac disease found in the elderly, including HF [151]. Findings from the Framingham Heart Study in a prospective, community-based investigation indicated that serum IGF-1 level was inversely related to the risk for HF in elderly people without a previous MI, suggesting that the maintenance of an optimal IGF-1 levels in the elderly may reduce the risk for HF [152]. In addition, this study revealed that greater levels or production of the catabolic cytokines TNF-α and interleukin 6 were associated with increased mortality in community-dwelling elderly adults, whereas IGF-1 levels had the opposite effect [153].

In aged animals and humans the secretion of GH, and the response of GH to the administration of GH-releasing hormone (GHRH) are lower than in young adults [154]. In rodents, a two-fold increase in GH receptors has been observed with age but this increase fails to compensate for the reduction in GH secretion [155, 156] Further investigation revealed that the apparent size of the GH receptor was not altered with age, whereas the capacity of GH to induce *IGF-1* gene expression and secretion was 40–50 % less in old than in young animal [157]. GH administration to old animals and humans raises plasma IGF-1 levels and results in increases in skeletal muscle and lean body mass, a decrease in adiposity, increased immune function, improvements in learning and memory, and increases in cardiovascular function. Furthermore, administration of GH can induce improvement in hemodynamic and clinical status in some patients with chronic HF, largely resulting from the ability of GH to increase cardiac mass [158]. On the other hand, disappointing results have been reported in patients with DCM undergoing infusion of GH [159]. This may be related to the choice of the incorrect agent (GH instead of IGF-1) and/or the failure to selectively target patients with low IGF-1 levels [160].

Interestingly, the Klotho protein which functions as a circulating hormone binds to a cell-surface receptor and represses intracellular signals of insulin and IGF-1. Amelioration of the aging-like phenotypes in Klotho-deficient mice was observed by perturbing insulin and IGF-1 signaling, suggesting that Klotho-mediated inhibition of insulin and IGF-1 signaling contributes to its anti-aging properties [161]. On the other hand, because Klotho induces IGF-1 and insulin resistance, it has been suggested that the above findings seem to contradict previous evidence for increased life span of dwarf mice with reduced IGF-1 and insulin levels and enhanced insulin sensitivity. Nevertheless, since activation of signaling molecules downstream from IGF-1 and insulin receptors is reduced in both Klotho and dwarf mice, a common mechanisms of delayed aging is suggested [162]. Furthermore, it has been reported that the Klotho protein increases resistance to OS at the cellular and organismal level in mammals thru activation of the FoxO forkhead transcription factors that are negatively regulated by insulin/IGF-1 signaling, thereby inducing expression of MnSOD. This facilitates the removal of ROS and confers OS resistance, likely contributing to the anti-aging properties of Klotho [163].

Autophagy and CV Aging

Cells faced with a short supply of nutrients in their extracellular fluid begin to engulf specific, often defective organelles (e.g., mitochondria) and to re-use their components. Autophagy comes from the Greek "self-digestion", which is a process for the turnover and recycling of "old" macromolecules and organelles thru the lysosomal degradative pathway that is involved in maintaining cellular homeostasis, cell differentiation, and tissue remodeling. This process involves formation of a double membrane within the cell, confinement of the material to be degraded into an autophagosome, fusion of the autophagosome with a lysosome, and the subsequent enzymatic degradation of the materials.

During development, autophagy occurs in many types of cells, including cardiomyocytes. Moreover, in cardiac diseases associated with aging such as ischemic heart disease and cardiomyopathy, intralysosomal degradation of cells plays an essential role in the renewal of cardiac myocytes. The interaction of mitochondria and lysosomes in cellular homeostasis is of great significance, since both organelles suffer significant age-related alterations in post-mitotic cells [164]. Many mitochondria undergo enlargement and structural disorganization, and since lysosomes responsible for mitochondrial turnover experience a loss of function the rate of total mitochondrial protein turnover declines with age [165]. Coupled mitochondrial and lysosomal defects contribute to irreversible functional impairment and cell death.

Under pathophysiological conditions, autophagy may have a protective role or may contribute to cell damage [166]. Nutrient depletion classically induces autophagy in order to provide amino acids for the synthesis of essential proteins, thus prolonging cell survival [167], and may up to a point neutralize the apoptotic or programmed cell death stimuli (PCD type I) [168, 169]. However, other observations suggest that autophagy can act as an alternative form of programmed cell death, termed PCD type II [170]. Apoptosis and autophagy are closely regulated biological processes that play a central role in tissue homeostasis, development, and disease [171, 172]. Pattingre et al. have shown that the antiapoptotic protein, Bcl-2, interacts with the evolutionarily conserved autophagy protein, Beclin 1, and that the wild-type Bcl-2 antiapoptotic proteins, but not Beclin 1 binding defective mutants of Bcl-2, inhibit Beclin 1-dependent autophagy in yeast and mammalian cells. Moreover, cardiac Bcl-2 transgenic expression inhibited autophagy in mouse heart muscle. In addition, Beclin 1 mutants that cannot bind to Bcl-2 induce more autophagy than wild-type Beclin 1, and differently from the wild-type Beclin 1, promote cell death [171] Besides its function as an antiapoptotic protein Bcl2 also operates as an antiautophagy protein thru its inhibitory interaction with Beclin 1. This latter function of Bcl-2 may be helpful to keep autophagy in check, at levels that are compatible with cell survival, rather than cell death.

Furthermore, mitochondrial interaction with other functional compartments of the cardiac cell (e.g., the ER for Ca^{2+} metabolism, peroxisomes for the interchange of antioxidant enzymes essential in the production and decomposition of H_2O_2) must be kept in check since defects in communication between these organelles may accelerate autophagy and the aging process.

Cardiac Function in Aging

The association of age and declining heart function has been amply documented. For example, the Baltimore Longitudinal Study on Aging found that even in the absence of disease, there is still a significant loss of cardiac reserve manifested by a reduction in maximum achievable heart rate during stress. At rest in the sitting position, age-associated decline in heart rate (HR) and increased systolic blood pressure occurred in both sexes. When hemodynamics were expressed as the change from rest to peak effort (upright cycle exercise) as an index of cardiovascular reserve function, both sexes demonstrated age-associated increases in end-diastolic volume index and end-systolic volume index (ESVI), and reductions in ejection fraction, HR, and cardiac index (CI). However, the exercise-induced reduction in ESVI and the increases in ejection fraction, CI, and stroke work index at rest were greater in men than in women [173]. Thus, age and gender each have a significant impact on the cardiac response to exhaustive upright cycle exercise. That age and gender are important factors in cardiovascular remodeling were also confirmed by Redfield et al. Using a cross-sectional sample of Olmsted County, Minnesota (Rochester Epidemiology) they found that advancing age and female gender are associated with increases in vascular and ventricular systolic and diastolic stiffness even in the absence of CVD [174]. This combined ventricular-vascular stiffening may contribute to the increased prevalence of HF with normal ejection fraction in elderly persons and particularly in elderly women. On the other hand, in the Honolulu Heart Program, it was noted that in the absence of hypertension the risk of developing CAD is significantly higher in elderly men, with the incidence of CAD increasing from 1.8 % in younger adults (45–54 years) to 8.1 % in the elderly (75–93 years). In the later group, alcohol intake was unrelated to CAD, while the effects of sedentary life-styles on promoting CAD seemed to be stronger than in those who were younger [175].

Genetic Make-up in Cardiac Aging

As we have noted, heritable genetic components exist that are important determinants in the duration of life span in human, analogous to the inherited factors operative in the incidence of certain CVDs such as congenital heart defects (CHD), cardiomyopathies and CAD. Genes, that otherwise may remain in a quiescent state, are stimulated with aging under adequate environmental conditions, to express transcription factors/proteins that may facilitate the development of cardiac pathologies, e.g., upon physiological stress families of stress-response genes are activated as natural defense mechanisms. Induction of specific inflammatory genes is significantly deregulated and altered in the heart of aged versus young mice when challenged with the bacterial endotoxin lipopolysaccharide (LPS), suggesting that endotoxin-mediated induction of specific inflammatory genes in cardiovascular tissues is abnormal with aging, and this may be causally related to the increased susceptibility of aged animals to endotoxic stress [176].

The aforementioned *Klotho*-deficient mice (discussed with reference to IGF-1 and GH signaling) develop a syndrome resembling accelerated human aging, with significant and accelerated atherosclerosis [177]. Moreover, it has been demonstrated that a number of advanced aging-like KL(-/-) phenotypes could be restored to normal whenever Klotho expression was induced. On the other hand, decreasing Klotho expression in these rescued KL(-/-) mice induced several aging-like KL(-/-) phenotypes. Therefore, Klotho may be effective in the prevention and treatment of age-related disorders [178]. The *Klotho* gene encodes a single-pass transmembrane protein that function in signaling pathways that suppress aging and which has β-glucuronidase activity. In humans, a functional variant of *Klotho* termed *KL-VS* has been found, common in the general population (frequency 0.157) and individuals homozygous for *KL-VS* manifest reduced human longevity [179]. The *KL-VS* variant harbors three mutations in the coding region, of which one is silent, and two code for missense mutations F352V and C370S, which substantially alter Klotho metabolism. The *KL-VS* allele influences the trafficking and catalytic activity of Klotho, and the variations in Klotho function contributed to heterogeneity in the onset and severity of human age-related phenotypes [179], and early-onset of occult CAD [180]. Furthermore, recent cross-sectional and prospective studies have confirmed a genetic model in which the *KL-VS* allele confers a heterozygous advantage in conjunction with a marked homozygous disadvantage for HDL-C levels, systolic blood pressure, stroke, and longevity [181].

As previously discussed in Chapter 1 *Drosophila melanogaster* has served as a valuable model/organism for the study of aging, and increasingly it appears a particularly promising genetic model to assess age-depending decline in cardiac function. Similar to human, maximal heart rate in aging *Drosophila* is reduced, and the incidence of cardiac dysrhythmias increases [182]. These findings suggest that cardiac performance declines with age in this organism, and it may serve as a good model to undergo genome-wide mutational screening for potential genes that cause or protect against cardiac aging. Wessells et al. have reported that characteristic age-related changes in *Drosophila* decreased or are absent in long-lived flies when systemic levels of insulin-like peptides are reduced by mutations of the receptor, InR, or its substrate, chico [183]. Furthermore, the age-related decline in cardiac performance was prevented by interfering with InR signaling exclusively in the heart, by overexpressing the phosphatase dPTEN or the forkhead transcription factor dFOXO. Taken together, this suggests that in addition to its systemic effect on life span, insulin-IGF signaling influences age-dependent organ physiology and senescence directly and autonomously.

Recently, Ocorr et al. evaluated heart function in *Drosophila* and found that the fly's cardiac performance, as in human, deteriorates with age. The aging fruit flies exhibit a progressive increase in electrical pacing-induced HF as well as in dysrhythmias [184]. In *Drosophila*, while it is clear that the insulin receptor and associated pathways have a dramatic and heart-autonomous influence on age-related cardiac performance, altered KCNQ and K_{ATP} ion channel functions, (besides their conserved role in protecting against dysrhythmias and hypoxia/ischemia respectively), also seem to contribute to the decline in heart performance in the aging flies. It is possible that both mechanisms may be operative in the regulation of cardiac aging in vertebrates.

Epigenetic and Environmental Factors in Cardiac Aging

A number of epigenetic factors may contribute to the development of diverse cardiac pathologies (e.g., CAD, hypertension, etc.) in aging, including increased caloric intake, inadequate diet, alcohol intake, smoking, obesity, and lack of adequate aerobic exercise. While an extensive discussion on the effect of caloric intake/diet on the aging heart will be presented in Chapter 15, at this time it may suffice to comment on some of the effects that aerobic exercise may have on cardiac aging. Intrinsically, in the normal human aging heart there is a significant decrease in the chronotropic and inotropic responses to catecholamine stimulation, compromising cardiac function. An age-associated reduction in cardiovascular β-adrenergic (β-AR) responsiveness has been noted in Fischer 344 rats, corresponding with alterations in post-receptor adrenergic signaling rather than with a decrease in LV β-AR receptor number [185]. Interestingly, chronic dynamic exercise partially attenuated these reductions through alterations in post-receptor elements of cardiac signal transduction. Moreover, exercise training improves the aging-induced downregulation of myocardial PPARα-mediated metabolic pathways, and contributes to an amelioration in fatty acid metabolic enzyme activity in rats [186].

Moreover, endothelial function deteriorates with aging in human, and exercise training appears to improve the function of vascular endothelial cells. Regular aerobic-endurance exercise has been found to reduce plasma ET-1 concentration and to increase NO production in previously sedentary older women, with probable beneficial effects on the cardiovascular system, i.e., prevention of progression of hypertension and/or atherosclerosis by endogenous ET-1 and the potent vasodilatory effects of NO [187, 188]. Also, regular aerobic exercise may prevent the age-associated loss in endothelium-dependent vasodilation and restore the levels in previously sedentary middle aged and older healthy men. This may be an important mechanism by which aerobic exercise lowers CVD risk in this population [189]. Furthermore, endothelial release of tissue-type plasminogen activator (t-PA), a primary regulator of fibrinolysis and part of the endogenous defense mechanism against thrombosis, decreases with age in sedentary men, and regular aerobic exercise may not only prevent it, but could also reverse the age-related loss in endothelial fibrinolytic function [190]. In obesity, which is associated with an increased risk of atherothrombosis, significant endothelial fibrinolytic dysfunction may be present; but regular aerobic exercise can increase the capacity of endothelium to release t-PA [191]. On the other hand, the endothelium-release of NO was not compromised in overweight and obese adults under basal conditions [192].

Endurance exercise provides cardioprotection (CP) against I/R-induced necrotic cell death, not only in young but also in aged Fischer 344 rats, by reducing I/R-induced myocardial apoptosis [193]. The mechanisms for this exercise-induced CP against I/R-induced apoptosis may be mediated by improved myocardial antioxidant capacity and the prevention of calpain and caspase-3 activation [193]. Similarly, French et al. found that exercise training prevented the I/R-induced rise in calpain activity and improved cardiac work in a working heart preparation from adult male rats compared to sedentary animals [194]. Pharmacological inhibition of calpain activity resulted in comparable CP against I/R injury. This exercise-induced protection against I/R-induced calpain activation was not due to abnormal myocardial protein levels of calpain or calpastatin. Interestingly, exercise training was also associated with increased levels of myocardial MnSOD, catalase and OS reduction. In addition, exercise training also prevented the I/R-induced degradation of SERCA2a, apparently by increasing levels of endogenous antioxidants.

Exercise intolerance has long been recognized as an important symptom of HF, but it also may develop in aged individuals without cardiac pathology. A number of non-specific factors such as skeletal muscle dysfunction (likely secondary to mitochondrial bioenergetics defects), ventilatory abnormalities, and endothelial dysfunction, individually or in association, may contribute to limitation in exercise capacity. An important contributing factor for skeletal muscle catabolism (e.g., elevated cytokine expression) can be found in both normal, healthy aging, and in patients with HF [195]. This commonality of aging and HF-associated changes in the skeletal muscle may explain the more severe clinical presentation of the HF syndrome observed among elderly patients. A decline in maximal aerobic capacity and the ability to sustain submaximal exercise with advancing age was demonstrated in young (6–8 months) and old (27–29 months) Fischer 344 x Brown Norway rats [196]. Besides heart rate and mean arterial pressure, blood flow (BF) to different organs (e.g., kidneys, splanchnic organs, and 28 hind limb muscles) was measured at rest and during submaximal treadmill exercise using radiolabeled microspheres. BF to the total hind limb musculature increased during exercise, but was similar for both young and old animals. However, in old compared to young rats, the BF was reduced in 6 (highly oxidative) and elevated in 8 (highly glycolytic) of the 28 individual hindquarter muscles or muscle parts examined, suggesting that although there were similar increases in total hind limb BF in young and old rats during submaximal exercise, there was a profound BF redistribution from highly oxidative to highly glycolytic muscles. Using the same animal model, the effect of aging on muscle BF with similar degrees of MI-induced LV dysfunction, was evaluated [197]. A significant age-related redistribution of BF from the highly oxidative to the highly glycolytic muscles of the hind limb was found during exercise in old compared to young rats.

Epidemiology of CV Aging and Population Differences

With population-based and intervention studies, evidence for interactions between dietary factors, genetic variants and biochemical markers of CVDs has been reported. Such studies may ultimately permit the characterization of individuals and ethnic factors, which may respond better to one type of dietary recommendation than another (nutrigenomics). For instance, a low-fat low-cholesterol strategy may be particularly efficacious in lowering the plasma cholesterol levels of those subjects carrying the apoE4 allele at the APOE gene. Similarly, interactions have been increasingly sought between drug/pharmacological agents, genetic variants and biochemical markers of CVD, which can predict which treatments might be most efficacious for an individual with a specific background (pharmacogenomics/ genetics). The role of age adds a further important variable in these equations.

That genetics is of paramount significance in aging has been confirmed by observations on offspring of centenarians showing markedly reduced prevalence of diseases associated with aging and in particular for cardiovascular disease and cardiovascular risk factors. Terry et al. [198] have assessed the prevalence of age-related diseases in the offspring (177) of 192 centenarians and compared to controls consisting of offspring whose parents were born in the same years as the centenarians but at least 1 of whom died at an average life expectancy. Prevalence of age-related diseases including heart disease, hypertension, diabetes were compared between the two groups with centenarian offspring exhibiting a 55–66 % reduced prevalence of heart disease, hypertension and diabetes. Subsequent studies found the offspring of centenarians also had median ages of onset for CAD, hypertension, diabetes and stroke which were significantly delayed by 5.0, 2.0, 8.5, and 8.5 years, respectively, compared with the age-matched controls [198]. A striking finding from this study was that the marked delay in the age of onset for cardiovascular disease, diabetes, hypertension, and stroke was not found for other age-related diseases such as cancer, osteoporosis, and thyroid disease in this centenarian offspring cohort. We concur with these investigators that, together with their parents, the centenarian offspring, with ages between 70s and 80s, may prove to be a valuable resource to further define both genetic and environmental factors contributing to cardiovascular health and the ability to live to very old age in good health.

The recent discovery of a genetic locus on chromosome 4 linked to exceptional longevity is a good indicator of the powerful potential of studying centenarians as well as their siblings and offspring to identify genetic factors, which significantly modulate aging and susceptibility to age-related diseases as well aging biomarkers [199]. Siblings of centenarians have a higher propensity to achieve exceptional old age and also have half the mortality risk of their birth cohort from young adulthood through extreme old age. In a recent study, which was part of the Longevity Genes Project at Albert Einstein College of Medicine in New York [200], parents of centenarians (born in approximately 1870) had a dramatically greater (approximately sevenfold) chance for reaching longevity (ages 90–99), reinforcing the significant role of genetics in aging while the offspring of long-lived parents had significantly lower prevalence of hypertension, diabetes mellitus, heart attacks, and strokes compared to several age-matched control groups. A number of the gene variants have been reported in these centenarian groups as described both in the previous chapter and further in Chapter 6. Interestingly, marked reduction in the circulating serum concentration of the stress chaperone HSP70 (nearly 10-fold) were found in a small group of centenarian offspring (n=20) compared to age-matched controls, perhaps as an indicator of less tissue destruction/damage as a function of lower cardiovascular/autoimmune disease [201]. Recent studies have confirmed the finding of lower serum HSP70 levels in a larger group of both centenarians (n=87) and their offspring (n=94) compared to controls (126), albeit no significant genetic associations were found with two SNPs within two HSP70 genes [202]. While the significance of lower circulating HSP70 in centenarian offspring is not clear, these results are suggestive that levels of circulating serum HSP70 may be a biomarker for longevity.

On the other hand, populations in developing countries not only still have a high prevalence of infectious diseases but also an increasing incidence of CVD reaching epidemic proportions The later has been linked to lifestyle and demographic changes including an increased aging population. As pointed out, by Dominguez et al. the current increase in longevity prolongs the time for exposure to risk factors, therefore resulting in a greater probability of CVD [203]. Moreover, increased longevity due to improved social and economical conditions associated with lifestyle changes such as a rich diet and sedentary habits, are factors that contributes to the incremental trend in CVD. This study makes recommendations for promoting specific strategies to control smoking, weight control, healthy diet and an active lifestyle. Clearly, increased longevity and economic well-being have less value when accompanied by an increasing burden of CVD and other chronic diseases affecting the quality of life and we concur with these authors that emphasis placed on increased longevity with good quality of life is an important and achievable goal.

Aging is Not a Disease, Rather a Risk Factor

Aging (and its deleterious effects) is not a disease, however it can predispose to disease. As the human population ages and the average life span increases, so does the burden of CVDs. Aging in general, and cardiac aging in particular is a very complex phenomenon encompassing a series of progressive degenerative processes affecting molecules, cells and to the whole organism, and ending with the cessation of life. Genetic or programmed factors and the combination of a variety of interacting environmental influences are key determinants in the development of the cardiovascular pathology of aging, with *advancing age* unequivocally remaining the most significant predictor of cardiac disease.

From a cardiovascular standpoint, some of these mechanisms appear to be more operative than others; for example changes in macromolecules caused by oxygen free radicals, non-enzymatic glycosylation and programmed cell death (apoptosis) play critical roles in the pathophysiology of aging which impacts specific cell function, as well as survival, in particular the molecular stresses that defective mitochondrial bioenergetics and biogenesis may bring to cardiomyocytes, hormonal and inflammatory signals, and telomere shortening as will be discussed later. A combination of genetic/programmed events modulated by environmental factors, such as irradiation, toxic chemicals, metal ions, and free radicals can result in a stochastic pattern of damage with aging affecting the integrity and functioning of membrane phospholipids, enzymatic proteins, DNA and phenotypic damage encompassing a number of fundamental cellular processes such as metabolism, cell responses to stimuli, and even survival. All of this is particularly evident in the aging-mediated changes on the cardiovascular system. Identification of the totality of the mechanisms/pathways contributing to cardiac aging is a rather difficult problem to solve, and may be an unattainable goal, although important work in this regard is going on.

Cardiovascular disease of old age should be distinguished from the changes to the cardiovascular system/heart *per se* occurring with aging. Although changes in old age increase the frequency of diseases, there is an overlap in the aging and diseased phenotypes. Those changes of aging associated with an increase in mortality (but not with specific disease), qualify as biomarkers of aging and may allow one to distinguish the biological from the chronological age (passage of time). Emerging pathological evidence indicates that major chronic aging-related diseases such as atherosclerosis, arthritis, dementia, osteoporosis, and cardiovascular diseases, are inflammation-related. Inflammation is a possible underlying basis for the molecular alterations that link aging and age-related pathological processes. The development of OS and redox derangement that appears to be inextricably linked with aging is a critical risk factor for age-related inflammation [104]. Much of this is mediated by the activation of redox-sensitive transcription factors and dysregulated gene expression in the nucleus by age-related OS as well as age-related upregulation of NF-κB, IL-1β, IL-6, TNF-α, cyclooxygenase-2, adhesion molecules, and inducible NO synthase.

As we shall further discuss in later chapters, aging unleashes a series of profound subcellular changes in cardiovascular cells both in the transcriptional agenda and chromatin organization in the nucleus as well as outside the nucleus, in the membranes, and membrane-bound organelles (e.g., mitochondria, lysosomes) which dictate the electrophysiological and metabolic functioning of the cardiovascular cells, as well as to the control (and generation) of OS. In contrast to the effects of traditional and recently established cardiovascular risk factors, further research will be necessary to unequivocally establish what the effect of aging is in the human heart.

Modifying/Delaying CV Aging

The scientific evidence regarding the efficacy, cost effectiveness, strengths, and limitations of a range of pharmacologic and lifestyle approaches to CVD prevention – both primary and secondary were recently reviewed by Daviglus et al [204]. Clinical trials aimed at primary and secondary prevention of CVD have documented the efficacy and cost effectiveness of various drugs in lowering individual risk factor levels and in reducing clinical CVD events. The idea of a "polypill" containing low doses of multiple drugs has generated great interest, with proponents arguing that, given the high prevalence of CVD risk factors and the effectiveness of pharmacologic interventions, such a drug combination would reduce CAD mortality by 88 % if taken by all individuals aged > or = 55 years. However, current treatments to control high BP and serum cholesterol, while effective, do not typically reduce morbidity and mortality to levels observed in low-risk individuals, i.e. those with favorable levels of all readily measured major risk factors. Rather, primary prevention of all major risk factors starting early in life is critical. Prospective population-based research has delineated multiple long-term benefits associated with low-risk status in young adulthood and middle age, i.e., markedly lower age-specific CVD and total mortality rates, increased life expectancy, lower healthcare costs, lower medication use and prevalence of chronic diseases, and higher self-reported quality of life at older ages. Data have also showed that adverse levels of one or more major risk factors precede clinical CAD in 90 % or more of all cases, undermining the assertion that major CVD risk factors account for "no more than 50 %" of CAD cases. Hence, while numerous treatment options exist for secondary prevention of CVD, strategies that focus on progressively increasing the proportion of low-risk individuals could greatly reduce the need for secondary prevention in the first place. Public health policies must focus on prevention of all major risk factors simultaneously, using lifestyle approaches from early ages onwards to reduce population CVD risk to endemic levels, rather than current epidemic levels.

For women, the impact of cardiovascular risk factors measured in young adulthood, particularly favorable (low-risk) profile, on mortality has been difficult to assess due to low short-term death rates. In a large prospective study of a cohort of 7302 young women aged 18–39 years, Daviglus et al. [205] found that for women with favorable levels for all five major risk factors (risk groups were defined using national guidelines for values of systolic and diastolic blood pressure, serum cholesterol level, body mass index, presence of diabetes, and smoking status) at younger ages, the incidence of CAD and CVD (ascertained over a 30 year follow-up) was rare, and the long-term and all-cause mortality were much lower compared with others.

Stem Cells and CV Aging

In the aging heart there is not only a decrease in the functional reserve and capacity to adapt to sudden increases in pressure and volume loads but also myocyte loss, and when this loss reaches a threshold (variable with the presence or absence of other pathologies), HF will follow. Cell-based therapy in the aging failing heart is becoming a definitive alternative to other modalities, i.e., drugs and diet, and will likely become more prevalent since currently heart transplant is mostly off-limits beyond 60 years of age. The attraction of stem cell-aging research lies in the ability of the body to use its own stem cells to repair damaged organs. In a recent study, mice with induced heart damage upon injection with cytokines and granulocyte-colony stimulating factor (G-CSF) stimulated the mice's own primitive bone marrow cells to migrated to the heart, differentiate several different types of cardiac cells, and contributed to repair of the damaged tissue, improving both heart function and survival of the treated mice [206]. While similar findings have been achieved by direct transfer of a variety of stem cells in numerous studies, many questions remain concerning the details, mechanism and efficiency of differentiation, the stability of the new cardiomyocytes and most importantly the relevance and clinical applicability of this approach with human subjects with both cardiovascular disease and aging dysfunction. Several small clinical trials of cell therapy in patients with MI and ischemic cardiomyopathy have recapitulated a modest level of beneficial effects in humans with infarct size reduction and improvement in ejection fraction, myocardial perfusion, and wall motion. In a study of human heart transplant patients, scientists found that primitive cells from heart transplant recipients can migrate to and become a functioning part of the donated heart [207]. Nevertheless, these results are extremely preliminary, and further research is needed. However, the findings from these studies challenge the conventional wisdom that damaged heart tissue cannot be regenerated, and suggest that the body's own naturally occurring stem cells may be able to repair tissue damage and fight disease. For further discussion on this topic, as well as on gene therapies and pharmacogenomics the reader is addressed to Chapters 13 and 14.

Dietary and Lifestyle Change

Diet could significantly modify aging heart substrate at the level of mitochondrial and other cardiac cell membranes. While the aging process results in defective membrane lipid composition in qualitative terms, lipid-protein interactions and pathological outcomes are altered due to modified production of lipid metabolites and their interactions with ROS, which modify proteins (adducts) to diminish energy metabolism, and to trigger pathological signaling and outcomes. A major effect of aging at the mitochondrial membrane level is deficiency in omega-3 PUFA and this can be modified by increased dietary intake of omega-3 PUFA [67]. This could potentially prevent atrial fibrillation when the follow-up data of this population will be available. This is one of the first solid reports showing that some effects of aging can be, to a certain extent, limited.

Conclusion

The etiology of CV aging is under intense scrutiny. Its mechanisms involve cumulative cellular and molecular damage mediated through a variety of insults. OS, non-enzymatic glycation, inflammation and changes in cardiovascular gene expression all seem to influence CV aging. The critical involvement of mitochondrial pathways in myocardial bioenergetic regulation, the balance of oxidant and antioxidants and the progression of apoptosis, are being increasingly reported as contributory to the cardiac dysfunction and remodeling found both in the aging and in the failing heart. These pathways involve considerable cross-talk between both nuclear and mitochondrial components that represent potential targets for the treatment of HF and for reversing the cardiac dysfunction occurring with aging. Furthermore, the development of novel strategies, by either targeting these factors directly (e.g., apoptotic factors), promoting or redirecting bioenergetic resources, or activating mitochondrial responses against apoptosis and/or OS, holds great promise for providing cardioprotection in HF and in the aging heart.

Current progress in pharmacogenomics and new discoveries in pharmacology may bring new ways to influence the CV aging process. Therapies that can reduce age-associated arterial stiffness, cardiac fibrosis and ventricular hypertrophy should prove useful. Antioxidants modalities will continue to be a topic of great interest and need further research. Conditioning through endurance may be an effective way to improve cardiovascular function in the elderly. Furthermore, early recognition and treatment of diseases that are distinguishable from normal aging, including hypertension and atherosclerosis, together with preventive efforts, should reduce cardiovascular morbidity and mortality in aging.

Summary

- The aging human heart displays alterations in the histology of the vasculature and hemodynamics, include the development of large resistance vessels with intima-media-thickening and increasing deposition of matrix substance, which ultimately will lead to reduced compliance and increased vessel stiffness and endothelial dysfunction.
- With aging, there is increased left ventricular mass relative to chamber volume, decreased diastolic function and decreased β-adrenergic sympathetic responsiveness.
- Cellular mechanisms including prolonged action potential (AP) duration, altered myosin heavy chain (MHC) isoform expression and sarcoplasmic reticulum (SR) function, all of which may lead to changes in cardiac excitation–contraction (E-C) coupling which is prolonged with increased age, likely as a result of cytosolic Ca^{2+} overload-induced dysregulation.
- Accumulation of nuclear and mtDNA damage will result in senescent cardiomyocytes in the aging heart since DNA is easily oxidized and damaged by insults from diet, toxins, pollution, environment, as well as other epigenetic influences.
- Despite extensive DNA repair systems, DNA damage including base modification, large-scale rearrangements single-strand and double-strand breaks and mutations produced over a lifetime accumulate in aging. This aging-associated DNA damage is most evident in mtDNA probably because of its proximity to ROS, and decreased protection of the mitochondrial-based DNA repair systems.
- Significant changes in telomere structure, overall length, DNA and function have been found in cardiovascular cells including endothelial cells, vascular SMCs, EPCs and cardiomyocytes, associated with replicative senescence both *in vivo* and *in vitro*. Changes in telomeric length and function have also been reported in association with cardiovascular diseases associated with aging including atherosclerosis and CAD.
- Oxidative stress (OS) and ROS can mediate both telomeric dysfunction and length (in part by regulating telomerase presence in the nucleus) leading to replicative senescence as well as can trigger senescence by telomere-independent pathways.
- Cell loss and remodeling in the heart occurs in aging in part due to increased apoptosis. Data from both animal models and human clinical studies indicate that apoptosis also plays a contributory

role in aging-associated CVDs including cardiomyopathy and heart failure (HF), increased susceptibility to ischemia and MI, and atherosclerosis.

- Apoptosis involves an extrinsic signaling pathway triggered by multiple stimuli targeting death receptors and stimulating a cascade of caspase activation.
- An intrinsic signaling pathway mediated largely by mitochondrial permeabilization via MAC formation, PT pore activation, release of mitochondrial peptide factors (e.g., AIF, endoG, smac/Diablo and cytochrome *c*) to the cytosol lead to caspase activation and nuclear DNA degradation as well as mitochondrial bioenergetic dysfunction. The intrinsic pathway is regulated by proxidants and ROS, intracellular and mitochondrial calcium, proapoptotic factors of the BH3-family, and antiapoptotic factors of the Bcl-2 family.
- Both apoptotic pathways exhibit extensive cross-talk, involve multiple organelles (nucleus, mitochondria, ER) and are highly regulated by both proapoptotic factors such as BH3-proteins and specific endogenous apoptotic inhibitors (e.g., XIAP, ARC). Factors such as p53 and p66Shc also can impact on apoptotic progression, and survival-promoting pathways promoted by stimuli such as IGF-1 can attenuate apoptotic progression.
- Increased level of mtDNA mutations (such as generated in transgenic mice containing proofreading deficient DNA polymerase γ) result in both accelerated aging and increased apoptosis.
- Accumulation of ROS, ROS-mediated damage to protein, DNA, and membrane lipids are significantly increased in aging. Age-mediated oxidative damage including nitration has been described in specific residues of cardiac proteins (SERCA, ANT) as well as more globally affecting proteins (e.g., protein carbonyl modification). Both point mutations and deletions in mtDNA have been reported to increase with age and may impact on further mitochondrial energetic dysfunction.
- Antioxidants to stem ROS accumulation and neutralize their effects may modulate cardiovascular dysfunction associated with aging and aging-associated diseases as well as overall longevity. Transgenic mice containing increased mitochondrial catalase live longer with lower levels of oxidative damage and cardiovascular dysfunction.
- Inflammatory mediators and neuroendocrine regulators including adrenergic, cholinergic and thyroid hormone receptors, G-proteins and signaling modulators (kinases and associated anchoring proteins) are altered in aging underlying significant changes in cardiac responsiveness to multiple hormonal and physiological stimuli and downstream changes in components of calcium signaling pathways (e.g., SERCA).
- Aging-mediated changes in IGF/GH signaling not only affects longevity but also are associated with marked changes in cardiovascular function.
- The removal of the increased load of oxidative damaged macromolecules and organelles by autophagy, lysosomal and proteosomal degradation becomes less efficient in aging. Moreover, autophagy in aging can lead to elevated cell death.
- Studies with centenarians, their siblings and children clearly demonstrate genetic components to altered cardiovascular health and susceptibility to CVD in aging. Moreover, several polymorphic gene variants have been identified which result in altered longevity and cardiovascular aging.
- Epigenetic and environmental influences including diet and exercise not only play a critical role in determining cardiovascular aging and longevity phenotypes but also can reverse age-mediated damage and dysfunction.

References

1. Wolf MJ, Amrein H, Izatt JA, Choma MA, Reedy MC, Rockman HA. Drosophila as a model for the identification of genes causing adult human heart disease. Proc Natl Acad Sci USA 2006;103:1394–1399
2. Roman MJ, Ganau A, Saba PS, Pini R, Pickering TG, Devereux RB. Impact of arterial stiffening on left ventricular structure. Hypertension 2000;36:489–494

3. Taddei S, Virdis A, Mattei P, Ghiadoni L, Gennari A, Fasolo CB, Sudano I, Salvetti A. Aging and endothelial function in normotensive subjects and patients with essential hypertension. Circulation 1995;91: 1981–1987
4. Lakatta EG, Gerstenblith G, Angell CS, Shock NW, Weisfeldt ML. Prolonged contraction duration in aged myocardium. J Clin Invest 1975;55:61–68
5. Schulman SP, Lakatta EG, Fleg JL, Lakatta L, Becker LC, Gerstenblith G. Age-related decline in left ventricular filling at rest and exercise. Am J Physiol 1992;263:H1932–H1938
6. Merillon JP, Motte G, Masquet C, Azancot I, Aumont MC, Guiomard A, Gourgon R. Changes in the physical properties of the arterial system and left ventricular performance with age and in permanent arterial hypertension: their interrelation. Arch Mal Coeur Vaiss 1982;75:127–132
7. Lakatta EG. Cardiovascular regulatory mechanisms in advanced age. Physiol Rev 1993;73:413–467
8. Edo MD, Andrés V. Aging, telomeres, and atherosclerosis. Cardiovasc Res 2005;66:213–221
9. Aviv H, Khan MY, Skurnick J, Okuda K, Kimura M, Gardner J, Priolo L, Aviv A. Age dependent aneuploidy and telomere length of the human vascular endothelium. Atherosclerosis 2001;159:281–287
10. Chang E, Harley CB. Telomere length and replicative aging in human vascular tissues. Proc Natl Acad Sci USA 1995;92:11190–11194
11. Okuda K, Khan MY, Skurnick J, Kimura M, Aviv H, Aviv A. Telomere attrition of the human abdominal aorta: relationships with age and atherosclerosis. Atherosclerosis 2000;152:391–398
12. Matthews C, Gorenne I, Scott S, Figg N, Kirkpatrick P, Ritchie A, Goddard M, Bennett M. Vascular smooth muscle cells undergo telomere-based senescence in human atherosclerosis: effects of telomerase and oxidative stress. Circ Res 2006;99:156–164
13. Samani NJ, Boultby R, Butler R, Thompson JR, Goodall AH. Telomere shortening in atherosclerosis. Lancet 2001;358:472–473
14. Benetos A, Gardner JP, Zureik M, Labat C, Xiaobin L, Adamopoulos C, Temmar M, Bean KE, Thomas F, Aviv A. Short telomeres are associated with increased carotid atherosclerosis in hypertensive subjects. Hypertension 2004;43:182–185
15. Collerton J, Martin-Ruiz C, Kenny A, Barrass K, von Zglinicki T, Kirkwood T, Keavney B. Telomere length is associated with left ventricular function in the oldest old: the Newcastle 85+ study. Eur Heart J 2007;28:172–176
16. von Zglinicki T. Oxidative stress shortens telomeres. Trends Biochem Sci 2002;27:339–344
17. Kurz DJ, Decary S, Hong Y, Trivier E, Akhmedov A, Erusalimsky JD. Chronic oxidative stress compromises telomere integrity and accelerates the onset of senescence in human endothelial cells. J Cell Sci 2004;117: 2417–2426
18. Haendeler J, Hoffmann J, Diehl JF, Vasa M, Spyridopoulos I, Zeiher AM, Dimmeler S. Antioxidants inhibit nuclear export of telomerase reverse transcriptase and delay replicative senescence of endothelial cells. Circ Res 2004;94:768–775
19. Spyridopoulos I, Haendeler J, Urbich C, Brummendorf TH, Oh H, Schneider MD, Zeiher AM, Dimmeler S. Statins enhance migratory capacity by upregulation of the telomere repeat-binding factor TRF2 in endothelial progenitor cells. Circulation 2004;110:3136–3142
20. Imanishi T, Hano T, Nishio I. Estrogen reduces endothelial progenitor cell senescence through augmentation of telomerase activity. J Hypertens 2005;23:1699–1706
21. Simoncini T, Hafezi-Moghadam A, Brazil DP, Ley K, Chin WW, Liao JK. Interaction of oestrogen receptor with the regulatory subunit of phosphatidylinositol-3-OH kinase. Nature 2000;407:538–541
22. Vasa M, Breitschopf K, Zeiher AM, Dimmeler S. Nitric oxide activates telomerase and delays endothelial cell senescence. Circ Res 2000;87:540–542
23. Imanishi T, Hano T, Sawamura T, Nishio I. Oxidized low-density lipoprotein induces endothelial progenitor cell senescence, leading to cellular dysfunction. Clin Exp Pharmacol Physiol 2004;31:407–413
24. Serrano AL, Andres V. Telomeres and cardiovascular disease: does size matter? Circ Res 2004;94:575–584
25. von Zglinicki T, Pilger R, Sitte N. Accumulation of single-strand breaks is the major cause of telomere shortening in human fibroblasts. Free Radic Biol Med 2000;28:64–74
26. Forsyth NR, Evans AP, Shay JW, Wright WE. Developmental differences in the immortalization of lung fibroblasts by telomerase. Aging Cell 2003;2:235–243
27. Serra V, von Zglinicki T, Lorenz M, Saretzki G. Extracellular superoxide dismutase is a major antioxidant in human fibroblasts and slows telomere shortening. J Biol Chem 2003;278:6824–6830
28. Saretzki G, Murphy MP, von Zglinicki T. MitoQ counteracts telomere shortening and elongates life span of fibroblasts under mild oxidative stress. Aging Cell 2003;2:141–143
29. Passos JF, von Zglinicki T. Mitochondria, telomeres and cell senescence. Exp Gerontol 2005;40:466–472
30. Kirkwood TB. Understanding the odd science of aging. Cell 2005;120:437–447
31. Cook SA, Sugden PH, Clerk A. Regulation of Bcl-2 family proteins during development and in response to oxidative stress in cardiac myocytes: association with changes in mitochondrial membrane potential. Circ Res 1999;85:940–949

32. Long X, Goldenthal MJ, Wu GM, Marín-García J. Mitochondrial Ca^{2+} flux and respiratory enzyme activity decline are early events in cardiomyocyte response to H_2O_2. J Mol Cell Cardiol 2004;37:63–70
33. Pollack M, Phaneuf S, Dirks A, Leeuwenburgh C. The role of apoptosis in the normal aging brain, skeletal muscle, and heart. Ann NY Acad Sci 2002;959:93–107
34. Marin-Garcia J, Pi Y, Goldenthal MJ. Mitochondrial-nuclear cross-talk in the aging and failing heart. Cardiovasc Drugs Ther 2006;20:477–491
35. Narula J, Haider N, Arbustini E, Chandrashekhar Y. Mechanisms of disease: apoptosis in heart failure–seeing hope in death. Nat Clin Pract Cardiovasc Med 2006;3:681–688
36. Madamanchi NR, Runge MS. Mitochondrial dysfunction in atherosclerosis. Circ Res 2007;100:460–473
37. Webster KA, Graham RM, Thompson JW, Spiga MG, Frazier DP, Wilson A, Bishopric NH. Redox stress and the contributions of BH3-only proteins to infarction. Antioxid Redox Signal 2006;8:1667–1676
38. Danial NN, Korsmeyer SJ. Cell death: critical control points. Cell 2004;116:205–219
39. Li LY, Luo X, Wang X. Endonuclease G is an apoptotic DNase when released from mitochondria. Nature 2001;412:95–99
40. Susin SA, Lorenzo HK, Zamzami N, Marzo I, Snow BE, Brothers GM, Mangion J, Jacotot E, Costantini P, Loeffler M, Larochette N, Goodlett DR, Aebersold R, Siderovski DP, Penninger JM, Kroemer G. Molecular characterization of mitochondrial apoptosis-inducing factor. Nature 1999;397:441–446
41. Joza N, Oudit GY, Brown D, Benit P, Kassiri Z, Vahsen N, Benoit L, Patel MM, Nowikovsky K, Vassault A, Backx PH, Wada T, Kroemer G, Rustin P, Penninger JM. Muscle-specific loss of apoptosis-inducing factor leads to mitochondrial dysfunction, skeletal muscle atrophy, and dilated cardiomyopathy. Mol Cell Biol 2005;25:10261–10272
42. Vahsen N, Cande C, Briere JJ, Benit P, Joza N, Larochette N, Mastroberardino PG, Pequignot MO, Casares N, Lazar V, Feraud O, Debili N, Wissing S, Engelhardt S, Madeo F, Piacentini M, Penninger JM, Schagger H, Rustin P, Kroemer G. AIF deficiency compromises oxidative phosphorylation. EMBO J 2004;23:4679–4689
43. Bahi N, Zhang J, Llovera M, Ballester M, Comella JX, Sanchis D. Switch from caspase-dependent to caspase-independent death during heart development: essential role of endonuclease G in ischemia-induced DNA processing of differentiated cardiomyocytes. J Biol Chem 2006;281:22943–22952
44. Liu X, Kim CN, Yang J, Jemmerson R, Wang X. Induction of apoptotic program in cell-free extracts: requirement for dATP and cytochrome c. Cell 1996;86:147–157
45. Acehan D, Jiang X, Morgan DG, Heuser JE, Wang X, Akey CW. Three-dimensional structure of the apoptosome: implications for assembly, procaspase-9 binding, and activation. Mol Cell 2002;9:423–432
46. Kinnally KW, Antonsson B. A tale of two mitochondrial channels, MAC and PTP, in apoptosis. Apoptosis 2007 Feb 6
47. Kroemer G. Mitochondrial control of apoptosis: an introduction. Biochem Biophys Res Commun 2003;304:433–435
48. Correa F, Soto V, Zazueta C. Mitochondrial permeability transition relevance for apoptotic triggering in the post-ischemic heart. Int J Biochem Cell Biol 2007 Jan 21
49. Marzo I, Brenner C, Zamzami N, Susin SA, Beutner G, Brdiczka D, Remy R, Xie ZH, Reed JC, Kroemer G. The permeability transition pore complex: a target for apoptosis regulation by caspases and Bcl-2 related proteins. J Exp Med 1998;187:1261–1267
50. Scorrano L, Ashiya M, Buttle K, Weiler S, Oakes S, Mannella CA, Korsmeyer SJ. A distinct pathway remodels mitochondrial cristae and mobilizes cytochrome c during apoptosis. Dev Cell 2002;2:55–67
51. Ekhterae D, Lin Z, Lundberg MS, Crow MT, Brosius FC 3rd, Nunez G. ARC inhibits cytochrome c release from mitochondria and protects against hypoxia-induced apoptosis in heart-derived H9c2 cells. Circ Res 1999;85:e70–e77
52. Scorrano L, Oakes SA, Opferman JT, Cheng EH, Sorcinelli MD, Pozzan T, Korsmeyer SJ. BAX and BAK regulation of endoplasmic reticulum Ca2+: a control point for apoptosis. Science 2003;300:135–139
53. Hajnoczky G, Csordas G, Das S, Garcia-Perez C, Saotome M, Sinha Roy S, Yi M. Mitochondrial calcium signalling and cell death: approaches for assessing the role of mitochondrial Ca2+ uptake in apoptosis. Cell Calcium 2006;40:553–560
54. Jacobson J, Duchen MR. Mitochondrial oxidative stress and cell death in astrocytes—requirement for stored Ca2+ and sustained opening of the permeability transition pore. J Cell Sci 2002;115:1175–1188
55. Migliaccio E, Giorgio M, Mele S, Pelicci G, Reboldi P, Pandolfi PP, Lanfrancone L, Pelicci PG. The p66shc adaptor protein controls oxidative stress response and life span in mammals. Nature 1999;402:309–313
56. Orsini F, Migliaccio E, Moroni M, Contursi C, Raker VA, Piccini D, Martin-Padura I, Pelliccia G, Trinei M, Bono M, Puri C, Tacchetti C, Ferrini M, Mannucci R, Nicoletti I, Lanfrancone L, Giorgio M, Pelicci PG. The life span determinant p66Shc localizes to mitochondria where it associates with mitochondrial heat shock protein 70 and regulates trans-membrane potential, J Biol Chem 2004;279:25689–25695
57. Trinei M, Giorgio M, Cicalese A, Barozzi S, Ventura A, Migliaccio E, Milia E, Padura IM, Raker VA, Maccarana M, Petronilli V, Minucci S, Bernardi P, Lanfrancone L, Pelicci PG. A p53–p66Shc signalling

pathway controls intracellular redox status, levels of oxidation-damaged DNA and oxidative stress-induced apoptosis. Oncogene 2002;21:3872–3878
58. Giorgio M, Migliaccio E, Orsini F, Paolucci D, Moroni M, Contursi C, Pelliccia G, Luzi L, Minucci S, Marcaccio M, Pinton P, Rizzuto R, Bernardi P, Paolucci F, Pelicci PG. Electron transfer between cytochrome c and p66Shc generates reactive oxygen species that trigger mitochondrial apoptosis. Cell 2005;122:221–233
59. Zaccagnini G, Martelli F, Fasanaro P, Magenta A, Gaetano C, Di Carlo A, Biglioli P, Giorgio M, Martin-Padura I, Pelicci PG, Capogrossi MC. p66ShcA modulates tissue response to hindlimb ischemia. Circulation 2004;109:2917–2923
60. Napoli C, Martin-Padura I, de Nigris F, Giorgio M, Mansueto G, Somma P, Condorelli M, Sica G, De Rosa G, Pelicci P. Deletion of the p66Shc longevity gene reduces systemic and tissue oxidative stress, vascular cell apoptosis, and early atherogenesis in mice fed a high-fat diet. Proc Natl Acad Sci USA 2003;100:2112–2116
61. Torella D, Rota M, Nurzynska D, Musso E, Monsen A, Shiraishi I, Zias E, Walsh K, Rosenzweig A, Sussman MA, Urbanek K, Nadal-Ginard B, Kajstura J, Anversa P, Leri A. Cardiac stem cell and myocyte aging, heart failure, and insulin-like growth factor-1 overexpression. Circ Res 2004; 94:514–524
62. Kujoth GC, Hiona A, Pugh TD, Someya S, Panzer K, Wohlgemuth SE, Hofer T, Seo AY, Sullivan R, Jobling WA, Morrow JD, Van Remmen H, Sedivy JM, Yamasoba T, Tanokura M, Weindruch R, Leeuwenburgh C, Prolla TA. Mitochondrial DNA mutations, oxidative stress, and apoptosis in mammalian aging. Science 2005;309:481–484
63. Ball AJ, Levine F. Telomere-independent cellular senescence in human fetal cardiomyocytes. Aging Cell 2005;4:21–30
64. Uhrbom L, Nister M, Westermark B. Induction of senescence in human malignant glioma cells by p16INK4A. Oncogene 1997;15:505–514
65. Melov S. Mitochondrial oxidative stress. Physiologic consequences and potential for a role in aging. Ann NY Acad Sci 2000;908:219–225
66. Lenaz G, D'Aurelio M, Merlo Pich M, Genova ML, Ventura B, Bovina C, Formiggini G, Parenti Castelli G. Mitochondrial bioenergetics in aging. Biochim Biophys Acta 2000;1459:397–404
67. Pepe S. Effect of dietary polyunsaturated fatty acids on age related changes in cardiac mitochondrial membranes. Exp Gerontol 2005;40:751–758
68. Hansford RG, Tsuchiya N, Pepe S. Mitochondria in heart ischaemia and aging. Biochem Soc Symp 1999; 66:141–7; Harper ME, Bevilacqua L, Hagopian K, Weindruch R, Ramsey JJ. Ageing, oxidative stress, and mitochondrial uncoupling. Acta Physiol Scand 2004;182:321–331
69. Di Lisa F, Bernardi P. Mitochondrial function and myocardial aging. A critical analysis of the role of permeability transition. Cardiovasc Res 2005;66:222–232
70. Jahangir A, Ozcan C, Holmuhamedov EL, Terzic A. Increased calcium vulnerability of senescent cardiac mitochondria: protective role for a mitochondrial potassium channel opener. Mech Ageing Dev 2001;122:1073–1086
71. Russell LK, Finck BN, Kelly DP. Mouse models of mitochondrial dysfunction and heart failure. J Mol Cell Cardiol 2005;38:81–91
72. Chakravarti B, Chakravarti DN. Oxidative modification of proteins: age-related changes. Gerontology 2006;53:128–139
73. Levine RL, Stadtman ER. Oxidative modification of proteins during aging. Exp Gerontol 2001;36:1495–1502
74. Stadtman ER, Levine RL. Protein oxidation. Ann. NY Acad.Sci 2000;899:191–208
75. Yarian CS, Rebrin I, Sohal RS. Aconitase and ATP synthase are targets of malondialdehyde modification and undergo an age-related decrease in activity in mouse heart mitochondria. Biochem Biophys Res Commun 2005;330:151–156
76. Yan LJ, Sohal RS. Mitochondrial adenine nucleotide translocase is modified oxidatively during aging. Proc Natl Acad Sci USA 1998;95:12896–12890
77. Choksi KB, Boylston WH, Rabek JP, Widger WR, Papaconstantinou J. Oxidatively damaged proteins of heart mitochondrial electron transport complexes. Biochim Biophys Acta 2004;1688:95–101
78. Vasquez-Vivar J, Kalyanaraman B, Kennedy MC. Mitochondrial aconitase is a source of hydroxyl radical. An electron spin resonance investigation. J Biol Chem 2000;2751:4064–4069
79. Viner RI, Ferrington DA, Williams TD, Bigelow DJ, Schoneich C. Protein modification during biological aging: selective tyrosine nitration of the SERCA2a isoform of the sarcoplasmic reticulum Ca2+-ATPase in skeletal muscle. Biochem J 1999;340:657–669
80. Knyushko TV, Sharov VS, Williams TD, Schoneich C, Bigelow DJ. 3-Nitrotyrosine modification of SERCA2a in the aging heart: a distinct signature of the cellular redox environment. Biochemistry 2005;44:13071–13081
81. Xu S, Ying J, Jiang B, Guo W, Adachi T, Sharov V, Lazar H, Menzoian J, Knyushko TV, Bigelow D, Schoneich C, Cohen RA. Detection of sequence-specific tyrosine nitration of manganese SOD and SERCA in cardiovascular disease and aging. Am J Physiol Heart Circ Physiol 2006;290:H2220–H2227
82. Murray J, Taylor SW, Zhang B, Ghosh SS, Capaldi RA. Oxidative damage to mitochondrial complex I due to peroxynitrite: identification of reactive tyrosines by mass spectrometry. J Biol Chem 2003;278:37223–37230

83. Kanski J, Behring A, Pelling J, Schoneich C. Proteomic identification of 3-nitrotyrosine-containing rat cardiac proteins: effects of biological aging. Am J Physiol Heart Circ Physiol 2005;288:H371–H381
84. LeDoux SP, Wilson GL. Base excision repair of mitochondrial DNA damage in mammalian cells. Prog Nucleic Acid Res Mol Biol 2001;68:273–284
85. Yakes FM, Van Houten B. Mitochondrial DNA damage is more extensive and persists longer than nuclear DNA damage in human cells following oxidative stress. Proc Natl Acad Sci USA 1997;94:514–519
86. Yowe DL, Ames BN. Quantitation of age-related mitochondrial DNA deletions in rat tissues shows that their pattern of accumulation differs from that of humans. Gene 1998;209:23–30
87. Zhang C, Bills M, Quigley A, Maxwell RJ, Linnane AW, Nagley P. Varied prevalence of age-associated mitochondrial DNA deletions in different species and tissues: a comparison between human and rat. Biochem Biophys Res Commun 1997;230:630–635
88. Muscari C, Giaccari A, Stefanelli C, Viticchi C, Giordano E, Guarnieri C, Caldarera CM. Presence of a DNA-4236 bp deletion and 8-hydroxy-deoxyguanosine in mouse cardiac mitochondrial DNA during aging. Aging (Milano) 1996;8:429–433
89. Wanagat J, Wolff MR, Aiken JM. Age-associated changes in function, structure and mitochondrial genetic and enzymatic abnormalities in the Fischer 344 -Brown Norway F(1) hybrid rat heart. J Mol Cell Cardiol 2002;34:17–28
90. Pak JW, Vang F, Johnson C, McKenzie D, Aiken JM. MtDNA point mutations are associated with deletion mutations in aged rat. Exp Gerontol 2005;40:209–218
91. Wang Y, Michikawa Y, Mallidis C, Bai Y, Woodhouse L, Yarasheski KE, Miller CA, Askanas V, Engel WK, Bhasin S, Attardi G. Muscle-specific mutations accumulate with aging in critical human mtDNA control sites for replication. Proc Natl Acad Sci USA 2001;98:4022–4027
92. Michikawa Y, Mazzucchelli F, Bresolin N, Scarlato G, Attardi G. Aging-dependent large accumulation of point mutations in the human mtDNA control region for replication. Science 1999;286:774–779
93. Marín-García J, Zoubenko O, Goldenthal MJ. Mutations in the cardiac mtDNA control region associated with cardiomyopathy and aging. J Card Fail 2002;8:93–100
94. Song X, Deng JH, Liu CJ, Bai Y. Specific point mutations may not accumulate with aging in the mouse mitochondrial DNA control region. Gene 2005;350:193–199
95. Trifunovic A, Wredenberg A, Falkenberg M, Spelbrink JN, Rovio AT, Bruder CE, Bohlooly-Y M, Gidlof S, Oldfors A, Wibom R, Tornell J, Jacobs HT, Larsson NG. Premature ageing in mice expressing defective mitochondrial DNA polymerase. Nature 2004;27:417–423
96. Trifunovic A, Hansson A, Wredenberg A, Rovio AT, Dufour E, Khvorostov I, Spelbrink JN, Wibom R, Jacobs HT, Larsson NG. Somatic mtDNA mutations cause aging phenotypes without affecting reactive oxygen species production. Proc Natl Acad Sci USA 2005;102:17993–17998
97. Loeb LA, Wallace DC, Martin GM. The mitochondrial theory of aging and its relationship to reactive oxygen species damage and somatic mtDNA mutations. Proc Natl Acad Sci USA 2005;102:18769–18770
98. Suh JH, Heath SH, Hagen T. Two subpopulations of mitochondria in the aging rat heart display heterogenous levels of oxidative stress. Free Radic Biol Med 2003;35:1064–1072
99. Judge S, Jang YM, Smith A, Hagen T, Leeuwenburgh C. Age-associated increases in oxidative stress and antioxidant enzyme activities in cardiac interfibrillar mitochondria: implications for the mitochondrial theory of aging. FASEB J 2005;19:419–421
100. Zhao K, Zhao GM, Wu D, Soong Y, Birk AV, Schiller PW, Szeto HH. Cell-permeable peptide antioxidants targeted to inner mitochondrial membrane inhibit mitochondrial swelling, oxidative cell death and reperfusion injury. J Biol Chem 2004;279:34682–34690
101. Smith RA, Porteous CM, Gane AM, Murphy MP. Delivery of bioactive molecules to mitochondria in vivo. Proc Natl Acad Sci USA 2003;100:5407–5412
102. Schriner SE, Linford NJ, Martin GM, Treuting P, Ogburn CE, Emond M, Coskun PE, Ladiges W, Wolf N, Van Remmen H, Wallace DC, Rabinovitch PS. Extension of murine life span by overexpression of catalase targeted to mitochondria. Science 2005;308:1909–1911
103. Ren J, Li Q, Wu S, Li SY, Babcock SA. Cardiac overexpression of antioxidant catalase attenuates aging-induced cardiomyocyte relaxation dysfunction. Mech Ageing Dev 2007;128:276–285
104. Chung HY, Sung B, Jung KJ, Zou Y, Yu BP. The molecular inflammatory process in aging. Antioxid Redox Signal 2006;8:572–581
105. Kritchevsky SB, Cesari M, Pahor M. Inflammatory markers and cardiovascular health in older adults. Cardiovasc Res 2005;66:265–275
106. Deten A, Marx G, Briest W, Volz HC, Zimmer H-G. Heart function and molecular biological parameters are comparable in young adult and aged rats after chronic myocardial infarction. Cardiovasc Res 2005;66:364–373
107. Antonicelli R, Olivieri F, Bonafe M, Cavallone L, Spazzafumo L, Marchegiani F, Cardelli M, Recanatini A, Testarmata P, Boemi M, Parati G, Franceschi C. The interleukin-6 −174 G>C promoter polymorphism is

associated with a higher risk of death after an acute coronary syndrome in male elderly patients. Int J Cardiol 2005;103:266–271
108. White M, Roden R, Minobe W, Khan MF, Larrabee P, Wollmering M, Port JD, Anderson F, Campbell D, Feldman AM. Age-related changes in beta-adrenergic neuroeffector systems in the human heart. Circulation 1994;90:1225–1238
109. Brodde OE, Konschak U, Becker K, Ruter F, Poller U, Jakubetz J, Radke J, Zerkowski H. Cardiac muscarinic receptors decrease with age. In vitro and in vivo studies. J Clin Invest 1998;101:471–478
110. Giraldo E, Martos F, Gomez A, Garcia A, Vigano MA, Ladinsky H, Sanchez de la Cuesta F. Characterization of muscarinic receptor subtypes in human tissues. Life Sci 1988;43:1507–1515
111. Deighton NM, Motomura S, Borquez D, Zerkowski, HR, Doetsch N, Brodde OE. Muscarinic cholinoceptors in the human heart: demonstration, subclassification, and distribution. Naunyn-Schmiedeberg's Arch Pharmacol 1990;341:414–421
112. Böhm M, Gierschik P, Jakobs KH, Piesk B, Schnabel P, Ungerer PM, Erdmann E. Increase of Gi in human hearts with dilated but not ischemic cardiomyopathy. Circulation 1990;82:1249–1265
113. Von Scheidt W, Böhm M, Stäblein A, Autenrieth G, Erdmann E. Antiadrenergic effect of M-cholinoceptor stimulation on human ventricular contractility in vivo. Am J Physiol 1992;263:H1927–H1931
114. Landzberg JS, Parker JD, Gauthier DF, Colucci WS. Effect of intracoronary acetylcholine and atropine on basal and dobutamine-stimulated left ventricular contractility. Circulation 1994;89:164–168
115. Turner MJ, Mier CM, Spina RJ, Ehsani AA.Effects of age and gender on cardiovascular responses to phenylephrine. J Gerontol A Biol Sci Med Sci 1999;54:M17–M24
116. Hees PS, Fleg JL, Mirza ZA, Ahmed S, Siu CO, Shapiro EP. Effects of normal aging on left ventricular lusitropic, inotropic, and chronotropic responses to dobutamine. J Am Coll Cardiol 2006;47:1440–1447
117. Korzick DH, Holiman DA, Boluyt MO, Laughlin MH, Lakatta EG. Diminished alpha1-adrenergic-mediated contraction and translocation of PKC in senescent rat heart. Am J Physiol Heart Circ Physiol 2001;281: H581–H589
118. Korzick DH, Hunter JC, McDowell MK, Delp MD, Tickerhoof MM, Carson LD. Chronic exercise improves myocardial inotropic reserve capacity through alpha1-adrenergic and protein kinase C-dependent effects in Senescent rats. J Gerontol A Biol Sci Med Sci 2004;59:1089–1098
119. Hunter JC, Korzick DH. Age- and sex-dependent alterations in protein kinase C (PKC) and extracellular regulated kinase 1/2 (ERK1/2) in rat myocardium. Mech Ageing Dev 2005;126:535–550
120. Montagne O, Le Corvoisier P, Guenoun T, Laplace M, Crozatier B. Impaired alpha1-adrenergic responses in aged rat hearts. Fundam Clin Pharmacol 2005;19:331–339
121. Esler M, Kaye D. Sympathetic nervous system activation in essential hypertension, cardiac failure and psychosomatic heart disease. J Cardiovasc Pharmacol 2000;35:S1–S7
122. Kaye D, Esler M. Sympathetic neuronal regulation of the heart in aging and heart failure. Cardiovasc Res 2005;66:256–64
123. Kilts JD, Akazawa T, El-Moalem HE, Mathew JP, Newman MF, Kwatra MM. Age increases expression and receptor-mediated activation of Galpha i in human atria. J Cardiovasc Pharmacol 2003;42:662–670
124. Kilts JD, Akazawa T, Richardson MD, Kwatra MM. Age increases cardiac Galpha (i2) expression, resulting in enhanced coupling to G protein-coupled receptors. J Biol Chem 2002;277:31257–31262
125. Brodde O-E, Michel MC. Adrenergic and muscarinic receptors in the human heart. Pharmacol Rev 1999;51:651–689
126. Richardson MD, Kilts JD, Kwatra MM. Increased expression of Gi-coupled muscarinic acetylcholine receptor and Gi in atrium of elderly diabetic subjects. Diabetes 2004;53:2392–2396
127. Brodde O-E, Konschack U, Becker K, Rüter F, Poller U, Jakubetz J, Radke J, Zerkowski H-R. Cardiac muscarinic receptors decrease with age:in vitro and in vivo studies. J Clin Invest 1998;101:471–478
128. Oberhauser V, Schwertfeger E, Rutz T, Beyersdorf F, Rump LC. Acetylcholine release in human heart atrium: influence of muscarinic autoreceptors, diabetes, and age. Circulation 2001;103:1638–1643
129. Halls ML, van der Westhuizen ET, Bathgate RA, Summers RJ. Relaxin Family Peptide Receptors – former orphans reunite with their parent ligands to activate multiple signalling pathways. Br J Pharmacol. 2007 Feb 12
130. Hisaw FL. Experimental relaxation of the pubic ligament of the guinea pig. Proc Soc Exp Biol Med 1926;23:661–663
131. Bathgate RAD, Hsueh AJW, Sherwood OD. Physiology and molecular biology of the relaxin peptide family. In: Neill JD, editor. Knobil and Neill's physiology of reproduction 3rd edn. New York: Academic Press; 2006.
132. Bathgate RA, Ivell R, Sanborn BM, Sherwood OD, Summers RJ. International Union of Pharmacology LVII: recommendations for the nomenclature of receptors for relaxin family peptides. Pharmacol Rev 2006;58:7–31
133. Long X, Boluyt MO, O'Neill L, Zheng JS, Wu G, Nitta YK, Crow MT, Lakatta EG. Myocardial retinoid X receptor, thyroid hormone receptor, and myosin heavy chain gene expression in the rat during adult aging. J Gerontol A Biol Sci Med Sci 1999;54:B23–B27

134. Iemitsu M, Miyauchi T, Maeda S, Tanabe T, Takanashi M, Matsuda M, Yamaguchi I. Exercise training improves cardiac function-related gene levels through thyroid hormone receptor signaling in aged rats. Am J Physiol Heart Circ Physiol 2004;286:H1696–H1705
135. Tang F. Effect of sex and age on serum aldosterone and thyroid hormones in the laboratory rat. Horm Metab Res 1985;17:507–509
136. Buttrick P, Malhotra A, Factor S, Greenen D, Leinwand L, Scheuer J. Effect of aging and hypertension on myosin biochemistry and gene expression in the rat heart. Circ Res 1991;68:645–652
137. Schmidt U, del Monte F, Miyamoto MI, Matsui T, Gwathmey JK, Rosenzweig A, Hajjar RJ. Restoration of diastolic function in senescent rat hearts through adenoviral gene transfer of sarcoplasmic reticulum Ca(2+)-ATPase. Circulation 2000;101:790–796
138. Cain BS, Meldrum DR, Joo KS, Wang JF, Meng X, Cleveland JC Jr, Banerjee A, Harken AH. Human SERCA2a levels correlate inversely with age in senescent human myocardium. J Am Coll Cardiol 1998;32:458–467
139. Tatar M, Bartke A, Antebi A. The endocrine regulation of aging by insulin-like signals. Science 2003;299:1346–1351
140. Muller EE, Cella SG, De Gennaro Colonna V, Parenti M, Cocchi D, Locatelli V. Aspects of the neuroendocrine control of growth hormone secretion in ageing mammals. J Reprod Fertil Suppl 1993;46:99–114
141. Bartke A. Minireview: role of the growth hormone/insulin-like growth factor system in mammalian aging. Endocrinology 2005;146:3718–3723
142. Brown-Borg HM, Borg KF, Meliska CJ, Bartke A. Dwarf mice and the ageing process. Nature 1996;384:33
143. Hsieh CC, de Ford JH, Flurkey K, Harrison DE, Papaconstantinou J. Effects of the Pit1 mutation on the insulin signaling pathway: implication on the longevity of the long lived Snell dwarf mouse. Mech Ageing Dev 2002;123:1254–1255
144. Barbieri M, Bonafe M, Franceschi C, Paolisso G. Insulin/IGF-1-signaling pathway: an evolutionarily conserved mechanism of longevity from yeast to humans. Am J Physiol Endocrinol Metab 2003;285:E1064–E1071
145. Bluher M, Kahn BB, Kahn CR. Extended longevity in mice lacking the insulin receptor in adipose tissue. Science 2003;299:572–574
146. Steger RW, Bartke A, Cecim M. Premature ageing in transgenic mice expressing different growth hormone genes. J Reprod Fertil Suppl 1993;46:61–75
147. Muller F. Growth hormone receptor knockout (Laron) mice. http://sageke.sciencemag.org/cgi/content/full/sageke;2002/8/tg1
148. Holzenberger M, Dupont J, Ducos B, Leneuve P, Geloen A, Even PC, Cervera P, Le Bouc Y. IGF-1 receptor regulates life span and resistance to oxidative stress in mice. Nature 2003;421:182–186
149. Goodman-Gruen D, Barrett-Connor E. Epidemiology of insulin-like growth factor-I in elderly men and women. The Rancho Bernardo Study. Am J Epidemiol 1997;145:970–976
150. Lieberman SA, Mitchell AM, Marcus R, Hintz RL, Hoffman AR. The insulin-like growth factor I generation test: resistance to growth hormone with aging and estrogen replacement therapy. Horm Metab Res 1994;26:229–233
151. Khan AS, Sane DC, Wannenburg T, Sonntag WE. Growth hormone, insulin-like growth factor-1 and the aging cardiovascular system. Cardiovasc Res 2002;54:25–35
152. Vasan RS, Sullivan LM, D'Agostino RB, Roubenoff R, Harris T, Sawyer DB, Levy D, Wilson PW. Serum insulin-like growth factor I and risk for heart failure in elderly individuals without a previous myocardial infarction: the Framingham Heart Study. Ann Intern Med 2003;139:642–648
153. Roubenoff R, Parise H, Payette HA, Abad LW, D'Agostino R, Jacques PF, Wilson PW, Dinarello CA, Harris TB. Cytokines, insulin-like growth factor 1, sarcopenia, and mortality in very old community-dwelling men and women: the Framingham Heart Study. Am J Med 2003;115:429–435
154. Ghigo E, Arvat E, Gianotti L, Ramunni J, DiVito L, Maccagno B, Grottoli S, Camanni F. Human aging and the GH-IGF-1 axis. J Pediatr Endocrinol Metab 1996;9:271–278
155. Takahashi S, Meites J. GH binding to liver in young and old female rats: relation to somatomedin-C secretion. Proc Soc Exp Biol Med 1987;186:229–233
156. Xu X, Bennett SA, Ingram RL, Sonntag WE. Decreases in growth hormone receptor signal transduction contribute to the decline in insulin-like growth factor I gene expression with age. Endocrinology 1995;136:4551–4557
157. Khan AS, Sane DC, Wannenburg T, Sonntag WE. Growth hormone, insulin-like growth factor-1 and the aging cardiovascular system. Cardiovasc Res 2002;54:25–35
158. Colao A, Marzullo P, Di Somma C, Lombardi G. Growth hormone and the heart. Clin Endocrinol 2001;54:137–154
159. Osterziel KJ, Strohm O, Schuler J, Friedrich M, Hänlein D, Willenbrock R, Anker SD, Poole-Wilson PA, Ranke MB, Dietz R. Randomised, double-blind, placebo-controlled trial of human recombinant growth hormone in patients with chronic heart failure due to dilated cardiomyopathy. Lancet 1998;351:1233–1237

160. Wang PH. Roads to survival: insulin-like growth factor-1 signaling pathways in cardiac muscle. Circ Res 2001;88:552–554
161. Kurosu H, Yamamoto M, Clark JD, Pastor JV, Nandi A, Gurnani P, McGuinness OP, Chikuda H, Yamaguchi M, Kawaguchi H, Shimomura I, Takayama Y, Herz J, Kahn CR, Rosenblatt KP, Kuro-o M. Suppression of aging in mice by the hormone Klotho. Science 2005;309:1829–1833
162. Bartke A. Long-lived Klotho mice: new insights into the roles of IGF-1 and insulin in aging. Trends Endocrinol Metab 2006;17:33–35
163. Yamamoto M, Clark JD, Pastor JV, Gurnani P, Nandi A, Kurosu H, Miyoshi M, Ogawa Y, Castrillon DH, Rosenblatt KP, Kuro-o M. Regulation of oxidative stress by the anti-aging hormone klotho. J Biol Chem 2005;280:38029–33834
164. Brunt UT, Terman A. The mitochondrial-lysosomal axis theory of aging: accumulation of damaged mitochondria as a result of imperfect autophagocytosis. Eur J Biochem 2002;269:1996–2002
165. Rooyackers OE, Adey DB, Ades PA, Nair KS. Effect of age on in vivo rates of mitochondrial protein synthesis in human skeletal muscle. Proc Natl Acad Sci USA 1996;93:15364–15369
166. Hamacher-Brady A, Brady NR, Gottlieb RA. The interplay between pro-death and pro-survival signaling pathways in myocardial ischemia/reperfusion injury: apoptosis meets autophagy. Cardiovasc Drugs Ther 2006;20:445–462
167. Klionsky DJ, Emr SD. Autophagy as a regulated pathway of cellular degradation. Science 2000;290:1717–1721
168. Breckenridge DG, Germain M, Mathai JP, Nguyen M, Shore GC. Regulation of apoptosis by endoplasmic reticulum pathways. Oncogene 2003;22:8608–8618
169. Ravikumar B, Berger Z, Vacher C, O'Kane CJ, Rubinsztein DC. Rapamycin pre-treatment protects against apoptosis. Hum Mol Genet 2006;15:1209–1216
170. Canu N, Tufi R, Serafino AL, Amadoro G, Ciotti MT, Calissano P. Role of the autophagic-lysosomal system on low potassium-induced apoptosis in cultured cerebellar granule cells. J Neurochem 2005;92:1228–1242
171. Pattingre S, Tassa A, Qu X, Garuti R, Liang XH, Mizushima N, Packer M, Schneider MD, Levine B. Bcl-2 antiapoptotic proteins inhibit Beclin 1-dependent autophagy. Cell 2005;122:927–939
172. Shimizu S, Kanaseki T, Mizushima N, Mizuta T, Arakawa-Kobayashi S, Thompson CB, Tsujimoto Y. Role of Bcl-2 family proteins in a non-apoptotic programmed cell death dependent on autophagy genes. Nat Cell Biol 2004;6:1221–1228
173. Fleg JL, O'Connor F, Gerstenblith G, Becker LC, Clulow J, Schulman SP, Lakatta EG. Impact of age on the cardiovascular response to dynamic upright exercise in healthy men and women. J Appl Physiol 1995;78: 890–900
174. Redfield MM, Jacobsen SJ, Borlaug BA, Rodeheffer RJ, Kass DA. Age- and gender-related ventricular-vascular stiffening: a community-based study. Circulation 2005;112:2254–2262
175. Abbott RD, Curb JD, Rodriguez BL, Masaki KH, Yano K, Schatz IJ, Ross GW, Petrovitch H. Age-related changes in risk factor effects on the incidence of coronary heart disease. Ann Epidemiol 2002;12:173–181
176. Saito H, Papaconstantinou J. Age-associated differences in cardiovascular inflammatory gene induction during endotoxic stress. J Biol Chem 2001;276:29307–29312
177. Kuro-o M, Matsumura Y, Aizawa H, Kawaguchi H, Suga T, Utsugi T, Ohyama Y, Kurabayashi M, Kaname T, Kume E, Iwasaki H, Iida A, Shiraki-Iida T, Nishikawa S, Nagai R, Nabeshima YI. Mutation of the mouse klotho gene leads to a syndrome resembling aging. Nature 1997;390:45–51
178. Masuda H, Chikuda H, Suga T, Kawaguchi H, Kuro-o M. Regulation of multiple ageing-like phenotypes by inducible klotho gene expression in klotho mutant mice. Mech Ageing Dev 2005;126:1274–1283
179. Arking DE, Krebsova A, Macek M Sr, Macek M Jr, Arking A, Mian IS, Fried L, Hamosh A, Dey S, McIntosh I, Dietz HC. Association of human aging with a functional variant of klotho. Proc Natl Acad Sci USA 2002;99:856–861
180. Arking DE, Becker DM, Yanek LR, Fallin D, Judge DP, Moy TF, Becker LC, Dietz HC. KLOTHO allele status and the risk of early-onset occult coronary artery disease. Am J Hum Genet 2003;2:1154–1161
181. Arking DE, Atzmon G, Arking A, Barzilai N, Dietz HC. Association between a functional variant of the KLOTHO gene and high-density lipoprotein cholesterol, blood pressure, stroke, and longevity. Circ Res 2005;96:412–418
182. Paternostro G, Vignola C, Bartsch DU, Omens JH, McCulloch AD, Reed JC. Age-associated cardiac dysfunction in Drosophila melanogaster. Circ Res 2001;88:1053–1058
183. Wessells RJ, Fitzgerald E, Cypser JR, Tatar M, Bodmer R. Insulin regulation of heart function in aging fruit flies. Nat Genet 2004;36:1275–1281
184. Ocorr K, Akasaka T, Bodmer R. Age-related cardiac disease model of Drosophila. Mech Ageing Dev 2007;128:112–116
185. Roth DA, White CD, Podolin DA, Mazzeo RS. Alterations in myocardial signal transduction due to aging and chronic dynamic exercise. J Appl Physiol 1998;84:177–184

186. Iemitsu M, Miyauchi T, Maeda S, Tanabe T, Takanashi M, Irukayama-Tomobe Y, Sakai S, Ohmori H, Matsuda M, Yamaguchi I. Aging-induced decrease in the PPAR-alpha level in hearts is improved by exercise training. Am J Physiol Heart Circ Physiol 2002;283:H1750–H1760
187. Maeda S, Tanabe T, Miyauchi T, Otsuki T, Sugawara J, Iemitsu M, Kuno S, Ajisaka R, Yamaguchi I, Matsuda M. Aerobic exercise training reduce plasma endothelin-1 concentration in older women. J Appl Physiol 2003;95: 336–341
188. Maeda S, Tanabe T, Otsuki T, Sugawara J, Iemitsu M, Miyauchi T, Kuno S, Ajisaka R, Matsuda M. Moderate regular exercise increases basal production of nitric oxide in elderly women. Hypertens Res 2004;27:947–953
189. DeSouza CA, Shapiro LF, Clevenger CM, Dinenno FA, Monahan KD, Tanaka H, Seals DR. Regular aerobic exercise prevents and restores age-related declines in endothelium-dependent vasodilation in healthy men. Circulation 2000;102:1351–1357
190. Smith DT, Hoetzer GL, Greiner JJ, Stauffer BL, DeSouza CA. Effects of ageing and regular aerobic exercise on endothelial fibrinolytic capacity in humans. J Physiol 2003;546:289–298
191. DeSouza CA, Van Guilder GP, Greiner JJ, Smith DT, Hoetzer GL, Stauffer BL. Basal endothelial nitric oxide release is preserved in overweight and obese adults. Obes Res 2005;13:1303–1306
192. Van Guilder GP, Hoetzer GL, Smith DT, Irmiger HM, Greiner JJ, Stauffer BL, Desouza CA. Endothelial t-PA release is impaired in overweight and obese adults but can be improved with regular aerobic exercise. Am J Physiol Endocrinol Metab 2005;289:E807–E813
193. Quindry J, French J, Hamilton K, Lee Y, Mehta JL, Powers S. Exercise training provides cardioprotection against ischemia-reperfusion induced apoptosis in young and old animals. Exp Gerontol 2005;40:416–425
194. French JP, Quindry JC, Falk DJ, Staib JL, Lee Y, Wang KK, Powers SK. Ischemia-reperfusion induced calpain activation and SERCA2a degradation are attenuated by exercise training and calpain inhibition. Am J Physiol Heart Circ Physiol 2005;290:H128–H136
195. Gielen S, Adams V, Niebauer J, Schuler G, Hambrecht R. Aging and heart failure – similar syndromes of exercise intolerance? Implications for exercise-based interventions. Heart Fail Monit 2005;4:130–136
196. Musch TI, Eklund KE, Hageman KS, Poole DC. Altered regional blood flow responses to submaximal exercise in older rats. J Appl Physiol 2004;96:81–88
197. Eklund KE, Hageman KS, Poole DC, Musch TI. Impact of aging on muscle blood flow in chronic heart failure. J Appl Physiol 2005;99:505–514
198. Terry DF, Wilcox M, McCormick MA, Lawler E, Perls TT. Cardiovascular advantages among the offspring of centenarians. J Gerontol A Biol Sci Med Sci 2003;58:M425–M431
199. Perls T, Terry D. Genetics of exceptional longevity. Exp Gerontol 2003;38:725–730
200. Atzmon G, Schechter C, Greiner W, Davidson D, Rennert G, Barzilai N. Clinical phenotype of families with longevity. J Am Geriatr Soc 2004;52:274–277
201. Terry DF, McCormick M, Andersen S, Pennington J, Schoenhofen E, Palaima E, Bausero M, Ogawa K, Perls TT, Asea A. Cardiovascular disease delay in centenarian offspring: role of heat shock proteins. Ann NY Acad Sci 2004;1019:502–505
202. Terry DF, Wyszynski DF, Nolan VG, Atzmon G, Schoenhofen EA, Pennington JY, Andersen SL, Wilcox MA, Farrer LA, Barzilai N, Baldwin CT, Asea A. Serum heat shock protein 70 level as a biomarker of exceptional longevity. Mech Ageing Dev 2006;127:862–868
203. Dominguez LJ, Galioto A, Ferlisi A, Pineo A, Putignano E, Belvedere M, Costanza G, Barbagallo M. Ageing, lifestyle modifications, and cardio-vascular disease in developing countries. J Nutr Health Aging 2006;10: 143–149
204. Daviglus ML, Lloyd-Jones DM, Pirzada A. Preventing cardiovascular disease in the 21st century: therapeutic and preventive implications of current evidence. Am J Cardiovasc Drugs 2006;6:87–101
205. Daviglus ML, Stamler J, Pirzada A, Yan LL, Garside DB, Liu K, Wang R, Dyer AR, Lloyd-Jones DM, Greenland P. Favorable cardiovascular risk profile in young women and long-term risk of cardiovascular and all-cause mortality. JAMA 2004;292:1588–1592
206. Orlic D, Kajstura J, Chimenti S, Limana F, Jakoniuk I, Quaini F, Nadal-Ginard B, Bodine DM, Leri A, Anversa P. Mobilized bone marrow cells repair the infarcted heart, improving function and survival. Proc Natl Acad Sci USA 2001;98:10344–10349
207. Quaini F, Urbanek K, Beltrami AP, Finato N, Beltrami CA, Nadal-Ginard B, Kajstura J, Leri A, Anversa P. Chimerism of the transplanted heart. N Engl J Med 2002;346:5–15

Part II
Methodologies, Cardiac Phenotypes and Adaptation

Chapter 3
Molecular and Cellular Methodologies: A Primer

Overview

During the last decade we have experienced a revolution in molecular and cellular technology. The number of techniques available to the cardiovascular scientist continues unabatedly to proliferate today. In this chapter, we will present a number of methodological approaches in molecular and cellular biology that have been used as well as currently available and developing techniques that could be deployed in future studies of the cardiovascular system and the aging heart. When possible, salient findings achieved with these techniques with representative citations are also discussed. Intentionally, the topics covered have been limited to: cell culture (with isolated cardiomyocytes and vascular cell models of senescence such as endothelial and smooth muscle cells), gene transfection, transgenic knock-out models, transcriptional and proteomic gene profiling, assessment of aging-mediated DNA damage, including mutation as well as DNA repair, telomeric analysis, cell and tissue engineering.

Introduction

Examination and manipulation of the cells comprising the cardiovascular system has greatly furthered our understanding of the molecular and cellular basis of both their normal function during growth and development and dysfunction in disease, and has proved extremely informative in defining changes and mechanisms of cardiovascular aging. In particular, analysis of cultured cells derived from both animal and human tissues provides an opportunity to assess both the diverse effects of aging-accumulated cellular damage in the heart and the vasculature, assessment of the numerous molecular and cellular signaling pathways that are involved in replicative senescence, aging-associated metabolic dysfunction, their capacity to respond to insults such as hypoxia, as well as to evaluate overall changes in cellular programming occurring in the aging phenotype. Cellular models may also provide an opportunity for molecular re-engineering (by gene transfection and gene silencing methodologies) to modulate specific gene expression, and to reverse aspects of the aging phenotype responsible for cardiac and cardiomyocyte dysfunction. As we shall see, transgenic animal models also offer the opportunity to assess the effects of specific gene knockouts or overexpression on the aging cardiovascular phenotype, as well as the added ability to assess the effects of specific genes on the overall longevity of the organism and on organ interaction. Moreover, these types of studies have significantly contributed to the identification of potential therapeutic targets for the treatment of aging-associated cardiovascular disease (CVD) and aging dysfunction, and the developmemt of novel treatment modalities involving gene-based, cell-based and tissue engineering.

J. Marín-García, *Aging and the Heart*,

Cell Culture: Studying Isolated Cardiomyocytes and Vascular Cells in Aging

A large proportion (estimated at over 70%) of the cells comprising the ventricular myocardium are not cardiac myocytes. This heterogeneous group of cells consists primarily of fibroblasts but also includes endothelial cells (ECs), smooth muscle cells (SMCs), and macrophages. This cardiac cell heterogeneity complicates the biochemical and molecular assessment of the intact heart. This has made extremely difficult to assess the many phenomena happening in the heart driven by receptors, kinases and signaling cascade pathways such as myocardial hypertrophy and responses to growth factors. The development of well-defined cardiac myocyte culture systems can markedly reduce the heterogeneity and complexity involved with *in vivo* myocardial studies. With a defined approach in cell culture with growth media supplemented with the DNA synthesis inhibitor, bromodeoxyuridine (BrdU), over 90% of the cells obtained represent cardiomyocytes while contaminating fibroblasts can be reduced to <10% of the cell population.

In general, growth serum is not used after the period of cell attachment so as to eliminate non-defined growth factors. With serum-free media, non-myocyte proliferation is also reduced eliminating the need for BrdU, and changes in myocyte size and contractility in response to defined signals can be carefully monitored. Increased cellular size is defined as hypertrophy. Cardiomyocyte cultures can be prepared from either neonatal or adult hearts, and their morphological integrity can be mantained for 2–3 days (adult cardiomyocytes, longer for neonatal cells). Moreover, the major functional aspects of both adult and neonatal cardiomyocytes, including excitation-contraction coupling and receptor-mediated signaling remain intact, while contraction kinetics are somewhat diminished in the adult cells. Furthermore, gene delivery via recombinant adenoviral infection has proved to be highly efficient and reproducible in both neonatal and adult cardiomyocytes [1].

With myocytes derived from neonatal rat heart, insulin stimulated DNA and protein synthesis in cells cultured on a fibronectin-coated surface in serum-free medium [2]. Moreover, IGF-1 stimulated both DNA synthesis and cell proliferation in neonatal myocytes cultured in serum-free medium, without inducing cellular hypertrophy [3]. These findings were somewhat unexpected since it is well established that cardiac myocytes terminate their mitotic activity in the neonatal period, and regeneration of cardiac muscle does not occur after myocardial injury in adult hearts. Even embryonic myocytes, which actively proliferate *in vivo,* quickly lose mitotic activity when placed in cell culture.

Growth factors, including platelet derived growth factor (PDGF), both acidic and basic fibroblast growth factor (FGF), and transforming growth factor (TGF) have been documented in embryonic hearts as well as in neonatal cardiomyocytes and they alter myocyte terminal differentiation in culture [4, 5]. While early studies found no demonstrable growth factor-mediated increases in cell division in postmitotic myocytes [6], a variety of factors have been shown to stimulate proliferative growth of cardiomyocytes derived from either neonatal or embryonic hearts, and other factors can inhibit this growth program. Moreover, there is evidence to support that proliferative pathways in the neonatal cardiomyocyte can be reactivated. Several studies have shown an increased proliferation of cardiomyocytes containing overexpressed genes (to be further discussed in the following section) such as FGF-2, FGF-receptor, cyclin D2, and cyclin D1 [7–10].

Interestingly, cultured neonatal cardiomyocyte has been employed as a model of aging by Terman and Brunk [11–13]. Essentially their experiments attempted to phenocopy aspects of aging cells, such as the accumulation of the nondegradable pigment lipofuscin (often denoted by the term, age pigment) and of large senescent mitochondria induced with specific cellular treatments. Long-term (but not short-term) exposure of cultured neonatal rat cardiac myocytes to the thiol protease-inhibitor leupeptin, causes an accumulation of numerous electron-dense autophagic lysosomes within the cells; these inclusions contained lipofuscin-like autofluorescent material [12]. These observations suggested that lipofuscin accumulation occurs not by protease inhibition itself and that prolonged time is needed for the autophagocytosed material to become peroxidized, autofluorescent and undegradable. Inhibition of autophagocytosis in cultured neonatal rat cardiac myocytes treated with 3-methyladenine (3-MA) resulted in abnormal accumulation of mitochondria within myocytes, loss of contractility, and reduced survival time in culture [13]. While some of these changes occurring with pharmacological inhibition of autophagocytosis reflect the aging phenotype, a dramatic accumulation of small mitochondria was noted with a moderate accumulation of large-senescent type mitochondria, the latter more typical of normal aging. Accumulation of this subset of abnormally large mitochondria was irreversible and became the major form over time (with 3-MA removal). The results suggested that under normal conditions, when autophagy is not blocked but is imperfect, large mitochondria accumulate with age, presumably because they are less effectively autophagocytosed than smaller mitochondria.

Induction of proliferative growth has also been recently reported in adult cardiomyocytes containing overexpression of the cyclin B1-CDC2 (cell division cycle 2 kinase) genes [14]. Previously, it has been shown that basic FGF and IGF can modestly stimulate DNA synthesis and cell proliferation in adult cardiomyocytes [15]. Transgenic mouse models in which IGF-1 is overexpressed in a cardiac-specific manner lead to increased cardiomyocyte number in adult hearts, consistent with a role of the IGF/IGFR pathway in adult cardiomyocyte proliferative growth [16].

The demonstration of reactivation of a proliferative phenotype in quiescent adult cardiomyocytes is especially of interest from the standpoint of aging studies [17]. Moreover, both pulse-labeling and saturation labeling studies have shown that cardiomyocytes derived from adult hearts maintain similar rates and overall capacity of protein synthesis in culture over a month, as in the adult heart *in vivo* [18]. In addition, cultured cardiomyocytes treated with a variety of stimuli (i.e., hormones, cytokines, growth factors, vasoactive peptides, and catecholamines) may develop a hypertrophic phenotype [19–21]. Increased cell size and protein content in both neonatal and adult cardiomyocytes result from treatment with stimuli such as IGF-1, β-FGF, triiodothyronine (T3). The hypertrophic signaling pathways triggered by these stimuli contain both common elements and distinct features, and have provided valuable information delineating the development of myocardial hypertrophy, which also can be triggered in aging.

Observations in Endothelial and Smooth Muscle Cells

Aging of cells other than cardiomyocytes can also be reproduced in monolayer cultures, revealing the phenotype of replicative senescence, a phenotype that has been well-characterised in cell culture, but whose occurrence *in vivo* has only recently begun to be appreciated. The importance of aging and senescence phenotype of vascular cells is also underlined by the recognition that changes in the proliferative capacities of vascular SMCs and ECs play a contributory role in vascular pathophysiologies frequently associated with aging, including atherosclerosis.

It is well established that diploid human fibroblasts enter a stable growth arrest phenotype at the end of their life span and, in particular, these cells are resistant to various apoptotic stimuli [22]. In contrast, human ECs from the umbilical vein (HUVECs) acquire a proapoptotic phenotype when reaching senescence and this probably results from reactive oxygen species (ROS) induced damage and associated signaling. Both these cell-types in culture treated with regulators of apoptotic cell death, such as exogenous ceramides, displayed apoptosis. However, while ceramide can efficiently induce apoptosis in both young and senescent cells of either histotype, quantitative evaluation of the data show that senescent fibroblasts are more resistant to apoptosis induction when compared to their young counterparts, whereas in the case of senescent ECs, there is an increased susceptibility for apoptosis [23].

Several studies have also assessed the proliferation activity in cultures of vascular SMCs from human subjects of different ages [24]. Using cells derived from arteries of 12 donors of both sexes from 45 to 91 years of age, the "proliferation rate" (i.e., cells grown per day in the different culture passages), measured in each passage, was inversely related to donor age, with regression analysis exhibiting a negative slope. Similarly, the mean time of passage duration for reaching the maximum of proliferation, as well as its "efficiency" (maximum of proliferation rate/mean time of passage duration), exhibited a statistically significant dependence on the age of the donor with a similar negative slope obtained on regression. These results suggest that with advancing donor age there is an increasing number of senescent SMCs in the culture; extrapolation of these data suggests that vascular SMCs of extremely old individuals would be nearly entirely senescent, and therefore show extremely low proliferation rates in the culture.

Notwithstanding, there is increasing recognition of the limited relationship of the present cell models to the aging phenotype *in vivo* [25], and ample evidence that cell culture does not mimic the conditions cells encounter *in vivo.* Cells *in vitro* are exposed to higher O_2 levels and pH variation than in *vivo* cells. With each passage *in vitro,* cells are exposed to proteolytic insult by trypsin which likely has consequences on cellular function, by degrading receptors and other molecules with extracellular domains. Furthermore, cells in culture are also deprived of interactions with other cell types, which are crucial for the regulation of cell proliferation, differentiation, and apoptosis. For instance, recent electrophysiological, immunohistochemical, and dye-coupling data revealed the presence of direct electrical coupling between cardiac myocytes and cardiac fibroblasts in normal cardiac tissue (such as the sinoatrial node), and suggested that similar interactions may occur in post-infarct scar tissue [26]. This heterogeneous coupling of cells and its effect on *in vivo* electrical impulse conduction and the transport of small molecules or ions may become even more critical in the aging heart with its decreased population of myocytes and increased number of fibroblasts. The next-generation of cell models that attempt to mimic aging events and the cardiac microenvironment should reflect this important interaction.

The use of 3-D culture techniques may provide an alternative to study cellular aging *in vitro.* Recent experiments have used explanted cultures of embryonic chick heart tissue, which initially thrive as beating 3-D tissue aggregates and lose their contractility, flatten and progress to dedifferentiation over one week in culture. Upon co-culture with a non-cardiac cell layer obtained from adult bone marrow, the cardiac aggregates maintained their contractile function, 3-D tissue morphology, and myocyte phenotype for a full month of incubation [27].

Cell and Tissue Transfection and Gene Transfer in Cardiovascular Studies

Largely because they are post-mitotic in nature, cardiomyocytes have limited growth in culture, and are difficult to re-implant. In contrast to transfections of most cell lines, which can be successfully performed using a variety of methods, delivering genes into adult cardiomyocytes and ECs, both *in vivo,* as well as in primary cells in culture, is rather difficult. However, these difficulties can be circumvented by a careful selection of gene transfer vectors (see Table 3.1) and delivery techniques (e.g., catheters and stents).

Both viral and plasmid DNAs have been employed as vectors in cardiovascular gene transfer studies with mammalian cells and tissues, and have been used in a variety of investigative studies involving the transfer of genes of interest to isolated cardiomyocytes, ECs, and to both vascular and cardiac tissues as potential targets for gene therapy. Some of the relative advantages and disadvantages posed by each approach are enumerated in Table 3.1. These features relate to the efficiency of vector transduction, the range of cell-type effectively targeted, the levels and duration of the gene expression provided by the vector, the long-term stability of the vector and of great importance, the nature of the host response (e.g., immunogenic response to adenoviral proteins) and potential harm to the host organism provided by the vector (e.g., insertional mutagenesis posed by some viruses).

Table 3.1 Comparison of vectors for gene transfer and expression

Vector	Targeted tissue/cell-type	Transfer efficiency/level of expression and its duration	Advantages	Disadvantages
Adenovirus	Cardiac myocytes	++++/++++; Transient	Rapid and high levels of transgene expression	Decreased efficiency of gene transfer *in vivo* aging rat myocardium; Immunogenic
AAV	Quiescent and dividing cells	+++/+++; Longterm	Non-immunogenic; longterm transgene expression; high levels of AAV-mediated transduction of mature/aged myofibers	Insertional mutagenesis
Lentivirus	Cardiac myocytes (neonatal and adult- both *in vivo* and *in vitro*)	+++/+++; Longterm	Infect non-dividing cells, have long-term transgene expression + absence of induced host immune/ inflammatory response	Insertional mutagenesis
Retrovirus	Dividing cells	++/+++; Longterm	Rapid and long term transgene expression	Oncogenic potential
Plasmid	Quiescent and dividing cells	+/+; Transient	Non-viral	Low efficiency of transduction

These features of course are of particular concern in potential gene transfer/transplantation aimed at modifying clinical phenotypes in human.

Adenoviral vectors, which can effectively transduce both dividing and non-dividing cells, are particularly efficient in transducing post-mitotic cells including cardiomyocytes and have been widely used in experimental transfection studies. However, adenoviral vectors provide transient rather than long-term transgene expression and often provoke inflammatory and immunogenic responses from the host, which can further limit transgene expression, promote myocardial necrosis and therefore pose numerous safety concerns in a clinical setting. Previously, several studies have suggested that *in vivo* gene transfer by adenoviral vectors in the aging myocardium may be less efficient. Several observations have shown that the transgene expression of SERCA and of a reporter gene (EGFP), on adenoviral constructs, are much higher in primary cultures of myocytes derived from neonates compared to adult rat hearts [28]. This difference was found to be related to the cardiomyocyte level of coxsackie adenovirus receptor (CAR) involved in the viral penetration of the cell and expression level of exogenous genes. Furthermore, Communal et al. have reported a significant decrease in adenoviral infectivity in aging rat cardiomyocytes, which was correlated with aging-mediated downregulation of expression of integrins (particularly $\alpha_3\beta_1$) that are involved in viral internalization [29]. Interestingly, this study demonstrated that CAR expression in the aging cardiomyocyte was upregulated, as gauged by western blot and immunoprecipitation analysis, suggesting that CAR levels are unlikely to be involved in the attenuated infectivity of the adenovirus with aging.

Michele et al. have found that the efficiency of adenoviral-mediated gene transfer of parvalbumin, a cytoplasmic calcium-binding protein, to adult cardiac myocytes *in vitro* was identical in young and old rats, suggesting that the basic processes of adenovirus binding and internalization are unaffected by aging, but that adenoviral-mediated gene transfer to the myocardium *in vivo* was reduced in old rats compared to young rats [30]. Nonetheless, parvalbumin gene transfer and expression *in vivo* were sufficient to improve *tau*, a load-independent indicator of diastolic function, in the aged myocardium. Similarly, adenoviral vectors containing specific genes have been shown to effectively transduce aging or senescent myocardium and impact significantly on the phenotype. In 26 month old senescent rat hearts, effective adenoviral-mediated gene transfer of parvalbumin reversed age-mediated diastolic dysfunction and improved relaxation parameters, dramatically increasing both the rate of calcium transient decay and the rate of myocyte relengthening, in senescent myocytes [31]. Similar results have been obtained in two different rat models of aging: the Fischer 344 and the Fischer 344 x Brown Norway F1 hybrid. *In vivo* overexpression of adenoviral-delivered parvalbumin in both rat aging models markedly reduced LV diastolic pressure and the time course of pressure decline, and improved the force frequency relationship in senescent rats [32].

In addition, adenoviral-mediated transfer of diverse genes has been used to effectively transduce ECs and vascular SMCs both *in vivo* and *in vitro*, albeit in regard to aging limited studies have been carried out. Brown et al. have noted that adenoviral-mediated transfer of human extracellular superoxide dismutase (ECSOD) results in marked improvement of the aortic relaxation response to acetylcholine in 30 month senescent Fischer 344 rats, in parallel with reduced superoxide levels in the aorta [33]. Furthermore, recently, van der Veer et al. demonstrated that the viral-mediated transfer of the human gene for nicotinamide phosphoribosyltransferase (Nampt/Visfatin), the rate-limiting enzyme for NAD^+ salvage from nicotinamide into aging human SMCs, resulted in delayed senescence and substantially lengthened the cell life span together with enhanced resistance to oxidative stress (OS); [34] the increase in SMC life span and replicative growth is in part achieved by SIRT1 activation and p53 degradation.

Using the aforementioned vectors, a varied assortment of genes have been used in cardiovascular gene transfer and myocardial therapy in relation to the aging phenotype, a representative list (the actual list is over 50 and needs to be continually updated) is presented in Table 3.2. These genes range from antioxidant enzymes (e.g., catalase, metallotheinein, thioredoxin), growth factors (e.g., VEGF, IGF-1), calcium signaling and handling pathway components (e.g., SERCA, parvalbumin, calsequestrin) to genes encoding adenosine receptor and ADH. The transgene product, usually a protein, can be produced at normal cellular levels or can be produced in greater amounts than normal (i.e., overexpressed). Dependent on the function of the protein, in some cases overexpression can trigger a toxic reaction in the cell. The addition of appropriate regulatory sequences within the genetic construct to be introduced can be used to modulate transgene expression. These can include the use of constitutive promoters or regulatable promoter elements and enhancers that are inducible in response to a variety of endogenous or exogenous molecular signals (e.g., steroid hormones, cytokines, growth factors). The incorporation of regulatable promoters offers the advantage of allowing gene expression to be switched on and off. Moreover, cardiac-specific or cardiomyocyte specific promoters, such as myocyte-specific promoter sequences of *mlc-v* (ventricle-specific myosin light chain-2), and *cTNT* (cardiac troponin T), can be used to limit tissue/cell-type gene expression. Targeting of the gene product to the appropriate sub-cellular compartment (e.g., nucleus, mitochondria) can also be regulated by the addition of specific peptide presequences to the transgene. For example, recent studies targeting a catalase transgene to the mitochondrial compartment resulted in enhanced longevity in the transgenic mouse [40].

In addition to transgene overexpression and activation, a number of gene transfer approaches that are presently available, can be used to negatively modulate gene expression, involving the use of antisense strategies such as ribozymes, antisense oligonucleotides, or RNA interference (RNAi). These approaches can downregulate the transcription or translation of targeted endogenous

Table 3.2 Specific gene overexpression and cardiovascular phenotype in aging

Gene	Target	Cellular role	Phenotype	Refs
ADH	Cardiac myocytes *in vivo*	Alcohol Dehydrogenase	Rescued aging-associated diastolic dysfunction	35
Metallotheinein	Cardiac myocytes *in vivo*	Antioxidant	Reduced changes in oxidative stress (e.g., aconitase activity); myocytes ↑ resistant to induce ROS generation and apoptosis	36
SERCA	Cardiac myocytes *in vivo*	Calcium handling/ Contraction	Improved rate-dependent contractility and diastolic function in senescent hearts.	37
Parvalbumin	Cardiac myocytes *in vivo*	Calcium-binding protein in cytosol	No effect on systolic parameters but ↓ LV diastolic pressure, time course of pressure decline and improved force frequency relationship in senescent rats	30–32
VEGF	Blood vessel *in vivo*	Growth factor	Enhanced blood vessel and fibrovascular tissue growth, and endothelial cell proliferation	38
Calsequestrin	Cardiac myocytes *in vivo*	Calcium signaling	↓ LV performance and fractional shortening with ventricular geometry changes, left atrial enlargement and mineralization; no progressive ↓ in LV contractility, HF nor LV fibrosis	39
Catalase	Mitochondrial targeted	Antioxidant enzyme	↑ Life span; delayed cataract development and cardiac pathology; ↓ ROS damage, H_2O_2 production and aconitase inactivation,	40
IGF-1	Cardiac myocyte targeted	Signaling	↑ Telomerase activity and nuclear Akt levels; delayed myocyte apoptosis + DNA damage	41
Thioredoxin	Global	Redox factor Antioxidant	↑ Life span, and enhanced resistance to oxidative stress	42
Adenosine receptor (A1AR)	Cardiac myocyte targeted	Signaling receptor	Improved tolerance to ischemic insult and restored adenosine-mediated CP (↓ with aging)	43

genes, and selectively inhibit their expression in both cultured cells and in specific animals and humans tissues. Thus far, these potent gene silencing techniques have been rarely used in studies of mammalian aging but have been used extensively in *C. elegans* aging (described in a later chapter).

Knock-out Transgenic Animal Models

Methods used for the creation of transgenic animals include DNA microinjection, embryonic stem (ES) cell-mediated gene transfer and retrovirus-mediated gene transfer. While animals containing deliberate modification of their genome (i.e., transgenics) have been generated in many species (primarily by DNA microinjection), including rats, rabbits, sheep, pigs, birds, and fish, mice have become the primary species for transgenic analysis mainly because their small size and low cost of housing in comparison to larger vertebrates, their short generation time, and their well defined genetics. Moreover, unique to the transgenic mouse is the ability to generate null mutations of specific genes either in all the cells of the organism (global knock-out) or an organ-specific knock-out (tissue-specific). Nevertheless, progress is being made to develop transgenic knock-outs in other species.

Table 3.3 Transgenic mouse: specific gene knock-outs as models of aging

Gene	Function	Phenotype	Refs
P66SHC	A cytoplasmic signal transducer involved in transmitting mitogenic signals from activated receptors to Ras and in regulating stress resistance	↑ Resistance to oxidative stress (i.e., paraquat); 30% ↑ in life span; ↑ Cardiomyocyte number and myocardial hyperplasia; null strains resistant to proapoptotic/ hypertrophic action of Ang II and have a marked ↑ in cardiac progenitor cells, which expand, form new myocytes preserving cardiac homeostasis	44–46
eNOS	Signaling	Premature aging with ↑ cardiac dilatation and dysfunction in male eNOS-null mice	47
PPAR-α	Metabolic regulator of fatty acid β oxidation (primarily in mitochondria)	↓ Longevity; age-dependent cardiac toxicity featuring ↓ mitochondrial fatty acid utilization and myocardial fatty acid transport, ↓ ATP levels after exposure to stress, abnormal mitochondrial cristae, abnormal caveolae, and extensive fibrosis	48,49
Caveolin- 1	Membrane subcompartments/ signaling	↓ Life span with ↑ progressive cardiac hypertrophy and sudden cardiac death	50
Klotho	Circulating anti-aging hormone that inhibits insulin and IGF-1 signaling	Knockouts with multiple age-related disorders and premature death; sudden death associated with sinoatrial node dysfunction	51
Connexin 43 (Cx43)	Predominant ventricular gap junction protein	Premature and sudden death; ↓ Cx43 levels were associated with slowing of impulse propagation and a dramatic ↑ in susceptibility to inducible ventricular dysrhythmias.	52
Relaxin	A naturally occurring inhibitor of collagen deposition and fibrosis	Age-related ↑ in interstitial collagen (fibrosis) in heart (+ numerous other organs); With aging, progressive ↑ heart size and collagen deposition with ↑ ventricular chamber stiffness	53
STAT3	Signal transducer and activator of transcription	Spontaneous heart dysfunction with advancing age; show a dramatic ↑ in cardiac fibrosis in aged mice	54

The knock-out technology most often uses ES cell-mediated gene transfer, which involves insertion of the desired DNA sequence by homologous recombination into ES cells *in vitro*, and subsequent incorporation of the modified ES cells into an embryo at the blastocyst stage of development resulting in a chimeric animal. Using appropriate genetic crosses, these null alleles can be produced either in heterozygous or homozygous form, and genetic backgrounds can be well-manipulated (allowing the presence of more than one mutant allele). These animals have been powerful tools to examine the effects of specific genes on aging phenotypes including, enhanced or shortened longevity, premature or accelerated aging and increased (or decreased) susceptibility to aging-associated disorders such as cardiomyopathy, atherosclerosis and heart failure (HF). In Table 3.3, we show representative examples of transgenic mice with defined gene knock-out and relevant information to their aging phenotypes. Many of the mouse models featured in Table 3.3 will also be discussed in further depth in later sections of this book.

Gene Profiling: Transcriptome and Proteomic Analysis

Recent methodological advances have made it possible to simultaneously assess the entire profile of expressed genes in affected tissues e.g., myocardium, using only a very limited amount of tissue (endomyocardial biopsy). Gene expression profiling (also termed transcriptome analysis), to comprehensively evaluate which genes are increased and which decreased in expression, has been achieved by several methods. In this chapter, we will briefly discuss the methodological approaches being currently used and salient findings emerging from their use, while a more comprehensive discussion of the results of these gene profiling studies will be presented in Chapter 13.

Although the techniques of differential display, subtractive hybridization and the serial analysis of gene expression (SAGE), a method that efficiently quantifies large numbers of mRNA transcripts by sequencing short tags, have been used in a number of studies of gene profiling in aging, increasingly, most investigators have employed DNA microarray analysis. These methods make use of DNA chips, in which either cDNA clones or oligonucleotides are spotted at high density on a membrane, appropriately treated glass slide or other appropriate material to analyze a cellular transcriptome after hybridization with labelled probes generated from total RNA or mRNA transcripts.

In aging studies, examination of gene expression in specific tissues by microarray profiling has been performed primarily in rodent models (although some have been performed in monkeys) and human subjects. In a study focusing on gene expression profiles in mouse heart, Lee et al. have found a significant modulation of gene expression with aging, with over 10% of myocardial transcripts significantly changed by aging [55]. Genes exhibiting increased expression with age included, structural genes involved in extracellular matrix (ECM) components, collagen deposition, cell adhesion, and cell growth; this is consistent with previous findings that the aging heart undergoes ECM protein deposition, fibrosis and cardiomyocyte hypertrophy. Downregulated expression was found with genes of energy metabolism, including genes associated with fatty acid transport and metabolism, and genes involved in mitochondrial function and turnover. Interestingly, an aging-induced shift in myocardial energy metabolism was suggested by increased expression of genes involved in carbohydrate metabolism, in particular glycolysis and glucose uptake [55].

The study of Lee et al. also examined the effects of a caloric restriction (CR) dietary regimen on transcript profiles initiated in middle-age in a second cohort of aging animals, and identified an altered transcriptional pattern (compared to the untreated aging animals) which was rather broad-based (over 20% of profiled genes showed significant changes), with over 75% of the changes associated with myocardial aging being either completely or partially reversed [55]. The CR-mediated changes included suppression of the structural genes (e.g., collagen and ECM proteins), downregulation of DNA damage-inducible transcripts (suggesting less endogenous DNA damage) and of proapoptotic factors, upregulation of both DNA repair and antiapoptotic factors, and a reversal of expression programming leading to upregulated glycolysis and downregulated fatty acid metabolism consistent with a CR-mediated reduction of aging-induced endogenous damage, and induction of a metabolic shift in the heart [56]. Further microarray studies of long-term CR effects on cardiac gene expression also revealed a pattern of altered murine gene expression consistent with reduced myocardial remodeling and fibrosis, and enhanced contractility and energy production via fatty acid β-oxidation [57]. In contrast to the extensive "reprogramming" of the myocardial transcriptome revealed by these studies, in a gene profiling analysis of isolated ventricular cardiomyocytes of aging mice compared to cardiomyocytes from young mice, Bodyak et al. identified only 43 gene transcripts that accumulated at significantly different levels with age [58]. These included decreased transcript levels of several stress response proteins including, heat shock proteins (e.g., HSP70 and HSP25) and heme oxygenase (HO-1), decreased levels of mitochondrial ETC transcripts and mitochondrial creatine kinase (Mi-CK), decreased transcript levels of proteins involved in contraction (e.g., dystrophin, tropomyosin, troponin I, α-MHC, skeletal actin and sarcoplasmic reticulum Ca^{2+}-ATPase [SERCA2]), and more uniquely, reduced mRNA levels of several transcription factors (e.g., Nkx2.5, GATA-4, c-jun, JunB) were noted.

These disparate findings suggest that a large subset of age-associated changes in myocardial transcript abundance, described by Lee et al. [55] may be associated with non-cardiomyocytes, strain differences or altered transcript abundance associated with isolation procedures and not aging. Also, altered gene expression in specific cell sub-populations (e.g., myocytes) including, changes in less-abundant transcription factors might be obscured by transcript levels in neighboring cells (e.g., fibroblasts). Moreover, these findings highlight both the necessity of taking into account biological diversity when performing studies of aging, as well as underlining the point that transcriptome (as well as proteomic) analysis of heart tissue is complicated by diverse factors such as tissue and cellular heterogeneity, genetic variability, disease state and pharmacological intervention.

Not unexpectedly, microarray gene profiling analysis of murine and monkey skeletal muscle transcripts revealed a number of striking tissue-specific differences, with regards to aging, as well as sharing some commonalities with the profiles obtained from myocardial/cardiomyocyte analysis [56, 59]. A lower proportion of genes appear to be affected overall in murine skeletal muscle aging compared to heart. A large percentage (nearly 20%) of the aging-associated upregulated genes in gastrocnemius muscle are involved in induction of genes involved in stress response including, heat shock response, with the notable exception of HSP70 which is downregulated, and genes induced by OS and DNA damage (e.g., GADD45). Another class of genes with elevated transcripts in muscle aging are involved with neuronal growth and remodeling, which may reflects the loss of motor neurons in skeletal muscle aging followed by reinnervation of muscle fibers by the remaining intact neuronal units. Genes involved in energy metabolism were downregulated with aging, including genes associated with mitochondrial function and turnover, as were genes associated with glycogen metabolism and glycolysis (the latter in marked contrast with their upregulation in the myocardium).

In a similar profiling analysis conducted with skeletal muscle derived from Rhesus monkeys, genes involved in OS responses and neuronal death, remodeling, and repair were induced with aging, while genes involved in energy metabolism, such as mitochondrial electron transport and oxidative phosphorylation, were downregulated [60]. In contrast to the CR-mediated reversal of the majority of age-related alterations in skeletal muscle in the aging mouse including, reprogramming energy metabolism, increased biosynthesis, macromolecular turnover, and reduced oxidative damage, beneficial aspects of CR at the transcriptional level in monkey skeletal muscle were not found suggesting potential problems with the timing of CR initiation, or differential species-specificity regarding the CR mechanism.

Thus far, microarray profiling studies with biopsied skeletal muscle from both older human male and female subjects have also demonstrated decreased expression of genes involved in energy metabolism and mitochondrial protein synthesis [61]. Interestingly, no consistent pattern on the activation of OS response genes has been found in human DNA microarray studies.

Studies comparing gene expression patterns across species have begun to prove informative in identifying shared transcriptional elements that appear to be conserved in the aging process [62]. Studies of the aging skeletal muscle transcriptome in mice, rat, monkey and man have all reported a large differential expression between young and old (in both male and female) in the expression of the cell cycle regulator p21 (an inhibitor of cyclin-dependent kinases) [56, 60, 63, 64]. Accordingly, the age-related upregulation of p21 is a evolutionarily conserved component of an age-related transcriptional program induced in skeletal muscle. It will be interesting to see if similar patterns emerge from comparative studies of heart muscle or cardiomyocyte-specific gene transcription. Of significance, the upregulation of p21 is associated with cell cycle arrest at the G_1/S boundary in human fibroblasts, and occurs with downregulation of Klotho [65], concomitant with the transition in the postnatal heart from hyperplasia to hypertrophy [66].

These studies also suggest that aging transcription profiling can be used to elucidate a panel of transcriptional biomarkers, which can be evaluated with interventions that delay or reverse aging phenotypes. Gene profiling by microarray has also proved to be highly informative in specific animal models of premature aging including the recently described mtDNA mutator strains (to be discussed in depth in Chapter 4).

Rigorously performed DNA microarray analysis has been highly informative in documenting gene expression patterns associated with diverse aging-related cardiac pathologies such as cardiac hypertrophy [67], myocardial ischemia [68], dilated cardiomyopathy [67], coronary artery disease [69], atrial fibrillation [70] and HF [71], in both animal models and human. This analytical approach has also been revealing establishing profiles in vascular cells of genes involved (or altered) in aging-associated neointimal formation, apoptotic progression and proinflammatory events [72, 73].

A number of limitations inherent in the transcriptome analysis of aging should be considered. The correlation between mRNA and protein levels for a particular gene can be highly variable, and since proteins are the primary effectors of most cellular processes, altered gene transcription are often not related to phenotype changes, or to altered protein levels. Moreover, most studies rely on a single timepoint (or endpoint) for their analysis, which may miss significant transcriptional events in the aging pathways. In addition, in myocardial studies there are numerous examples showing that the biological activity of proteins are subject to regulation by post-translational modifications, including their subcellular localization, with subsequent effects on the cardiac phenotype, which will not be detected by transcriptional analysis. For instance, oxidative and nitrosative damage to proteins, including the effects of lipid peroxidation, nitrotyrosines, and protein carbonylation are prevalent in aging cells and tissues, including the heart (this will be discussed more thoroughly in Chapter 4).

Progressive development and refinement in microarray techniques requires the normalization of microarray data, to remove thru filtering the "noise from signal", as well as the availability of computational software, and statistical analysis [74]. Given the numerous studies and models undergoing evaluation of aging gene expression, tissues diversity, organisms and populations being undertaken, an increased effort is currently in place to standardize approaches for normalization and statistical treatment of microarray data that may allow direct and informative comparison between experiments. Moreover, further validation of specific gene expression patterns ascertained by microarray data, is often necessary by either quantitative RT-PCR, RNAse protection or Northern blot analysis. Awareness of these limitations underscores the need for complementary approaches (e.g., proteomic analysis) to advance our understanding of complex cardiac disorders and cardiovascular aging.

Proteomic Analysis

Proteomic analysis also provides the opportunity to evaluate gene expression in aging tissues in a global fashion. Increased interest has emerged in the application of proteomic analysis in the identification of cardiovascular and cardiac-specific biomarkers of aging [75]. The traditional proteomic approach involves two-dimensional polyacrylamide gel electrophoresis (2-DE) to resolve and identify thousands of proteins in a single gel. This technique can resolve >5000 proteins simultaneously (2000 proteins routinely) and can detect <1 ng of protein per spot [76]. Developments over the last few years, particularly those involving the use of narrow-range immobilized pH gradients (IPGs) for the first-dimension isoelectric focusing (IEF) separation, have resulted in increased resolving power and high reproducibility with relative simplicity of use [77]. On the other hand, an important limitation of this technique is that specific classes of proteins, such as transmembrane-spanning proteins, high-molecular-weight proteins, and very acidic or basic proteins, which may be difficult to solubilize, are frequently excluded or underrepresented by these analyses. Furthermore, alternative methods are increasingly being employed, including different mass spectrometry based approaches following both one-dimensional SDS-PAGE and gel-free approaches, and blue native gel electrophoresis (BN-PAGE).

There have been very few studies of myocardial proteomics in aging at the global level. One recent study employed a proteomic analysis in the aging heart of both males and females in a primate (*Macaca fascicularis*), a model which is phylogenetically close to 60 year old humans and does not have the associated diseases of aging. After 2D gel comparison in the different groups of monkeys, 20 proteins, which showed different expression among the groups, were identified by mass spectrometry. A large number of the affected proteins were involved in glycolytic and mitochondrial electron transport protein expression and function, and were primarily affected in older male monkeys [78]. Another method under development is the use of protein microarrays with immobilized antibodies. This method offers a suitable alternative for the rapid screening of the expression levels of known proteins, which could provide high sensitivity and specificity. However, presently, this technique is limited by the availability (and expense) of suitable antibodies [79].

Proteome simplification by subcellular fractionation and organelle enrichment and affinity chromatography has allowed a higher resolution analysis of targeted organelles (e.g., mitochondria). Recently, a novel technique of continuous-flow ultracentrifugation using a sucrose gradient allowed effective high-yield separation, accumulation, and enrichment of bovine heart mitochondria in a single step (bypassing the multiple, time-consuming, and potentially artifact-inducing series of many small centrifugation steps that traditionally comprise organelle fractionation) facilitating a subsequent evaluation of the aging heart mitochondrial proteome [80]. This technique has also recently been applied to the separation and enrichment of other organelles including the Golgi apparatus and endoplasmic reticulum followed by 2D gel electrophoresis, digitized imaging of 2D gel electrophoresis and mass spectrometry enabling analysis of these organelle proteomes in aging tissues [81].

Evaluation of proteomes for evidence of specific protein modifications (e.g., phosphorylation or oxidative changes) has been facilitated by the use of specific antibodies to phosphorylated residues (e.g., phosphoserine or phosphotyrosine), protein carbonyls or nitrotyrosine. For instance, proteomic analysis of cardiac proteins in aging rat utilized separation of proteins by one- and two-dimensional gel electrophoresis, subsequent immunoblot analysis using an anti-nitrotyrosine antibody to detect specific proteins (which show an age-related increase in immunoresponse) followed by their identification using nanoelectrospray ionization-tandem mass spectrometry (NSI-MS/MS) [82]. 48 proteins were identified in this study, including enzymes responsible for energy production and metabolism as well as proteins involved in the structural integrity of the cells. Similarly, a hydrazide biotin-streptavidin methodology (coupled with liquid chromatography tandem mass spectrometry) has been employed in sensitively identifying protein carbonylation in aged mice tissues, including several low-abundance receptor proteins, mitochondrial proteins involved in glucose and energy metabolism, and a series of receptors and tyrosine phosphatases known to be associated with insulin and insulin-like growth factor metabolism and cell-signaling pathways [83].

In contrast to the complexity of heart tissues and their cellular heterogeneity, cell culture systems are attractive models for proteomic analysis because they can provide highly defined systems with much lower inherent variability between samples. There have been relatively few published proteomic investigations of isolated adult cardiac myocytes, and none that we are aware of with aging studies.

Proteomic investigations have been carried out with ECs undergoing replicative senescence [84]. As we shall discuss in later chapters, the aging of ECs and vascular SMCs is thought to play a significant role in the pathophysiology of age-related vascular diseases, including atherosclerosis; however, the precise mechanisms responsible for senescence have not been elucidated. Proteomic analysis has also been applied to analyze aging–associated protein profiles in the vascular SMC [85].

Interestingly, another promising methodological approach, which should be applied to aging or senescent cardiovascular cells (e.g., cardiomyocyte or ECs) combines proteomic and metabolomic techniques to reveal protein and metabolite alterations [86]. This combined approach has been applied to both specific gene-knockout mice and in cultured vascular SMCs derived from these animals [87].

DNA Damage and Mutations in Aging

The involvement of genetic instability, DNA damage and repair, and DNA mutation are important aspects of the aging process as both suggested by studies in model organisms (including premature-aging models), human progeroid phenotypes and senescent cells (to be discussed in Chapter 4). In this section we will describe a number of techniques used for the evaluation of DNA damage and mutations. In those cases where these techniques have yet to be applied in cardiovascular aging studies, mention will be made.

Types of DNA Damage

Microsatellite Instability

Microsatellites are repetitive genetic sequences, in which the repeating unit is from one to six bases. The number of tracts containing repetitive sequences in the human genome is rather abundant, comprising over 100,000 CA/GT repeats, each with a chain length >24 [88]. Microsatellites are particularly prone to slippage during DNA replication, resulting in a number of base repeats in the newly replicated strand differing from the original resulting in a small loop in either the template or the new DNA strand. Despite the tendency to mistakes (microsatellite instability) occurring in all dividing cells, microsatellites remain stable in length, due to the efficiency of the mismatch repair system [89].

Small pool PCR (SP-PCR) is a sensitive method for the detection and quantification of microsatellite instability (MSI) in somatic cells [90]. In normal human somatic cells (peripheral blood lymphocytes) there is evidence that mutant microsatellite fragments accumulate at 6 microsatellite loci with age and that this increase in MSI can be quantified by SP-PCR. However, to the best of our knowledge, this technique has not yet been applied for the analysis of aging in cardiovascular cells.

Single-Strand versus Double-Strand Damage

A variety of molecular methods including gel electrophoresis, pulsed-field gel electrophoresis, filter elution method, sedimentation analysis, electron microscopy and most recently, atomic force microscropy [91] have been applied to the analysis of single-strand (SSBs) and double-strand breaks (DSBs) in DNA.

Early studies of SSBs, which are often generated by oxidative damage, utilized single-strand specific nucleases, alkaline electrophoresis and Southern blotting or alkaline sucrose gradient sedimentation. These techniques are rather time-consuming with relatively low sensitivity. The assessment of SSBs and their repair has been recently updated with the development of a fast micromethod using a quick fluorometric microplate assay [92]. This method measures the rate of unwinding of cellular DNA on exposure to alkaline conditions, using a fluorescent dye which preferentially binds to double-strand DNA, but not to single-strand DNA or protein. The method requires only minute amounts of material (30 ng of DNA or about 3000 cells per single well), allows simultaneous measurements of multiple samples (e.g., 96 well format), and can be performed within 3 hours or less.

The neutral (or nondenaturing) filter elution assay at pH 7.2 or 9.6 has long been a standard method for the measurement of double-strand breakage and rejoining in eukaryotic cells, with a threshold dose for detection of DSBs ranging from 5–10 Gy. In addition, pulsed-field electrophoresis (PFGE) has become one of the most widely used methods for the evaluation of radiation-induced DSBs since it can detect DSBs induced by as little as 1 Gy of ionizing radiation. In most studies a simple quantification of DNA migration from the well in the gel has been used as a correlate of DSB formation. A modified PFGE-based system represents an extremely sensitive tool for measuring DSB induction and repair after low doses of X rays, using as few as 125 cells with no DNA labeling necessary [93]. To quantify the DSBs after electrophoresis, the DNA was transferred to nylon membranes and hybridized with ^{32}P-labeled chromosomal DNA.

Comet Assay

The comet assay or single-cell gel test is a microgel electrophoresis technique that measures DNA damage at the level of single cells. This assay involves suspension of a small number of cells in a thin agarose gel on a microscope slide, lysis *in situ*, electrophoresis, and staining with a fluorescent DNA binding dye (usually ethidium bromide) [94]. Cells harboring elevated levels of DNA damage display increased migration of chromosomal DNA from the nucleus toward the anode, which resembles the shape of a comet. Under alkaline conditions, DNA DSBs, alkali-labile sites, and SSBs associated with incomplete excision repair sites cause increased DNA migration. On the other hand, intermolecular crosslinks (either DNA-DNA or DNA-protein) can lead to decreased DNA migration. Variations of the comet assay have been established for the detection of specific DNA base modifications. The neutral comet assay can be applied to detect double-strand DNA fragments resulting from apoptosis and has been used to effectively distinguish necrotic from apoptotic cell death in both single cell models and in parenchymal tissues, such as skeletal and cardiac muscle after ischemia-reperfusion [95].

The presence of DSBs can also be indirectly inferred by analysis of the levels of specific markers or DNA damage sensors including ATM, p53 and phosphorylated histone 2AX, which can be quantitatively determined by immunoblotting with specific antibodies. Phosphorylation of histone H2AX occurs in megabase chromatin domains around DSBs and this modification (termed gamma-H2AX) has proven to be a useful marker of genome damage as well as DNA repair in terminally differentiated cells. Using immunohistochemistry, analysis of the kinetics of gamma-H2AX formation and elimination in the X-irradiated mouse heart revealed that levels of gamma-H2AX-positive cells increased from 3 to 5% in unradiated heart to between 20 and 30% after 3 Gy irradiation. Time-course analysis indicated that after 3 Gy of irradiation, maximal induction of gamma-H2AX in heart is observed 20 min after irradiation and then is decreased slowly with about half remaining 23 h later, suggesting repair of 50% of the lesions [96]. The utility of this approach, to quantitate levels of DNA damage (or more precisely DNA damage signaling) in human cardiomyocytes under controlled conditions of ischemia-reperfusion, has been recently demonstrated [97]. In this model, LV samples taken from 20 patients undergoing elective valve surgery before aortic cross-clamping, 20 min after brief ischemia, 58 min after the cross-clamping period (prolonged ischemia), and 20 min after reconstitution of coronary blood flow (reperfusion) were evaluated for specific DNA damage sensor protein levels. This study found that prolonged ischemia induced extensive DNA damage (increased p53 and phosphorylation of histone H2AX) and the activation of ATM checkpoint, whereas reperfusion triggered the repair of the DNA lesions and salvage of ischemic cells. Analysis of this signaling pathway in aging cardiomyocytes may prove useful when applied to analysis of cardiomyocyte-specific levels of DNA damage and responses to DNA damage during aging.

DNA Repair Enzymes in Aging

Similar to the inference of double-strand DNA damage by increased levels of DNA sensor proteins as discussed above, DNA SSBs induce the catalytic activation of two isoforms of poly ADP-ribose polymerases (PARP-1 and PARP-2) which catalyze the post-translational modification of proteins containing poly ADP-ribose and is pivotally involved in DNA repair pathways, including base-excision repair. Poly ADP-ribosylation is an immediate cellular response to genotoxic insults induced by ionizing radiation, alkylating agents, and OS. PARP-1 mediates the repair of DNA single-strand breaks in mammalian cells in concert with DNA ligase IIIα, and XRCC1 and plays a critical role in maintaining genome stability [98].

Recently, a novel real-time assay has been reported to assess an imbalance of DNA SSB repair by indirectly measuring PARP-1 activation through the depletion of intracellular NAD(P)H [99]. This assay employs a water-soluble tetrazolium salt to monitor the amount of NAD(P)H in living cells through its reduction to a yellow colored water-soluble formazan dye, and while not a direct method of SSB determination, it requires neither DNA extraction nor alkaline treatment, both of which can cause artifactual induction of SSBs.

In vitro studies with human cell extracts have demonstrated that PARP-1 is involved in repair of a uracil-containing oligonucleotide and that it binds to the damaged DNA during the early stages of repair. Furthermore, excessive poly ADP-ribosylation was found when repair intermediates containing SSBs were in excess of the repair capacity of the cell extract, indicating that repeated binding of PARP-1 to the nicked DNA occurs [100]. In addition, increased sensitivity of repair intermediates to nuclease cleavage has been reported in PARP-deficient mouse fibroblasts and after depletion of PARP-1 from HeLa whole cell extracts. This further highlights PARP's protective effects stemming nucleolytic deterioration from DNA breaks.

Correlative data suggest a critical link between DNA-damage induced poly ADP-ribosylation and mammalian longevity. Significant positive correlation has been reported between poly ADP-ribosylation capacity of mononuclear blood cells and longevity of 13 mammalian species, including human [101]. This has been further reinforced by recent evidence demonstrating physical and functional interactions between PARP-1 and the Werner syndrome protein (WRN), as well as with the Cockayne syndrome protein (CSB) [102, 103]. Deficiencies in these proteins cause segmental premature aging phenotypes in humans (as discussed in the following chapter). Furthermore, PARP-2 as well as PARP-1 have been found in association with telomeric DNA and are able to poly ADP-ribosylate the telomere-binding proteins TRF-1 and TRF-2, thus blocking their DNA-binding activity and controlling telomere extension by telomerase [104]. Another important signaling factor interacting with PARP is the tumor suppressor protein p53, which serves as a substrate for direct modification by poly ADP-ribose, with attendant changes in its DNA-binding properties, and can also bind to the PARP polymer in a noncovalent fashion.

The beneficial functions of poly ADP-ribosylation, under conditions of genotoxic stress, have been illustrated by inhibiting PARP activity through treatment of cells or organisms with low-molecular-weight compounds (mainly NAD^+ analogs), by expression of *PARP-1* antisense RNA, or of dominant negative derivatives of PARP-1, supporting its role in genomic instability reduction and cytoprotection. This has been assessed by measurement of several biological markers such as chromosomal aberrations, gene amplification, sister chromatid exchange, or mutagenesis.

While impaired PARP activity can lead to less effective repair of DNA damage, and induction of mutations, gene amplification, or apoptosis, PARP overactivity has been implicated in cell destruction. Severe DNA damage can trigger either acute overactivation or sustained activity of the energy-consuming PARP coupled with inadequate regeneration capacity for NAD^+. This has been shown to lead to excessive NAD^+ and ATP consumption, and subsequent cell death secondary to energy depletion (as documented in several nonproliferative cell types *in vivo* as well as in cell culture) [105]. The susceptible cells include neurons and cardiomyocytes exposed to ischemia-reperfusion damage, and ECs leading to vascular dysfunction. A protective effect of pharmacological inhibition of PARP or lack of the PARP gene in abrogating cardiovascular dysfunction has been demonstrated in experimental models of endotoxic shock [106], reperfusion injury [107, 108], diabetes [109], myocardial infarction [110], and HF [111]. Moreover, the use of a new PARP inhibitor (INO-1001) in Fischer rats, attenuated the cardiac and endothelial dysfunction associated with advanced aging, resulting in marked improvement of both systolic and diastolic cardiac function and in acetylcholine-induced, nitric oxide-mediated vascular relaxation of the endothelium [112]. Cardiac and endothelial function were assessed using a pressure-volume conductance catheter system and isolated aortic rings respectively.

Analysis of the *in vivo* interaction of damaged regions of DNA (e.g., DSBs) or telomeric regions with proteins involved in specific DNA repair, replication and transcription has been greatly enhanced by using chromatin immunoprecipitation (ChIP) as shown in Fig. 3.1. In this methodology, a gentle formaldehyde treatment of living intact cells results in DNA-bound proteins being cross-linked to the chromatin on which they are situated. After fixation, the cells are lysed, the chromatin is fragmented, and the DNA broken into pieces 0.2–1 kb in length by sonication. This is followed by protein-DNA complex immunoprecipitation using an antibody specific for the protein in question. Once the complex is isolated, cross-linking can be reversed releasing the protein (for further identification and characterization) and the DNA from the isolated protein/DNA fraction. Then the

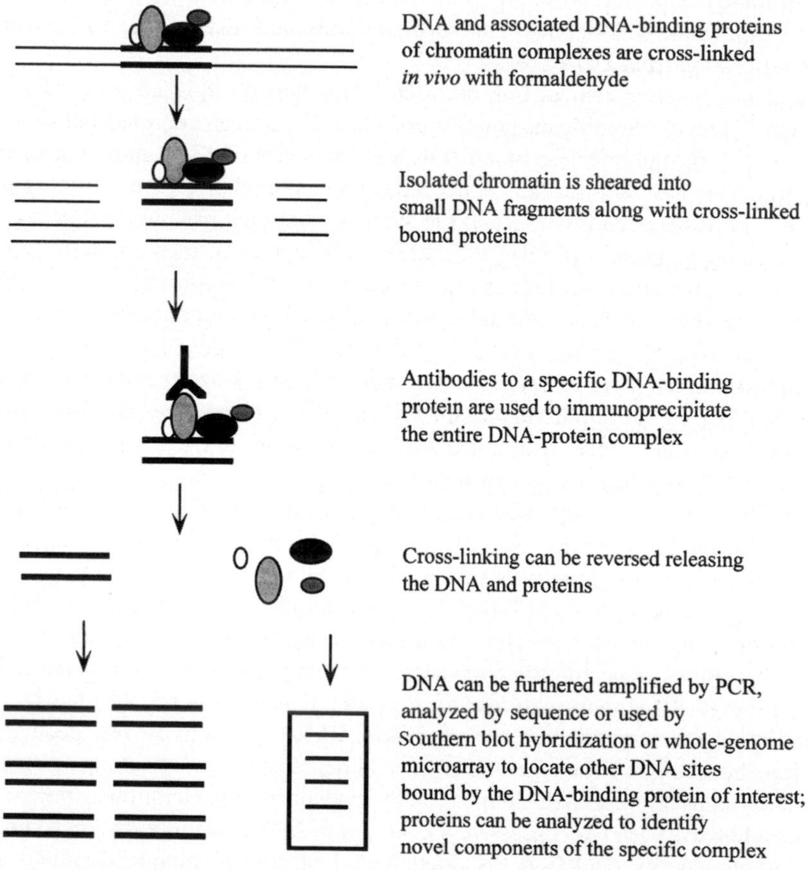
DNA and associated DNA-binding proteins of chromatin complexes are cross-linked *in vivo* with formaldehyde
Isolated chromatin is sheared into small DNA fragments along with cross-linked bound proteins
Antibodies to a specific DNA-binding protein are used to immunoprecipitate the entire DNA-protein complex
Cross-linking can be reversed releasing the DNA and proteins
DNA can be furthered amplified by PCR, analyzed by sequence or used by Southern blot hybridization or whole-genome microarray to locate other DNA sites bound by the DNA-binding protein of interest; proteins can be analyzed to identify novel components of the specific complex

Fig. 3.1 Chromatin immunoprecipitation (ChIP)

DNA can be purified and identified by PCR using primers specific for the DNA regions where the protein in question may bind. Furthermore, for identification of regions across the whole genome, to which a specific protein binds, a DNA microarray can be used (ChIP on chip or ChIP-chip). ChIP can also be used to screen specific chromatin regions for epigenetic changes, including methylation and acetylation.

This technique has also been useful for identification of chromatin changes in premature-aging syndromes with genomic instability, including Bloom syndrome, which is caused by loss of function of a 3′–5′ RecQ DNA helicase, BLM. Chromatin immunoprecipitation of BLM complexes recovered telomere and ribosomal DNA repeats and identified these elements as chromosomal targets for the BLM DNA helicase during the S/G_2 phase of the cell cycle [113].

Mutation Analysis

There is evidence that with age DNA damage and mutations accumulate in somatic cells. In a cross sectional *ex-vivo* study, mutation frequency in the HPRT locus was increased in human lymphocytes from middle age individuals compared to young [114]. Furthermore, Southern blotting and loss of heterozygosity at the HLA-A locus have been used to detect increased mutation frequency in human lymphocytes with aging [115].

Since the detection and quantitation of somatic mutations in different organs and tissues have often proved difficult, particularly postmitotic tissues *in vivo*, probing the role that DNA mutation accumulation plays during mammalian aging has also been problematic. An alternative approach is the use of transgenic mouse strains that possess chromosomally integrated plasmids harboring reporter genes that can be easily recovered from genomic DNA and transferred into a suitable *Escherichia coli* host for subsequent mutant detection and analysis. Vijg et al. have used plasmids containing the *lacZ* reporter gene in which a wide range of aging-mediated somatic mutations, including large rearrangements, have been reported to be generated in a tissue-specific manner; these observations show that the heart displayed extensive mutations, and in particular large-scale rearrangements [116–119]. Vijg et al. noted that point mutations do not accumulate at the level needed to affect function, whereas large-scale rearrangements could seriously affect normal gene regulation (by positional effects), changes in gene dosage (leading to random alterations of gene expression profiles in individual cells), and a pattern of gradual molecular change consistent with both heterogeneous gene expression profile (found in a cell to cell analysis in the aging heart) [120], as well as with the relatively subtle phenotypic changes that are typical for aging individuals [116].

A number of observations have implicated mtDNA as a particular "hotspot" for mutagenesis in aging. This might be expected given its proximity to a primary site of mitochondrial ROS generation and oxidative damage (i.e., ETC), the limited protection by proteins (i.e., no chromatin) and DNA repair systems (for further discussion see Chapter 4) Several methods of mtDNA mutation detection are currently in use, including single strand conformation polymorphism (SSCP) analysis, allelic specific oligonucleotides (ASO), restriction fragment length polymorphism (RFLP) analysis, mismatch detection/cleavage and denaturing gradient gel electrophoresis (DGGE). SSCP is based on the differences in secondary structure of single-strand DNA molecules, differing in a single nucleotide and gauged by an alteration of their electrophoretic mobility in nondenaturing gels. Hybridization with radioactively labeled *allelic specific oligonucleotides* (ASO) utilizes differences in the melting temperature of short DNA fragments differing by a single nucleotide.

High-density Oligonucleotide Arrays (HDOA) is a high-throughput technique, which has been used in combination with sequencing to construct a MITOCHIP. Maitra et al [121]. reported that in matched fluid samples (urine and pancreatic juice) obtained from seven patients with head/neck cancer, the MitoChip detected at least one cancer-associated mitochondrial mutation in four samples [122].

Techniques for examining mtDNA deletions include PCR, which can detect very low levels of specific deletions (utilizing specific primers), as in cases in which the mutant allele represents <1% of the total mtDNA; long-range PCR in which the entire 16 kB mtDNA genome can be effectively screened for rearrangement events, and Southern blot analysis which are used for more abundant deletions (>15% of the total mtDNA).

Amplification, plasmid cloning and sequence revealed increased levels of mtDNA point mutations in aging mice [123], in human lymphocytes, and in skeletal muscle from aging individuals [124–126]. These studies have focused on mutations in the D-loop region, which contains the regulatory sites for mtDNA transcription and replication. Levels of mutant allele heteroplasmy, mtDNA deletions and copy-number can also be rapidly and efficiently determined using real-time quantitative PCR [127–130].

Telomere Analysis

The length of telomeres is believed to be critical in cellular aging as noted in Chapter 2, and as more extensively discussed in later chapters. The repetitive sequences of these DNA-protein complexes progressively shorten with each mitosis and when the critical length is bridged, telomeres trigger DNA repair and cell cycle checkpoint mechanisms that result in chromosomal fusions, cell cycle arrest, senescence and/or apoptosis. While telomere lengths of human chromosomes within the same cell are generally heterogenous [131, 132], lengths of specific chromosome arms in different tissues within the same individual tend to be similar compared to those of other individuals. For example, the mean telomeric length of human hematopoietic progenitor cells from fetal blood cord, peripheral blood and bone marrow are 11, 7.6 and 7.4 kb respectively [133]. In the absence of telomerase activity, the telomere loses 30 to 150 bp per successive division; with aging, human senescent cells (at phase M1) can exhibit telomeres with as low as 5 kb in length. With successive telomere shortenings, cells enter the crisis stage (M2) in which telomere length has been reported to range from 1.5 to 2 kb [134]. In order to reliably monitor telomere length, a number of techniques have been used and they are shown in Table 3.4.

The most common technique of telomere analysis, Southern blotting/hybridization [135, 136] can resolve up to 300 bp and requires minimally 1ug of purified high molecular weight DNA; however, this method is time consuming and the smeared pattern of the bands generated (a function of the heterogeneity) can lead to inaccuracy. Utilization of the hybridization protection assay (HPA) is more rapid and requires only small amounts of DNA, which does not have to be intact (sheared DNA can be utilized) [137], and does not involve radioactivity; however, HPA does not provide information concerning the direct telomere size or its chromosomal location that can be provided by Southern

Table 3.4 Methods of telomere analysis

Technique	Refs
Southern blot	135, 136
Hybridization protection assay (HPA)	137
Fluorescence *in situ* hybridization (FISH)	138
Primed *in situ*	143, 144
Quantitative PCR	139
Single telomere length analysis (STELA)	140
Primer extension/nick translation	141
Oligononucleotide ligation assay	142

blot. More direct measures of telomeric lengths can be obtained from quantitative-fluorescence *in situ* hybridization (Q-FISH) using a fluorescein-labeled peptide nucleic acid (PNA) (CCCTAA)3 probe and DNA staining with propidium iodide [138]. Q-FISH can be performed separately (primarily in proliferating cells) or combined with flow cytometry (in either cycling or non-cycling) cells. A significant breakthrough in telomere analysis has been the development of quantitative PCR approaches; [139, 140] these methods are extremely fast, and require less DNA. The ratio of telomere repeat copy number to a single gene copy number is determined and the relative telomeric length can be detected quantitatively. In a PCR-modified technique known as STELA (single telomere length analysis), telomere length at the individual chromosome level is assessed [140]. In addition to these techniques, which either directly or indirectly measure telomere length, several techniques have been developed to quantitatively measure the G-rich telomere 3′ overhang; these include primer extension/nick translation, telomeric-oligonucleotide ligation and electron microscopy [141, 142].

Cell-Engineering and Transplantation

Early studies have found that fetal cardiomyocytes could be grown in culture and reintroduced into an injured heart where they could form stable grafts, electrically couple with the resident cardiomyocytes and assist in the generation of action potential [145, 146]. However, the yield of cardiomyocytes at the sites of ischemic injury were low, and they decreased over time primarily as a result of their vulnerability to apoptosis [147]. Initial studies from embryonic stem cells (ESCs) cultured *in vitro* have shown that these cells can differentiate to cardiomyocytes *in situ*, and electrically couple [148–152]. Also, recent studies have shown that cultured mouse embryonic stem cells marked with transfected green fluorescent protein (GFP), injected into the myocardium of aging Fischer 344 rats resulted in both increased myocyte numbers (i.e., myogenesis) and enhanced perfusion of the left ventricle (i.e., angiogenesis) 6 weeks after transplant, and improved heart function in response to isoproteronol [153]. Moreover, the characteristic phenotype of engrafted ESCs was identified in the transplanted heart by GFP-markers and their differentiation into cardiac tissue gauged by cardiac α-MHC expression. However, the present legal/ethical maelstrom surrounding the generation and use of human ESCs has severely affected research to develop useful sources of ESCs, to overcome the difficulties associated with their use (e.g., development of potential teratomas) and also the development of long-term studies of their functional effects and stability to repair the damaged or aged human heart.

Several other types of stem cells have shown promise in restoring contractility to the ischemic-damaged heart. Skeletal myoblasts derived from adults can be robustly grown in culture, can be delivered (by catheter or direct injection) to the heart, and can ameliorate contractile dysfunction. This has been shown both in animal models and in clinical trials [154, 155]. However, while the transplanted myoblasts do show evidence of acclimation to the cardiac milieu and appear to be more resistant to the damaging effects of apoptosis, the introduced cells do not become cardiomyocytes and do not electrically couple with the resident myocardial cells, and may be also potential sources of cardiac dysrhythmias [156, 157].

Bone marrow cells (BMCs) primarily mesenchymal cells, also derived from adult human, can be introduced into the infarcted myocardium. Such BMCs can be easily generated from the same individual on which the cell therapy will be directed; this may avoid eliciting an immune response that can negate the effects of cell transplant (another problem with the ESCs). Several animal studies (primarily in mouse) have shown clear evidence of BMC-mediated cardiovascular benefits, [158–160]. albeit large-scale clinical studies performed thus far have shown less compelling effects [161–163]. The mechanism by which these benefits occur is hotly debated. One camp has presented considerable evidence showing BMCs transdifferentiating to cardiomyocytes, [164–167] while the other camp has found little evidence of transdifferentiation, rather that cell fusion with existing cardiomyocytes is the primary mechanism [168–171]. Data obtained by Fazel et al. suggest that the primary cardioprotective effect of recruited BMCs appears to be largely of paracrine nature, due to the secretion of growth factors and cytokines, which stimulate cardiomyocytes as well as endothelial proliferation/angiogenic process [172]. The recruited c-kit+ cells established a proangiogenic milieu in the infarct border zone by increasing VEGF and by reversing the cardiac ratio of angiopoietin-1 to angiopoietin-2. This had led to increase the focus on the use of growth factor/cytokine cocktails to mediate cardioprotection and myocardial repair. On the other hand, it remains largely undetermined whether such a paracrine effect, elicited by stem cells, has a beneficial value in treating injured myocardium in aging. Recent observations indicated that the therapeutic efficacy of granulocyte colony-stimulating factor (G-CSF) and stem cell factor (SCF) in ameliorating post-myocardial infarction (post-MI) remodeling is impaired in old rats (20 month) compared to young adult rats (6 month) [173]. Furthermore, adult stem cells have proved to be a useful platform for the delivery of therapeutic genes and proteins. For instance, transplanted MSCs appear to be effective delivery platforms for introducing channel proteins involved in pacemaking activity (e.g., channel protein HCN2), resulting in modifying the heart rhythm *in vivo* [174].

Another recent development in the search for stem cells with potential for cardiac repair has been the identification of a small group of resident cardiac stem cells. At least 4 different groups of investigators have identified small sub-populations of multipotent cells in the myocardium. One group has reported the existence of a self-renewing cardiac stem cell subpopulation consisting of Lin^{-}c-kit^{+} cells in adult rat myocardium [175]. When injected into the ischemic heart, these cells contribute to the formation of endothelium and vascular smooth muscle and to the regeneration of myocardium in the region of necrosis, improving its pump function and the geometry of the ventricular chamber [175, 176]. Oh et al. have reported the isolation and characterization of a small population of adult heart-derived progenitor cells (from post-natal mouse myocardium), which express the surface marker stem cell antigen-1 (Sca-1^{+}) and telomerase activity associated with self-renewal potential [177, 178]. This sub-population of Sca-1^{+} cardiac stem cells can differentiate *in vitro* in response to treatment with either oxytocin or the DNA demethylating agent 5′-azacytidine, forming beating cardiomyocytes, as well as expressing genes of cardiac transcription factors (GATA-4, MEF-2C, TEF-1) and contractile proteins [179]. Laugwitz et al. have described a population of cardioblasts in both embryonic and postnatal heart (in mouse, rats and human) numbering just a few hundred per heart, which were identified on the basis of their expression of a LIM-homeodomain transcription factor, Isl1 [180]. These myocardial-derived stem cells were primarily localized in the atria, right ventricle, and ventricular outflow tract regions (where Isl1 is most prevalently expressed during cardiac organogenesis) and they could be isolated, transplanted, survive and replicate in the damaged heart showing evidence of functional improvement [180, 181].

At present, these non-abundant putative cardiac stem cells populations often appear to be heterogeneous, and there is little consensus on the phenotypic markers that would allow their unambiguous identification. Gude et al. have recently shown that nuclear targeting of Akt (by cardiac-specific overexpression) promotes the proliferative expansion of the presumptive cardiac progenitor cell population, as assessed by immunolabeling for c-kit^{+} cells in combination with myocyte-specific markers Nkx 2.5 or MEF 2C [182]. Furthermore, recent data indicate that the c-kit^{+} population of cardiac stem cells are primary targets of aging/senescence with attendant telomeric dysfunction leading to replicative senescence and increased apoptosis [183]. Building on these data, Anversa et al. proposed that the loss of these stem cells in the aging myocardium is central to the inability of the aging heart to replace lost parenchymal cells, and likely underlies reduced cardiac function in aging [184].

Clearly, more research is needed to define these stem cells, their origin, the stability of their differentiated phenotype and their role in the aging heart. Interestingly, the study of Fazel et al.

Table 3.5 Myocardial transplant: cell-type specific advantages and limitations

Cell-type	Source	Features
Embryonic stem cell (ESCs)	Allogenic blastocyst (inner mass)	1. Pluripotency, easily propagated. Can differentiate to form cardiomyocytes, which after transplant can be electrically coupled *in vivo* to myocardial cells. 2. Limitations include potential for tumor formation and immune rejection (allogenic), limited donor availability and numerous legal and ethical issues.
Skeletal myoblast	Autologous skeletal muscle biopsy	1. Proliferate robustly *in vitro* allowing for autologous transplant), more ischemia-resistant than cardiomyocytes, upon transplant can significantly reduce progressive ventricular dilatation and improve cardiac function 2. No formation of new cardiomyocytes *in vivo*; limited electrical coupling to host myocardial cells (may cause dysrhythmias)
Adult bone marrow stem cell	Autologous bone marrow stromal cells (mesenchymal)	1. Pluripotent, easy to isolate, grow well in culture, and can be derived from autologous source; they can develop into cardiomyocyte and vascular cells (although transdifferentiation to cardiomy ocytes is controversial)
	Bone marrow (endothelial progenitor cells)	2. Upon transplant, neovascularization can occur at site of myocardial scar reducing ischemia. Improvement in myocardial contractility; it is unclear whether this derives from paracrine effects. 3. Limitations include uncertainties as to efficiency and long-term stability of differentiated adult cardiomyocytes
Cardiac progenitor cells	Allogenic fetal, neonatal or adult heart	1. Efficient recognition of myocardial growth factors, myocardial recruitment and *in vivo* electrical coupling 2. Limited availability, growth *in vitro* and demonstrable long-term survival 3. Benefits of transplantation may derive from paracrine effects.

presented evidence that that the c-kit$^+$ sub-populations of cardiac stem cells are actually of bone marrow origin and provide a source of paracrine stimulation to the heart [172].

A comparative synopsis of the advantages and limitations of the various stem cell types currently used in cardiac transplantation is presented in Table 3.5. Although no clear-cut choice has yet emerged as to the best cell type to transplant for myocardial repair, there are reasons to believe that a multiplicity of approaches in the application of cell engineering will be required for effective cardioprotection. While preclinical studies with stem cell and myoblast transplantation have shown similar levels of efficacy thus far, there is a critical need for a comprehensive evaluation of the relative benefits, adverse effects and efficiency of the various stem cell transplants in the clinical setting, in particular in the aging patient. It is possible that the long-term repair to achieve a fully functioning myocardium, may require the incorporation of more than a single cell type (e.g., the addition of cardiomyocytes, fibroblasts, and ECs) for the integration and generation of a stable and responsive cardiac graft.

Tissue Engineering

The identification of features of the cardiac milieu that contribute to the growth and development of transplanted cells *in vivo* has been advanced by the use of 3-dimensional matrices designed as a novel *in vitro* system to mimic aspects of the electrical and biochemical environment of the native myocardium. This approach can provide a finer resolution of electrical and biochemical signals that may be involved in cell proliferation and plasticity. Myoblasts have been grown on 3-D polyglycolic acid mesh scaffolds in the presence of cardiac-like electrical current fluxes, and in the presence of culture medium that had been conditioned by mature cardiomyocytes [185]. The scaffolds generally employ an immunocompatible biodegradable material such as collagen or gelatin which can be degraded shortly after grafting. Such scaffolds containing either fetal or neonatal aggregates of contracting cardiac cells have been used to generate artificial cardiac grafts transplanted into injured myocardium with rescue of ventricular function, and formation of functional gap junctions between the grafted cells and the myocardium.

As previously noted, the co-culture of cardiac fibroblasts and non-cardiac tissue (adult bone marrow cells) in the generation of this 3-D aggregate appears to increase the functional longevity of the cardiac explant [27].

Similarly fabricated 3-D scaffolds and cardiac grafts might be used to replace cardiovascular parts worn-out during the aging process. For instance, the tissue engineering of blood vessels and formation of a microvascular network can be achieved by promoting vasculogenesis *in situ,* initiated by seeding vascular ECs within a biopolymeric scaffolding construct; the inclusion of human SMCs seeded with human endothelial progenitor-derived ECs can form capillary-like microvessel structures throughout the scaffold [186, 187].

Particular interest has been centered on the reengineering of heart valves [188]. Utilizing collagen scaffolds produced by a novel process termed rapid prototyping, valve interstitial cells isolated from three human aortic valves seeded on the scaffolds and cultured for up to 4 weeks remained viable and proliferated; an important step in the tissue engineering of an aortic valve. Repopulation of a scaffold of a decellularized valve matrix (usually porcine) *in vitro* using valve interstitial cells or mesenchymal stem cells, has also been an area of intensive investigation [189]. Engineering of autologous semilunar heart valves *in vitro* with mesenchymal stem cells, and a biodegradable scaffold, has been recently achieved following their implantation, under cardiopulmonary bypass, into the pulmonary valve position of the sheep. These valves were shown to undergo extensive remodeling *in vivo,* resembling the native heart valves, and functioned satisfactorily for periods of >4 months [190]. These promising advances in valves engineering may have a particular application in the management of the valvular pathology that may be present in the aging heart.

Conclusion

In addition to the enormous contributions that molecular and cellular approaches have already made to the study of aging, including modulation of gene function in cells and transgenic animals, the unraveling of the subcellular pathways leading to aging-mediated macromolecular damage, cellular reprogramming and phenotypic dysfunction, new discoveries will undoubtedly lead to further identification of cardiac and cardiovascular biomarkers of aging and aging-related diseases. Furthermore, advances in the identification of genes and genetic variants, involved directly in the aging process and underlying susceptibility to disease may have, in the very near future, great implications in the diagnosis and management of cardiovascular diseases and aging-associated cardiac dysfunction. Much remains to be found from the interaction of molecular analysis of gene and environmental factors, and in the delineation of epigenetic changes involved in aging and disease. Another nascent area of extreme interest in aging studies is the further development of gene-transfer and cell-based platforms for increasing gene expression, as well as for targeting localized defective functions. The further molecular and cellular elucidation of stem cells and their transplantation is clearly an area in which new techniques will be needed to advance their enormous potential in applied therapies of aging-related dysfunction. Novel techniques remain to be developed to promote these studies particularly adapted to use in larger mammals and in humans. Of particular important is the development of non-invasive techniques to gauge cardiac and cardiovascular macromolecular damage, as well as the development and incorporation of new algorithms for integrating the huge database of molecular, physiological, morphological and clinical findings to elaborate testable models of aging with a global system biology-type approach.

Summary

- Cultured cells derived from the aging heart (e.g., cardiac myocytes and fibroblasts) and vasculature (e.g., endothelial and smooth muscle cells [SMCs] have provided critical information about the mechanism of replicative senescence, the signaling pathways involved in aging and aging-associated diseases, and the different responses of aging cells to a variety of physiological stimuli.
- Introduction and expression of novel genes into a wide range of cardiac and cardiovascular cells can be effectively mediated by the use of vectors including viral constructs (e.g., adenoviral, retroviral, lentiviral and AAV) and DNA-containing plasmids.
- Gene transfer leading to either overexpression or silencing of specific genes has been performed both with target tissues *in vivo* and with cells *in vitro* and has been shown to reverse aging-mediated cardiovascular dysfunction at either the cell or tissue level.
- The creation of transgenic animals containing modulation of specific gene function has provided important information about aging pathways and has also provided informative models of age-related cardiovascular disease.
- Transgenic models (primarily available with mice) can furnish information concerning multi-systemic interactions in aging phenotype not possible with cellular models and can also provide a substrate for testing diverse therapeutic modalities. Null alleles generated by homologous recombination can be used (with genetic crosses) to generate either heterozygous or homozygous mouse strains including either global knock-out or tissue-specific knock-out strains.
- Gene transcript profiling by either microarray or SAGE analysis allows the possibility of examining a large number of age or disease-related transcripts at the same time. As such it can be informative about the overall nature of gene programming in specific tissues with aging or age-related diseases.
- Changes in the profile occurring with interventions such as caloric restriction (CR) can be informative about the pathways critical to aging phenotypes. To circumvent confounding effects on this analysis promoted by the marked heterogeneity of cell-types in the heart, this analysis can also be conducted with isolated cardiomyocytes or fibroblasts derived from the aging heart.
- Proteomic analysis can also be informative in the analysis of aging programming in cardiovascular tissues or isolated cell-types. In addition to a global analysis which attempts to gauge all the proteins in a particular cell/tissue, increasing attention has focused on investigation of cellular sub-proteomes including organelle-specific proteomes and even proteomes of specific aging-mediated post-translational modifications such as protein nitration. Proteomic analysis can also be effectively combined with transcriptome and metabolomic analysis to provide a more detailed picture of the overall phenotypic context.
- A variety of types of DNA damage and techniques to detect them have been discovered and utilized in aging studies. These include the detection of single strand breaks (SSBs), double strand breaks (DSBS) and a variety of oxidative DNA lesions. Analyses of the frequency of mutation, microsatellite instability, point mutations, and large DNA rearrangements have shown age-specific patterns in both animal studies and human subjects that often are tissue-specific.
- MtDNA mutations are particularly prevalent in aging and a host of PCR-related techniques have proved useful in determining age-mediated changes in mtDNA integrity (e.g., deletions) and overall copy number.

- Factors involved in DNA repair are significantly affected in aging, and in some cases are indirect manifestations of the presence of DNA damage. Mutations in repair proteins can affect accumulation of DNA damage and aging phenotypes, including the development of premature aging in humans and in animal models.
- Changes in telomere DNA size and in telomere-associated proteins are found in aging and can be evaluated by a variety of techniques including Southern blot analysis, hybridization protection assay, *in situ* hybridization, primer extension, and PCR-based quantitative assay and single telomeric length assay (e.g., STELA)
- Stem cells from embryos (e.g., ESC) and adults (e.g., skeletal myoblasts, bone marrow cells, cardiac stem cells) can be transplanted into defective/dysfunctional heart and can enhance contractility, and repair injured myocardium dependent on the particular cell type. These findings have been replicated primarily in animal models but a more modest phenotypic effect has been demonstrated in preliminary clinical studies.
- Many of the details concerning long-range stability, the extent of differentiation to cardiomyocytes and the paracrine-associated effects of cells transplantation have not yet been elucidated. Stem cells can also serve as platforms to introduce genes in the rescue of cardiac function in aging.

References

1. Zhou YY, Wang SQ, Zhu WZ, Chruscinski A, Kobilka BK, Ziman B, Wang S, Lakatta EG, Cheng H, Xiao RP. Culture and adenoviral infection of adult mouse cardiac myocytes: methods for cellular genetic physiology. Am J Physiol Heart Circ Physiol 2000;279:H429–H436
2. Suzuki T, Ohta M, Hoshi H. Serum-free, chemically defined medium to evaluate the direct effects of growth factors and inhibitors on proliferation and function of neonatal rat cardiac muscle cells in culture. In Vitro Cell Dev Biol 1989;25:601–606
3. Kajstura J, Cheng W, Reiss K, Anversa P. The IGF-1-IGF-1 receptor system modulates myocyte proliferation but not myocyte cellular hypertrophy in vitro. Exp Cell Res 1994;215:273–283
4. Weiner HL, Swain JL. Acidic fibroblast growth factor mRNA is expressed by cardiac myocytes in culture and the protein is localized to the extracellular matrix. Proc Natl Acad Sci USA 1989;86:2683–2687
5. Long CS, Kariya K, Karns L, Simpson PC. Trophic factors for cardiac myocytes. J Hypertens 1990;8: S219–S224
6. Mima T, Ueno H, Fischman DA, Williams LT, Mikawa T. Fibroblast growth factor receptor is required for in vivo cardiac myocyte proliferation at early embryonic stages of heart development. Proc Natl Acad Sci USA 1995;92:467–471
7. Pasumarthi KB, Kardami E, Cattini PA. High and low molecular weight fibroblast growth factor-2 increase proliferation of neonatal rat cardiac myocytes but have differential effects on binucleation and nuclear morphology. Evidence for both paracrine and intracrine actions of fibroblast growth factor-2. Circ Res 1996;78: 126–136
8. Sheikh F, Fandrich RR, Kardami E, Cattini PA. Overexpression of long or short FGFR-1 results in FGF-2-mediated proliferation in neonatal cardiac myocyte cultures. Cardiovasc Res 1999;42:696–705
9. Busk PK, Hinrichsen R, Bartkova J, Hansen AH, Christoffersen TE, Bartek J, Haunso S. Cyclin D2 induces proliferation of cardiac myocytes and represses hypertrophy. Exp Cell Res 2005;304:149–161
10. Tamamori-Adachi M, Ito H, Sumrejkanchanakij P, Adachi S, Hiroe M, Shimizu M, Kawauchi J, Sunamori M, Marumo F, Kitajima S, Ikeda MA. Critical role of cyclin D1 nuclear import in cardiomyocyte proliferation. Circ Res 2003;92:e12–e19
11. Terman A, Dalen H, Eaton JW, Neuzil J, Brunk UT. Aging of cardiac myocytes in culture: oxidative stress, lipofuscin accumulation, and mitochondrial turnover. Ann NY Acad Sci 2004;1019:70–77
12. Terman A, Brunk UT. On the degradability and exocytosis of ceroid/lipofuscin in cultured rat cardiac myocytes. Mech Ageing Dev 1998;100:145–156
13. Terman A, Dalen H, Eaton JW, Neuzil J, Brunk UT. Mitochondrial recycling and aging of cardiac myocytes: the role of autophagocytosis. Exp Gerontol 2003;38:863–876
14. Bicknell KA, Coxon CH, Brooks G. Forced expression of the cyclin B1-CDC2 complex induces proliferation in adult rat cardiomyocytes. Biochem J 2004;382:411–416

15. Kardami E. Stimulation and inhibition of cardiac myocyte proliferation in vitro. Mol Cell Biochem 1990;92:129–135
16. Reiss K, Cheng W, Ferber A, Kajstura J, Li P, Li B, Olivetti G, Homcy CJ, Baserga R, Anversa P. Overexpression of insulin-like growth factor-1 in the heart is coupled with myocyte proliferation in transgenic mice. Proc Natl Acad Sci USA 1996;93:8630–8635
17. Pasumarthi KBS, Field LJ. Cardiomyocyte cell cycle regulation. Circ Res 2002;90:1044–1054
18. Clark WA, Rudnick SJ, Simpson DG, LaPres JJ, Decker RS. Cultured adult cardiac myocytes maintain protein synthetic capacity of intact adult hearts. Am J Physiol 1993;264:H573–H582
19. Bell D, McDermott BJ. Contribution of de novo protein synthesis to the hypertrophic effect of IGF-1 but not of thyroid hormones in adult ventricular cardiomyocytes. Mol Cell Biochem 2000;206:113–124
20. Guo W, Kamiya K, Hojo M, Kodama I, Toyama J. Regulation of Kv4.2 and Kv1.4 K+ channel expression by myocardial hypertrophic factors in cultured newborn rat ventricular cells. J Mol Cell Cardiol 1998;30: 1449–1455
21. Schaub MC, Hefti MA, Harder BA, Eppenberger HM. Various hypertrophic stimuli induce distinct phenotypes in cardiomyocytes. J Mol Med 1997;75:901–920
22. Erusalimsky JD, Kurz DJ. Cellular senescence in vivo: its relevance in ageing and cardiovascular disease. Exp Gerontol 2005;40:634–642
23. Hampel B, Malisan F, Niederegger H, Testi R, Jansen-Durr P. Differential regulation of apoptotic cell death in senescent human cells. Exp Gerontol 2004;39:1713–1721
24. Ruiz-Torres A, Gimeno A, Melon J, Mendez L, Munoz FJ, Macia M. Age-related loss of proliferative activity of human vascular smooth muscle cells in culture. Mech Ageing Dev 1999;110:49–55
25. Moon SK, Thompson LJ, Madamanchi N, Ballinger S, Papaconstantinou J, Horaist C, Runge MS, Patterson C. Aging, oxidative responses, and proliferative capacity in cultured mouse aortic smooth muscle cells. Am J Physiol Heart Circ Physiol 2001;280:H2779–H2788
26. Camelliti P, Green CR, Kohl P. Structural and functional coupling of cardiac myocytes and fibroblasts. Adv Cardiol 2006;42:132–149
27. Eisenberg LM, Eisenberg CA. Embryonic myocardium shows increased longevity as a functional tissue when cultured in the presence of a noncardiac tissue layer. Tissue Eng 2006;12:853–865
28. Sumbilla C, Ma H, Seth M, Inesi G. Dependence of exogenous SERCA gene expression on coxsackie adenovirus receptor levels in neonatal and adult cardiac myocytes. Arch Biochem Biophys 2003;415:178–183
29. Communal C, Huq F, Lebeche D, Mestel C, Gwathmey JK, Hajjar RJ. Decreased efficiency of adenovirus-mediated gene transfer in aging cardiomyocytes. Circulation 2003;107:1170–1175
30. Michele DE, Szatkowski ML, Albayya FP, Metzger JM. Parvalbumin gene delivery improves diastolic function in the aged myocardium in vivo. Mol Ther 2004;10:399–403
31. Huq F, Lebeche D, Iyer V, Liao R, Hajjar RJ. Gene transfer of parvalbumin improves diastolic dysfunction in senescent myocytes. Circulation 2004;109:2780–2785
32. Schmidt U, Zhu X, Lebeche D, Huq F, Guerrero JL, Hajjar RJ. In vivo gene transfer of parvalbumin improves diastolic function in aged rat hearts. Cardiovasc Res 2005;66:318–323
33. Brown KA, Chu Y, Lund DD, Heistad DD, Faraci FM. Gene transfer of extracellular superoxide dismutase protects against vascular dysfunction with aging. Am J Physiol Heart Circ Physiol 2006;290:H2600–H2605
34. van der Veer E, Ho C, O'Neil C, Barbosa N, Scott R, Cregan SP, Pickering JG. Extension of human cell lifespan by nicotinamide phosphoribosyltransferase. J Biol Chem 2007 Feb 16; [Epub ahead of print]
35. Guo KK, Ren J. Cardiac overexpression of alcohol dehydrogenase (ADH) alleviates aging-associated cardiomyocyte contractile dysfunction: role of intracellular Ca^{2+} cycling proteins. Aging Cell 2006;5:259–265
36. Yang X, Doser TA, Fang CX, Nunn JM, Janardhanan R, Zhu M, Sreejayan N, Quinn MT, Ren J. Metallothionein prolongs survival and antagonizes senescence-associated cardiomyocyte diastolic dysfunction: role of oxidative stress. FASEB J 2006;20:1024–1026
37. Schmidt U, del Monte F, Miyamoto MI, Matsui T, Gwathmey JK, Rosenzweig A, Hajjar RJ. Restoration of diastolic function in senescent rat hearts through adenoviral gene transfer of sarcoplasmic reticulum Ca^{2+}-ATPase. Circulation 2000;101:790–796
38. Wang H, Keiser JA, Olszewski B, Rosebury W, Robertson A, Kovesdi I, Gordon D. Delayed angiogenesis in aging rats and therapeutic effect of adenoviral gene transfer of VEGF. Int J Mol Med 2004;13: 581–587
39. Sato Y, Schmidt AG, Kiriazis H, Hoit BD, Kranias EG. Compensated hypertrophy of cardiac ventricles in aged transgenic FVB/N mice overexpressing calsequestrin. Mol Cell Biochem 2003;242:19–25
40. Schriner SE, Linford NJ, Martin GM, Treuting P, Ogburn CE, Emond M, Coskun PE, Ladiges W, Wolf N, Van Remmen H, Wallace DC, Rabinovitch PS. Extension of murine life span by overexpression of catalase targeted to mitochondria. Science 2005;308:1909–1911
41. Torella D, Rota M, Nurzynska D, Musso E, Monsen A, Shiraishi I, Zias E, Walsh K, Rosenzweig A, Sussman MA, Urbanek K, Nadal-Ginard B, Kajstura J, Anversa P, Leri A. Cardiac stem cell and myocyte aging, heart failure, and insulin-like growth factor-1 overexpression. Circ Res 2004;94:514–524

42. Mitsui A, Hamuro J, Nakamura H, Kondo N, Hirabayashi Y, Ishizaki-Koizumi S, Hirakawa T, Inoue T, Yodoi J. Overexpression of human thioredoxin in transgenic mice controls oxidative stress and life span. Antioxid Redox Signal 2002;4:693–696
43. Headrick JP, Willems L, Ashton KJ, Holmgren K, Peart J, Matherne GP. Ischaemic tolerance in aged mouse myocardium: the role of adenosine and effects of A1 adenosine receptor overexpression. J Physiol 2003;549:823–833
44. Migliaccio E, Giorgio M, Mele S, Pelicci G, Reboldi P, Pandolfi PP, Lanfrancone L, Pelicci PG. The p66shc adaptor protein controls oxidative stress response and life span in mammals. Nature 1999;402:309–313
45. Graiani G, Lagrasta C, Migliaccio E, Spillmann F, Meloni M, Madeddu P, Quaini F, Padura IM, Lanfrancone L, Pelicci P, Emanueli C. Genetic deletion of the p66Shc adaptor protein protects from angiotensin II-induced myocardial damage Hypertension 2005;46:433–440
46. Rota M, LeCapitaine N, Hosoda T, Boni A, De Angelis A, Padin-Iruegas ME, Esposito G, Vitale S, Urbanek K, Casarsa C, Giorgio M, Luscher TF, Pelicci PG, Anversa P, Leri A, Kajstura J. Diabetes promotes cardiac stem cell aging and heart failure, which are prevented by deletion of the p66shc gene. Circ Res 2006;99:42–52
47. Li W, Mital S, Ojaimi C, Csiszar A, Kaley G, Hintze TH. Premature death and age-related cardiac dysfunction in male eNOS-knockout mice. J Mol Cell Cardiol 2004;37:671–680
48. Howroyd P, Swanson C, Dunn C, Cattley RC, Corton JC. Decreased longevity and enhancement of age-dependent lesions in mice lacking the nuclear receptor peroxisome proliferator-activated receptor alpha (PPAR-alpha). Toxicol Pathol 2004;32:591–599
49. Watanabe K, Fujii H, Takahashi T, Kodama M, Aizawa Y, Ohta Y, Ono T, Hasegawa G, Naito M, Nakajima T, Kamijo Y, Gonzalez FJ, Aoyama T. Constitutive regulation of cardiac fatty acid metabolism through peroxisome proliferator-activated receptor alpha associated with age-dependent cardiac toxicity. J Biol Chem 2000;275:22293–22299
50. Park DS, Cohen AW, Frank PG, Razani B, Lee H, Williams TM, Chandra M, Shirani J, De Souza AP, Tang B, Jelicks LA, Factor SM, Weiss LM, Tanowitz HB, Lisanti MP. Caveolin-1 null (-/-) mice show dramatic reductions in life span. Biochemistry 2003;42:15124–15131
51. Takeshita K, Fujimori T, Kurotaki Y, Honjo H, Tsujikawa H, Yasui K, Lee JK, Kamiya K, Kitaichi K, Yamamoto K, Ito M, Kondo T, Iino S, Inden Y, Hirai M, Murohara T, Kodama I, Nabeshima Y. Sinoatrial node dysfunction and early unexpected death of mice with a defect of klotho gene expression. Circulation 2004;109:1776–1782
52. Danik SB, Liu F, Zhang J, Suk HJ, Morley GE, Fishman GI, Gutstein DE. Modulation of cardiac gap junction expression and arrhythmic susceptibility. Circ Res 2004;95:1035–1041
53. Samuel CS, Zhao C, Bathgate RA, DU XJ, Summers RJ, Amento EP, Walker LL, McBurnie M, Zhao L, Tregear GW. The relaxin gene-knockout mouse: a model of progressive fibrosis. Ann NY Acad Sci 2005;1041:173–181
54. Jacoby JJ, Kalinowski A, Liu MG, Zhang SS, Gao Q, Chai GX, Ji L, Iwamoto Y, Li E, Schneider M, Russell KS, Fu XY. Cardiomyocyte-restricted knockout of STAT3 results in higher sensitivity to inflammation, cardiac fibrosis, and heart failure with advanced age. Proc Natl Acad Sci USA 2003;100:12929–12934
55. Lee CK, Allison DB, Brand J, Weindruch R, Prolla TA. Transcriptional profiles associated with aging and middle age-onset caloric restriction in mouse hearts. Proc Natl Acad Sci USA 2002;99:14988–14993
56. Park SK, Prolla TA. Gene expression profiling studies of aging in cardiac and skeletal muscles. Cardiovasc Res 2005;66:205–212
57. Dhahbi JM, Tsuchiya T, Kim HJ, Mote PL, Spindler SR. Gene expression and physiologic responses of the heart to the initiation and withdrawal of caloric restriction. J Gerontol A Biol Sci Med Sci 2006;61:218–231
58. Bodyak N, Kang PM, Hiromura M, Sulijoadikusumo I, Horikoshi N, Khrapko K. Gene expression profiling of the aging mouse cardiac myocytes. Nucleic Acids Res 2002;30:3788–3794
59. Lee CK, Klopp RG, Weindruch R, Prolla TA, Gene expression profile of aging and its retardation by caloric restriction. Science 1999;285:1390–1393
60. Kayo T, Allison DB, Weindruch R, Prolla TA. Influences of aging and caloric restriction on the transcriptional profile of skeletal muscle from rhesus monkeys. Proc Natl Acad Sci USA 2001;98:5093–5098
61. Welle S, Brooks AI, Delehanty JM, Needler N, Thornton CA. Gene expression profile of aging in human muscle. Physiol Genomics 2003;14:149–159
62. McCarroll SA, Murphy CT, Zou S, Pletcher SD, Chin CS, Jan YN, Kenyon C, Bargmann CI, Li H. Comparing genomic expression patterns across species identifies shared transcriptional profile in aging. Nat Genet 2004;36:197–204
63. Machida S, Booth FW. Increased nuclear proteins in muscle satellite cells in aged animals as compared to young growing animals. Exp Gerontol 2004;39:1521–1525
64. Welle S, Brooks AI, Delehanty JM, Needler N, Bhatt K, Shah B, Thornton CA. Skeletal muscle gene expression profiles in 20–29 year old and 65–71 year old women. Exp Gerontol 2004;39:369–377

65. de Oliveira RM. Klotho RNAi induces premature senescence of human cells via a p53/p21 dependent pathway. FEBS Lett 2006 Sep 27; [Epub ahead of print]
66. Horky M, Kuchtickova S, Vojtesek B, Kolar F. Induction of cell-cycle inhibitor p21 in rat ventricular myocytes during early postnatal transition from hyperplasia to hypertrophy. Physiol Res 1997;46:233–235
67. Hwang JJ, Allen PD, Tseng GC, Lam CW, Fananapazir L, Dzau VJ, Liew CC. Microarray gene expression profiles in dilated and hypertrophic cardiomyopathic end-stage heart failure. Physiol Genomics 2002;10: 31–44
68. Stanton LW, Garrard LJ, Damm D, Garrick BL, Lam A, Kapoun AM, Zheng Q, Protter AA, Schreiner GF, White RT. Altered patterns of gene expression in response to myocardial infarction. Circ Res 2000:86:939–945
69. Archacki SR, Angheloiu G, Tian XL, Tan FL, DiPaola N, Shen GQ, Moravec C, Ellis S, Topol EJ, Wang Q. Identification of new genes differentially expressed in coronary artery disease by expression profiling. Physiol Genomics 2003;15:65–74
70. Kim YH, Lim do S, Lee JH, Shim WJ, Ro YM, Park GH, Becker KG, Cho-Chung YS, Kim MK. Gene expression profiling of oxidative stress on atrial fibrillation in humans. Exp Mol Med 2003;35:336–349
71. Ueno S, Ohki R, Hashimoto T, Takizawa T, Takeuchi K, Yamashita Y, Ota J, Choi YL, Wada T, Koinuma K, Yamamoto K, Ikeda U, Shimada K, Mano H. DNA microarray analysis of in vivo progression mechanism of heart failure. Biochem Biophys Res Commun 2003;307:771–777
72. Vazquez-Padron RI, Lasko D, Li S, Louis L, Pestana IA, Pang M, Liotta C, Fornoni A, Aitouche A, Pham SM. Aging exacerbates neointimal formation, and increases proliferation and reduces susceptibility to apoptosis of vascular smooth muscle cells in mice. J Vasc Surg 2004;40:1199–1207
73. Csiszar A, Ungvari Z, Koller A, Edwards JG, Kaley G. Proinflammatory phenotype of coronary arteries promotes endothelial apoptosis in aging. Physiol Genomics 2004;17:21–30
74. Ishihata A, Katano Y. Investigation of differentially expressed genes in the ventricular myocardium of senescent rats. Ann NY Acad Sci 2006;1067:142–151
75. McGregor E, Dunn MJ. Proteomics of the heart: unraveling disease. Circ Res 2006;98:309–321
76. Fu Q, Van Eyk JE. Proteomics and heart disease: identifying biomarkers of clinical utility. Expert Rev Proteomics 2006;3:237–249
77. Westbrook JA, Wheeler JX, Wait R, Welson SY, Dunn MJ. The human heart proteome: Two-dimensional maps using narrow-range immobilised pH gradients. Electrophoresis 2006;27:1547–1555
78. Yan L, Ge H, Li H, Lieber SC, Natividad F, Resuello RR, Kim SJ, Akeju S, Sun A, Loo K, Peppas AP, Rossi F, Lewandowski ED, Thomas AP, Vatner SF, Vatner DE. Gender-specific proteomic alterations in glycolytic and mitochondrial pathways in aging monkey hearts. J Mol Cell Cardiol 2004;37:921–929
79. Lal SP, Christopherson RI, dos Remedios CG. Antibody arrays: an embryonic but rapidly growing technology. Drug Discov Today 2002;7:S143–S149
80. Kiri AN, Tran HC, Drahos KL, Lan W, McRorie DK, Horn MJ. Proteomic changes in bovine heart mitochondria with age: using a novel technique for organelle separation and enrichment. J Biomol Tech 2005;16: 371–379
81. Drahos KL, Tran HC, Kiri AN, Lan W, McRorie DK, Horn MJ. Comparison of Golgi apparatus and endoplasmic reticulum proteins from livers of juvenile and aged rats using a novel technique for separation and enrichment of organelles. J Biomol Tech 2005;16:347–355
82. Kanski J, Behring A, Pelling J, Schoneich C. Proteomic identification of 3-nitrotyrosine-containing rat cardiac proteins: effects of biological aging. Am J Physiol Heart Circ Physiol 2005;288:H371–H381
83. Soreghan BA, Yang F, Thomas SN, Hsu J, Yang AJ. High-throughput proteomic-based identification of oxidatively induced protein carbonylation in mouse brain. Pharm Res 2003;20:1713–1720
84. Kamino H, Hiratsuka M, Toda T, Nishigaki R, Osaki M, Ito H, Inoue T, Oshimura M. Searching for genes involved in arteriosclerosis: proteomic analysis of cultured human umbilical vein endothelial cells undergoing replicative senescence. Cell Struct Funct 2003;28:495–503
85. Cremona O, Muda M, Appel RD, Frutiger S, Hughes GJ, Hochstrasser DF, Geinoz A, Gabbiani G. Differential protein expression in aortic smooth muscle cells cultured from newborn and aged rats. Exp Cell Res 1995;217:280–287
86. Mayr M, Siow R, Chung YL, Mayr U, Griffiths JR, Xu Q. Proteomic and metabolomic analysis of vascular smooth muscle cells: role of PKCdelta. Circ Res 2004;94:e87–e96
87. Mayr M, Chung YL, Mayr U, McGregor E, Troy H, Baier G, Leitges M, Dunn MJ, Griffiths JR, Xu Q. Loss of PKC-delta alters cardiac metabolism. Am J Physiol Heart Circ Physiol 2004;287:H937–H945
88. Weber JL, May PE. Abundant class of human DNA polymorphisms which can be typed using the polymerase chain reaction. Am J Hum Genet 1989;44:388–396
89. Ben Yehuda A, Globerson A, Krichevsky S, Bar On H, Kidron M, Friedlander Y, Friedman G, Ben Yehuda D. Ageing and the mismatch repair system. Mech Ageing Dev 2000;121:173–179
90. Coolbaugh-Murphy MI, Xu J, Ramagli LS, Brown BW, Siciliano MJ. Microsatellite instability (MSI) increases with age in normal somatic cells. Mech Ageing Dev 2005;126:1051–1059

91. Murakami M, Hirokawa H, Hayata I. Analysis of radiation damage of DNA by atomic force microscopy in comparison with agarose gel electrophoresis studies. J Biochem Biophys Methods 2000;44:31–40
92. Schroder HC, Batel R, Schwertner H, Boreiko O, Muller WE. Fast micromethod DNA single-strand-break assay. Methods Mol Biol 2006;314:287–305
93. Longo JA, Nevaldine B, Longo SL, Winfield JA, Hahn PJ. An assay for quantifying DNA double-strand break repair that is suitable for small numbers of unlabeled cells. Radiat Res 1997;147:35–40
94. Speit G, Hartmann A. The comet assay: a sensitive genotoxicity test for the detection of DNA damage. Methods Mol Biol 2005;291:85–95
95. Yasuhara S, Zhu Y, Matsui T, Tipirneni N, Yasuhara Y, Kaneki M, Rosenzweig A, Martyn JA. Comparison of comet assay, electron microscopy, and flow cytometry for detection of apoptosis. J Histochem Cytochem 2003;51:873–885
96. Gavrilov B, Vezhenkova I, Firsanov D, Solovjeva L, Svetlova M, Mikhailov V, Tomilin N. Slow elimination of phosphorylated histone gamma-H2AX from DNA of terminally differentiated mouse heart cells in situ. Biochem Biophys Res Commun 2006;347:1048–1052
97. Corbucci GG, Perrino C, Donato G, Ricchi A, Lettieri B, Troncone G, Indolfi C, Chiariello M, Avvedimento EV. Transient and reversible deoxyribonucleic acid damage in human left ventricle under controlled ischemia and reperfusion. J Am Coll Cardiol 2004;43:1992–1999
98. Leppard JB, Dong Z, Mackey ZB, Tomkinson AE. Physical and functional interaction between DNA ligase IIIalpha and poly(ADP-Ribose) polymerase 1 in DNA single-strand break repair. Mol Cell Biol 2003;23: 5919–5927
99. Nakamura J, Asakura S, Hester SD, de Murcia G, Caldecott KW, Swenberg JA. Quantitation of intracellular NAD(P)H can monitor an imbalance of DNA single strand break repair in base excision repair deficient cells in real time. Nucleic Acids Res 2003;31:e104
100. Parsons JL, Dianova II, Allinson SL, Dianov GL. Poly(ADP-ribose) polymerase-1 protects excessive DNA strand breaks from deterioration during repair in human cell extracts. FEBS J 2005;272: 2012–2021
101. Grube K, Burkle A. Poly(ADP-ribose) polymerase activity in mononuclear leukocytes of 13 mammalian species correlates with species-specific life span. Proc Natl Acad Sci USA 1992;89:11759–11763
102. Thorslund T, von Kobbe C, Harrigan JA, Indig FE, Christiansen M, Stevnsner T, Bohr VA. Cooperation of the Cockayne syndrome group B protein and poly(ADP-ribose) polymerase 1 in the response to oxidative stress. Mol Cell Biol 2005;25:7625–7636
103. von Kobbe C, Harrigan JA, May A, Opresko PL, Dawut L, Cheng WH, Bohr VA. Central role for the Werner syndrome protein/poly(ADP-ribose) polymerase 1 complex in the poly(ADP-ribosyl)ation pathway after DNA damage. Mol Cell Biol 2003;23:8601–8613
104. Burkle A, Diefenbach J, Brabeck C, Beneke S. Ageing and PARP. Pharmacol Res 2005;52:93–99
105. Virág L, Szabó C. The therapeutic potential of poly(ADP-ribose) polymerase inhibitors. Pharmacol Rev 2002;54:375–429
106. Pacher P, Cziraki A, Mabley JG, Liaudet L, Papp L, Szabo C. Role of poly(ADP-ribose) polymerase activation in endotoxin-induced cardiac collapse in rodents. Biochem Pharmacol. 2002;64:1785–1791
107. Thiemermann C, Bowes J, Myint FP, Vane JR. Inhibition of the activity of poly(ADP ribose) synthetase reduces ischemia-reperfusion injury in the heart and skeletal muscle. Proc Natl Acad Sci USA 1997;94: 679–683
108. Pieper AA, Walles T, Wei G, Clements EE, Verma A, Snyder SH, Zweier JL. Myocardial postischemic injury is reduced by polyADPribose polymerase-1 gene disruption. Mol Med 2000;6:271–282
109. Burkart V, Wang ZQ, Radons J, Heller B, Herceg Z, Stingl L, Wagner EF, Kolb H. Mice lacking the poly(ADP-ribose) polymerase gene are resistant to pancreatic beta-cell destruction and diabetes development induced by streptozotocin. Nat Med 1999;5:314–319
110. Murthy KG, Xiao CY, Mabley JG, Chen M, Szabo C. Activation of poly(ADP-ribose) polymerase in circulating leukocytes during myocardial infarction. Shock 2004;21:230–234
111. Pacher P, Liaudet L, Mabley J, Komjati K, Szabo C. Pharmacologic inhibition of poly(adenosine diphosphate-ribose) polymerase may represent a novel therapeutic approach in chronic heart failure. J Am Coll Cardiol 2002;40:1006–1016
112. Pacher P, Vaslin A, Benko R, Mabley JG, Liaudet L, Hasko G, Marton A, Batkai S, Kollai M, Szabo C. A new, potent poly(ADP-ribose) polymerase inhibitor improves cardiac and vascular dysfunction associated with advanced aging. J Pharmacol Exp Ther 2004;311:485–491
113. Schawalder J, Paric E, Neff NF. Telomere and ribosomal DNA repeats are chromosomal targets of the bloom syndrome DNA helicase. BMC Cell Biol 2003;4:15
114. Barnett YA, Barnett CR. DNA damage and mutation: contributors to the age-related alterations in T cell-mediated immune responses? Mech Ageing Dev 1998;102:165–175
115. Grist SA, McCarron M, Kutlaca A, Turner DR, Morley AA. In vivo human somatic mutation: frequency and spectrum with age. Mutat Res 1992;266:189–196

116. Vijg J, Busuttil RA, Bahar R, Dolle ME. Aging and genome maintenance. Ann NY Acad Sci 2005;1055:35–47
117. Dolle ME, Vijg J. Genome dynamics in aging mice. Genome Res 2002;12:1732–1738
118. Vijg J, Dolle ME. Large genome rearrangements as a primary cause of aging. Mech Ageing Dev 2002;123: 907–915
119. Dolle ME, Snyder WK, Gossen JA, Lohman PH, Vijg J. Distinct spectra of somatic mutations accumulated with age in mouse heart and small intestine. Proc Natl Acad Sci USA 2000;97:8403–8408
120. Bahar R, Hartmann CH, Rodriguez KA, Denny AD, Busuttil RA, Dolle ME, Calder RB, Chisholm GB, Pollock BH, Klein CA, Vijg J. Increased cell-to-cell variation in gene expression in ageing mouse heart. Nature 2006;441:1011–1014
121. Maitra A, Cohen Y, Gillespie SE, Mambo E, Fukushima N, Hoque MO, Shah N, Goggins M, Califano J, Sidransky D, Chakravarti A. The Human MitoChip: a high-throughput sequencing microarray for mitochondrial mutation detection. Genome Res 2004;14:812–819
122. Zhou S, Kassauei K, Cutler DJ, Kennedy GC, Sidransky D, Maitra A, Califano J. An oligonucleotide microarray for high-throughput sequencing of the mitochondrial genome. J Mol Diagn 2006;8:476–482
123. Khaidakov M, Heflich RH, Manjanatha MG, Myers MB, Aidoo A. Accumulation of point mutations in mitochondrial DNA of aging mice. Mutat Res 2003;526:1–7
124. Michikawa Y, Mazzucchelli F, Bresolin N, Scarlato G, Attardi G. Aging-dependent large accumulation of point mutations in the human mtDNA control region for replication. Science 1999;286:774–779
125. Wang Y, Michikawa Y, Mallidis C, Bai Y, Woodhouse L, Yarasheski KE, Miller CA, Askanas V, Engel WK, Bhasin S, Attardi G. Muscle-specific mutations accumulate with aging in critical human mtDNA control sites for replication. Proc Natl Acad Sci USA 2001;98:4022–4027
126. Zhang J, Asin-Cayuela J, Fish J, Michikawa Y, Bonafe M, Olivieri F, Passarino G, De Benedictis G, Franceschi C, Attardi G. Strikingly higher frequency in centenarians and twins of mtDNA mutation causing remodeling of replication origin in leukocytes. Proc Natl Acad Sci USA 2003;100:1116–1121
127. Bai RK, Wong LJ. Detection and quantification of heteroplasmic mutant mitochondrial DNA by real-time amplification refractory mutation system quantitative PCR analysis: a single-step approach. Clin Chem 2004;50: 996–1001
128. Mohamed SA, Hanke T, Erasmi AW, Bechtel MJ, Scharfschwerdt M, Meissner C, Sievers HH, Gosslau A. Mitochondrial DNA deletions and the aging heart. Exp Gerontol 2006;41:508–517
129. He L, Chinnery PF, Durham SE, Blakely EL, Wardell TM, Borthwick GM, Taylor RW, Turnbull DM. Detection and quantification of mitochondrial DNA deletions in individual cells by real-time PCR. Nucleic Acids Res 2002;30:e68
130. Masuyama M, Iida R, Takatsuka H, Yasuda T, Matsuki T. Quantitative change in mitochondrial DNA content in various mouse tissues during aging. Biochim Biophys Acta 2005;1723:302–308
131. Londono-Vallejo JA, DerSarkissian H, Cazes L, Thomas G. Differences in telomere length between homologous chromosomes in humans. Nucleic Acids Res 2001;29:3164–3171
132. de Lange T, Shiue L, Myers RM, Cox DR, Naylor SL, Killery AM, Varmus HE. Structure and variability of human chromosome ends. Mol Cell Biol 1990;10:518–527
133. Engelhardt M, Kumar R, Albanell J, Pettengell R, Han W, Moore MA. Telomerase regulation, cell cycle, and telomere stability in primitive hematopoietic cells. Blood 1997;90:182–193
134. Lin KW, Yan J. The telomere length dynamic and methods of its assessment. J Cell Mol Med 2005;9:977–989
135. Allshire RC, Dempster M, Hastie ND. Human telomeres contain at least three types of G-rich repeat distributed non-randomly. Nucleic Acids Res 1989;17:4611–4627
136. Norwood D, Dimitrov DS. Sensitive method for measuring telomere lengths by quantifying telomeric DNA content of whole cells. Biotechniques 1998;25:1040–1045
137. Nakamura Y, Hirose M, Matsuo H, Tsuyama N, Kamisango K, Ide T. Simple, rapid, quantitative, and sensitive detection of telomere repeats in cell lysate by a hybridization protection assay. Clin Chem 1999;45: 1718–1724
138. Hultdin M, Gronlund E, Norrback K, Eriksson-Lindstrom E, Just T, Roos G. Telomere analysis by fluorescence in situ hybridization and flow cytometry. Nucleic Acids Res 1998;26:3651–3656
139. Cawthon RM. Telomere measurement by quantitative PCR. Nucleic Acids Res 2002;30:e47
140. Baird DM, Rowson J, Wynford-Thomas D, Kipling D. Extensive allelic variation and ultrashort telomeres in senescent human cells. Nat Genet 2003;33:203–207
141. Huffman KE, Levene SD, Tesmer VM, Shay JW, Wright WE. Telomere shortening is proportional to the size of the G-rich telomeric 3′-overhang. J Biol Chem 2000;275:19719–19722
142. Cimino-Reale G, Pascale E, Battiloro E, Starace G, Verna R, D'Ambrosio E. The length of telomeric G-rich strand 3'-overhang measured by oligonucleotide ligation assay. Nucleic Acids Res 2001;29:E35
143. Yan J, Chen BZ, Bouchard EF, Drouin R. The labeling efficiency of human telomeres is increased by double-strand PRINS. Chromosoma 2004;113:204–209

144. Therkelsen AJ, Nielsen A, Koch J, Hindkjaer J, Kolvraa S. Staining of human telomeres with primed in situ labeling (PRINS). Cytogenet Cell Genet 1995;68:115–118
145. Reinecke H, Zhang M, Bartosek T, Murry CE. Survival, integration, and differentiation of cardiomyocyte grafts: a study in normal and injured rat hearts. Circulation 1999;100:193–202
146. Etzion S, Battler A, Barbash IM, Cagnano E, Zarin P, Granot Y, Kedes LH, Kloner RA, Leor J. Influence of embryonic cardiomyocyte transplantation on the progression of heart failure in a rat model of extensive myocardial infarction. J Mol Cell Cardiol 2001;33:1321–1330
147. Zhang M, Methot D, Poppa V, Fujio Y, Walsh K, Murry CE. Cardiomyocyte grafting for cardiac repair: graft cell death and anti-death strategies. J Mol Cell Cardiol 2001;33:907–921
148. Kehat I, Khimovich L, Caspi O, Gepstein A, Shofti R, Arbel G, Huber I, Satin J, Itskovitz-Eldor J, Gepstein L. Electromechanical integration of cardiomyocytes derived from human embryonic stem cells. Nat Biotechnol 2004;22:1237–1238
149. Doetschman T, Shull M, Kier A, Coffin JD. Embryonic stem cell model systems for vascular morphogenesis and cardiac disorders. Hypertension 1993;22:618–629
150. He JQ, Ma Y, Lee Y, Thomson JA, Kamp TJ. Human embryonic stem cells develop into multiple types of cardiac myocytes: action potential characterization. Circ Res 2003;93:32–39
151. Muller M, Fleischmann BK, Selbert S, Ji GJ, Endl E, Middeler G, Muller OJ, Schlenke P, Frese S, Wobus AM, Hescheler J, Katus HA, Franz WM. Selection of ventricular-like cardiomyocytes from ES cells in vitro. FASEB J 2000;14:2540–2548
152. Wobus AM, Boheler KR. Embryonic stem cells: prospects for developmental biology and cell therapy. Physiol Rev 2005;85:635–678
153. Min JY, Chen Y, Malek S, Meissner A, Xiang M, Ke Q, Feng X, Nakayama M, Kaplan E, Morgan JP. Stem cell therapy in the aging hearts of Fisher 344 rats: synergistic effects on myogenesis and angiogenesis. J Thorac Cardiovasc Surg 2005;130:547–553
154. Kessler PD, Byrne BJ. Myoblast cell grafting into heart muscle: cellular biology and potential applications. Annu Rev Physiol 1999;61:219–42
155. Menasche P. Cell transplantation for the treatment of heart failure. Semin Thorac Cardiovasc Surg 2002;14: 157–66
156. Leobon B, Garcin I, Menasche P, Vilquin JT, Audinat E, Charpak S. Myoblasts transplanted into rat infarcted myocardium are functionally isolated from their host. Proc Natl Acad Sci USA 2003;100:7808–7811
157. Menasche P, Hagege AA, Vilquin JT, Desnos M, Abergel E, Pouzet B, Bel A, Sarateanu S, Scorsin M, Schwartz K, Bruneval P, Benbunan M, Marolleau JP, Duboc D. Autologous skeletal myoblast transplantation for severe postinfarction left ventricular dysfunction. J Am Coll Cardiol 2003;41:1078–1083
158. Orlic D, Kajstura J, Chimenti S, Limana F, Jakoniuk I, Quaini F, Nadal-Ginard B, Bodine DM, Leri A, Anversa P. Mobilized bone marrow cells repair the infarcted heart, improving function and survival. Proc Natl Acad Sci USA 2001;98:10344–10349
159. Orlic D, Kajstura J, Chimenti S, Jakoniuk I, Anderson SM, Li B, Pickel J, McKay R, Nadal-Ginard B, Bodine DM, Leri A, Anversa P. Bone marrow cells regenerate infarcted myocardium. Nature 2001;410:701–705
160. Orlic D, Hill JM, Arai AE. Stem cells for myocardial regeneration. Circ Res 2002;91:1092–1102
161. Wollert KC, Meyer GP, Lotz J, Ringes-Lichtenberg S, Lippolt P, Breidenbach C, Fichtner S, Korte T, Hornig B, Messinger D, Arseniev L, Hertenstein B, Ganser A, Drexler H. Intracoronary autologous bone-marrow cell transfer after myocardial infarction: the BOOST randomised controlled clinical trial. Lancet 2004;364:141–148
162. Lee MS, Makkar RR. Stem-cell transplantation in myocardial infarction: a status report. Ann Intern Med 2004;140:729–737
163. Strauer BE, Brehm M, Zeus T, Kostering M, Hernandez A, Sorg RV, Kogler G, Wernet P. Repair of infarcted myocardium by autologous intracoronary mononuclear bone marrow cell transplantation in humans. Circulation 2002;106:1913–1918
164. Badorff C, Brandes RP, Popp R, Rupp S, Urbich C, Aicher A, Fleming I, Busse R, Zeiher AM, Dimmeler S. Transdifferentiation of blood-derived human adult endothelial progenitor cells into functionally active cardiomyocytes. Circulation 2003;107:1024–1032
165. Toma C, Pittenger MF, Cahill KS, Byrne BJ, Kessler PD. Human mesenchymal stem cells differentiate to a cardiomyocyte phenotype in the adult murine heart. Circulation 2002;105:93–98
166. Kajstura J, Rota M, Whang B, Cascapera S, Hosoda T, Bearzi C, Nurzynska D, Kasahara H, Zias E, Bonafe M, Nadal-Ginard B, Torella D, Nascimbene A, Quaini F, Urbanek K, Leri A, Anversa P. Bone marrow cells differentiate in cardiac cell lineages after infarction independently of cell fusion. Circ Res 2005;96:127–137
167. Eisenberg CA, Burch JB, Eisenberg LM. Bone marrow cells transdifferentiate to cardiomyocytes when introduced into the embryonic heart. Stem Cells 2006 Jan 12; [Epub ahead of print]
168. Matsuura K, Wada H, Nagai T, Iijima Y, Minamino T, Sano M, Akazawa H, Molkentin JD, Kasanuki H, Komuro I. Cardiomyocytes fuse with surrounding noncardiomyocytes and reenter the cell cycle. J Cell Biol 2004;167:351–363

169. Murry CE, Field LJ, Menasche P. Cell-based cardiac repair: reflections at the 10year point. Circulation 2005;112: 3174–3183
170. Reinecke H, Minami E, Poppa V, Murry CE. Evidence for fusion between cardiac and skeletal muscle cells. Circ Res 2004;94:e56–e60
171. Murry CE, Soonpaa MH, Reinecke H, Nakajima H, Nakajima HO, Rubart M, Pasumarthi KB, Virag JI, Bartelmez SH, Poppa V, Bradford G, Dowell JD, Williams DA, Field LJ. Haematopoietic stem cells do not transdifferentiate into cardiac myocytes in myocardial infarcts. Nature 2004;428:664–668
172. Fazel S, Cimini M, Chen L, Li S, Angoulvant D, Fedak P, Verma S, Weisel RD, Keating A, Li RK. c-kit+ cells are from the bone marrow and regulate the myocardial balance of angiogenic cytokines. J Clin Invest 2006;116:1865–1877
173. Lehrke S, Mazhari R, Durand DJ, Zheng M, Bedja D, Zimmet JM, Schuleri KH, Chi AS, Gabrielson KL, Hare JM. Aging impairs the beneficial effect of granulocyte colony-stimulating factor and stem cell factor on post-myocardial infarction remodeling. Circ Res 2006;99:553–560
174. Potapova I, Plotnikov A, Lu Z, Danilo P Jr, Valiunas V, Qu J, Doronin S, Zuckerman J, Shlapakova IN, Gao J, Pan Z, Herron AJ, Robinson RB, Brink PR, Rosen MR, Cohen IS. Human mesenchymal stem cells as a gene delivery system to create cardiac pacemakers. Circ Res 2004;94:952–959
175. Beltrami AP, Barlucchi L, Torella D, Baker M, Limana F, Chimenti S, Kasahara H, Rota M, Musso E, Urbanek K, Leri A, Kajstura J, Nadal-Ginard B, Anversa P. Adult cardiac stem cells are multipotent and support myocardial regeneration. Cell 2003;114:763–776
176. Dawn B, Stein AB, Urbanek K, Rota M, Whang B, Rastaldo R, Torella D, Tang XL, Rezazadeh A, Kajstura J, Leri A, Hunt G, Varma J, Prabhu SD, Anversa P, Bolli R. Cardiac stem cells delivered intravascularly traverse the vessel barrier, regenerate infarcted myocardium, and improve cardiac function. Proc Natl Acad Sci USA 2005;102:3766–3771
177. Oh H, Chi X, Bradfute SB, Mishina Y, Pocius J, Michael LH, Behringer RR, Schwartz RJ, Entman ML, Schneider MD. Cardiac muscle plasticity in adult and embryo by heart-derived progenitor cells. Ann NY Acad Sci 2004;1015:182–189
178. Oh H, Bradfute SB, Gallardo TD, Nakamura T, Gaussin V, Mishina Y, Pocius J, Michael LH, Behringer RR, Garry DJ, Entman ML, Schneider MD. Cardiac progenitor cells from adult myocardium: homing, differentiation, and fusion after infarction. Proc Natl Acad Sci USA 2003;100:12313–12318
179. Matsuura K, Nagai T, Nishigaki N, Oyama T, Nishi J, Wada H, Sano M, Toko H, Akazawa H, Sato T, Nakaya H, Kasanuki H, Komuro I. Adult cardiac Sca-1-positive cells differentiate into beating cardiomyocytes. J Biol Chem 2004;279:11384–11391
180. Laugwitz KL, Moretti A, Lam J, Gruber P, Chen Y, Woodard S, Lin LZ, Cai CL, Lu MM, Reth M, Platoshyn O, Yuan JX, Evans S, Chien KR. Postnatal isl1+ cardioblasts enter fully differentiated cardiomyocyte lineages. Nature 2005;433:647–653
181. Messina E, De Angelis L, Frati G, Morrone S, Chimenti S, Fiordaliso F, Salio M, Battaglia M, Latronico MV, Coletta M, Vivarelli E, Frati L, Cossu G, Giacomello A. Isolation and expansion of adult cardiac stem cells from human and murine heart. Circ Res 2004;95:911–921
182. Gude N, Muraski J, Rubio M, Kajstura J, Schaefer E, Anversa P, Sussman MA. Akt promotes increased cardiomyocyte cycling and expansion of the cardiac progenitor cell population. Circ Res 2006;99:381–388
183. Chimenti C, Kajstura J, Torella D, Urbanek K, Heleniak H, Colussi C, Di Meglio F, Nadal-Ginard B, Frustaci A, Leri A, Maseri A, Anversa P. Senescence and death of primitive cells and myocytes lead to premature cardiac aging and heart failure. Circ Res 2003;93:604–613
184. Anversa P, Kajstura J, Leri A, Bolli R. Life and death of cardiac stem cells: a paradigm shift in cardiac biology. Circulation 2006;113:1451–1463
185. Pedrotty DM, Koh J, Davis BH, Taylor DA, Wolf P, Niklason LE. Engineering skeletal myoblasts: roles of three-dimensional culture and electrical stimulation. Am J Physiol Heart Circ Physiol 2005;288:H1620–H1626
186. Wu X, Rabkin-Aikawa E, Guleserian KJ, Perry TE, Masuda Y, Sutherland FW, Schoen FJ, Mayer JE Jr, Bischoff J. Tissue-engineered microvessels on three-dimensional biodegradable scaffolds using human endothelial progenitor cells. Am J Physiol Heart Circ Physiol 2004;287:H480–H487
187. Shen G, Tsung HC, Wu CF, Liu XY, Wang XY, Liu W, Cui L, Cao YL. Tissue engineering of blood vessels with endothelial cells differentiated from mouse embryonic stem cells. Cell Res 2003;13:335–341
188. Taylor PM, Sachlos E, Dreger SA, Chester AH, Czernuszka JT, Yacoub MH. Interaction of human valve interstitial cells with collagen matrices manufactured using rapid prototyping. Biomaterials 2006;27:2733–2737
189. Knight RL, Booth C, Wilcox HE, Fisher J, Ingham E. Tissue engineering of cardiac valves: re-seeding of acellular porcine aortic valve matrices with human mesenchymal progenitor cells. J Heart Valve Dis 2005;14:806–813
190. Sutherland FWH, Perry TE, Yu Y, Sherwood MC, Rabkin E, Masuda Y, Garcia GA, McLellan DL, Engelmayr GC Jr, Sacks MS, Schoen FJ, Mayer JE Jr. From stem cells to viable autologous semilunar heart valve. Circulation 2005;111:2783–2791

Chapter 4
Molecular and Cellular Phenotypes of Cardiovascular Aging

Overview

Whereas in Chapter 2 we have presented a general overview of the cardiovascular changes associated with aging, in this chapter we will discuss more specifically the structural changes occurring in the aging heart, and the underlying mechanisms leading to myocardial dysfunction in both aging and diseased state. The molecular and subcellular changes underlying cardiac fibrosis and remodeling, including cell loss that are characteristic of the aging processes as well as age-mediated alterations in mitochondrial ETC, ROS production and accumulation, mtDNA damage, dysregulation of autophagy and cellular degradative mechanisms in lysosomes will be presented. In addition, aging-related nuclear changes, including altered telomere length and structural integrity, accumulated DNA damage and genomic instability, and changes in DNA maintenance and repair will be laid out.

Introduction: Morphological Changes in the Aging Heart

With advanced age, the heart and the vasculature undergo subtle but progressive changes resulting in altered structure and function as depicted in Table 4.1. The endocardium becomes thicker and more opaque (most prominently in the left atria) and increasingly exhibits endocardial plaques. The myocardium develops increased thickness, mainly in the left ventricular wall, and the left atrium exhibits hypertrophy and increased interstitial fibrosis. There is a loss of cardiac myocytes as well as conduction cells, although remaining myocytes often increase in size. Increases in the levels of fat, collagen and elastic tissue with increased fibrosis are prevalent throughout the heart including muscle and conduction system, and are considered to be contributory (along with the cell loss) to cardiac dysfunction, increased incidence of dysrhythmias and conduction defects.

Amyloid deposition and calcification are also frequently found in the heart of elderly individuals. In subjects over 80 years of age, detectable levels of atrial amyloid were found in over 80% of the subjects [1]. Moreover, amyloid restrictive cardiomyopathy is primarily found in elderly patients, and senile systemic amyloidosis contributes to both infiltrative cardiomyopathy and heart failure (HF) in individuals over 80 years old [2].

Calcification involving the AV conduction system and valves is seen in most elderly individuals and may predispose to the common dysrhythmias of old age. Mitral annular calcification, aortic annular calcification, and aortic valve sclerosis are often present in aging human [3]. There is evidence that aortic valve and coronary artery calcification are neither random nor passive degenerative processes but rather active highly-regulated processes similar to calcification in bone associated with the acquisition of cells, either osteoblast-like or chrondoblast phenotypes [4–7]. The mechanism of these phenotypic changes, including the multiple physiological stimuli (e.g., inflammation, shear, oxidative stress [OS], and hyperphosphatemia), morphogens and signaling factors (e.g., bone

J. Marín-García, *Aging and the Heart*,

Table 4.1 Structural and functional changes in the aging heart

Structural changes	Functional changes
Increased LV wall thickness	Decreased early diastolic filling rate
Increased endocardial plaque	Increased late diastolic rate
Thicker and more opaque endocardium	Decreased maximum achievable heart rate
Increased left atrial hypertrophy	Diminished β-adrenergic contractile response
Increased interstitial fibrosis in myocardium and pericardium	Prolonged contraction
Decreased number of myocytes	Increased action potential
Increased size of myocytes	Reduced acute response to stress
Increased amyloid deposition	Increased myocardial stiffness
Increased calcification in the AV and semilunar valves (mainly mitral and aortic valves), and coronary arteries	
Decreased cell number in the sinoatrial and AV nodes	

morphogenetic protein-2 [BMP] and BMP4 and Wnt) that promote calcification will be further examined in Chapter 6 when addressing vascular aging phenotypes.

Age-dependent degenerative changes in the myocyte revealed by ultrastructural analysis include lipid and lipofuscin deposition, and diminished levels of protein synthesis impacting the replacement of myocyte contractile proteins. Increased OS is associated with declining function of mitochondrial bioenergetic capacity and damage to a variety of myocyte macromolecules (e.g., DNA, protein and lipids). Changes in gene expression programming have been reported with age, which alter the myocyte responses to hemodynamic and neurohormonal stimuli as well as responses to insults and stresses.

Numerous studies in rodent models have shown that with aging changes in cardiac structure occur, including increase in LV mass (secondary to ventricular myocyte enlargement) and proliferation of the matrix (where the myocytes reside), which may be linked to alterations in cardiac fibroblast number or function. Reduction in the number of cardiac myocytes is related to necrosis or apoptosis [8]. Many of these changes are thought to be adaptive in response to arterial changes occurring with aging (described in Chapter 5) [9]. Stimuli that promote cardiac cell enlargement in aging rodents include an age-associated increase in vascular load (due largely to arterial stiffening) and stretching of cells caused by the death and loss of neighboring myocytes [10]. Stretching of cardiac myocytes and fibroblasts also initiates growth-factor-dependent signaling (by angiotensin II or TGF-β), and, in some cases, apoptosis [11].

Aging in humans is associated with structural and functional changes in cardiac muscle (Table 4.1), including increased myocyte size and decreased sensitivity to β-adrenergic stimulation [12]. In addition, there is a prolongation of cardiac contraction produced, at least in part, by an increase in the time course of the diastolic relaxation. A decrease in myocardial sarcoplasmic reticulum (SR) content, in particular in the sarcoplasmic reticulum Ca^{2+} ATPase (SERCA2), assessed by immunoblot, has been reported in humans [13] that in part contributes to the prolongation of contraction by slowing the post-contraction removal of Ca^{2+}. Studies in animal models including the Wistar and Fischer 344 rat indicate that the excitation-contraction coupling cycle is prolonged with aging [14, 15]. Except for the prolonged time course, the contraction characteristics, when normalized for cell length and sarcomere number in isolated unloaded ventricular myocytes contracting over a range of sarcomere lengths, do not change appreciably with age [15]. The decreases in relaxation capacity seen in these studies is likely to be due to prolonged Ca^{2+} transient produced by compromised SR function, due to either reduced SERCA content [16] or decreased SERCA activity [17, 18]. A pronounced age-associated reduction in transcription of the SERCA2 gene, coding for the SR Ca^{2+} pump, accounts in part for a decrease in the SR pump site density [19]. These observations also showed a shift in the myosin heavy chain (MHC) isoform in rats from α-MHC to the slower β-MHC, which is also expected to contribute to a prolongation of contraction.

Furthermore, coordinated changes in gene expression and in sarcolemmal ion channel function with aging result in prolonged action potential (AP), Ca^{2+} (i) transient, and contraction [20–22]. With advancing age, there are increases in the number and activity of cardiac L-type Ca^{2+} channels that inactivate more slowly, and reduction in outwardly-directed K^{+} currents, likely contributing to the AP-prolongation. This is further discussed in Chapter 11.

In this chapter, the cellular and molecular basis of the changes in cardiac structure occurring in aging will be presented, and in particular the events leading to apoptosis and remodeling, increases in aging-associated fibrosis and alteration of the extracellular matrix, defects in cardiac bioenergetic reserves and the generation of OS and its potent effect on molecules (e.g., DNA, proteins and lipids) of the aging cardiac cell.

Fibrosis

Aging-associated remodeling of the myocardium and pericardium are characterized by the development of fibrosis. In addition to the characteristic loss of the cardiomyocytes, which impact both heart geometry and pump function, aging affects fibroblasts, the heart's most prevalent cell-type whose major role is deposition of the extracellular matrix (ECM), of which collagen is the principal component. Histopathologic analysis of the aging human heart revealed a maladaptive remodeling of the interstitium, resulting in an increase in interstitial collagen content. Given the critical role of the ECM in maintaining the heart structural and functional integrity, and contributing to coordinated mechanical action, excessive collagen deposition or pathological fibrosis is an important factor in LV dysfunction and an important problem in the aging heart, in hypertension and HF. Significantly, interstitial fibrosis occurs in the aging heart independently of the clinical pathology and appears to be a primary correlate to the aging process [23].

The interstitium also plays a critical role in the generation of early diastolic dysfunction. Excessive increases in the volume of collagen and fibrinogen in the myocardium will increase the viscoelastic burden to the functioning heart, which can lead to increased diastolic pressure with ensuing LV diastolic dysfunction. Neurohumoral abnormalities associated with diastolic dysfunction include activation of the renin-angiotensin-aldosterone system with increased production of myocardial aldosterone, which plays a major role in the development of myocardial fibrosis [24].

Excessive accumulation of fibrillar collagen type I occurs in the aging heart where collagen fibers increase in both number and in thickness (as a result of increased intermolecular cross-linking of collagen which also increases with age) [25]. The mechanism responsible for elevated myocardial fibrosis and collagen deposition in the senescent myocardium is presently unknown, although it appear to involve a combination of responses to cardiomyocyte loss **(replacement fibrosis)** and an interstitial response to a variety of stimuli **(reactive fibrosis),** including some elicited by chronic cardiovascular diseases.

Activation of cardiac fibroblasts can be regulated by diverse autocrine and paracrine factors, such as angiotensin II, aldosterone, endothelins, cytokines, and growth factors [26]. The regulation of collagen biosynthesis can occur at pre-translational levels with regulatory elements involved in this process, including growth factors such as TGF-β, hormones and neurotransmitters [25]. Aging-dependent modulation of gene expression in cardiac fibroblasts is also likely to be modified by the activity of the cAMP-dependent signaling pathway, including the cAMP response element binding protein (CREB) [27].

In addition to collagen synthesis, other constituents of the ECM have recently been evaluated in aging mice [28]. Levels of specific matrix metalloproteinases (MMPs), including MMP-3, MMP-8, MMP-9, MMP-12, and MMP-14 were increased in aging, while specific tissue inhibitor of metalloproteinase (TIMPs) including TIMP-3 and TIMP-4 decreased in the insoluble fraction of old mice, suggesting increased ECM degradative capacity with age.

A deficiency in murine TIMP-3 may be sufficient to cause progressive maladaptive cardiac remodeling and dysfunction, similar to human HF. In a study examining TIMP-3 deficiency in aging, mice containing TIMP-3 deficiency developed a phenotype of spontaneous LV dilatation, cardiomyocyte hypertrophy, and contractile dysfunction at 21 months of age, similar to human dilated cardiomyopathy (DCM) not present in age-matched wild-type controls [29]. TIMP-3 absence also resulted in interstitial matrix disruption with elevated MMP-9 activity, and activation of tumor necrosis factor-α (TNF-α), a hallmark of human myocardial remodeling. The authors concluded that TIMP-3 deficiency appears to disrupt matrix homeostasis and the balance of inflammatory mediators, eliciting the transition to cardiac dilation and dysfunction. It is possible that therapeutic restoration of myocardial TIMP-3 may limit or reverse the cardiac remodeling and progressive failure that often develop in aging patients with DCM.

Another regulatory aspect of ECM that may be targeted in aging is the ECM binding to membrane-bound receptors, or integrins, which normally links ECM directly to cardiac muscle and fibroblast cells, allowing modulation of heart function. Advancing age was associated with not only greater levels of collagen and fibronectin protein in the left ventricle but also with marked increases of $\alpha 1$ and $\alpha 5$ integrin protein content coincident with lower levels of $\beta 1$ integrin content in senescent mice (compared to young or middle-aged animals) suggesting that these matrix proteins are coordinately regulated in the aging heart [30]. The differential modulation of integrin expression and ECM protein content also suggests a role for regulatory signaling to fibroblasts in maintaining cardiac ECM.

In addition to its effects on both myocardial stiffness and diastolic function, interstitial fibrosis reduces cardiomyocyte electrical coupling. Fibroblasts produce collagenous septa, which electrically insulate cardiac cells or muscle bundles thereby disrupting the normal myocardial substrate with multiple insulating barriers impeding the uniform spread of the depolarization wave [31]. Poor electrical coupling between cardiac myocytes and fibroblasts associated with slower impulse conduction has been demonstrated *in vitro* with cultured cells [32], and there has been considerable debate about its occurrence *in vivo* [33].

Furthermore, several studies using a variety of models have demonstrated that myocardial fibrosis can play an important role in the development of a substrate for reentrant dysrhythmias. Li et al. have found that atrial fibrosis was associated with an increase in heterogeneity of conduction and stability of atrial fibrillation (AF) in the canine model of pacing-induced congestive HF [34]. In addition, in atria of older dogs, progressive fibrosis with aging was correlated with an increased vulnerability to AF [35]. Similarly, heterogeneous atrial interstitial fibrosis (as well as increased atrial cell hypertrophy) were coincident with the aging-related increase in atrial conduction slowing, conduction block, and inducible AF in the 24 month old Fischer 344 rat [36].

Apoptosis (Programmed Cell Death), Necrosis and Myocardial Remodeling

The cardiac remodeling described in aging has been increasingly associated with extensive cell loss primarily attributed to the activity of two cell death processes, necrosis and apoptosis. Olivetti et al. [37] have estimated that nearly one-third of the cardiomyocytes are lost from the human heart between the ages of 17 and 90, a phenomenon that is strikingly more evident in males than females [38, 39].

Apoptosis can be initiated by several diverse pathways that possess overlapping or convergent elements. In one pathway, apoptosis represents the execution of an ATP-dependent death program primarily initiated by extracellular death ligand/death receptor interactions, such as Fas ligand with

Fas, which leads to a cysteine protease (caspase) activation cascade. Alternatively, in response to several proapoptotic signals, mitochondria release caspase-activating factors, that initiate an escalating caspase cascade and commit the cell to die. These proteases selectively cleave vital cellular substrates, which results in the onset of a characteristic apoptotic morphology including shrinkage of the cell, its fragmentation into membrane-bound apoptotic bodies and relatively rapid phagocytosis by neighboring cells as well as internucleosomal fragmentation of nuclear DNA by selectively activated DNAses [40]. The DNA fragmentation of apoptotic cells constitutes the basis of the apoptotic detection assay termed TUNEL (transferase-mediated dUTP nick end labeling). This assay while employed in a large number of studies has been more recently viewed as a limited apoptotic indicator since without rigorous handling procedures false-positives can arise from a variety of tissue fixation artifacts. In addition, both DNA repair and RNA synthesis/splicing events in living cells can contribute to a positive-TUNEL reaction in myocytes leading to the potential over-estimation of the incidence of apoptosis [41, 42]. The development of more specific assays of apoptosis based on analysis of DNA fragmentation (i.e., the DNA laddering technique) and the demonstration of caspase activation (e.g., the immunohistochemical detection of the activated form of caspase 3 using selective antibodies) have proved to be useful and reliable independent apoptotic markers, or at least complementary to TUNEL findings [43, 44]. In addition, gathered observations have exploited the finding that phosphatidylserine, normally found only on the inner leaflet of the cell membrane double layer, is actively transported to the outer layer as an early event in apoptosis and becomes available for annexin binding; hence, the externalization of phosphatidylserine (gauged using labeled annexin V) has been used to identify apoptotic cells [45]. It is noteworthy that appraisal of the extent of myocardial apoptosis is also limited by its relative short duration and the removal of most apoptotic cells by phagocytosis, rendering a single-point determination of apoptosis less informative. Cell death by autophagy (which often involves apoptotic pathways) will be discussed in a later section of this chapter.

Cell death by necrosis is typically the consequence of acute metabolic perturbations resulting in extensive ATP depletion, such as occurs in myocardial ischemia/reperfusion and acute drug-induced toxicity. Necrosis is a rapid and irreversible process that occurs when cells are severely damaged. Characteristic features include swelling of the cell and its organelles, extensive disruption of mitochondria, plasma membrane blebbing and rupture, and cell lysis [46]. Unlike apoptosis which as we shall shortly see is a highly-regulated and energy-dependent process, necrosis is passive and unregulated [47]. Also, in contrast to apoptosis, disruption of the plasma membrane in necrosis leads to the release of cellular content into the extracellular space (e.g., release of creatine kinase from necrotic myocardial cells) which further promotes inflammatory reactions and subsequent damage or death to neighboring cells. Plasma-membrane disruption underlies the basis of various necrosis detection assays involving the use of exclusion dyes or the deployment of large myosin-antibody both to detect and quantify necrosis. Many of the morphological differences between apoptotic and necrotic processes may result from the action of the caspases. Nevertheless, there is a rather fine line between apoptosis and necrosis which also complicates their discrimination. Honda et al have demonstrated that in the absence of phagocytic cells (to remove damaged apoptotic cells), disruption of the plasma membrane of the apoptotic cell can occur leading to secondary necrosis [45]. Recent observations have also demonstrated that the early phase of apoptosis and of some types of necrosis may involve common signaling events. For instance, a common event leading to both apoptosis and necrosis is mitochondrial permeabilization and dysfunction (i.e., both involve opening of the mitochondrial permeability transition [PT] pore), although the mechanistic basis of mitochondrial injury appears to vary in different settings [48]. Evidence has been presented that ATP levels are key factors determining which type of cell death will proceed [49–51]. If ATP levels fall profoundly, plasma membrane permeabilization and cell rupture ensue leading to necrosis. If ATP levels are partially maintained, apoptosis (which requires ATP for its progression) follows the opening of the PT pore. In neonatal rat cardiomyocytes subjected to hypoxia in conditions of glucose deprivation, ATP levels dropped precipitously and cell death occurred exclusively by necrosis [52]. However, when hypoxic cardiomyocytes were supplemented with increasing glucose concentrations, cellular ATP levels increased correspondingly, and apoptosis progressively replaced necrosis until it became the sole form of cell death, as determined by nuclear morphology, and caspase-3 activation. Hence ATP supplied by glycolysis is a critical determinant of the form of cell death in hypoxic cardiomyocytes.

Given the rather large number of caveats concerning the appraisal of apoptosis and its discrimination from other types of cell death, it is not entirely surprising that the actual burden of chronic cell loss attributable to apoptosis in aging (or in HF) remains unclear at this time despite the critical importance and potential relevance of myocardial cell death to cardiac function in aging. Measures of actual rates of myocardial apoptosis have been highly variable and dependent on species investigated, type of injury, timing, location, and method of assessment. Moreover, few studies have actually simultaneously gauged both forms of cell death in the aging and failing heart. In 24 month old Fischer 344 rats, cell loss due to cardiomyocyte necrosis occurred in both the LV free wall and the right ventricle and was over 10-fold greater than the cell loss due to myocyte apoptosis which was restricted to the LV [53]. Studies with catecholamine-induced cardiomyocyte death and HF have demonstrated a 4–10 fold increase in necrosis compared to myocyte apoptosis [54]. Understanding the mechanism of cell death may reveal important information about how the cell attrition rate might be attenuated or reversed in aging by attacking specific targets within these pathways.

When viewed in absolute terms, the rate of myocyte apoptosis at any given time is rather low, rarely exceeding 1% of examined cells, however, when viewed in the context of time, it is entirely plausible that the accumulative apoptotic burden could in fact be significant. Unfortunately, the timing of the apoptotic process is not well defined and the assessment of the true rates and their cumulative consequences remain speculative.

In general, apoptosis is mediated by two highly-regulated, evolutionarily conserved death pathways: The extrinsic pathway, which utilizes a number of cell surface death receptors; and the intrinsic pathway, which involve the mitochondria and the ER, both of which are depicted in Fig. 4.1. In the extrinsic pathway, death ligands (e.g., FasL, TNF-α) initiate apoptosis by binding to their cognate receptors (Fas and TNF receptor [TNFR] respectively) [55]. This binding stimulates the recruitment of the adaptor protein Fas-associated via death domain (FADD), which then recruits procaspase-8 into the death-inducing signaling complex (DISC) [56]. Procaspase-8 is activated by dimerization within this complex and subsequently cleaves and activates procaspase-3 and other downstream procaspases [57]. While both Fas ligand and its receptor have been reported to increase in experimental models of myocardial infarction (MI), ischemia and hypoxia [58, 59] and in patients with congestive HF [60], appraisal of their levels has not been reported in conjunction with myocardial aging. Observations showing increased levels of TNF-α and its receptor in patients in HF [61], and also that TNF-α treatment can induce apoptosis in cardiomyocytes *in vitro* [62], have been tempered by reports showing that TNF-α under some conditions can promote antiapoptotic pathways [63], and can even provide cardioprotection against myocardial ischemia [64]. As with Fas, levels of TNF-α and its receptor have not been ascertained in the aging heart.

The intrinsic pathway has been demonstrated to transduce a wide variety of extracellular and intracellular stimuli, including loss of survival/trophic factors, toxins, radiation, hypoxia, OS, myocardial ischemia/reperfusion (I/R) injury and DNA damage. A dynamic and complex interaction of numerous prosurvival and prodeath signals regulating apoptosis is largely mediated by the Bcl-2 family of proteins, which may be antiapoptotic (Bcl-2, Bcl-xL) or proapoptotic (Bax, Bid), and which exert their effects primarily at the level of mitochondria and the ER [65]. The proapoptotic proteins, including the Bcl-2 related proteins that possess only Bcl-2 homology domain 3 (BH3-only proteins) and the proapoptotic multidomain Bcl-2 proteins Bax and Bak undergo activation through diverse mechanisms to trigger the release of mitochondrial apoptogenic proteins, such as cytochrome *c*, Smac, EndoG and AIF into the cytoplasm [66–69]. Once in the cytoplasm, cytochrome *c* binds Apaf-1 along with dATP. This stimulates Apaf-1 to homo-oligomerize and recruit procaspase-9 into the multiprotein complex called the apoptosome [70–73]. Within the apoptosome, procaspase-9 is

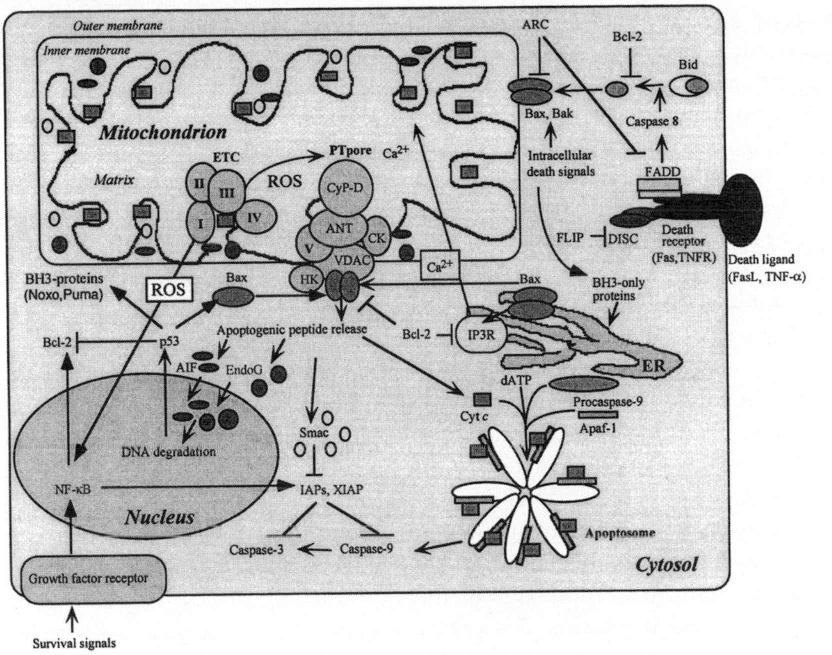

Fig. 4.1 The intrinsic and extrinsic pathways of apoptosis
An array of extracellular and intracellular signals trigger the intrinsic apoptotic pathway regulated by proapoptotic proteins (e.g., Bax, Bid and Bak) binding to outer mitochondrial membrane leading to mitochondrial outer-membrane permeabilization and PT pore opening. Elevated levels of mitochondrial Ca^{2+} as well as ETC-generated ROS also promote PT pore opening. This is followed by the release of cytochrome c (Cyt*c*), Smac, endonuclease G (Endo G), and apoptosis-inducing factor (AIF) from the mitochondrial intermembrane space to the cytosol, and apoptosome formation (with Cyt*c*) leading to caspase 9 activation, DNA fragmentation (with nuclear translocation of AIF and EndoG) and inhibition of IAP (by Smac) further stimulating activation of caspases-9 and Bax and Bid mediate mitochondrial membrane permeabilization, and antiapoptogenic proteins (e.g., Bcl-2) prevent apoptogen release. Also depicted are major proteins comprising the PT pore including hexokinase (Hx), adenine nucleotide translocator (ANT), creatine kinase (CK), cyclophilin-D (CyP-D), and porin (VDAC). The extrinsic pathway is initiated by ligand binding to death receptors leading to recruitment of FADD and DISC which stimulates the activation of caspase-8 resulting in caspase-3 activation and Bid cleavage (a C-terminal fragment of Bid targets mitochondria). FLIP and ARC can stem this pathway's progression at specific points. Intracellular stimuli trigger ER release of Ca^{2+} through both Bax and BH3-protein interactions. Also shown is the survival pathway triggered by survival stimuli, mediated by growth factor receptors, transcription factor activation (e.g., NF-κB) and enhanced expression of IAPs and Bcl-2.

activated by dimerization, after which it cleaves and activates downstream procaspases. Bid, a BH3-only protein, unites the extrinsic and intrinsic pathways; following cleavage by caspase-8, the Bid's C-terminal portion translocates to the mitochondria and triggers further apoptogen release [74, 75].

Given the high density of mitochondria in the functioning cardiomyocyte, it has been proposed that to prevent accidental apoptosis resulting from the leakage of proapoptotic factors into the cytosol, mitochondrial-dependent stimulation of apoptosis may be down-regulated in the cardiomyocyte, possibly by increased levels of endogenous inhibitors or by a lack of an essential component of the apoptotic pathway [47]. Indeed, both the extrinsic and intrinsic pathways are regulated by a variety of endogenous inhibitors of apoptosis. For instance, FLICE-like (Fas-associated death domain protein-like-interleukin-1 – converting enzyme – like) inhibitory protein (FLIP), whose expression is highly enriched in striated muscle, binds to and inhibits procaspase-8 in the DISC [76]. Imanishi et al demonstrated that FLIP RNA and protein are abundantly expressed in cardiomyocytes, and that FLIP protein was downregulated in TUNEL-positive cardiomyocytes [77]. Moreover, the same study noted that FLIP-positive cardiomyocytes in failing human hearts rarely showed evidence of apoptosis, indicating that this regulatory mechanism is likely operative in the heart.

Antiapoptotic proteins, such as Bcl-2 and Bcl-xL, inhibit mitochondrial apoptogen release through biochemical mechanisms that are still incompletely understood. The X-linked inhibitor of apoptosis (XIAP) and related proteins that contain baculovirus inhibitor of apoptosis repeats bind to and inhibit already activated caspases-9, −3, and −7, and interfere with procaspase-9 dimerization and activation [78, 79]. In explanted terminally human failing hearts, significant accumulation of cytosolic cytochrome *c* was associated with activation of caspase-9 and downregulation of FLIP inhibitory protein and the XIAP caspase inhibitor, implicating modulation of the regulatory inhibition of both intrinsic and extrinsic apoptotic pathways in the failing heart [80].

Findings with the apoptosis repressor with a caspase recruitment domain (CARD [ARC]), which is expressed preferentially in striated and cardiac muscle and in some neurons, have shown that this single inhibitor has the capacity to antagonize both the intrinsic and extrinsic apoptosis pathways [81]. The extrinsic pathway is inhibited by ARC's direct interactions with Fas, FADD, and procaspase-8, which prevent DISC assembly, while the intrinsic pathway is inhibited by ARC's direct binding and inhibition of Bax's interaction with the mitochondrial membrane [81, 82]. Furthermore, ARC inhibits cytochrome *c* release from mitochondria and protects against hypoxia-induced apoptosis, suggesting that ARC may be a key regulator of apoptosis in the heart [83]. The role of these endogenous inhibitors of apoptosis in cardiac aging remains to be determined.

Recently, the endoplasmic reticulum (ER) has been recognized as an important organelle in the intrinsic apoptosis pathway. In addition to its role in mediating cellular responses to traditional ER stresses, such as misfolded proteins, this organelle appears to be critical in mediating cell death elicited by a subset of stimuli originating outside of the ER, such as OS [84]. Similar to their roles in transducing upstream signals to the mitochondria, BH3-only proteins appear to relay upstream death signals to the ER [85]. Gathered observations have suggested a contributory role of the ER stress response pathway(s) in cardiac myocyte apoptosis [65].

During aging, mitochondrial dysfunction and ROS generation may promote increased apoptosis leading to myocyte cell loss. There is accumulated evidence that mitochondrial OS and declining mitochondrial bioenergetic production can lead to apoptotic pathway activation *in vitro*; whether this also occurs in the *in vivo* aging heart is presently unknown. Experimental data have shown that the activation of the intrinsic pathway of cardiomyocyte apoptosis occurs in the aging heart with the release of cytochrome *c* from heart mitochondria of senescent rats, decreased levels of Bcl-2 and unchanged Bax levels [86, 87]. Furthermore, myocytes derived from the heart of old mice displayed markedly increased levels of markers of cell death and senescence as compared to myocytes from younger animals [88].

As suggested by a number of experimental models, mitochondria-related apoptosis is likely contributory to the mechanisms of aging. In recent transgenic studies in which mice expressing a proofreading-deficient version of the mitochondrial DNA polymerase γ (POLG) accumulate mtDNA mutations and display features of accelerated aging, the accumulation of mtDNA mutations was found to be correlated with the induction of apoptotic markers [89]. In other studies, mice containing an IGF-1 transgene exhibited attenuated levels of senescence-associated gene products (e.g., p27Kip1, p53, p16INK4a, and p19ARF), Akt phosphorylation in myocytes and compared to wild-type mice exhibited decreased levels of myocyte DNA damage and cell death [88]. These studies have provided important information which may allow, in the near future, the therapeutic targeting of cardiomyocyte apoptosis in the aging heart.

Mitochondria, ETC and ROS

Under normal physiological conditions, the primary source of ROS is the mitochondrial electron transport chain (ETC), where O_2 can be activated to form superoxide radicals by a nonenzymatic process. The production of ROS is primarily a by-product of normal metabolism and occurs from electrons produced (or leaked) from the ETC primarily at complexes I and III. There is evidence that semiquinones generated within complexes I and III are the most likely donors of electrons to molecular oxygen, providing a constant source of superoxide; however, a supportive role for complex II in ROS production has also been suggested [90–92]. Mitochondrial ROS generation can be amplified in cells with abnormal respiratory chain function as well as under both physiological and pathological conditions, where oxygen consumption is increased. In addition to mitochondria, other cellular sources for the generation of superoxide radicals include the reactions of O_2 with microsomal cytochrome p450 and with reduced flavins (e.g., NADPH), usually in the presence of metal ions.

The production of ROS and OS is a function of both the inefficiency of electron transfer through the mitochondria respiratory chain and the overall level of antioxidant defenses in the cell [93]. Because ROS are the result of normal metabolic processes, the more active tissues, such as the heart, suffer the most damage. In addition, the mitochondrial bioenergetic dysfunction occurring with aging will further increase ROS accumulation. Among its many targets, ROS can reduce the inner-membrane fluidity by attacking polyunsaturated fatty acids (forming reactive lipid peroxides) and the anionic phospholipid cardiolipin, an important inner membrane constituent which can substantially affect protein transport and ETC function, in particular respiratory complex IV activity. Cardiolipin (which is only found in mitochondrial membranes) is particularly vulnerable to attack by oxidative damage due to the high degree of unsaturation in its fatty acids.

There is evidence of ROS-mediated oxidative damage to lipids and proteins in the aging heart, and both myocardial mtDNA and nuclear DNA damage will result in further accumulation of oxidative species. In addition, the highly reactive peroxynitrite, formed from the reaction of superoxide with nitric oxide (NO), irreversibly impairs mitochondrial respiration [94] since it inhibits complex I activity, largely by tyrosine nitration of several targeted subunits [95, 96], modifies cytochrome *c* structure and function [97], affects cytochrome *c* oxidase activity, inhibits mitochondrial aconitase [98], and causes induction of the PT pore [99]. Cardiomyocytes from aged hearts are highly susceptible to PT pore opening [100]. Some of the effects of peroxynitrite on its mitochondrial targets (e.g., the PT pore) are potentiated by increased Ca^{2+} levels [101]. The effects of peroxynitrite on mitochondria can be clearly distinguished from the effects of NO, which often are reversible [94].

In the aging heart, neutralization of ROS by mitochondrial antioxidants such as superoxide dismutase (SOD2 or MnSOD), glutathione peroxidase (GPx) and glutathione as well as cytosolic ROS-scavenging enzymes (e.g., catalase and CuSOD) becomes of critical significance (Fig. 4.2). Moreover, in the aging heart, a marked decline in mitochondrial ascorbate levels and reduced glutathione (GSH) is found in interfibrillar (but not sarcolemmal) mitochondria, and the levels of myocardial GPx and glutathione reductase [102], as well as MnSOD are increased [103]. The basis of the selective increases of antioxidant activities in specific mitochondrial subpopulations in aging has not yet been determined but may reflect an adaptive mechanism to cope with the increased ROS generation.

The uncoupling of mitochondrial respiration from oxidative phosphorylation (OXPHOS) ATP production—mediated by treatment with either artificial uncouplers such as 2,4-dinitrophenol (e.g., DNP) or natural uncouplers (e.g., laurate), fatty acids, and mitochondrial uncoupling (UCP) proteins—strongly inhibits superoxide and H_2O_2 formation in mitochondria [104, 105]. ROS production is favored when the mitochondrial membrane potential is above a specific threshold. Under conditions where the mitochondrial membrane potential is at its peak (e.g., state 4 respiration), ROS production is augmented. Significantly, increased mitochondrial membrane potential slows electron transport through the respiratory chain, resulting in increased half-life of the ubiquinone free radical and increasing the likelihood that electrons will interact with O_2 to form ROS [106]. Uncouplers prevent the transmembrane electrochemical H^+ potential difference ($\Delta\psi\mu$) from being above a threshold critical for ROS formation by respiratory complexes I and III. The status of UCP proteins which may promote protection against the accumulation of ROS in the aging heart has been recently

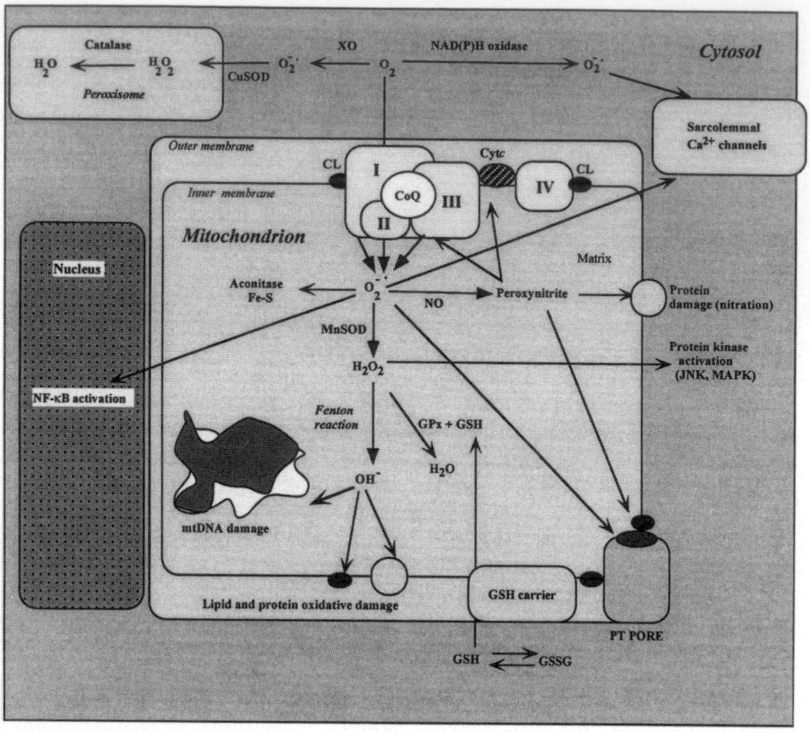

Fig. 4.2 ROS generation, antioxidant response and signaling
Mitochondrial bioenergetic activity generates reactive oxygen species (ROS) including superoxide, hydroxyl radicals and hydrogen peroxide (H_2O_2). Sites of mitochondrial superoxide $O_2^{-\cdot}$ radical (via respiratory complexes I, II, and III) and cytosolic $O_2^{-\cdot}$ generation (by NADPH oxidase or xanthine oxidase) are depicted. Also shown are reactions of the $O_2^{\bullet -}$ radical with NO to form the highly reactive peroxynitrite, which can target PT pore opening and the inactivation of mitochondrial aconitase by $O_2^{-\cdot}$. MnSOD (in mitochondria) and CuSOD (in cytosol) to form H_2O_2 are also displayed. The H_2O_2 is then either further neutralized in the mitochondria by glutathione peroxidase (GPx) and glutathione, in the peroxisome by catalase, or in the presence of Fe^{++} via the Fenton reaction, which forms the highly reactive OH^- radical, which can cause severe lipid peroxidation and extensive oxidative damage to proteins and mtDNA. Superoxide radicals produced in mitochondria can be delivered to the cytosol through anion channels and may impact sites far from their generation, including activation of nuclear transcription factor NF-κB.

addressed [107]. Intriguingly, levels of UCP3 transcript were upregulated in the hearts of mice with increased longevity due to caloric restriction [108].

Studies from several laboratories have suggested that cardiac aging (not unlike HF) is accompanied by changes in bioenergetic substrate utilization and overall capacity. Data from several animal models of aging as well as human subjects have demonstrated significant alterations in the myocardial TCA cycle, ETC and OXPHOS [109–111]. However, these observations have generated increasing controversy among investigators with some finding that the aging heart has either a modest, nonsignificant reduction or no overt effect on either ETC or OXPHOS function [112–116] while others found significant alterations in ETC, in which single respiratory complexes were more affected than others, i.e., complex I [117, 118], complex IV [119, 120] or complex V [121, 122] Recently, in our laboratory we have found a modest decrease in complex I and IV activities, and a more severe decline in complex V activity in the hearts of 30-month Fischer 344 rats. A potential reason underlying these discordant findings is that heart muscle mitochondria are composed of two distinct subpopulations: one beneath the sarcolemma (subsarcolemmal mitochondria [SSM]), and another along the myofilaments (interfibrillar mitochondria [IFM]). A preferential loss of IFM function with age has been reported, including a significant reduction of complex III [123, 124] and complex IV [125] activities; hence the variability may arise from the existence of disparate mitochondrial subpopulations with different susceptibilities to damage.

Autophagy and Cardiac Aging

The continuous renewal of cellular components requires the removal of worn-out and damaged macromolecules and defective organelles (e.g., mitochondria) for recycling and replacement with newly synthesized ones. Several complementary degradation systems are employed in the turnover of cellular components. Proteins are digested by a variety of proteases including calcium-dependent neutral proteases (calpains), multicatalytic proteinase complexes (proteasomes) with some organelles such as mitochondria possessing their own proteolytic systems including matrix-associated Lon protease and the membrane-bound AAA proteases. More long-lived proteins, other macromolecules, cell membranes and entire organelles are turned over by a highly conserved process involving intralysosomal degradation termed autophagy [126]. Interestingly, in the senescent heart while autophagy targets defective mitochondria, the myofibril proteins are targeted by non-lysosomal proteases such as calpain [127].

A number of steps are involved in autophagy including: (1) formation of a double -membrane enclosed vacuole (autophagosome) within the cell; (2) sequestering of the material to be degraded into an autophagosome; (3) fusion of the autophagosome with a lysosome or a late endosome and (4) the enzymatic degradation of the sequestered materials by a large spectrum of lysosomal enzymes (acid hydrolases) [126]. Variations on this theme include the lysosomal incorporation of cytoplasmic components without a preliminary sequestration through invaginations of the membrane (microautophagy as compared to macroautophagy), and a process termed chaperone-mediated autophagy in which particular cytosolic proteins are selectively transported to lysosomes by molecular chaperones, including several HSP proteins [128, 129]. Many signaling pathway components, including target of rapamycin (TOR) or mammalian target of rapamycin (mTOR), phosphatidylinositol 3-kinase PI3K, PKB/Akt, GTPases, calcium and protein synthesis have contributory roles in regulating autophagy. A number of proteins involved in autophagosome formation and function originally described in yeast have been identified (Atg proteins) and orthologs and their corresponding genes (ATG genes) in worms, fruit-flies and mammals have been subsequently reported [130]. Two Atg proteins (Atg 12 and Atg8) involved in autophagosome formation have also been found to be ubiquitin-like proteins indicating that ubiquitin tagging may be involved in autophagic degradation in addition to its well-documented role targeting proteins for degradation by the proteasome [131]. In yeast, a mitochondrial outer membrane protein Uth1p has been found to be essential for autophagy of these organelles [132]. This finding has prompted the suggestion that autophagy of mitochondria, peroxisomes, and possibly other organelles may be selective rather than random. It will be of great interest to find out if this selective mechanism increases with aging and whether it may play a role in retarding the accumulation of somatic mutations in mtDNA with aging by selective degradation of mitochondria containing high levels of these mutant alleles [133].

Autophagy occurs in many types of cells during development, including in cardiomyocytes, as an adaptive response to cell stresses including OS, radiation, toxins, starvation, and for survival when either extracellular or intracellular nutrients are limited. Moreover, intralysosomal degradation of cells plays an essential role in the renewal of cardiac myocytes in cardiac diseases associated with aging such as ischemic heart disease [134]. In a porcine model of chronically instrumented pigs subjected to repetitive myocardial ischemia, levels of autophagic proteins including cathepsin B, heat shock cognate protein HSP 73 (a key protein marker for chaperone-mediated autophagy), beclin 1 (a mammalian autophagy gene), and the processed form of microtubule-associated protein 1 light chain 3 (a marker for autophagosomes), were increased, as was the accumulation of autophagic vacuoles in myocytes as detected by electron microscopy [135]. In a hamster model of cardiomyopathy, myocardial autophagy-related proteins i.e., ubiquitin, cathepsin D and Rab7-were upregulated and autophagy-dependent degeneration was found to be an important contributor to the loss of cardiomyocyte function in the cardiomyopathic hamster [136]. These studies also suggested a link between autophagic degeneration and elevated levels of cardiomyocyte death. Treatment with granulocyte colony-stimulating factor (G-CSF) significantly improved survival, cardiac function and remodeling in these animals, and such beneficial effects were accompanied by a reduction in autophagy, an increase in cardiomyocyte size, and a reduction in myocardial fibrosis.

An interaction between deficient mitochondria and lysosomes has recently received attention as a potentially critical element of aging, since both organelles appear to suffer significant age-related alterations in post-mitotic cells. In a number of aging cell-types, an increasing number of senescent mitochondria undergo both enlargement and gradual structural alterations including loss of cristae and swelling associated with decreased capacity to produce energy. In addition, aging markedly increases the amount of oxidatively damaged cytosolic proteins and resulted in a surfeit of increasingly undigestable (due to cross-linking) macromolecules which comprise the lysosomal substrate including the aging-related deposition of the undegradable pigment lipofuscin, most of which is refractory to removal by exocytosis [137]. Moreover, lysosomal degradative function including the activities of both the proteasomal system and the lysosomal proteases has been shown to markedly decrease in post-mitotic human fibroblasts cultured under hyperoxic conditions to facilitate age-related oxidative senescence [138]. Lysosomes from 22-month-old rats show lower rates of chaperone-mediated autophagy, and both substrate binding (due to lower levels of specific receptors) to the lysosomal membrane and transport into lysosomes decline with age [129]. Therefore given that lysosomes responsible for mitochondrial turnover experience a loss of function, it is not surprising that the rate of total mitochondrial protein turnover declines with age [139].

Several mechanisms may potentially contribute to the age-related accumulation of damaged mitochondria following initial oxidative injury, including the clonal expansion of defective mitochondria, a reduction in the number of mitochondria targeted for autophagocytosis, suppressed autophagy because of the increased load of undegradable and irreversibly oxidized substrate, and decreased efficiency of specific proteases [140]. Abnormal autophagic degradation of damaged macromolecules and organelles, termed biological "garbage", is also considered an important contributor to aging and the death of post-mitotic cells, including cardiomyocytes. Evidence that enlarged mitochondria can interfere with autophagocytosis was demonstrated in studies in which cultured neonatal rat cardiac myocytes were treated with 3-methyladenine (3-MA) to inhibit autophagocytosis. A dramatic accumulation of small mitochondria was found in these 3-MA treated myocytes whereas the number of large organelles increased only slightly suggesting that the majority of normally autophagocytosed mitochondria are small, while larger mitochondria are less efficiently autophagocytosed. However, the mechanism of how mitochondria are selected for autophagocytosis remains to be determined. In a recent study of cultured neonatal rat cardiac myocytes, Terman et al found that the content of the intralysosomal undegradable pigment lipofuscin, which varied drastically between cells, positively correlated with mitochondrial damage (evaluated by decreased membrane potential), as well as with ROS production [141, 142]. These data suggest that both lipofuscin accumulation and mitochondrial damage have common underlying mechanisms, including imperfect autophagy with limited lysosomal degradation of oxidatively damaged mitochondria and other organelles. Lipofuscin-loaded lysosomes in aging cells have been proposed to act as sinks for newly synthesized enzymes which diminishes the ability to degrade and clear out oxidatively damaged materials, organelles and cellular debris leaving them to accumulate increasing damage as well as limiting the needed recycling of mitochondrial components [140]. This view has been borne out by experiments showing that lipofuscin loading of human fibroblasts does decrease their autophagocytotic capacity [143]. However, further confirmation of the hypothesis concerning the mitochondrial-lysosomal axis of diminished autophagy and mitochondrial recycling in aging will require these experiments to be conducted in aging post-mitotic tissues and cells.

A further consequence of aging-induced accumulation of oxidized substrates is lysosomal rupture. Due to autophagy and degradation of iron containing proteins (such as iron-containing metalloproteins, including cytochromes and ferritin), lysosomes contain a pool of redox-active iron, which makes these organelles particularly susceptible to oxidative damage; chelation of the intralysosomal pool of redox-active iron prevents these effects. In addition, lipofuscin-loaded cells appear highly sensitive to oxidant-induced damage as a result of their enlarged lysosomal compartment and the presence of iron bound to lipofuscin [144]. OS above a certain limit causes lysosomal rupture due to intralysosomal iron-catalyzed peroxidative reactions [145]. Moderate release of hydrolytic lysosomal enzymes to the cytosol can promote apoptosis in a variety of ways; after the initiating lysosomal rupture, cytochrome *c* is released from mitochondria and caspases are activated. Subsequently, mitochondrial damage follows the release of lysosomal hydrolases, which may act either directly or indirectly, through activation of phospholipases or proapoptotic proteins such as Bid. A more pronounced release of lysosomal enzymes results in necrotic cell death [146]. This interrelated mitochondrial and lysosomal damage eventually results in functional failure and death of cells, including cardiac myocytes. Hence, while under some conditions (e.g., ischemia), autophagy may provide cardioprotection and stress resistance to chronic ischemic insult [147], autophagy can also lead to cell death. In fact, autophagy-associated cell death has increasingly been reported as a third major type of cell death (although with considerable overlap with the apoptotic and necrotic pathways). While autophagic cell death has been recently documented in myocardial cells from hypertrophied, failing, and hibernating myocardium, its role in the aging heart remains to be determined and quantitated [148].

Post-translational Changes Associated with Aging

The interaction and subsequent modification of specific peptides and proteins with nitric oxide and its metabolites (including the reactive nitrosative species, peroxynitrite) has been shown to be elevated in aging, consistent with elevations of age-dependent OS and accumulation of free radical-dependent damage of proteins. One such common aging-mediated modification is the conversion of tyrosine to 3-nitrotyrosine (3-NT); nitration of tyrosine can compromise the functional and/or structural integrity of target proteins. The differential accumulation of nitrated proteins at a faster rate in older tissues may indicate either a higher yield of nitrating species in the old or a reduced rate of protein turnover (or both).

An age-related increase in 3-nitrotyrosine in targeted cardiac proteins, was recently reported in the 26 month old Fischer rat [149]. Among the targeted proteins identified by reaction with an anti-nitrotyrosine antibody were pivotal enzymes responsible for energy production and metabolism including cytosolic proteins of glycolysis (i.e., α-enolase, α-aldolase, GAPDH), and mitochondrial proteins involved in electron transport, TCA cycle, fatty acid β-oxidation and OXPHOS (i.e., 3-ketoacyl-CoA thiolase, acetyl-CoA acetyltransferase, malate dehydrogenase, creatine kinase, electron-transfer flavoprotein, F1-ATPase and the voltage-dependent anion channel/porin), as well as proteins involved in myocyte structural integrity (i.e., desmin). This study also reported nitration at Y105 of the electron-transfer flavoprotein using MS/MS analysis and revealed that many highly abundant cardiac proteins exhibit no aging-mediated nitration, suggesting a specificity of targeting.

It is well-established that polyunsaturated fatty acids of membrane lipids are highly susceptible to peroxidation by oxygen radicals, giving rise to various aldehydes, alkenals, and hydroxyalkenals such as malonaldehyde and 4-hydroxy-2-nonenal (HNE) [150]. HNE, the most reactive of these compounds and critical mediator of free radical damage reacts with protein at the sulfhydryl group of cysteine, the imidazole nitrogen(s) of histidine, and/or the ε-amine of lysine, often resulting in enzyme inactivation

Recent studies employing proteomic analysis, found both evidence of increased nitration and HNE-modified serum proteins in older Fischer 344 rats [151]. Moreover, Lucas and Szweda have found that HNE modification of specific mitochondrial proteins was present exclusively in hearts isolated from senescent rats subjected to ischemia and reperfusion with concomitant decline in enzyme function [152]. While there is increasing evidence that HNE adducts comprise a reliable marker of increasing protein oxidation in the aging heart, their physiological significance is not so clear. For instance, *in vitro* studies documented that HNE, a product of omega-6 polyunsaturated fatty acid peroxidation, reduced mitochondrial respiration by adducting α-ketoglutarate dehydrogenase complex and inhibiting its activity; in contrast, *in vivo* studies have later reported increased levels of HNE-modified subunits of α-ketoglutarate dehydrogenase in the aging myocardium, resulting in an increased level of enzyme activity in older rats [153]. On the other hand, recent observations in the spontaneously hypertensive rat suggest that other mitochondrial metabolic enzymes (i.e., $NADP^+$-isocitrate dehydrogenase) are modified by HNE with age resulting in decline of enzyme function [154].

In cardiac muscle, the function of the SERCA2a isoform declines by over 60 % during aging, in part as a result of reduced SERCA protein levels (estimated at roughly 20 %) and in part as a result of the nitration of selected tyrosines. Nitration in the senescent heart was found to increase by more than two nitrotyrosines on average per Ca^{2+} ATPase molecule, coinciding with the appearance of partially nitrated Tyr(294), Tyr(295) and Tyr(753) residues [155]. The age-related loss-of-function of these critical calcium regulatory proteins are consistent with the observed increases in intracellular calcium levels within senescent cells.

Attacks of ROS on proteins have been shown to increase their carbonyl content because of the formation of aldehydes and ketones in certain amino acid residues. Because the generation of carbonyl derivatives occurs by many different mechanisms, the level of carbonyl groups in proteins is widely used as a marker of oxidative protein damage. Age-associated increases in protein carbonyls have been reported in cultured human fibroblasts [156] and in a variety of tissues [157]. Moreover, cells obtained from patients with diseases of accelerated aging have dramatically higher levels of protein carbonyls [156]. Evidence suggests that age-associated oxidative damage to proteins, detected as carbonyl modifications, is a selectively targeted rather than a randomly directed process. In studies gauging whether oxidative damage to proteins in the aging process occurs randomly or selectively in the flight muscles of the housefly, adenine nucleotide translocase (ANT) was found to be the only protein in the mitochondrial membranes exhibiting a detectable age-associated increase in carbonyls [158], while aconitase was found to be the only protein in the mitochondrial matrix that exhibited an age-associated increase in carbonylation [159]. The accrual of oxidative damage was accompanied by a significant loss in aconitase and ANT activities. Interestingly, mild protein oxidation has been shown to be a marking step in the preferential degradation of oxidized proteins, whereas severe oxidative damage may lead to cross-linking and resistance to proteolysis [160]. Inefficient removal of oxidized proteins by proteolytic cleavage, may also promote the accumulation of specific protein carbonyls with aging.

While aging-associated oxidation of selective proteins can lead to the nitration of aromatic amino acid residues and the conversion of some amino acid residues to carbonyl derivatives, other types of protein modifications have also been reported including hydroxylation of aromatic groups and aliphatic amino acid side chains, nitrosylation of sulfhydryl groups, sulfoxidation of methionine residues, and chlorination of aromatic groups and primary amino groups. The oxidation of particularly vulnerable sulfhydryl surface-exposed methionine and cysteine residues of proteins is frequently reversible, unlike other kinds of oxidation [161], and the variable modification of S-nitrosylation has been increasingly associated with signal transduction pathways. Nevertheless, irreversible oxidation of protein sulfhydryls is more extensive in aged tissues, and may be prevented by the presence of an adequate pool of glutathione. Furthermore, increased levels of irreversible protein sulfhydryl damage have been proposed to have a critical impact on the function of signal-transduction and transcription events that utilize proteins containing these reactive sites [162].

Glycation

Glycation (also called the Maillard reaction, or non-enzymatic glycosylation) is a reaction by which reducing sugars become attached to proteins without the assistance of an enzyme. This attachment occurs via the formation of a double-bond between the glucose aldehyde-group and the free amino group of either lysine or arginine. The resultant formation of the imine group (and its rearranged version known as the Amadori product) is completely reversible, but Amadori products subjected to further oxidation form Advanced Glycation End-products (AGEs) that are irreversible.

Collagen, elastin and basement membrane are among the proteins most vulnerable to cross-linking and AGE formation because they are the most long-lived proteins, with a slow rate of turnover. Both the accumulation of interstitial collagen (reported in both the diabetic and in the aging heart) [163, 164] and the development of increasing glucose-crosslinks by AGE have been proposed as a primary basis for increased left ventricle stiffness and consequently, diastolic dysfunction in the aging heart. This hypothesis is supported by the fact that hyperglycemia produces a greatly accelerated stiffening of the myocardium of young diabetic animals. Further evidence supporting a role for AGE in myocardial stiffening comes from the observation that regimens that specifically inhibit AGE formation such as diet restriction [165], and treatment with aminoguanidine [166], effectively prevent the pathological stiffening process associated with diabetes and aging. Furthermore, a class of thiazolium derivatives able to break established AGE cross-links was developed, exemplified by the cross-link breaker phenyl-4,5-dimethylthazolium chloride (ALT-711), which was found to significantly reduce left ventricle chamber stiffness and to ameliorate cardiac function in both older dogs [167], and in an aging dog model of diabetes (alloxan-induced) [168].

The interaction of AGEs with a number of specific cellular binding sites or receptors has also been reported to lead to the production of pro-inflammatory cytokines and free radical formation. These receptors include the receptor for AGE (termed RAGE), an integral membrane protein of the immunoglobulin superfamily acting as a multiligand receptor and present in numerous tissues, including cardiac myocytes, neural tissues and vascular cells (e.g., SMCs, endothelial cells and macrophages) and in the expanded intima of human atherosclerotic plaques [169]. Myocardial levels of RAGE have been found to be significantly upregulated with hyperglycemia, with increasing age and reduced cardiac function [170], and most recently as a result of ischemic insult in rats [171]. Data with overexpressed RAGE targeted to hearts of transgenic mice have suggested a role for AGE/RAGE in modulating myocardial calcium homeostasis [172]. RAGE overexpression was found to reduce systolic and diastolic intracellular calcium concentration, which is likely contributory to diabetes-induced cardiac dysfunction.

DNA Damage

Types of Damage

A large body of evidence supports the view that DNA damage and mutations accumulate with age in a variety of mammalian tissues. The kinds of DNA damage and their extent show considerable variation in different tissues which appear to reflect tissue-specific characteristics, including mitotic rate, transcriptional activity, metabolic activity and the DNA repair pathways available [173]. Defects in DNA including single-strand and double-strand breaks (DSBs), base damage and modification (including 8-oxoguanosine formation), and a number of adducts can be caused by a variety of exogenous physical and chemical agents such as ionizing radiation and genotoxic drugs. In addition to external sources of DNA damage, there are also endogenous sources of DNA damage including replication errors, spontaneous chemical changes to the DNA, and endogenous DNA damaging agents including ROS, such as superoxide anion, hydroxyl radical, hydrogen peroxide, NO, and others. Gathered observations have also directly demonstrated that the nonenzymatic Maillard glycation reaction can lead to oxidative DNA damage and is genotoxic [174, 175]. These diverse defects in DNA can result in the generation of point mutations, deletions, insertions and a variety of genomic re-arrangements, including translocations which also accumulate in aging mammalian cells. Increased levels of somatic mutations occurring at a number of specific genetic loci have been shown to accumulate with age in both humans and animal models [176–178]. Senescence-accelerated mice, which have been bred to have a shortened life span, show accelerated accumulation of somatic mutations [179]. Conversely, dietary restriction, which prolongs life span, results in slowed accumulation of spontaneous HPRT mutations in mice [180].

As previously discussed in Chapters 1 and 2, a central tenet of the free radical theory of aging, (also termed the OS aging hypothesis) relates to the contributory role of ROS resulting in oxidative damage to DNA (and in particular mtDNA) and that the progressive accumulation of ROS and its attendant irreversible oxidative damage, occurring with age, leads to a decline in the function of organ systems that eventually will result in failure and death [181, 182]. As we shall shortly see, there is evidence both supporting and challenging this model.

There is considerable evidence, mostly derived from studies with cultured cells, that oxidative damage affects nucleic acids, and in particular mtDNA, by the induction of single-and double-strand breaks, base damage, and modification resulting in the generation of point mutations and deletions [183–185]. In addition, in rat liver it has been found that the normal levels of the oxidized base, 8-oxo-2′ deoxyguanosine (oxo8dG) are present at 1 per 130,000 bases in nuclear DNA and 1 per 8000 bases in mtDNA and that mtDNA sustained more than ten-fold increase in oxidative damage as compared to nuclear DNA in this tissue [186]. Since oxidative damage to DNA primarily arises from ROS produced as by-products of normal metabolism, as well as other sources such as radiation, the accumulation of damaged DNA in aging tissues might be expected. In support of this conclusion is the strong direct correlation of specific metabolic rate with oxidative DNA damage found in the analysis of several mammalian species, as gauged by the presence of altered deoxynucleosides and bases (e.g., thymidine and thymidine glycols) [187]. Observations by Ames et al revealed a 2-3 fold increase in oxo8dG levels in nuclear DNA isolated from liver, kidney, and intestine in older Fischer 344 male rats (24 months of age), compared to younger rats [188]. Levels of oxo8dG in cerebellar and cerebral cortex samples from human brain were reported to significantly increase with aging in both nuclear DNA and mtDNA, with a greater than 10-fold increase in mtDNA compared to nuclear DNA; [189] these studies were conducted in tissues from a limited number of normal individuals (n=10) ranging in age from 42–97 years. Hayakawa et al have reported the accumulation of 8-OH-dG in mtDNA in the diaphragm muscle and also in the heart of aging patients [190, 191].

The proximity of mtDNA to the major source of cellular ROS (i.e., the ETC) in part underlies its primacy as a target for oxidative damage. In addition, mtDNA may be more susceptible to oxidative damage since unlike nuclear DNA, mtDNA is not enveloped (and protected) by histone proteins, and as we shall see in a later section of this chapter is associated with a more limited DNA repair capacity.

However, the high levels of aging-mediated oxidative DNA damage reported by most of the aforementioned investigators is at odds with other observations of much lower estimates in the amount of oxidatively damaged DNA highlighting the difficulty of accurately measuring ROS and oxidative damage experimentally [192, 193]. An explanation for these contradictory results may lie with artifactual DNA oxidation, which can be produced during the isolation and analysis of DNA samples, in particular arising from the common use of phenol during DNA extraction; [194] this indicates that a reassessment was required for evaluating the *in vivo* levels of oxo8dG in DNA. Nevertheless, Hamilton et al. by carefully avoiding nuclear DNA extraction oxidation (using the NaI extraction technique) have found significant aging-related increases in the levels of oxo8dG (although lower absolute levels of oxo8dG than previously reported) in a number of tissues including heart, liver, kidney, brain, skeletal muscle and spleen from both aging Fischer 344 rats and mice [192]. Higher levels of oxo8dG accumulation were also found in the mtDNA in the liver of 24 month old Fischer 344 rat, but the extent of aging-mediated increase in mtDNA oxidative damage was comparable to nuclear DNA levels. These findings suggest that while the steady-state levels of oxo8dG are relatively small in the genome of rodent cells, the *de novo* formation of oxo8dG lesions is considerable in both nuclear DNA and mtDNA, implying that oxidative damage to DNA arising from normal cellular metabolism may be highly relevant in aging. Moreover, if ROS are indeed an important source of aging-associated damage, both nuclear and mtDNA appear to be functional targets, albeit which of the two is the most relevant functional target in aging is not clear. Increased interest in the role of OS on nuclear genes in aging has come from recent assessment of gene profiling in human frontal cortex where it was found that many nuclear genes, involved in critical neural functions, showed reduced expression after age 40 and concomitantly sustained elevated levels of oxo8dG and DNA damage in their promoters [195]. Moreover, these gene promoters were selectively damaged by OS in cultured human neurons, and exhibited reduced base-excision DNA repair.

Data collected from a number of animal studies have shown that with aging there is a progressive accumulation of other types of mtDNA damage, which tend to be tissue-specific such as elevated levels of large-scale mtDNA deletions in heart and brain. Studies with brain (cerebellum and caudate regions), skeletal muscle and heart DNA derived from human subjects have shown the accumulation of age-dependent, tissue specific mtDNA deletions [196, 197]. The increase (in number and variety) of a subset of specific large-scale deletions produced over a lifetime was more pronounced in skeletal muscle or heart [198]. Recent studies employing a cell-by-cell analysis in human cardiomyocytes and neurons have demonstrated a clonal origin for these mtDNA deletions; molecules with deletions were found to primarily originate from a single deleted mtDNA molecule that had expanded clonally [196, 199]. For instance, while most of the cells examined contain no deletions, in a small subset of cardiomyocytes derived from the hearts of old donors a significant portion of the mtDNA molecules carried one particular deletion [200]. In addition, studies with individual skeletal muscle fibres isolated by laser-capture microdissection from aging rats found the presence of specific mtDNA deletions in strict correlation with a ragged red phenotype (often associated with certain mitochondrial-based cytopathies) including cytochrome *c* oxidase deficiency, indicative of the clonal expansion of deleted mtDNA genomes in ETC- abnormal regions of muscle fibers [201].

The mechanisms driving these clonal expansions remain largely unknown, as does the precise mechanism of their somatic generation. However, a number of factors have been implicated in the mechanism including ROS formation [202], recombination between flanking sequences including short direct repeats [203–204], and DSBs [205]. Multiple mtDNA deletions have been associated with mutations in the nuclear genes for the mtDNA polymerase γ, adenine nucleotide translocator and the helicase Twinkle [206, 207]. The increased level of both point mutations and deletions in mtDNA from post-mitotic tissues in individuals bearing either mutation in the mitochondrial helicase Twinkle or in Polγ suggests a critical role for the activity of proteins involved in mtDNA replication, which may be selectively targeted in aging.

A model of slip-mispairing replication involving direct repeats has been proposed to mediate the origin of most common clonal mtDNA deletions [208, 209], although recent observations suggest that DSBs (promoted by ROS or produced during stalled mtDNA replication) may be involved in the formation of multiple deletions containing either no repeats or small homologies at the deletion breakpoint region [205, 206].

The tissue-specific pattern of mtDNA deletion accumulation also appears to be species-specific. While several types of myocardial mtDNA deletions increase with aging in rats, their relative incidence appears to be significantly lower in rats compared to humans [210, 211]. Nevertheless, significant accumulation of a 4.2kb mtDNA deletion has been found in the myocardium of senescent mice in comparison to young or middle-aged animals [212]. Similarly, in Fischer 344 x Brown Norway F1 hybrid rats of ages 5, 18 and 36 months, specific mtDNA deletions of 8–9 kb have been detected in the right and left ventricle and their abundance increased with age [213]. Interestingly, recent observations have shown that over 40 % of cardiac mtDNA deletions in the aging rat heart contain unique point mutations located near the deletion breakpoints [214].

Over the last decade, a number of investigators have reported the accumulation of a significant number of mtDNA point mutations in humans above a certain age. Increased levels of age-associated mutations in the mtDNA non-coding control region (termed the D-loop) have been reported in skin fibroblasts and skeletal muscle from human subjects at critical sites for mtDNA replication [215]. More recently, mutation screening of the mtDNA control region in leukocytes from subjects of an Italian population found a homoplasmic C150T mutation in the D-loop near a replication origin for the mtDNA heavy strand [216]. This mutation was detected in approximately 17 % of 52 subjects 99–106 years old, and was present at strikingly lower levels (3.4 %) in 117 younger individuals. Subsequent molecular analysis of individuals with the C150T mutation revealed that the 5′ end of nascent heavy mtDNA strands contained a new replication origin at position 149, substituting for that at 151, and suggesting a remodeled replication origin of mtDNA that may provide a survival advantage in the aging process.

As noted with the mtDNA deletions, a tissue-specific pattern of accumulation of mtDNA point mutations in the control region appears to be operative. Marin-Garcia et al. [217] in their study using DNA sequence analysis of the incidence and location of D-loop mutations as a function of age, found no evidence of an age-related correlation in the accumulation of mutations (either homoplasmic or heteroplasmic) in either a group of patients with cardiomyopathy or in a group of normal controls. Neither was there an age-related accumulation in mitochondrial structural gene mutations (e.g., cytochome *b* gene). Similarly, no significant accumulation of specific mutations in the mtDNA control region was detected in the aging (26 month old mouse) heart, brain and skeletal muscle [218]. In contrast, evaluation of the D-loop region in the 22 month old mouse liver shows a significant increase in the level of base substitutions with a frequency ranging from 11–25 mutations per 100,000 nucleotides [219].

Recent evidence supports the concept that like mtDNA deletions, somatic mtDNA point mutations also are frequently clonal expansions in normal human tissues. Cell-to-cell analysis of proliferating epithelial cells and post-mitotic cardiomyocytes revealed that a significant proportion of cells contained high levels of clonal mutant mtDNAs expanded from single initial mutant mtDNA molecules; these clonal expansions were only present in tissues derived from aging individuals, confirming their somatic origin [220]. Qualitative differences between the mutational spectra of clonally expanded mutations suggest that either the processes generating these mutations or mechanisms driving them to homoplasmy are likely to be fundamentally different between the two tissues. For instance, a mutational hotspot in epithelial cells was located in the homopolymeric C-tract located between base pairs 303 and 309 or 310, which was rarely found in cardiomyocytes. While the majority of mutations in the cardiomyocyte mtDNA fell within a 30 bp area between base pairs 16,025–16,055 of the control region, no mutations were mapped to this area in the epithelial cells.

The role of point mutations and deletions in mtDNA in aging has been further addressed experimentally by two groups of investigators utilizing transgenic mice that express a proof-reading-deficient version of Polγ, the nuclear-encoded catalytic subunit of mtDNA polymerase [89, 221]. In these studies, homozygous mice developed a mtDNA mutator phenotype characterized by the acquisition of between a 3-fold and 8-fold increase in the levels of accumulated mtDNA mutations compared to wild-type strains; primarily base substitution mutations were reported with evidence of mtDNA deletion events. In both mtDNA mutator mouse strains, the increase in somatic mtDNA mutations was associated with a significantly reduced life span and the premature onset of aging-related phenotypes, including cardiomegaly, sarcopenia, osteoporosis, hair loss, cardiomyopathy, anemia, and fertility problems suggesting a causative link between mtDNA mutations and aging. However, these studies with mtDNA mutator mice were unable to detect a significant accumulation of ROS, changes of antioxidant enzymes or markers of OS (including neither generalized oxidative damage to proteins in either heart or liver nor reduced levels of mitochondrial aconitase activity). While no evidence was found for ROS production in embryonic fibroblasts derived from the mtDNA mutator mice, severe respiratory deficiency was described in one of these mutant strains, which may be the primary inducer of aging, rather than ROS [222]. One of these models also exhibited a marked induction of apoptotic markers as noted earlier, particularly in tissues characterized by rapid cellular turnover [89]. A potential explanation for the lack of detectable OS in these mice may be that the accumulation of mtDNA mutations are located downstream of ROS effects in the aging pathway (i.e., in normal aging, ROS stimuli may be needed or are contributory to the formation of mtDNA mutations). Alternatively, introduction of an error-prone DNA polymerase may cause extensive mutations throughout the mitochondrial genome that prevent the generation of ROS [223]. This is consistent with the 95 % reduction in oxygen consumption reported in transgenic mouse embryo fibroblasts.

While the transgenic mtDNA mutator mouse model is the first to directly demonstrate a role for mtDNA mutations in aging, it remains to be seen whether these findings are truly relevant to higher organisms. The level of mtDNA mutation accumulation in these strains is more than an order of magnitude higher than that found with aging human tissues [224]. In addition, mtDNA mutations in the mutator mouse strains are primarily point mutations which start to accumulate rapidly early in embryogenesis and thus distribute at high levels among most if not all tissues whereas large-scale mtDNA deletions, which account for a majority of the mitochondrial defects in human heart and skeletal muscle [225], and brain [196], are clearly tissue-specific and accumulate much later in life [226]. Another issue that has been raised with these mice is that the premature-aging phenotype is more similar to the aging phenotype found in humans and is markedly dissimilar to events in natural mouse aging. Therefore findings with the mtDNA mutator mice, in which the rapid generation and enormous accumulation of mtDNA mutations in a relatively small number of progenitor cells beginning at the earliest stages of mouse embryonic development have a disproportionately large effect on the mutant load in postnatal life, likely do not recapitulate the slow and tissue-specific accumulation of mutations seen either in normal human or mouse aging and further suggest important limitations with the model as defined.

Interestingly, a related transgenic mouse model which also employs a proofreading-deficient mitochondrial DNA polymerase but which is selectively targeted for expression solely in the heart may prove to be informative in aging studies [227]. These mutator mice generate increased levels of cardiac mtDNA mutations and eventually (over several weeks) develop increased fibrosis and severe DCM, often leading to HF. It is noteworthy that the levels of elevated mtDNA mutations in these tissue-targeted mutator strains are much lower (2 mutations per mitochondrial genome) compared to the aforementioned mutator models, and the resultant phenotype may be more relevant to natural aging events. Notably, in the cardiac-specific mutator strain, mitochondrial respiratory function and mitochondrial number and ultrastructure remained normal suggesting that the cardiac dysfunction does not result from impaired mitochondrial bioenergetic function. Significantly, increased levels of apoptotic markers, including the release of cytochrome *c* from mitochondria, and histological evidence of apoptotic cell death occurring in all regions of the heart suggest that the elevated frequency of mtDNA mutations might trigger the initiation of apoptosis. Interestingly, activation of myocardial programmed cell death pathway precedes (and may itself trigger) a vigorous prosurvival response including the upregulation of antiapoptotic proteins such as Bcl-2, Bcl-xl, Bfl1, and heat shock protein 27 [228]. Gene expression profiling using microarray analysis confirmed that the cardiomyopathy caused by mtDNA mutations was largely characterized by gene expression changes indicative of increased fibrosis and cardiac remodeling of the extracellular matrix [229]. Moreover, minimal changes were found in the expression of genes involved in either mitochondrial energy production or generation of increased OS.

It remains unclear how increased mitochondrial DNA mutations activate the apoptotic pathway at levels lower than required to affect respiration or increase OS. Surprisingly, Mott et al. [230] have recently reported that cardiac mitochondria from mutator transgenic mice that develop mitochondrial DNA mutations have a marked inhibition of the calcium-induced PT pore opening accompanied by increased levels of Bcl-2 protein recruitment to the mitochondrial membrane; temporally, inhibited pore opening coincides with the onset of cardiac dysfunction, a rather unexpected finding. The authors conclude that mitochondrial DNA mutations induce an adaptive-protective response in the heart that inhibits opening of the mitochondrial permeability pore, while increasing other aspects of apoptotic signaling [230].

Due to difficulties in detecting, quantifying and characterizing somatic mutations *in vivo* in different organs and tissues particularly post-mitotic tissues, it has proved difficult to test the premise that mutations accumulate during the aging of mammals in a sufficiently high number to cause some of the pathophysiological signs and symptoms of aging. To address this problem, transgenic mouse models have been developed. These mice contain chromosomally integrated plasmids harboring reporter genes that can be efficiently recovered from genomic DNA and transferred into a suitable *Escherichia coli* host for subsequent mutant selection, quantitation, and characterization [231]. One of these models, based on plasmids containing the *lacZ* reporter gene allows the detection of a wide range of somatic mutations, including large rearrangements and has been extensively used in Vijg's laboratory. Animals harboring these constructs have been studied over their lifetime to test the hypothesis that mutations accumulate with age, as predicted in the original somatic mutation theories of aging.

Using this *lacZ*-plasmid transgenic reporter mouse model, early studies of Vijg et al. reported an age-related increase in mutation frequency in the liver but not in the brain [232]. Interestingly, a substantial fraction of the spontaneous mutations in the liver were large genome rearrangements, whereas in the brain mainly point mutations were detected. These findings suggested that post-mitotic tissue is more resistant to mutation accumulation in the nuclear genome with aging-dependent cytogenetic alterations limited to cells that are still mitotically active. However, this conclusion was not supported by subsequent studies from the same group in which the aging-associated mutational spectra were compared in an actively proliferating organ (i.e., small intestine) and a post-mitotic organ (i.e., heart) from young and old mice [233]. Both organs showed significantly increased levels of mutation accumulation with age, albeit the small intestine had increased age-related mutation frequency relative to the heart. The pattern of mutations was strikingly different in the two organs with the small intestine harboring primarily point mutations, including G-C to T-A, G-C to C-G, and A-T to C-G transversions and G-C to A-T transitions. In contrast, over half of the mutations accumulated in the aging heart were comprised of large genome rearrangements, involving up to as much as 34 centimorgans of chromosomal DNA with nearly all other mutations being G-C to A-T transitions at CpG sites. It is noteworthy that OS has been found in other studies to be associated with increased multilocus DNA deletions and gross chromosomal rearrangements [234–235], and that the G-C to A-T transition is considered as a potential oxygen radical signature, albeit a large variety of DNA lesions that can be induced by oxygen free radicals were not detected in aging tissues in these studies.

Another approach to assessing aging-related mutation accumulation in transgenic mouse models using a different reporter systems (i.e., bacteriophage λ rather than plasmid vector based) documented a similar propensity for increased G-C to A-T transitions at CpG sites in the aging heart (which may reflect increased deamination events), while not detecting large-scale rearrangements and deletions [236]. This difference suggests that the relatively smaller integrating plasmid vector might be more useful in detecting aging-associated genome rearrangement events compared to the larger bacteriophage vectors, whose insertion/removal from the chromosome might be expected to impact mutagenesis and/or repair. In order to explain how mutations can be formed and accumulate during aging in a post-mitotic organ in the absence of DNA replication, it is necessary to invoke the involvement of a process such as error-prone DNA repair (discussed further below). For instance, the increase in large genome rearrangements in the old heart may arise from misrepair or misannealing of DSBs or cross-links by nonhomologous end-joining (NHEJ), a recombinational DNA repair system notorious for being error-prone.

Role of DNA Repair

Modulation of the multiple pathways that provide genomic maintenance including DNA replication enzymes and associated factors, DNA repair proteins, and transcription factors can markedly impact the overall accumulation of mutations in both chromosomal and mtDNA and thereby contribute to genomic instability and aging phenotypes. Mutant mice defective in individual DNA repair pathways frequently show increased genomic instability as well as hypersensitivity to specific DNA-damaging agents. Mutations in certain DNA repair genes in mice and humans lead to phenotypes that, in some respects, mimic aging including premature-aging or segmental progeroids. Defects in NHEJ, homologous recombination (HR), and nucleotide excision repair (NER) have been shown to cause aging-like phenotypes in mice (shown in Table 4.2) and humans.

Mammals employ various pathways to repair specific types of DNA damage. There are four broad classes of DNA repair, direct reversal repair, excision repair, mismatch repair and recombinational repair (RER), distinguished primarily by their general mechanisms of action.

Table 4.2 Features of selected models of premature aging in the mouse

Mutant	Cellular process	Accelerated fibroblast senescence
ATM	DSB signaling/repair	Yes
Bub1bH/H	Spindle assembly checkpoint	Yes
BRCA1D11/D11/p53+/−	DSB repair	Yes
DNA-PKcs	NHEJ	No
Ercc1, XPF	Nucleotide excision repair, cross-link repair	Yes
Ku80	NHEJ, other	Yes
Dysfunctional p53 (p44 Tg)	DNA damage response	Yes
PASG/Lsh	DNA methylation	Yes
Polg	Mitochondrial DNA polymerase	ND
Rad50S/S	DSB repair	No
Terc	Telomere maintenance	Yes
Terc/Atm	Telomere maintenance/DSB signaling/repair	Yes
Terc/DNA-PKcs	Telomere maintenance/NHEJ	ND
Terc/Parp-1	Telomere maintenance/ DNA repair	ND
Terc/Ku80	Telomere maintenance/NHEJ	ND
Terc/Wrn	Telomere maintenance/DNA repair	Yes
Terc/Wrn/Blm	Telomere maintenance/DNA repair	Yes
TopIIIbeta	Topoisomerase	ND
Wrn	DNA repair	YES
XPA/CSB	NER, transcription	ND
XPDTTD	NER, transcription	ND
XPDTTD/XPA	NER, transcription	ND

ND: Not determined

The direct reversal pathway consists of repair proteins that act directly on a damaged base and re-establish the correct structure without removing the damaged nucleotide. For example, direct repair of photoproducts and UV-induced cyclobutane pyrimidine dimers is carried out by photolyase described in yeast, *Xenopus* and *Drosophila.* In mammalian cells, direct reversal of O6 adducts caused by chemotherapy agents is accomplished by the alkyltransferase protein O6-methylguanine DNA methyltransferase (MGMT).

Single-stranded DNA lesions are repaired via nucleotide excision repair (NER) or base excision repair (BER), depending on the type of lesion. Bulky photodimer single-strand lesions induced by UV irradiation are primarily repaired by NER, whereas more simple types of single-stranded lesions usually are repaired by BER. BER is the primary pathway for repairing spontaneously occurring single-strand DNA lesions, such as those arising from endogenous alkylation (usually methylation), base oxidation, and deamination events, as well as small, nonhelix-distorting DNA lesions induced by chemical mutagens such as the alkylating agent methyl-methane sulphonate (MMS) [237]. BER is also the main pathway for the repair of 8-oxodG. The BER pathway may repair up to one million nucleotides per cell per day [238]. BER involves the removal of relatively short stretches of DNA, between 1 and 13 nucleotides. The general scheme of the BER pathway entails removal of the damaged base by a glycosylase, cleavage of the phosphodiester backbone by an apyrimidinic/apurinic (AP) endonuclease or glycosylase/lyase, insertion of the complementary nucleotides by a polymerase with the removal of the phospho-deoxyribose group, and ligation of the DNA backbone restoring the native structure and sequence [239].

Consistent with the view that declining DNA repair capacity with age may contribute to the accumulation of DNA damage, a decline in BER capacity concomitant with decreased levels of DNA polymerase β (both activity levels and content) were reported in all tissues examined in 24 month old compared to 4 month old mice [240]. Nuclear 8-oxodG incision activity showed no significant change with age in contrast to the mitochondrial 8-oxodG incision activity which increased with age in the mouse liver [241]. Moreover, this study also found that the aging-induced elevation in mitochondrial BER activity in mice (which has also been reported in rat heart and liver) was not due to a general upregulation of BER/DNA-metabolizing enzymes since no change with aging was found in either uracil glycosylase or endonuclease G in either mitochondria or nucleus. Interestingly, a general upregulation of nuclear BER occurs in mice with caloric restriction, which was not seen in most tissues examined with mitochondrial BER activities indicating differential aging-mediated regulation in these organelles [242].

Among the transgenic mouse models with mutations in DNA excision repair, only those that affect NER display symptoms of accelerated aging. Germline deletion in mice of any gene essential for BER function is embryonic lethal, consistent with the high frequency of BER lesions and necessity for their rapid removal. On the other hand, germline deletion of one of the many glycosylase genes, which repair only a subset of BER substrates, generally confer no obvious phenotype [243], probably as a result of functional redundancy. Similarly, hereditary defects in essential BER components have not been found in humans, most likely because they are embryonic lethal.

MMR (mismatch repair) a highly evolutionarily conserved pathway is a post-replicative DNA repair system which has been estimated to contribute a 1000-fold increase to the fidelity of replication [244]. MMR corrects errors made during DNA copying, such as the mispairing of an adenosine base with an guanosine; correction of A-C and T-C mismatches is more efficient than G-A and T-C mismatches. While DNA methylation is used to distinguish which base should be corrected in prokaryotic organisms, this appears not to be case in multi-cellular organisms and the means of mismatch detection is unknown. Mismatch repair differs from BER primarily in the first glycosylase, which recognizes and removes *mispaired* bases in contrast to BER which recognizes and removes *defective* bases. In MMR, removal of the mispaired base leaves an AP site which can then be repaired by the subsequent BER pathway enzymes. Importantly, failures in MMR directly results in mutations, whereas failures in BER result in DNA damage which may or may not lead to mutations. MMR corrects not only single mispaired base, but also insertion/deletion loops (IDLs) that result from strand misalignments, and which can produce frameshift mutations. MMR also plays a significant role in protecting against incorporation of 8-OHdG/8-oxoG into DNA.

NER is activated by a wide range of helix-distorting DNA lesions, including UV-induced photoproducts, bulky chemical adducts, and certain oxidative lesions. The NER pathway repairs DNA lesions irrespective of genome location and point in the cell cycle [245, 246]. Through a two-step recognition process, NER recognizes a broad spectrum of base alterations. The initial process depends on the broad capability of XPC-hR23B to recognize and bind to a large number of DNA lesions based on the ability of this protein complex to distinguish unusual DNA conformations and to recruit the multisubunit, basal transcription factor TFIIH allowing assembly of the larger NER complex. In subsequent steps in the NER pathway, the helicase subunits XPB and XPD of TFIIH unwind DNA allowing the XPA-RPA heterodimer to interact directly with the lesion while simultaneously XPC-hR23B leaves the repair complex. XPA verifies the presence of a chemically altered base and the initial damage recognition. If base alterations are identified a repair tract of 25–32 nucleotides is removed by XPG and XPF-ERCC1 endonucleases. XPG (present in the repair complex prior to damage verification) is activated only subsequent to XPF-ERCC1 has been positioned 5′ to the nick. After positive damage verification by XPA, activated XPG cuts 3′ to the lesion. Following incision, most of the NER complex leaves the repair site and the remaining single-strand DNA tract is stabilized and protected by RPA. Resynthesis is carried out by the replicative polymerases Polδ and Polε, assisted by their processivity factor PCNA and RFC, and DNA ligase I (LIGI) seals the remaining nick.

In an alternate pathway, NER can also be coupled with transcription, hence the term "transcription-coupled repair" pathway (TCR), in which NER repairs bulky lesions of transcribed genes. TCR occurs in response to the RNA polymerase II stalling such as occurs when this transcriptional enzyme encounters an altered base incapable of normal hydrogen bonding, which acts as damage recognition trigger. Two additional proteins CSA and CSB are necessary for the assembly of the NER complex and contribute to the removal of the stalled RNA polymerase II to create access for repair proteins [247].

Mammalian NER has been reconstituted *in vitro* and involves at least 25 different proteins, including seven factors involved in the human disease Xeroderma Pigmentosum (XPA to XPG) as well as two involved in Cockayne's syndrome (CSA and CSB) [247]. Mutations in some NER pathway factors can lead to premature aging syndromes in mice and humans [248].

Double-strand breaks (DSBs) are primarily due to ionizing radiation or very high doses of alkylating carcinogens such as nitrogen mustards. Even with ionizing radiation, DSBs tend to be relatively rare, produced with lower frequency than single strand breaks. DSBs are difficult to repair and can be very injurious for dividing somatic cells. It is noteworthy that repair of double-strand damage in mammals can best occur in the meiotic division of germ cells when complementary pairs of chromosomes line-up, whereas complementary pairs don't typically line-up as well in somatic cells. The potential consequences of unrepaired or improperly repaired DSBs are severe including cell death, senescence and genomic instability, since such lesions frequently lead to extensive genome rearrangements, including translocations, inversions, and large deletions.

DSBs are primarily repaired by NHEJ or HR pathways. An initial step in both repair pathways involves the detection of the lesion, and this step primarily involves the ataxia-telangiectasia mutated (ATM) kinase, other related phosphatidylinositol 3-kinase-like kinases (PIKKs), as well as proteins (such as the Ku proteins) described below and illustrated in Fig. 4.3. ATM functions as a master regulator of the response to DSBs induced by exogenous and endogenous factors, by phosphorylating and activating a large number of downstream proteins that are involved in DNA repair and checkpoint signaling, and also by activating p53 which in turn can stimulate or repress transcription of many target genes and coordinate the progression of checkpoint, senescence, and apoptosis pathways in response to DSBs and other signals.

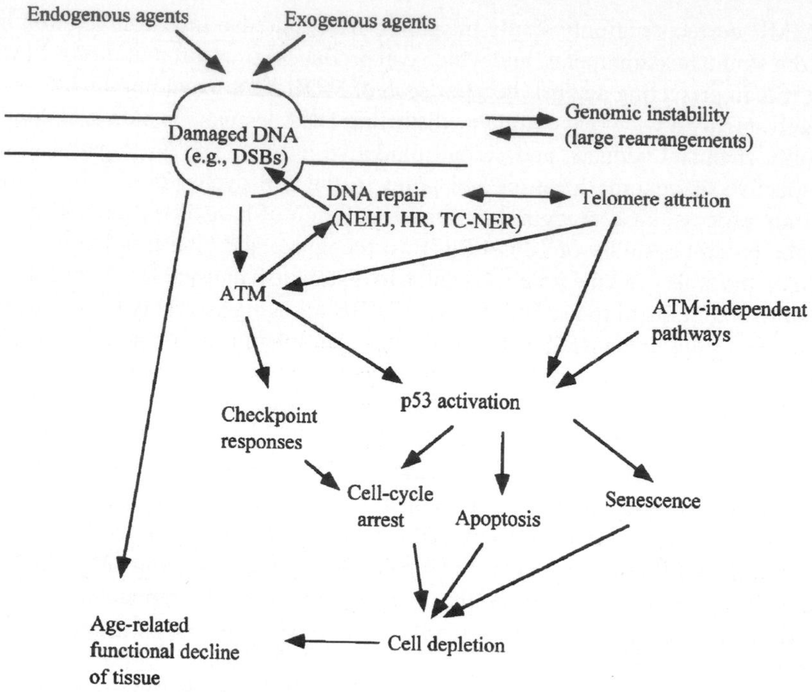

Fig. 4.3 DNA and telomere damage in aging and DNA repair pathways leading to senescence, apoptosis and functional decline

The different outcomes set in motion by this signaling pathway are determined by multiple factors (many not yet completely characterized) that appear to vary with the cell type, as well as the kind, intensity, and duration of the damage [249].

NHEJ is the simplest and most common means of DSB repair in mammalian cells, but it is the least accurate and error-prone. In NHEJ the two broken ends are rejoined without regard to the presence of deletions or rearrangements. Since NHEJ can delete a few nucleotides at sites of DSB repair, this process often will lead to mutation accumulation and may contribute to a decline of cell function and aging [250]. NHEJ typically occurs in the G_1 phase of the cell-cycle when a second copy of the relevant chromosome is not available.

NHEJ is initiated by the Ku protein heterodimer (Ku70/Ku86) binding to broken DNA ends and bringing them together, and recruiting the assembly of a DNA-dependent Protein Kinase complex (DNA-PKcs) and the WRN helicase protein (defective in Werner's syndrome). WRN unwinds the DNA strands and then Ku attachment to WRN and DNA-PKcs strongly stimulates subsequent endonuclease activity (Artemis) to process ends that cannot be rejoined. Finally XRCC4 and the ligase activity (Ligase IV) are enlisted to the repair complex and function together to catalyze end ligation. It is also noteworthy, that in addition to their roles in DSB repair, at least three NHEJ factors, including Ku70, Ku80, and DNA-PKcs, localized to telomeres appear to be operative in telomere maintenance. Recent observations have suggested that ATM kinase may functions in the same pathways as DNA-PK for survival at collapsed replication forks and contribute to NHEJ [251].

Cells such as mouse embryonic fibroblasts deficient in either XRCC4, Ligase IV, Ku70, or Ku80 (but not DNA-PKcs or Artemis) senesce prematurely in culture. In addition, mice deficient for each of these four factors are very small and show widespread neuronal apoptosis during embryogenesis. The demonstration that both premature senescence and neuronal apoptosis can be relieved in strains harboring p53 deficiency suggests that these phenotypes occur as a response to unrepaired DSBs, rather than as a direct consequence of their presence [252].

Phenotypes resembling accelerated aging have been reported in Ku80- and DNA-PKcs-deficient mice [253, 254]. One line of Ku80-deficient mice prematurely exhibits age-specific changes including osteopenia, atrophic skin, liver lesions, and shortened life span [253]. Similarly, a strain of DNA-PKcs-deficient mice was noted to exhibit age-related pathologies, with osteopenia, intestinal atrophy, thymic lymphoma, and reduced longevity [254].

While these findings suggest a potential role for NEHJ in delaying aging, this conclusion is not supported by findings that Ku70- and Artemis-deficient mice do not exhibit premature aging phenotypes. Null Ligase IV and XRCC4 mice display embryonic lethality, precluding analyses of their role in aging. Available data suggest that the aging phenotypes likely do not arise from a failure of DSB repair alone but may rather be mediated by a loss of other functions or combinations of functions of these proteins, including their involvement in telomere function or in checkpont signaling.

NHEJ has been proposed to play a causative role in the aging process. In addition, genetic studies support the notion that NHEJ plays an important role in the repair of ROS-induced DNA lesions. Moreover, in the absence of NHEJ, DSBs often are repaired concomitant with large deletions and/or translocations; thus, absent or even decreased levels of NHEJ also might contribute to accelerated aging.

In contrast to error-prone repair, the less frequently used HR pathway is characterized by a more precise reconstitution of the original DNA sequence using the sister chromatid for information, and is the dominant method used in the S and G_2 phases of the cell-cycle, after a sister chromatid has been created [255, 256]. In HR repair, the ends of the DSB are processed by a exonuclease, such as the Mre11/RAD50/Nbs1 (MRN) protein complex, which clears additional damage to DNA and generates free 3′ single-strand DNA overhangs [257]. This process is accompanied by the binding of number of factors including RAD52 and RPA and followed by strand invasion initiated by RAD51 [257]. Rad52 protein recognizes the DSB and adheres to the free ends of the break while Rad51 searches the undamaged sister chromatid for a homologous repair template. Once bound to DNA, RAD51 directs strand invasion and pairing with undamaged sequences on the homologous strand, a process that is aided by the RAD54 protein. Once strand invasion is completed, DNA polymerases extend the 3′ end using the homologous sequence as a template [258]. Subsequent branch migration leads to the formation of Holliday junctions, in which two double strand DNA duplexes are intertwined and this must be resolved before the sister chromatids can be separated. The identity of the resolvase (mediating the resolution of the strands) in humans is presently unknown, however, Mus81 has been proposed as a candidate [259].

Several other factors yet to be identified also contribute to the homologous recombination repair pathway. The multi-functional tumor suppressor protein BRCA1 complexes and co-localizes with Rad51 during HR repair, and contributes significantly to its activity. BRCA1 deficiency leads to impaired HR-mediated repair of chromosomal DSBs. Activation of BRCA1 has been also implicated in controlling the fidelity of DNA end-joining by precise NHEJ, suggesting that these proteins can be operative in more than one repair pathway [260]. In mammalian cells phosphorylated histone (γ-H2AX) facilitates post-replicational repair of DSBs by recruiting cohesin, a protein complex that holds sister chromatids together [261].

Defects in proteins involved in the HR pathway can lead to aberrant aging. Defects in Rad50 or BRCA1 cause progeroid phenotypes in mice. Mouse strains homozygous for a Rad50 hypomorphic allele show a shortened life span with cells from this strain exhibiting pronounced genomic instability [262]. Mice homozygous for a BRCA1 hypomorphic allele have many features reminiscent of accelerated aging including wasting, skin atrophy, osteopenia, and malignancy [263]. The signs of premature aging in both Rad50 and BRCA1-defective transgenic strains have been shown to occur primarily as a consequence of the p53-mediated responses to unrepaired DNA damage. However, loss of other functions beyond their DNA repair roles may contribute to these aging-like mutant phenotypes since BRCA1 and Rad50 are multi-functional and involved in multiple cellular pathways.

Targeting histone 2AX in mice results in a growth-retarded phenotype with marked chromosomal instability and repair defects [264]. Furthermore, perturbations in ATM function can also lead to symptoms of accelerated aging. Individuals with mutations in the ATM gene suffer from Ataxia-Telangiectasia (AT), a disorder characterized by a prematurely aged appearance, immunodeficiency, cerebellar degeneration, and cancer. Similarly, ATM deficiency in mice recapitulates many of these phenotypes, although the progeroid features in the mouse model are less prominent than in the human phenotype. Given the many targets of ATM, it is difficult to trace the progeroid appearance of AT patients to one specific function of this protein although genomic instability and defective DNA repair may be contributory. The phenotype of premature senescence in mice is reversed in ATM-deficient strains containing p53 deficiency, indicating that downstream p53 function is likely contributory to the premature-aging phenotype in mice [265]. Another pivotal role of ATM is in telomere maintenance with cells from AT patients undergoing premature senescence displaying abnormal telomere regulation [264]. Moreover, mice doubly null for ATM and the telomerase RNA component (Terc) displayed increased telomere erosion and genomic instability, proliferative defects in all cell types and tissues examined and evidence of premature aging [266].

Mitochondrial DNA Repair

In the foregoing discussion, it was noted that alterations of the mitochondrial genome as a result of its high susceptibility to oxidative damage appear to be prominently involved in aging as well as in CVDs associated with aging including cardiomyopathy. Some of the burden of accumulated mtDNA mutations may be directly attributed to limited mtDNA repair capacity compared to nuclear DNA repair.

A number of studies have documented a rather extensive set of BER pathways in mitochondria [267], not entirely surprising since these pathways are most extensively used in the removal of simple oxidative lesions which are prevalent in mtDNA. Gathered observations have documented representative components of mitochondrial BER including glycosylase, AP endonuclease, DNA polymerase and ligase and confirmed the importance of these pathways in repair of mtDNA. While proteins with central roles in MMR, NER and RER pathways are present in mitochondria, which might suggest that some form(s) of these pathways may also exist in the organelle, available evidence has mainly showed that classic NER lesions such as thymine dimers, cisplatin intrastrand cross-links and complex alkyl damage are not able to be repaired in mammalian mitochondria [268, 269]. Evidence of a limited MMR pathway in mammalian mitochondria has also been reported; [270] however, these MMR activities appear unique in that they lack strand discrimination, (i.e., preference for the nicked strand). This could contribute to the observed increased mutation frequencies of mtDNA compared to nuclear DNA.

Support for the presence of recombinational repair pathways in mammalian mitochondria is provided by the fact that both homologous recombination and NHEJ activity are present *in vitro*. *In vitro* analysis demonstrated that mitochondrial extracts from human fibroblasts catalyze homologous recombination between closed plasmid substrates [271]. Data have also shown that mammalian mitochondria were capable of rejoining both cohesive and blunt-ended linearized plasmid DNA suggesting NHEJ activity in the organelle [272]. Interestingly, the nature of deletions obtained in this study was similar to deletions found in Kearns-Sayre (KSS) and Pearson syndromes suggesting that these mitochondrial diseases may originate from defects in the repair of DSBs.

Mitochondrial transcription factor (TFAM) appears to play a role in the protection of mtDNA by binding damaged mtDNA [273]. *In vitro,* TFAM binds to oligonucleotides containing cisplatin adducts and 8-oxoG DNA lesions with a higher affinity than to undamaged DNA. Increased affinity to heavily damaged DNA may allow TFAM to block transcription and replication of damaged mtDNA molecules, and also may mark damaged mtDNA for selective degradation [267]. Furthermore, TFAM is present at levels sufficient to cover the entire mtDNA (900 molecules of TFAM have been estimated for every mtDNA molecule), suggesting that TFAM could act as a physical shield protecting mtDNA [274, 275].

It has been suggested that TFAM may play a role in the initiation of apoptosis in response to DNA damage. Mice with a cardiac-specific knockout of TFAM display a higher rate of apoptosis in the affected tissue, in concert with a progressive mosaic of cardiac-specific mitochondrial ETC defects, mtDNA depletion and the development of DCM and atrioventricular conduction blocks, resulting in early HF [276, 277]. Moreover, during p53-dependent apoptosis, direct interaction between TFAM and p53 has been reported [278]. The mitochondrial localization of p53 leads to a significant increase in the affinity of TFAM for cisplatin damaged DNA, whereas its affinity for oxidative damaged DNA remains unaffected. Delay in the onset of apoptosis, arising in part from the interaction between TFAM and p53, may underlie the higher rate of myocardial apoptosis noted in TFAM-deficient mice.

DNA Repair and Human Diseases of Aging

In humans, several heritable mutations accelerate the onset of multiple aging phenotypes (Table 4.3). Disorders caused by these mutations are termed segmental progeroid syndromes, because they accelerate some but not all signs of normal aging. Mutations giving rise to the symptoms of accelerated aging in these patients partially or wholly inactivate proteins that sense or repair DNA damage highlighting that failure to maintain genomic integrity underlies at least some aging phenotypes [250]. It is important to emphasize that as segmental progerias, premature aging models fail to recapitulate all aspects of aging as it occurs in wild-type animals. In this regard, the myriad of histopathologic changes of normal aging corresponds poorly with the changes that occur in models of premature aging. Nevertheless, the importance of these progeroid models as informative models with relevance to the role of genome maintenance in normal aging process has been underscored by recent demonstration that progeroid syndromes, to varying degrees, accelerate an age-associated transcription pattern strikingly similar to that found with normal aging and thereby the aging phenotype [279]. Microarray analysis of transcription profiles in primary human fibroblasts from normally aged individuals, Werner syndrome (WS) patients and young control individuals, revealed that 91 % of the annotated genes showed similar expression changes in WS and normal aging while 3 % were unique to WS, and 6 % were unique to normal aging [280]. In this study, the largest functional group effected in both WS and normal aging fibroblasts included genes related to DNA and RNA processing, 75 % of which were downregulated. Among the most severely downregulated genes were several genes involved in the RNA polymerase II (RNAP II) complex, which transcribes protein-encoding genes and interacts with the promoter regions as well as with a variety of transcription factors, including RNAP II polypeptide A (*POLR2A*), a second RNAP II subunit, polypeptide J (*POLR2J*), transcription factor Dp-2 (*TFDP2*), a component of the drtf1/e2f transcription factor complex which regulates genes encoding proteins required for the cell cycle progression of S-phase, the *FOXM1 (HFH-11)* transcription factor gene (previously reported to decline in both elderly patients and patients with Hutchinson-Gilford progeria) and downregulated *SMARCA1* and *SMARCB1* products that contribute to chromatin remodeling, providing access for the transcriptional machinery. This analysis also showed a major shared downregulation of cell-cycle regulatory and growth related genes, including reduced expression of *BRF2* (a nuclear transcription factor regulating the response to growth factors), *CSF3R* (a receptor that transduces signals regulating the proliferation, differentiation, and survival of myeloid cells), *INSR* (the insulin receptor gene), *IGF2* (insulin-like growth factor 2 gene), and the *IGF2R* (IGF2 receptor) correlating with the reduced replicative potential of both WS cells and cells from normal old donors. These findings suggest that WS causes acceleration

Table 4.3 Human segmental progeroid disorders

Syndrome	Phenotype	Cellular defect	Gene defect	Mean lifespan
Werner	Gray hair, skin atrophy, cataracts, diabetes, atherosclerosis, malignancies, regional fibrosis, lipid metabolic defects, osteoporosis, hypogonadism, autoimmunity, vascular disease	Transcription, DNA repair (HR, NHEJ, BER), DNA replication + recombination, chromosome defects, telomere metabolism, apoptosis	Loss of function of WRN/DNA helicase	48 yrs
Cockayne	Neurodegeneration, atherosclerosis, diabetes, lipid metabolic disorder, thin hair, poor growth, deafness, hypogonadism, hypertension, cataracts, regional fibrosis, osteoporosis	Transcription, apoptosis, DNA repair: NER (TCR), BER of some types of oxidative damage	Loss of function mutations in CSA and CSB, DNA helicase	20 yrs
Rothmund-Thomson	Alopecia, cataracts, malignancies, gray hair poikiloderma, osteoporosis, hypogonadism	Recombination	DNA helicase	Normal
Trichothio-dystrophy	Cachexia, cataracts, osteoporosis, fragile hair, neurodegeneration (cerebellar ataxia)	DNA repair, basal transcription	Defect in XPD DNA helicase	10 yrs
Bloom	Cancer, hypogonadism, regional fibrosis, growth deficiency, diabetes mellitus, cataracts	Transcription, DNA repair, replication, and recombination, apoptosis, chromosome defects	DNA helicase	28 yrs
Hutchinson-Guilford	Atherosclerosis, sarcopenia, alopecia, sclerosis, osteolysis, reduced adipose tissue	Nuclear stability and transcription	Dominant negative mutations in *LMNA* (Lamin A), nuclear envelope defect	12 yrs
Ataxia telangiectasia	Dermal sclerosis, gray hair, malignancies, immunodeficiency, ataxia	Decreased genome maintenance	Loss of function mutation in ATM	20 yrs

of a normal aging mechanism and implies that the phenotypic manifestations of both WS and aging may be secondary to specific transcriptional defects contributing to cellular degeneration.

The stochastic deregulation of gene expression and the extreme heterogeneity that appears to be fundamental to the aging phenotype in post-mitotic tissues have been recently reported [281]. Analysis of single cardiomyocytes dissociated from samples of both young and old mice, global mRNA amplification and quantification of mRNA levels of a panel of housekeeping and heart-specific genes revealed a striking pattern of heterogeneity in aging. These observations are consistent with a mosaic model of aging in which cell-to-cell differences become increasingly pronounced.

The role of transcriptional defect in aging is also highlighted by defects in several transcription-coupled NER-specific factors CSA or CSB that lead to Cockayne syndrome (CS) in humans, a severely debilitating disorder with striking progeroid features. In addition, CSA- and CSB-deficient mice show much milder phenotypes than their human counterparts [248]. Patients with specific mutations in XPD suffer from trichothiodystrophy (TTD), a disease characterized by photosensitivity, brittle hair, skin defects, and a shortened life span. These patients show defects in transcription of hair- and skin-specific transcripts. In addition, cells derived from TTD patients exhibit NER defects, suggesting that multiple functions of XPD are defective in these individuals. Mice bearing a targeted mutation in XPD, which recapitulates a human TTD mutation, show manifestations similar to human TTD patients and of aging-associated changes such as wasting, scoliosis, osteoporosis, and melanocyte loss [282].

The aging-like phenotypes in human CS patients and in XPDTTD, XPDTTD/XPA, and CSB/XPA mouse mutants may be explained by failure to repair lesions in transcribed genes that can result in cell death, leading to tissue attrition and aging. Stalled RNA polymerase provides a signal for activation of p53-dependent apoptosis [283]. In this regard, it will be of interest to determine whether p53 deficiency rescues the aging-like features of XPDTTD, XPDTTD/XPA, and CSB/XPA mice. Alternatively, the involvement of XPD and the CSB proteins in transcription suggests that impaired transcription of critical genes may play a role in causing these progeroid phenotypes, perhaps by interacting with repair defects in a complicated fashion.

While the role of genome instability and defective DNA repair clearly are contributory to aging phenotypes, many questions remain as to how they are actually involved. The multifunctional nature of many of the repair proteins active in several pathways has made it difficult to ascertain which functions/pathways are critical to aging. The commonality in aging phenotypes elicited by mutations in diverse repair systems suggests that not the lesion itself but the signaling pathways affected may be more critical in the actual aging pathways. A model depicting some of the salient interactions of factors in the aging pathway including genomic instability, mutation accumulation and senescence is shown in Fig. 4.4.

Telomeres and Telomere-related Proteins

As we have previously noted, telomeres are specialized structures that consist of tandem repeats of the DNA sequence TTAGGG and several proteins located at the end of chromosomes, which shorten with each replication unless they are preserved by the action of the enzyme telomerase reverse transcriptase (TERT) [284]. The telomerase enzyme employs an RNA template (TERC) to extend telomeres during the S phase of the cell cycle. Most human somatic cells contain very low levels of telomerase activity. Telomerase access to its DNA substrate is regulated by a rather large group of diverse telomere-associated proteins, some required for replication others involved in the formation of a protective end structure, i.e., "capping" (Fig. 4.5). Particularly notable amongst these proteins are the telomeric repeat-binding factors (TRFs) [285]. TRF1 has been shown to regulate telomere length, assisting the telomerase enzyme while TRF2 has been implicated in modeling the telomere into the T-loop structure, protecting the single-stranded 3′-end overhang from degradation, and binding to the ATM kinase protein to prevent the ATM-dependent DNA damage response. In addition, TRF2 stimulates the helicase activity of both WRN (of Werner's Syndrome) and BLM (of Bloom Syndrome), which are thought to play a role in telomere maintenance. As we have previously noted, other DNA repair factors including DNA damage signaling molecules such as PARP-1, DNA-PKcs, Ku70/80, XRCC4 and ATM have been associated with telomere function. Mice deficient in a DNA-break sensing molecule, PARP (poly [ADP]-ribopolymerase), have increased levels of chromosomal instability associated with extensive telomere shortening while Ku80 null cells showed a telomere shortening associated with extensive chromosome end fusions [286].

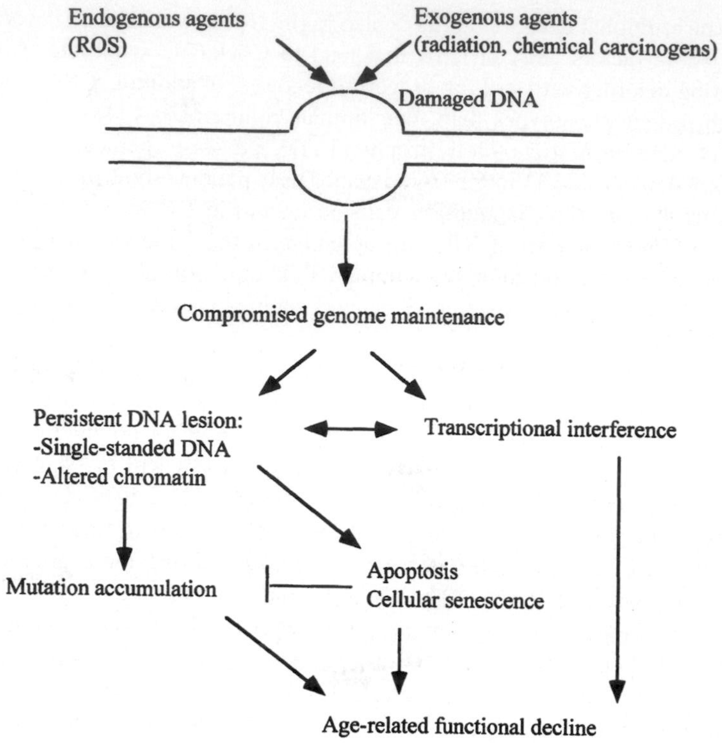

Fig. 4.4 Model depicting interactions of genomic instability, mutation accumulation and senescence in aging

During aging with each successive generation, telomere length is progressively reduced in most somatic cells; after a number of cell cycles, upon reaching a critical size, cellular replication stops and the cell becomes senescent. Age-dependent telomere shortening in most somatic cells, including vascular endothelial cells, smooth muscle cells (SMCs) and cardiomyocytes, appears to impair cellular function and the viability of the aged organism triggering a phenotype of cellular senescence. This phenotype is generally accompanied by a loss of protective proteins termed telomere uncapping, which appears to be a potent signal recognized by cell cycle checkpoint sensors and triggers pathways leading to cell cycle arrest.

Most human somatic cells can undergo only limited replication *in vitro*, a state originally termed replicative senescence, more recently cellular senescence. This state of irreversible cell cycle arrest can be triggered by ROS and diverse DNA damaging agents and is accompanied by a number of characteristic functional and morphological changes. Replicative senescence in human cell lines can be triggered when telomeres can not carry out their normal protective functions. Senescent human fibroblasts display a range of molecular markers characteristic of cells bearing DNA double-strand breaks. The inactivation of DNA damage checkpoint kinases in senescent cells may restore the cell-cycle progression into S phase [287]. Hence, telomere-initiated senescence may reflect a DNA damage checkpoint response that is activated with a direct contribution from dysfunctional telomeres. Transfection of telomerase activity into human cells including retinal pigment epithelial cells and foreskin fibroblasts halted telomere loss and prevented the subsequent proliferation block, which characterizes *in vitro* replicative senescence [288].

Unlike human fibroblasts, mouse embryonic fibroblasts possess high levels of telomerase and long telomeres, and generally do not senesce as a function of telomere attrition [289]. However, despite the apparent absence of telomere shortening, most mouse cells cease dividing after only 10–15 doublings with factors other than telomere length contributing to their senescence. The

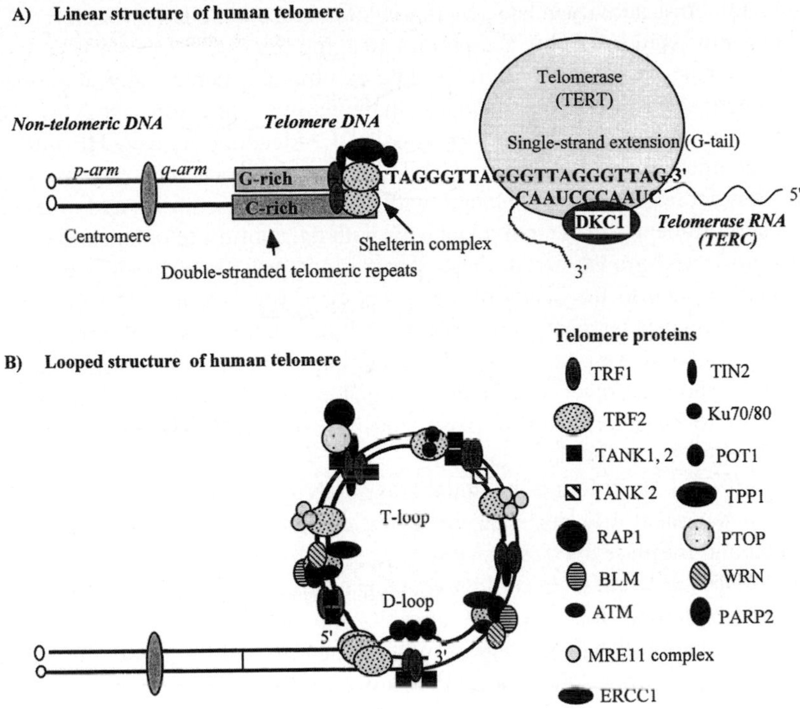

Fig. 4.5 Telomere structure with associated proteins
Linear structure of a human telomere including the telomeric DNA with relative location of double-stranded repeats, associated proteins (shelterin complex) and the telomere RNA (TERC), telomerase (TERT) complex with the single-strand extension (G-tail) noted. B. Looped structure of the telomere indicating relative positions of the telomere D-loop and T-loop and the telomere binding proteins as indicated in the key.

differences in telomerase expression between humans and mice may be a limitation to employ mouse models to study the role of human telomere shortening in age-associated conditions.

Roles for many of the telomere factors in senescence and aging have been established by molecular studies with cells containing mutant TRF2 alleles (e.g., dominant negative). Loss of TRF2 activity and resultant telomere malfunction promoted apoptosis in some mammalian cell-types [290]. These observations also demonstrated that this effect was mediated by the ATM kinase and p53 activation, consistent with activation of a DNA damage checkpoint. Furthermore, TRF2 inhibition in neurons (primary embryonic hippocampal neurons) and mitotic neural cells (astrocytes and neuroblastoma cells) induced by adenovirus-mediated expression of dominant-negative TRF2 triggered a DNA damage response involving the formation of nuclear foci containing phosphorylated histone H2AX and activated ATM in each cell type [291]. A potential explanation for these findings is that telomeres that lack TRF2 signal the onset of apoptosis, because they contain (or expose) regions of damaged DNA. The involvement of ATM suggests that inappropriately exposed telomeric DNA might be like a double-strand break, which is the predominant initiating signal for ATM-mediated p53 activation [266].

Despite its role in replicative senescence in some human cells, the role of telomerase in aging remains largely controversial and undefined. A lack of correlation between telomerase activity and aging of cells *in vivo*, and between telomere length in cells and the maximum life span of the species from which the cells were derived has been well-documented [292]. However, telomerase knock-out mice exhibit some aspects of accelerated aging after three generations including premature greying of the hair, hair loss, impaired wound healing, and compromised hematopoiesis [293]. Furthermore, re-introducing telomerase activity in late generation telomerase-deficient mice, $Terc^{-}/^{-}$ reversed the phenotype of chromosomal instability and premature aging [294].

As with other tissues, the heart in Terc-/- mice exhibits an increasingly abnormal phenotype, progressive telomere shortening, and a reduction in the numbers of cardiomyocytes with successive generations. However, these mice also develop classic DCM leading to severe HF with abnormalities in both cardiac contractility and relaxation [295]. Analysis of isolated cardiomyocytes from these mice demonstrates decreasing telomere length with successive generations and upregulation of p53 expression, most prominently in the individual cells with the shortest telomeres. Since p53 signaling can induce apoptosis and growth arrest, these observations provide a potential explanation for the reduced cell number seen in the hearts of late-generation Terc-/- mice. The finding of increased levels of myocyte apoptosis but comparatively little cellular necrosis is consistent with the view that increased p53 expression is responsible for the reduction in the number of cardiomyocytes [296]. However, the contribution of other tissue abnormalities in the telomerase-null mouse to the cardiac phenotype remains to be determined. The availability of a cardiac-specific telomerase knockout might prove to be informative in that regard.

Previously, Leri et al. have found that telomerase activity was detectable in young adult, fully mature adult, and senescent rat ventricular myocytes, challenging the dogma that this cell population is permanent and irreplaceable [297]. Moreover, these investigators found that aging decreased telomerase activity (by 31%) in male cardiomyocytes, whereas in aging female cardiomyocytes the telomerase activity increased (by 72 %.) These results may underlie the observed myocyte loss that occurs in men as a function of age, in contrast to the preservation of myocyte number in women.

Gathered observations support the concept that the average telomere length is better maintained in conditions of low OS. Selective targeting of antioxidants directly to the mitochondria can counteract telomere shortening and increase life span in fibroblasts under mild OS. As noted in Chapter 2, mitochondrial dysfunction can lead to a loss of cellular proliferative capacity through telomere shortening, and the generation of ROS may signal the nucleus to limit cell proliferation through telomere shortening and telomeres as sensors to damaged mitochondria [298].

In addition to the direct effects of telomeres on aging, it is evident that telomere dysfunction is emerging as an important factor in the pathogenesis of human cardiovascular diseases associated with aging, including hypertension, atherosclerosis, and HF [299, 300]. The implications of these findings for the development of potential cardiovascular therapeutics will be discussed in Chapter 14.

Conclusion

At first glance it would appear that the aging heart is morphologically and functionally compromised by a striking array of defects stemming from diverse sources. The lengthy list of defects, many evident at the cellular and subcellular level, includes amyloid deposition, calcification, fibrosis, cell death and remodeling, mitochondrial dysfunction, production of ROS leading to elevated OS and damaged macromolecules, difficulties with cellular turnover and waste/defect removal, accumulation of DNA and chromosome damage including telomeres, leading to changes in gene expression, genomic instability and a non-proliferative senescent phenotype. In actuality, careful scrutiny of molecular and sub-cellular changes occurring in aging cells has identified some striking inter-relationships between many of these defects, although the actual sequence of events remains speculative.

Although mitochondrial-derived ROS play a central role in a considerable proportion of age-mediated cardiac defects proof that this damage is causative remains unclear. The ROS-mediated defects in DNA, proteins and lipids lead to extensive cardiac remodeling, AGE-glycation and calcium alterations, deficits in mitochondrial bioenergetics and chromosomal abnormalities (e.g., telomeric dysfunction) and may add an excessive burden to the cell maintenance systems, including lysosomal degradation and DNA repair. The most compelling support for the role of mitochondrial dysfunction in aging has emerged from recent transgenic studies, although the resulting picture is by no means clear at this time with some pieces of the puzzle likely missing (e.g., in many analyses the element of time has been lacking). Interestingly, interventions that reverse aging-mediated cardiac defects (e.g., caloric restriction, antioxidants) have begun to be utilized in the identification of gene expression and signaling pathways that are required for the onset of the aging heart phenotypes.

Summary

- With aging the heart develops increasing myocardium and endocardium thickness, left atrial hypertrophy and increased interstitial fibrosis.
- Loss of cardiac myocytes as well as conduction cells and increased levels of fat, collagen and elastic tissue with increased fibrosis are prevalent in the aging heart and are likely contributory to dysrhythmias, conduction defects and defects in cardiac contractility.
- Amyloid deposition and calcification are increasingly found in the aging heart. Also fibrosis, mediated largely by aging effects on cardiac fibroblasts, is a primary correlate of the aging heart characterized by excessive collagen deposition and extracellular matrix defects. These changes contribute to LV dysfunction (primarily diastolic), myocardial stiffness and atrial fibrillation (AF).
- Central to aging-mediated cardiac remodeling is cardiac myocyte cell death arising from apoptosis and necrosis processes, both of which are increased in the aging heart.
- Cardiac aging is associated with mitochondrial generation of ROS leading to an accumulation of cellular and mitochondrial macromolecular damage, including lipid peroxidation altering membrane fluidity and function, protein modifications (e.g., protein nitration and carbonylation) and enzyme function (including the mitochondrial bioenergetic enzymes) and a variety of both nuclear and mtDNA defects.
- The cellular mechanisms to remove/degrade of damaged-worn out organelles, membrane components, defective mitochondria and proteins including lysosomes and proteasomes are less effective in aging cells. Mechanisms leading to this inefficiency while in part involving accumulated non-degradable substrates (e.g., lipofuscin) are not yet known.
- DNA damage, including mtDNA defects, is clearly a primary factor in aging. Defects in DNA can lead to mutations compromising function, chromosomal damage and rearrangement, diminished gene expression and genomic instability.
- Mutational defects in mtDNA can lead to premature aging, cardiomyopathy and heart failure in both animal models and in aging humans, and appear to be linked to increased apoptotic activation.
- Mutations in DNA repair proteins (primarily involved in the nucleotide excision repair and recombination pathways) may cause premature aging syndromes in animals and humans.
- Changes in telomere DNA size and structure are associated with aging and the onset of replicative senescence; these changes can be mediated in the heart by increased OS.

References

1. Kawamura S, Takahashi M, Ishihara T, Uchino F. Incidence and distribution of isolated atrial amyloid: histologic and immunohistochemical studies of 100 aging hearts. Pathol Int 1995;45:335–342
2. Kyle RA, Spittell PC, Gertz MA, Li CY, Edwards WD, Olson LJ, Thibodeau SN. The premortem recognition of systemic senile amyloidosis with cardiac involvement. Am J Med 1996;101:395–400

3. Barasch E, Gottdiener JS, Larsen EK, Chaves PH, Newman AB, Manolio TA. Clinical significance of calcification of the fibrous skeleton of the heart and aortosclerosis in community dwelling elderly. The Cardiovascular Health Study (CHS). Am Heart J 2006;151:39–47
4. Srivatsa SS, Harrity PJ, Maercklein PB, Kleppe L, Veinot J, Edwards WD, Johnson CM, Fitzpatrick LA. Increased cellular expression of matrix proteins that regulate mineralization is associated with calcification of native human and porcine xenograft bioprosthetic heart valves. J Clin Invest 1997;99:996–1009
5. Rajamannan NM, Subramaniam M, Rickard D, Stock SR, Donovan J, Springett M, Orszulak T, Fullerton DA, Tajik AJ, Bonow RO, Spelsberg T. Human aortic valve calcification is associated with an osteoblast phenotype. Circulation 2003;107:2181–2184
6. Vattikuti R, Towler DA. Osteogenic regulation of vascular calcification: an early perspective. Am J Physiol Endocrinol Metab 2004;286:E686–E696
7. Fitzpatrick LA, Turner RT, Ritman ER. Endochondral bone formation in the heart:a possible mechanism of coronary calcification. Endocrinology 2003;144:2214–2219
8. Anversa P, Palackal T, Sonnenblick EH, Olivetti G, Meggs LG, Capasso JM. Myocyte cell loss and myocyte cellular hyperplasia in the hypertrophied aging rat heart. Circ Res 1990;67:871–885
9. Lakatta EG. Cardiovascular aging research: The next horizons. J Am Geriatr Soc 1999;47:613–625
10. Lakatta EG. Changes in cardiovascular function with aging. Eur Heart J 1990;11:22–29
11. Cigola E, Kajstura J, Li B, Meggs LG, Anversa P. Angiotensin II activates programmed myocyte cell death in vitro. Exp. Cell Res 1997;231:363–371
12. Lakatta EG, Levy D. Arterial and cardiac aging: major shareholders in cardiovascular disease Enterprises: part II: the aging heart in health: links to heart disease. Circulation 2003;107:346–354
13. Cain BS, Meldrum DR, Joo KS, Wang J-F, Meng X, Cleveland JC, Banerjee A, Harken AH. Human SERCA2a levels correlate inversely with age in senescent human myocardium. J Am Coll Cardiol 1998;32:458–467
14. Anversa P, Puntillo E, Nikitin P, Olivetti G, Capasso JM, Sonnenblick EH. Effects of age on mechanical and structural properties of myocardium of Fischer 344 rats. Am J Physiol 1989;256:H1440–H1449
15. Fraticelli A, Josephson R, Danziger R, Lakatta E, Spurgeon H. Morphological and contractile characteristics of rat cardiac myocytes from maturation to senescence. Am J Physiol 1989;257:H259–H265
16. Taffet GE, Tate CA. Ca^{2+} ATPase content is lower in cardiac sarcoplasmic reticulum isolated from old rats. Am J Physiol Heart Circ Physiol 1993;264:H1609–H1614
17. Jiang M-T, Narayanan N. Effects of aging on phospholamban phosphorylation and calsium transport in rat cardiac sarcoplasmic reticulum. Mech Ageing Dev 1990;54:87–101
18. Xu A, Narayanan N. Effects of aging on sarcoplasmic reticulum Ca^{2+}-cycling proteins and their phosphorylation in rat myocardium. Am J Physiol Heart Circ Physiol 1998;275:H2087–H2094
19. Lompre AM, Lambert F, Lakatta EG, Schwartz K. Expression of sarcoplasmic reticulum Ca(2+)-ATPase and calsequestrin genes in rat heart during ontogenic development and aging. Circ Res 1991;69:1380–1388
20. Zhou YY, Lakatta EG, Xiao RP. Age-associated alterations in calcium current and its modulation in cardiac myocytes. Drugs Aging 1998;13:159–171
21. Walker KE, Lakatta EG, Houser SR. Age associated changes in membrane currents in rat ventricular myocytes. Cardiovasc Res 1993;27:1968–1977
22. Lakatta EG. Myocardial adaptations in advanced age. Basic Res Cardiol 1993;88:125–133
23. Klima M, Burns TR, Chopra A. Myocardial fibrosis in the elderly. Arch Pathol Lab Med 1990;114:938–942
24. Burlew BS. Diastolic dysfunction in the elderly—the interstitial issue. Am J Geriatr Cardiol 2004;13:29–38
25. de Souza RR. Aging of myocardial collagen. Biogerontology 2002;3:325–335
26. Manabe I, Shindo T, Nagai R. Gene expression in fibroblasts and fibrosis: involvement in cardiac hypertrophy. Circ Res 2002;91:1103–1113
27. Husse B, Isenberg G. CREB expression in cardiac fibroblasts and CREM expression in ventricular myocytes. Biochem Biophys Res Commun 2005;334:1260–1265
28. Lindsey ML, Goshorn DK, Squires CE, Escobar GP, Hendrick JW, Mingoia JT, Sweterlitsch SE, Spinale FG. Age-dependent changes in myocardial matrix metalloproteinase/tissue inhibitor of metalloproteinase profiles and fibroblast function. Cardiovasc Res 2005;66:410–419
29. Fedak PW, Smookler DS, Kassiri Z, Ohno N, Leco KJ, Verma S, Mickle DA, Watson KL, Hojilla CV, Cruz W, Weisel RD, Li RK, Khokha R. TIMP-3 deficiency leads to dilated cardiomyopathy. Circulation 2004;110: 2401–2409
30. Burgess ML, McCrea JC, Hedrick HL. Age-associated changes in cardiac matrix and integrins. Mech Ageing Dev 2001;122:1739–1756
31. Allessie M, Schotten U, Verheule S, Harks E. Gene therapy for repair of cardiac fibrosis: a long way to Tipperary. Circulation 2005;111:391–393
32. Fast VG, Darrow BJ, Saffitz JE, Kleber AG. Anisotropic activation spread in heart cell monolayers assessed by high-resolution optical mapping. Role of tissue discontinuities. Circ Res 1996;79:115–127

33. Camelliti P, Green CR, Kohl P. Structural and functional coupling of cardiac myocytes and fibroblasts. Adv Cardiol 2006;42:132–149
34. Li D, Shinagawa K, Pang L, Leung TK, Cardin S, Wang Z, Nattel S. Effects of angiotensin-converting enzyme inhibition on the development of the atrial fibrillation substrate in dogs with ventricular tachypacing-induced congestive heart failure. Circulation 2001;104:2608–2614
35. Anyukhovsky EP, Sosunov EA, Plotnikov A, Gainullin RZ, Jhang JS, Marboe CC, Rosen MR. Cellular electrophysiologic properties of old canine atria provide a substrate for arrhythmogenesis. Cardiovasc Res 2002;54:462–469
36. Hayashi H, Wang C, Miyauchi Y, Omichi C, Pak HN, Zhou S, Ohara T, Mandel WJ, Lin SF, Fishbein MC, Chen PS, Karagueuzian HS. Aging-related increase to inducible atrial fibrillation in the rat model. J Cardiovasc Electrophysiol 2002;13:801–808
37. Olivetti G, Melissari M, Capasso JM, Anversa P. Cardiomyopathy of the aging human heart. Myocyte loss and reactive cellular hypertrophy. Circ Res 1991;68:1560–1568
38. Olivetti G, Giordano G, Corradi D, Melissari M, Lagrasta C, Gambert SR, Anversa P. Gender differences and aging: effects on the human heart. J Am Coll Cardiol 1995;26:1068–1079
39. Mallat Z, Fornes P, Costagliola R, Esposito B, Belmin J, Lecomte D, Tedgui A. Age and gender effects on cardiomyocyte apoptosis in the normal human heart. J Gerontol A Biol Sci Med Sci 2001;56:M719–M723
40. Saraste A, Pulkki K. Morphologic and biochemical hallmarks of apoptosis. Cardiovasc Res 2000;45:528–537
41. Kanoh M, Takemura G, Misao J, Hayakawa Y, Aoyama T, Nishigaki K, Noda T, Fujiwara T, Fukuda K, Minatoguchi S, Fujiwara H. Significance of myocytes with positive DNA in situ nick end-labeling (TUNEL) in hearts with dilated cardiomyopathy: not apoptosis but DNA repair. Circulation 1999;99:2757–2764
42. Kockx MM, Muhring J, Knaapen MW, de Meyer GR. RNA synthesis and splicing interferes with DNA in situ end labeling techniques used to detect apoptosis. Am J Pathol 1998;152:885–888
43. Duan WR, Garner DS, Williams SD, Funckes-Shippy CL, Spath IS, Blomme EA. Comparison of immunohistochemistry for activated caspase-3 and cleaved cytokeratin 18 with the TUNEL method for quantification of apoptosis in histological sections of PC-3 subcutaneous xenografts. J Pathol 2003;199:221–228
44. Dumont EA, Hofstra L, van Heerde WL, van den Eijnde S, Doevendans PA, DeMuinck E, Daemen MA, Smits JF, Frederik P, Wellens HJ, Daemen MJ, Reutelingsperger CP. Cardiomyocyte death induced by myocardial ischemia and reperfusion: measurement with recombinant human annexin-V in a mouse model. Circulation 2000;102:1564–1568
45. Honda O, Kuroda M, Joja I, Asaumi J, Takeda Y, Akaki S, Togami I, Kanazawa S, Kawasaki S, Hiraki Y. Assessment of secondary necrosis of Jurkat cells using a new microscopic system and double staining method with annexin V and propidium iodide. Int J Oncol 2000;16:283–288
46. Searle J, Kerr JF, Bishop CJ. Necrosis and apoptosis: distinct modes of cell death with fundamentally different significance. Pathol Ann 1982;17:229–259
47. Gill C, Mestril R, Samali A. Losing heart: the role of apoptosis in heart disease—a novel therapeutic target. FASEB J 2002;16:135–146
48. Malhi H, Gores GJ, Lemasters JJ. Apoptosis and necrosis in the liver: a tale of two deaths? Hepatology 2006;43:S31–S44
49. Kim JS, He L, Lemasters JJ. Mitochondrial permeability transition: a common pathway to necrosis and apoptosis. Biochem Biophys Res Commun 2003;304:463–470
50. Lemasters JJ, Nieminen AL, Qian T, Trost LC, Elmore SP, Nishimura Y, Crowe RA, Cascio WE, Bradham CA, Brenner DA, Herman B. The mitochondrial permeability transition in cell death: a common mechanism in necrosis, apoptosis and autophagy. Biochim Biophys Acta 1998;1366:177–196
51. Zamzami N, Hirsch T, Dallaporta B, Petit PX, Kroemer G. Mitochondrial implication in accidental and programmed cell death: apoptosis and necrosis. J Bioenerg Biomembr 1997;29:185–193
52. Tatsumi T, Shiraishi J, Keira N, Akashi K, Mano A, Yamanaka S, Matoba S, Fushiki S, Fliss H, Nakagawa M. Intracellular ATP is required for mitochondrial apoptotic pathways in isolated hypoxic rat cardiac myocytes. Cardiovasc Res 2003;59:428–440
53. Kajstura J, Cheng W, Sarangarajan R, Li P, Li B, Nitahara JA, Chapnick S, Reiss K, Olivetti G, Anversa P. Necrotic and apoptotic myocyte cell death in the aging heart of Fischer 344 rats. Am J Physiol 1996;271:H1215–H1228
54. Goldspink DF, Burniston JG, Tan LB. Cardiomyocyte death and the ageing and failing heart. Exp Physiol 2003;88:447–458
55. Ashkenazi A, Dixit VM. Death receptors: signaling and modulation. Science 1998;281:1305–1308
56. Muzio M, Chinnaiyan AM, Kischkel FC, O'Rourke K, Shevchenko A, Ni J, Scaffidi C, Bretz JD, Zhang M, Gentz R, Mann M, Krammer PH, Peter ME, Dixit VM. FLICE, a novel FADD-homologous ICE/CED-3-like protease, is recruited to the CD95 (Fas/APO-1) death—inducing signaling complex. Cell 1996;85: 817–827

57. Boatright KM, Renatus M, Scott FL, Sperandio S, Shin H, Pedersen IM, Ricci JE, Edris WA, Sutherlin DP, Green DR, Salvesen GS. A unified model for apical caspase activation. Mol Cell 2003;11:529–541
58. Kajstura J, Cheng W, Reiss K, Clark WA, Sonnenblick EH, Krajewski S, Reed JC, Olivetti G, Anversa P. Apoptotic and necrotic myocyte cell deaths are independent contributing variables of infarct size in rats. Lab Invest 1996;74:86–107
59. Tanaka M, Ito H, Adachi S, Akimoto H, Nishikawa T, Kasajima T, Marumo F, Hiroe M. Hypoxia induces apoptosis with enhanced expression of Fas antigen messenger RNA in cultured neonatal rat cardiomyocytes. Circ Res 1994;75:426–433
60. Yamaguchi S, Yamaoka M, Okuyama M, Nitoube J, Fukui A, Shirakabe M, Shirakawa K, Nakamura N, Tomoike H. Elevated circulating levels and cardiac secretion of soluble Fas ligand in patients with congestive heart failure. Am J Cardiol 1999;83:1500–1503
61. Torre-Amione G, Kapadia S, Lee J, Durand JB, Bies RD, Young JB, Mann DL. Tumor necrosis factor-alpha and tumor necrosis factor receptors in the failing human heart. Circulation 1996;93:704–711
62. Krown KA, Page MT, Nguyen C, Zechner D, Gutierrez V, Comstock KL, Glembotski CC, Quintana PJ, Sabbadini RA. Tumor necrosis factor alpha-induced apoptosis in cardiac myocytes. Involvement of the sphingolipid signaling cascade in cardiac cell death. J Clin Invest 1996; 98:2854–2865
63. Sack MN, Smith RM, Opie LH. Tumor necrosis factor in myocardial hypertrophy and ischaemia—an anti-apoptotic perspective. Cardiovasc Res 2000;45:688–695
64. Kurrelmeyer KM, Michael LH, Baumgarten G, Taffet GE, Peschon JJ, Sivasubramanian N, Entman ML, Mann DL. Endogenous tumor necrosis factor protects the adult cardiac myocyte against ischemic-induced apoptosis in a murine model of acute myocardial infarction. Proc Natl.Acad Sci USA 2000;97:5456–5461
65. Crow MT, Mani K, Nam YJ, Kitsis RN. The mitochondrial death pathway and cardiac myocyte apoptosis. Circ Res 2004;95:957–970
66. Du C, Fang M, Li Y, Li L, Wang X. Smac, a mitochondrial protein that promotes cytochrome c-dependent caspase activation by eliminating IAP inhibition. Cell 2000;102:33–42
67. Li LY, Luo X, Wang X. Endonuclease G is an apoptotic DNase when released from mitochondria. Nature 2001;412:95–99
68. Liu X, Kim CN, Yang J, Jemmerson R, Wang X. Induction of apoptotic program in cell-free extracts: requirement for dATP and cytochrome c. Cell 1996;86:147–157
69. Susin SA, Lorenzo HK, Zamzami N, Marzo I, Snow BE, Brothers GM, Mangion J, Jacotot E, Costantini P, Loeffler M, Larochette N, Goodlett DR, Aebersold R, Siderovski DP, Penninger JM, Kroemer G. Molecular characterization of mitochondrial apoptosis-inducing factor. Nature 1999;397:441–446
70. Acehan D, Jiang X, Morgan DG, Heuser JE, Wang X, Akey CW. Three-dimensional structure of the apoptosome: implications for assembly, procaspase-9 binding, and activation. Mol Cell 2002;9:423–432
71. Hu Y, Ding L, Spencer DM, Nunez G. WD-40 repeat region regulates Apaf-1 self-association and procaspase-9 activation. J Biol Chem 1998;273:33489–33494
72. Qin H, Srinivasula SM, Wu G, Fernandes-Alnemri T, Alnemri ES, Shi Y. Structural basis of procaspase-9 recruitment by the apoptotic protease-activating factor 1. Nature 1999;399:549–557
73. Zou H, Henzel WJ, Liu X, Lutschg A, Wang X. Apaf-1, a human protein homologous to C. elegans CED-4, participates in cytochrome c-dependent activation of caspase-3. Cell 1997;90:405–413
74. Gross A, Yin XM, Wang K, Wei MC, Jockel J, Milliman C, Erdjument-Bromage H, Tempst P, Korsmeyer SJ. Caspase cleaved BID targets mitochondria and is required for cytochrome c release, while BCL-XL prevents this release but not tumor necrosis factor-R1/Fas death. J Biol Chem 1999;274:1156–1163
75. Luo X, Budihardjo I, Zou H, Slaughter C, Wang X. Bid, a Bcl2 interacting protein, mediates cytochrome c release from mitochondria in response to activation of cell surface death receptors. Cell 1998;94:481–490
76. Peter ME. The flip side of FLIP. Biochem J 2004;382:e1–e3
77. Imanishi T, Murry CE, Reinecke H, Hano T, Nishio I, Liles WC, Hofsta L, Kim K, O'Brien KD, Schwartz SM, Han DK. Cellular FLIP is expressed in cardiomyocytes and down-regulated in TUNEL-positive grafted cardiac tissues. Cardiovasc Res 2000;48:101–110
78. Shiozaki EN, Chai J, Rigotti DJ, Riedl SJ, Li P, Srinivasula SM, Alnemri ES, Fairman R, Shi Y. Mechanism of XIAP-mediated inhibition of caspase-9. Mol Cell 2003;11:519–527
79. Sun C, Cai M, Meadows RP, Xu N, Gunasekera AH, Herrmann J, Wu JC, Fesik SW. NMR structure and mutagenesis of the third Bir domain of the inhibitor of apoptosis protein XIAP. J Biol Chem 2000;275: 33777–33781
80. Scheubel RJ, Bartling B, Simm A, Silber RE, Drogaris K, Darmer D, Holtz J. Apoptotic pathway activation from mitochondria and death receptors without caspase-3 cleavage in failing human myocardium: fragile balance of myocyte survival? J Am Coll Cardiol 2002;39:481–488
81. Nam YJ, Mani K, Ashton AW, Peng CF, Krishnamurthy B, Hayakawa Y, Lee P, Korsmeyer SJ, Kitsis RN. Inhibition of both the extrinsic and intrinsic death pathways through nonhomotypic death-fold interactions. Mol Cell 2004;15:901–912

82. Gustafsson AB, Tsai JG, Logue SE, Crow MT, Gottlieb RA. Apoptosis repressor with caspase recruitment domain protects against cell death by interfering with Bax activation. J Biol Chem 2004;279:21233–21238
83. Ekhterae D, Lin Z, Lundberg MS, Crow MT, Brosius FC 3rd, Nunez G. ARC inhibits cytochrome c release from mitochondria and protects against hypoxia-induced apoptosis in heart-derived H9c2 cells. Circ Res 1999;85:e70–e77
84. Scorrano L, Oakes SA, Opferman JT, Cheng EH, Sorcinelli MD, Pozzan T, Korsmeyer SJ. BAX and BAK regulation of endoplasmic reticulum Ca2+: a control point for apoptosis. Science 2003;300:135–139
85. Morishima N, Nakanishi K, Tsuchiya K, Shibata T, Seiwa E. Translocation of Bim to the endoplasmic reticulum (ER) mediates ER stress signaling for activation of caspase-12 during ER stress-induced apoptosis. J Biol Chem 2004;279:50375–50381
86. Phaneuf S, Leeuwenburgh C. Cytochrome c release from mitochondria in the aging heart: a possible mechanism for apoptosis with age. Am J Physiol Integr Comp Physiol 2002;282:R423–R430
87. Pollack M, Phaneuf S, Dirks A, Leeuwenburgh C. The role of apoptosis in the normal aging brain, skeletal muscle, and heart. Ann NY Acad Sci 2002;959:93–107
88. Torella D, Rota M, Nurzynska D, Musso E, Monsen A, Shiraishi I, Zias E, Walsh K, Rosenzweig A, Sussman MA, Urbanek K, Nadal-Ginard B, Kajstura J, Anversa P, Leri A. Cardiac stem cell and myocyte aging, heart failure, and insulin-like growth factor-1 overexpression. Circ Res 2004;94:514–524
89. Kujoth GC, Hiona A, Pugh TD, Someya S, Panzer K, Wohlgemuth SE, Hofer T, Seo AY, Sullivan R, Jobling WA, Morrow JD, Van Remmen H, Sedivy JM, Yamasoba T, Tanokura M, Weindruch R, Leeuwenburgh C, Prolla TA. Mitochondrial DNA mutations, oxidative stress, and apoptosis in mammalian aging. Science 2005;309:481–484
90. Chen Q, Vazquez EJ, Moghaddas S, Hoppel CL, Lesnefsky EJ. Production of reactive oxygen species by mitochondria: Central role of complex III. J Biol Chem 2003;278:36027–36031
91. Herrero A, Barja G. Localization of the site of oxygen radical generation inside the complex I of heart and nonsynaptic brain mammalian mitochondria. J Bioenerg Biomembr 2000;32:609–615
92. McLennan HR, Degli Esposti M. The contribution of mitochondrial respiratory complexes to the production of reactive oxygen species. J Bioenerg Biomembr 2000;32:153–162
93. Melov S. Mitochondrial oxidative stress. Physiologic consequences and potential for a role in aging. Ann NY Acad Sci 2000;908:219–225
94. Brown GC. Nitric oxide and mitochondrial respiration. Biochim Biophys Acta 1999;1411:351–369
95. Riobo NA, Clementi E, Melani M, Boveris A, Cadenas E, Moncada S, Poderoso JJ. Nitric oxide inhibits mitochondrial NADH: ubiquinone reductase activity through peroxynitrite formation. Biochem J 2001;359: 139–151
96. Murray J, Taylor SW, Zhang B, Ghosh SS, Capaldi RA. Oxidative damage to mitochondrial complex I due to peroxynitrite: identification of reactive tyrosines by mass spectrometry. J Biol Chem 2003;278:37223–37230
97. Cassina AM, Hodara R, Souza JM, Thomson L, Castro L, Ischiropoulos H, Freeman BA, Radi R. Cytochrome c nitration by peroxynitrite. J Biol Chem 2000;275:21409–21415
98. Castro L, Rodriguez M, Radi R. Aconitase is readily inactivated by peroxynitrite, but not by its precursor, nitric oxide. J Biol Chem 1994;269:29409–29415
99. Packer MA, Scarlett JL, Martin SW, Murphy MP. Induction of the mitochondrial permeability transition by peroxynitrite. Biochem Soc Trans 1997;25:909–914
100. Di Lisa F, Bernardi P. Mitochondrial function and myocardial aging. A critical analysis of the role of permeability transition. Cardiovasc Res 2005;66:222–232
101. Brookes PS, Darley-Usmar VM. Role of calcium and superoxide dismutase in sensitizing mitochondria to peroxynitrite-induced permeability transition. Am J Physiol Heart Circ Physiol 2004;286:H39–H46
102. Suh JH, Heath SH, Hagen T. Two subpopulations of mitochondria in the aging rat heart display heterogenous levels of oxidative stress. Free Radic Biol Med 2003;35:1064–1072
103. Judge S, Jang YM, Smith A, Hagen T, Leeuwenburgh C. Age-associated increases in oxidative stress and antioxidant enzyme activities in cardiac interfibrillar mitochondria: implications for the mitochondrial theory of aging. FASEB J 2005;19:419–421
104. Okuda M, Lee HC, Kumar C, Chance B. Comparison of the effect of a mitochondrial uncoupler, 2,4-dinitrophenol and adrenaline on oxygen radical production in the isolated perfused rat liver. Acta Physiol Scand 1992;145:159–168
105. Korshunov SS, Korkina OV, Ruuge EK, Skulachev VP, Starkov AA. Fatty acids as natural uncouplers preventing generation of O_2^- and H_2O_2 by mitochondria in the resting state. FEBS Lett 1998;435:215–218
106. Casteilla L, Rigoulet M, Penicaud L. Mitochondrial ROS metabolism: modulation by uncoupling proteins. IUBMB Life 2001;52:181–188
107. Harper ME, Bevilacqua L, Hagopian K, Weindruch R, Ramsey JJ. Ageing, oxidative stress, and mitochondrial uncoupling. Acta Physiol Scand 2004;182:321–333
108. Lee CK, Allison DB, Brand J, Weindruch R, Prolla TA. Transcriptional profiles associated with aging and middle age-onset caloric restriction in mouse hearts. Proc Natl Acad Sci USA 2002;99:14988–14993

109. Hansford RG, Castro F. Age-linked changes in the activity of enzymes of the tricarboxylate cycle and lipid oxidation, and of carnitine content, in muscles of the rat. Mech Ageing Dev 1982;19:191–200
110. Papa S. Mitochondrial oxidative phosphorylation changes in the life span. Molecular aspects and physiopathological implications. Biochim Biophys Acta 1996;1276:87–105
111. Wei YH, Lu CY, Lee HC, Pang CY, Ma YS. Oxidative damage and mutation to mitochondrial DNA and age-dependent decline of mitochondrial respiratory function. Ann NY Acad Sci 1998; 854:155–170
112. Maklashina E, Ackrell BA. Is defective electron transport at the hub of aging? Aging Cell 2004;3:21–27
113. Miro O, Casademont J, Casals E, Perea M, Urbano-Marquez A, Rustin P, Cardellach F. Aging is associated with increased lipid peroxidation in human hearts, but not with mitochondrial respiratory chain enzyme defects. Cardiovasc Res 2000;47:624–631
114. Marin-Garcia J, Ananthakrishnan R, Goldenthal MJ. Human mitochondrial function during cardiac growth and development. Mol Cell Biochem 1998;179:21–26
115. Torii K, Sugiyama S, Takagi K, Satake T, Ozawa T. Age-related decrease in respiratory muscle mitochondrial function in rats. Am J Respir Cell Mol Biol 1992;6:88–92
116. Barazzoni R, Short KR, Nair KS. Effects of aging on mitochondrial DNA copy number and cytochrome c oxidase gene expression in rat skeletal muscle, liver, and heart. J Biol Chem 2000;275:3343–3347
117. Lenaz G, D'Aurelio M, Merlo Pich M, Genova ML, Ventura B, Bovina C, Formiggini G, Parenti Castelli G. Mitochondrial bioenergetics in aging. Biochim Biophys Acta 2000;1459:397–404
118. Genova ML, Castelluccio C, Fato R, Parenti Castelli G, Merlo Pich M, Formiggini G, Bovina C, Marchetti M, Lenaz G. Major changes in complex I activity in mitochondria from aged rats may not be detected by direct assay of NADH:coenzyme Q reductase. Biochem J 1995;311:105–109
119. Muller-Hocker J. Cytochrome-c-oxidase deficient cardiomyocytes in the human heart—an age-related phenomenon. A histochemical ultracytochemical study. Am J Pathol 1989;134:1167–1173.
120. Paradies G, Ruggiero FM, Petrosillo G, Quagliariello E. Age-dependent decline in the cytochrome c oxidase activity in rat heart mitochondria: role of cardiolipin. FEBS Lett 1997;406:136–138
121. Guerrieri F, Capozza G, Kalous M, Zanotti F, Drahota Z, Papa S. Age-dependent changes in the mitochondrial F0F1 ATP synthase. Arch Gerontol Geriatr 1992;14:299–308
122. Davies SM, Poljak A, Duncan MW, Smythe GA, Murphy MP. Measurements of protein carbonyls, ortho- and meta-tyrosine and oxidative phosphorylation complex activity in mitochondria from young and old rats. Free Radic Biol Med 2001;31:181–190
123. Hoppel CL, Moghaddas S, Lesnefsky EJ. Interfibrillar cardiac mitochondrial comples III defects in the aging rat heart. Biogerontology 2002;3:41–44
124. Lesnefsky EJ, Gudz TI, Moghaddas S, Migita CT, Ikeda-Saito M, Turkaly PJ, Hoppel CL. Aging decreases electron transport complex III activity in heart interfibrillar mitochondria by alteration of the cytochrome c binding site. J Mol Cell Cardiol 2001;33:37–47
125. Fannin SW, Lesnefsky EJ, Slabe TJ, Hassan MO, Hoppel CL. Aging selectively decreases oxidative capacity in rat heart interfibrillar mitochondria. Arch Biochem Biophys 1999;372:399–407
126. Terman A, Brunk UT. Autophagy in cardiac myocyte homeostasis, aging, and pathology. Cardiovasc Res 2005;68:355–365
127. Yoshida K, Hanafusa T, Matoba R, Wakasugi C. Proteolysis of myosin and troponin in human myocardium of elderly subjects. Jpn Heart J 1990;31:683–691
128. Cuervo AM, Dice JF. Age-related decline in chaperone-mediated autophagy. J Biol Chem 2000;275: 31505–31513
129. Cuervo AM. Autophagy: many paths to the same end. Mol Cell Biochem 2004;263:55–72
130. Levine B, Klionsky DJ. Development by self-digestion: molecular mechanisms and biological functions of autophagy. Dev Cell 2004;6:463–477
131. Ohsumi Y, Mizushima N. Two ubiquitin-like conjugation systems essential for autophagy. Semin Cell Dev Biol 2004;15:231–236
132. Kissova I, Deffieu M, Manon S, Camougrand N. Uth1p is involved in the autophagic degradation of mitochondria. J Biol Chem 2004;279:39068–39074
133. Lemasters JJ. Selective mitochondrial autophagy, or mitophagy, as a targeted defense against oxidative stress, mitochondrial dysfunction, and aging. Rejuvenation Res 2005;8:3–5
134. Terman A, Brunk UT. The aging myocardium: roles of mitochondrial damage and lysosomal degradation. Heart Lung Circ 2005;14:107–114
135. Yan L, Vatner DE, Kim SJ, Ge H, Masurekar M, Massover WH, Yang G, Matsui Y, Sadoshima J, Vatner SF. Autophagy in chronically ischemic myocardium. Proc Natl Acad Sci USA 2005;102:13807–13812
136. Takemura G, Miyata S, Kawase Y, Okada H, Maruyama R, Fujiwara H. Autophagic degeneration and death of cardiomyocytes in heart failure. Autophagy 2006;2:212–214
137. Terman A, Brunk UT. On the degradability and exocytosis of ceroid/lipofuscin in cultured rat cardiac myocytes. Mech Ageing Dev 1998;100:145–156

138. Grune T, Merker K, Jung T, Sitte N, Davies KJ. Protein oxidation and degradation during postmitotic senescence. Free Radic Biol Med 2005;39:1208–1215
139. Rooyackers OE, Adey DB, Ades PA, Nair KS. Effect of age on in vivo rates of mitochondrial protein synthesis in human skeletal muscle. Proc Natl Acad Sci USA 1996;93:15364–15369
140. Brunk UT, Terman A. The mitochondrial-lysosomal axis theory of aging: accumulation of damaged mitochondria as a result of imperfect autophagocytosis. Eur J Biochem 2002;269:1996–2002
141. Terman A, Dalen H, Eaton JW, Neuzil J, Brunk UT. Aging of cardiac myocytes in culture: oxidative stress, lipofuscin accumulation, and mitochondrial turnover. Ann NY Acad Sci 2004;1019:70–77
142. Terman A, Brunk UT. Myocyte aging and mitochondrial turnover. Exp Gerontol 2004;39:701–705
143. Terman A, Dalen H, Brunk UT. Ceroid/lipofuscin-loaded human fibroblasts show decreased survival time and diminished autophagocytosis during amino acid starvation. Exp Gerontol 1999;34:943–957
144. Terman A, Abrahamsson N, Brunk UT. Ceroid/lipofuscin-loaded human fibroblasts show increased susceptibility to oxidative stress. Exp Gerontol 1999;34:755–770
145. Brunk UT, Neuzil J, Eaton JW. Lysosomal involvement in apoptosis. Redox Report 2001;6:91–97
146. Terman A, Gustafsson B, Brunk UT. The lysosomal-mitochondrial axis theory of postmitotic aging and cell death. Chem Biol Interact. 2006 May 1
147. Yan L, Sadoshima J, Vatner DE, Vatner SF. Autophagy: a novel protective mechanism in chronic ischemia. Cell Cycle 2006;5:1175–1177
148. Kunapuli S, Rosanio S, Schwarz ER. "How do cardiomyocytes die?" apoptosis and autophagic cell death in cardiac myocytes. J Card Fail 2006;12:381–391
149. Kanski J, Behring A, Pelling J, Schoneich C. Proteomic identification of 3-nitrotyrosine-containing rat cardiac proteins: effects of biological aging. Am J Physiol Heart Circ Physiol 2005;288:H371–H381
150. Esterbauer H, Schaur RJ, Zollner H. Chemistry and biochemistry of 4-hydroxynonenal, malonaldehyde and related aldehydes. Free Radic Biol Med 1991;11:81–128
151. Kim CH, Zou Y, Kim DH, Kim ND, Yu BP, Chung HY. Proteomic analysis of nitrated and 4-hydroxy-2-nonenal-modified serum proteins during aging. J Gerontol A Biol Sci Med Sci 2006;61:332–338
152. Lucas DT, Szweda LI. Cardiac reperfusion injury: aging, lipid peroxidation, and mitochondrial dysfunction. Proc Natl Acad Sci USA 1998;95:510–514
153. Moreau R, Heath SH, Doneanu CE, Lindsay JG, Hagen TM. Age-related increase in 4-hydroxynonenal adduction to rat heart alpha-ketoglutarate dehydrogenase does not cause loss of its catalytic activity. Antioxid Redox Signal 2003;5:517–527
154. Benderdour M, Charron G, Comte B, Ayoub R, Beaudry D, Foisy S, Deblois D, Des Rosiers C. Decreased cardiac mitochondrial NADP+-isocitrate dehydrogenase activity and expression: a marker of oxidative stress in hypertrophy development. Am J Physiol Heart Circ Physiol 2004;287:H2122–H2131
155. Knyushko TV, Sharov VS, Williams TD, Schoneich C, Bigelow DJ. 3-Nitro-tyrosine modification of SERCA2a in the aging heart: a distinct signature of the cellular redox environment. Biochemistry 2005;44:13071–13081
156. Oliver CN, Ahn BW, Moerman EJ, Goldstein S, Stadtman ER. Age-related changes in oxidized proteins. J Biol Chem 1987;262:5488–5491
157. Berlett BS, Stadtman ER. Protein oxidation in aging, disease, and oxidative stress. J Biol Chem 1997;272:20313–20316
158. Yan LJ, Sohal RS. Mitochondrial adenine nucleotide translocase is modified oxidatively during aging. Proc Natl Acad Sci USA 1998;95:12896–12901
159. Das N, Levine RL, Orr WC, Sohal RS. Selectivity of protein oxidative damage during aging in Drosophila melanogaster. Biochem J 2001;360:209–216
160. Stadtman ER, Berlett BS. Reactive oxygen-mediated protein oxidation in aging and disease. Chem Res Toxicol 1997;10:485–494
161. Stadtman ER, Levine RL. Free radical-mediated oxidation of free amino acids and amino acid residues in proteins. Amino Acids 2003;25:207–218
162. Thomas JA, Mallis RJ. Aging and oxidation of reactive protein sulfhydryls. Exp Gerontol 2001;36:1519–1526
163. Avendano GF, Agarwal RK, Bashey RI, Lyons MM, Soni BJ, Jyothirmayi GN, Regan TJ. Effects of glucose intolerance on myocardial function and collagen-linked glycation. Diabetes 1999;48:1443–1447
164. Burgess ML, McCrea JC, Hedrick HL. Age-associated changes in cardiac matrix and integrins. Mech Ageing Dev 2001;122:1739–1756
165. Reiser KM. Influence of age and long-term dietary restriction on enzymatically mediated crosslinks and nonenzymatic glycation of collagen in mice. J Gerontol 1994;49:B71–B79
166. Norton GR, Candy G, Woodiwiss AJ. Aminoguanidine prevents the decreased myocardial compliance produced by streptozotocin-induced diabetes mellitus in rats. Circulation 1996;93:1905–1912
167. Asif M, Egan J, Vasan S, Jyothirmayi GN, Masurekar MR, Lopez S, Williams C, Torres RL, Wagle D, Ulrich P, Cerami A, Brines M, Regan TJ. An advanced glycation endproduct cross-link breaker can reverse age-related increases in myocardial stiffness. Proc Natl Acad Sci USA 2000;97:2809–2813

222. Trifunovic A, Hansson A, Wredenberg A, Rovio AT, Dufour E, Khvorostov I, Spelbrink JN, Wibom R, Jacobs HT, Larsson NG. Somatic mtDNA mutations cause aging phenotypes without affecting reactive oxygen species production. Proc Natl Acad Sci USA 2005;102:17993–17998
223. Loeb LA, Wallace DC, Martin GM. The mitochondrial theory of aging and its relationship to reactive oxygen species damage and somatic mtDNA mutations. Proc Natl Acad Sci USA 2005;102:18769–18770
224. Khrapko K, Kraytsberg Y, de Grey AD, Vijg J, Schon EA. Does premature aging of the mtDNA mutator mouse prove that mtDNA mutations are involved in natural aging? Aging Cell 2006;5:279–282
225. Gokey NG, Cao Z, Pak JW, Lee D, McKiernan SH, McKenzie D, Weindruch R, Aiken JM. Molecular analyses of mtDNA deletion mutations in microdissected skeletal muscle fibers from aged rhesus monkeys. Aging Cell 2004;3:319–326
226. Soong NW, Hinton DR, Cortopassi G, Arnheim N. Mosaicism for a specific somatic mitochondrial DNA mutation in adult human brain. Nat Genet 1992;2:318–323
227. Zhang D, Mott JL, Farrar P, Ryerse JS, Chang SW, Stevens M, Denniger G, Zassenhaus HP. Mitochondrial DNA mutations activate the mitochondrial apoptotic pathway and cause dilated cardiomyopathy. Cardiovasc Res 2003;57:147–157
228. Zhang D, Mott JL, Chang SW, Stevens M, Mikolajczak P, Zassenhaus HP. Mitochondrial DNA mutations activate programmed cell survival in the mouse heart. Am J Physiol Heart Circ Physiol 2005;288:H2476–H2483
229. Zhang D, Ezekiel UR, Chang SW, Zassenhaus HP. Gene expression profile in dilated cardiomyopathy caused by elevated frequencies of mitochondrial DNA mutations in the mouse heart. Cardiovasc Pathol 2005;14: 61–69
230. Mott JL, Zhang D, Chang SW, Zassenhaus HP. Mitochondrial DNA mutations cause resistance to opening of the permeability transition pore. Biochim Biophys Acta 2006;1757:596–603
231. Vijg J, Dolle ME, Martus HJ, Boerrigter ME. Transgenic mouse models for studying mutations in vivo: applications in aging research. Mech Ageing Dev 1997;98:189–202
232. Dolle ME, Giese H, Hopkins CL, Martus HJ, Hausdorff JM, Vijg J. Rapid accumulation of genome rearrangements in liver but not in brain of old mice. Nat Genet 1997;17:431–434
233. Dolle ME, Snyder WK, Gossen JA, Lohman PH, Vijg J. Distinct spectra of somatic mutations accumulated with age in mouse heart and small intestine. Proc Natl Acad Sci USA 2000;97:8403–8408
234. Hsie AW, Recio L, Katz DS, Lee CQ, Wagner M, Schenley RL. Evidence for reactive oxygen species inducing mutations in mammalian cells. Proc Natl Acad Sci USA 1986;83:9616–9620
235. Gille JJ, van Berkel CG, Joenje H. Mutagenicity of metabolic oxygen radicals in mammalian cell cultures. Carcinogenesis.1994;15:2695–2699
236. Ono T, Ikehata H, Nakamura S, Saito Y, Hosoi Y, Takai Y, Yamada S, Onodera J, Yamamoto K. Age-associated increase of spontaneous mutant frequency and molecular nature of mutation in newborn and old lacZ-transgenic mouse. Mutat Res 2000;447:165–177
237. Barnes DE, Lindahl T. Repair and genetic consequences of endogenous DNA base damage in mammalian cells. Annu Rev Genet 2004;38:445–476
238. Holmquist GP. Endogenous lesions, S-phase-independent spontaneous mutations, and evolutionary strategies for base excision repair. Mutat Res 1998;400:59–68
239. Lindahl T, Karran P, Wood RD. DNA excision repair pathways. Curr Opin Genet Dev 1997;7:158–169
240. Cabelof DC, Raffoul JJ, Yanamadala S, Ganir C, Guo Z, Heydari AR. Attenuation of DNA polymerase beta-dependent base excision repair and increased DMS-induced mutagenicity in aged mice. Mutat Res 2002;500:135–145
241. de Souza-Pinto NC, Hogue BA, Bohr VA. DNA repair and aging in mouse liver: 8-oxodG glycosylase activity increase in mitochondrial but not in nuclear extracts. Free Radic Biol Med 2001;30:916–923
242. Stuart JA, Karahalil B, Hogue BA, Souza-Pinto NC, Bohr VA. Mitochondrial and nuclear DNA base excision repair are affected differently by caloric restriction. FASEB J 2004;18:595–597
243. Hasty P, Campisi J, Hoeijmakers J, van Steeg H, Vijg J. Aging and genome maintenance: lessons from the mouse? Science 2003;299:1355–1359
244. Schofield MJ, Hsieh P. DNA mismatch repair: molecular mechanisms and biological function. Annu Rev Microbiol 2003;57 :579–608
245. Sancar A, Lindsey-Boltz LA, Unsal-Kacmaz K, Linn S. Molecular mechanisms of mammalian DNA repair and the DNA damage checkpoints. Annu Rev Biochem 2004;73:39–85
246. Gillet LC, Scharer OD. Molecular mechanisms of mammalian global genome nucleotide excision repair. Chem Rev 2006;106:253–276
247. Costa RM, Chigancas V, Galhardo Rda S, Carvalho H, Menck CF. The eukaryotic nucleotide excision repair pathway. Biochimie 2003;85:1083–1099
248. Mitchell JR, Hoeijmakers JH, Niedernhofer LJ. Divide and conquer: nucleotide excision repair battles cancer and ageing. Curr Opin Cell Biol 2003;15:232–240

249. Bassing CH, Alt FW. The cellular response to general and programmed DNA double strand breaks. DNA Repair (Amst.) 2004;3:781–796
250. Karanjawala ZE, Lieber MR. DNA damage and aging. Mech Ageing Dev 2004;125:405–416
251. Bryant HE, Helleday T. Inhibition of poly (ADP-ribose) polymerase activates ATM which is required for subsequent homologous recombination repair. Nucleic Acids Res 2006;34:1685–1691
252. Ferguson DO, Alt FW. DNA double strand break repair and chromosomal translocation: lessons from animal models. Oncogene 2001;20:5572–5579
253. Vogel H, Lim DS, Karsenty G, Finegold M, Hasty P. Deletion of Ku86 causes early onset of senescence in mice. Proc Natl Acad Sci USA 1999;96:10770–10775
254. Espejel S, Martin M, Klatt P, Martin-Caballero J, Flores JM, Blasco MA. Shorter telomeres, accelerated ageing and increased lymphoma in DNA-PKcs-deficient mice. EMBO Rep 2004;5:503–509
255. Mills KD, Ferguson DO, Essers J, Eckersdorff M, Kanaar R, Alt FW. Rad54 and DNA Ligase IV cooperate to maintain mammalian chromatid stability. Genes Dev 2004;18:1283–1292
256. Takata M, Sasaki MS, Sonoda E, Morrison C, Hashimoto M, Utsumi H, Yamaguchi-Iwai Y, Shinohara A, Takeda S. Homologous recombination and non-homologous end-joining pathways of DNA double-strand break repair have overlapping roles in the maintenance of chromosomal integrity in vertebrate cells. EMBO J 1998;17: 5497–5508
257. Helleday T. Pathways for mitotic homologous recombination in mammalian cells. Mutat Res 2003;532:103–115
258. Scharer OD. Chemistry and biology of DNA repair. Angew Chem Int Ed Engl 2003;42:2946–2974
259. West SC. Molecular views of recombination proteins and their control. Nat Rev Mol Cell Biol 2003;4:435–445
260. Wang HC, Chou WC, Shieh SY, Shen CY. Ataxia telangiectasia mutated and checkpoint kinase 2 regulate BRCA1 to promote the fidelity of DNA end-joining. Cancer Res 2006;66:1391–1400
261. Lowndes NF, Toh GW. DNA repair: the importance of phosphorylating histone H2AX. Curr Biol 2005;15: R99–R102
262. Bender CF, Sikes ML, Sullivan R, Huye LE, Le Beau MM, Roth DB, Mirzoeva OK, Oltz EM, Petrini JH. Cancer predisposition and hematopoietic failure in Rad50(S/S) mice. Genes Dev 2002;16:2237–2251
263. Cao L, Li W, Kim S, Brodie SG, Deng CX. Senescence, aging, and malignant transformation mediated by p53 in mice lacking the Brca1 full-length isoform. Genes Dev 2003;17:201–213
264. Celeste A, Petersen S, Romanienko PJ, Fernandez-Capetillo O, Chen HT, Sedelnikova OA, Reina-San-Martin B, Coppola V, Meffre E, Difilippantonio MJ, Redon C, Pilch DR, Olaru A, Eckhaus M, Camerini-Otero RD, Tessarollo L, Livak F, Manova K, Bonner WM, Nussenzweig MC, Nussenzweig A. Genomic instability in mice lacking histone H2AX. Science 2002;296:922–927
265. Y, Yang EM, Brugarolas J, Jacks T, Baltimore D. Involvement of p53 and p21 in cellular defects and tumorigenesis in Atm-/- mice. Mol Cell Biol 1998;18:4385–4390
266. Wong KK, Maser RS, Bachoo RM, Menon J, Carrasco DR, Gu Y, Alt FW, DePinho RA. Telomere dysfunction and Atm deficiency compromises organ homeostasis and accelerates ageing. Nature 2003;421:643–648
267. Larsen NB, Rasmussen M, Rasmussen LJ. Nuclear and mitochondrial DNA repair: similar pathways? Mitochondrion 2005;5:89–108
268. Clayton DA, Doda JN, Friedberg EC. The absence of a pyrimidine dimer repair mechanism in mammalian mitochondria. Proc Natl Acad Sci USA 1974;71:2777–2781
269. LeDoux SP, Wilson GL, Beecham EJ, Stevnsner T, Wassermann K, Bohr VA. Repair of mitochondrial DNA after various types of DNA damage in Chinese hamster ovary cells. Carcinogenesis 1992;13:1967–1973
270. Mason PA, Matheson EC, Hall AG, Lightowlers RN. Mismatch repair activity in mammalian mitochondria. Nucleic Acids Res 2003;31:1052–1058
271. Thyagarajan B, Padua RA, Campbell C. Mammalian mitochondria possess homologous DNA recombination activity. J Biol Chem 1996;271:27536–27543
272. Lakshmipathy U, Campbell C. Double strand break rejoining by mammalian mitochondrial extracts. Nucleic Acids Res 1999;27:1198–1204
273. Yoshida Y, Izumi H, Ise T, Uramoto H, Torigoe T, Ishiguchi H, Murakami T, Tanabe M, Nakayama Y, Itoh H, Kasai H, Kohno K. Human mitochondrial transcription factor A binds preferentially to oxidatively damaged DNA. Biochem Biophys Res Commun 2002;295:945–951
274. Alam TI, Kanki T, Muta T, Ukaji K, Abe Y, Nakayama H, Takio K, Hamasaki N, Kang D. Human mitochondrial DNA is packaged with TFAM. Nucleic Acids Res 2003;31:1640–1645
275. Kanki T, Ohgaki K, Gaspari M, Gustafsson CM, Fukuoh A, Sasaki N, Hamasaki N, Kang D. Architectural role of mitochondrial transcription factor A in maintenance of human mitochondrial DNA. Mol Cell Biol 2004;24:9823–9834
276. Wang J, Wilhelmsson H, Graff C, Li H, Oldfors A, Rustin P, Bruning JC, Kahn CR, Clayton DA, Barsh GS, Thoren P, Larsson NG. Dilated cardiomyopathy and atrioventricular conduction blocks induced by heart-specific inactivation of mitochondrial DNA gene expression. Nat Genet 1999;21:133–137

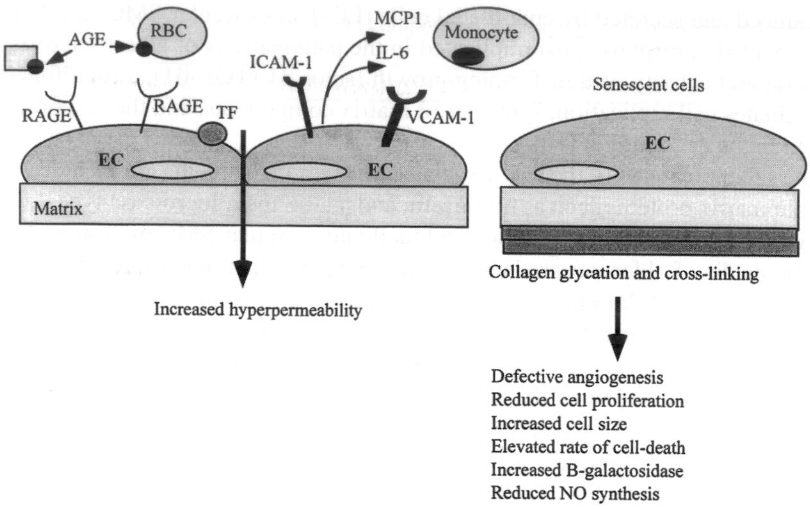

Fig. 5.1 The effect of glycation and age on endothelial cell (EC) dysfunction

While central arteries stiffen progressively with age, stiffness of muscular arteries changes little with age [23]. Interestingly, recent studies have documented a similar alteration of the mechanical properties of cardiac myocytes with aging in cells from 4-month and 30-month male Fischer 344 x Brown Norway F1 hybrid rats using atomic force microscopy (AFM), which determines cellular mechanical property changes at nanoscale resolution. A significant increase was found in the apparent elastic modulus (i.e., a measure of stiffness) of single, aging cardiac myocytes [24].

In addition, arterial stiffness seems to have a genetic component, which is largely independent of the influence of blood pressure and other cardiovascular risk factors. In studies of several monogenic connective tissue diseases including Marfan, Williams, and Ehlers-Danlos syndromes and in the corresponding animal models, a precise characterization of the arterial phenotype has underscored the influence of abnormal genetically determined wall components on arterial stiffness. It also highlighted the role of extracellular matrix signaling in the vascular wall and revealed that elastin and collagen not only modulate vessel elasticity or rigidity but also are critically involved in control of vascular SMC function [25]. A number of studies have also suggested that arterial stiffness can be further influenced by the presence of specific gene polymorphisms (as shown in Table 5.2). Studies have focused on the involvement of genes encoding components of the renin-angiotensin-aldosterone system, which are involved in blood pressure control, as well as cell proliferation, matrix production, signaling and vascular hypertrophy, and play a key role in arterial stiffness. Significant associations with arterial stiffness have been found for specific gene variants of angiotensinogen (AGT), angiotensin converting enzyme (ACE) and angiotensin II type 1 receptor, AT1 [26–29]. The T344C polymorphism of the aldosterone synthase (CYP11B2) gene has also been shown to be associated with an increase in arterial stiffness in several independent studies [30–32], but not in others [27]. A potential explanation for this discrepancy lies in the recent demonstration that sodium intake (i.e., diet) can serve as an epigenetic modulator of CYP11B2 phenotypic expression [31].

Genotype–phenotype studies have also focused on extracellular matrix proteins, primarily elastin and collagens. Elevated carotid stiffness was reported in elderly subjects (> 55 year old) carrying the A allele of the Ser422Gly polymorphism of the elastin gene [33]. In patients with CAD, the 2–3 tandem repeat genotype of the fibrillin-1 gene has been shown to be associated with greater aortic stiffness than the 2–2 and 2–4 genotypes [34, 35]. Variants of MMPs have also been investigated

Table 5.2 Human gene polymorphisms and aortic stiffness

Genetic loci	Polymorphism	Arterial phenotype	Ref
Angiotensin II type 1 receptor (AT1)	A1166C	Carriers of the AT1 1166C allele had ↑ aortic stiffness	26, 27
	−153A/G	Carriers of the AT 1 −153G allele (> 55 yr) had ↑ aortic stiffness	27
Angiotensin converting enzyme (ACE)	Insertion/deletion (I/D)	Subjects with ID and DD genotype had higher carotid stiffness compared to subjects with II genotype	28
Angiotensinogen (AGT)	M235T	Reduced carotid distensibility and ↑ carotid stiffness in subjects with T allele homozygosity	29
Aldosterone synthase (CYP11B2)	T344C	Presence of the −344C allele was associated with ↑ levels of plasma aldosterone and arterial stiffness in patients with essential hypertension	30, 31, 32
Elastin	Ser422Gly (A-> G)	Subjects (> 50 yr) carrying the A allele had a significant decline in distensibility for the carotid but not radial artery	33
Fibrillin-1	The 2–3 Tandem repeat genotype	In CAD patients, 2-3 genotype had ↑ input impedance and carotid pulse pressure compared with 2-2 and 2-4 genotypes	34, 35
Stromelysin-1 (MMP-3)	Homozygous for 5A allele	↑ aortic stiffness in subjects > than 60 yr	36
MMP-9	−1562C>T R279Q	In healthy individuals, ↑ aortic stiffness, serum MMP-9 and elastase activity in carriers of rare alleles for−1562C>T and R279Q polymorphisms; age was contributory	37, 38
Endothelial nitric oxide synthase (eNOS)	G894T	The T allele was associated with significantly lower values of arterial stiffness and elastic modulus (YEM) in African Americans	39
Endothelin receptors	ETA-R −231A/G ETB-R 30G/A	Increased arterial stiffness was associated with −231G and 30G alleles in women and the ETB-R 30G/A receptor gene variant in men,	40
G-protein beta3 subunit (GNB3)	C825T	C825T is associated with ↑arterial stiffness in healthy males	41

for their association with arterial stiffness because they are involved in matrix homeostasis and arterial wall remodeling. Variants of the MMP-3 gene encoding stromelysin-1 [36], which acts on a variety of substrates, including fibronectin, elastin, and collagens, and MMP-9 have shown significant association with arterial stiffness [37, 38]. In addition, consistent with the critical roles of endothelial function and signaling on vascular arterial changes, it is not unexpected that specific polymorphic variants of genes involved in NO synthesis (eNOS) [39], endothelin receptors (ETA-R and ETB-R) [40], and G-protein β3 subunit (GNB3)[41] have shown a significant association with arterial stiffness. Recent studies have also implicated the involvement of specific variants of both ETA-R and ETB-R in mediating arterial stiffness in response to exercise [42].

Gene expression analysis has also proved to be informative in elucidating the molecular underpinnings of arterial stiffness. A microarray analysis of genes whose expression correlates with arterial stiffness in human aortic specimens, identified 2 distinct groups of genes, those associated with cell signaling and those associated with the mechanical regulation of vascular structure (e.g., cytoskeleton, cell membrane and extracellular matrix) [43]. Differentially expressed genes involved in the mechanical regulation of vascular structure included integrins (α2b, α6, β3 and β5), proteoglycans (decorin, osteomodulin, etc.), chondroitin sulfate proteoglycan-5, fibulin-1, thrombospondin and fascin. Several signaling proteins including the catalytic subunit B isoform of protein phosphatase-1 (PPP1CB) and Yotiao, a protein kinase A (PRKA) anchor protein that targets PPP1CB were negatively correlated with arterial stiffness and were dramatically downregulated in the stiff vessel wall. In contrast, transcript levels of the regulatory subunit polypeptide-1 (p85-α) of phosphoinositide-3-kinase (PI3K) were positively correlated with arterial stiffness and significantly upregulated by >3-fold. In addition to growth regulation, PI3K has multiple effects on the vascular system including its involvement in the signaling pathway of vasoconstrictors such as angiotensin II [44], activation of vascular SMC calcium channels [45], cell adhesion and cytoskeletal organization through activation of focal adhesion kinase [46], and in isolated smooth muscle strips, PI3K inhibition leads to relaxation [47].

Other studies have examined the effects of metalloproteinase gene expression and arterial stiffness. In a study demonstrating that the MMP-3 5A/6A promoter polymorphism contributes to age-related large artery stiffening, homozygotes (of either 5A/5A or 6A/6A genotype) had higher aortic input and characteristic impedance, i.e., higher stiffness, compared to 5A/6A heterozygotes [36]. In dermal biopsies in randomly selected older men from the same cohort, MMP-3 gene expression was 4-fold higher in 5A homozygotes and in 6A homozygotes, 2-fold lower compared with the heterozygotes. Clearly, MMP-3 genotype and expression may be an important determinant of vascular remodeling and age-related arterial stiffening, with the heterozygote maintaining the optimal balance between matrix accumulation and deposition. Similarly, studies analyzing the role of MMP-9 genotype (e.g., C-1562T promoter polymorphism) on large artery stiffening and aortic MMP-9 gene and protein expression found that T-allele carriers (C/T and T/T) had stiffer large arteries (higher input and characteristic impedance) and higher carotid pulse and systolic blood pressure than C/C homozygotes [37]. Aortic gene expression exhibited 5-fold elevation in MMP-9 transcripts and > 2-fold higher in active protein levels in T-allele carriers suggesting that the more extensive large artery stiffness in T-allele carriers may be attributable to excessive degradation of the arterial elastic matrix by upregulated metalloproteinases.

The use of gene expression profiling has also proved to be informative with respect to understanding the mechanism of reversing aortic stiffness by exercise-training [48]. Arterial stiffness was higher in the abdominal aorta and systemic arterial compliance was lower in the sedentary control rats (8 week old) compared to the exercise-trained rats (8 week old, treadmill running for 4 weeks). Global gene expression analysis revealed that the prostaglandin EP2 receptor (PGE-EP2R), prostaglandin EP4 receptor (PGE-EP4R), C-type natriuretic peptide (CNP), and endothelial nitric oxide synthase (eNOS) genes were expressed at significantly higher levels in the abdominal aorta of exercise-trained animals compared with untrained controls and correlated with levels of arterial stiffness.

As we shall shortly see, ECs play a pivotal role in regulating several arterial properties, including vascular tone, vascular permeability, angiogenesis, and inflammatory response. Endothelial-derived substances (e.g., NO, endothelin-1) are critical determinants of large arterial compliance, suggesting that ECs may also modulate central arterial stiffness [49]. In the brachial artery, endothelial function, as assessed by agonist- or flow-mediated vasoreactivity, has been shown to decline with advancing age in both men and women [50, 51]. However, since a direct correlation between endothelial function and definitive measures of arterial stiffness and wave reflections in larger central arteries had not previously been described in healthy individuals, a recent study undertook assessment of whether endothelial function is inversely correlated with aortic pulse wave velocity, central pulse pressure, and augmentation index in healthy individuals [52]. Global endothelial function was significantly and inversely correlated with aortic stiffness and central and peripheral pulse pressure.

Endothelial Cell Function and Remodeling

A number of alterations in the structure and function of ECs accompany advancing age including a higher prevalence of cells with polyploid nuclei, increased endothelial permeability, alterations in the arrangement and integrity of the cytoskeleton, the appearance of senescence-associated (SA) β-galactosidase staining, and the expression of several inhibitors of the cell cycle. Senescent ECs of aged arteries secrete more plasminogen activator inhibitor-1, favoring thrombosis formation. Furthermore, with aging, EC production of vasoconstriction growth factors such as angiotensin II (Ang II) and endothelin increases, and that of vasodilatory factors (e.g., NO, prostacyclin, and endothelium-derived hyperpolarizing factor) is reduced. Moreover, the interaction between monocytes and ECs is enhanced by EC senescence as well as largely mediated by the upregulation of adhesion molecules (e.g., ICAM-1) and pro-inflammatory cytokines as well as the decrease in the production of NO in senescent ECs. Elevated glycation in aging not only increases arterial stiffness but markedly impacts endothelial function as depicted in Fig. 5.1. These age-associated alterations in the arterial wall create a milieu conducive for the initiation or progression of superimposed vascular diseases (e.g., atherosclerosis) as well as for the development of generalized endothelial dysfunction [53, 54].

Role of Cell Senescence

A critical element in the effect of aging on the EC is the development of the senescent phenotype, which has a significant impact of vascular integrity, function, and overall homeostasis. ECs both *in vitro* and *in vivo*, are known to undergo replicative senescence. While senescent ECs are viable and metabolically active, they display altered gene and protein expression compared to proliferating cells. Senescent cells, including ECs, possess a characteristic enlarged, flattened cell morphology, increased granularity and vacuolization, contain polymorphic nuclei and express senescence-associated acidic β-galactosidase activity. This activity, which is detected when cells are incubated with the chromogenic substrate 5-bromo-4-chloro-3-indolyl-β-d-galactopyranoside (X-gal) at pH 6.0, is a manifestation of an increase in lysosomal mass in the senescent cell [55], and has been widely used as a marker of senescence.

Under normal conditions ECs rarely divide and are in effect quiescent, exhibiting a turnover rate estimated at approximately 3 years. Both physiological and pathological processes, such as endothelial injury, wound healing or angiogenesis are known to initiate endothelial proliferation [56], and consequently, the impaired wound healing and angiogenesis typically observed in the elderly, have been attributed to endothelial senescence [57]. Moreover, it has been reported that senescent human ECs show a reduced ability to form capillaries *in vitro* [58].

Bone marrow–derived circulating endothelial progenitor cells (EPCs) are known to participate in postnatal neovascularization and vascular repair [59, 60]. Several studies have revealed that both the growth and function of cultured bone marrow–derived EPCs are impaired in patients with coronary artery disease (CAD) and show a negative correlation with various risk factors for coronary atherosclerosis, including age [61, 62]. Thus, aging may also promote the senescence of EPCs as well as vascular ECs, resulting in a decline of angiogenesis and vascular healing. Observations from Edelberg et al. indicated that dysregulation in platelet-derived growth factor (PDGF)-B is a factor in the age-related decline in angiogenesis [63]. *In vitro* studies found that young 3-month-old murine bone marrow–derived EPCs recapitulated the cardiac myocyte–induced expression of PDGF-B, whereas EPCs from the bone marrow of aging 18-month-old mice did not express PDGF-B when cultured in the presence of cardiac myocytes. These studies also demonstrated that transplantation of young but not old bone-marrow derived EPCs were able to be successfully incorporated into the vasculature of aging mice and restored both angiogenic function and the PDGF-B induction pathway suggesting a possible therapeutic modality.

In human ECs, senescence has largely been thought to be a consequence of the progressive shortening and eventual dysfunction of telomeres. Senescence is reached when the telomeres are shortened below a critical length [64]. In ECs obtained from different regions of the vasculature and from donors of different ages [65, 66], telomeres have been found to shorten with age. This telomere erosion is in part due to a downregulation in the activity of the telomerase reverse transcriptase (TERT) activity. While most somatic cells do not display detectable telomerase activity, normal human ECs and vascular SMCs both express telomerase activity, which is markedly activated by mitogenic stimuli via a protein kinase C (PKC)-dependent pathway;[67] this activity significantly declines with *in vitro* aging of vascular cells due to a decrease in TERT expression leading to telomere shortening and cellular senescence [68, 69].

Loss of telomere function was recently shown to induce endothelial dysfunction in vascular ECs, whereas inhibition of telomere shortening was shown to suppress the age-associated dysfunction in these cells [70]. Moreover, introduction of TERT has been shown to extend the cell life span of human ECs (and vascular SMCs as well) further supporting the critical role of telomere shortening in vascular cell senescence as well [58, 71]. Introduction of TERT also prevented endothelial dysfunction associated with senescence, including decrease in eNOS activity and an increase in monocyte binding to ECs [70, 72].

Other factors have been shown to contribute to the loss of telomere integrity. Studies with cultured cells have shown that a relatively mild chronic oxidative stimulus can accelerate telomere erosion, in part attributed to the increased generation of single strand breaks in the telomeric DNA resulting from oxidative damage [73], and the downregulation of telomerase activity [74]. Haendler et al. demonstrated that ECs cultured *in vitro* accumulate ROS, which induces both mtDNA damage and results in the export of TERT from the nucleus into the cytoplasm as well as leading to the activation of the Src-kinase [75]. Incubation of EC cells with the antioxidant N-acetylcysteine, or with low doses of the statin, atorvastatin resulted in reducing the intracellular ROS formation, preventing mtDNA damage and delaying the nuclear export of TERT protein, loss in the overall telomerase activity, and the onset of replicative senescence.

Increasing evidence suggests that these mechanisms may also operate *in vivo*. In a provocative study, Epel and co-workers demonstrated that psychological stress evaluated in healthy women with both perceived stress and in women with chronic stress (i.e., caregivers to chronically ill-children) was significantly associated with higher OS, significantly lower telomerase activity, and shorter telomere length, assessed in peripheral blood mononuclear cells [76]. Many questions have arisen from this study including whether shorter telomeres in leukocytes lead to earlier immune senescence and whether these dynamics also occur in other proliferative cells, such as vascular ECs. However, subsequent studies from this group have demonstrated that telomerase activity in human blood leukocytes (which can precede telomere length changes) can also be used as an early marker of CVD risk. Significantly reduced telomerase activity was associated with the major risk factors for vascular disease including smoking, poor lipid profile, high systolic blood pressure, high fasting glucose, and greater abdominal adiposity [77]. In a similar vein, Ogami et al. found significant levels of telomere shortening in coronary ECs obtained from patients with CAD compared to age-matched non-CAD patients [78]. This latter study gauged telomeric DNA content in ECs by DNA-DNA hybridization with a telomere-specific oligonucleotide [TTAGGG] standardized relative to centromeric DNA content (T/C ratio) to estimate telomere length. Moreover, in a subset of the CAD patients, the T/C ratio at the site of the atherosclerotic lesion was significantly smaller than that at the non-atherosclerotic portion, suggesting that focal replicative senescence and telomere shortening of ECs may play a critical role in the development and perhaps in the early diagnosis of coronary atherogenesis and CAD.

In addition, there is considerable evidence that the maintenance of telomere integrity requires functional telomere-binding proteins of which an increasing number have been identified. For instance, disruption/inactivation of the gene for one of these proteins, the telomere repeat binding factor-2 (TRF2), has been shown to cause telomere dysfunction and replicative senescence in either human or mouse cells *in vitro* albeit different downstream pathways appear to be activated in these different species [79]. TRF2 inhibition in mice also impacted telomere dysfunction *in vivo* and could lead either to the induction of senescence or apoptosis depending on the cellular level of telomere dysfunction and TRF2 expression levels [80]. In addition, the reduction of POT1 (protection of telomeres 1) a highly conserved telomere-specific single-stranded DNA-binding protein by RNA interference led to the loss of telomeric single-stranded overhangs and induced apoptosis, chromosomal instability, and senescence in human cells [81].

It has been recognized that the senescence response can also be induced by a number of stressful stimuli, including those causing intracellular OS or persistent mitogenic stimulation which appears to be unrelated to telomere damage [82]. This process has been called stress-induced premature senescence (SIPS) [83], or alternatively 'stress or aberrant signaling-induced senescence' (STASIS) [84]. A telomere-independent pathway for triggering vascular cell senescence was found with the constitutive activation of mitogenic stimuli by expression of oncogenic Ras or E2F [85, 86]. The constitutive activation of Ras-promoted senescence in vascular cells, was associated with accumulation of the proteins p53 and p16 [87], activation of extracellular signal-regulated kinase (ERK) [88], and p38 mitogen-activated protein kinase (MAPK) [89].

It has also been recognized that senescence-like phenotypic changes in ECs can also be induced in the absence of telomere length changes through collagen glycation [90]. Advanced glycation end (AGE) products, which accumulate with aging, increase the production of superoxide anion through the activation of NADPH oxidase as discussed below.

Mechanisms of Cell Senescence

Although diverse stimuli can induce senescence, they appear to converge mainly on either or both of 2 pathways that establish and maintain the process of cellular senescence. As shown in the Fig. 5.2, these senescence-signaling pathways are regulated by the tumor suppressor proteins p53 and Rb [91]. Both proteins are transcriptional regulators, and each lies at the center of signaling pathways responsible for cell cycle regulation, DNA repair, and cell death, involving a number of upstream regulators and downstream effectors. Rb is found at senescence in its active, hypophosphorylated form, in which it binds to the E2F protein repressing its transcriptional targets [92]. p53 is a mediator of the response to DNA damage, and it induces the cyclin-dependent inhibitor p21 [93]. This DNA damage-response pathway, is mediated by the ATM/ATR and Chk1/Chk2 proteins, which cause the post-translational stabilization of p53 through its phosphorylation [94, 95]. Moreover, dysfunctional telomeres resemble damaged DNA and trigger a p53-dependent response. A number of studies have shown that nuclear foci containing markers of double-strand DNA breaks form in cells with critically short or dysfunctional telomeres. The p53 pathway is also important for senescence occurring in response to oncogenic stimuli such as activation of Ras [96]. Oncogenic Ras may trigger a p53-dependent damage response by increasing the production of ROS, which are required for the mitogenic effects of Ras activation, which can be independent of telomere dysfunction.

The alternative products of the *INK4a* locus, p16 and ARF are key players in the vascular senescence pathway *in vivo* [97, 98]. ARF (p19ARF in mouse or p14ARF in human) acts by sequestering the E3 ubiquitin ligase Mdm2 to the nucleolus, preventing the proteolytic degradation of p53, which in turn participates in the induction of senescence through upregulation of its transcriptional target p21, a CDK inhibitor, which in turn activates Rb, keeps it in a hypophosphorylated state that prevents the binding of E2F to its targeted gene promoters. While stress-inducible, ARF is generally considered to play a critical role in mouse cell senescence; its significance in human cell senescence has not yet been ascertained.

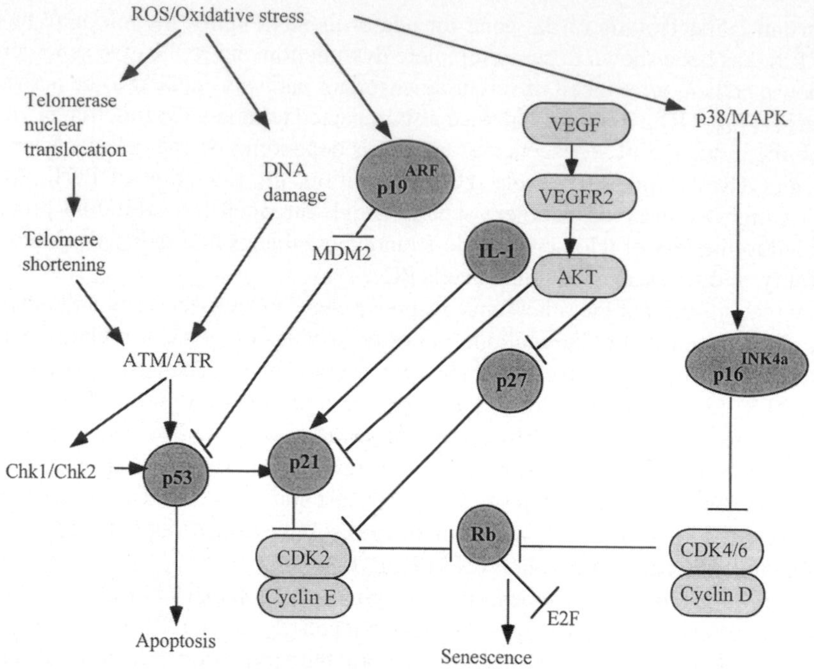

Fig. 5.2 Senescence signaling pathways

p16 also acts as a positive regulator of Rb-induced senescence by inhibiting the activity of the cyclin-dependent kinases CDK4 and CDK6, which would otherwise phosphorylate and inactivate the tumour suppressor Rb. The p16 protein is induced by a variety of stress stimuli, including the overexpression of oncogenes such as Ras [99]. In some cell-types, p16 expression is silenced by the methylation of its promoter [100], and in such cells the senescence response depends primarily on the p53-dependent pathway. Vascular ECs show markedly increased expression of p16 during replicative senescence [101, 102]. Overexpression of p16 has been shown to prevent the reversal of senescence caused by inactivation of p53 [103]. Thus, the p16/Rb pathway can provide a formidable barrier to cell proliferation that cannot be overcome by loss of p53. p16 functions in both murine and human cells, although it appears to be much more active in the latter. It has been implicated in both stress-induced premature senescence and also in the response to telomere damage that occurs during replicative senescence.

Studies have shown that the p16/Rb pathway induces chromatin remodeling and affects the expression of cell cycle regulators [104]. Senescent cells develop dense foci of heterochromatin that repress the E2F target genes encoding positive cell cycle regulators in a Rb-dependent manner. Senescence occurs via the p53 pathway in response to DNA damage and telomere dysfunction, whereas the p16/Rb pathway mediates senescence in response to oncogenic stimuli, chromatin disruption, and other cellular stresses as shown in Fig. 5.2.

Functional Effects of Endothelial Cell Senescence

Both eNOS activity and NO production decline in senescent human vascular ECs [70, 105]. The extent of NO production in response to shear stress is also less in senescent vascular ECs [72]. ROS production is increased in senescent ECs[106, 107] leading to a decline in NO bioavailability as well as increased formation of peroxynitrite [108]. In addition, with *in vitro* aging of vascular ECs, prostacyclin production is reduced [109], while the generation of thromboxane A2 and endothelin-1 is augmented [110, 111], and the plasminogen activator inhibitor-1 is upregulated [112, 113]. All of these age-associated changes are likely to be involved in the impairment of endothelium-dependent vasodilation, as well as favoring an increased tendency for thrombogenesis that occurs in human atherosclerosis. Also, the interaction between monocytes and vascular ECs is enhanced by EC senescence, and contributes to the promotion of atherogenesis [114]. This enhanced EC-cell interaction appears to be mediated by upregulation of adhesion molecules and proinflammatory cytokines, as well as through decreased NO production by senescent ECs.

The relationship of EC apoptosis and senescence is not clear. Early studies reported that as ECs age in culture, the number of senescent cells increases in the population but overall levels of apoptosis did not change [115]. Wagner et al. have found that senescent ECs arrested in the G_1 phase of the cell cycle and accumulated G_1 cyclins (cyclin D1 and cyclin E), hypophosphorylated Rb, and the cyclin dependent kinase inhibitors p16, p21 and p27 [116]. At senescence, the ECs increased in size, demonstrated polyploidy, and SA-β-galactosidase activity was detected in over 90% of the cells. Moreover, this growth arrest was not stable as many cells underwent significant spontaneous apoptosis gauged by detection of significant sub-G_0 DNA content within the EC population and the presence of TUNEL (terminal deoxynucleotide transferase dUTP nick end labeling) and annexin V positive cells. This enhanced apoptosis in senescent vascular ECs may contribute to plaque erosion and thrombosis in human atherosclerosis. In contrast to the senescent ECs, senescent fibroblasts entered a stable G_1 growth arrest and were resistant to apoptosis as previously described [117]. Furthermore, it has been found that the senescent population of ECs had enhanced levels of ROS, as detected by using the redox-sensitive dye dihydrorhodamine 123 [107]. Similarly, increased apoptosis has been found in senescent porcine pulmonary artery ECs cultured *in vitro* for prolonged times [118].

To elucidate the mechanisms underlying EC senescence and age-associated apoptosis, gene expression profiling was undertaken and revealed upregulation of genes coding for extracellular proteins in senescent HUVECs including significant upregulation of interleukin-8, vascular endothelial growth inhibitor (VEGI), and the IGF-binding proteins 3 and 5, confirmed by both RT-PCR and Western immunoblot analysis. In the case of interleukin-8, a roughly 50-fold upregulation of the protein was also found in cellular supernatants. The extracellular proteins encoded by these genes are well known for their ability to modulate the apoptotic response of human cells, and in the case of interleukin-8, a link to the establishment of atherosclerotic lesions was defined [119].

These findings in addition to confirming the relevance of cellular senescence to cardiovascular dysfunction *in vivo* have also allowed the identification of potential biomarkers that can be used to monitor changes in the vascular cells in both disease and aging. Nevertheless, the role and relevance of cellular senescence and telomere dysfunction in the aging vasculature *in vivo* remains somewhat unclear and confusing and has been recently debated in several excellent reviews [120–122]. Telomerase-deficient mice generated by targeting the telomerase RNA subunit develop senescence-related organ failure in many systems including highly proliferative tissues such as the hematopoietic system, male reproductive organs, the skin and the intestinal epithelium as well as liver but do not develop a spontaneous vascular phenotype [123–125] This may be in part explained by the fact that mice have extremely long telomeres and it takes several generations to shorten them to the point of triggering some phenotypic effects. In fact, late-generation telomerase-deficient mice exhibited reduced angiogenesis in matrigel implants [126]. Furthermore, in mouse models of premature aging resulting from deletions of genes involved in genome maintenance, an increase in cellular senescence has been observed, but anomalies of the vascular system have generally not been reported [127]. A number of human premature aging disorders are associated with abnormal telomere homeostasis but show little evidence of *in vivo* cellular senescence, although cells derived from these patients undergo premature senescence when grown *in vitro* [128–131]. Moreover, while severe atherosclerosis is a conspicuous pathological feature of Werner and Hutchinson-Gilford Progeria syndromes, other well-characterised inherited disorders associated with short telomeres and features of premature aging, dyskeratosis congenital and ataxia teleangiectasia, do not feature accelerated development of atherosclerosis arguing against a requisite role for telomere-based cell senescence in atherogenesis.

Endothelial Aging and Oxidative Stress

As we have previously noted, aging is associated with increased OS and oxidative damage. The endothelium appears to be an important source of superoxide in the vascular wall [132–135]. This effect seems to increase with age and leads to an endothelium-dependent attenuation of nitrovasodilator reactivity. Removal of the endothelium, as well as inhibition of the NADPH oxidase and eNOS reduce vascular superoxide generation in aorta of aged Wistar–Kyoto rats [132].

However, the sources of the free radical generation in vascular aging have not been fully determined. As we have previously noted, it is widely believed that leakage of superoxide and of H_2O_2 from mitochondria and mitochondrial dysfunction increases with age. The continuous production of O_2 during the life span leads to an ever-increasing amount of mtDNA damage. Consequences in endothelial cells include reduction in the number of EC mitochondria [136], distinct alterations in overall mitochondrial morphology and fine structure and loss of membrane potential [137], impaired expression and formation of dysfunctional mitochondrial proteins [138, 139], which leads to cellular energy depletion and further ROS generation. For instance, senescent EC cells exhibit diminished levels of mitochondrial cytochrome *c* oxidase (complex IV) leading to OS [138]. Moreover, in the rat aorta, peroxynitrite-dependent inactivation of the mitochondrial MnSOD isoform by tyrosine-nitrosylation occurs with vascular aging, which further promotes mitochondrial superoxide accumulation [139]. Nevertheless, recent studies suggest that there are other significant sources of ROS in human ECs in addition to mitochondria including NADPH oxidase [140].

Several other non-mitochondrial enzymes are thought to be involved in aging-induced radical formation. Uncoupled endothelial NO synthases can be transformed into radical generating enzymes [141], an OS-generating process that can be induced in ECs by homocysteine [142]. A critical component of the transformation of eNOS to a superoxide-producing pro-atherosclerotic enzyme is the peroxynitrite-mediated oxidation of the essential NOS cofactor, 6R-5, 6, 7, 8-tetrahydrobiopterin (BH4). Diminished levels of the BH4 cofactor promote superoxide production by eNOS. While this transformation of eNOS from a protective enzyme to a contributor to OS has been observed in several *in vitro* models, in animal models of cardiovascular diseases, and in patients with cardiovascular risk factors [143], its role in aging has not been ascertained and it may be secondary to ROS production by mitochondrial ETC and by NADPH oxidase.

Xanthine oxidase (XO) is another potential source of superoxide formation in vascular disease. Oxypurinol, a non-competitive XO inhibitor has been reported to reduce superoxide production and improve endothelium-dependent vascular relaxations to acetylcholine in blood vessels from hyperlipidemic animals [144]. This suggests a contribution of XO to endothelial dysfunction in early hypercholesterolemia. However, the general importance of xanthine oxidase for endothelial dysfunction in aging or cardiovascular disease is uncertain. Recent reports found that XO activity was increased as well as XO expression in the aorta of 18-month old aging male Sprague Dawley rats in parallel with a 2-fold increase in free radical generation and unchanged vascular NADPH levels [145]. Another study found that XO does not contribute to the decline in OS-associated peripheral conduit artery endothelium-dependent dilatation that occurs with aging in humans [146]. This may be related to the absence of age-associated upregulation of endothelial XO in these tissues. Moreover, while some improvement in endothelial vasodilation function were reported in hypercholesterolemic patients treated with the XO inhibitor oxypurinol, no salutary effects were found in hypertensive patients [147], and other have failed to show an effect in patients treated with the common XO inhibitor allopurinol [148].

Studies have shown that a major source of endothelial superoxide involved in redox signaling is a multicomponent phagocyte-type NADPH oxidase (NOX) that is subject to specific regulation by stimuli such as oscillatory shear stress, hypoxia, angiotensin II, growth factors, cytokines, and hyperlipidemia [149]. It has been shown that incubation of aortic vessels derived from 1-year-old rats with the NOX inhibitors diphenyleneiodonium (DPI) and apocynin resulted in a significant decrease in superoxide production [132], albeit the specificity of these inhibitors is not well defined. This study also demonstrated that aortic rings from older rats had increased superoxide levels (primarily in the endothelium) and lower NO bioavailability concomitant with increased levels of the p22phox subunit of NADPH oxidase. Moreover, Oudot et al. recently found that the activity and expression of NOX in the aorta of Wistar rats increased with age, and was localized to ECs [150]. In addition, this study documented an age-related increase in the expression of endothelial angiotensin AT(1) receptor suggesting involvement of one of the regulators of vascular NOX activity, the renin-angiotensin system, in modulating vascular superoxide production during aging. This involvement is further suggested by studies showing that aging-related endothelial dysfunction in rats can be prevented by treatment with ACE inhibitors [151]. *In vitro* studies with cultured human dermal microvessel ECs found that angiotensin II treatment promoted OS as gauged by a decline in glutathione (GSH) levels and increased oxidative DNA damage as evaluated by the comet assay [152]. Stimulation or overexpression of a retroviral human heme oxygenase (HO-1) gene in these ECs was protective against angiotensin-mediated OS and effectively attenuated both the DNA damage and GSH decline.

Endothelial cells constitutively express a superoxide generating NOX enzyme similar in many respects to the well-characterized neutrophil NADPH oxidase composed of two membrane components, the p22phox subunit and the gp91phox (NOX1-5) subunit and several cytosolic regulatory subunits including p47phox (p41nox), p40phox and p67phox (p51nox) [149]. A family of gp91phox-related proteins termed the NOX proteins (NOX1-5) are present in vascular ECs and SMCs [153]. ECs contain NOX1, NOX2, NOX4 and NOX5, whereas vascular SMCs express NOX1, NOX4 and NOX5. While p22phox mRNA and protein were detected in both ECs and SMCs, the expression of gp91phox was confined to ECs [134]. Interestingly, NOX4, a homologue of gp91phox/NOX2, is more abundantly expressed in ECs than NOX2. Downregulation of NOX4 mediated by deployment of an antisense oligonucleotide resulted in reduced superoxide production in ECs both *in vivo* and *in vitro* suggesting that NOX4 may function as the major catalytic component of the endothelial NOX [154]. The NOX molecular composition differed in veins and arteries; veins expressed more NOX2 and p22phox, whereas the relative expression of NOX4 was greater in arteries [155]. However in contrast to the neutrophil NADPH oxidase enzyme, in which superoxide generation occurs primarily in the extracellular compartment, a substantial proportion of superoxide generated by the EC NOX enzyme is produced intracellularly, and is primarily located subcellularly in the vicinity of the endoplasmic reticulum [156] or in association with the cytoskeleton [157]. A role for PKC activated by translocation from the cytosol to the membrane in activating NADPH oxidase in vascular aging was ruled out in a study of 32–35 month old rats [158]. This study also found that the aortic expression of the cytosolic NOX subunits, p47(phox) and p67(phox), assessed by RT-PCR remained unchanged with age in senescent rats.

Evidence for an activation of vascular NOX has been provided in animal models including angiotensin II-mediated hypertension [159], and spontaneously hypertensive rats (SHRs) [160], as well as in early stages of experimental hypercholesterolemia [161]. Increased expression of gp91phox (NOX2) and NOX4 has also been reported in atherosclerotic coronary arteries from patients with NOX4 found primarily in non-phagocytic vascular cells [162]. Upregulation of the AT1 receptor in vessels from hypercholesterolemic animals [163], and in platelets from hypercholesterolemic patients [164], along with findings that angiotensin II stimulate NOX activity strongly suggest that an activated (local or systemic) renin-angiotensin system can cause vascular dysfunction [165].

Both NOX-mediated OS and angiotensin II also impact EPCs as well as resulting in senescence. This is in spite of the fact that circulating EPCs are thought to have enhanced protection against OS since they have a lower basal ROS level, show a minor increase in ROS and apoptosis when exposed to exogenous H_2O_2 and exhibit significantly higher expression of the intracellular antioxidative enzymes catalase, glutathione peroxidase and MnSOD as compared to either mature umbilical vein ECs or human microvascular ECs [166]. The exposure of cultured EPCs to angiotensin II (100 nmol/l) significantly accelerated the rate of senescence compared to untreated controls during 14 days in culture as determined by acidic β-galactosidase staining [167]. This *in vitro* model of angiotensin II-mediated EPC senescence was accompanied by elevated levels of gp91phox expression as gauged by RT-PCR and Western immunoblot analysis, OS as gauged by peroxynitrite levels and by impaired cell proliferative activity. The angiotensin II-induced EPC senescence was significantly inhibited by pre-treatment of the EPC s with either valsartan, an angiotensin II type 1 (AT1) receptor antagonist or SOD confirming the importance of OS in the induction of senescence. Further studies from this group demonstrated that estrogen (17 β-estradiol) treatment also could attenuate the angiotensin II-mediated EPC senescence in part through downregulation of AT1R expression [168]. In addition to angiotensin II, EPCs subjected to hyperglycemia show significant acceleration in the rate of *in vitro* senescence partially mediated by the p38 MAP kinase [169], impaired EPC function and elevated OS [170].

In vivo studies with an angiotensin II-infusion model, showed that bone marrow derived EPCs obtained from rat tibias and femurs contained a significantly greater level of senescent cells, less functional activity and decreased differentiation, effects reversed by valsartin treatment [171]. Similarly, the quantity, proliferation, migration and functional activity of bone marrow derived EPCs were reduced in aging mice [172].

Endothelial Dysfunction is Central to the Vascular Aging Phenotype

Endothelial dysfunction, which mainly arises from the onset of senescent pathways, is central to the vascular aging phenotype. It affects a wide array of interacting pathways including hemodynamics, angiogenic vascular remodeling, metabolic, synthetic, anti-inflammatory, and antithrombogenic processes. Its centrality in the regulation of neointimal, intimal and media interactions, cell proliferation and migration, changes in vascular permeability and tonicity, neovascularization and angiogenesis, thrombosis and atheroma formation is depicted in Fig. 5.3.

Aging and Vascular Smooth Muscle Cells (SMCs)

As aging proceeds, SMCs progressively migrate from the vessel media and accumulate into the intima. Intimal SMC accumulation is characterized by a switch from a differentiated to a synthetic phenotype with reduced cytoskeletal markers and the expression of new proteins, and possibly the reinitiation of their embryonic gene expression programs [173]. Aging also alters SMC proliferative and apoptotic behavior and enhanced the response to mitogenic growth factors, such as transforming growth factor-β1. The aging-mediated alterations of SMC properties including the altered expression of matrix metalloproteinases such as MMP-2 and MMP-9 [174, 175], increased ICAM-1 expression and ROS generation [176], represent crucial event in the pathobiology of arterial wall, since they contributes to the vascular remodeling and decline of function with aging and favors the progression of atherosclerosis. Interestingly, the effects of aging on arterial SMC proliferation (*in vivo* and *in vitro*) have yielded conflicting results with different models. For instance, SMCs of aging rats displayed a higher proliferative rate *in vitro* than SMCs from young rats, in association with increased PDGF activity, decreased heparin-like activity[177] and enhanced migration rates [178].

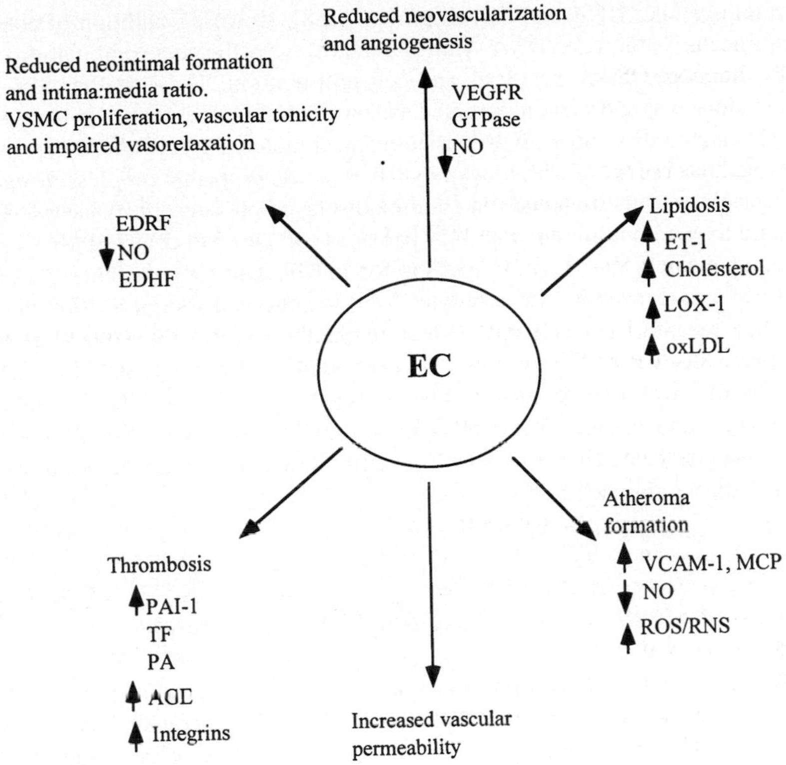

Fig. 5.3 Centrality of endothelial cell dysfunction in vascular aging phenotype

Similar findings of age-mediated proliferation were obtained with mice aortic SMCs [174, 176]. In addition to exacerbated neointimal formation and increased proliferation, vascular SMCs from aging mice also displayed a reduced susceptibility to apoptosis when subjected to either serum starvation or NO, compared to SMCs from younger mice [179]. In contrast, cultured SMC migration and proliferative activity from arteries of human subjects grown under basal conditions and after IGF-1 or insulin treatment decrease with increased subject age [180, 181]. Decreased migration of human aortic SMCs has been attributed to decreased MMP-2 and upregulated levels of tissue inhibitor of metalloproteinases (TIMPs) in aged cells [182]. This discrepancy may be in part due to the development of senescent vascular SMCs, even in the presence of a proliferative SMC subpopulation with an exaggerated response to growth factors and cytokines and may be responsible for intimal SMC accumulation and enhanced expression of TGF-β1, MMP-2 and ICAM-1 [175]. Both proliferative and senescent SMCs have been reported to coexist within the same vascular layer [183].

There is also evidence that senescence-associated functional changes occur in vascular SMCs. Gathered observations revealed that the *in vitro* response of vascular SMCs to NO and β-adrenoreceptor stimulation is decreased by aging, and such changes may contribute to impairment of endothelium-dependent (as well as endothelium-independent) vasodilation in the elderly [184, 185]. Moreover, production of elastase by senescent vascular SMCs is increased [186]. Vascular SMCs of aging rats also exhibit increased levels in monocyte chemotactic protein-1 (MCP-1) and its receptor CCR2, which enhance vascular SMC migration and invasion and appear to play a role in age-associated arterial remodeling [187].

Age-related impaired responses to serum mitogens may be contributory to the senescent vascular SMC phenotype. *In vitro* studies with rabbit arterial vascular SMCs found that PDGF (10 ng/ml), IGF-1 (20 ng/ml), and EGF (10 ng/ml) when added alone, produced minimal effects on BrdU incorporation into cellular DNA and on cell growth [188]. However, addition of combined PDGF and IGF-1 significantly stimulated DNA synthesis and cell growth and a combination of all 3 factors synergistically stimulated DNA synthesis and cell proliferation. These studies also revealed that PDGF addition alone was sufficient to initiate DNA synthesis in quiescent secondary cultured SMC (G_{1B} phase), although IGF-1 and EGF were required to complete DNA synthesis. Interestingly, arterial SMCs derived from patients with moyamoya disease, an idiopathic progressive cerebrovascular occlusive disease that occurs frequently in children,displayed poor responsiveness to PDGF as well as a significantly longer doubling time at early passages compared to control SMCs [189].

Age-related changes in the receptor systems for PDGF may be contributory to the failure of DNA synthesis in senescent SMCs. In a study of 3 different human arterial SMC strains, the number of specific PDGF receptors per cell-surface area markedly decreased *in vitro* with increasing age as did the apparent K_d for PDGF binding [190]. In addition, the internalization and degradation of PDGF per receptor were significantly reduced in senescent SMCs and the amount of PDGF that escaped degradation, and was recycled back to the cell surface, was significantly greater in senescent SMCs than in young cells. Furthermore, PDGF receptor downregulation was significantly greater in senescent SMCs than young cells.

Mechanisms and Significance of Vascular SMC Senescence

Vascular SMCs are an important component of atherosclerotic plaques, responsible for promoting plaque stability in advanced lesions. In contrast, vascular SMC apoptosis has been implicated in a number of deleterious consequences of atherosclerosis, including plaque rupture, vessel remodeling, coagulation, inflammation and calcification. In studies using transgenic mice with selective induction of vascular SMC apoptosis, examination of the direct consequences of apoptosis in both normal vessels and atherosclerotic plaques showed that while normal arteries are able to withstand extensive cell losses with little change, vascular SMC apoptosis alone was sufficient to induce vulnerability to rupture in plaques [191]. Moreover, vascular SMCs derived from human plaques show numerous features of senescence both in culture and *in vivo*.[192] Compared with SMCs from normal vessels, SMCs from human atherosclerotic plaques proliferate more slowly, undergo earlier senescence, and demonstrate higher levels of apoptosis in culture. In addition, compared with normal vascular SMCs, plaque SMCs showed a higher ratio of the active (hypophosphorylated) to the inactive (phosphorylated) form of Rb and a lower level of E2F transcriptional activity [193]. This defect in Rb phosphorylation may underlie the slower rate of cell proliferation and earlier onset of senescence in human plaque SMCs.

In an analysis of normal human vessels and plaques, vascular SMCs in fibrous caps expressed markers of senescence (SA-β-galactosidase and the cyclin-dependent kinase inhibitors p16 and p21) not seen in normal vessels [194]. Moreover, in matched samples from the same individual, plaques showed markedly shorter telomeres than normal vessels, with telomere shortening closely associated with increasing severity of atherosclerosis. In addition, changes in cyclins D/E, p16, p21, and Rb were mediated by vascular SMC senescence. *In vivo*, plaque vascular SMCs exhibited extensive oxidative DNA damage, suggesting that telomere damage may be induced by OS. Furthermore, oxidants induced premature senescence *in vitro*, with accelerated telomere shortening and reduced telomerase activity. These findings suggested that human atherosclerosis is characterized by senescence of vascular SMCs, accelerated by OS-induced DNA damage, inhibition of telomerase and marked telomere shortening.

Angiotensin II (Ang II) significantly induced premature senescence of human vascular SMCs via the p53/p21-dependent pathway *in vitro*.[195] Inhibition of this signaling pathway effectively suppressed induction of proinflammatory cytokines and the premature senescence of vascular SMCs by Ang II. Ang II also significantly increased the number of senescent vascular SMCs and promoted vascular inflammation by inducing the expression of proinflammatory molecules and of p21 in a mouse model of atherosclerosis *in vivo*. Disruption of p21 markedly ameliorated the induction of proinflammatory molecules by Ang II, thereby preventing the development of atherosclerosis suggesting a direct role of p21 in its pathogenesis.

Introduction of a retroviral-based construct containing an activated ras allele (H-rasV12) into human SMCs induced a growth arrest with features characteristic of a cellular senescence phenotype, including enlarged cell shapes and increases in expression levels of cyclin-dependent kinase (CDK) inhibitors and SA-β-galactosidase activity [196]. Moreover, Ras-mediated SMC senescence was associated with the increased expression of proinflammatory cytokines, in part through ERK activation. Further experiments, in which an adenoviral vector containing H-rasV12 was transduced into rat carotid arteries injured by a balloon catheter, have shown enhanced vascular inflammation and senescence compared with mock-infected injured arteries. Similarly, SA-β-galactosidase positive vascular SMCs were detected in the intima of advanced human atherosclerotic lesions and exhibited increased levels of ERK activity and proinflammatory cytokine expression

There is evidence that cellular injury and subsequent intimal proliferative response (primarily of vascular SMCs) leads to increased replicative senescence. In rabbit carotid arteries subjected to single and double balloon denudation, an accumulation of senescent cells (i.e., SA-β-galactosidase-positive cells) in the neointima and media of all injured vessels has been reported, in contrast to the near absence of such cells in control vessels [183]. The majority of SA-β-galactosidase-positive cells were vascular SMCs and a minority were ECs. SMCs, the most numerous cells in the vascular wall, are capable to respond to injury through their ability to synthesize extracellular matrix molecules and protease inhibitors. Moreover, vascular SMCs exhibit an extraordinary capacity to undergo phenotypic changes during development and during insult. In response to injury, contractile vascular SMCs can be induced to change phenotype, proliferate and migrate to effect repair and after repair is completed, the SMCs return to a nonproliferating contractile phenotype. In the context of atherosclerosis, vascular SMCS contribute to the formation of a protective fibrous cap maintained at sites of injury, primarily by providing collagen and components of the ECM including proteoglycans; stability of these caps is known to require greater collagen and ECM content than the adjacent intima. In some cases, this phenotypic transition is dysregulated and vascular SMCs are induced to undergo inappropriate differentiation into cells with features of other mesenchymal lineages such as osteoblasts, chondrocytes and adipocytes. This differentiation of the SMCs may be contributory to vascular calcification, which appears to increase with aging, and can also contribute to vessel stiffness as well as to coronary atherosclerotic plaque burden, increased risk of myocardial infarction, and plaque instability [197, 198].

In some pathologies such as aortic aneurysm, the SMC responsive capacity is overcome and the quantity of extracellular matrix decreases [199]. In support of this view, it has been proposed that abdominal aortic aneurysms arise largely through a degenerative process characterized in part by depletion of medial SMCs, implying that generalized aging and SMC senescence contribute to aneurysmal degeneration [200]. SMCs derived from patients' aneurysm vascular wall exhibited a distinct morphologic appearance in culture (i.e., larger and rounder), a diminished proliferative capacity compared to SMCs from the adjacent regions, and a limited *in vitro* life span; however, they displayed no differences with respect to necrosis, apoptosis or cell viability.

Markers of SMC in Aging and Aging-Related Diseases

Markers of cell senescence have been identified in the vascular wall of patients with atherosclerosis. In particular, SMCs from human plaques show numerous features of senescence including reduced proliferative growth in culture, shorter telomeres, increased ICAM-1 and SA β-galactosidase, as well as altered patterns of gene expression of cell-cycle regulators and matrix metalloproteinases, many of these changes are detectable in SMCs *in vivo* as well [201].

In SMCs cultured from old animals, Li and co-workers found alterations in cytoskeletal proteins including decreased levels of smooth muscle myosin, α-smooth muscle actin, and vimentin [12]. Further observations in aging rats revealed decreased desmin levels [202]. Jones et al. found that aortic vascular SMC polyploidy (primarily tetraploidy) is a biomarker for aging and that the augmented DNA dosage modulates selective gene-specific transcript expression [203]. Over 60% of the SMCs in the wall of the thoracic aorta of 36-month-old Norway rats are tetraploid compared with 8% in 3-month-old rats. However, a select group of mRNAs assessed by microarray analysis were reduced in tetraploid compared with diploid cells, including transcripts of guanine deaminase, the matrix proteins rat glypican 3 (OCI-5) and decorin, and the inflammation-associated transcripts such as insulin-like growth factor-binding protein 6, macrophage inflammatory protein 2 precursor, macrophage galactose N-acetylgalactoseamine-specific lectin, and complement component C4. A dramatic attenuation of clock gene expression in senescent human vascular SMCs, compared with their young counterparts, has been also documented. The molecular mechanisms underlying the loss of circadian rhythmicity in senescent cells have been related, at least in part, to telomere shortening and impaired activation of the CREB/ERK pathway [204, 205].

Thrombosis, Fibrinolysis and Inflammation in Aging

A dramatic increase in the rates of venous and arterial thrombotic events has been reported with aging [206, 207]. Contributory to increased thrombosis are vascular hypercoagubility due to significant elevation in procoagulant factors, including fibrinogen, factors VIII and IX (Table 5.3), without a proportional increase in anticoagulant factors, some of which show only a marginal increase (e.g., protein C), while others decline (e.g., heparin factor) in aging [208, 209].

A number of genomic elements involved in controlling age-related expression of some coagulation proteins have been identified. For instance, one of the key genes for aging-associated thrombosis is plasminogen activator inhibitor-1 (PAI-1), a principal inhibitor of fibrinolysis. The expression of PAI-1 is not only elevated in the elderly but also significantly induced in a variety of aging-associated pathologies including obesity, insulin resistance, emotional stress, immune responses, and vascular sclerosis/remodeling. Several cytokines and hormones, including tumor necrosis factor-α, transforming growth factor-β, angiotensin II, and insulin, positively regulate the gene expression of PAI-1 [210].

Another key procoagulant factor upregulated in aging is factor IX (FIX), a plasma protease precursor occupying a key position in the blood coagulation cascade, where the intrinsic and extrinsic initiation pathways merge. FIX is synthesized in the liver with high tissue specificity, its deficiency results in the bleeding disorder hemophilia B. With advancing age, the circulatory levels of FIX increase to approximately two fold in comparison to those found at young ages with concomitant increases in the liver FIX transcript level and blood coagulation potential in both, human subjects and in mice [211, 212].

Two essential age-regulatory elements in the human X-linked FIX gene, AE5' (or more recently ASE) and AE3' (AIE), have been identified (depicted in Fig. 5.4) that are required and sufficient for normal age regulation of factor IX expression. ASE, a PEA-3 related element present in the long interspersed repetitive element–derived sequence of the 5′ upstream region is responsible for FIX age-stable expression and functions in a position-independent manner. AIE, in the middle of the 3′ untranslated region, is responsible for age-associated elevation in liver FIX mRNA levels.

Table 5.3 Hemostatic changes during aging

Coagulation system proteins	
Fibrinogen	↑
Factor V	↑
Factor VII	↑
Factor VIII	↑
Factor IX	↑
Factor XIII	↑
Prekallikrein levels	↑
von Willebrand factor	↑
High molecular-weight kininogen	↑
Markers of coagulation activation	↑
Anticoagulant proteins	
Antithrombin	↑(F); ↓(M)
Tissue factor pathway inhibitor	↑
Protein C	=
Heparin Cofactor II	↓
Fibrinolytic system proteins	
Plasminogen activator inhibitor-1	↑
Plasminogen activator activity	↓
Plasmin-antiplasmin complex	↑
Thrombin-activable fibrinolysis inhibitor	↑
Platelet function	
β-Thromboglobulin	↑
Platelet factor 4	↑
Aggregation to ADP and collagen	↑
Vascular endothelium	
Rigidity of vessel wall	↑
Endothelial angiotensin II	↑
Endothelial nitric oxide	↓
Endothelial nitric oxide synthase	↓
Endothelial prostacyclin	↓

F: Female; M: Male

Transgenic mouse model studies revealed that ASE and AIE act in a concerted manner to recapitulate natural patterns of the advancing age-associated increase in factor IX gene expression [213].

Interestingly, molecular analysis revealed that the human anticoagulant factor protein C (PC) contains a functional age-related stability element (hPC ASE) in the 5′-upstream proximal region but it was found to lack any age-related increase element [214]. The ASE in the PC gene (shown in Fig. 5.4) is located in nearly the same position with respect to the start site (near −800) and contains a sequence CAGGAAG similar to the hFIX ASE sequence GAGGAAG. Expression analysis in the transgenic gene revealed that the ASE regulatory sequences are responsible for the stable expression of PC with age, in contrast with the age-mediated induction of FIX gene expression.

In addition, enhanced platelet activity as well as molecular and anatomic/sclerotic changes in the vessel wall both contribute to an enhanced propensity for thrombosis in aging. Elevated levels of interleukin-6 (IL-6) and C-reactive protein (CRP) are also indicative of a potent role of inflammation, as a stimulus for thrombus formation in the elderly. Nevertheless, despite evidence of a prothrombotic state, many elderly people do not experience clinical thrombotic events [215]. In centenarians, biochemical signs of marked hypercoagulability are associated with a healthy state. Moreover, the increase in coagulation proteins and activation markers conveys a survival advantage, such as inhibiting tumor angiogenesis [216]. Increased obesity may heighten thrombotic risks in the elderly since adipose tissue is an important source of inflammatory cytokines and PAI-1.

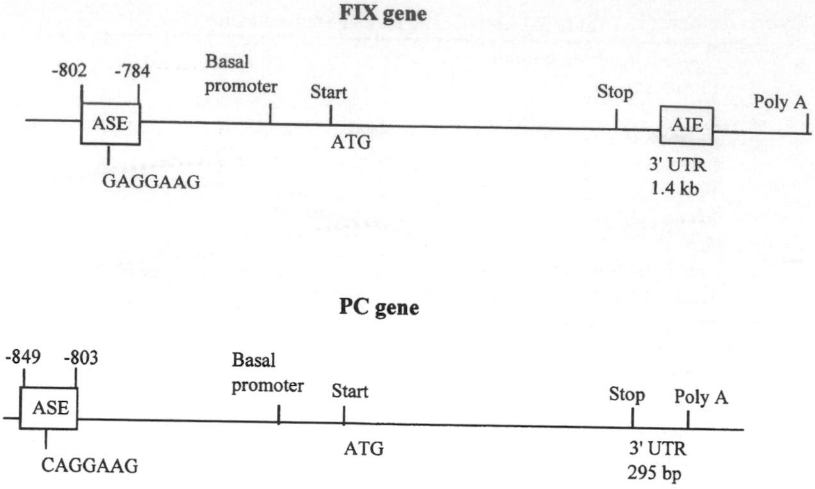

Fig. 5.4 Age-sensitive regulatory elements in hemostatic genes

Besides alterations in the thrombotic pathways, changes in the vascular endothelium occurring with aging are also closely linked to inflammatory pathway induction. Shelton et al. [217] using microarray analysis documented the induction of adhesion molecule, ICAM-1 (CD54), normally expressed at low levels in resting ECs. The binding partners for ICAM-1 are the integrins CD11a/CD18 (leukocyte function-associated antigen 1, LFA-1) and CD11b/CD18 (complement receptor 3, CR3 or αM integrin). Both CD11a/CD18 and CD11b/CD18 are abundantly expressed on inflammatory cells (including monocytes, neutrophils, and macrophages), thus, the induction of ICAM-1 on senescent ECs can enhance the binding of inflammatory cells that may damage the vessel and surrounding tissues such as seen in atherosclerosis.

Angiogenesis/Neovascularization in Aging

Aging-mediated changes in angiogenesis have been noted at the molecular, cellular, and physiological levels of regulation. Age-sensitive components of the neovascular process include ECs and their proliferative pathways, including neuro-chemical mediators, as well as growth factors and their cognate receptors and hemostatic pathway elements as shown in Fig. 5.5. In addition, structural and regulatory components of the matrix scaffold that surround newly formed vessels are also altered in aged tissues. Cell-matrix interactions are primarily mediated by membrane-spanning integrins capable of cell or matrix component recognition and involved in two-way intracellular signal transduction. Alterations in cell-matrix interactions associated with aging largely result from quantitative and qualitative changes in matrix macromolecules and the integrins that bind them [218].

These myriad changes result in delayed and impaired neovascularization. Edelberg and Reed have pointed out that the clinical consequences of the decreased potential of aged tissues to form new vessels are particularly likely to be detrimental during the revascularization of the ischemic heart and during the repair of injured tissues, but may provide some benefit in slowing the growth of tumors in aging individuals [219, 220].

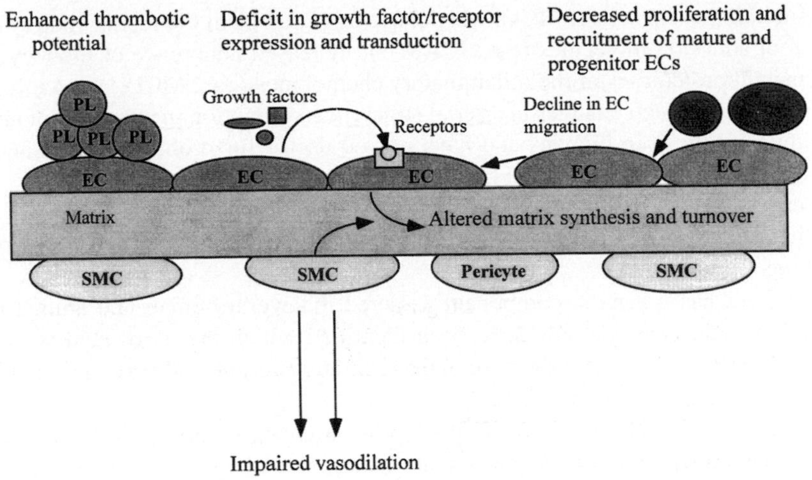

Fig. 5.5 Age-mediated damage in elements of the angiogenic response
The involvement of PL (platelets), SMC (smooth muscle cells) and ECs (endothelial cells) is shown

Conclusion

Senescence of the ECs and vascular smooth muscle whether occurring naturally in the course of cellular aging, initiated by telomere shortening, or prematurely by DNA damage, results in significant changes in the cellular phenotype including a variety of vascular and arterial defects. In addition to the aging-mediated marked reduction in endothelial NO production that has striking effects on vascular dilation, vascular tone and thrombotic promotion, there are also enhanced interactions with inflammatory cells via signaling, and critical changes in vascular cell proliferation, migration and cell death that underlie the extensive vascular remodeling that occurs both in aging and in aging-related vascular diseases such as atherosclerosis, CAD and hypertension. At the present time, molecular tools are being successfully deployed in unraveling the molecular mechanisms responsible for EC and SMC aging and senescence, including a delineation of the corresponding changes in gene/protein expression profiles occurring in aging vascular cells, and in identifying genes and genomic elements that play a role in determining both normal aging vascular gene expression, as well as factors predisposing to pathological changes such as arterial stiffness. This area of research has begun to provide valuable information for both diagnostic and novel effective therapeutic approaches in treating aging related vascular disease some of which are discussed in Chapter 14.

Summary

- Aging is associated with alterations in a number of structural and functional properties of large arteries, including diameter, wall thickness, wall stiffness, and endothelial function.
- Evidence indicates that arterial changes are also accelerated in age-associated cardiovascular diseases including hypertension, coronary artery disease, congestive heart failure, and stroke. These changes themselves can be risk factors for the appearance and/or progression of these diseases.
- Age-associated increase in arterial wall thickening is caused primarily by an increase in intimal thickening.
- The thickened intima in aging contains matrix proteins, collagen, fibronectin, proteoglycans and

vascular smooth muscle cells (SMCs), which have migrated from the media and exhibit elevated expression of adhesion molecules (e.g., ICAM-1), increased adherence of monocytes, elevated levels of metalloproteinases of the inflammatory chemokines (e.g., MCP-1) and receptors.

- Patterns of age-associated changes in arterial structure and function in a number of animals models are similar to those in humans and have proved useful for probing cellular and molecular determinants of age-mediated arterial remodeling.
- Age-associated increases in thickness of the arterial wall are accompanied by an increase in arterial stiffness in part mediated by elastin depletion, increased collagen and glycation-mediated cross-linking.
- Arterial stiffness has a genetic component as noted in several human and animal genetic disorders, and specific gene variants have been identified which are associated with phenotypic expression. Genes involved include those in the renin-aldosterone pathway, endothelin receptors, matrix remodeling and NO production.
- Age-mediated endothelial cell (EC) dysfunction is associated with a marked reduction in NO production that has striking effects on vascular dilation, vascular tone, thrombotic promotion and enhanced binding to inflammatory cells.
- Aging causes profound changes in both EC and vascular SMC proliferation, migration and cell death that underlie the extensive vascular remodeling that occurs both in aging and in aging-related vascular diseases, such as atherosclerosis, CAD and hypertension.
- Elements of the highly conserved senescence pathways are present in both ECs and vascular SMCs. Senescence and its effect on vascular cell function have been documented in both *in vivo* and *in vitro* studies.
- In addition to changes in proliferative cell growth, specific markers of vascular cell senescence include specific gene expression profiles, elevated levels of senescence-associated β-galactosidase, telomere shortening and changes in cell-cycle regulators.
- Primary triggers in vascular senescence include telomere dysfunction, oncogenic stimulation (e.g., Ras), DNA damage and oxidative stress.
- Both angiotensin II treatment and increased glycation accumulation also lead to vascular cell senescence.
- The source of OS mediating both vascular cell senescence and aging-associated EC and SMC dysfunction, includes mitochondrial ROS production, uncoupled endothelial NO synthase (eNOS), vascular xanthine oxidase and NADPH oxidase (NOX).

References

1. Najjar SS, Scuteri A, Lakatta EG. Arterial aging: is it an immutable cardiovascular risk factor? Hypertension 2005;46:454–462
2. Lakatta EG. Cardiovascular regulatory mechanisms in advanced age. Physiol Rev 1993;73:413–467
3. Nagai Y, Metter EJ, Earley CJ, Kemper MK, Becker LC, Lakatta EG, Fleg JL. Increased carotid artery intimal-medial thickness in asymptomatic older subjects with exercise-induced myocardial ischemia. Circulation 1998;98:1504–1509
4. Virmani R, Avolio AP, Mergner WJ, Robinowitz M, Herderick EE, Cornhill JF, Guo SY, Liu TH, Ou DY, O'Rourke M. Effect of aging on aortic morphology in populations with high and low prevalence of hypertension and atherosclerosis. Comparison between occidental and Chinese communities. Am J Pathol 1991;139:1119–1129
5. Li Z, Froehlich J, Galis ZS, Lakatta EG. Increased expression of matrix metalloproteinase-2 in the thickened intima of aged rats. Hypertension 1999;33:116–123
6. Asai K, Kudej RK, Shen YT, Yang GP, Takagi G, Kudej AB, Geng YJ, Sato N, Nazareno JB, Vatner DE, Natividad F, Bishop SP, Vatner SF. Peripheral vascular endothelial dysfunction and apoptosis in old monkeys. Arterioscler Thromb Vasc Biol 2000;20:1493–1499
7. Orlandi A, Marcellini M, Spagnoli LG. Aging influences development and progression of early aortic atherosclerotic lesions in cholesterol-fed rabbits. Arterioscler Thromb Vasc Biol 2000;20:1123–1136

8. Spinetti G, Wang M, Monticone R, Zhang J, Zhao D, Lakatta EG. Rat aortic MCP-1 and its receptor CCR2 increase with age and alter vascular smooth muscle cell function. Arterioscler Thromb Vasc Biol 2004;24:1397–1402
9. Boring L, Gosling J, Cleary M, Charo IF. Decreased lesion formation in CCR2–/–mice reveals a role for chemokines in the initiation of atherosclerosis. Nature 1998;394:894–897
10. Wang M, Lakatta EG. Altered regulation of matrix metalloproteinase-2 in aortic remodeling during aging. Hypertension 2002;39:865–887
11. Wang M, Takagi G, Asai K, Resuello RG, Natividad FF, Vatner DE, Vatner SF, Lakatta EG. Aging increases aortic MMP-2 activity and angiotensin II in nonhuman primates. Hypertension 2003;41:1308–1316
12. Li Z, Cheng H, Lederer WJ, Froehlich J, Lakatta EG. Enhanced proliferation and migration and altered cytoskeletal proteins in early passage smooth muscle cells from young and old rat aortic explants. Exp Mol Pathol 1997;64:1–11
13. Hariri RJ, Hajjar DP, Coletti D, Alonso DR, Weksler ME, Rabellino E. Aging and arteriosclerosis. Cell cycle kinetics of young and old arterial smooth muscle cells. Am J Pathol 1988;131:132–136
14. Torella D, Leosco D, Indolfi C, Curcio A, Coppola C, Ellison GM, Russo VG, Torella M, Li Volti G, Rengo F, Chiariello M. Aging exacerbates negative remodeling and impairs endothelial regeneration after balloon injury. Am J Physiol Heart Circ Physiol 2004;287:H2850–H2860
15. Hofmann CS, Wang X, Sullivan CP, Toselli P, Stone PJ, McLean SE, Mecham RP, Schreiber BM, Sonenshein GE. B-Myb represses elastin gene expression in aortic smooth muscle cells. J Biol Chem 2005;280: 7694–7701
16. Duca L, Floquet N, Alix AJ, Haye B, Debelle L. Elastin as a matrikine. Crit Rev Oncol Hematol 2004;49:235–244
17. Vaitkevicius PV, Lane M, Spurgeon H, Ingram DK, Roth GS, Egan JJ, Vasan S, Wagle DR, Ulrich P, Brines M, Wuerth JP, Cerami A, Lakatta EG. A cross-link breaker has sustained effects on arterial and ventricular properties in older rhesus monkeys. Proc Natl Acad Sci USA 2001;98:1171–1175
18. O'Rourke MF, Nichols WW. Aortic diameter, aortic stiffness, and wave reflection increase with age and isolated systolic hypertension. Hypertension 2005;45:652–658
19. Susic D, Varagic J, Ahn J, Frohlich ED. Collagen cross-link breakers: a beginning of a new era in the treatment of cardiovascular changes associated with aging, diabetes, and hypertension. Curr Drug Targets Cardiovasc Haematol Disord 2004;4:97–101
20. Bakris GL, Bank AJ, Kass DA, Neutel JM, Preston RA, Oparil S. Advanced glycation end-product cross-link breakers. A novel approach to cardiovascular pathologies related to the aging process. Am J Hypertens 2004;17:23S–30S
21. Franklin SS, Gustin WIV, Wong ND, Larson MG, Weber MA, Kannel WB, Levy D. Hemodynamic patterns of age-related changes in blood pressure. The Framingham Heart Study. Circulation 1997;96:308–315
22. Wilkinson IB, Franklin SS, Hall IR, Tyrrell S, Cockcroft JR. Pressure amplification explains why pulse pressure is unrelated to risk in young subjects. Hypertension 2001;38:1461–1466
23. Benetos A, Laurent S, Hoeks AP, Boutouyrie PH, Safar ME. Arterial alterations with aging and high blood pressure. A noninvasive study of carotid and femoral arteries. Arterioscler Thromb 1993;13:90–97
24. Lieber SC, Aubry N, Pain J, Diaz G, Kim SJ, Vatner SF. Aging increases stiffness of cardiac myocytes measured by atomic force microscopy nanoindentation. Am J Physiol Heart Circ Physiol 2004;287:H645–H651
25. Laurent S, Boutouyrie P, Lacolley P. Structural and genetic bases of arterial stiffness. Hypertension 2005;45:1050–1055
26. Benetos A, Topouchian J, Ricard S, Gautier S, Bonnardeaux A, Asmar R, Poirier O, Soubrier F, Safar M, Cambien F. Influence of angiotensin II type 1 receptor polymorphism on aortic stiffness in never-treated hypertensive patients. Hypertension 1995;26:44–47
27. Lajemi M, Labat C, Gautier S, Lacolley P, Safar M, Asmar R, Cambien F, Benetos A. Angiotensin II type 1 receptor-153A/G and 1166A/C gene polymorphisms and increase in aortic stiffness with age in hypertensive subjects. J Hypertens 2001;19:407–413
28. Mattace-Raso FU, van der Cammen TJ, Sayed-Tabatabaei FA, van Popele NM, Asmar R, Schalekamp MA, Hofman A, van Duijn CM, Witteman JC. Angiotensin-converting enzyme gene polymorphism and common carotid stiffness. The Rotterdam study. Atherosclerosis 2004;174:121–126
29. Bozec E, Lacolley P, Bergaya S, Boutouyrie P, Meneton P, Herisse-Legrand M, Boulanger CM, Alhenc-Gelas F, Kim HS, Laurent S, Dabire H. Arterial stiffness and angiotensinogen gene in hypertensive patients and mutant mice. J Hypertens 2004;22:1299–1307
30. Pojoga L, Gautier S, Blanc H, Guyene TT, Poirier O, Cambien F, Benetos A. Genetic determination of plasma aldosterone levels in essential hypertension. Am J Hypertens 1998;11:856–860
31. Wojciechowska W, Staessen JA, Stolarz K, Nawrot T, Filipovsky J, Ticha M, Bianchi G, Brand E, Cwynar M, Grodzicki T, Kuznetsova T, Struijker-Boudier HA, Svobodova V, Thijs L, Van Bortel LM, Kawecka-Jaszcz K. European Project on Genes in Hypertension (EPOGH) Investigators. Association of peripheral and central

arterial wave reflections with the CYP11B2 -344C allele and sodium excretion. J Hypertens 2004;22: 2311–2319
32. Safar ME, Cattan V, Lacolley P, Nzietchueng R, Labat C, Lajemi M, de Luca N, Benetos A. Aldosterone synthase gene polymorphism, stroke volume and age-related changes in aortic pulse wave velocity in subjects with hypertension. J Hypertens 2005;23:1159–1166
33. Hanon O, Luong V, Mourad JJ, Bortolotto LA, Jeunemaitre X, Girerd X. Aging, carotid artery distensibility, and the Ser422Gly elastin gene polymorphism in humans. Hypertension 2001;38:1185–1189
34. Medley TL, Cole TJ, Gatzka CD, Wang WY, Dart AM, Kingwell BA. Fibrillin-1 genotype is associated with aortic stiffness and disease severity in patients with coronary artery disease. Circulation 2002;105:810–815
35. Powell JT, Turner RJ, Sian M, Debasso R, Lanne T. Influence of fibrillin-1 genotype on the aortic stiffness in men. J Appl Physiol 2005;99:1036–1040
36. Medley TL, Kingwell BA, Gatzka CD, Pillay P, Cole TJ. Matrix metalloproteinase-3 genotype contributes to age-related aortic stiffening through modulation of gene and protein expression. Circ Res 2003;92: 1254–1261
37. Medley TL, Cole TJ, Dart AM, Gatzka CD, Kingwell BA. Matrix metalloproteinase-9 genotype influences large artery stiffness through effects on aortic gene and protein expression. Arterioscler Thromb Vasc Biol 2004;24:1479–1484
38. Yasmin, McEniery CM, O'Shaughnessy KM, Harnett P, Arshad A, Wallace S, Maki-Petaja K, McDonnell B, Ashby MJ, Brown J, Cockcroft JR, Wilkinson IB. Variation in the human matrix metalloproteinase-9 gene is associated with arterial stiffness in healthy individuals. Arterioscler Thromb Vasc Biol 2006;26:1799–1805
39. Chen W, Srinivasan SR, Bond MG, Tang R, Urbina EM, Li S, Boerwinkle E, Berenson GS. Nitric oxide synthase gene polymorphism (G894T) influences arterial stiffness in adults: The Bogalusa Heart Study. Am J Hypertens 2004;17:553–559
40. Lajemi M, Gautier S, Poirier O, Baguet JP, Mimran A, Gosse P, Hanon O, Labat C, Cambien F, Benetos A. Endothelin gene variants and aortic and cardiac structure in never-treated hypertensives. Am J Hypertens 2001;14:755–760
41. Nurnberger J, Opazo Saez A, Mitchell A, Buhrmann S, Wenzel RR, Siffert W, Philipp T, Schafers RF. The T-allele of the C825T polymorphism is associated with higher arterial stiffness in young healthy males. J Hum Hypertens 2004;18:267–271
42. Iemitsu M, Maeda S, Otsuki T, Sugawara J, Tanabe T, Jesmin S, Kuno S, Ajisaka R, Miyauchi T, Matsuda M. Polymorphism in endothelin-related genes limits exercise-induced decreases in arterial stiffness in older subjects. Hypertension 2006;47:928–936
43. Durier S, Fassot C, Laurent S, Boutouyrie P, Couetil JP, Fine E, Lacolley P, Dzau VJ, Pratt RE. Physiological genomics of human arteries: quantitative relationship between gene expression and arterial stiffness. Circulation 2003;108:1845–1851
44. Saward L, Zahradka P. Angiotensin II activates phosphatidylinositol 3-kinase in vascular smooth muscle cells. Circ Res 1997;81:249–257
45. Quignard JF, Mironneau J, Carricaburu V, Fournier B, Babich A, Numberg B, Mironneau C, Macrez N. Phosphoinositide 3-kinase gamma mediates angiotensin II–induced stimulation of L-type calcium channels in vascular myocytes. J Biol Chem 2001;276:32545–32551
46. Shen TL, Guan JL. Differential regulation of cell migration and cell cycle progression by FAK complexes with Src, PI3K, Grb7 and Grb2 in focal contacts. FEBS Lett 2001;499:176–181
47. Zheng XL, Renaux B, Hollenberg MD. Parallel contractile signal transduction pathways activated by receptors for thrombin and epidermal growth factor–urogastrone in guinea pig gastric smooth muscle: blockade by inhibitors of mitogen-activated protein kinase-kinase and phosphatidyl inositol 3'-kinase. J Pharmacol Exp Ther 1998;285:325–334
48. Maeda S, Iemitsu M, Miyauchi T, Kuno S, Matsuda M, Tanaka H. Aortic stiffness and aerobic exercise: mechanistic insight from microarray analyses. Med Sci Sports Exerc 2005;37:1710–1716
49. Wilkinson IB, Franklin SS, Cockcroft JR. Nitric oxide and the regulation of large artery stiffness: from physiology to pharmacology. Hypertension 2004;44:112–116
50. Celermajer DS, Sorensen KE, Spiegelhalter DJ, Georgakopoulos D, Robinson J, Deanfield JE. Aging is associated with endothelial dysfunction in healthy men years before the age-related decline in women. J Am Coll Cardiol 1994;24:471–476
51. Gerhard M, Roddy MA, Creager SJ, Creager MA. Aging progressively impairs endothelium-dependent vasodilation in forearm resistance vessels of humans. Hypertension 1996;27:849–853
52. McEniery CM, Wallace S, Mackenzie IS, McDonnell B, Yasmin, Newby DE, Cockcroft JR, Wilkinson IB. Endothelial function is associated with pulse pressure, pulse wave velocity, and augmentation index in healthy humans. Hypertension 2006;48:602–608
53. Brandes RP, Fleming I, Busse R. Endothelial aging. Cardiovasc Res 2005;66:286–294
54. Goligorsky MS. Endothelial cell dysfunction: can't live with it, how to live without it. Am J Physiol Renal Physiol 2005;288:F871–F880

55. Kurz DJ, Decary S, Hong Y, Erusalimsky JD. Senescence-associated (beta)-galactosidase reflects an increase in lysosomal mass during replicative ageing of human endothelial cells. J Cell Sci 2000;113:3613–3622
56. Foreman KE, Tang J. Molecular mechanisms of replicative senescence in endothelial cells. Exp Geronto 2003;38:1251–1257
57. Rivard A, Fabre JE, Silver M, Chen D, Murohara T, Kearney M, Magner M, Asahara T, Isner JM. Age-dependent impairment of angiogenesis. Circulation 1999;99:111–120
58. Yang J, Chang E, Cherry AM, Bangs CD, Oei Y, Bodnar A, Bronstein A, Chiu CP, Herron GS. Human endothelial cell life extension by telomerase expression. J Biol Chem 1999;274:26141–26148
59. Asahara T, Murohara T, Sullivan A, Silver M, van der Zee R, Li T, Witzenbichler B, Schatteman G, Isner JM. Isolation of putative progenitor endothelial cells for angiogenesis. Science 1997;275:964–967
60. Werner N, Nickenig G. Clinical and therapeutical implications of EPC biology in atherosclerosis. J Cell Mol Med 2006;10:318–332
61. Hill JM, Zalos G, Halcox JP, Schenke WH, Waclawiw MA, Quyyumi AA, Finkel T. Circulating endothelial progenitor cells, vascular function, and cardiovascular risk. N Engl J Med 2003;348:593–600
62. Vasa M, Fichtlscherer S, Aicher A, Adler K, Urbich C, Martin H, Zeiher AM, Dimmeler S. Number and migratory activity of circulating endothelial progenitor cells inversely correlate with risk factors for coronary artery disease. Circ Res 2001;89:e1–e7
63. Edelberg JM, Tang L, Hattori K, Lyden D, Rafii S. Young adult bone marrow-derived endothelial precursor cells restore aging-impaired cardiac angiogenic function. Circ Res 2002;90:E89–E93
64. Buys CH. Telomeres, telomerase, and cancer. N Engl J Med 2000;342:1282–1283
65. Aviv H, Khan MY, Skurnick J, Okuda K, Kimura M, Gardner J, Priolo L, Aviv A. Age dependent aneuploidy and telomere length of the human vascular endothelium. Atherosclerosis 2001;159:281–287
66. Chang E, Harley CB. Telomere length and replicative aging in human vascular tissues. Proc Natl Acad Sci USA 1995;92:11190–11194
67. Minamino T, Kourembanas S. Mechanisms of telomerase induction during vascular smooth muscle cell proliferation. Circ Res 2001;89:237–243
68. Hsiao R, Sharma HW, Ramakrishnan S, Keith E, Narayanan R. Telomerase activity in normal human endothelial cells. Anticancer Res 1997;17:827–832
69. Minamino T, Mitsialis SA, Kourembanas S. Hypoxia extends the life span of vascular smooth muscle cells through telomerase activation. Mol Cell Biol 2001;21:3336–3342
70. Minamino T, Miyauchi H, Yoshida T, Ishida Y, Yoshida H, Komuro I. Endothelial cell senescence in human atherosclerosis:role of telomere in endothelial dysfunction. Circulation 2002;105:1541–1544
71. Young AT, Lakey JR, Murray AG, Mullen JC, Moore RB. In vitro senescence occurring in normal human endothelial cells can be rescued by ectopic telomerase activity. Transplant Proc 2003;35:2483–2485
72. Matsushita H, Chang E, Glassford AJ, Cooke JP, Chiu CP, Tsao PS. eNOS activity is reduced in senescent human endothelial cells: preservation by hTERT immortalization. Circ Res 2001;89:793–798
73. von Zglinicki T. Oxidative stress shortens telomeres. Trends Biochem Sci 2002;27:339–344
74. Kurz DJ, Decary S, Hong Y, Trivier E, Akhmedov A, Erusalimsky JD. Chronic oxidative stress compromises telomere integrity and accelerates the onset of senescence in human endothelial cells. J Cell Sci 2004;117:2417–2426
75. Haendeler J, Hoffmann J, Diehl JF, Vasa M, Spyridopoulos I, Zeiher AM, Dimmeler S. Antioxidants inhibit nuclear export of telomerase reverse transcriptase and delay replicative senescence of endothelial cells. Circ Res 2004;94:768–775
76. Epel ES, Blackburn EH, Lin J, Dhabhar FS, Adler NE, Morrow JD, Cawthon RM. Accelerated telomere shortening in response to life stress. Proc Natl Acad Sci USA 2004;101:17312–17315
77. Epel ES, Lin J, Wilhelm FH, Wolkowitz OM, Cawthon R, Adler NE, Dolbier C, Mendes WB, Blackburn EH. Cell aging in relation to stress arousal and cardiovascular disease risk factors. Psychoneuroendocrinology 2006;31:277–287
78. Ogami M, Ikura Y, Ohsawa M, Matsuo T, Kayo S, Yoshimi N, Hai E, Shirai N, Ehara S, Komatsu R, Naruko T, Ueda M. Telomere shortening in human coronary artery diseases. Arterioscler Thromb Vasc Biol 2004;24:546–550
79. Smogorzewska A, de Lange T. Different telomere damage signaling pathways in human and mouse cells. EMBO J 2002;21:4338–4348
80. Lechel A, Satyanarayana A, Ju Z, Plentz RR, Schaetzlein S, Rudolph C, Wilkens L, Wiemann SU, Saretzki G, Malek NP, Manns MP, Buer J, Rudolph KL. The cellular level of telomere dysfunction determines induction of senescence or apoptosis in vivo. EMBO Rep 2005;6:275–281
81. Yang Q, Zheng YL, Harris CC. POT1 and TRF2 cooperate to maintain telomeric integrity. Mol Cell Biol 2005;25:1070–1080
82. Serrano M, Blasco MA. Putting the stress on senescence. Curr Opin Cell Biol 2001;13:748–753
83. Toussaint O, Medrano EE, von Zglinicki T. Cellular and molecular mechanisms of stress-induced premature senescence (SIPS) of human diploid fibroblasts and melanocytes. Exp Gerontol 2000;35:927–945

84. Drayton S, Peters G. Immortalisation and transformation revisited. Curr Opin Genet Dev 2002;12:98–104
85. Serrano M, Lin AW, McCurrach ME, Beach D, Lowe SW. Oncogenic ras provokes premature cell senescence associated with accumulation of p53 and p16 INK4a. Cell 1997;88:593–602
86. Dimri GP, Itahana K, Acosta M, Campisi J. Regulation of a senescence checkpoint response by the E2F1 transcription factor and p14(ARF) tumor suppressor. Mol Cell Biol 2000;20:273–285
87. Minamino T, Yoshida T, Tateno K, Miyauchi H, Zou Y, Toko H, Komuro I. Ras induces vascular smooth muscle cell senescence and inflammation in human atherosclerosis. Circulation 2003;108:2264–2269
88. Lin AW, Barradas M, Stone JC, van Aelst L, Serrano M, Lowe SW. Premature senescence involving p53 and p16 is activated in response to constitutive MEK/MAPK mitogenic signaling. Genes Dev 1998;12:3008–3019
89. Wang W, Chen JX, Liao R, Deng Q, Zhou JJ, Huang S, Sun P. Sequential activation of the MEK-extracellular signal-regulated kinase and MKK3/6-p38 mitogen-activated protein kinase pathways mediates oncogenic ras-induced premature senescence. Mol Cell Biol 2002;22:3389–3403
90. Chen J, Brodsky SV, Goligorsky DM, Hampel DJ, Li H, Gross SS, Goligorsky MS. Glycated collagen I induces premature senescence-like phenotypic changes in endothelial cells. Circ Res 2002;90:1290–1298
91. Ben-Porath I, Weinberg RA. When cells get stressed: an integrative view of cellular senescence. J Clin Invest 2004;113: 8–13
92. Narita M, Nunez S, Heard E, Lin AW, Hearn SA, Spector DL. Rb-mediated heterochromatin formation and silencing of E2F target genes during cellular senescence. Cell 2003;113:703–716
93. Kulju KS, Lehman JM. Increased p53 protein associated with aging in human diploid fibroblasts. Experimental Cell Research 1995;217:336–345
94. Wahl GM, Carr AM. The evolution of diverse biological responses to DNA damage: insights from yeast and p53. Nature Cell Biology 2001;3:E277–E286
95. d'Adda di Fagagna F, Reaper PM, Clay-Farrace L, Fiegler H, Carr P, Von Zglinicki T, Saretzki G, Carter NP, Jackson SP. A DNA damage checkpoint response in telomere-initiated senescence. Nature 2003;426:194–198
96. Serrano M, Lin AW, McCurrach ME, Beach D, Lowe SW. Oncogenic ras provokes premature cell senescence associated with accumulation of p53 and p16 INK4a. Cell 1997;88:593–602
97. Krishnamurthy J, Torrice C, Ramsey MR, Kovalev GI, Al-Regaiey K, Su L, Sharpless NE. Ink4a/Arf expression is a biomarker of aging. J Clin Invest 2004;114:1299–1307
98. Alcorta DA, Xiong Y, Phelps D, Hannon G, Beach D, Barrett JC. Involvement of the cyclin-dependent kinase inhibitor p16 (INK4a) in replicative senescence of normal human fibroblasts. Proc Natl Acad Sci USA 1996;93:13742–13747
99. Malumbres M, Perez De Castro I, Hernandez MI, Jimenez M, Corral T, Pellicer A. Cellular response to oncogenic ras involves induction of the Cdk4 and Cdk6 inhibitor p15(INK4b). Mol Cell Biol 2000;20:2915–2925
100. Robertson KD, Jones PA. The human ARF cell cycle regulatory gene promoter is a CpG island which can be silenced by DNA methylation and down-regulated by wild-type p53. Mol Cell Biol 1998;18:6457–6473
101. Freedman DA, Folkman J. CDK2 translational down-regulation during endothelial senescence. Exp Cell Res 2005;307:118–130
102. Tang J, Gordon GM, Nickoloff BJ, Foreman KE. The helix-loop-helix protein id-1 delays onset of replicative senescence in human endothelial cells. Lab Invest 2002;82:1073–1079
103. Beausejour CM, Krtolica A, Galimi F, Narita M, Lowe SW, Yaswen P, Campisi J. Reversal of human cellular senescence: roles of the p53 and p16 pathways. EMBO J 2003;22:4212–4222
104. Narita M, Nunez S, Heard E, Narita M, Lin AW, Hearn SA, Spector DL, Hannon GJ, Lowe SW. Rb-mediated heterochromatin formation and silencing of E2F target genes during cellular senescence. Cell 2003;113:703–716
105. Sato I, Morita I, Kaji K, Ikeda M, Nagao M, Murota S. Reduction of nitric oxide producing activity associated with in vitro aging in cultured human umbilical vein endothelial cell. Biochem Biophys Res Commun 1993;195:1070–1076
106. Deshpande SS, Qi B, Park YC, Irani K. Constitutive activation of rac1 results in mitochondrial oxidative stress and induces premature endothelial cell senescence. Arterioscler Thromb Vasc Biol 2003;23:e1–e6
107. Unterluggauer H, Hampel B, Zwerschke W, Jansen-Durr P. Senescence-associated cell death of human endothelial cells: the role of oxidative stress. Exp Gerontol 2003;38:1149–1160
108. van der Loo B, Labugger R, Skepper JN, Bachschmid M, Kilo J, Powell JM, Palacios-Callender M, Erusalimsky JD, Quaschning T, Malinski T, Gygi D, Ullrich V, Luscher TF. Enhanced peroxynitrite formation is associated with vascular aging. J Exp Med 2000;192:1731–1744
109. Nakajima M, Hashimoto M, Wang F, Yamanaga K, Nakamura N, Uchida T, Yamanouchi K. Aging decreases the production of PGI2 in rat aortic endothelial cells. Exp Gerontol 1997;32:685–693
110. Sato I, Kaji K, Morita I, Nagao M, Murota S. Augmentation of endothelin-1, prostacyclin and thromboxane A2 secretion associated with in vitro ageing in cultured human umbilical vein endothelial cells. Mech Ageing Dev 1993;71:73–84
111. Neubert K, Haberland A, Kruse I, Wirth M, Schimke I. The ratio of formation of prostacyclin/thromboxane A2 in HUVEC decreased in each subsequent passage. Prostaglandins 1997;54:447–462

112. Comi P, Chiaramonte R, Maier JA. Senescence-dependent regulation of type 1 plasminogen activator inhibitor in human vascular endothelial cells. Exp Cell Res 1995;219:304–308
113. West MD, Shay JW, Wright WE, Linskens MH. Altered expression of plasminogen activator and plasminogen activator inhibitor during cellular senescence. Exp Gerontol 1996;31:175–193
114. Maier JA, Statuto M, Ragnotti G. Senescence stimulates U937-endothelial cell interactions. Exp Cell Res 1993;208:270–274
115. Kalashnik L, Bridgeman CJ, King AR, Francis SE, Mikhalovsky S, Wallis C, Denyer SP, Crossman D, Faragher RG. A cell kinetic analysis of human umbilical vein endothelial cells. Mech Ageing Dev 2000;120:23–32
116. Wagner M, Hampel B, Bernhard D, Hala M, Zwerschke W, Jansen-Durr P. Replicative senescence of human endothelial cells in vitro involves G1 arrest, polyploidization and senescence-associated apoptosis. Exp Gerontol 2001;36:1327–1347
117. Wang, E. Senescent human fibroblasts resist programmed cell death, and failure to suppress Bcl2 is involved. Cancer Res 1995;55:2284–2292
118. Zhang J, Patel JM, Block ER. Enhanced apoptosis in prolonged cultures of senescent porcine pulmonary artery endothelial cells. Mech Ageing Dev 2002;123:613–625
119. Hampel B, Fortschegger K, Ressler S, Chang MW, Unterluggauer H, Breitwieser A, Sommergruber W, Fitzky B, Lepperdinger G, Jansen-Durr P, Voglauer R, Grillari J. Increased expression of extracellular proteins as a hallmark of human endothelial cell in vitro senescence. Exp Gerontol 2006;41:474–481
120. Cristofalo VJ, Lorenzini A, Allen RG, Torres C, Tresini M. Replicative senescence: a critical review. Mech Ageing Dev 2004;125:827–848
121. Minamino T, Komuro I. Vascular cell senescence: contribution to atherosclerosis. Circ Res 2007;100:15–26
122. Erusalimsky JD, Kurz DJ. Cellular senescence in vivo: its relevance in ageing and cardiovascular disease. Exp Gerontol 2005;40:634–642
123. Blasco MA, Lee HW, Hande MP, Samper E, Lansdorp PM, DePinho RA, Greider CW. Telomere shortening and tumor formation by mouse cells lacking telomerase RNA. Cell 1997;91:25–34
124. Satyanarayana A, Wiemann SU, Buer J, Lauber J, Dittmar KE, Wustefeld T, Blasco MA, Manns MP, Rudolph KL. Telomere shortening impairs organ regeneration by inhibiting cell cycle re-entry of a subpopulation of cells. EMBO J 2003;22:4003–4013
125. Lee HW, Blasco MA, Gottlieb GJ, Horner JW, Greider RA, DePinho RA. Essential role of mouse telomerase in highly proliferative organs. Nature 1998;392:569–574
126. Franco S, Segura I, Riese HH, Blasco MA. Decreased B16F10 melanoma growth and impaired vascularization in telomerase-deficient mice with critically short telomeres. Cancer Res 2002;62:552–559
127. Hasty P, Campisi J, Hoeijmakers J, van Steeg H, Vijg J. Aging and genome maintenance: lessons from the mouse? Science 2003;299:1355–1359
128. Allsopp RC, Vaziri H, Patterson C, Goldstein S, Younglai EV, Futcher AB, Greider CW, Harley CB. Telomere length predicts replicative capacity of human fibroblasts. Proc Natl Acad Sci USA 1992;89:10114–10118
129. Marciniak RA, Johnson FB, Guarente L. Dyskeratosis congenita, telomeres and human ageing. Trends Genet 2000;16:193–195
130. Tchirkov A, Lansdorp PM. Role of oxidative stress in telomere shortening in cultured fibroblasts from normal individuals and patients with ataxia-telangiectasia, Hum Mol Genet 2003:12:227–232
131. Crabbe L, Verdun RE, Haggblom CI, Karlseder J. Defective telomere lagging strand synthesis in cells lacking WRN helicase activity. Science 2004;306:1951–1953
132. Hamilton CA, Brosnan MJ, McIntyre M, Graham D, Dominiczak AF. Superoxide excess in hypertension and aging: a common cause of endothelial dysfunction. Hypertension 2001;37:529–534
133. Brandes RP, Barton M, Philippens KM, Schweitzer G, Mugge A. Endothelial-derived superoxide anions in pig coronary arteries: evidence from lucigenin chemiluminescence and histochemical techniques. J Physiol 1997;500:331–342
134. Gorlach A, Brandes RP, Nguyen K, Amidi M, Dehghani F, Busse R. A gp91phox containing NADPH oxidase selectively expressed in endothelial cells is a major source of oxygen radical generation in the arterial wall. Circ Res 2000;87:26–32
135. Jung O, Schreiber JG, Geiger H, Pedrazzini T, Busse R, Brandes RP. gp91phox-containing NADPH oxidase mediates endothelial dysfunction in renovascular hypertension. Circulation 2004;109:1795–1801
136. Burns EM, Kruckeberg TW, Comerford LE, Buschmann MT. Thinning of capillary walls and declining numbers of endothelial mitochondria in the cerebral cortex of the aging primate. Macaca nemestrina. J Gerontol 1979;34:642–650
137. Jendrach M, Pohl S, Voth M, Kowald A, Hammerstein P, Bereiter-Hahn J. Morpho-dynamic changes of mitochondria during ageing of human endothelial cells. Mech Ageing Dev 2005;126:813–821
138. Xin MG, Zhang J, Block ER, Patel JM. Senescence-enhanced oxidative stress is associated with deficiency of mitochondrial cytochrome c oxidase in vascular endothelial cells. Mech Ageing Dev 2003;124:911–919

139. van der Loo B, Labugger R, Skepper JN, Bachschmid M, Kilo J, Powell JM, Palacios-Callender M, Erusalimsky JD, Quaschning T, Malinski T, Gygi D, Ullrich V, Luscher TF. Enhanced peroxynitrite formation is associated with vascular aging. J Exp Med 2000;192:1731–1744
140. Bellin C, de Wiza DH, Wiernsperger NF, Rosen P. Generation of reactive oxygen species by endothelial and smooth muscle cells: influence of hyperglycemia and metformin. Horm Metab Res 2006;38: 732–739
141. Forstermann U. Janus-faced role of endothelial NO synthase in vascular disease: uncoupling of oxygen reduction from NO synthesis and its pharmacological reversal. Biol Chem 2006;387:1521–1533
142. Topal G, Brunet A, Millanvoye E, Boucher JL, Rendu F, Devynck MA, David-Dufilho M. Homocysteine induces oxidative stress by uncoupling of NO synthase activity through reduction of tetrahydrobiopterin. Free Radic Biol Med 2004;36:1532–1541
143. Forstermann U, Munzel T. Endothelial nitric oxide synthase in vascular disease: from marvel to menace. Circulation 2006;113:1708–1714
144. Ohara Y, Peterson TE, Harrison DG. Hypercholesterolemia increases endothelial superoxide anion production. J Clin Inves 1993;91:2546–2551
145. Newaz MA, Yousefipour Z, Oyekan A. Oxidative stress-associated vascular aging is xanthine oxidase-dependent but not NAD(P)H oxidase-dependent. J Cardiovasc Pharmacol 2006;48:88–94
146. Eskurza I, Kahn ZD, Seals DR. Xanthine oxidase does not contribute to impaired peripheral conduit artery endothelium-dependent dilatation with ageing. J Physiol 2006;571:661–668
147. Cardillo C, Kilcoyne CM, Cannon RO 3rd, Quyyumi AA, Panza JA. Xanthine oxidase inhibition with oxypurinol improves endothelial vasodilator function in hypercholesterolemic but not in hypertensive patients. Hypertension 1997;30:57–63
148. O'Driscoll JG, Green DJ, Rankin JM, Taylor RR. Nitric oxide-dependent endothelial function is unaffected by allopurinol in hypercholesterolaemic subjects. Clin Exp Pharmacol Physiol 1999;26:779–783
149. Li JM, Shah AM. Endothelial cell superoxide generation: regulation and relevance for cardiovascular pathophysiology. Am J Physiol Regul Integr Comp Physiol 2004;287:R1014–R1030
150. Oudot A, Martin C, Busseuil D, Vergely C, Demaison L, Rochette L. NADPH oxidases are in part responsible for increased cardiovascular superoxide production during aging. Free Radic Biol Med 2006;40:2214–2222
151. Goto K, Fujii K, Onaka U, Abe I, Fujishima M. Angiotensin-converting enzyme inhibitor prevents age-related endothelial dysfunction. Hypertension 2000;36:581–587
152. Mazza F, Goodman A, Lombardo G, Vanella A, Abraham NG. Heme oxygenase-1 gene expression attenuates angiotensin II-mediated DNA damage in endothelial cells. Exp Biol Med (Maywood) 2003;228:576–583
153. Cai H, Griendling KK, Harrison DG. The vascular NAD(P)H oxidases as therapeutic targets in cardiovascular diseases. Trends Pharmacol Sci 2003;24:471–478
154. Ago T, Kitazono T, Ooboshi H, Iyama T, Han YH, Takada J, Wakisaka M, Ibayashi S, Utsumi H, Iida M. Nox4 as the major catalytic component of an endothelial NAD(P)H oxidase. Circulation 2004;109:227–233
155. Guzik TJ, Sadowski J, Kapelak B, Jopek A, Rudzinski P, Pillai R, Korbut R, Channon KM. Systemic regulation of vascular NAD(P)H oxidase activity and nox isoform expression in human arteries and veins. Arterioscler Thromb Vasc Biol 2004;24:1614–1620
156. Bayraktutan U, Blayney L, Shah AM. Molecular characterization and localization of the NAD(P)H oxidase components gp91-phox and p22-phox in endothelial cells. Arterioscler Thromb Vasc Biol 2000;20: 1903–1911
157. Li JM, Shah AM. Intracellular localization and preassembly of the NADPH oxidase complex in cultured endothelial cells. J Biol Chem 2002;277:19952–19960
158. Bachschmid M, van der Loo B, Schuler K, Labugger R, Thurau S, Eto M, Kilo J, Holz R, Luscher TF, Ullrich V. Oxidative stress-associated vascular aging is independent of the protein kinase C/NAD(P)H oxidase pathway. Arch Gerontol Geriatr 2004;38:181–90
159. Rajagopalan S, Kurz S, Munzel T, Tarpey M, Freeman BA, Griendling KK, Harrison DG. Angiotensin II-mediated hypertension in the rat increases vascular superoxide production via membrane NADH/NADPH oxidase activation: contribution to alterations of vasomotor tone. J Clin Invest 1996;97:1916–1923
160. Li H, Witte K, August M, Brausch I, Gödtel-Armbrust U, Habermeier A, Closs EI, Oelze M, Münzel T, Förstermann U. Reversal of eNOS uncoupling and upregulation of eNOS expression lowers blood pressure in hypertensive rats. J Am Coll Cardiol 2006;47:2536–2544
161. Warnholtz A, Nickenig G, Schulz E, Macharzina R, Brasen JH, Skatchkov M, Heitzer T, Stasch JP, Griendling KK, Harrison DG, Bohm M, Meinertz T, Munzel T. Increased NADH-oxidase-mediated superoxide production in the early stages of atherosclerosis: evidence for involvement of the renin-angiotensin system. Circulation 1999;99:2027–2033
162. Sorescu D, Weiss D, Lassegue B, Clempus RE, Szocs K, Sorescu GP, Valppu L, Quinn MT, Lambeth JD, Vega JD, Taylor WR, Griendling KK. Superoxide production and expression of Nox family proteins in human atherosclerosis. Circulation 2002;105:1429–1435

163. Vergnani L, Hatrik S, Ricci F, Passaro A, Manzoli N, Zuliani G, Brovkovych V, Fellin R, Malinski T. Effect of native and oxidized low-density lipoprotein on endothelial nitric oxide and superoxide production: key role of L-arginine availability. Circulation 2000;101:1261–1266
164. Nickenig G, Baumer AT, Temur Y, Kebben D, Jockenhovel F, Bohm M. Statin-sensitive dysregulated AT1 receptor function and density in hypercholesterolemic men. Circulation 1999;100:2131–2134
165. Griendling KK, Sorescu D, Ushio-Fukai M. NAD(P)H oxidase: role in cardiovascular biology and disease. Circ Res 2000;86:494–501
166. Dernbach E, Urbich C, Brandes RP, Hofmann WK, Zeiher AM, Dimmeler S. Antioxidative stress-associated genes in circulating progenitor cells: evidence for enhanced resistance against oxidative stress. Blood 2004;104:3591–3597
167. Imanishi T, Hano T, Nishio I. Angiotensin II accelerates endothelial progenitor cell senescence through induction of oxidative stress. J Hypertens 2005;23:97–104
168. Imanishi T, Hano T, Nishio I. Estrogen reduces angiotensin II-induced acceleration of senescence in endothelial progenitor cells. Hypertens Res 2005;28:263–271
169. Kuki S, Imanishi T, Kobayashi K, Matsuo Y, Obana M, Akasaka T. Hyperglycemia accelerated endothelial progenitor cell senescence via the activation of p38 mitogen-activated protein kinase. Circ J 2006;70:1076–1081
170. Callaghan MJ, Ceradini DJ, Gurtner GC. Hyperglycemia-induced reactive oxygen species and impaired endothelial progenitor cell function. Antioxid Redox Signal 2005;7:1476–1482
171. Kobayashi K, Imanishi T, Akasaka T. Endothelial progenitor cell differentiation and senescence in an angiotensin II-infusion rat model. Hypertens Res 2006;29:449–455
172. Zhang W, Zhang G, Jin H, Hu R. Characteristics of bone marrow-derived endothelial progenitor cells in aged mice. Biochem Biophys Res Commun 2006;348:1018–1023
173. Orlandi A, Bochaton-Piallat ML, Gabbiani G, Spagnoli LG. Aging, smooth muscle cells and vascular pathobiology: implications for atherosclerosis. Atherosclerosis 2006;188:221–230
174. Moon SK, Cha BY, Lee YC, Nam KS, Runge MS, Patterson C, Kim CH. Age-related changes in matrix metalloproteinase-9 regulation in cultured mouse aortic smooth muscle cells. Exp Gerontol 2004;39:123–131
175. Li Z, Froehlich J, Galis ZS, Lakatta EG. Increased expression of matrix metalloproteinase-2 in the thickened intima of aged rats. Hypertension 1999;33:116–123
176. Moon SK, Thompson LJ, Madamanchi N, Ballinger S, Papaconstantinou J, Horaist C, Runge MS, Patterson C. Aging, oxidative responses, and proliferative capacity in cultured mouse aortic smooth muscle cells. Am J Physiol Heart Circ Physiol 2001;280:H2779–H2788
177. McCaffrey TA, Nicholson AC, Szabo PE, Weksler ME, Weksler BB. Aging and arteriosclerosis. The increased proliferation of arterial smooth muscle cells isolated from old rats is associated with increased platelet-derived growth factor-like activity. J Exp Med 1988;167:163–174
178. Li Z, Cheng H, Lederer WJ, Froehlich J, Lakatta EG. Enhanced proliferation and migration and altered cytoskeletal proteins in early passage smooth muscle cells from young and old rat aortic explants. Exp Mol Pathol 1997;64:1–11
179. Vazquez-Padron RI, Lasko D, Li S, Louis L, Pestana IA, Pang M, Liotta C, Fornoni A, Aitouche A, Pham SM. Aging exacerbates neointimal formation, and increases proliferation and reduces susceptibility to apoptosis of vascular smooth muscle cells in mice. J Vasc Surg 2004;40:1199–1207
180. Ruiz-Torres A, Gimeno A, Melon J, Mendez L, Munoz FJ, Macia M. Age-related loss of proliferative activity of human vascular smooth muscle cells in culture. Mech Ageing Dev 1999;110:49–55
181. Ruiz-Torres A, Lozano R, Melon J, Carraro R. Age-dependent decline of in vitro migration (basal and stimulated by IGF-1 or insulin) of human vascular smooth muscle cells. J Gerontol A Biol Sci Med Sci 2003;58:B1074–B1077
182. Vigetti D, Moretto P, Viola M, Genasetti A, Rizzi M, Karousou E, Pallotti F, De Luca G, Passi A. Matrix metalloproteinase 2 and tissue inhibitors of metalloproteinases regulate human aortic smooth muscle cell migration during in vitro aging. FASEB J 2006;20:1118–1130
183. Fenton M, Barker S, Kurz DJ, Erusalimsky JD. Cellular senescence after single and repeated balloon catheter denudations of rabbit carotid arteries. Arterioscler Thromb Vasc Biol 2001;21:220–226
184. Marin J. Age-related changes in vascular responses: a review. Mech Ageing Dev 1995;79:71–114
185. Crass MF 3rd, Borst SE, Scarpace PJ. Beta-adrenergic responsiveness in cultured aorta smooth muscle cells. Effects of subculture and aging. Biochem Pharmacol 1992;43:1811–1815
186. Robert L, Robert AM, Jacotot B. Elastin-elastase-atherosclerosis revisited. Atherosclerosis 1998;140:281–295
187. Spinetti G, Wang M, Monticone R, Zhang J, Zhao D, Lakatta EG. Rat aortic MCP-1 and its receptor CCR2 increase with age and alter vascular smooth muscle cell function. Arterioscler Thromb Vasc Biol 2004;24:1397–1402
188. Yamamoto M, Yamamoto K. Growth regulation in primary culture of rabbit arterial smooth muscle cells by platelet-derived growth factor, insulin-like growth factor-I, and epidermal growth factor. Exp Cell Res 1994;212:62–68

Chapter 6
Aging and the Cardiovascular-Related Systems

Overview

While the focus of this book is on aging and the cardiovascular system, changes in the function of other related systems also occur with aging. In this chapter we will discuss salient features of the aging process focusing on the immune/inflammatory system, in particular its cellular components (e.g., macrophage, neutrophil and lymphocyte) and molecular analysis, as well as on the hormonal/neuroendocrine and renal systems, and skeletal muscle. A number of changes in these systems occur with aging, including a myriad of cellular and molecular alterations that will affect the synthesis and degradation of specific proteins and also alter the cell signaling behavior. In response to a variety of physiological stresses and neuroendocrine-based stimuli, these changes play an important role in the onset/development of normal cardiovascular aging and have been implicated in the development of aging-associated cardiovascular diseases, including hypertension, coronary artery disease, atherosclerosis and heart failure as well as other diseases associated with aging such as Alzheimer Disease (AD). Although in brief, we will also discuss the aging blood-brain barrier, primarily in relation to its role mediating vascular signaling dysfunction. Finally, the implications of these findings on future therapeutic applications for the treatment of aging-associated cardiac dysfunction will be examined.

Introduction

In understanding the aging process, the involvement of highly conserved features such as insulin signaling pathways and transcriptional regulation has been demonstrated, an important paradigm for aging analysis as noted in several chapters of this book. Findings from animal models ranging from the more simple (yeast and *C. elegans*) to rodent have revealed critical aspects of aging pathways that are relevant to human aging. Notwithstanding this, the analysis of the effects of aging on many of the critical regulatory interactions and integration between pathways of highly evolved specialized cells comprising different functional systems will be of limited value in very simple model organisms, and requires analysis in more evolved models. In discussing some of the features of aging in this chapter, it is noteworthy that despite many problems inherent to humans (e.g., genetic heterogeneity, difficult-to-control confounding elements including diet and exercise), investigations in certain human population (e.g., centenarian populations) have provided valuable information which appears to be at least in part unique to human aging, or at least better tailored for understanding human aging. For instance, increased levels of systemic inflammation characteristic of human aging, a phenomena recently termed "inflamm-aging" by Franceschi et al. [1] has prefaced the identification of inflammation-related biomarkers as useful predictors of frailty and mortality in the elderly [2]. Furthermore, by careful examination of the subcellular events occurring in various

J. Marín-García, *Aging and the Heart,*

cellular components of these immune responses we may unravel the paradox (and cellular mechanism) of immunodeficiency and hyperactive inflammation that is characteristic of human aging.

The role of genetic and molecular analysis may be useful in the supplementation of a large body of biochemical information already available on aging. For instance, gene variants appear to play a significant role in modulating the delicate balance between pro-inflammatory and anti-inflammatory factors that both play an important role in the adaptation to increasing insults in aging and serve as critical markers of healthy aging process. Gene expression profiling can serve to identify molecular signatures or specific gene expression profiles that may underlie a specific aging phenotype (e.g., sarcopenia), in some cases in concert with specific genotypes or resulting from specific aging-modulating treatments (e.g., exercise, anti-oxidants).

The Aging Immune System

It is well recognized that as one ages the overall immune function becomes compromised. In comparison to the young, the aged immune system is less able to mount an effective immune response after challenges with infectious pathogens because of a series of aging-mediated cellular changes often referred to as immunosenescence. This condition contributes to morbidity and mortality due in part to a greater incidence or reactivation of infectious diseases, and also because of potentially enhanced susceptibility to autoimmune diseases and cancer [3].

Due to a combination of intrinsic and extrinsic factors, in both rodent models and humans, adaptive immunity suffers severe deterioration with age [4]. Specific features of adaptive immunity affected by aging are shown in Table 6.1. For instance, the decline in naive T lymphocytes number in the elderly is in part due to thymic involution and reduced T cell output [5], but it is also multifactorial in origin, involving changes in growth factors and hormones, hematopoietic progenitor cells, and their surrounding micro-environment. In contrast, the aging-associated accumulation of $CD8^+$ T memory cells has been considered an adaptive response to the loss of the naïve lymphocytes, as well as to life-long chronic antigenic stress resulting from immunosurveillance against persistent viruses, especially cytomegalovirus (CMV) [6]. The marked reduction in both the T cell and B cell antigen-recognition repertoire observed with age has been attributed to both a declining number and function

Table 6.1 Age-associated changes in the adaptive immune system

Cellular
Decreased naïve peripheral T cells
Decreased diversity of antigen-recognition repertoire
Increased number of memory T and B cells
Oligoclonal expansion of functionally incompetent memory lymphocytes
Decreased generation and efficacy of differentiation of common lymphoid precursors and T cell progenitors
Functional
Decreased antigen presentation
Antibody responses are delayed and blunted and antibody affinity (and affinity maturation) is impaired
T cell receptor and co-stimulatory signaling pathways are blunted
Decline in naïve CD4+ T cell responsiveness to T cell receptor stimulation
Decline in helper function of naïve CD4+ T cells for antibody production by B cells
Accumulation of CD28− CD8+ T cells
Subcellular/Molecular
Alteration of cell-surface receptor expression with elevated expression of chemokines and cytokine receptors
Downregulation of proliferative regulators (*myc*)
Constitutive cytokine secretion is generally elevated, whereas that in response to antigen or pathogen stimulation is reduced (i.e. IL-2 secretion by stimulated naive T cells is drastically reduced)
Alteration in immunoglobulin generation (through class switch) in B cells

of naïve lymphocytes, fewer bone marrow early progenitor B cells, as well as the accumulation of clonally expanded and functionally incompetent memory lymphocytes. Aging-associated clonal expansion of CD28-CD8$^+$ T cells (presumably a compensatory mechanism) also leads to reduction in the diversity of the T cell repertoire, compromises the ability of immune protection against new infections, and may be directly responsible for increased infections and reduced response to vaccines in the elderly [7]. Interestingly, latent CMV infection also decreases the naive CD8$^+$ T-cell pool and increases the CD28$^-$ CD8$^+$ effector T cell number leading to reduced diversity of CD8 responses.

As a consequence of decreased generation of early progenitor B cells, the output of new naïve B cells decreases in old mice with associated decline in the antigen-recognition repertoire of B cells [8]. Moreover, alteration in immunoglobulin generation in B cells (through class switch recombination mediated by the aging-related downregulation of E2A-encoded transcription factor E47) has been reported in both aged mice and humans[9] that likely contributes to a decline in the quality of humoral response in the elderly.

Intrinsic changes in naïve CD4$^+$ T cell lymphocytes from older humans and aging mice include decreased *in vitro* responsiveness to T cell receptor stimulation, altered profiles of cytokine secretion and decreased helper function for antibody production by B cells [10]. Some of these defects have been attributed to modifications in signaling pathways including altered recruitment of signaling proteins and receptors as well as changes in fluidity of lipid rafts. In addition to their reduced number, CD28$^+$ T cells from old donors display significantly shorter telomeres and have a restricted T cell receptor repertoire. Interestingly, the aging defects in the naïve CD4$^+$ T cells are due to their chronological age rather than the chronological age of the individual [10]. Naïve CD4$^+$ T cells that have undergone cell divisions proliferate less and produce less IL-2 in response to antigen stimulation than do naïve CD4$^+$ T cells that have not undergone previous homeostatic divisions; moreover, newly generated naïve CD4$^+$ T cells from old mice exhibit robust proliferation, IL-2 secretion, and helper functions in response to antigen both in *ex vivo* and *in vivo* conditions.

In contrast to naïve cells, long-lived memory CD4$^+$ T cells are maintained by homeostatic cytokines, and are relatively competent with age displaying normal antigen-induced proliferation *in vitro* [11]. Also in contrast to naïve T cells, memory CD4$^+$ T cells generated at a young age respond well to antigens over time, whereas memory CD4$^+$ T cells derived in old age respond poorly suggesting that age-associated memory CD4$^+$ T cell defects may stem from defects of aged naïve CD4$^+$ T cells, which have reduced diversity and proliferative capacity [12]. In addition, changes in the composition of CD4$^+$ T cell memory cells with age have also been implicated in the impaired immune response to influenza virus infection and to vaccines [13].

There are multiple causes for elevated inflammation in aging. Alterations in the production of inflammatory mediators in the elderly can be caused by a number of preexisting conditions such as autoimmune or degenerative diseases, cancer, or other factors that diminish the ability to combat infections. Moreover, such alterations may also result from age-associated defects in the innate immune system, which normally maintain cytokine balance and control inflammation and which represents the body's first line of defense against environmental insults such as microbial infection and other physical injuries.

Among the array of cell-types utilized by the innate immunity system,neutrophils, macrophages and related dendritic cells and the Natural Killer (NK) cells are the most important. Specific aging-associated changes have been reported in each type as depicted in Table 6.2.

Neutrophils, also known as polymorphonuclear neutrophilic leukocytes (PMN) are rapid responders to bacterial and fungal infection, and their capabilities of chemotactic migration, adhesion, phagocytosis, production of bacteriostatic and bacteriocidal products are critical to their function. Their activity requires specific functions driven by specific receptors, including formyl methionyl leucyl peptide (FMLP), granulocyte macrophage colony stimulating factor (GM-CSF) and interleukin-8 (IL-8) receptors [14]. In addition, pattern recognition receptors including at

marked decrease in VEGF production by stimulated peritoneal macrophages from aged mice, and contributed to impaired angiogenesis [34]. Although other cell-types (e.g., connective tissues and endothelial cells [ECs]) are likely involved in both the VEGF levels and diminished angiogenic response, an impaired inflammatory response (diminished macrophage levels) precedes the delay in angiogenesis in wound repair in aged animals suggesting that altered macrophage response provides a key upstream pathway for affecting angiogenic responses in aged tissues [35].

Another antigen-presenting cell component of the innate immunity system is the dendritic cell (DC). Activation of DCs through pattern recognition receptors such as TLRs is involved in inducing their maturation and migration to secondary lymphoid organs, where they present antigens to T cells and initiate an immune response. The majority of observations on age-associated changes in the phenotype and function of DCs have focused on the characteristics of Langerhans cells (LCs) in the skin and found a decrease in the number of these cells in elderly people and old mice. In contrast to macrophages, DCs from healthy elderly people seem to retain their capacity to efficiently present antigen to T cells. Age-related changes in the T cell compartment in the healthy elderly may be compensated by a boost in DC function [36]. In contrast, DCs from frail elderly people may have decreased expression of co-stimulatory molecules and IL-12 production, and therefore exhibit an impaired ability to induce T cell proliferation. In addition, the production of IL-10 is elevated in the elderly and it may inhibit DC maturation and macrophage function [36].

The function of NK cells, another key cellular mediator of innate defense, is regulated by the dynamic balance between activating and inhibitory signals delivered by specific membrane receptors. NK killing of target cells requires not only the interaction of activating NK receptors with their ligands on specific targets but also the lack of inhibitory signals initiated by interaction of NK inhibitory receptors with target MHC class I molecules. A variety of NK receptors have been implicated in the effective recognition and regulation of cytotoxic tumor cells and virally infected cells [37].

An increased overall percentage of NK cells is found in elderly subjects, largely arising in response to decreased levels of T cells and increases in the absolute number of NK cells. Several studies have reported that NK cytoxicity is either normal or moderately increased in centenarians and in healthy elderly subjects [38], but others have shown that the majority of the elderly population will experience some deficit in NK cell activity. Elderly individuals suffering from chronic diseases and those who are frail, but without apparent disease, are characterized by lower NK cytotoxicity. Low NK activity tends to be associated with the development of infections and death, secondary not only to infection but also by association with other diseases such as atherosclerosis [39]. High NK cell cytotoxicity tends to be related to better health status and lower incidence of respiratory tract infections in elderly individuals, as well as better development of protective antibody titers in response to influenza vaccination [40]. Together, these results support the theory that high NK cytotoxicity can be useful as a biomarker of healthy aging and longevity, whereas low NK cytotoxicity is a predictor of morbidity and mortality due to infections.

Interestingly, when cytotoxicity is examined at the cell level, there is a decrease in cytotoxicity per NK cell in the aged, which likely arises due to inefficient signal transduction [38]. Additionally, NK cells from aging individuals may be less prepared to carry out their assumed function, as there is a significant increase in the number of agranular cells in humans and a decrease in the adherence to tumor cells in mice [41].

While the information available concerning the changes in the expression and function of activating and inhibitory NK receptors in the elderly is limited, a delay in phosphatidylinositol biphosphate hydrolysis, coupled with a failure of inositol triphosphate to increase above basal levels has been reported in aging NKs with respect to spontaneous cytolytic activity [42]. However, NK cell activation mediated by CD16, seems unaffected by aging, indicating that NK activation and cytotoxic granule release remain largely intact [38, 39, 43]. As the per-cell cytotoxicity against conventional NK targets is significantly decreased in the elderly, the maintenance of CD16-mediated killing supports the view that either other NK-activating receptors are defective in the elderly, or that there is overexpression of inhibitory receptors. NK cells from elderly individuals present an age-related increase in killer cell immunoglobulin-like receptor expression and a reciprocal decrease in CD94-NKG2A expression, although the CD94-NKG2A inhibitory signaling pathway is intact [43]. The ability of IFN-α and IFN-β to enhance cytotoxicity of NK cells is also decreased with age both in mice and humans. In addition, the secretion of IFN-γ after stimulating purified NK cells with IL-2 also declines, which can be overcome by prolonging the incubation time [44].

NK cells from healthy elderly subjects retain the ability to synthesize chemokines and express the corresponding chemokine receptors. IL-12 or IL-2 can upregulate chemokine production although to a significantly lesser extent than that observed in young subjects [42]. Collectively, these findings suggest that NK cells exhibit an age-associated defect in their response to cytokines with a subsequent attenuation in their capacity both to kill target cells and to synthesize cytokines and chemokines. This is further supported from studies demonstrating that NK cells from the elderly are also unable to properly proliferate following IL-2 stimulation. In human- and murine-derived NK cells, the proliferative response to IL-2 is decreased by 40–60% among the elderly with decline in proliferative response paralleled by an age-specific decrease in Ca^{2+} mobilization [45]. Lower Ca^{2+} levels prevented the upregulation of CD69 on elderly human NK cells, an early activator of NK cell proliferation and cytotoxicity. The consequences of the combined diminished proliferative responses and cytotoxic activity of NK cells are that elderly persons are more prone to developing longer lasting infections and a decreased ability to rid the body of tumor cells [46].

In addition to the demonstrable modulation of elements of both adaptive and innate immunity in aging, there is also evidence that these immunity elements play crucial roles in aging-associated cardiovascular diseases including atherosclerosis and myocardial infarction (MI). The considerable cross-talk between these different cell-based inflammatory and immune elements in atherosclerosis is illustrated in Fig. 6.1.

Demonstration of these interactions have emerged most strikingly in studies of polymorphic variants and their relationship to disease and longevity in human studies, a number of which are depicted in Table 6.3 and are also indicated in Fig. 6.1.

The pattern recognition receptor, Toll-like receptor 4 (TLR4) is involved in the innate immune response to various microorganisms and other exogenous and endogenous stress factors. Recent information has emerged that important inflammatory processes operative in human atherogenesis are mediated in part via the TLR4/NF-κB pathway. Polymorphisms such as the Asp299Gly TLR4 attenuate receptor signaling, thereby enhancing the risk of acute infections, but appear to have an opposite effect on atherogenesis in an Italian population, being associated with both a lower risk of atherosclerosis and smaller intima-media thickness in the common carotid artery [47]. Moreover, among a cohort of symptomatic men with documented coronary artery disease (CAD), carriers of the TLR4 Asp299Gly polymorphism had significantly more benefit from pravastatin treatment than non-carriers [61]. A potential linkage between TLR4 genotype and statin treatment was further suggested by the findings of a significant association of 299Gly bearing genotypes with lower susceptibility to MI in a cohort of patients with angiographically documented CAD (observed only in patients receiving statin treatment) [62]. These results suggested that TLR4 and statin therapy may have a synergistic interaction on reducing susceptibility to coronary ischemic events.

A large-scale study (the PRIME Study) prospectively investigating a cohort of 9758 healthy men aged 50–59 years recruited in France and Northern Ireland however found no association of the TLR4/Asp299Gly variant with the risk of CAD [63]. Similarly, no significant association of the TLR4/Asp299Gly variant with MI was found in a large recent study of a Caucasian population including 3657 patients with MI and the control group comprised 1211 individuals with angiographically normal coronary arteries and without signs or symptoms of MI [64].

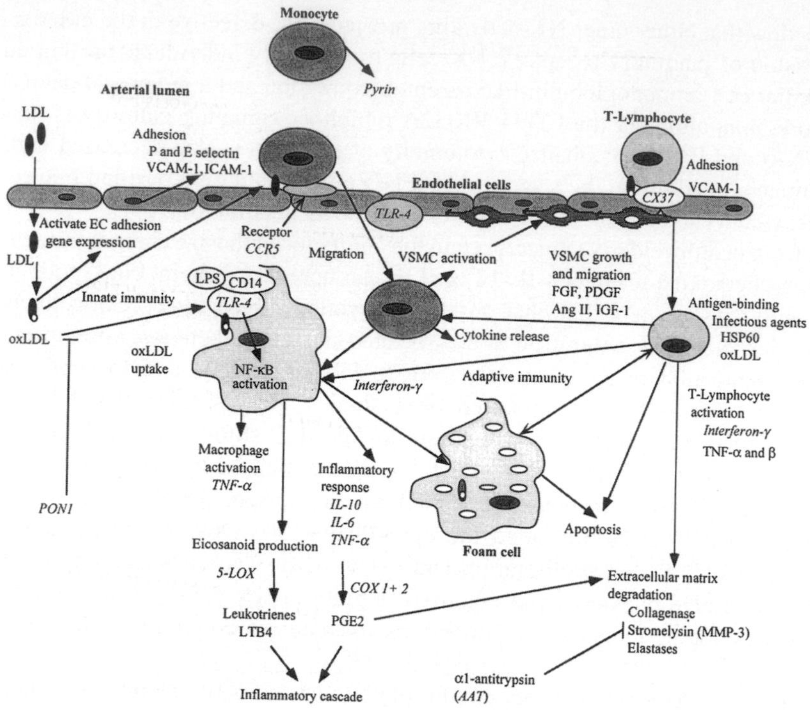

Fig. 6.1 Cross-talk of immune cells involved in aging-associated diseases such as atherosclerosis
Formation of lesions of atherosclerosis initiated at the endothelium. Changes include increased endothelial permeability to lipoproteins and other plasma constituents, upregulation of leukocyte adhesion molecules, upregulation of endothelial adhesion molecules, which include E-selectin, P-selectin, ICAM-1, and vascular-cell adhesion molecule 1; migration of leukocytes into the artery wall, which is mediated by oxidized low-density lipoprotein (oxLDL) and an array of chemokines. Monocytes and macrophages (foam cells) together with T lymphocytes are recruited to form the fatty streak. The fatty streaks progress to intermediate and advanced lesions, with formation of a fibrous cap covering a mixture of leukocytes, lipid, and debris formed as a result of increased activity of growth factors, inflammatory cytokines, and decreased connective-tissue degradation. The necrotic core represents the results of apoptosis and necrosis, increased proteolytic activity, and lipid accumulation. Specific markers are shown in plain text. Polymorphic gene variants, which impact aging and aging-associated cardiovascular disease progression in humans, are shown in italic.

Given their involvement with cardiovascular diseases such as atherosclerosis and MI, it is not surprising that polymorphic variants of genes encoding proinflammatory cytokines have been found associated with increased risk of CAD and acute MI. Therefore, it might be predicted that alleles associated with susceptibility to acute MI would be less represented in genetic backgrounds that favor longevity. Nevertheless, large-scale studies examining allelic variants of inflammatory cytokine IL-1, a primary mediator of systemic inflammatory responses for their association with longevity, demonstrated no significant differences in polymorphic IL-1 allele distribution in 250 Finnish nonagenarians compared to 400 younger subjects[65] or in 134 centenarians in an analysis of over 1100 Italian subjects [66].

Published reports have shown an age-related increase in serum levels of IL-6, a pleiotropic cytokine involved in acute phase and stress responses, and in the balancing of the pro-inflammatory/anti-inflammatory pathways, from elderly people devoid of any overt age-related disease [67], being more prominent among men [68]. Furthermore, since estrogen and testosterone downregulate IL-6 gene expression, following menopause or andropause, IL-6 levels are elevated, even in the absence of infection, trauma, or stress [69]. In addition, IL-6 dysregulation has

Table 6.3 Immune gene variants in aging and aging-associated diseases

Gene	Allele	Phenotypic effects	References
TLR4	ASP299GLY (+896A→G)	Reduced risk of atherosclerosis but increased risk of age-related macular degeneration. Overrepresented in male Sicilian centenarians	47, 48, 49
IL-10	−1082G→A	Increased GG genotype among male centenarians; also decreased GG genotype found among patients with AD. Findings nor replicated in either Irish or Finnish nonagenarians	50, 51, 52, 53
IL-6	−174C	Increased in Italian male centenarians along with lower serum levels of IL-6; decreased levels of GG homozygotes were found in different populations of centenarians and in a group of nonagenarian and octogenarian subjects; GG homozygotes were significantly more prevalent in subjects with peripheral artery occlusive disease; ACS patients carrying the IL-6 −174 C-(GG) genotypes showed a marked increase in mortality rate at 1yr follow-up	54, 55, 56
IFN-γ	+874A	Found more frequently in female centenarians	57
MEFV (pyrin)	M694V (A2080G)	Over-represented in CHD/AMI patients and under-represented in Sicilian centenarians	58
PON1 (Paraoxonasel)	192 R	Increased frequency of R allele in both Italian and Irish nonagenarians/ centenarians	59, 60

been implicated in the inflammatory pathogenesis found in age-related diseases, such as diabetes and atherosclerosis, and has been proposed to contribute to characteristic phenotypic changes of advanced age, particularly those that resemble chronic inflammatory disease including decreased lean body mass, osteopenia, low-grade anemia, decreased serum albumin and cholesterol, and increased inflammatory proteins such as C-reactive protein (CRP) and serum amyloid A.

A C/G polymorphism located in the promoter region of IL-6 (−174 C/G locus) has been associated with different IL-6 plasma levels in healthy subjects and with different rate of IL-6 gene transcription [70]. Subjects carrying either CC or CG genotypes were defined as C^+ and those carrying the GG genotype as C^-. In a study of 700 Italian subjects with similar genetic background, including 323 centenarians, male centenarians had increased C allele frequency, with the C^-genotype (as well as high IL-6 serum levels) significantly under-represented [54]. This difference was not found in women, implying that genetic variability at IL-6 −174 locus has a gender-dependent impact on longevity and that the C^+genotype is favorable for longevity in some populations, at least in men. Similarly, decreased frequency of IL-6 −174 C^-carriers in Irish octogenarian and nonagenarian subjects from the BELFAST elderly longitudinal ageing study have been recently reported [53, 56]. These findings, although in conflict with other observations, are consistent with data showing an increased frequency of IL-6 high production (C^-subjects) among those affected by age-related diseases including diabetes, atherosclerosis and CAD, and osteoporosis, which have a substantial inflammatory pathogenesis [71, 72]. In a longitudinal study of 324 relatively healthy 80-year-old people, Bruunsgaard et al. reported that the IL-6 C allele was associated with elevated serum levels of IL-6 at baseline and the CC genotype had a high prevalence of CVD and increased mortality risk [73].

Other studies have reported that C^{+} carriers have an increased risk of aging-associated neurodegenerative disease, such as Alzheimer disease (AD) [74]. Interestingly, when gender was taken into account the −174 CC genotype (and high IL-6 levels in both blood and brain) were associated with a high risk of the disease in women, further suggesting the importance of taking gender into account in these analyses. However, other recent large-scale studies in various populations have been unable to demonstrate a consistent relationship between AD, dementia and IL-6 genotype [75, 76].

Significantly, polymorphic variants of gene encoding anti-inflammatory elements have shown different allelic distribution with aging and aging-associated diseases. For instance, the frequency of the genotype associated with interleukin 10 (−1082GG) is associated with significant increased production of the antiinflammatory cytokine IL-10 in Italian centenarian men but not women [50]. In an analysis of two different populations from north and south Italy, Lio et al. [77, 78] found that IL-10 genotype distribution exhibited a significantly higher frequency of the −1082GG genotype among the centenarian subgroup compared to controls and patients with acute MI. Conversely, the frequency of the −1082AA genotype, associated with low production of IL-10, was significantly higher in patients with acute MI than in either controls or the centenarian subjects. The fact that the frequency of the −1082AA genotype, associated with low production of interleukin 10, was significantly higher in patients with acute MI compared to controls and oldest subjects suggests that not only is IL-10 genotype nonrandomly distributed with respect to longevity but it can also be cardioprotective against acute myocardial infarction. In contrast, no association was found between IL-10 genotype and aging in a study of 250 Finnish nonagenarians (52 men and 198 women)[52] nor with an aged Irish population[53] or centenarians from the island of Sardinia, whose population shows a genetic background quite different from that of mainland Italy [79], even when analyzed by gender. Nevertheless, the impact of the genetic background on this genotypic expression remains to be determined.

Polymorphic variants of the PON1 gene, encoding paraoxonase, play a critical role in atherogenesis and inflammation and impact on aging and longevity. It is well-established that peroxidation of low density lipoproteins (LDL) in atherogenesis by oxygen free radicals impacts the capability of lipoprotein-associated proteins, such as ApoE and Lpa, of modulating local inflammatory response. Paraoxonase removes lipoperoxides from oxidized LDL and has been implicated in the protective antiatherogenic effects of HDL. A common polymorphism of the PON1 gene, located at amino acid position 192 in exon 6 and due to a glutamine (Q allele) to arginine (R allele) interchange has been found to impact aging-associated MI [80]. A decline of PON1 activity levels with advancing age was found in subjects carrying the low-activity QQ genotype, particularly in MI patients. Furthermore, PON1 activity and age negatively correlated in MI patients but not in controls, and the effect of PON1-192 genotypes on the association of age and MI risk was related to gene-dosage. An analysis of 308 Italian centenarians, compared to 509 young subjects, revealed that the frequency of R allele, and consequently of R+ carriers (QR + RR individuals) increased significantly from young people to centenarians, suggesting that this allele decreases mortality risk in carriers [81, 82]. These observations have been confirmed in other studies including a pooled statistical analysis incorporating data from a large combined group of Italian centenarians and octo/nonagenarians from Northern Ireland demonstrating a modest but significant survival advantage for octo/nonagenarian/centenarian subjects who carried the R allele [60]. Moreover, being homozygous for 192 RR further enhanced survival advantage; this effect was not found to be sex specific suggesting a gene-dosage effect. In addition, the PON1 192 allele polymorphism may be protective against AD development in Chinese Han populations [83]. The presence of at least one of PON1 R alleles (Q/R or R/R) was lower in AD patients than in controls suggesting that the PON1 R allele might be a protective factor for AD in Chinese subjects.

Aging and Neurohormonal Regulation

The role of neurohormonal regulation in modulating both longevity and aging-mediated cardiovascular function is clearly of great importance but remains not well understood. There is evidence that both hormone levels and target organ responsivity are altered in the aging endocrine-cardiovascular system and are unique for each hormone. Table 6.4 depicts some of the better characterized neuroendocrine changes occurring with aging. For instance, serum levels of vasopressor hormones can increase with age (e.g., norepinephrine) or decrease (e.g., renin, aldosterone). Due to postreceptor changes, target organ response to β-adrenergic stimulation in the heart, and probably also in vascular smooth muscle, decreases. These effects may contribute to the clinical problems of hypertension and orthostatic hypotension, frequently encountered in the elderly. Aging produces mild carbohydrate intolerance and a minimal increase in fasting serum glucose in healthy, non-obese individuals, primarily due to decreasing postreceptor responsiveness to insulin. While significant alterations of thyroid hormone (TH) levels do not occur, aging decreases the metabolism of TH, including its conversion to triiodothyronine, and reduced levels of the thyroid hormone receptor (TR). Changes in the end-organ response to thyroid hormones, however, significantly alter the clinical presentation of thyroid diseases in aging subjects.

In addition, aging has been found to profoundly impact the hypothalamo-neurohypophysial system (HNS) and the hypothalamo-pituitary-adrenocortical (HPA) axis in rodents as well as in humans. The HPA axis, which coordinates multiple neuroendocrine and metabolic responses to stressors is primarily regulated by the hypothalamic peptide hormone corticotropin-releasing factor (CRF), arginine vasopressin, and glucocorticoid (GC) feedback; it has been described as hyperactive in both aging animals and humans and is characterized in part by prolonged GC secretion in response to a challenge [84, 85]. Increased HPA activation and elevated GC are a critical adaptation to short-term stress; they mobilize energy stores and increased cardiovascular tone by increasing serum glucose and lipids, eliciting immunosuppression and mediating cardiovascular changes.

Table 6.4 Neuroendocrine changes in aging

Hormone/receptor	Change in aging
Dopamine	↓
Dopamine receptor 2	↓
Noradrenalin	↓
Serotonin	↓; Nc
Muscarinic receptor	↓
Choline acyltransferase	↓
Nicotinic receptor	↓
Adrenocorticotrophic hormone	↓
Follicle-stimulating hormone	↑
Luteinizing hormone	↑
Luteinizing hormone-releasing hormone	↓
Aldosterone	↓
Growth hormone	↓
Thyroid-stimulating hormone	↓; Nc
Thyroxin	Nc
Antidiuretic hormone	↑; Nc
Oxytocin	↓
Prolactin	↑; Nc
Melatonin	↓
Testosterone	↓; Nc

Nc: No change

One characteristic of advancing aging is a loss of hormonal responsiveness, which may be attributable to a loss of hormone receptor sensitivity, and/or a reduction in the output of the target endocrine gland.

Glucocorticoid action is mediated by both glucocorticoid (GR) and mineralocorticoid (MR) receptors. HPA hyperactivity is associated with a loss of resiliency and reduced sensitivity to the negative glucocorticoid feedback, which mainly reflects hippocampal receptor damage. Reduced levels of MR as well as an oscillation in the pattern of receptor function during aging have been reported in liver from senescent rats [86]. Furthermore, reduction of MR number in the hippocampus and of GR number in the hypothalamus and the pituitary have been found in 30 month old Brown Norway rats suggesting a linkage to increased neuroendocrine responsiveness and negative feedback following stress. The observed changes in receptor binding did not parallel the changes in the amount of MR and GR transcripts, as gauged by hybridization suggesting that the aging-mediated tissue-specific regulation *in situ* is mediated at the receptor processing level rather than at transcriptional level [87].

A significant increase in the basal release of arginine vasopressin (AVP) within the hypothalamic paraventricular nucleus (PVN) was reported in aged male Wistar rats. With increasing age the rise in intra-PVN release of both AVP and OXT was blunted in response to forced swimming[88]. Interestingly, studies in 24 month-old Fischer 344 rats reported that CRF mRNA levels and content in the hypothalamic PVN and secreted CRF levels were progressively and significantly reduced with age, whereas the steady state levels of AVP mRNA were significantly increased with age [89]. The elevation of both AVP mRNA expression and CRF-induced ACTH release in aged rats, suggest that HPA hyperactivity is mediated by enhanced AVP action and increased pituitary responsiveness to CRF. In contrast, other studies using F344 rats of comparable age found elevated basal CRF levels in portal blood, and decreased pituitary CRF receptor expression, consistent with enhanced CRF release [90, 91].

Significant reduction in the density of CRF-binding receptors in both the anterior pituitary and hypothalamus of 24 month-old rats have been demonstrated [92], and thus far two receptors to CRF have been identified and cloned. CRFR1 encodes a 415 amino acid protein comprising seven putative membrane-spanning domains and is structurally related to the calcitonin/vasoactive intestinal peptide/growth hormone-releasing hormone subfamily of G-protein-coupled receptor; CRFR2 encodes a 411 amino acid rat brain protein with approximately 70% homology to CRFR1. Observations in aging rats have documented a downregulation of the CRFR1 mRNA localized in the anterior pituitary contrasting with increased levels in the intermediate lobe [93]. Stress increases hypothalamic CRF secretion which, in turn, downregulates CRF receptors in the anterior pituitary [94]. Recently, Herman et al. in a study conducted with F344/BN F1 hybrid rats, found that 30 month old rats displayed evidence of central HPA hyperactivity, including elevated ACTH levels and decreased pituitary proopiomelanocortin (POMC) and CRFR1 mRNA expression, consistent with increased activity of hypophysiotrophic PVN neurons [95]. In this age group, responses to acute stress are also more severe, with aged rats showing enhanced corticosterone secretion in response to new or unusual spatial location. The responses to chronic stress in 30 month old rats was similarly exaggerated with PVN CRF immunoreactivity and pituitary POMC levels increasing disproportionately, consistent with differential activation of CRF neurons in this age group.

A CRF binding protein (CRF-BP) has also been identified which binds CRF in plasma, rendering it inactive and unable to bind to its receptor. It has been shown that pituitary and amygdla-localized CRF-BP mRNA levels increase in response to acute restraint stress, antagonizing CRF-induced ACTH release *in vitro*, providing an additional feedback mechanism to maintain the homeostasis of the stress response. Furthermore, adrenalectomy attenuates CRF-BP synthesis indicating that glucocorticoids play a significant role in this positive regulation [96]. Recently, cells in the basolateral and lateral nucleus of the amygdala were found to have lower CRF-BP levels in the 24 month old rats compared to 4 month old rats [97].

Recent studies of clinically healthy elderly human and age-matched demented Alzheimer disease (AD) patients, including both the degenerative and the vascular type, found significantly higher cortisol levels at nighttime in both elderly subjects and demented patients when compared to young controls. At the same time, an age- and disease-dependent reduction of DHEAS secretion was found. The cortisol to DHEAS molar ratio was significantly higher in healthy old subjects, and even more in demented patients, when compared to young controls, and significantly linked to both age and cognitive impairment [98]. Increased cortisol/DHEA ratio has been considered a determinant of immunological changes (termed immunosenescence), including thymic involution, lower number of naive T cells, reduced cell-mediated immunity, and poor vaccination response to new antigens during aging.

Moreover, there is evidence that when compared with young subjects, healthy elders are more stressed and show activation of the HPA axis [99]. Since a number of studies have suggested that glucocorticoid (GC) levels in the human are essentially unaltered by age, both the beneficial and undesirable effects of GCs ultimately depend on the target tissue sensitivity to these steroids. Recent data indicate that peripheral lymphocytes from elders respond poorly to GC treatment *in vitro*. Chronically stressed elderly subjects may be particularly at risk of stress-related pathology because of further alterations in GC-immune signaling.

A particularly critical hypothalamic hormone affected in aging with consequences for the heart and cardiovascular system is growth hormone peptide (GH) [100]. Episodic GH secretion is markedly impaired in aging, particularly during sleep. It has been proposed that decreased GH release contributes to the age-related decline in protein synthesis. Moreover, a negative correlation was found between the density of GH-binding sites in several areas of the human brain (e.g. hippocampus, choroid plexus, hypothalamus, putamen, and the pituitary) with increasing age [101]. Some evidence suggests that catecholaminergic alterations in the hypothalamus in old age are in part responsible for the reduced GH release.

The decrease in both GH and IGF-1 (whose plasma levels decline as a function of both age and adiposity) is likely in part responsible for the loss of muscle and bone mass characteristic of older people. This is supported by the strong association of decreased IGF-1 serum levels with increased risk of bone fracture in postmenopausal women [102]. Moreover, GH supplementation several times a week resulted in increase in lean body mass, decrease in fat mass and bone density in healthy older males [103]. Both non-muscle and muscle protein synthesis increased in subjects with GH supplementation [104, 105, 106], as did markers of bone remodeling activation [107].

Given GH's beneficial effect on myocardial contractility, cardiac tissue growth, and myocardial energetics and on peripheral vascular resistance, GH deficiency in older patients may contribute to the development of heart failure (HF). Aging in GH deficient patients was associated with a marked depression of LV ejection fraction at peak exercise compared to age-matched controls indicating severely reduced exercise capacity [108]. In healthy subjects, GH administration increased heart rate, cardiac output and contractility [109]. However, recent preclinical studies of the effects of long-term GH supplementation in senescent rats indicate GH treatment preserved diastolic function and significantly attenuated the LV remodeling that occurs during normal aging [110]. As compared to the low IGF-1 levels, impaired diastolic left ventricular filling (as gauged by Doppler), increased cardiac angiotensin II (Ang II) and reduced plasma Ang II levels, and elevated cardiac collagen exhibited by 30 month-old male Brown Norway x F344 rats receiving saline-injections, GH administration in 30 month-old rats restored IGF-1 and diastolic indices to values comparable to those of adults, reduced cardiac Ang II and attenuated accumulation in cardiac collagen. These findings suggested that age-related decreases in GH and IGF-1 may contribute to the decline in diastolic function of aging, in part through alterations in renin-angiotensin system-mediated ventricular remodeling and that GH supplementation might provide adjunct benefits in some cases of cardiac dysfunction. An early double-blind study of a recombinant GH trial found no significant beneficial effects on cardiac structure or function in 22 patients with congestive HF [111]. More recent studies have demonstrated some clinical benefits in treating HF with GH, depending on both the dose and consistency of application (at least every other day). One recent study found that high doses of GH improved left ventricular fraction from 23 to 38 with extended treatment in patients with decompensated congestive HF and cardiac cachexia [112].

Several studies have begun to focus on the potential clinical application of GH peptide secretagogues (e.g., hexarelin and ghrelin) in lowering peripheral resistance, improvement of contractility and providing cardioprotection [113]. A recent small scale clinical study found that a three-week administration of ghrelin to 10 patients with congestive HF resulted in a significant decrease in plasma norepinephrine, increased LV ejection fraction, increased LV mass and decreased LV end-systolic volume. Furthermore, ghrelin treatment increased peak workload and peak oxygen consumption during exercise and markedly improved muscle wasting, as indicated by increases in muscle strength and lean body mass [114]. Use of recombinant GH to provide life extension and improved cardiovascular function in aging individuals has neither been demonstrated and is not presently recommended since there are potential adverse effects and the risk/benefit have not been fully ascertained [115].

In addition to its effect on the myocardium, GH and IGF-1 have multiple effects on the vascular function and structure in aging. Sonntag et al. [116] found that cerebral arteriolar density significantly decreased as did arteriolar anastomoses in 29 month-old rats with no changes in venular density; the number of cortical surface arterioles was positively correlated with plasma IGF-1 levels at the time of vascular mapping. Injection of bovine GH (0.25 mg/kg, twice daily for 35 days) to 30-month-old animals increased both plasma IGF-1 and the number of cortical arterioles implicating GH and IGF-1 in the decline in vascular density with age. Subsequent studies by this group found that a similar regimen of treatment with bovine GH of 30 month-old old rats significantly reversed a marked age-mediated decline in coronary blood flow and decreased capillary density in the apex and middle segments of the LV suggesting that GH can enhance regional blood flow in the aging heart in part due to increasing capillary density [117]. Other studies have reported that GH treatment of old female rats increased the aorta diameter and cross-section of the aortic lumen concomitant to elevated collagen content and an increased amount of type I collagen relative to type III collagen [118]. Moreover, the age-mediated increase in aortic media found in 20-month old female Wistar rats was significantly reduced by GH treatment [119]. Similar findings were obtained with 20 month-old rats which also exhibited impairment in the vasodilatory response to acetylcholine and isoproterenol; GH treatment significantly improved the vasodilatation induced by isoproterenol, whereas the response to acetylcholine was not significantly enhanced [120]. These findings confirmed that GH treatment has beneficial effects on vascular function and structure in both old male and female rats.

It should be noted that the very close relationship between GH and IGF-1 (whose synthesis is elevated with GH) has made it difficult at times to ascertain which molecule is directly responsible in reversing vascular dysfunction of aging. A vascular protective role for IGF-1 has been suggested because of its ability to stimulate NO production from endothelial and vascular smooth muscle cells [121]. The decline in IGF-1 levels in aging are thought to play a significant role in the development of a wide range of aging-associated pathologies including cardiovascular diseases such as atherosclerosis and hypertension as well as cognitive decline, dementia, sarcopenia and frailty. Low IGF-1 levels have been associated in cross sectional studies with unfavorable CVD risk factors such as atherosclerosis, abnormal lipoprotein levels and hypertension, while in prospective studies, lower IGF-1 levels have been shown to predict future development of ischemic heart disease.

Aging and Skeletal Muscle

Increasing age is associated with significant structural and functional changes in skeletal muscle in a wide range of species, including humans. These changes are thought to contribute to the development of many aging associated cardiovascular and metabolic disorders including insulin resistance, type 2 diabetes, hypertension, and hyperlipidemia, which result in an increased incidence of cardiovascular death [122].

In humans, an age-related decrease in muscle mass and quality appears to begin in the fourth decade of life with a parallel decline in both muscle strength and maximal oxygen uptake [123–125]. The decrease in muscle mass and muscle strength, combined with reduced endurance, will result in reduced physical activity and decreased total energy expenditure in the elderly. The decline in overall energy expenditure can lead to changes in body composition resulting in an increased prevalence of obesity, especially abdominal fat accumulation, insulin resistance, which contributes to the development of a high prevalence of type 2 diabetes, hyperlipidemia, and hypertension in a genetically susceptible population, with increased risk of further cardiovascular disease and death as depicted in Fig. 6.2.

One underlying mechanism that causes a decrease in muscle fibers, muscle mass, and muscle function, which has been documented in aging studies in many species including human, involves an overall decrease in the skeletal muscle protein synthesis rate [122]. Interestingly, Balagopal et al. have shown that the age-mediated decline in muscle protein is not truly global since the synthesis rate of some sarcoplasmic proteins is actually higher in aging subjects while other proteins including mitochondrial proteins and myosin heavy chain (MHC) are markedly reduced [126]. A reduction in the synthesis rate of MHC, the key protein in the contractile apparatus, is likely to be a primary contributory factor in the development of muscle weakness. However, it is unclear whether the

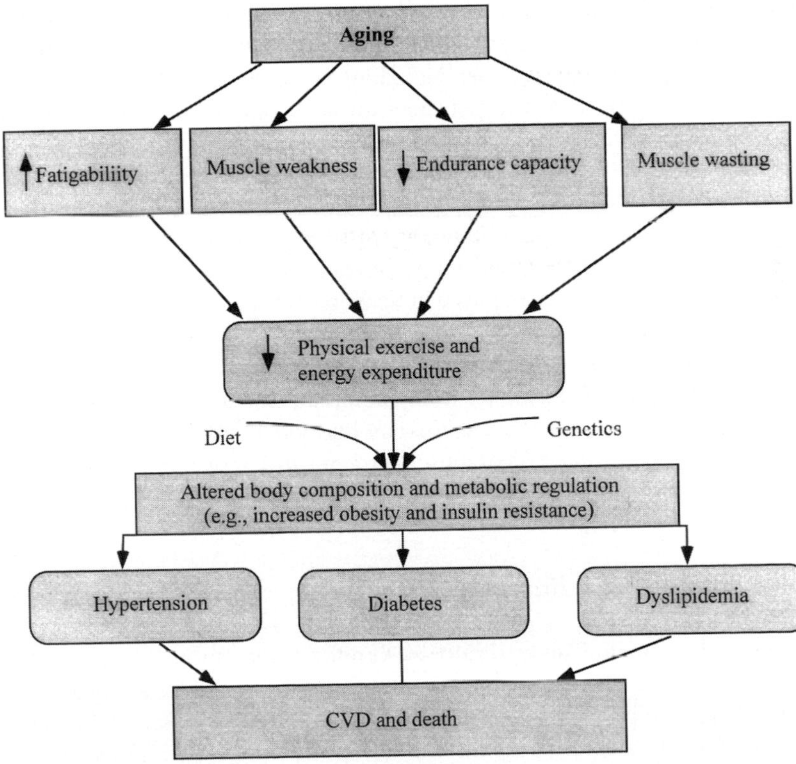

Fig. 6.2 Aging-associated functional changes in skeletal muscle
Changes with age are a major contributor to obesity, insulin resistance and hypertension, all the components of metabolic syndrome leading to further cardiovascular disease (CVD) and death.

concentration of myosin and other key proteins involved in muscle contraction are reduced with aging in humans.

Another characteristic of aging skeletal muscle is a shift of muscle fibers toward type 1 (slow-twitch) fibers. Moreover, there is a significant decline in fiber size in type II (fast-twitch) with increased aging whereas type I fibers are less affected [127, 128]. However, the relative increase in type 1 fibers does not make older muscle fatigue resistant, in contrast to type 1 fibers in athletes and endurance trained animal [129]. An aging-mediated reduction in overall mitochondrial content and bioeneregetic capacity in these muscle fibers might underlie the lack of fatigue resistance and may contribute to the muscle weakness with age. There is considerable evidence from both rat studies[130] and human studies[131] that skeletal muscle mitochondrial dysfunction occurs with age. This includes a decline in mtDNA copy number, reduced transcript levels encoding muscle mitochondrial proteins, reduced muscle mitochondrial oxidative enzyme activities, and reduced mitochondrial protein synthesis rates. Recent studies with aging rat soleus muscle, found a significant decrease in complex IV activity with age occurring in parallel with an age-related muscle atrophy starting at about 28 months [132]. This muscle atrophy was also accompanied by a decrease in the amount and integrity of mtDNA with a significant increase in the number of large-scale mtDNA deletions. There are conflicting data as to whether skeletal muscle mitochondrial ATP production decreases with age [122, 133]. There is also increasing evidence from studies with senescent rats that the sarcopenia that accompanies skeletal muscle aging is associated with a significant increase in fibers with defective electron transport chain activity and increased levels of mtDNA damage including an increasing abundance of large-scale mtDNA deletions [134]. These authors have subsequently proposed that as a result of both the decline in energy production and the increase in oxidative damage in the region, the muscle fiber is no longer capable of self-maintenance, resulting in the observed intrafiber atrophy and fiber breakage [135]. In addition, since mitochondria play an integral role in apoptosis initiation via both inner and outer membrane permeabilization and the release of specific apoptogenic peptides including Smac/diablo, AIF, cytochrome *c* and endo G, apoptosis activation may be in part responsible for the initiation of muscle protein degradation, loss of muscle nuclei associated with local atrophy, and myocyte cell death in aging muscle [136]. Recent studies examining the regulation of apoptotic mediators in the extensor digitorum longus and soleus muscles of 30 and 36 month-old senescent rats found that the expression of Bax, Bcl-2, caspase-3 and caspase-9 was regulated differently with aging between muscle types and in a manner not consistent with mitochondria-mediated apoptosis suggesting that mitochondrial-dependent apoptosis pathways may not play a requisite role in the loss of muscle nuclei with aging and sarcopenia [137].

Sarcopenia has been attributed to other factors as listed in Table 6.5. Moreover, Fig. 6.3 illustrates the extensive cross-talk between subcellular (mitochondrial, calcium regulators, ubiquitin degradation systems and plasma membrane) and numerous hormonal/neuroendocrine/cytokine inputs in regulating the synthesis and degradation of muscle proteins in sarcopenia.

Aging and the Blood-Brain Barrier

Aging of the cerebral microcirculation results in significant alteration in the blood-brain barrier. Most evidence indicates that the barrier function remains intact in older animals, although it may be more susceptible to disruption by external factors (e.g., hypertension), and drugs (e.g., haloperidol). Moreover, in humans, infectious agents with relatively long incubation period and a chronic progressive course (e.g., viral or prions) may enter the central nervous system by transcytosis across blood-brain barrier cells therefore increasing in frequency with age. While altered overall transport processes have not been reported with age, several studies have documented abnormal blood-brain

Table 6.5 Factors leading to sarcopenia with aging

Extrinsic factors
Malnutrition and aging-associated anorexia
Inadequate exercise
Disuse atrophy (e.g., limb immobilization)
Traumatic injury
Disease
Intrinsic factors
Reduced metabolism with nitrogen imbalance and impaired glucose metabolism
Slowdown of muscle protein synthesis and turnover
Reduction of enzyme activities and energy reserves
Decreased mitochondrial function and increased oxidative stress and ROS
Changes in CNS functioning and neural stimulation
Changes in cytokine and neuroendocrine secretion and regulation including decreased anabolic hormones (e.g. testosterone, DHEA, growth hormone, IGF-1) and increased catabolic factors such as inflammatory cytokines (e.g. IL-6)
Reduction in blood supply and capillary beds
Reduction in mediating factors involved in activation of progenitor myoblasts
Imbalance between degradation and removal of "old" damaged muscle proteins

barrier function of select carrier-mediated transport systems, including the transport of choline, glucose, butyrate and triiodothyronine in aging animals and humans. Such age-related changes are the consequence of either alteration in the carrier molecules or the physiochemical properties of the cerebral microvessels. At the present time, it is not clear whether changes in the barrier contribute

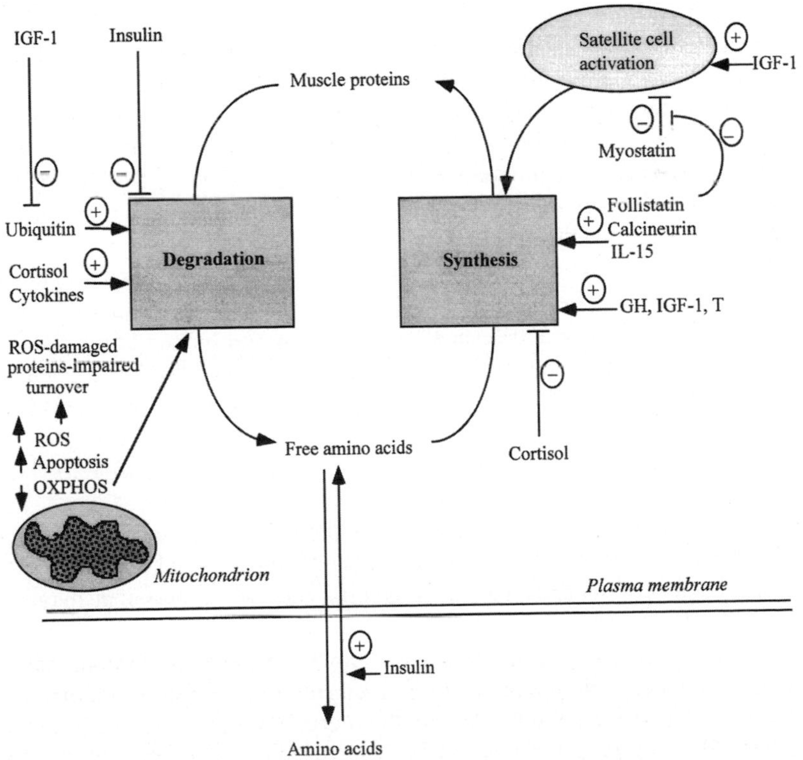

Fig. 6.3 Cross-talk of cellular and extracellular stimuli in regulating skeletal muscle protein degradation and synthesis in aging

to the age-related neurodegenerative diseases, suggested by the link between ischemic cerebral small-vessel disease, and several apparently clinically distinct dementia syndromes or are simply epiphenomena of aging. Proof that blood-brain barrier failure is integral to the development of aging-associated cerebrovascular dysfunction including lacunar stroke and dementia could provide an important target for novel interventions to reduce the effects of vascular disease on the brain and prevent cognitive decline and dementia [138].

Conclusion

Age-mediated changes in multiple cellular and molecular stimuli impact the overall homeostatic regulation (e.g., neuroendocrine controls) as well as the components of the immune defense system, including the inflammatory responses. These changes also appear to interface with defects in normal cardiovascular aging and may contribute to the onset and severity of age-associated cardiovascular diseases. Significantly, these discoveries may provide new targets and novel approaches to reverse both the cardiac and vascular structural/remodeling and dysfunction that occur with disease and aging. These new approaches may include both gene-based and cell-based therapies or a combination thereof. The use of stem cells to replenish specific cell populations, as well as to provide a platform for increasing angiogenic and proliferative factors may prove particularly valuable in aging-damaged and cell-diminished tissues, including immune cell-types and skeletal muscle. As many of the relevant targets are delineated, care needs to be exercised in defining the most effective, and perhaps less global, more highly targeted types of therapies. For instance, concerns have been raised with the use of growth hormone, IGF-1, or even changes in signaling transducers such as β-adrenergic receptors, in cardiovascular-targeted therapies because of potentially devastating side-effects that may include aberrant cell proliferation and constitutive activation of receptors. This may lead to unwanted myocardial hypertrophy and downstream signaling deficits. Furthermore, the discovery that age-alterations in physical exercise and overall energy expenditure, with skeletal muscle acting as a critical sensor/target, may play a significant role in the development of a range of cardiovascular diseases has important implications for the use (and potential limitations) of lifestyle therapeutic approaches, such as dietary and exercise to reverse aging-associated cardiovascular dysfunction, improve health and modulate longevity.

Evidently, better delineation of the cross-talk between the signaling components in these cardiovascular-related homeostatic systems is needed, focusing in particular on human studies. For instance, the relationship between elevated inflammation and human aging needs to be better defined, including not just an unraveling of the minutia (albeit important) of biochemical/signaling pathways but detailed examination as to what are the overall benefits for these pathways, i.e., cell-types and specific stressors vis a vis survival and function. Furthermore, detection of mitochondrial dysfunction in a variety of cell-types ranging from skeletal and cardiac muscle to vascular cells in aging may prove to be helpful in the identification of therapies.

Genetics is the other side of the coin to define both the susceptibility to age-associated disease and the impact of homeostatic/signaling pathways on health and survival. As previously discussed, association studies have only recently begun to identify genetic variants that may play a role in both disease susceptibility and longevity. More candidate loci for association testing will certainly be unveiled in the near future as the sensitivity and power of gene expression analysis to define age-specific transcripts in specific human cell-types are improved. Moreover, some of the genetic variants thus far identified also respond differentially to drug therapies indicating that pharmacogenomics may eventually also have a critical role to improve the care of the elderly. The discovery that many of these gene variant effects are specific to ethnic populations, and in some cases are gender-specific underlines the overall cross-talk between a variety of homeostatic/regulatory loci, some involving potentially reproductive factors, others thus far unidentified acting as modulators of genotype/phenotype expression of specific gene variants.

Summary

- Elevated levels of systemic inflammation are characteristic of human aging, a phenomena recently termed "inflamm-aging".
- Identification of inflammation-related biomarkers, are useful predictors of frailty and mortality in the elderly.
- Aging in rodent models and elderly humans is associated with severe deterioration of adaptive immunity due to a combination of intrinsic and extrinsic factors. These include a decline in naive T lymphocytes cell number and function, fewer bone marrow early progenitor B cells, with associated decline in the antigen-recognition repertoire of B cells, as well as accumulation of clonally expanded and functionally incompetent memory lymphocytes.
- Diminished adaptive immunity in the elderly contributes to a decline in the quality of humoral response, to reduction in the diversity of the T cell repertoire, compromises the ability to battle new infection and may be directly responsible for increased infections and failed response to vaccines.
- Elements of innate immunity also are markedly affected by aging. The response of neutrophils and macrophages to important signaling pathways involved in immune defense, including ROS production, response to cytokines and chemokines and toll-like receptor (TLR) function diminish with age leading to reduced phagocytosis, cytotoxic and chemotactic behavior of these cellular components of immunity.
- With aging there is diminished capacity of natural killer (NK) cells and dendritic cells to provide additional innate immunity.
- Defects in components of innate and adaptive immunity have been also implicated in the onset of aging-associated cardiovascular diseases such as atherosclerosis and myocardial infarction.
- Studies with centenarians and elderly subjects have documented a significant association of specific polymorphic variants in genes encoding key signaling components of immune response, such as TLR4, proinflammatory factors like interleukin-6 (IL-6) and anti-inflammatory elements, such as interleukin-10 (IL-10), with altered longevity and the risk and/or susceptibility of developing cardiovascular dysfunction; however, this association appears to be operative in specific ethnic populations and are frequently gender-specific.
- Polymorphisms in the PON1 gene, which encodes a key enzyme in the modulation of lipid peroxidation in response to oxidative damage and the inflammatory response, have been implicated in both cardiovascular dysfunction and increased survival in specific ethnic populations.
- Aging affects multiple aspects of neuroendocrine components including hormone synthesis and release, receptor function and expression, postreceptor signaling. These changes in hypothalamic, pituitary, adrenal and thyroid function involving both the hypothalamo-neurohypophysial system (HNS) and the hypothalamo-pituitary-adrenocortical (HPA) axis can impact many aspects of cardiovascular function in aging including marked changes in stress response and metabolic regulation in aging tissues. This has been demonstrated in both rodent models and elderly human subjects.
- Decline in growth hormone (GH) and IGF-1 levels have been found in the elderly and similarities between the dysfunction present in GH deficient and aging subjects have been reported.
- Supplementation of animal models with GH has shown significant benefits reversing normal heart and vascular aging-mediated dysfunction as well as the cardiac dysfunction in animal models of heart failure.

- Clinical studies have also shown significant cardiovascular benefits with supplementation of GH and other GH released peptides (e.g., hexarelin and ghrelin) including lowering peripheral resistance, improvement of contractility and providing cardioprotection in patients with severe cardiovascular dysfunction.
- In numerous species, including humans, increasing age is associated with significant structural and functional changes in skeletal muscle, which are contributory to aging associated cardiovascular and metabolic disorders including insulin resistance, type 2 diabetes, hypertension, and hyperlipidemia. Underlying the aging-mediated loss of muscle strength and mass (including sarcopenia) are decreased levels of muscle protein synthesis, changes in neural stimulation, cytokine and neurohormone secretion and regulation, aberrant regulation of protein degradation and metabolic function, including energetic production and expenditure, and disturbed mitochondrial function with increased OS, ROS production and oxidative damage.
- In sarcopenia there is extensive cross-talk between subcellular components (mitochondrial, calcium regulators, ubiquitin degradation systems and plasma membrane) and numerous hormonal/neuroendocrine/cytokine inputs in the synthesis, regulation and degradation of muscle proteins.

References

1. Franceschi C, Bonafe M, Valensin S, Olivieri F, De Luca M, Ottaviani E, De Benedictis G. Inflamm-aging. An evolutionary perspective on immunosenescence. Ann NY Acad Sci 2000;908:244–254
2. De Martinis M, Franceschi C, Monti D, Ginaldi L. Inflammation markers predicting frailty and mortality in the elderly. Exp Mol Pathol 2006;80:219–227
3. Solana R, Pawelec G, Tarazona R. Aging and innate immunity. Immunity 2006;24:491–494
4. Weng N. Aging of the immune system: how much can the adaptive immune system adapt? Immunity 2006;24:495–499
5. Linton PJ, Dorshkind K. Age-related changes in lymphocyte development and function. Nat Immunol 2004;5:133–139
6. Tarazona R, Delarosa O, Alonso C, Ostos B, Espejo J, Pena J, Solana R. Increased expression of NK cell markers on T lymphocytes in aging and chronic activation of the immune system reflects the accumulation of effector/senescent T cells. Mech Ageing Dev 2000:121:77–88
7. Almanzar G, Schwaiger S, Jenewein B, Keller M, Herndler-Brandstetter D, Wurzner R, Schonitzer D, Grubeck-Loebenstein B. Long-term cytomegalovirus infection leads to significant changes in the composition of the CD8+ T-cell repertoire, which may be the basis for an imbalance in the cytokine production profile in elderly persons. J Virol 2005;79:3675–3683
8. Allman D, Miller JP. B cell development and receptor diversity during aging. Curr Opin Immunol 2005;17:463–467
9. Frasca D, Riley RL, Blomberg BB. Humoral immune response and B-cell functions including immunoglobulin class switch are downregulated in aged mice and humans. Semin Immunol 2005;17:378–384
10. Swain S, Clise-Dwyer K, Haynes L. Homeostasis and the age-associated defect of CD4 T cells. Semin Immunol 2005;17:370–377
11. Kovaiou RD, Weiskirchner I, Keller M, Pfister G, Cioca DP, Grubeck-Loebenstein B. Age-related differences in phenotype and function of CD4+ T cells are due to a phenotypic shift from naive to memory effector CD4+ T cells. Int Immunol 2005;17:1359–1366
12. Haynes L., Eaton SM, Burns EM, Randall TD, Swain SL. CD4 T cell memory derived from young naive cells functions well into old age, but memory generated from aged naive cells functions poorly. Proc Natl Acad Sci USA 2003;100:15053–15058
13. Kang I, Hong MS, Nolasco H, Park SH, Dan JM, Choi JY, Craft J. Age-associated change in the frequency of memory CD4+ T cells impairs long term CD4+ T cell responses to influenza vaccine. J Immunol 2004;173:673–681
14. Fulop T Jr, Seres I. Signal transduction changes in granulocytes and lymphocytes with aging. Immunol Lett 1994;40:259–268
15. Medzhitov R. Toll-like receptors and innate immunity. Nat Rev Immunol 2001;1:135–145
16. Fulop T, Larbi A, Douziech N, Fortin C, Guerard KP, Lesur O, Khalil A, Dupuis G. Signal transduction and functional changes in neutrophils with aging. Aging Cell 2004;3:217–226

17. Fu Y-K, Arkins S. Li Y, Dantzer R, Kelley KW. Reduction in superoxide anion secretion and bactericidal activity of neutrophils from aged rats: reversal by combination of interferon and growth hormone. Infect Immun 1994;62:1–8
18. Seres I, Csongor J, Mohacsi A, Leovey A, Fulop T. Age-dependent alterations of human recombinant GM-CSF effects on human granulocytes. Mech Ageing Dev 1993;71:143–154
19. Varga Z, Jacob MP, Csongor J, Robert L, Leovey A, Fulop T Jr. Altered phosphatidylinositol breakdown after K-elastin stimulation in PMNLs of elderly. Mech Ageing Dev 1990;52:61–70
20. Babior BM. Phagocytes and oxidative stress. Am J Med 2000;109:33–44
21. Shao D, Segal AW, Dekker LV. Lipid rafts determine efficiency of NADPH oxidase activation in neutrophils. FEBS Lett 2003;550:101–106
22. Fulop T Jr, Fouquet C, Allaire P, Perrin N, Lacombe G, Stankova J, Rola-Pleszczynski M, Gagne D, Wagner JR, Khalil A, Dupuis G. Changes in apoptosis of human polymorphonuclear granulocytes with aging. Mech Ageing Dev 1997;96:15–34
23. Fulop T Jr, Larbi A, Linteau A, Desgeorges S, Douziech N. The role of Mcl-1 and Bax expression alteration in the decreased rescue of human neutrophils from apoptosis by GM-CSF with aging. Ann NY Acad Sci 2002;973:305–308
24. Fortin CF, Larbi A, Lesur O, Douziech N, Fulop T. Impairment of SHP-1 down-regulation in the lipid rafts of human neutrophils under GM-CSF stimulation contributes to their age-related, altered functions. J. Leukoc Biol 2006;79:1061–1072
25. Alvarez E, Ruiz-Guttierrez V, Sobrino F, Santa-Maria C. Age-related changes in membrane lipid composition, fluidity and respiratoty burst in rat peripheral neutrophils. Clin Exp Immunol 2001;124:95–102
26. Rao KMK. Age-related decline in ligand-induced actin polymerization in human leukocytes and platelets. J Gerontol 1986;41:561–566
27. Rao KMK, Currie MS, Padmanabhan J, Cohen HJ. Age-related alteration in actin cytoskeleton and receptor expression in human leukocytes. J Gerontol 1992;47:B37–B44
28. Plowden J, Renshaw-Hoelscher M, Engleman C, Katz J, Sambhara S. Innate immunity in aging: impact on macrophage function. Aging Cell 2004;3:161–167
29. Ding A, Hwang S, Schwab R. Effect of aging on murine macrophages. Diminished response to IFN-γ for enhanced oxidative metabolism. J Immunol 1994;153:2146–2152
30. Renshaw M, Rockwell J, Engleman C, Gewirtz A, Katz J, Sambhara S. Cutting edge: impaired Toll-like receptor expression and function in aging. J Immunol 2002;169:4697–701
31. Boehmer ED, Meehan MJ, Cutro BT, Kovacs EJ. Aging negatively skews macrophage TLR2- and TLR4-mediated pro-inflammatory responses without affecting the IL-2-stimulated pathway. Mech Ageing Dev 2005;126:1305–1313
32. Plackett TP, Boehmer ED, Faunce DE, Kovacs EJ. Aging and innate immune cells. J Leukoc Biol 2004;76: 291–299
33. Herrero C, Marques L, Lloberas J, Celada A. IFN-gamma-dependent transcription of MHC class II IA is impaired in macrophages from aged mice. J Clin Invest 2001;107:485–493
34. Swift ME., Kleinman HK, DiPietro LA. Impaired wound repair and delayed angiogenesis in aged mice. Lab Invest 1999;79:1479–1487
35. Sadoun E, Reed MJ. Impaired angiogenesis in aging is associated with alterations in vessel density, matrix composition, inflammatory response, and growth factor expression. J Histochem Cytochem 2003;51:1119–1130
36. Uyemura K, Castle SC, Makinodan T. The frail elderly: role of dendritic cells in the susceptibility of infection. Mech Ageing Dev 2002;123:955–962
37. Bottino C, Moretta L, Moretta A. NK cell activating receptors and tumor recognition in humans. Curr Top Microbiol Immunol 2006;298:175–182
38. Solana R, Mariani E. NK and NK/T cells in human senescence. Vaccine 2000;18:1613–1620
39. Bruunsgaard H, Pedersen AN, Schroll M, Skinhoj P, Pedersen BK. Decreased natural killer cell activity is associated with atherosclerosis in elderly humans. Exp Gerontol 2001;37:127–136
40. Mysliwska J, Trzonkowski P, Szmit E, Brydak LB, Machala M, Mysliwski A. Immunomodulating effect of influenza vaccination in the elderly differing in health status. Exp Gerontol 2004;39:1447–1458
41. Dussault I, Miller SC. Decline in natural killer cell-mediated immunosurveillance in aging mice–a consequence of reduced cell production and tumor binding capacity. Mech Ageing Dev 1994;75:115–129
42. Mariani E, Meneghetti A, Neri S, Ravaglia G, Forti P, Cattini L, Facchini A. Chemokine production by natural killer cells from nonagenarians. Eur J Immunol 2002;32:1524–1529
43. Lutz CT, Moore MB, Bradley S, Shelton BJ, Lutgendorf SK. Reciprocal age related change in natural killer cell receptors for MHC class I. Mech Ageing Dev 2005;126:722–731
44. Murasko DM, Jiang J. Response of aged mice to primary virus infections. Immunol Rev 2005;205:285–296
45. Borrego F, Alonso MC, Galiani MD, Carracedo J, Ramirez R, Ostos B, Pena J, Solana R. NK phenotypic markers and IL2 response in NK cells from elderly people. Exp Gerontol 1999;34:253–265

46. Albright JW, Albright JF. Impaired natural killer cell function as a consequence of aging. Exp Gerontol 1998;33:13–25
47. Kiechl S, Lorenz E, Reindl M, Wiedermann CJ, Oberhollenzer F, Bonora E, Willeit J, Schwartz DA. Toll-like receptor 4 polymorphisms and atherogenesis. N Engl J Med 2002;347:185–192
48. Zareparsi S, Buraczynska M, Branham KE, Shah S, Eng D, Li M, Pawar H, Yashar BM, Moroi SE, Lichter PR, Petty HR, Richards JE, Abecasis GR, Elner VM, Swaroop A. Toll-like receptor 4 variant D299G is associated with susceptibility to age-related macular degeneration. Hum Mol Genet 2005;14:1449–1455
49. Balistreri CR, Candore G, Colonna-Romano G, Lio D, Caruso M, Hoffmann E, Franceschi C, Caruso C. Role of Toll-like receptor 4 in acute myocardial infarction and longevity. JAMA 2004;292:2339–2340
50. Lio D, Scola L, Crivello A, Colonna-Romano G, Candore G, Bonafe M, Cavallone L, Franceschi C, Caruso C. Gender-specific association between -1082 IL-10 promoter polymorphism and longevity. Genes Immun 2002;3:30–33
51. Lio D, Licastro F, Scola L, Chiappelli M, Grimaldi LM, Crivello A, Colonna-Romano G, Candore G, Franceschi C, Caruso C. Interleukin-10 promoter polymorphism in sporadic Alzheimer's disease. Genes Immun 2003;4:234–238
52. Wang XY, Hurme M, Jylha M, Hervonen A. Lack of association between human longevity and polymorphisms of IL-1 cluster, IL-6, IL-10 and TNF-alpha genes in Finnish nonagenarians. Mech Ageing Dev 2001;123:29–38
53. Ross OA, Curran MD, Meenagh A, Williams F, Barnett YA, Middleton D, Rea IM. Study of age-association with cytokine gene polymorphisms in an aged Irish population. Mech Ageing Dev 2003;124:199–206
54. Bonafe M, Olivieri F, Cavallone L, Giovagnetti S, Mayegiani F, Cardelli M, Pieri C, Marra M, Antonicelli R, Lisa R, Rizzo MR, Paolisso G, Monti D, Franceschi C. A gender—dependent genetic predisposition to produce high levels of IL-6 is detrimental for longevity. Eur J Immunol 2001;31:2357–2361
55. Flex A, Gaetani E, Pola R, Santoliquido A, Aloi F, Papaleo P, Dal Lago A, Pola E, Serricchio M, Tondi P, Pola P. The -174 G/C polymorphism of the interleukin-6 gene promoter is associated with peripheral artery occlusive disease. Eur J Vasc Endovasc Surg 2002;24:264–268
56. Rea IM, Ross OA, Armstrong M, McNerlan S, Alexander DH, Curran MD, Middleton D. Interleukin-6-gene C/G 174 polymorphism in nonagenarian and octogenarian subjects in the BELFAST study. Reciprocal effects on IL-6, soluble IL-6 receptor and for IL-10 in serum and monocyte supernatants. Mech Ageing Dev 2003;124:555–561
57. Lio D, Scola L, Crivello A, Bonafe M, Franceschi C, Olivieri F, Colonna-Romano G, Candore G, Caruso C. Allele frequencies of +874T–>A single nucleotide polymorphism at the first intron of interferon-gamma gene in a group of Italian centenarians. Exp Gerontol 2002;37:315–319
58. Grimaldi MP, Candore G, Vasto S, Caruso M, Caimi G, Hoffmann E, Colonna-Romano G, Lio D, Shinar Y, Franceschi C, Caruso C. Role of the pyrin M694V (A2080G) allele in acute myocardial infarction and longevity: a study in the Sicilian population. J Leukoc Biol 2006;79:611–615
59. Bonafe M, Marchegiani F, Cardelli M, Olivieri F, Cavallone L, Giovagnetti S, Pieri C, Marra M, Antonicelli R, Troiano L, Gueresi P, Passeri G, Berardelli M, Paolisso G, Barbieri M, Tesei S, Lisa R, De Benedictis G, Franceschi C. Genetic analysis of Paraoxonase (PON1) locus reveals an increased frequency of Arg192 allele in centenarians. Eur J Hum Genet 2002;10:292–296
60. Rea IM, McKeown PP, McMaster D, Young IS, Patterson C, Savage MJ, Belton C, Marchegiani F, Olivieri F, Bonafe M, Franceschi C. Paraoxonase polymorphisms PON1 192 and 55 and longevity in Italian centenarians and Irish nonagenarians. A pooled analysis. Exp Gerontol 2004;39:629–635
61. Boekholdt SM, Agema WR, Peters RJ, Zwinderman AH, van der Wall EE, Reitsma PH, Kastelein JJ, Jukema JW. REgression GRowth Evaluation Statin Study Group. Variants of toll-like receptor 4 modify the efficacy of statin therapy and the risk of cardiovascular events. Circulation 2003;107:2416–2421
62. Holloway JW, Yang IA, Ye S. Variation in the toll-like receptor 4 gene and susceptibility to myocardial infarction. Pharmacogenet Genomics 2005;15:15–21
63. Morange PE, Tiret L, Saut N, Luc G, Arveiler D, Ferrieres J, Amouyel P, Evans A, Ducimetiere P, Cambien F, Juhan-Vague I. PRIME Study Group. TLR4/Asp299Gly, CD14/C-260T, plasma levels of the soluble receptor CD14 and the risk of coronary heart disease: the PRIME Study. Eur J Hum Genet 2004;12:1041–1049
64. Koch W, Hoppmann P, Pfeufer A, Schomig A, Kastrati A. Toll-like receptor 4 gene polymorphisms and myocardial infarction: no association in a Caucasian population. Eur Heart J 2006;27:2524–2529
65. Wang XY, Hurme M, Jylha M, Hervonen A. Lack of association between human longevity and polymorphisms of IL-1 cluster, IL-6, IL-10 and TNF-alpha genes in Finnish nonagenarians. Mech Ageing Dev 2001;123:29–38
66. Cavallone L, Bonafe M, Olivieri F, Cardelli M, Marchegiani F, Giovagnetti S, Di Stasio G, Giampieri C, Mugianesi E, Stecconi R, Sciacca F, Grimaldi LM, De Benedictis G, Lio D, Caruso C, Franceschi C. The role of IL-1 gene cluster in longevity: a study in Italian population. Mech Ageing Dev 2003;124:533–538
67. Fagiolo U, Cossarizza A, Scala E, Fanales-Belasio E, Ortolani C, Cozzi E, Monti D, Franceschi C, Paganelli R. Increased cytokine production in mononuclear cells of healthy elderly people. Eur J Immunol 1993;23:2375–2378

68. Young DG, Skibinski G, Mason JI, James K. The influence of age and gender on serum dehydroepiandrosterone sulphate (DHEA-S), IL-6, IL-6 soluble receptor (IL-6 sR) and transforming growth factor beta 1 (TGF-beta1) levels in normal healthy blood donors. Clin Exp Immunol 1999;117:476–481
69. Ershler WB, Keller ET. Age-associated increased interleukin-6 gene expression, late-life diseases, and frailty. Annu Rev Med 2000;51:245–270
70. Terry CF, Loukaci V, Green FR. Cooperative influence of genetic polymorphisms on interleukin 6 transcriptional regulation. J Biol Chem 2000;275:18138–18144
71. Ross R. Atherosclerosis is an inflammatory disease. Am. Heart J 1999;138:S419–S420
72. Basso F, Lowe GD, Rumley A, McMahon AD, Humphries SE. Interleukin-6-174G > C polymorphism and risk of coronary heart disease in west of Scotland coronary prevention study (WOSCOPS). Arterioscler Thromb Vasc Biol 2002;22:599–604
73. Bruunsgaard H, Christiansen L, Pedersen AN, Schroll M, Jorgensen T, Pedersen BK. The IL-6 -174G>C polymorphism is associated with cardiovascular diseases and mortality in 80-year-old humans. Exp Gerontol 2004;39:255–261
74. Licastro F, Grimaldi LM, Bonafe M, Martina C, Olivieri F, Cavallone L, Giovanietti S, Masliah E, Franceschi C. Interleukin-6 gene alleles affect the risk of Alzheimer's disease and levels of the cytokine in blood and brain. Neurobiol Aging 2003;24:921–926
75. van Oijen M, Arp PP, de Jong FJ, Hofman A, Koudstaal PJ, Uitterlinden AG, Breteler MM. Polymorphisms in the interleukin 6 and transforming growth factor beta1 gene and risk of dementia. The Rotterdam Study. Neurosci Lett 2006;402:113–117
76. Ravaglia G, Paola F, Maioli F, Martelli M, Montesi F, Bastagli L, Bianchin M, Chiappelli M, Tumini E, Bolondi L, Licastro F. Interleukin-1beta and interleukin-6 gene polymorphisms as risk factors for AD: a prospective study. Exp Gerontol 2006;41:85–92
77. Lio D, Scola L, Crivello A, Colonna-Romano G, Candore G, Bonafe M, Cavallone L, Marchegiani F, Olivieri F, Franceschi C, Caruso C. Inflammation, genetics, and longevity: further studies on the protective effects in men of IL-10 -1082 promoter SNP and its interaction with TNF alpha -308 promoter SNP. J Med Genet 2003;40: 296–9
78. Lio D, Candore G, Crivello A, Scola L, Colonna-Romano G, Cavallone L, Hoffmann E, Caruso M, Licastro F, Caldarera CM, Branzi A, Franceschi C, Caruso C. Opposite effects of interleukin 10 common gene polymorphisms in cardiovascular diseases and in successful ageing: genetic background of male centenarians is protective against coronary heart disease. J Med Genet 2004;41:790–794
79. Pes GM, Lio D, Carru C, Deiana L, Baggio G, Franceschi C, Ferrucci L, Oliveri F, Scola L, Crivello A, Candore G, Colonna-Romano G, Caruso C. Association between longevity and cytokine gene polymorphisms. A study in Sardinian centenarians. Aging Clin Exp Res 2004;16:244–248
80. Senti M, Tomas M, Vila J, Marrugat J, Elosua R, Sala J, Masia R. Relationship of age-related myocardial infarction risk and Gln/Arg 192 variants of the human paraoxonase1 gene: the REGICOR study. Atherosclerosis 2001;156:443–449
81. Franceschi C, Olivieri F, Marchegiani F, Cardelli M, Cavallone L, Capri M, Salvioli S, Valensin S, De Benedictis G, Di Iorio A, Caruso C, Paolisso G, Monti D. Genes involved in immune response/inflammation, IGF1/insulin pathway and response to oxidative stress play a major role in the genetics of human longevity: the lesson of centenarians. Mech Ageing Dev 2005;126:351–361
82. Marchegiani F, Marra M, Spazzafumo L, James RW, Boemi M, Olivieri F, Cardelli M, Cavallone L, Bonfigli AR, Franceschi C. Paraoxonase activity and genotype predispose to successful aging. J Gerontol A Biol Sci Med Sci 2006;61:541–546
83. He XM, Zhang ZX, Zhang JW, Zhou YT, Tang MN, Wu CB, Hong Z. Gln192Arg polymorphism in paraoxonase 1 gene is associated with Alzheimer disease in a Chinese Han ethnic population. Chin Med J (Engl) 2006;119:1204–1209
84. Sapolsky RM, Krey LC, McEwen B. The neuroendocrinology of stress and aging: the glucocorticoid cascade hypothesis. Endocr Rev 1986;7:284–301
85. Seeman TE, Robbins RJ. Aging and hypothalamic-pituitary-adrenal response to challenge in humans. Endocr Rev 1994;15:233–260
86. Djordjevic-Markovic R, Radic O, Jelic V, Radojcic M, Rapic-Otrin V, Ruzdijic S, Krstic-Demonacos M, Kanazir S, Kanazir D. Glucocorticoid receptors in ageing rats. Exp Gerontol 1999;34:971–982
87. van Eekelen JA, Rots NY, Sutanto W, Oitzl MS, de Kloet ER. Brain corticosteroid receptor gene expression and neuroendocrine dynamics during aging. J Steroid Biochem Mol Biol 1991;40:679–683
88. Keck ME, Hatzinger M, Wotjak CT, Landgraf R, Holsboer F, Neumann ID. Ageing alters intrahypothalamic release patterns of vasopressin and oxytocin in rats. Eur J Neurosci 2000;12:1487–1494
89. Cizza G, Calogero AE, Brady LS, Bagdy G, Bergamini E, Blackman MR, Chrousos GP, Gold PW. Male Fischer 344/N rats show a progressive central impairment of the hypothalamic-pituitary-adrenal axis with advancing age. Endocrinology 1994;134:1611–1620

90. Tizabi YG, Aguilera G, Gilad GM. Age-related reduction in pituitary corticotropin-releasing hormone receptors in two rat strains. Neurobiol Aging 1992;13:227–230
91. Hauger RL, Thrivikraman KV, Plotsky PM. Age-related alterations of hypothalamic-pituitary-adrenal axis function in male Fischer 344 rats. Endocrinology 1994;134:1528–1536
92. Heroux JA, Grigoriadis DE, De Souza EB. Age-related decreases in corticotropin-releasing factor (CRF) receptors in rat brain and anterior pituitary gland. Brain Res 1991;542:155–158
93. Ceccatelli S, Calza L, Giardino L. Age-related changes in the expression of corticotropin-releasing hormone receptor mRNA in the rat pituitary. Brain Res Mol Brain Res 1996;37:175–180
94. De Souza EB. Corticotropin-releasing factor receptors: physiology, pharmacology, biochemistry and role in central nervous system and immune disorders. Psychoneuroendocrinology 1995;20:789–819
95. Herman JP, Larson BR, Speert DB, Seasholtz AF. Hypothalamo-pituitary-adrenocortical dysregulation in aging F344/Brown-Norway F1 hybrid rats. Neurobiol Aging 2001;22:323–332
96. McClennen SJ, Cortright DN, Seasholtz AF. Regulation of pituitary corticotropin-releasing hormone-binding protein messenger ribonucleic acid levels by restraint stress and adrenalectomy. Endocrinology 1998;139:4435–4441
97. Xiao C, Sartin J, Mulchahey JJ, Segar T, Sheriff S, Herman JP, Kasckow JW. Aging associated changes in amygdalar corticotropin-releasing hormone (CRH) and CRH-binding protein in Fischer 344 rats. Brain Res 2006;1073–1074:325–331
98. Magri F, Cravello L, Barili L, Sarra S, Cinchetti W, Salmoiraghi F, Micale G, Ferrari E. Stress and dementia: the role of the hypothalamicpituitary-adrenal axis. Aging Clin Exp Res 2006;18:167–170
99. Bauer ME. Stress, glucocorticoids and ageing of the immune system. Stress 2005;8:69–83
100. Rehman HU, Masson EA. Neuroendocrinology of ageing. Age Ageing 2001;30:279–287
101. Lai Z, Roos P, Zhai O, Olsson Y, Fholenhag K, Larsson C, Nyberg F. Age-related reduction of human growth hormone-binding sites in the human brain. Brain Res 1993;621:260–266
102. Garnero P, Sornay-Rendu E, Delmas PF. Low serum IGF-1 and occurrence of osteoporotic fractures in postmenopausal women. Lancet 2000;355:898–899
103. Rudman D, Feller AG, Nagraj HS, Gergans GA, Lalitha PY, Goldberg AF, Schlenker RA, Cohn L, Rudman IW, Mattson DE. Effects of human growth hormone in men over 60 years old. N Engl J Med 1990;323:1–6
104. Copeland KC, Nair KS. Acute growth hormone effects on amino acid and lipid metabolism. J Clin Endocrinol Metab 1994;78:1040–1047
105. Fryburg DA, Louard RJ, Gerow KE, Gelfand RA, Barrett EJ. Growth hormone stimulates skeletal muscle protein synthesis and antagonizes insulin's antiproteolytic action in humans. Diabetes 1992;41:424–429
106. Fryburg DA, Gelfand RA, Barrett EJ. Growth hormone acutely stimulates forearm muscle protein synthesis in normal humans. Am J Physiol 1991;260:E499–E504
107. Binnerts A, Swart GR, Wilson JH, Hoogerbrugge N, Pols HA, Birkenhager JC, Lamberts SW. The effect of growth hormone administration in growth hormone deficient adults on bone, protein, carbohydrate and lipid homeostasis, as well as on body composition. Clin Endocrinol (Oxf) 1992;37:79–87
108. Colao A, Cuocolo A, Di Somma C, Cerbone G, Della Morte AM, Nicolai E, Lucci R, Salvatore M, Lombardi G. Impaired cardiac performance in elderly patients with growth hormone deficiency. J Clin Endocrinol Metab 1999;84:3950–3955
109. Thuesen L, Christiansen JS, Sorensen KE, Jorgensen JO, Orskov H, Henningsen P. Increased myocardial contractility following growth hormone administration in normal man. An echocardiographic study. Dan Med Bull 1988;35:193–196
110. Groban L, Pailes NA, Bennett CD, Carter CS, Chappell MC, Kitzman DW, Sonntag WE. Growth hormone replacement attenuates diastolic dysfunction and cardiac angiotensin II expression in senescent rats. J Gerontol A Biol Sci Med Sci 2006;61:28–35
111. Isgaard J, Bergh CH, Caidahl K, Lomsky M, Hjalmarson A, Bengtsson BA. A placebo-controlled study of growth hormone in patients with congestive heart failure. Eur Heart J 1998;19:1704–1711
112. Bocchi E, Moura L, Guimaraes G, Conceicao Souza GE, Ramires JA. Beneficial effects of high doses of growth hormone in the introduction and optimization of medical treatment in decompensated congestive heart failure. Int J Cardiol 2006;110:313–317
113. Isgaard J, Johansson I. Ghrelin and GHS on cardiovascular applications/functions. J Endocrinol Invest 2005;28:838–842
114. Nagaya N, Moriya J, Yasumura Y, Uematsu M, Ono F, Shimizu W, Ueno K, Kitakaze M, Miyatake K, Kangawa K. Effects of ghrelin administration on left ventricular function, exercise capacity, and muscle wasting in patients with chronic heart failure. Circulation 2004;110:3674–3679
115. Harman SM, Blackman MR. Use of growth hormone for prevention or treatment of effects of aging. J Gerontol A Biol Sci Med Sci 2004;59:652–658
116. Sonntag WE, Lynch CD, Cooney PT, Hutchins PM. Decreases in cerebral microvasculature with age are associated with the decline in growth hormone and insulin-like growth factor 1. Endocrinology 1997;138:3515–3520

117. Khan AS, Lynch CD, Sane DC, Willingham MC, Sonntag WE. Growth hormone increases regional coronary blood flow and capillary density in aged rats. J Gerontol A Biol Sci Med Sci 2001;56:B364–B371
118. Bruel A, Oxlund H. Growth hormone influences the content and composition of collagen in the aorta from old rats. Mech Ageing Dev 2002;123:627–635
119. Castillo C, Cruzado M, Ariznavarreta C, Gil-Loyzaga P, Lahera V, Cachofeiro V, Tresguerres JA. Body composition and vascular effects of growth hormone administration in old female rats. Exp Gerontol 2003;38:971–979
120. Castillo C, Cruzado M, Ariznavarreta C, Gil-Loyzaga P, Lahera V, Cachofeiro V, Tresguerres JA. Effect of recombinant human growth hormone administration on body composition and vascular function and structure in old male Wistar rats. Biogerontology 2005;6:303–312
121. Ceda GP, Dall'Aglio E, Maggio M, Lauretani F, Bandinelli S, Falzoi C, Grimaldi W, Ceresini G, Corradi F, Ferrucci L, Valenti G, Hoffman AR. Clinical implications of the reduced activity of the GH-IGF-I axis in older men. J Endocrinol Invest 2005;28:96–100
122. Nair KS. Aging muscle. Am J Clin Nutr 2005;81:953–963
123. Lexell J, Taylor CC, Sjostrom M. What is the cause of the ageing atrophy? Total number, size and proportion of different fiber types studied in whole vastus lateralis muscle from 15- to 83-year-old men. J Neurol Sci 1988;84:275–294
124. Short KR, Vittone J, Bigelow ML, Proctor DN, Nair KS. Age and aerobic exercise training effects on whole body and muscle protein metabolism. Am J Physiol 2004;286:E92–E101
125. Lindle RS, Metter EJ, Lynch NA, Fleg JL, Fozard JL, Tobin JD, Roy TA, Hurley BF. Age and gender comparisons of muscle strength in 654 women and men aged 20–93 yr. J Appl Physiol 1997;83:1581–1587
126. Balagopal P, Rooyackers OE, Adey DB, Ades PA, Nair KS. Effects of aging on in vivo synthesis of skeletal muscle myosin heavy-chain and sarcoplasmic protein in humans. Am J Physiol 1997;273:E790–E800
127. Thompson LV. Effects of age and training on skeletal muscle physiology and performance. Phys Ther 1994;74:71–81
128. Lexell J. Human aging, muscle mass, and fiber type composition. J Gerontol A Biol Sci Med Sci 1995;50:11–16
129. Wang YX, Zhang CL, Yu RT, Cho HK, Nelson MC, Bayuga-Ocampo CR, Ham J, Kang H, Evans RM. Regulation of muscle fiber type and running endurance by PPARdelta. PLoS Biol 2004;2:e294
130. Barazzoni R, Short KR, Nair KS. Effects of aging on mitochondrial DNA copy number and cytochrome *c* oxidase gene expression in rat skeletal muscle, liver, and heart. J Biol Chem 2000;275:3343–3347
131. Rooyackers OE, Adey DB, Ades PA, Nair KS. Effect of age in vivo rates of mitochondrial protein synthesis in human skeletal muscle. Proc Natl Acad Sci USA 1996;93:15364–15369
132. Yarovaya NO, Kramarova L, Borg J, Kovalenko SA, Caragounis A, Linnane AW. Age-related atrophy of rat soleus muscle is accompanied by changes in fibre type composition, bioenergy decline and mtDNA rearrangements. Biogerontology 2002;3:25–27
133. Short KR, Bigelow ML, Kahl J, Singh R, Coenen-Schimke J, Raghavakaimal S, Nair KS. Decline in skeletal muscle mitochondrial function with aging in humans. Proc Natl Acad Sci USA 2005;102:5618–5623
134. Wanagat J, Cao Z, Pathare P, Aiken JM. Mitochondrial DNA deletion mutations colocalize with segmental electron transport system abnormalities, muscle fiber atrophy, fiber splitting, and oxidative damage in sarcopenia. FASEB J 2001;15:322–332
135. McKenzie D, Bua E, McKiernan S, Cao Z, Aiken JM, Wanagat J. Mitochondrial DNA deletion mutations: a causal role in sarcopenia. Eur J Biochem 2002;269:2010–2015
136. Dirks AJ, Leeuwenburgh C. The role of apoptosis in age-related skeletal muscle atrophy. Sports Med 2005;35:473–483
137. Rice KM, Blough ER. Sarcopenia-related apoptosis is regulated differently in fast- and slow-twitch muscles of the aging F344/N x BN rat model. Mech Ageing Dev 2006;127:670–679
138. Wardlaw JM, Sandercock PA, Dennis MS, Starr J. Is breakdown of the blood-brain barrier responsible for lacunar stroke, leukoaraiosis, and dementia? Stroke 2003;34:806–812

Table 7.1 Common etiologies of heart failure in the aged population

1. Hypertensive heart disease
2. Coronary artery disease
Acute myocardial infarction
Chronic ischemic cardiomyopathy
3. Age-related diastolic dysfunction
4. Valvular heart disease
Aortic stenosis or insufficiency
Mitral regurgitation
Prosthetic valve malfunction
5. Cardiomyopathy
Hypertrophic
Non-ischemic (dilated)
Restrictive

In addition to determining the etiologies, it is important to identify factors that commonly precipitate or contribute to HF exacerbation in the elderly (Table 7.2). As discussed below, non-compliance with medications and diet is the most common cause of HF exacerbation [9]. Other contributory factors include myocardial ischemia, volume overload owing to excess fluid intake, dysrhythmias (especially atrial fibrillation), intercurrent infections, anemia and various toxins including alcohol.

Clinical Presentation and Diagnostic Challenges

Accurate diagnosis of the HF syndrome at older age is complicated by the increasing prevalence of atypical symptoms and signs. Exertional dyspnea, orthopnea, lower extremities edema and impaired exercise tolerance are the cardinal symptoms of HF. However, with increasing age, often accompanied by reduced physical activity, exertional symptoms become less prominent [10]. Although most clinical trials of therapy have studied patients with an average age in the mid 60's, HF is most common in the elderly, who bear a greater burden of co-morbidity and polypharmacy[11] as well as psychogeriatric co-morbidities, health service utilization, functional decline, and frailty [12]. Frailty characterizes elderly persons in whom the ability to independently perform activities of daily living, such as bathing, toileting, dressing, grooming, and feeding, is progressively eroded and these associations have ramifications on the diagnosis and prognosis of HF [10, 13].

Table 7.2 Common precipitants of heart failure exacerbations in the aged population

Myocardial ischemia or infarction
Uncontrolled hypertension
Dietary sodium excess
Non-compliance with medications
Dysrhythmias
Supraventricular: atrial fibrillation
Ventricular Bradydysrhythmias
Intercurrent illness
Fever
Infection, especially pneumonia
Anemia
Renal insufficiency
Drugs and toxins
Alcohol
Antidysrhythmic agents
Nonsteroidal anti-inflammatory agents

Table 7.3 Atypical clinical features of heart failure in the frail elderly

Symptoms	Signs
Delirium	Ankle edema: may reflect venous insufficiency, drug effects and malnutrition
Falls	Sacral edema
Sudden functional decline	Rales/crackles are nonspecific
Sleep disturbances	
Nocturia	

A prominent feature that distinguishes HF in the elderly from the younger individuals is the much higher frequency of HF occurring in the absence of systolic dysfunction i.e., diastolic HF or HF with preserved systolic function. Indeed, heart failure with preserved systolic function accounts for less than 10% of HF cases in persons under age of 65 but more than 50% of cases over the age of 75 [14, 15].

Elderly patients with HF often have clinical presentations that are not commonly encountered in younger patients, which may confound the diagnosis (Table 7.3) [13]. HF is also associated with cognitive impairment in the domains of attention, short-term memory, and executive function (insight, judgment, problem solving and decision-making) and these attributes have been associated with non-adherence to treatment, accelerated functional decline, and even mortality [16]. Acute and fluctuating cognitive impairment, or delirium, can be precipitated by decompensated HF. Generally under-recognized by health care providers, delirium is usually reversible, though it may persist well beyond hospital discharge [17]. Cognitive impairment can occur in patients with stable HF and is called dementia if it impinges upon independent function such as adherence to prescribed therapy. Symptoms of depression are also common in HF patients [18]. Depression reduces quality of life, increases the risk of functional impairment, re-hospitalization and mortality, and may reduce adherence to prescribed therapy. Depression and HF share common clinical features in elderly patients, including weight gain, sleep disturbances, fatigue, poor energy, and cognitive disturbances [19]. Because of the atypical presentations, the use of biomarkers such as B-type natriuretic peptide in the diagnosis of HF in the elderly may be particularly useful [20].

Pharmacotherapy of Heart Failure in the Elderly

A small number of randomized trials of therapies conducted specifically in elderly populations, in conjunction with a multitude of data from observational data sets, suggest that most recommendations on HF therapies are applicable to elderly patients. Observational data suggests that ACE inhibitor use in elderly HF patients may preserve cognition, slow functional decline, and reduce hospitalizations and perhaps even mortality, even in patients with relative contraindications such as mild to moderate renal impairment [21]. The β-blocker nebivolol has been studied in over 2000 patients ≥ 70 years with clinical evidence of HF, regardless of ejection fraction (EF) [22]. After follow up of less than 2 years, a significant benefit for nebivolol was seen with reduction of the combined primary endpoint of mortality and cardiovascular hospitalization. Results of the ongoing Japanese Diastolic Heart Failure Study will further evaluate the effects of the β-blocker carvedilol in 800 elderly Japanese patients with HF and documented EF > 40% [23].

Elderly patients are vulnerable to adverse drug events (ADE), due to the growing complexity of medication regimens, age-related physiologic changes, and a higher burden of co-morbid illnesses. Cardiovascular medications are frequently associated with ADE in the elderly [24]. Digitalis toxicity can occur at therapeutic serum levels [25]. Falls constitute common clinical presentations of ADE in the elderly, often from postural hypotension. In randomized trials of drug treatment for HF, titration to target doses is less frequently successful in older patients due to higher side effect rates. As such, care must be taken with titration of medications to target doses in order to avoid ADE. In particular, orthostatic hypotension is a frequent side effect in elderly patients, but if recognized, and managed, can be controlled in order to allow for use of evidence-based therapies. Cardiovascular medications in general, and HF medications specifically, are under-prescribed in the elderly patients, despite the observation that as a result of a higher baseline incidence of cardiovascular events, the absolute benefit of evidence-based therapies is greatest in the elderly [26].

Disease Management Programs for Heart Failure in the Elderly

Several systematic reviews support the role of HF management programs in elderly HF patient populations [27]. While active involvement of caregivers in patient monitoring and medication adjustment is common to studies showing benefit, the optimal way of providing HF management remains controversial. The precise design of such care delivery systems depends in part upon local resources and infrastructure. Comprehensive geriatric assessment, shown to improve function, prevent hospitalization and institutionalization, reduce the risk of adverse drug reactions, and improve sub-optimal prescribing, may have a role to play in the management of frail elderly patients with HF.

The occurrence of diabetes mellitus and renal insufficiency in older HF patients portends a significantly worse prognosis and a greater likelihood of adverse drug events. The potential for contradictory recommendations may arise when these co-morbidities are managed in separate settings. Conflicting advice from multiple care providers can result in patient confusion, non-adherence and adverse outcomes. For example, recommendations to limit diuretic use in order to maintain renal function, or dietary advice for controlling blood glucose that results in increased sodium intake, may lead to worsening HF symptoms. An integrative approach to care is required, based on shared therapeutic goals and involving all care providers, including the primary care physician and the patient.

Device and Replacement Therapy in the Elderly

Cardiac resynchronization therapy (CRT) with or without concurrent use of implantable cardioverter defibrillator (ICD) is now a widely used treatment modality both for primary and secondary prevention in patients HF. There are still limited data on the impact of this type of device therapy in the elderly as most large-scale efficacy trials either excluded the very elderly patients or the number of elderly patients was small. A recent study has evaluated the effects of CRT in elderly patients [28]. The study included 170 consecutive patients whose clinical and echocardiographic improvements were evaluated after 6 months of follow-up. Survival was evaluated up to 2 years. The effects of CRT in elderly patients (age >70 years) were compared with those in younger patients (age <70 years). After 6 months of follow-up, CRT was beneficial in both groups, as reflected by improvements in clinical and echocardiographic parameters. Moreover, the magnitude of improvement was comparable between the 2 groups in clinical (NYHA class, quality-of-life score, and 6-minute walking distance) and echocardiographic parameters (improvement in the LV ejection fraction and extent of LV reverse remodeling). In addition, the number of non-responders was comparable between the patients aged <70 years (25%) and those aged ≥70 years (22%). Survival was not different between the two groups.

Heart transplantation has become a highly successful therapeutic option for patients with end-stage cardiomyopathy. Consequently, the criteria for patient selection, including recipients' upper age limits, have been expanded, with an increasing number of people older than 60 years of age now undergoing transplantation. Several studies have now reported similar long-term survival rate

Table 7.4 Key effects of aging on cardiovascular function

1. Increased blood vessel stiffness, increased impedance to ventricular ejection and increased pulse wave velocity
2. Impaired left ventricular relaxation and diastolic compliance
3. Myocyte loss
4. Attenuated response to β_1 and β_2 adrenergic stimulation
5. Altered myocardial energy metabolism and impaired mitochondrial function
6. Reduced sinus node pacemaker cells and impaired sinoatrial function

in patients transplanted at age > 60 versus patients transplanted at younger age [29–31]. Older transplant recipients have equal or less rejection episodes [31, 32] but may have equal or higher rate of infection and transplant CAD [29].

Pathophysiologic Considerations

Aging is associated with significant alterations in cardiac structure and function; some of these changes may predispose an individual to the development of HF [6]. The changes at a whole-organ level, which are listed in Table 7.4, include reduced vascular compliance, which increases the impedance to left ventricular ejection, and impaired ventricular diastolic performance [33]. It has been estimated that about one third of the cardiomyocytes are lost from the human heart between the ages of 17–90 years [34]. Attenuated β-adrenergic responsiveness to inotropic stimulation and degenerative changes in the sinoatrial node limit cardiac reserve and in particular its response to stress. The latter impairment is exacerbated by impaired mitochondrial dysfunction with reduced capacity to generate high-energy phosphates [33, 35].

Basic Mechanisms Mediating Aging-Related Cardiac Dysfunction and Heart Failure

Biological aging is a fundamental process that represents the major risk factor with respect to the development of cancer, neurodegenerative, as well as cardiovascular diseases. It is therefore not surprising that the molecular mechanisms of aging are fundamentally involved in many disease processes and critically important to understand. Some of the basic mechanisms that have been proposed for cardiac aging that may lead to cardiac dysfunction (most of which have been extensively discussed in this text) include prolonged action potential duration, myosin isozyme switch, impaired intracellular Ca^{2+} homeostasis, altered membrane structure and permeability, accumulation of reactive oxygen species (ROS) and cell loss through apoptosis, all of which may lead to abnormal cardiac contractile function and contribute to the development to HF [35, 36]. A model illustrating the triggering stimuli and cellular pathways involved in the onset and progression of HF is shown in Fig. 7.1.

Myocardial Remodeling and Aging

To determine the effects of aging on the human myocardium, hearts from individuals (aged 17–90 years) who died from causes other than cardiovascular disease were studied [34].. The aging process was characterized by a loss of 38 million and 14 million nuclei/year in the left and right ventricle respectively. This loss in muscle mass was accompanied by a progressive increase in myocyte cell volume per nucleus, resulting in a preservation of ventricular wall thickness. However, the

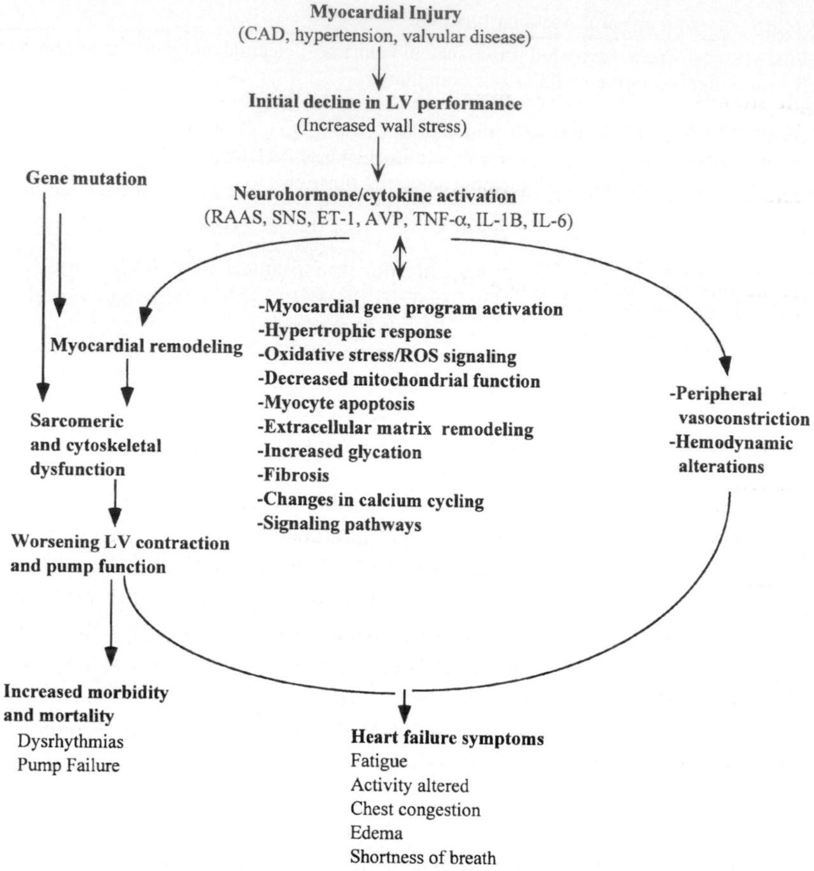

Fig. 7.1 Model of triggers and cellular pathways leading to heart failure

cellular hypertrophic response was unable to maintain normal cardiac mass. Left and right ventricular weights decreased by 0.70 and 0.21 g/year, respectively. It is therefore proposed that about one third of the cardiomyocytes are lost from the human heart between the ages of 17–90 years [34].

Recent studies, however, have challenged the widely-held but unproven paradigm that describes the heart as a post-mitotic organ [7]. Moreover, recent developments in the field of stem cell biology have led to the recognition that the possibility exists for extrinsic and intrinsic regeneration of myocytes and coronary vessels, leading to reevaluation of cardiac homeostasis and myocardial aging [37]. A newer paradigm views the adult mammalian heart as composed of non-dividing (primarily terminally differentiated) myocytes and a small and continuously renewed subpopulation of cycling myocytes produced by the differentiation of cardiac stem cells. A dynamic balance between myocyte death and the formation of new myocytes by cardiac stem cells is an important regulator of myocardial maintenance of function and mass from birth to adulthood and very critical in old age. Increasing evidence suggests that numerous pathological or physiological stimuli can activate the stem cells to enter the cell cycle and differentiate into new myocytes and in some cases vasculature which significantly contribute to changes in cardiac output and myocardial mass [38].

Telomere length is a useful marker of these processes. Studies in fetal, neonatal and senescent (27 month-old) Fischer 344 rats found that while the loss of telomeric DNA was minimal in fetal and neonatal myocytes, telomeric shortening increased with age in a subgroup of myocytes that constituted nearly 20% of the myocyte population, suggesting that this population reflects the most actively dividing myocyte class in the organ. Early studies found in the remaining nondividing rat myocytes, the progressive accumulation of another marker of cellular senescence, senescent associated nuclear protein, p16(INK4) [39].

More recent studies with myocytes from aging individuals with age-related HF compared to myocytes from individuals with idiopathic dilated cardiomyopathy (DCM) observed several differences in heart and myocyte phenotype [40]. While aged diseased hearts exhibited moderate hypertrophy and dilation, they also displayed an accumulation of p16INK4a positive primitive stem cells and myocytes. A marked increase in cell death was primarily limited to cells expressing p16INK4a with significant telomeric shortening. Importantly, this finding suggested that stem cells could also be targeted by senescence. While cell multiplication, mitotic index and telomerase increased in these aging hearts, evidence suggested that these regenerative events could not compensate for cell death or prevent telomeric shortening. This study also found that hearts from subjects with idiopathic DCM had more severe hypertrophy and dilation, more extensive cardiac interstitial fibrosis and tissue inflammatory injury, increased necrosis and a reduced level of myocytes with p16INK4a labeling. This is consistent with the involvement of p16INK4a with death signals linked to apoptosis in senescent myocardium in contrast to idiopathic DCM in which myocyte necrosis predominates and myocyte death is largely independent from the expression of the kinase inhibitor p16INK4a. Nevertheless, some important commonalities were also found: while idiopathic DCM had increased necrosis compared to aging tissues, hearts of aged diseased and idiopathic DCM subjects had similar levels of myocyte apoptosis. Moreover, extensive stem cell death was found in both tissues and not in healthy controls, suggesting that mechanisms (e.g., oxidative stress) that target stem cells may contribute to the phenotype of cardiac dysfunction in both the aging and cardiomyopathic heart. Moreover, Torella et al. have identified a population of cardiac stem cells in young and senescent mice that with increased age display increased evidence of senescence, i.e., p16ink4a expression, telomere shortening (indicative of reduced telomerase activity), and apoptosis [41]. Interestingly, the effect of murine aging on cardiac stem cells (including the expression of gene products implicated in growth arrest and senescence, such as p27Kip1, p53, p16INK4a, and p19ARF), and on the resulting cardiac dysfunction was remarkably attenuated in aged transgenic mice containing overexpressed IGF-1. It remains to be seen whether similar effects of IGF-1 on preserving stem cell regenerative function would be seen in strains with idiopathic DCM.

Besides stem cells and myocytes, another critical component of the heart milieu is the cardiac fibroblast, the predominant cell type in the heart. Fibroblasts activated by various autocrine and paracrine factors, such as angiotensin II, aldosterone, endothelins, cytokines, and growth factors likely play a key role in the formation and maintenance of fibrous tissue by the production of various extracellular-matrix (ECM) proteins, such as collagen, fibronectin and integrin proteins [42]. Cardiac fibrosis is characterized by excessive accumulation of fibrillar collagen in the extracellular space, in part arising as a loss of cardiomyocytes (replacement fibrosis) and as an interstitial response to various chronic cardiovascular diseases such as hypertension, myocarditis, and congestive HF (reactive fibrosis) and is generally considered to be elevated in the aging human heart [43, 44]. Evidence has documented an increase in collagen concentration (primarily collagen type 1) and the intermolecular cross-linking of collagen increase with age [45]. Nevertheless, several recent findings suggest that the fibroblast involvement in aging-associated myocardial fibrosis is more complex, and that the underlying mechanisms are undetermined. Surprisingly, both AngII stimulation of collagen synthesis and fibroblast proliferation are diminished in aging compared to young cardiac fibroblasts [46]. Moreover, enzymes involved in the degradation of ECM components including the matrix metalloproteinases (MMPS) such as MMP-3, MMP-8, MMP-9, MMP-12, and MMP-14 increased in concert with decreased insoluble collagen in aging mice, suggesting that the accumulated collagen and fibronectin are not attributable to aging-mediated decline in degradation [47, 48]. This suggests that the increased fibrosis and stiffness found in the aging heart must have another mechanism. Both age-mediated changes in glycation (as discussed extensively in Chapter 4) and integrin kinase signaling can contribute to accumulated collagen cross-interactions and fiber bundling, which can lead to fibrosis [49, 50].

Increased fibrosis with age leads to increased diastolic stiffness and contractile dysfunction in the heart and its larger vessels, and can also reduce electrical coupling between cardiac myocytes resulting in non-uniform depolarization, conduction delays and dysrhythmias. Excessive collagen deposition or pathological fibrosis is an important contributor to LV dysfunction and poor outcome in hypertension, myocardial infarction and HF.

Genomics

Cardiomyopathy, diseases of heart muscle can arise either as a primary myocardial disorder or secondary to a diverse array of factors including infection, inflammation, toxins and ischemic insult. Over the last decade, the importance of gene defects in the etiology of primary cardiomyopathies has been recognized. Numerous mutations identified as etiological factors have been identified in the more prevalent types of cardiomyopathy, i.e., hypertrophic cardiomyopathy (HCM) and dilated cardiomyopathy (DCM), and more recently in more uncommon phenotypes such as restrictive cardiomyopathy (RCM) and arrhythmogenic right ventricular dysplasia/cardiomyopathy (ARVD/ARVC). Moreover, genetic defects have been increasingly implicated in the pathogenesis of metabolic cardiomyopathies (often associated with extra-cardiac presentations) including the mitochondrial cardiomyopathies as well as the cardiomyopathy associated with diabetes.

HCM

Numerous chromosomal loci have been detected in association with clinical hypertrophic cardiomyopathy. A list of genes identified thus far and their respective chromosomal loci is presented in Table 7.5. Of the HCM-causing genes thus far identified, a significant proportion encode protein components of the cardiac sarcomere which were the first class of HCM genes to be identified and remain the most prevalent [51]. Mutations have been found in genes that encode components of the thick filament (i.e., β-MHC, essential MLC, regulatory MLC, and cMyBP-C), genes that encode thin filament proteins (i.e., cardiac actin, cardiac troponin T, cardiac troponin I, cardiac troponin C, and α-tropomyosin). HCM mutations have also been found in genes involved in the cytoskeleton including titin, telethonin, myozenin and cardiac muscle LIM protein. Mutations resulting in HCM have also been reported in genes encoding nonsarcomeric/non-cytoskeletal proteins including the γ2-regulatory subunit of an AMP-activated protein kinase (AMPK), LAMP-2, a lysosome-associated membrane glycoprotein, caveolin-3, a contributor to the caveolin micro-domains involved in cellular signaling [52, 53]. Another significant sub-group of mutant genes identified in patients with HCM are comprised of genes encoding proteins involved in mitochondrial bioenergetic metabolism. These include subunits of the mitochondrial respiratory chain (NDUFV2, NDUFS2), SCO2 encoding a copper metallochaperone, COX10 and COX15 involved in the assembly of the multi-subunit mitochondrial respiratory complex IV enzyme also known as cytochrome *c* oxidase; genes involved in fatty acid transport and oxidation (SLC22A4, ACADVL) and iron import (FRDA/frataxin); mutations in ANT encoding the adenine nucleotide translocator which also has been recently found to play a role in mtDNA maintenance. Moreover, numerous mutations in mtDNA have also been reported to be associated with the development of HCM often in conjunction with multisystemic disorders including a wide-spectrum of associated disorders, such as hypotonia, myopathies, muscle-weakness, lactic acidosis, deafness, ophthalmic disease and diabetes.

It is well-recognized that left ventricular remodeling and progressive increases in left ventricular wall thickness tend to increase with age [44]. Several of the HCM-associated alleles have been described primarily in the very young and show what is termed early-onset presentation; these often

Table 7.5 Genes implicated in clinical HCM

Gene	Protein	Function
TNNT2	Cardiac troponin T	Sarcomeric
TTN	Titin	Z disc
MYL3	Essential myosin light chain	Sarcomeric
TNNC1	Cardiac troponin C	Sarcomeric
MYBPC3	Cardiac myosin binding protein C	Sarcomeric
CSRP3	Cardiac muscle LIM protein	Cytoskeletal/Z disc
MYL2	Regulatory myosin light chain	Sarcomeric
MYH7	β-Myosin heavy chain	Sarcomeric
ACTC	Cardiac actin	Sarcomeric
TPM1	α -Tropomyosin	Sarcomeric
TNNI3	Cardiac troponin I	Sarcomeric
CAV3	Caveolin-3	Signaling
LAMP2	Lysosome associated membrane protein 2	Lysosome
TCAP	T-Cap (telethonin)	Cytoskeletal/Z disc
MYOZ2	Myozenin 2	Cytoskeletal/Z disc
PRKAG2	AMP-activated protein kinase (regulatory subunit)	Energy sensor
SCO2	COX assembly	Energy metabolism
NDUFV2	Respiratory complex I subunit	Energy metabolism
NDUFS2	Respiratory complex I subunit	Energy metabolism
ANT	Adenine nucleotide transporter/mtDNA maintenance	Energy metabolism
ACADVL	VLCAD activity (Fatty acid oxidation)	Energy metabolism
FRDA	Mitochondrial iron import	Energy metabolism
COX10	COX assembly	Energy metabolism
SLC22A4	Carnitine transporter (OCTN2)	Energy metabolism
COX15	COX assembly	Energy metabolism
GLA	Alpha galactosidase	Lysosomal storage

are associated with sudden cardiac death and are of great concern in neonates and young athletes (including specific mutations in β-MHC and cardiac troponin T). Several mutations in fatty acid metabolism (e.g., ACADVL, carnitine transport), and in bioenergetic metabolism (e.g., NDUFV2, COX 15) and a number of mtDNA mutations have also been primarily identified in neonates and children. Interestingly, while the relationship between genotype and phenotype with HCM mutations is often not clear-cut, the distribution of specific mutations in elderly-onset disease is often markedly different from specific mutations found in familial early onset HCM [54]. For instance, mutations in *MYBPC3* encoding cardiac myosin binding protein-C, show delayed onset of HCM and induce the disease predominantly in the fifth or sixth decade of life and along with specific troponin I, and α-myosin heavy chain alleles are more prevalent in elderly-onset HCM [55, 56]. Moreover, mutations which alter the charge of the encoded amino acid tend to affect patient survival more significantly than those that produce a conservative amino acid change [57]. The milder cardiac phenotype in many of the patients with elderly-onset HCM genes is also consistent with the observation that HCM is frequently well tolerated and compatible with normal life expectancy, and may remain clinically dormant for long periods of time with symptoms and initial diagnosis deferred until late in life [58].

Another genetic defect which shows a marked association with late-onset HCM is due to mutations in the X-linked defect GLA gene encoding the lysosomal enzyme α-galactosidase A causing α-galactosidase A deficiency leading to an inborn lysosomal storage disorder characterized by pathological intracellular glycosphingolipid deposition. Cardiac involvement, consisting of progressive left ventricular hypertrophy is very common and constitutes the most frequent cause of death. Mutations in this gene have been found in up to 6% of men with late-onset HCM, and in 12% of women with late-onset HCM [59, 60].

DCM and RCM

Although DCM was traditionally regarded as a sporadic nongenetic disorder, recent studies of large families with DCM have suggested that inherited gene defects comprise a significant subset of idiopathic DCM cases. Revised estimates gauged by careful screening of relatives of patients has documented a greater-than-expected prevalence of familial DCM, reflecting the contribution of inherited genes, ranging from 25 to 50% of the cases of idiopathic DCM [61]. It is also relevant to note that the incidence of idiopathic DCM has been reported to increase with age, males are afflicted at a higher rate than females and elderly patients tend to have a worse prognosis than their younger counterparts with this disease. Moreover, it is clear that age-related penetrance, i.e., absence of disease manifestations in genotype-positive individuals until after a particular age, and nonpenetrance, has contributed to the underestimation of the prevalence of familial disease [62, 63].

Mutations in a large assortment of genes with diverse functions can lead to DCM [51]. The identification of DCM-causing mutations (shown in Table 7.6) present at a wide variety of genetic loci has confirmed the assessment of DCM as highly heterogeneous genetically.

The first gene identified by candidate gene analysis in DCM was cardiac actin. Mutations in five other genes encoding sarcomere proteins have been implicated in DCM (all of which can also cause HCM) including β-MHC, cMyBP-C, cardiac troponin T, α-tropomyosin and titin. While a subset of HCM patients develop a dilated phenotype, DCM resulting from sarcomeric gene mutations often arises without previous HCM. Mutations were subsequently described in genes encoding cytoskeletal proteins including desmin, δ-sarcoglycan, muscle LIM protein, α-actinin-2, Cypher/Zasp, Tcap/telethonin and metavinculin which stabilize the myofibrillar apparatus and link the cytoskeleton to the contractile apparatus. Dystrophin is another critical gene involved in the

Table 7.6 Genes implicated in familial human dilated cardiomyopathy (DCM)

Gene	Protein	Function	Chromosomal locus	Inher.
ABCC9	SUR2A, regulatory subunit of cardiac K_{ATP} channel	Membrane channel	12p12.1	AD
ACTC	Cardiac α-actin	Sarcomeric	15q14	AD
ACTN2	α-actinin-2	Cytoskeletal	1q43	AD
DES	Desmin	Cytoskeletal	2q35	AD
DMD	Dystrophin	Cytoskeletal	Xp21	X-R
FOXD4	Forkhead Box D4	Transcription factor	9p11-q11	Nd
TAZ (G4.5)	Tafazzin	Metabolic	Xq28	X-R
LMNA	Lamins A and C	Nuclear membrane	1p1–q21	AD
CSRP3	muscle LIM protein	Cytoskeletal	11p15	AD
MYBPC3	Cardiac myosin binding protein C	Sarcomeric	11p11	AD
MYH6	α-Myosin heavy chain	Sarcomeric	14q12	AD
MYH7	β-Myosin heavy chain	Sarcomeric	14q12	AD
PLN	Phospholamban	Calcium cycling	6q22.1	AD
SCN5A	Cardiac sodium channel	Membrane channel	3p22–25	AD
SGCD	δ-sarcoglycan	Cytoskeletal	5q33	AD
STA	Emerin	Nuclear membrane	Xq28	X-R
TCAP	Tcap/telethonin	Cytoskeletal	17q12	AD
TNNC1	Cardiac troponin C	Sarcomeric	3p21.3–3p14.3	AD
TNNI3	Cardiac troponin I	Sarcomeric	19q13.4	AR
TNNT2	Cardiac troponin T	Sarcomeric	1q32	AD
TPM1	α-Tropomyosin	Sarcomeric	15q22	AD
TTN	Titin	Cytoskeletal	2q31	AD
VCL	Metavinculin	Cytoskeletal	10q22–q23	AD
ZASP	Cypher/Zasp	Cytoskeletal	10q22.3–q23.2	AD

AD: Autosomal dominant; AR: Autosomal recessive; X-R: X-linked recessive; Nd: Not determined intracellular cytoskeleton (linking it to the ECM and contributing to intracellular organization, force transduction, and membrane stability), whose mutation can lead to DCM either in association with Duchenne muscular dystrophy or result in an adult-onset X-linked DCM without skeletal myopathy. In addition, mutations in gene-products serving critical electrophysiological function in the heart have been associated with DCM in a limited number of cases including the ABCC9 gene encoding SUR2A, the regulatory subunit of the cardiac K_{ATP} channel and the SCN5A gene encoding the cardiac sodium channel involved in the generation of the action potential. Mutations in the phospholamban (PLN) gene encoding a transmembrane phosphoprotein that by inhibiting the cardiac sarcoplasmic reticular Ca^{2+} -adenosine triphosphatase (SERCA2a) pump is a critical regulator of calcium cycling have also been recently described in subjects with DCM [64–66]. A T116G point mutation, substituting a termination codon for Leu-39 (L39stop), and resulting in loss-of-function mutation (PLN null allele) was identified in two families with hereditary HF; subjects homozygous for L39stop developed DCM and HF, requiring cardiac transplantation [65].

DCM-causing mutations have also been found in proteins which appear to be involved in the maintenance of nuclear integrity as well as playing roles in other nuclear processes including gene transcription, cell cycle regulation and chromatin remodeling. For example, mutations in the LMNA gene encoding lamin A and the STA gene encoding emerin, both multifunctional nuclear membrane proteins, have been found to lead to DCM, the latter most commonly in association with Emery-Dreifuss muscular dystrophy. Recent studies have also identified a mutation disrupting an extremely highly conserved tryptophan residue in the forkhead domain of FOXD4, a nuclear transcription factor of the forkhead/winged helix box (FOX) gene family in a pedigree presenting with a complex phenotype including DCM [67].

Finally, mutations in proteins involved in energy metabolism can also lead to DCM. Mutations in the *TAZ/G4.5* gene encoding an acyltransferase involved in fatty acid metabolism have been associated with Barth's syndrome, an X-linked disorder characterized by infantile-onset DCM, skeletal myopathy, short stature, neutropenia, and abnormal mitochondria, as well as with isolated cases of X-linked DCM [51]. In addition to these defective nuclear loci, specific pathogenic mutations in mtDNA have been implicated in DCM (often in conjunction with multisystemic disorders) and these show maternal inheritance. Clearly, the wide spectrum of defective intracellular functions that can lead to DCM suggest that multiple pathophysiological mechanisms are likely involved in triggering this disorder, consistent with its frequently heterogeneous presentation.

A number of the forementoned genetic defects are associated with late-onset DCM and a higher incidence of presentation in the elderly. In a large-scale mutation analysis of European patients with DCM, carriers of mutations in the β-myosin heavy chain (MYH7) gene were significantly older (mean age at diagnosis was 48 years) compared to carriers of mutations in the cardiac T troponin (TNNT2) gene (mean age at diagnosis was 23 years) [68]. Moreover, several specific DCM-associated mutations are associated with a milder presentation and increased disease presentation with age. While mutations in the MyBP-C gene have been previously described in association with a favorable clinical course and with late onset HCM, late-onset DCM has been reported in association with an Arg820Gln mutation in the MyBP-C gene [69]. Similarly, carriers of the Arg71Thr mutation in the SGCD gene encoding the cytoskeletal δ-sarcoglycan protein had a relatively mild phenotype and a late onset of DCM [70].

Mutations in the DMD gene have been reported in both familial and sporadic cases of Duchenne (DMD) and Becker (BMD) muscular dystrophies [71, 72]. DMD usually presents in early childhood with progressive skeletal muscle weakness, mainly of the large proximal muscle groups, and loss of ambulation generally by early adolescence with DCM and conduction defects tend to present late in the disease with the majority of patients dying in their 20s, most commonly as a result of respiratory failure. Individuals with DMD usually have frameshift or nonsense DMD mutations that result in premature termination of translation, and a reduction or absence of dystrophin protein; typically, patients with DMD lack any detectable dystrophin expression in their skeletal muscles.

In contrast, BMD is a milder, allelic form of DMD with affected males presenting later in life, exhibiting a milder course and display a high incidence of cardiac involvement despite their milder skeletal muscle disease; the most common cause of death in BMD is HF. While clinical expression occurs primarily in the young adult, expression including severe DCM has also been reported in the older adult (>50 years old) [73, 74]. Subjects with BMD usually have DMD deletions that result in truncation or reduced levels of expression of dystrophin; skeletal muscle from patients with BMD contains dystrophin proteins of altered size and/or reduced abundance. Interestingly, female carriers of DMD and BMD experience a high incidence of cardiac involvement, that progresses with age and manifests primarily as cardiomyopathy.

A D626N mutation in the Cypher/ZASP encoding the Z-disc associated protein was found in all affected individuals in a family and was associated with late-onset DCM [75]. This mutation also proved interesting in that it alters the binding function of the Cypher/ZASP LIM domain and increased its interaction with protein kinase C (PKC), suggesting an association between DCM and an inherited abnormality involved in signal transduction.

Mutations in other signal transduction proteins appear to play a role in late-onset DCM. For instance, in one family with a deletion of arginine 14 in the PLN gene, individuals did not present with DCM until their seventh decade when they were only mildly symptomatic with congestive HF [64]. While this finding suggests that PLN mutations should be considered as a contributory factor in the development of late onset cardiomyopathy, the finding that other heterozygous individuals with the identical PLN Arg 14 mutation were reported to exhibit more severe disease at an earlier age (i.e., left ventricular dilation, contractile dysfunction, and episodic ventricular dysrhythmias, with overt HF by middle-age) suggests that other modulatory factors are likely involved in the expression of the DCM phenotype [76].

Another intriguing development in the connection between genes involved in DCM and aging phenotypes has emerged in the characterization of LMNA mutations affecting lamin A/C. In addition to a variety of laminopathies including DCM along with neuropathy, lipodystrophy, limb girdle muscular dystrophy (LGMD), and autosomal dominant Emery-Dreifuss muscular dystrophy (EDMD), mutations in LMNA can result in premature aging syndromes or progeria. LMNA mutations have been reported in segmental progerias: Hutchinson–Gilford Progeria Syndrome (HGPS) [77], and Atypical Werner Syndrome [78]. The age of onset is quite different in these aging diseases. In sharp contrast to Werner Syndrome, which becomes apparent at or shortly after puberty and early adulthood, HGPS manifests early in childhood. Growth retardation can be observed by three to 6 months of age, with degenerative changes in cutaneous, musculoskeletal and cardiovascular systems apparent shortly thereafter, baldness occurs by age 2 and median age of death is 13.5 years with mortality primarily attributable to myocardial infarction or congestive HF. While many of the diseases arising from LMNA mutations arise from dominant missense mutations (e.g., DCM type 1A, LGMD) some are autosomal recessive (e.g., Charcot-Marie-Tooth-disease) and others sporadic (e.g., HGPS, EDMD); it is clear (although largely unexplained) that different mutations in the same gene can lead to diverse dysfunctions with limited phenotypic overlap, with specific tissues targeted in each pathology [79]. An important unanswered question is why defects in nuclear envelope proteins that are found in most adult cell types should give rise to pathologies associated predominantly with skeletal and cardiac muscle and adipocytes.

Interestingly among three different LMNA-mediated myopathies (i.e., EDMD, DCM and LGMD), cardiomyopathy occurs with an underlying potential of sudden death due to cardiac dysrhythmia. Moreover, the cardiac disease of LMNA mutated patients is often defined by conduction system and rhythm disturbances occurring early in the course of the disease, followed by DCM and HF. One family comprised of members heterozygous for the same single nucleotide deletion in exon 6 of the LMNA gene, showed different presentations in affected individuals, one with LGMD, one with EDMD and another with DCM. The intrafamilial variability and mutational pleiotrophy observed in this (and other studies) suggests that other modifying factors (genetic, environmental or epigenetic) likely influence phenotypic expression [80].

While over 20 LMNA mutations (primarily missense defects localized in exons 1 and 3) have been reported to lead to autosomal dominant DCM (type 1A), evidence has been presented that different LMNA mutations can have substantially different age-expression. Molecular analysis of two 4-generation white families with autosomal dominant familial DCM and conduction system disease revealed novel mutations in the rod segment of LMNA [81]. A missense mutation (nucleotide G607A, amino acid E203K) was identified in 14 adult subjects of family A with cardiac disorder primarily manifested as progressive conduction disease occurring in the fourth and fifth decades with ensuing death by HF. In contrast, a nonsense mutation (nucleotide C673T, amino acid R225X) was identified in 10 adult subjects of family B with progressive conduction disease occurring with an earlier onset (third and fourth decades), accompanied by ventricular dysrhythmias, left ventricular enlargement, and systolic dysfunction and death caused by HF or sudden cardiac death.

Given the multiplicity of lamin A/C intracellular functions, a clear picture of the pathogenic mechanism by which LMNA mutations causes DCM (and conduction defects) is not yet evident [79–82]. One attractive hypothesis suggests that defective lamin A/C undermines the structural integrity of the nuclear envelope promoting a mechanical nuclear fragility and by its interactions with the cytoskeletal desmin, results in a whole cell-mechanical vulnerability particularly notable under conditions of constant mechanical stress typical of cardiac and skeletal muscle cells with resultant impairment of force transmission and contractile function. Other viable pathogenic mechanisms include loss or rearrangement of other LMNA-associated protein (e.g., emerin) and nuclear pore modification, changes in heterochromatin relative to the nuclear lamina, and altered gene expression due to disrupted interaction with RNA polymerases and transcription factors. We discuss these further in the section on animal models presented below.

Restrictive cardiomyopathy (RCM), the rarest form of cardiomyopathy, involves impaired ventricular filling and reduced diastolic volume in the presence of normal systolic function, and normal or near normal myocardial thickness. This condition is most frequently caused by pathological conditions that stiffen the myocardium by promoting infiltration or fibrosis, including endomyocardial disease, amyloidosis, sarcoidosis, scleroderma, storage diseases (e.g., hemochromatosis, Gaucher's disease, Fabry disease, glycogen storage disease), metastatic malignancy, anthracycline toxicity, or radiation damage. Several of the infiltrative diseases resulting in RCM can be inherited, including familial amyloidosis, hemochromatosis, Gaucher's disease, and glycogen storage disease. Most cases of congestive HF in the elderly are due to diastolic dysfunction with preserved systolic function suggesting that RCM is an important entity [83].

Amyloidosis is the most prevalent underlying cause of RCM [84]. RCM in cardiac amyloidosis results from replacement of normal myocardial contractile elements by infiltration and interstitial deposits of amyloid, leading to alterations in cellular metabolism, Ca^{2+} transport, receptor regulation, and cellular edema. Amyloid myocardium becomes firm, rubbery, and noncompliant, and can also involve the cardiac conduction system presenting with different types of conduction defects and dysrhythmias.

Familial amyloidosis, or hereditary amyloidosis, while overall less common than immunoglobin amyloidosis (AL), is more frequently associated with RCM, and is most often caused by an autosomal-dominant mutation in the serum protein transthyretin encoded by the TTR gene. This gene encodes a protein containing 127-amino acid residues of four identical, noncovalently linked subunits that dimerize in the plasma protein complex. Over 60 distinct amino acid substitutions distributed throughout the TTR sequence have been correlated with an increased amyloidogenicity of TTR [84]. The pattern of myocardial involvement varies according to the specific mutation and has distinct age-expression. A large number of these mutations have been associated with late-onset amyloid cardiomyopathy, as well as with polyneuropathy.

Patients with the Met 30 transthyretin variant, the most prevalent *TTR* mutation, primarily display conduction defects and often require pacemaker implantation [85]. In early-onset cases (i.e., patients younger than 50 years old), cardiac amyloid deposition was most prominent in the atrium and subendocardium but became evident throughout the myocardium in late-onset cases. The Tyr77 mutation, the second most prevalent TTR mutation was studied in a large family with 12 affected individuals over 4 generations; the clinical phenotype is characterized by an initial and sometimes prolonged carpal tunnel syndrome, beginning between the 6th and 7th decade, with subsequent RCM [86]. In addition, different ethnic groups have been shown to have varying degrees of susceptibility to cardiac amyloid deposition, while other groups do not have cardiac involvement. Substitution of isoleucine for valine at position 122 of the TTR gene has been reported to be more prevalent in African-Americans (estimated to be present in approximately 4% of the Black population) [87], and is also associated with the occurrence of late-onset RCM [88]. Molecular analysis has revealed that this isoleucine for valine substitution shifts the equilibrium toward monomer (indicating lower tetramer stability), and favors tetramer dissociation required for amyloid fibril formation resulting in accelerated amyloidosis [89].

RCM can also be associated with an iron-overload cardiomyopathy that manifests systolic or diastolic dysfunction primarily attributable to increased cardiac iron deposition, and occurs with common genetic disorders such as hemochromatosis [90]. While the precise mechanism of iron-induced HF has not yet been elucidated, the toxicity of iron in biological systems has largely been attributed to its ability to catalyze ROS generation. Hereditary hemochromatosis is a common autosomal recessive disorder among Caucasians with the genotype at risk accounting for 1:200–400 individuals of Northern European ancestry. Clinical complications appear late in life and often include cardiomyopathy (primarily but not necessarily restrictive) with development of subsequent congestive HF limited to homozygotes. As with many cardiomyopathies, phenotypic expression of the disease shows intrafamilial variabity, likely as a result of effects of modifier genes or environmental factors. Hereditary hemochromatosis has been linked to pathogenic mutations of the gene coding for HFE, an atypical HLA class I molecule on chromosome 6 (6p21.3), hemojuvelin (HJV or HFE2) on chromosome 1 (most often associated with the juvenile form of hemochromatosis) and more rarely, the gene coding for hepcidin (HAMP), on chromosome 19, and the gene encoding serum transferrin receptor 2 [90, 91, 92]. Two missense mutations in HFE have been found to be responsible for the majority of cases, C282Y and H63D; the C282Y mutation has a higher penetrance than the H63D mutation, and appears to result in a greater loss of HFE protein function [90]. Iron-overload in the heart resulting from HFE knockout in the mice can also lead to increased susceptibility to myocardial ischemia/reperfusion injury as indicated by increased postischemic ventricular dysfunction, increased myocardial infarct size and myocyte apoptosis with the degree of injury significantly elevated with high-iron diet [93].

Interestingly, while HFE mutations have also been reported to be involved in several age-related chronic diseases such as Alzheimer's disease and CAD, one study suggested that in some populations the same HFE mutations associated with CVDs paradoxically have also shown an increased prevalence (in the heterozygous state) in centenarians (primarily women) suggesting a beneficial role with respect to longevity [94]. This may be because individuals heterozygous for the C282Y mutation tend to have slightly but significantly higher values for serum iron and transferrin saturation and are therefore less likely to exhibit anemia because of iron deficiency. However, subsequent studies have failed to replicate this relationship in other populations [95, 96].

Animal Models of Cardiomyopathy and HF

A rather diverse assortment of animal models have been developed to study the pathophysiology of HF and cardiomyopathy as well as to test new therapeutic approaches to treat the complex syndrome of HF. Several of these models have also provided increased data about the genes involved in these diseases as well as providing significant information regarding their phenotypic expression in the elderly.

In particular, the effects of specific mutations on sarcomere and cytoskeletal structure and function, as well as on overall cardiac structure and function *in vivo* have been examined in genetically engineered mouse models. A large number of transgenic studies have provided a wealth of information including, the identification of new genetic targets, the confirmation of pathogenic mutations described in clinical studies, and in some cases elucidation of the role of these specific pathogenic mutations, and resultant proteins, in the progression of cardiac hypertrophy, fibrosis and onset of cardiomyopathy (either hypertrophic or dilated). Several specific alterations in genes involved in cytoskeletal and sarcomeric function, which generate cardiomyopathy (and often HF) in transgenic mice, are presented in Table 7.7.

The age-specific phenotypic expression of specific sarcomeric protein mutations was compared between heterozygous mice bearing a cardiac MHC missense mutation (α-MHC $^{403/+}$) and mice bearing a cardiac MyBP-C mutation (MyBP-C$^{t/+}$) [97]. While both mutant strains exhibited progressive LV hypertrophy, by 30 weeks of age α-MHC$^{403/+}$ mice showed considerably more LV hypertrophy than MyBP-C$^{t/+}$ mice. Moreover, there was increased expression of molecular markers of cardiac hypertrophy in hearts from 50 week-old α-MHC $^{403/+}$ mice while MyBP-C $^{t/+}$ mice did not demonstrate expression of these molecular cardiac markers until the mice were >125 weeks old. Electrophysiological assessment also indicated that MyBP-C $^{t/+}$ mice were not as likely to have inducible ventricular tachycardia as α-MHC $^{403/+}$ mice and significant cardiac dysfunction was noted in α-MHC $^{403/+}$ mice before the development of LV hypertrophy, whereas the cardiac function of MyBP-C$^{t/+}$ mice was not impaired even after the development of cardiac hypertrophy. Although

Table 7.7 Selected mouse models of cardiomyopathy and HF – sarcomeric and structural genes

Gene (protein)	Genetic Alteration	Function	Phenotype
α-MHC	S532P + F764L R403Q	Myosin heavy chain	DCM, HCM
cMyBP-C	Cardiac-specific KO; Truncated C-terminus	Cardiac myosin binding protein C	HCM
cTnT	R92Q, I79N	Cardiac troponin T	HCM
MLP	Null	Muscle LIM protein	DCM
SGCD	Null	δ-sarcoglycan	DCM, necrosis
Lamin A/C (LMNA)	Null; L85R + N195K	Nuclear membrane protein	DCM
TIMP-3	Null	Matrix metalloproteinases (MMP) inhibitor	DCM , hypertrophy
ABCA5	Null	Lysosomal ABC transporter	DCM
Desmin	Null	Cytoskeletal protein	DCM, fibrosis
Plakoglobin	Plakoglobin + /−	Desmosomal protein	ARVC
SERCA2a	Gene-replacement with SERCA2b (> Ca^{2+} affinity)	SR Ca^{2+} transport ATPase, calcium cycling	HCM
N-cadherin (Cdh2)	Cardiac-specific null or overexpression	Cell adhesion molecule in intercalated disc	DCM
Tmod	Cardiac-specific overexpression	Tropomodulin	DCM
Calsarcin	Null	Sarcomeric Z disc protein	Accelerated CM in response to pathological biomechanical stress
RLC	Cardiac-specific expression of E22K-RLC mutation	Myosin regulatory light-chain	Inter-ventricular septal hypertrophy and enlarged papillary muscles with no filament disarray

it is not yet clear as to the extent to which these murine models mimic their human counterparts of familial HCM, both the use of electrophysiological and cardiac function studies may enable more definitive risk stratification in older patients. Other studies with the R(403)Q mutation in cardiac α-MHC murine model of familial HCM showed gender-specific differences with age [98]. Cardiac hypertrophy was found to be significantly increased with age in female animals while male hearts exhibited severe dilation by 8 months of age, in the absence of increased mass.

In addition to mutations in the sarcomere and cytoskeleton which mediate cardiomyopathy, we have previously noted that mutations in the intermediate filament lamin proteins of the nuclear lamina (lamin A/C) underlying the inner nuclear membrane are associated with clinical DCM with conduction defects. A mouse line that might recapitulate this clinical phenotype was constructed using homologous recombination and expressed the LMNA -N195K lamin A variant analogous to the asparagine-to-lysine substitution at amino acid 195, which causes DCM in humans [99]. Several phenotypes observed in the $Lmna^{N195K/N195K}$ mice were consistent with DCM including heart chamber dilation, increased heart weight and interstitial fibrosis, upregulation of a fetal gene expression profile and progressive conduction defects albeit neither apoptosis in the ventricles nor ventricular myocyte hypertrophy were detected. Also, similarly to the human disorder, an age-dependent phenotypic progression was observed in the transgenic mouse. Despite a minor growth defect, $Lmna^{N195K/N195K}$ mice initially appeared healthy, with no diminished activity levels or behavioral defects, and were difficult to distinguish from littermates until just before their demise, which generally followed an acute period of deterioration. This tended to occur between 11 and 14 weeks of age, with most mutant homozygous animals dying in that period (average, 12 week), none surviving past 16 week. Similarly, although impulse propagation initially appeared normal, the conduction system showed a deficit with increasing age. Interestingly, the $Lmna^{N195K/N195K}$ mice live twice as long as Lmna null mice and show earlier mortality (3 months) compared to another Lmna mutant model (H222P) (4–9 months) despite the fact that all three Lmna-deficient murine strains have similar cardiovascular phenotypes (i.e., conduction defects, lack of hypertrophy, dilation of heart chambers and nuclear shape defects). The $Lmna^{N195K/N195K}$ strain does not exhibit the multiple tissue pathologies of the Lmna null mice nor the muscular dystrophy seen with the Lmna mutant model (H222P) [100, 101].

It is well-known that diverse neurohormonal stimuli acting through a series of interwoven signal transduction pathways contribute to pathological cardiac hypertrophy and HF. Many such agonists act on the myocardium through cell surface receptors coupled with G-proteins to mobilize intracellular Ca^{2+} with consequent activation of downstream kinases and the Ca^{2+} - and calmodulin-dependent phosphatase calcineurin. In addition, MAPK signaling pathways are interconnected at multiple levels with intracellular Ca^{2+} [102]. β-adrenergic agonists also influence cardiac growth and function through the generation of cAMP, which activates protein kinase A (PKA) and other downstream effectors [103]. These signaling pathways target a variety of substrates in the cardiomyocyte, including components of the contractile apparatus, intracellular Ca^{2+}, with consequent activation of downstream kinases, the Ca^{2+} channels and their regulatory proteins.

Mutations in proteins involved in a number of signal transduction pathways in the heart have also been found to lead to cardiomyopathy and HF in transgenic mice. A list of several identified gene mutations in cardiac signaling proteins, which can lead to cardiomyopathy and their phenotypic effects, is presented in Table 7.8. The functions of genes involved cover an extremely wide spectrum ranging from kinases (e.g., p38 MAPK, DMPK, PKA, the receptor tyrosine kinase ErbB2, integrin-linked kinase, ILK): growth factors (e.g., FGF-2), receptors [e.g., Angiotensin II type 2 receptor (AT2R), Bradykinin B2 receptor, α-adrenergic receptor 1B (α-AR 1B), β1-adrenergic receptors (e.g., β 2-AR, β 1-AR); transcription factors (e.g., CREB, CHF1/HEY2), G-proteins ($G_s\alpha$), caveolins (e.g., CAV1, CAV3), calcium regulatory factors (e.g., calcineurin) and splicing factors (e.g., CELF, SC35).

Table 7.8 Selected mouse models of cardiomyopathy and HF – signaling genes

Gene (protein)	Genetic Alteration	Function	Phenotype
CAV-1	Homozygous null	Caveolin signaling proteins	HCM, DCM
CAV-3	Null, P 104 L	Caveolin signaling proteins	HCM
DMPK	Overexpression	Protein kinase	HCM, fibrosis
p38 MAPK	Cardiac-specific dominant-negative	Mitogen-activated protein kinase	HCM
AGT	Null	Angiotensinogen	DCM
FGF-2	Null	Fibroblast growth factor	DCM
BK B2 receptor	Null	Bradykinin B2 signaling	DCM
AT2R	Cardiac-targeted overexpression	Angiotensin II type 2 receptor	DCM
CHF1 (Hey2)	Null	HLH transcription factor	DCM
Ena-VASP	Cardiac-specific dominant-negative	Vasodilator-stimulated phosphoprotein	DCM, hypertrophy
CELF	Cardiac-specific dominant-negative	RNA binding proteins involved in alternative splicing	DCM, hypertrophy
ABCA5	Null	Lysosomal ABC transporter	DCM
α-AR 1B	Cardiac-specific overexpressiom	Alpha-adrenergic receptor 1B	DCM
β2-AR	Overexpression	Beta2-adrenergic receptor	DCM. HF
β1-AR	Overexpression	Beta1-adrenergic receptor	DCM. HF
PKA	Cardiac-specific constitutive expression-catalytic subunit	Protein kinase A	DCM
SC35	Cardiac-specific null	Trans-acting splicing factor	DCM
ErbB2 (Her2)	Cardiac-specific conditional mutant allele	Receptor tyrosine kinase	DCM
Calcineurin	Cardiac-specific expression of constitutively active gene	Calcium signaling regulator	HCM/HF
CREB	Cardiac-specific dominant negative	Transcription factor	DCM
ILK	Cardiac-specific KO	Integrin-linked kinase	DCM, HF
iNOS	Cardiac-specific overexpression	Inducible nitric oxide synthase	Cardiac fibrosis, hypertrophy, and dilatation and sudden death
$G_s\alpha$	Cardiac-specific overexpression	Stimulatory G-protein	Hypertrophy, Fibrosis; DCM in older mice

Interestingly, transgenic mice with cardiac-specific overexpression of the stimulatory GTP-binding protein $G_s\alpha$ subunit exhibit increased cardiac contractility in response to β-adrenergic receptor stimulation. However, with aging, these mice develop a cardiomyopathy which involves induction of apoptosis of cardiac myocytes [104].

Overexpression of the G-protein Gαq or constitutively active components of its signaling pathway have been shown in transgenic studies to lead to increased cardiac mass, cardiomyocyte hypertrophy, contractile dysfunction and ventricular remodeling. These studies also demonstrated that massive cardiomegaly and extensive ventricular dilation were limited to animals with much elevated levels of Gαq and that a relatively modest overexpression of Gαq produced features of compensated LV hypertrophy with more extensive LV dilation and HF only arising as a consequence of hemodynamic overload or neurohormonal stress (e.g., occurs with pregnancy) [105]. Mende et al. in studying a transgenic mouse line containing a constitutively active Gαq allele (Gαq52) found that a cardiomyopathic phenotype including increased ventricular mass and dilation was present by 10 weeks of age [106]. Moreover, undetectable levels of the constitutively activated transgene product were found at 10 weeks suggesting that persistent expression of the transgene was not required for the progression of the cardiomyopathic phenotype. Another transgenic mouse line containing an epitope-tagged Gαq 44 allele expressed a lower level of transgene product, and ultimately displayed the same DCM phenotype with severely impaired left ventricular systolic function (assessed by M-mode and 2D echocardiography), but with a much delayed disease onset [107]. At 12–14 months, over 60% of mice with Gαq 44 still had normal cardiac function and ventricular weight/body weight ratio but manifested increased phospholipase C (PLC) levels compared to either wild-type mice or mice with the Gαq52 allele. This suggests that different Gαq alleles (in the same genetic background) can exert markedly different age-dependent phenotypes including disease onset, that PLC activation is not correlated with Gαq-determined phenotype and that environmental modifiers may be involved in the age-dependent phenotypic expression.

Cytokine signaling and inflammation are well-recognized for their involvement in HF pathogenesis. Several important components of these signaling pathways are the IL-6 family of cytokines, the extracellular gp130 receptor and the signal transducer and activator of transcription 3 (STAT3) activated through gp130 – all of which have integral roles in cardiac myocyte survival and hypertrophy. Mice containing a cardiomyocyte-restricted deletion of STAT3 are significantly more susceptible to cardiac injury after doxorubicin treatment than age-matched controls [108]. Moreover, suggestive of a potential role of STAT3 in protecting against inflammation-induced heart damage, STAT3-deficient mice treated with lipopolysaccharide (LPS) displayed significantly more apoptosis than their wild-type counterparts; cardiomyocytes with STAT3 deleted, secreted significantly more tumor necrosis factor (TNF) in response to LPS and cardiomyocyte-restricted STAT3-deficient mice exhibited a dramatic increase in cardiac fibrosis in aged mice. While no overt signs of HF were present in young STAT3-deficient mice, heart dysfunction develops with advancing age. Therefore, these studies reveal a crucial role for STAT3 in mediating cardiomyocyte resistance to inflammation and other acute injury and in the pathogenesis of age-related HF.

It is well-recognized that the adult heart is strongly reliant on fatty acids as its key fuel supply and a number of studies have shown that a variety of pathological conditions (e.g., cardiac hypertrophy) can shift the utilization of metabolic substrates [109, 110]. It has been proposed that initially this switch in metabolic substrate provides adequate energy to maintain normal cardiac function, however over time diastolic dysfunction and HF may arise associated with a depletion in high-energy phosphates. Moreover, the functioning of mitochondrial bioenergetic pathways (e.g., TCA cycle, FAO pathway and the ETC/OXPHOS) provides most of the cellular ATP necessary for contractile and electrophysiological function. Results from both animal and human studies have confirmed that a variety of cardiomyopathic disorders and HF can be an important consequence of compromised mitochondrial bioenergetic function [109–114].

The creation of transgenic mice with altered expression of genes involved in carbohydrate, lipid and mitochondrial metabolism has provided unique insights into the fine balance within the mouse heart to maintain energy status and cardiac function, as well as to explore the cause–effect relationships between mitochondrial function and myocardial disease. A list of transgenic models of metabolic modification in the heart that are associated with cardiac dysfunction and/or HF phenotype is shown in Table 7.9.

Loss-of-function model studies, which disrupt mitochondrial metabolism, can exhibit specific cardiac phenotypes. Mouse models demonstrating a causal relationship between a mitochondrial energetic defect and cardiomyopathy include the *Ant1* null and the TFAM null mice [115, 116].

Table 7.9 Selected mouse models of metabolic genes involved in CM and HF

Gene (protein)	Genetic Alteration	Function	Phenotype	Refs
MTPα	Null	FAO; Mitochondrial trifunctional protein	CM; sudden death	121
LCAD	Global ablation	FAO; long chain acyl-CoA dehydrogenase	CM, ↑ myocardial lipid + fibrosis	118
Frataxin	Cardiac-specific KO	Iron metabolism; FRDA	CM, hypertrophy	122
TFAM/mtTFA	Cardiac-specific KO	Mitochondrial transcription factor A	DCM, AV heart conduction block	116
LpL	Cardiac-specific LPL with a GPI anchor	Lipoprotein lipase	DCM; ↓ FAO;	123
PRKAG2	Cardiac-specific overexpression of N488I mutation	AMP kinase regulatory subunit	LV hypertrophy, ventricular preexcitation and sinus node dysfunction.	124
Polymerase γ	Cardiac-specific knock-in mutation	Mitochondrial DNA polymerase	DCM	125
Mito-CK	Null	Mitochondrial creatine kinase	Increased LV dilation and hypertrophy	117
AIF	Cardiac-specific null	Apoptosis inducing factor	DCM	126
TrxR2	Cardiac-specific null	Mitochondrial thioredoxin reductase	Fatal DCM	127
MnSOD/SOD2	Null	Mn superoxide dismutase	DCM	128
PGC-1α	Cardiac-specific inducible overexpression	Peroxisome proliferator-activated receptor gamma coactivator-1α	Cardiomyopathy and mitochondrial defects only in adult not neonate	129
5-HT2B receptor	Cardiac-specific overexpression	Serotonin receptor	HCM with mitochondrial proliferation	130
OCTN2	Heterozygous carriers of mutation	Carnitine transporter	Age-associated CM with lipid deposition, hypertrophy	131
ANT1	Null	Adenine nucleotide translocator	CM, cardiac hypertrophy with ↑ mitochondria	115
FATP1	Cardiac-specific overexpression	Fatty acid transport protein 1	Lipotoxic cardiomyopathy	132
PPAR-α	Cardiac-specific overexpression	Peroxisome proliferator-activated receptor-α	Diabetic CM with ↑ FAO, ↓ glucose uptake + use, cardiac hypertrophy	133
PPAR-δ	Cardiac-specific null	Peroxisome proliferator-activated receptor-δ	Lipotoxic CM with ↑ myocardial lipid, dysfunction, hypertrophy, HF	120
ACS	Cardiac-specific overexpression	Long chain acyl-CoA synthetase	Cardiac lipid accumulation + hypertrophy, LV dysfunction and HF	134

The affected proteins are critically involved in mitochondrial bioenergetics; the adenine-nucleotide-translocator (ANT) protein involved in mitochondrial nucleotide transport and the mitochondrial transcription factor (TFAM/mtTFA) which plays a variety of roles in mtDNA function (e.g., gene transcription, mtDNA replication and maintenance) and in mitochondrial biogenesis. In addition, null mutation of mitochondrial creatine kinase can lead to LV dilation and hypertrophy [11].

Transgenic models of specific defects in the mitochondrial fatty acid oxidation (FAO) pathways have also been established (also enumerated in Table 7.8). Two distinct mouse models with genetic deletion of the second step in the mitochondrial FAO pathway, a fatty acid chain-length-specific dehydrogenase enzyme (VLCAD and LCAD), display a cardiomyopathic phenotype [118, 119]. Furthermore, mice null for the PPAR-δ gene also exhibit diminished myocardial fat catabolic capacity and mild cardiomyopathic phenotype that accompanies aging [120]. A null mutation in the mitochondrial trifunctional protein (MTPα) encoding a multifunctional enzyme in the β oxidation of fatty acids also results in cardiomyopathy and can lead to increased incidence of sudden death [121].

Several studies have shown that loss-of-function of critical mitochondrial antioxidant proteins can lead to cardiac dysfunction and cardiomyopathy. Strains harboring null mutations in either the Mn superoxide dismutase (MnSOD) or in TrxR2 encoding the mitochondrial thioredoxin reductase exhibit DCM [127, 128]. Mouse strains with a null mutation in frataxin (FRDA), a mitochondrial protein thought to be involved in regulating iron accumulation and flux and a regulator of oxidative stress (OS), also develop cardiac hypertrophy and cardiomyopathy [122]. These strains appear to reliably recapitulate Friedreich ataxia, a human disorder with both neuropathic (e.g., ataxia) and cardiac involvement (e.g., HCM) caused by alterations in the gene for frataxin (most often trinucleotide repeats).

In addition to transgenic models with loss-of-function, studies utilizing "gain of function"/overexpression of a transgene have provided insights into the relation between mitochondrial dysfunction and cardiac dysfunction, particularly in cardiomyopathy associated with diabetes. Transgenic mice with cardiac-restricted overexpression of PPAR-α (the MHC-PPAR-α mice) exhibit increased expression of genes encoding enzymes involved in multiple steps of mitochondrial FAO with strong reciprocal downregulation of glucose transporter (GLUT4) and glycolytic enzyme gene expression [133]. This activation of FAO via the elevation of the cardiac PPAR-α/PGC-1α mimics events occurring in the diabetic heart in which this metabolic shift is associated with high levels of fatty acid import and oxidation and can eventually lead to pathological mitochondrial and cardiac remodeling typical of diabetic cardiomyopathy. Echocardiographic assessment identified LV hypertrophy and dysfunction in the MHC-PPAR-α mice in a transgene expression-dependent manner. Sequential studies showed that both HF diet and insulinopenia induced further remodeling accompanied by signs of HF.

Overexpression of several genes with roles in metabolic regulation also can lead to cardiomyopathy, HF and hypertrophy in these mouse models. These include overexpression of genes involved in fatty acid transport and utilization (e.g. ACS, FATP1) [133, 134], and of genes acting as global transcription regulators of metabolic regulation (PGC-1) [129]. The latter gene is of particular relevance with respect to aging since it appears to show little overall affect on the heart when overexpressed in neonates, while overexpression in adult mice leads to extensive mitochondrial defects and cardiomyopathy.

As we have repeatedly noted throughout this book, the age-mediated accumulation of ROS and their potent damaging effects on cellular macromolecules (particularly mitochondrial) and their function is particularly evident in aging cardiomyocytes, in the heart and appear also to be involved in aging of the vasculature. Accumulating data have shown that mitochondrial defects resulting in the accumulation of OS can lead to cardiomyopathy and HF [135]. Associated with the cardiomyopathy resulting from murine knock-out of MnSOD, thioredoxin and TFAM genes are increased levels of mtDNA damage and OS. While in some cases global overexpression of antioxidants have not proven able to reverse the OS and aging-mediated dysfunction in the heart, recent studies have demonstrated that cardiac targeted-overexpression of the antioxidant catalase can successfully interfere with aging-mediated cardiac dysfunction. The previously discussed findings of Schriner demonstrated that overexpression of catalase targeted to the mitochondria increased overall mouse longevity, diminished OS and mitochondrial protein and mtDNA damage, and delayed the onset of aging-mediated cardiac pathology [136]. Similar findings including significantly diminished levels of protein carbonyls, advanced glycation end-products (AGE) and of age-induced mechanical defects in myocyte contractility and increased life span have been demonstrated by Ren et al. in mice with cardiac-specific catalase overexpression [137]. Recent evidence from this group suggests that catalase overexpression exerts its attenuation of aging-induced contractile defect and cardiomyocyte relaxation dysfunction in part by improving intracellular Ca^{2+} cycling in particular restoring expression levels of the Na^{+}/Ca^{2+} exchanger (NCX) and the Kv1.2 K^{+} channel [138].

In addition to the wealth of molecular information concerning age-mediated cardiomyopathy and HF which has emerged from mouse transgenic models, studies with genetic models highlighting the involvement of specific genes in cardiomyopathic and HF pathways have also been provided by other species including rat, rabbit, hamster and even the fly *Drosophila* [139]. Studies with aging spontaneously hypersensitive (SHR) strains and with a rat strain prone to HF (SHHF) rats have contributed greatly to the understanding of signaling pathways involved in HF including generalized activation of the renin-angiotensin-aldosterone, endothelin, and ANP systems [140, 141]. For instance, left ventricular homogenates from SHHF rats, exhibited marked increases in Ca^{2+}-dependent NOS activity with age accompanied by enhanced expression of endothelial NOS (eNOS), a change not seen in SHR or wildtype rats [142]. In addition, the SHR strains have provided a useful model of the transition from stable compensated hypertrophy to decompensated HF in the context of aging and have allowed the identification of programmatic changes in myocardial gene expression including increased expression of genes encoding elements of the ECM associated with this transition [143]. Moreover, pharmacological treatments that prevent matrix gene expression in the SHR heart have been shown to improve myocardial function and survival, albeit with limited success in reversing myocardial tissue dysfunction [140].

Similarly, studies in cardiomyopathic-prone strains of hamsters have been shown to mimic many of the modifications occurring in otherwise healthy aged mammalian hearts [144]. These strains also exhibit age-associated changes in the ECM. Several hamster strains including CHF147 present progressive DCM due to a large deletion of the δ-sarcoglycan (δ-SG) gene that leads to HF [145, 146]. These strains have been useful in both elucidating the changes leading to cardiomyopathy and HF and in testing strategies for reversing this cardiac dysfunction. In addition to its hereditary origin in these strains, HF can be aggravated by treatment with catecholamines and ameliorated by the administration of some kinds of β-antagonist both in genetic cardiomyopathic hamsters and in humans. Moreover, short-term treatment with recombinant human IGF-1 slows down the evolution of the DCM in the CHF147 hamster while not significantly increasing IGF-1 serum levels and significantly increased overall CHF147 survival [147]. In addition, δ-SG null cardiomyopathic hamsters fed from weaning to death with an alpha-lipoic acid (ALA)-enriched diet had significantly increased viability with marked preservation of myocardium structure and function and attenuation of myocardial fibrosis. At the cellular level, ALA treatment resulted in an increased eicosapentaenoic/arachidonic acid ratio with preserved plasmalemma and mitochondrial membrane integrity, maintenance of proper cell/extracellular matrix contacts and signaling, as well as a normal gene expression profile (in terms of myosin heavy chain isoforms, ANP TGF-β1) and limited development of fibrotic areas within ALA-fed cardiomyopathic hearts [148]. In the TO-2 strain of hamsters with DCM, gene therapy for DCM was successfully achieved by intramural delivery of a δ-SG gene in a recombinant AAV vector into the cardiac apex and left ventricle and significantly improved the morphological and physiological deterioration of the heart [149].

4. O'Connell JB. The economic burden of heart failure. Clin Cardiol 2000;23:III6–III10
5. Kannel WB, Belanger AJ. Epidemiology of heart failure. Am Heart J 1991;121:951–957
6. Rich MW. Heart failure in the 21st century: a cardiogeriatric syndrome. J Gerontol A Biol Sci Med Sci 2001;56:M88–M96
7. Anversa P, Rota M, Urbanek K, Hosoda T, Sonnenblick EH, Leri A, Kajstura J, Bolli R. Myocardial aging—a stem cell problem. Basic Res Cardiol 2005;100:482–493
8. Gottdiener JS, Arnold AM, Aurigemma GP, Polak JF, Tracy RP, Kitzman DW, Gardin JM, Rutledge JE, Boineau RC. Predictors of congestive heart failure in the elderly: the cardiovascular health study. J Am Coll Cardiol 2000;35:1628–1637
9. Ghali JK, Kadakia S, Cooper R, Ferlinz J. Precipitating factors leading to decompensation of heart failure. Traits among urban blacks. Arch Intern Med 1988;148:2013–2016
10. Tresch DD. Clinical manifestations, diagnostic assessment, and etiology of heart failure in elderly patients. Clin Geriatr Med 2000;16:445–456
11. Heiat A, Gross CP, Krumholz HM. Representation of the elderly, women, and minorities in heart failure clinical trials. Arch Intern Med 2002;162:1682–1688
12. Incalzi AR, Capparella O, Gemma A, Porcedda P, Raccis G, Sommella L, Carbonin PU. A simple method of recognizing geriatric patients at risk for death and disability. J Am Geriatr Soc 1992;40:34–38
13. Arnold JM, Liu P, Demers C, Dorian P, Giannetti N, Haddad H, Heckman GA, Howlett JG, Ignaszewski A, Johnstone DE, Jong P, McKelvie RS, Moe GW, Parker JD, Rao V, Ross HJ, Sequeira EJ, Svendsen AM, Teo K, Tsuyuki RT, White M. Canadian Cardiovascular Society consensus conference recommendations on heart failure 2006: diagnosis and management. Can J Cardiol 2006;22:23–45
14. Vasan RS, Larson MG, Benjamin EJ, Evans JC, Reiss CK, Levy D. Congestive heart failure in subjects with normal versus reduced left ventricular ejection fraction: prevalence and mortality in a population-based cohort. J Am Coll Cardiol 1999;33:1948–1955
15. Kitzman DW. Heart failure with normal systolic function. Clin Geriatr Med 2000;16:489–512
16. Zuccala G, Pedone C, Cesari M, Onder G, Pahor M, Marzetti E, Lo Monaco MR, Cocchi A, Carbonin P, Bernabei R. The effects of cognitive impairment on mortality among hospitalized patients with heart failure. Am J Med 2003;115:97–103
17. Kelly KG, Zisselman M, Cutillo-Schmitter T, Reichard R, Payne D, Denman SJ. Severity and course of delirium in medically hospitalized nursing facility residents. Am J Geriatr Psychiatry 2001;9:72–77
18. Gottlieb SS, Khatta M, Friedmann E, Einbinder L, Katzen S, Baker B, Marshall J, Minshall S, Robinson S, Fisher ML, Potenza M, Sigler B, Baldwin C, Thomas SA. The influence of age, gender, and race on the prevalence of depression in heart failure patients. J Am Coll Cardiol 2004;43:1542–1549
19. Joynt KE, Whellan DJ, O'Connor CM. Why is depression bad for the failing heart? A review of the mechanistic relationship between depression and heart failure. J Card Fail 2004;10:258–271
20. Cournot M, Leprince P, Destrac S, Ferrieres J. Usefulness of in-hospital change in B-type natriuretic peptide levels in predicting long-term outcome in elderly patients admitted for decompensated heart failure. Am J Geriatr Cardiol 2007;16:8–14
21. Ahmed A, Kiefe CI, Allman RM, Sims RV, DeLong JF. Survival benefits of angiotensin-converting enzyme inhibitors in older heart failure patients with perceived contraindications. J Am Geriatr Soc 2002;50: 1659–1666
22. Flather MD, Shibata MC, Coats AJ, Van Veldhuisen DJ, Parkhomenko A, Borbola J, Cohen-Solal A, Dumitrascu D, Ferrari R, Lechat P, Soler-Soler J, Tavazzi L, Spinarova L, Toman J, Bohm M, Anker SD, Thompson SG, Poole-Wilson PA. Randomized trial to determine the effect of nebivolol on mortality and cardiovascular hospital admission in elderly patients with heart failure (SENIORS). Eur Heart J 2005;26:215–225
23. Hori M, Kitabatake A, Tsutsui H, Okamoto H, Shirato K, Nagai R, Izumi T, Yokoyama H, Yasumura Y, Ishida Y, Matsuzaki M, Oki T, Sekiya M. Rationale and design of a randomized trial to assess the effects of beta-blocker in diastolic heart failure; Japanese Diastolic Heart Failure Study (J-DHF). J Card Fail 2005;11:542–547
24. Gurwitz JH, Field TS, Harrold LR, Rothschild J, Debellis K, Seger AC, Cadoret C, Fish LS, Garber L, Kelleher M, Bates DW. Incidence and preventability of adverse drug events among older persons in the ambulatory setting. JAMA 2003;289:1107–1116
25. Miura T, Kojima R, Sugiura Y, Mizutani M, Takatsu F, Suzuki Y. Effect of aging on the incidence of digoxin toxicity. Ann Pharmacother 2000;34:427–432
26. Cleland JG, Cohen-Solal A, Aguilar JC, Dietz R, Eastaugh J, Follath F, Freemantle N, Gavazzi A, van Gilst WH, Hobbs FD, Korewicki J, Madeira HC, Preda I, Swedberg K, Widimsky J. Management of heart failure in primary care (the IMPROVEMENT of Heart Failure Programme): an international survey. Lancet 2002;360:1631–1639
27. Gonseth J, Guallar-Castillon P, Banegas JR, Rodriguez-Artalejo F. The effectiveness of disease management programmes in reducing hospital re-admission in older patients with heart failure: a systematic review and meta-analysis of published reports. Eur Heart J 2004;25:1570–1595

28. Bleeker GB, Schalij MJ, Molhoek SG, Boersma E, Steendijk P, van der Wall EE, Bax JJ. Comparison of effectiveness of cardiac resynchronization therapy in patients <70 versus > or = 70 years of age. Am J Cardiol 2005;96:420–422
29. Morgan JA, John R, Weinberg AD, Remoli R, Kherani AR, Vigilance DW, Schanzer BM, Bisleri G, Mancini DM, Oz MC, Edwards NM. Long-term results of cardiac transplantation in patients 65 years of age and older: a comparative analysis. Ann Thorac Surg 2003;76:1982–1987
30. Zuckermann A, Dunkler D, Deviatko E, Bodhjalian A, Czerny M, Ankersmit J, Wolner E, Grimm M. Long-term survival (>10 years) of patients > 60 years with induction therapy after cardiac transplantation. Eur J Cardiothorac Surg 2003;24:283–291
31. Potapov EV, Loebe M, Hubler M, Musci M, Hummel M, Weng Y, Hetzer R. Medium-term results of heart transplantation using donors over 63 years of age. Transplantation 1999;68:1834–1838
32. Blanche C, Kamlot A, Blanche DA, Kearney B, Magliato KE, Czer LS, Trento A. Heart transplantation with donors fifty years of age and older. J Thorac Cardiovasc Surg 2002;123:810–815
33. Wei JY. Age and the cardiovascular system. N Engl J Med 1992;327:1735–1739
34. Olivetti G, Melissari M, Capasso JM, Anversa P. Cardiomyopathy of the aging human heart. Myocyte loss and reactive cellular hypertrophy. Circ Res 1991;68:1560–1568
35. Lakatta EG. Cardiovascular aging in health. Clin Geriatr Med 2000;16:419–444
36. Kass DA, Shapiro EP, Kawaguchi M, Capriotti AR, Scuteri A, deGroof RC, Lakatta EG. Improved arterial compliance by a novel advanced glycation end-product crosslink breaker. Circulation 2001;104:1464–1470
37. Nadal-Ginard B, Kajstura J, Leri A, Anversa P. Myocyte death, growth, and regeneration in cardiac hypertrophy and failure. Circ Res 2003;92:139–150
38. Ellison GM, Torella D, Karakikes I, Nadal-Ginard B. Myocyte death and renewal: modern concepts of cardiac cellular homeostasis. Nat Clin Pract Cardiovasc Med 2007;4:S52–S59
39. Kajstura J, Pertoldi B, Leri A, Beltrami CA, Deptala A, Darzynkiewicz Z, Anversa P. Telomere shortening is an in vivo marker of myocyte replication and aging. Am J Pathol 2000;156:813–819
40. Chimenti C, Kajstura J, Torella D, Urbanek K, Heleniak H, Colussi C, Di Meglio F, Nadal-Ginard B, Frustaci A, Leri A, Maseri A, Anversa P. Senescence and death of primitive cells and myocytes lead to premature cardiac aging and heart failure. Circ Res 2003;93:604–613
41. Torella D, Rota M, Nurzynska D, Musso E, Monsen A, Shiraishi I, Zias E, Walsh K, Rosenzweig A, Sussman MA, Urbanek K, Nadal-Ginard B, Kajstura J, Anversa P, Leri A. Cardiac stem cell and myocyte aging, heart failure, and insulin-like growth factor-1 overexpression. Circ Res 2004;94:514–524
42. Jugdutt BI. Remodeling of the myocardium and potential targets in the collagen degradation and synthesis pathways. Curr Drug Targets Cardiovasc Haematol Disord 2003;3:1–30
43. Allessie M, Schotten U, Verheule S, Harks E. Gene therapy for repair of cardiac fibrosis: a long way to Tipperary. Circulation 2005;111:391–393
44. Lakatta EG. Cardiovascular regulatory mechanisms in advanced age. Physiol Rev 1993;73:413–467
45. de Souza RR. Aging of myocardial collagen. Biogerontology 2002;3:325–335
46. Shivakumar K, Dostal DE, Boheler K, Baker KM, Lakatta EG. Differential response of cardiac fibroblasts from young adult and senescent rats to ANG II. Am J Physiol Heart Circ Physiol 2003;284:H1454–R1459
47. Lindsey ML, Goshorn DK, Squires CE, Escobar GP, Hendrick JW, Mingoia JT, Sweterlitsch SE, Spinale FG. Age-dependent changes in myocardial matrix metalloproteinase/tissue inhibitor of metalloproteinase profiles and fibroblast function. Cardiovasc Res 2005;66:410–419
48. Li YY, McTiernan CF, Feldman AM. Interplay of matrix metalloproteinases, tissue inhibitors of metalloproteinases and their regulators in cardiac matrix remodeling. Cardiovasc Res 2000;46:214–224
49. Chen X, Li Z, Feng Z, Wang J, Ouyang C, Liu W, Fu B, Cai G, Wu C, Wei R, Wu D, Hong Q. Integrin-linked kinase induces both senescence-associated alterations and extracellular fibronectin assembly in aging cardiac fibroblasts. J Gerontol A Biol Sci Med Sci 2006;61:1232–1245
50. Brown RD, Ambler SK, Mitchell MD, Long CS. The cardiac fibroblast: therapeutic target in myocardial remodeling and failure. Annu Rev Pharmacol Toxicol 2005;45:657–687
51. Fatkin D, Graham RM. Molecular mechanisms of inherited cardiomyopathies. Physiol Rev 2002;82:945–980
52. Taylor MR, Carniel E, Mestroni L. Familial hypertrophic cardiomyopathy: clinical features, molecular genetics and molecular genetic testing. Expert Rev Mol Diagn 2004;4:99–113
53. Roberts R, Sidhu J. Genetic basis for hypertrophic cardiomyopathy: implications for diagnosis and treatment. Am Heart Hosp J 2003;1:128–134
54. Richard P, Villard E, Charron P, Isnard R. The genetic bases of cardiomyopathies. J Am Coll Cardiol 2006;48:A79–A89
55. Niimura H, Patton KK, McKenna WJ, Soults J, Maron BJ, Seidman JG, Seidman CE. Sarcomere protein gene mutations in hypertrophic cardiomyopathy of the elderly. Circulation 2002;105:446–451
56. Charron P, Dubourg O, Desnos M, Bennaceur M, Carrier L, Camproux AC, Isnard R, Hagege A, Langlard JM, Bonne G, Richard P, Hainque B, Bouhour JB, Schwartz K, Komajda M. Clinical features and prognostic

implications of familial hypertrophic cardiomyopathy related to the cardiac myosin-binding protein C gene. Circulation 1998;97:2230–2236

57. Anan R, Greve G, Thierfelder L, Watkins H, McKenna WJ, Solomon S, Vecchio C, Shono H, Nakao S, Tanaka H, Mares A, Towbin JA, Spirito P, Roberts R, Seidman JG, Seidman CE. Prognostic implications of novel beta cardiac myosin heavy chain gene mutations that cause familial hypertrophic cardiomyopathy. J Clin Invest 1994;93:280–285
58. Maron BJ, Casey SA, Hauser RG, Aeppli DM. Clinical course of hypertrophic cardiomyopathy with survival to advanced age. J Am Coll Cardiol 2003;42:882–888
59. Chimenti C, Pieroni M, Morgante E, Antuzzi D, Russo A, Russo MA, Maseri A, Frustaci A. Prevalence of Fabry disease in female patients with late-onset hypertrophic cardiomyopathy. Circulation 2004;110:1047–1053
60. Sachdev B, Takenaka T, Teraguchi H, Tei C, Lee P, McKenna WJ, Elliott PM. Prevalence of Anderson-Fabry disease in male patients with late onset hypertrophic cardiomyopathy. Circulation 2002;105:1407–1411
61. Dec GW, Fuster V. Idiopathic dilated cardiomyopathy. N Engl J Med 1994;331:1564–1575
62. Burkett EL, Hershberger RE. Clinical and genetic issues in familial dilated cardiomyopathy. J Am Coll Cardiol 2005;45:969–981
63. Mestroni L, Rocco C, Gregori D, Sinagra G, Di Lenarda A, Miocic S, Vatta M, Pinamonti B, Muntoni F, Caforio ALP, McKenna WJ, Falaschi A, Giacca M, Camerini F. Familial dilated cardiomyopathy: evidence for genetic and phenotypic heterogeneity. J Am Coll Cardiol 1999;34:181–190
64. DeWitt MM, MacLeod HM, Soliven B, McNally EM. Phospholamban R14 deletion results in late-onset, mild, hereditary dilated cardiomyopathy. J Am Coll Cardiol 2006;48:1396–1398
65. Haghighi K, Kolokathis F, Pater L, Lynch RA, Asahi M, Gramolini AO, Fan GC, Tsiapras D, Hahn HS, Adamopoulos S, Liggett SB, Dorn GW 2nd, MacLennan DH, Kremastinos DT, Kranias EG. Human phospholamban null results in lethal dilated cardiomyopathy revealing a critical difference between mouse and human. J Clin Invest 2003;111:869–876
66. Schmitt JP, Kamisago M, Asahi M, Li GH, Ahmad F, Mende U, Kranias EG, MacLennan DH, Seidman JG, Seidman CE. Dilated cardiomyopathy and heart failure caused by a mutation in phospholamban. Science 2003;299:1410–1413
67. Minoretti P, Arra M, Emanuele E, Olivieri V, Aldeghi A, Politi P, Martinelli V, Pesenti S, Falcone C. A W148R mutation in the human FOXD4 gene segregating with dilated cardiomyopathy, obsessive-compulsive disorder, and suicidality. Int J Mol Med 2007;19:369–372
68. Villard E, Duboscq-Bidot L, Charron P, Benaiche A, Conraads V, Sylvius N, Komajda M. Mutation screening in dilated cardiomyopathy: prominent role of the beta myosin heavy chain gene. Eur Heart J 2005;26:794–803
69. Konno T, Shimizu M, Ino H, Matsuyama T, Yamaguchi M, Terai H, Hayashi K, Mabuchi T, Kiyama M, Sakata K, Hayashi T, Inoue M, Kaneda T, Mabuchi H. A novel missense mutation in the myosin binding protein-C gene is responsible for hypertrophic cardiomyopathy with left ventricular dysfunction and dilation in elderly patients. J Am Coll Cardiol 2003;41:781–786
70. Karkkainen S, Miettinen R, Tuomainen P, Karkkainen P, Helio T, Reissell E, Kaartinen M, Toivonen L, Nieminen MS, Kuusisto J, Laakso M, Peuhkurinen K. A novel mutation, Arg71Thr, in the delta-sarcoglycan gene is associated with dilated cardiomyopathy. J Mol Med 2003;81:795–800
71. Bonne G, Mercuri E, Muchir A, Urtizberea A, Becane HM, Recan D, Merlini L, Wehnert M, Boor R, Reuner U, Vorgerd M, Wicklein EM, Eymard B, Duboc D, Penisson-Besnier I, Cuisset JM, Ferrer X, Desguerre I, Lacombe D, Bushby K, Pollitt C, Toniolo D, Fardeau M, Schwartz K, Muntoni F. Clinical and molecular genetic spectrum of autosomal dominant Emery-Dreifuss muscular dystrophy due to mutations of the lamin A/C gene. Ann Neurol 2000;48:170–180
72. Wehnert MS, Bonne G. The nuclear muscular dystrophies. Semin Pediatr Neurol 2002;9:100–107
73. Vandenhende MA, Bonnet F, Sailler L, Bouillot S, Morlat P, Beylot J. [Dilated cardiomyopathy and lipid-lowering drug muscle toxicity revealing late-onset Becker's disease] Rev Med Interne 2005;26:977–979
74. Yazaki M, Yoshida K, Nakamura A, Koyama J, Nanba T, Ohori N, Ikeda S. Clinical characteristics of aged Becker muscular dystrophy patients with onset after 30 years. Eur Neurol 1999;42:145–149
75. Arimura T, Hayashi T, Terada H, Lee SY, Zhou Q, Takahashi M, Ueda K, Nouchi T, Hohda S, Shibutani M, Hirose M, Chen J, Park JE, Yasunami M, Hayashi H, Kimura A. A Cypher/ZASP mutation associated with dilated cardiomyopathy alters the binding affinity to protein kinase C. J Biol Chem 2004;279:6746–6752
76. Haghighi K, Kolokathis F, Gramolini AO, Waggoner JR, Pater L, Lynch RA, Fan GC, Tsiapras D, Parekh RR, Dorn GW 2nd, MacLennan DH, Kremastinos DT, Kranias EG. A mutation in the human phospholamban gene, deleting arginine 14, results in lethal, hereditary cardiomyopathy. Proc Natl Acad Sci USA 2006;103:1388–1393
77. De Sandre-Giovannoli A, Bernard R, Cau P, Navarro C, Amiel J, Boccaccio I, Lyonnet S, Stewart CL, Munnich A, Le Merrer M, Levy N. Lamin a truncation in Hutchinson-Gilford progeria. Science 2003; 300:2055

78. Chen L, Lee L, Kudlow BA, Dos Santos HG, Sletvold O, Shafeghati Y, Botha EG, Garg A, Hanson NB, Martin GM, Mian IS, Kennedy BK, Oshima J. LMNA mutations in atypical Werner's syndrome. Lancet 2003;362:440–445
79. Capell BC, Collins FS. Human laminopathies: nuclei gone genetically awry. Nat Rev Genet 2006;7:940–952
80. Brodsky GL, Muntoni F, Miocic S, Sinagra G, Sewry C, Mestroni L. Lamin A/C gene mutation associated with dilated cardiomyopathy with variable skeletal muscle involvement. Circulation 2000;101:473–476
81. Jakobs PM, Hanson EL, Crispell KA, Toy W, Keegan H, Schilling K, Icenogle TB, Litt M, Hershberger RE. Novel lamin A/C mutations in two families with dilated cardiomyopathy and conduction system disease. J Card Fail 2001;7:249–256
82. Fatkin D, MacRae C, Sasaki T, Wolff MR, Porcu M, Frenneaux M, Atherton J, Vidaillet HJ Jr, Spudich S, De Girolami U, Seidman JG, Seidman C, Muntoni F, Muehle G, Johnson W, McDonough B. Missense mutations in the rod domain of the lamin A/C gene as causes of dilated cardiomyopathy and conduction-system disease. N Engl J Med 1999;341:1715–1724
83. Tresch DD, McGough MF. Heart failure with normal systolic function: a common disorder older people. J Amer Geriatr Soc 1995;43:1035–1042
84. Hassan W, Al-Sergani H, Mourad W, Tabbaa R. Amyloid heart disease. New frontiers and insights in pathophysiology, diagnosis, and management. Tex Heart Inst J 2005;32:178–184
85. Koike H, Misu K, Sugiura M, Iijima M, Mori K, Yamamoto M, Hattori N, Mukai E, Ando Y, Ikeda S, Sobue G. Pathology of early- vs late-onset TTR Met30 familial amyloid polyneuropathy. Neurology 2004;63:129–138
86. Blanco-Jerez CR, Jimenez-Escrig A, Gobernado JM, Lopez-Calvo S, de Blas G, Redondo C, Garcia Villanueva M, Orensanz L. Transthyretin Tyr77 familial amyloid polyneuropathy: a clinicopathological study of a large kindred. Muscle Nerve 1998;21:1478–85
87. Hamidi Asl K, Nakamura M, Yamashita T, Benson MD. Cardiac amyloidosis associated with the transthyretin Ile122 mutation in a Caucasian family. Amyloid 2001;8:263–269
88. Yamashita T, Asl KH, Yazaki M, Benson MD. A prospective evaluation of the transthyretin Ile122 allele frequency in an African-American population. Amyloid 2005;12:127–130
89. Jiang X, Buxbaum JN, Kelly JW. The V122I cardiomyopathy variant of transthyretin increases the velocity of rate-limiting tetramer dissociation, resulting in accelerated amyloidosis. Proc Natl Acad Sci USA 2001;98:14943–14948
90. Burke W, Press N, McDonnell SM. Hemochromatosis: genetics helps to define a multifactorial disease. Clin Genet 1998;54:1–9
91. Hanson EH, Imperatore G, Burke W. HFE gene and hereditary hemochromatosis: a HuGE review. Human Genome Epidemiology. Am J Epidemiol 2001;154:193–206
92. Papanikolaou G, Samuels ME, Ludwig EH, MacDonald ML, Franchini PL, Dube MP, Andres L, MacFarlane J, Sakellaropoulos N, Politou M, Nemeth E, Thompson J, Risler JK, Zaborowska C, Babakaiff R, Radomski CC, Pape TD, Davidas O, Christakis J, Brissot P, Lockitch G, Ganz T, Hayden MR, Goldberg YP. Mutations in HFE2 cause iron overload in chromosome 1q-linked juvenile hemochromatosis. Nat Genet 2004;36:77–82
93. Turoczi T, Jun L, Cordis G, Morris JE, Maulik N, Stevens RG, Das DK. HFE mutation and dietary iron content interact to increase ischemia/reperfusion injury of the heart in mice. Circ Res 2003;92:1240–1246
94. Lio D, Balistreri CR, Colonna-Romano G, Motta M, Franceschi C, Malaguarnera M, Candore G, Caruso C. Association between the MHC class I gene HFE polymorphisms and longevity: a study in Sicilian population. Genes Immun 2002;3:20–24
95. Coppin H, Bensaid M, Fruchon S, Borot N, Blanche H, Roth MP. Longevity and carrying the C282Y mutation for haemochromatosis on the HFE gene: case control study of 492 French centenarians. BMJ 2003;327: 132–133
96. Lio D, Pes GM, Carru C, Listi F, Ferlazzo V, Candore G, Colonna-Romano G, Ferrucci L, Deiana L, Baggio G, Franceschi C, Caruso C. Association between the HLA-DR alleles and longevity: a study in Sardinian population. Exp Gerontol 2003;38:313–317
97. McConnell BK, Fatkin D, Semsarian C, Jones KA, Georgakopoulos D, Maguire CT, Healey MJ, Mudd JO, Moskowitz IP, Conner DA, Giewat M, Wakimoto H, Berul CI, Schoen FJ, Kass DA, Seidman CE, Seidman JG. Comparison of two murine models of familial hypertrophic cardiomyopathy. Circ Res 2001;88: 383–389
98. Vikstrom KL, Factor SM, Leinwand LA. Mice expressing mutant myosin heavy chains are a model for familial hypertrophic cardiomyopathy. Mol Med 1996;2:556–567
99. Mounkes LC, Kozlov SV, Rottman JN, Stewart CL. Expression of an LMNA-N195K variant of A-type lamins results in cardiac conduction defects and death in mice. Hum Mol Genet 2005;14:2167–2180
100. Nikolova V, Leimena C, McMahon AC, Tan JC, Chandar S, Jogia D, Kesteven SH, Michalicek J, Otway R, Verheyen F, Rainer S, Stewart CL, Martin D, Feneley MP, Fatkin D. Defects in nuclear structure and function promote dilated cardiomyopathy in lamin A/C-deficient mice. J Clin Invest 2004;113:357–369

101. Arimura T, Helbling-Leclerc A, Massart C, Varnous S, Niel F, Lacene E, Fromes Y, Toussaint M, Mura AM, Keller DI, Amthor H, Isnard R, Malissen M, Schwartz K, Bonne G. Mouse model carrying H222P-Lmna mutation develops muscular dystrophy and dilated cardiomyopathy similar to human striated muscle laminopathies. Hum Mol Genet 2005;14:155–169
102. Sugden PH, Clerk A. "Stress-responsive" mitogen-activated protein kinases (c-Jun N-terminal kinases and p38 mitogen-activated protein kinases) in the myocardium. Circ Res 1998;83:345–352
103. Rockman HA, Koch WJ, Lefkowitz RJ. Seven-transmembrane-spanning receptors and heart function. Nature 2002;415:206–212
104. Geng YJ, Ishikawa Y, Vatner DE, Wagner TE, Bishop SP, Vatner SF, Homcy CJ. Apoptosis of cardiac myocytes in Gsalpha transgenic mice. Circ Res 1999;84:34–42
105. Adams JW, Sakata Y, Davis MG, Sah VP, Wang Y, Liggett SB, Chien KR, Brown JH, Dorn GW 2nd. Enhanced Galphaq signaling: a common pathway mediates cardiac hypertrophy and apoptotic heart failure. Proc Natl Acad Sci USA 1998;95:10140–10145
106. Mende U, Kagen A, Cohen A, Aramburu J, Schoen FJ, Neer EJ. Transient cardiac expression of constitutively active Galphaq leads to hypertrophy and dilated cardiomyopathy by calcineurin-dependent and independent pathways. Proc Natl Acad Sci USA 1998;95:13893–13898
107. Mende U, Semsarian C, Martins DC, Kagen A, Duffy C, Schoen FJ, Neer EJ. Dilated cardiomyopathy in two transgenic mouse lines expressing activated G protein alpha(q): lack of correlation between phospholipase C activation and the phenotype. J Mol Cell Cardiol 2001;33:1477–1491
108. Jacoby JJ, Kalinowski A, Liu MG, Zhang SS, Gao Q, Chai GX, Ji L, Iwamoto Y, Li E, Schneider M, Russell KS, Fu XY. Cardiomyocyte-restricted knockout of STAT3 results in higher sensitivity to inflammation, cardiac fibrosis, and heart failure with advanced age. Proc Natl Acad Sci USA 2003;100: 12929–12934
109. Russell LK, Finck BN, Kelly DP. Mouse models of mitochondrial dysfunction and heart failure. J Mol Cell Cardiol 2005;38:81–91
110. Carvajal K, Moreno-Sanchez R. Heart metabolic disturbances in cardiovascular diseases. Arch Med Res 2003;34:89–99
111. Smeitink J, van den HL, DiMauro S. The genetics and pathology of oxidative phosphorylation. Nat Rev Genet 2001;2:342–352
112. Wallace DC. Mitochondrial diseases in man and mouse. Science 1999;283:1482–1488
113. Larsson NG, Oldfors A. Mitochondrial myopathies. Acta Physiol Scand 2001;171:385–393
114. Kelly DP, Strauss AW. Inherited cardiomyopathies. N Engl J Med 1994;330:913–919
115. Graham BH, Waymire KG, Cottrell B, Trounce IA, MacGregor GR, Wallace DC. A mouse model for mitochondrial myopathy and cardiomyopathy resulting from a deficiency in the heart/muscle isoform of the adenine nucleotide translocator. Nat Genet 1997;16:226–234
116. Wang J, Wilhelmsson H, Graff C, Li H, Oldfors A, Rustin P, Bruning JC, Kahn CR, Clayton DA, Barsh GS, Thoren P, Larsson NG. Dilated cardiomyopathy and atrioventricular conduction blocks induced by heart-specific inactivation of mitochondrial DNA gene expression. Nat Genet 1999;21:133–137
117. Nahrendorf M, Spindler M, Hu K, Bauer L, Ritter O, Nordbeck P, Quaschning T, Hiller KH, Wallis J, Ertl G, Bauer WR, Neubauer S. Creatine kinase knockout mice show left ventricular hypertrophy and dilatation, but unaltered remodeling post-myocardial infarction. Cardiovasc Res 2005;65:419–427
118. Kurtz DM, Rinaldo P, Rhead WJ, Tian L, Millington DS, Vockley J, Hamm DA, Brix AE, Lindsey JR, Pinkert CA, O'Brien WE, Wood PA. Targeted disruption of mouse long-chain acyl-CoA dehydrogenase gene reveals crucial roles for fatty acid oxidation. Proc Natl Acad Sci USA 1998;95:15592–15597
119. Exil VJ, Gardner CD, Rottman JN, Sims H, Bartelds B, Khuchua Z, Sindhal R, Ni G, Strauss AW. Abnormal mitochondrial bioenergetics and heart rate dysfunction in mice lacking very-long-chain acyl-CoA dehydrogenase. Am J Physiol Heart Circ Physiol 2006;290:H1289–H1297
120. Cheng L, Ding G, Qin Q, Huang Y, Lewis W, He N, Evans RM, Schneider MD, Brako FA, Xiao Y, Chen YE, Yang Q. Cardiomyocyte-restricted peroxisome proliferator-activated receptor-delta deletion perturbs myocardial fatty acid oxidation and leads to cardiomyopathy. Nat Med 2004;10:1245–1250
121. Ibdah JA, Paul H, Zhao Y, Binford S, Salleng K, Cline M, Matern D, Bennett MJ, Rinaldo P, Strauss AW. Lack of mitochondrial trifunctional protein in mice causes neonatal hypoglycemia and sudden death. J Clin Invest 2001;107:1403–1409
122. Puccio H, Simon D, Cossee M, Criqui-Filipe P, Tiziano F, Melki J, Hindelang C, Matyas R, Rustin P, Koenig M. Mouse models for Friedreich ataxia exhibit cardiomyopathy, sensory nerve defect and Fe-S enzyme deficiency followed by intramitochondrial iron deposits. Nat Genet 2001;27:181–186
123. Yokoyama M, Yagyu H, Hu Y, Seo T, Hirata K, Homma S, Goldberg IJ. Apolipoprotein B production reduces lipotoxic cardiomyopathy: studies in heart-specific lipoprotein lipase transgenic mouse. J Biol Chem 2004;279:4204–4211
124. Arad M, Moskowitz IP, Patel VV, Ahmad F, Perez-Atayde AR, Sawyer DB, Walter M, Li GH, Burgon PG, Maguire CT, Stapleton D, Schmitt JP, Guo XX, Pizard A, Kupershmidt S, Roden DM, Berul CI, Seidman

CE, Seidman JG. Transgenic mice overexpressing mutant PRKAG2 define the cause of Wolff-Parkinson-White syndrome in glycogen storage cardiomyopathy. Circulation 2003;107:2850–2856

125. Zhang D, Mott JL, Farrar P, Ryerse JS, Chang SW, Stevens M, Denniger G, Zassenhaus HP. Mitochondrial DNA mutations activate the mitochondrial apoptotic pathway and cause dilated cardiomyopathy. Cardiovasc Res 2003;57:147–157
126. Joza N, Oudit GY, Brown D, Benit P, Kassiri Z, Vahsen N, Benoit L, Patel MM, Nowikovsky K, Vassault A, Backx PH, Wada T, Kroemer G, Rustin P, Penninger JM. Muscle-specific loss of apoptosis-inducing factor leads to mitochondrial dysfunction, skeletal muscle atrophy, and dilated cardiomyopathy. Mol Cell Biol 2005;25:10261–10272
127. Conrad M, Jakupoglu C, Moreno SG, Lippl S, Banjac A, Schneider M, Beck H, Hatzopoulos AK, Just U, Sinowatz F, Schmahl W, Chien KR, Wurst W, Bornkamm GW, Brielmeier M. Essential role for mitochondrial thioredoxin reductase in hematopoiesis, heart development, and heart function. Mol Cell Biol 2004;24:9414–9423
128. Huang TT, Carlson EJ, Kozy HM, Mantha S, Goodman SI, Ursell PC, Epstein CJ. Genetic modification of prenatal lethality and dilated cardiomyopathy in Mn superoxide dismutase mutant mice. Free Radic Biol Med 2001;31:1101–1110
129. Russell LK, Mansfield CM, Lehman JJ, Kovacs A, Courtois M, Saffitz JE, Medeiros DM, Valencik ML, McDonald JA, Kelly DP. Cardiac-specific induction of the transcriptional coactivator peroxisome proliferator-activated receptor gamma coactivator-1alpha promotes mitochondrial biogenesis and reversible cardiomyopathy in a developmental stage-dependent manner. Circ Res 2004;94:525–533
130. Nebigil CG, Jaffre F, Messaddeq N, Hickel P, Monassier L, Launay JM, Maroteaux L. Overexpression of the serotonin 5-HT2B receptor in heart leads to abnormal mitochondrial function and cardiac hypertrophy. Circulation 2003;107:3223–3229
131. Xiaofei E, Wada Y, Dakeishi M, Hirasawa F, Murata K, Masuda H, Sugiyama T, Nikaido H, Koizumi A. Age-associated cardiomyopathy in heterozygous carrier mice of a pathological mutation of carnitine transporter gene, OCTN2. J Gerontol A Biol Sci Med Sci 2002;57:B270–B278
132. Chiu HC, Kovacs A, Blanton RM, Han X, Courtois M, Weinheimer CJ, Yamada KA, Brunet S, Xu H, Nerbonne JM, Welch MJ, Fettig NM, Sharp TL, Sambandam N, Olson KM, Ory DS, Schaffer JE. Transgenic expression of fatty acid transport protein 1 in the heart causes lipotoxic cardiomyopathy. Circ Res 2005;96:225–233
133. Finck BN, Lehman JJ, Leone TC, Welch MJ, Bennett MJ, Kovacs A, Han X, Gross RW, Kozak R, Lopaschuk GD, Kelly DP. The cardiac phenotype induced by PPAR overexpression mimics that caused by diabetes mellitus. J Clin Invest 2002;109:121–130
134. Chiu HC, Kovacs A, Ford DA, Hsu FF, Garcia R, Herrero P, Saffitz JE, Schaffer JE. A novel mouse model of lipotoxic cardiomyopathy. J Clin Invest 2001;107:813–822
135. Marin-Garcia J, Pi Y, Goldenthal MJ. Mitochondrial-nuclear cross-talk in the aging and failing heart. Cardiovasc Drugs Ther 2006;20:477–491
136. Schriner SE, Linford NJ, Martin GM, Treuting P, Ogburn CE, Emond M, Coskun PE, Ladiges W, Wolf N, Van Remmen H, Wallace DC, Rabinovitch PS. Extension of murine life span by overexpression of catalase targeted to mitochondria. Science 2005;308:1909–1911
137. Wu S, Li Q, Du M, Li SY, Ren J. Cardiac-specific overexpression of catalase prolongs lifespan and attenuates ageing-induced cardiomyocyte contractile dysfunction and protein damage. Clin Exp Pharmacol Physiol 2007;34:81–87
138. Ren J, Li Q, Wu S, Li SY, Babcock SA. Cardiac overexpression of antioxidant catalase attenuates aging-induced cardiomyocyte relaxation dysfunction. Mech Ageing Dev 2007;128:276–285
139. Ocorr K, Akasaka T, Bodmer R. Age-related cardiac disease model of Drosophila. Mech Ageing Dev 2007;128:112–116
140. Bing OH, Conrad CH, Boluyt MO, Robinson KG, Brooks WW. Studies of prevention, treatment and mechanisms of heart failure in the aging spontaneously hypertensive rat. Heart Fail Rev 2002;7:71–88
141. Heyen JR, Blasi ER, Nikula K, Rocha R, Daust HA, Frierdich G, Van Vleet JF, De Ciechi P, McMahon EG, Rudolph AE. Structural, functional, and molecular characterization of the SHHF model of heart failure. Am J Physiol Heart Circ Physiol 2002;283:H1775–H1784
142. Khadour FH, Kao RH, Park S, Armstrong PW, Holycross BJ, Schulz R. Age-dependent augmentation of cardiac endothelial NOS in a genetic rat model of heart failure. Am J Physiol 1997;273: H1223–H1230
143. Boluyt MO, Bing OH. Matrix gene expression and decompensated heart failure: the aged SHR model. Cardiovasc Res 2000;46:239–249
144. Minieri M, Fiaccavento R, Carosella L, Peruzzi G, Di Nardo P. The cardiomyopathic hamster as model of early myocardial aging. Mol Cell Biochem 1999;198:1–6
145. Sakamoto A, Ono K, Abe M, Jasmin G, Eki T, Murakami Y, Masaki T, Toyo-oka T, Hanaoka F. Both hypertrophic and dilated cardiomyopathies are caused by mutation of the same gene, delta-sarcoglycan, in

hamster: an animal model of disrupted dystrophin-associated glycoprotein complex. Proc Natl Acad Sci USA 1997;94:13873–13878
146. Nigro V, Okazaki Y, Belsito A, Piluso G, Matsuda Y, Politano L, Nigro G, Ventura C, Abbondanza C, Molinari AM, Acampora D, Nishimura M, Hayashizaki Y, Puca GA. Identification of the Syrian hamster cardiomyopathy gene. Hum Mol Genet 1997;6:601–607
147. Serose A, Salmon A, Fiszman MY, Fromes Y. Short-term treatment using insulin like growth factor-1 (IGF-1) improves life expectancy of the delta-sarcoglycan deficient hamster. J Gene Med 2006;8:1048–1055
148. Fiaccavento R, Carotenuto F, Minieri M, Masuelli L, Vecchini A, Bei R, Modesti A, Binaglia L, Fusco A, Bertoli A, Forte G, Carosella L, Di Nardo P. Alpha-linolenic acid-enriched diet prevents myocardial damage and expands longevity in cardiomyopathic hamsters. Am J Pathol 2006;169:1913–1924
149. Toyo-oka T, Kawada T, Xi H, Nakazawa M, Masui F, Hemmi C, Nakata J, Tezuka A, Iwasawa K, Urabe M, Monahan J, Ozawa K. Gene therapy prevents disruption of dystrophin-related proteins in a model of hereditary dilated cardiomyopathy in hamsters. Heart Lung Circ 2002;11:174–181
150. McLean AJ, Le Couteur DG. Aging biology and geriatric clinical pharmacology. Pharmacol Rev 2004;56:163–184
151. Flather MD, Yusuf S, Kober L, Pfeffer M, Hall A, Murray G, Torp-Pedersen C, Ball S, Pogue J, Moye L, Braunwald E. Long-term ACE-inhibitor therapy in patients with heart failure or left-ventricular dysfunction: a systematic overview of data from individual patients. ACE-Inhibitor Myocardial Infarction Collaborative Group. Lancet 2000;355:1575–1581
152. Richardson LG, Rocks M. Women and heart failure. Heart Lung 2001;30:87–97

Chapter 8
Atherosclerosis, Hypertension and Aging

Overview

Aging is an independent risk factor for the development of atherosclerosis and CAD as well as for essential primary hypertension. In this chapter we present a discussion of the molecular genetic elements thus far identified in these diseases and what is known thus far in terms of their interaction with environmental determinants affecting their phenotypic expression. We present a brief review of the involvement of these genetic and environmental factors in the pathogenesis of the atherosclerotic disease, as well as their increased application in the identification and development of reliable biomarkers for more effective diagnostic evaluation and their impact on clinical medicine. We also survey the clinical issues these age-associated disorders present including present and future treatment modalities with particular focus where possible on the elderly.

Introduction

Aging is an independent risk factor for the development of atherosclerosis [1], a vascular abnormality that plays a significant role in the development of many cardiovascular disorders including Coronary Artery Disease (CAD). With advancing age, a series of structural, architectural and compositional modifications take place in the vasculature as we have discussed in Chapter 5. The diameter of the vessels tends to increase, and thickening of intimal and medial layers is often observed [2]. In the subendothelial space, blood-derived leukocytes and an increased amount of "activated" Smooth Muscle Cells (SMCs) are present. Extracellular matrix (ECM) accumulates and becomes particularly rich in glycosaminoglycans. Collagen content increases, while elastin fibers appear progressively disorganized, thinner, and fragmented. These changes in the architecture of the vessel wall, sometimes referred to as "the vasculopathy of aging" [2], are likely to be the consequence of adaptive mechanisms to maintain normal conditions of flow, mechanical stress and/or wall tension. Although many of these features are similar to the histological findings of the atherosclerotic vessels, atherosclerosis and age-related "vasculopathy" are likely to be distinct phenomena. Nonetheless, several experimental observations in animal models suggest a special link between "the vasculopathy of aging" and atherosclerotic disease, and suggest a particular predisposition of the old vessel to develop the atherosclerotic lesion. Compared to vessels from young animals, older ones show a greater reactivity to mechanical injury and to chronic insults. This may reflect changes in the biology of the vessels that are "intrinsic" to the aging process. Indeed, as we have previously noted, aging affects the function and responsiveness of the endothelium and vascular SMCs. Endothelial permeability is increased with age, while ability to produce vasoactive substances declines. SMCs from older individuals show a growth advantage over the young ones, and display an increased ability to migrate toward chemoattractants. Moreover, the accumulation of Advanced Glycation

J. Marín-García, *Aging and the Heart*,

End products (AGEs) occurring with aging can trigger a series of cellular events, such as cellular Oxidative Stress (OS), expression of leukocyte adhesion molecules, endothelial transmigration of monocytes, and SMC chemotaxis, all considered important pre-lesional events in the atherogenesis process. Although atherosclerotic lesion formation resulting from age-induced modifications has not been directly demonstrated, the changes occurring with aging are likely to accelerate the development of the atherosclerotic plaque and contribute to increased severity of vascular disease in the elderly.

Animal experiments have demonstrated that aging predisposes the vasculature to advanced atherosclerotic disease and vessel injury and that this predisposition is a function of age-associated changes in the vessel wall itself, as discussed in previous paragraph and in Chapter 5 [1, 2] Because vascular SMCs play important roles in the pathogenesis of many vascular disorders, identifying age-associated differences in the way these cells respond to extracellular stimuli has been an area of active research. The most notable differences in intracellular signaling between vascular SMCs isolated from young and old animals are related to the control of cell migration through the calcium/calmodulin-dependent protein kinase II (CamKII) pathways and the accelerated transition of older vascular SMCs from the contractile to the synthetic phenotype [2, 3]. These differences may be due to alternative signaling pathways revealed by the inability of older cells to respond to inhibitors, such as transforming growth factor (TGF)-β1, or to altered interactions with the extracellular matrix resulting from age-associated shifts in integrin expression or changes in the matrix composition of blood vessels. The exact role that these alterations have in explaining age-associated differences in the response of the vessel wall to injury and its increased susceptibility to developing advanced atherosclerotic lesions remains to be determined.

Atherosclerosis is a complex disease caused by multiple genetic and environmental factors and gene-environment interactions involving diverse physiological processes and a wide spectrum of cell types and organs even beyond the vasculature [4]. Molecular mechanisms of atherosclerosis involve lipid metabolism, inflammatory signaling and thrombosis as well as immunity and OS. Risk factors involved in these areas such as dyslipidemia and diabetes, pro- and anti-coagulant factors have provided information about genes, which play a significant role in establishing the risk of developing atherosclerosis. Over 100 genes have been identified thus far that influence the development of atherosclerotic lesions underlining the complex and polygenic nature of this disorder. While the genetic differences contributing to CAD and atherosclerosis are greatest in lipid metabolism as we shall shortly discuss, a large array of candidate genes has been examined in population-association studies. A number of these genes have common variations with significant (and convincing) association to CAD. A partial list of candidate genes is presented in Table 8.1.

While common atherosclerosis is primarily polygenic, critical molecular information concerning its pathogenic mechanism has been gleaned from rare monogenic forms of atherosclerosis and thrombosis [5]. Rare monogenic forms of dyslipidemia lead to atherosclerosis including familial hypercholesterolemia (FH), hypertriglyceridemia, Tangier disease, Fish-eye disease and sitosterolemia. These atherosclerotic disorders comprise single gene traits inherited in a Mendelian fashion as an autosomal dominant or recessive or X-linked disorder and are primarily a result of changes in specific lipoprotein content, metabolism and/or function. For instance, FH an autosomal dominant disorder characterized by elevated cholesterol, and premature CAD, provided strong evidence for the association between blood lipids and atherosclerosis, and is the result of mutations that affect the low-density lipoprotein receptor (LDLR) responsible for the binding of LDL, a cholesteryl-rich particle containing the apoB100 lipoprotein, and control of plasma LDL levels [6]. Over 800 LDLR mutations have been identified that alter LDLR function by a variety of mechanisms, including its synthesis, transportation, affinity to bind LDL-cholesterol (LDL-C), internalization, recycling and degradation of the receptors. Familial hypercholesterolemia can also arise from mutations in apoB the major protein of LDL [7], from mutations in the *PCSK9* gene encoding neural apoptosis- regulated convertase 1 (NARC-1), a member of the proteinase K family of subtilases [8],

Table 8.1 Candidate genes associated with CAD and atherosclerosis

Gene
Apo A-I (APOA1)
Apo A-V (APOA5)
ApoB (APOB)
ApoE (APOE)
Liver x receptor (LXR)
Myocyte enhancer factor 2A (MEF2A)
Lymphotoxin-α (LTA)
Endothelial nitric oxide synthase (eNOS)
Angiotensin-converting enzyme (ACE)
Cholesteryl ester transfer protein (CETP)
Paraoxonase-1 (PON1)
Lipoprotein lipase (LPL)
Upstream transcription factor-1 (USF-1)
Peroxisome proliferator-activator receptor-γ (PPAR-γ)
Plasminogen activator inhibitor (PAI)
Methylenetetrahydrofolate reductase (MTHFR)
5-lipoxygenase activating protein (ALOX5AP)
5-lipoxygenase (5-LO); also 5-LOX
Hepatic lipase
LDL receptor (LDLR)
Phosphodiesterase 4D (PDE4D)

from mutations in the ARH gene encoding an adaptor protein containing a phosphotyrosine binding domain targeting a specific motif (NPXY) in LDLR resulting in a autosomal recessive disorder [9, 10], and as a recessive deficiency of *CYP7A1* encoding cholesterol 7-hydroxylase, the first enzyme in the classical pathway for bile acid biosynthesis [11].

In addition to the important demonstration that increased plasma LDL-C levels arising from these disorders is involved in atherosclerosis, the atherogenic potential of LDL has been further suggested by numerous animal studies implicating circulating lipoproteins which strikingly resemble human LDL in producing atherosclerosis [12], by epidemiological studies in which LDL-C was independently associated with CAD [13], by pathological studies which have detected LDL in atherosclerotic lesions and plaques [14], as well as by studies showing a positive correlation between LDL levels and disease severity [15].

However, while these monogenic disorders and the genes involved have clearly demonstrated the effects of endogenously increased LDL on the evolution of atherosclerosis, most studies concur that excess serum LDL in individuals from western countries is largely related to environmental factors such as diet as compared to changes in HDL which are primarily genetic [16]. It is noteworthy that increased serum LDL and cholesterol levels have been reported in the elderly and have been in part attributed to the effects of aging-increased obesity (which stimulates hepatic overproduction of VDL and LDL) [17], aging-mediated downregulation of hepatic LDLR expression [18], and in postmenopausal women, the loss of estrogen-mediated stimulation of LDLR expression [15]. Interestingly, the rate at which the LDL-C concentration increases in women begins to accelerate between 40 and 50 years of age, and by 55–60 years, its concentration exceeds that in men [19].

In addition to atherosclerosis stemming from the accumulation of the "bad" cholesterol lipoproteins (i.e., aberrant LDL levels), reduced HDL levels have also been associated with atherosclerosis, particularly in several rare monogenic disorders. Tangier disease (TD) is an autosomal co-dominant disease characterized by the absence of HDL and very low plasma levels of apoA-I resulting in premature CAD. TD is caused by mutations in the ATP binding cassette transporter (ABCA1) gene encoding an integral membrane protein with 12 transmembrane domains involved in cholesterol and phospholipid efflux at the membrane [20–23]. In the absence of the ABCA1 transporter, free cholesterol is not transported extracellularly. Another rare autosomal dominant disorder effecting HDL levels called *Fish eye disease* [24, 25], arises from a deficiency in lecithin: cholesterol acyltransferase (LCAT). *LCAT* encodes a protein involved in the synthesis of HDL3 from pre-lipoprotein A-I and its conversion to HDL2 cholesterol and its deficiency leads to premature CAD, proteinuria, anemia and renal failure.

The antiatherogenic effects of HDL have been largely attributed to several well-documented HDL functions. These include the capacity of HDL to transport cholesterol from the periphery to the liver termed reverse cholesterol transport and thereby prevent cholesterol deposition in the arterial wall. Moreover, HDL has potent anti-oxidative, antithrombotic (i.e., inhibition of platelet activation and platelet aggregation) and anti-inflammatory properties. Apolipoprotein A-I (apo A-I), the major protein component of HDL, is associated with two antioxidant enzymes on HDL, paraoxonase and platelet-activating factor acetylhydrolase (also known as plasma lipoprotein-associated phospholipase A2, Lp-PLA2 [26, 27], which help diminish the formation of the highly atherogenic oxidized LDL, reducing its proatherogenic potential. Moreover, HDL has been implicated in downregulating the expression of cellular adhesion molecules (e.g., VCAM, ICAM and E-selectin) and cytokines (e.g., IL-8) involved in inflammatory events in leukocyte-mediated CAD. HDL also prevents endothelial apoptosis by mediating inhibition of caspase activation and prevents subsequent endothelial apoptosis as well as activates the protein kinase Akt, a mediator of antiapoptotic signaling. Both protein components of HDL (such as apolipoprotein A-I) and its lipid components (such as, lysosphingolipids) appear to mediate the antiatherogenic and anti-aging effects of HDL.

In the general population, declining HDL-C levels with aging have been attributed in part to increased body mass and menopause [28]. In addition, in recent studies of subjects older than 75 years, HDL-C levels, rather than total or LDL-C, were associated with increased mortality from ischemic coronary disease and stroke with these CVD events rising as the HDL-C levels fell [29, 30]. Interestingly, HDL has been shown to be not only a risk factor for CAD but also for frailty and disability in the elderly.

Studies of HDL-C levels in centenarian subjects have produced conflicting data, some reporting similar levels to middle-aged adults [31], others describing a decline in HDL-C levels [32]. Several studies using a variety of analytical techniques ranging from gel electrophoresis and ultracentrifugation to NMR spectroscopy have demonstrated that the predominance of the larger, more lipid-rich HDL2 subclass is a reproducible phenotype among centenarians [31–33]. Barzilai et al. also reported that the offspring of centenarians had an intermediate HDL particle size (between control and the centenarian groups) suggesting that these lipoprotein phenotypes might have a genetic basis [31]. Interestingly, Middelberg et al. in an analysis to gauge the genetic and environmental influences on serum lipid levels in premenopausal and postmenopausal women found that environmental influences on HDL levels tend to be significantly greater in premenopausal women and less so in older postmenopausal women who displayed greater genetic variance and were more impacted by genetic influences [34]. Furthermore, in a subsequent longitudinal study from this research group examining lipid levels in 415 twins followed over 10–17 years, multivariate modeling analysis suggested that more than one genetic factor influenced HDL and LDL components of cholesterol over time, and that different genes may affect the risk profile at different ages [35].

A number of molecular genetic studies have sought to demonstrate a significant association between genes involved in HDL metabolism, atherosclerosis and longevity. One pivotal candidate gene which has been the focus of several studies is the CETP gene encoding the cholesteryl ester transfer protein, a carrier protein involved in reverse cholesterol transport that mediates the transfer of cholesteryl esters from HDL to apoB-containing lipoproteins. The CETP gene is known to have many polymorphic variants (i.e., SNPs), which have been associated with altered CETP activity and plasma HDL-C concentrations. Mutations in CETP causing CETP deficiency have been demonstrated to lead to increased plasma HDL-C in Japanese subjects [36, 37]. Although some of these studies have shown that CETP deficiency can be associated with enhanced longevity, others have suggested a more complex picture. For instance, Hirano et al. reported in a study of 201 individuals with high HDL-C levels that reduced CETP function in conjunction with reduced hepatic lipase activity is associated with an increased risk for CAD [38]. This suggested that the metabolic setting of the individual might, at least in part, determine the ultimate effect of CETP on atherosclerosis. Although the role of CETP in atherosclerosis is not well defined and is likely dependent on the metabolic, genetic, and environmental context, an increasing number of potential therapies to treat atherosclerosis have centered on CETP as a therapeutic target to raise HDL-C levels [39]. For instance, the CETP inhibitor, Torcetrapib, when tested in human subjects provided a 50–100% increase in HDL-C [40].

Studies of different CETP alleles in centenarians also have emerged with a rather complex picture with respect to CETP's effect on longevity. In a study of Japanese centenarians, although heterozygous CETP deficiency and the B2 allele of the Taq1B polymorphism were consistently associated with higher plasma HDL C levels both in centenarians and controls, the allelic frequencies of those CETP polymorphisms did not differ between the two groups [41]. In contrast, in a case control study of 213 Ashkenazi Jewish probands with exceptional longevity (mean age, 98.2 years) and their offspring (n = 216; mean age, 68.3 years) compared to 253 age-matched controls, a I1405V mutation in CETP resulting in increased size of HDL particles in both the very old parents and their offspring was reported [31]. In addition, a significantly higher frequency of homozygosity for the 405 valine allele of CETP (VV genotype) was found in the probands and their offspring compared to the controls. One obvious difference between the effects of these two diverse findings is the ethnic background suggesting the potential involvement of modifier genes; another variable that needs to be assessed is diet. Interestingly, this same CETP polymorphic 405 valine variant when examined in Japanese men with hypertriglyceridemia, was found to be associated with increased prevalence of CAD despite elevated HDL-C, again suggesting that CETP can either be pro-or antiatherogenic, depending on the metabolic setting as well as the genetic background [42].

Similarly, studies with variants of the gene for lipoprotein lipase (LPL), a pivotal enzyme involved in regulating lipolysis of triglyceride-rich lipoproteins, assessed in Japanese centenarians have also found that despite a significant association of LPL(−/−) genotype with significantly higher HDL-C concentration, which was specific to centenarians (and not found in controls), there was no discernable association between this genetic polymorphism and longevity [41].

In addition, environmental factors including acute phase reactants such as C-reactive protein (CRP) have also been reported to be linked with HDL-C levels in both aging and in atheroscleosis [43]. An inverse relationship between CRP levels with HDL was reported in 3 elderly cohorts (aged 75, 80, and 85 years; n=455) of the population-based Helsinki Ageing [44]. Lower levels of HDL-C in a group of 75 Japanese centenarians were associated with decreased serum albumin, elevated CRP and IL-6 levels, and cognitive impairment [45]. In addition, analysis of a cohort of 130 subjects (average age 81 years) found increased circulating levels of tumor necrosis factor-α (TNF-α) and CRP and lower levels of HDL-C compared to a young adult control group. In the group with the highest TNF-α levels, a significant proportion had atherosclerosis [46].

Strandberg et al. have reported that treatment of 60 hypercholesterolemic coronary patients with hypolipidemic 3-hydroxy-3-methylglutaryl coenzyme A (HMG-CoA) reductase inhibitor (statin) found that LDL-C was substantially decreased and HDL-C increased during statin treatment [44]. Moreover, CRP levels decreased significantly during treatment, and were significantly associated with changes in HDL-C but not with changes in LDL-C; these results are consistent with indications that HDL has anti-inflammatory properties. While other large-scale studies have found that statin treatment impacted CRP levels, a significant association between CRP and HDL-C levels has not been replicated suggesting that statin effects on HDL and CRP may operate by independent mechanisms [47–49].

Lipoprotein Oxidation and Modification

Damage to endothelium structure and function is widely considered to be among the primary causes of atherosclerosis leading to the subsequent combination of inflammation, cell death, cell proliferation, fibrosis, and eventual calcification which contribute to the formation of an atheromatous plaque, which with stenosis or rupture, develops a thrombus resulting in clinical sequelae including myocardial infarction (MI). Possible causes of endothelial dysfunction injury leading to atherosclerosis include elevated and modified LDL, hypertension, smoking, diabetes mellitus, elevated plasma homocysteine, infectious microorganisms such as *Chlamydia pneumoniae*, and various combinations of these or other factors [50]. A pivotal factor in the initial endothelial damage is the infiltration of oxidized LDL (oxLDL) into the arterial endothelium. In addition, oxLDL appears to play a role in the chemotactic attraction of macrophages and their transformation into foam cells to form the developing atherosclerotic lesion ("the fatty streak"). Taken together, this is indicative that lipoprotein oxidation plays a central role in atherogenesis.

While the role of oxLDL is central in atherogenesis, there is little indication that aging itself modulates oxLDL levels. Mosinger reported an increase in oxLDL in post-menopausal compared to pre-menopausal women although no age-related effect was seen with men [51]. While increased plasma oxLDL has been found in a study of healthy elderly individuals with high risk for CAD [52], no consistent association of oxLDL has been reported in the limited studies available with aging [53]. Moreover, isolated LDL obtained from elderly healthy individuals (65–74 years) compared to young controls (18–30 years) revealed a decreased susceptibility to *in vitro* oxidation in the aged group with an increased lag time and decline in the maximal rate of LDL oxidation [54].

Oxidation of LDL phospholipids containing arachidonic acid result in the production of specific proinflammatory oxidized phospholipids. One type of phospholipid oxidation product mimics the structure of the potent inflammatory mediator platelet-activating factor (PAF), and these oxidation products activate the PAF receptor found on platelets, monocytes and leukocytes and can lead to platelet aggregation. Production of such PAF mimetics is not regulated thereby leading to aberrant inflammatory cell function. Moreover, production of nitric oxide (NO) in vascular SMCs, and PAF along with other phospholipid oxidation products has been detected in atherosclerotic lesions [55, 56]. Oxidation of phospholipid moieties as well as targeted amino acid residues (e.g., lysine) in the apolipoprotein B-100 component of LDL are largely generated by oxidants produced in the arterial wall and in macrophages by cell-associated lipoxygenase and myeloperoxidase. The phosphatidylcholine (PC) group is one of several active components of lipoproteins targeted by oxidation.

The integral role of oxLDL in the genesis of atherosclerosis also has been corroborated by molecular studies in animal models as well as by human genetic analysis. A number of studies have focused on paraoxonase (encoded by PON1 and PON2), a serum esterase associated with plasma HDLs which confers protection against atherosclerosis by reducing pro-inflammatory oxidized LDLs and hydrolyzing lipid peroxides. Transgenic mice containing a knock-out of serum paraoxonase (PON1) were more susceptible to atherosclerosis than their wild-type littermates when fed a high-fat, high-cholesterol diet [57]. Conversely, overexpression of protective genes such as PON1 in apoE deficient mice markedly reduced atherosclerosis [58]. Recent studies with one month old rabbits fed a high-fat diet which normally display enhanced LDL oxidation and the development of atherosclerotic lesions found that the local overexpression of PON1 (as a Sendai virus gene construct) in the arteries attenuated OS, thereby inhibiting the atherosclerotic process [59]. In this model, PON1 overexpression greatly reduced levels of the lectin-like oxidized LDL receptor-1 (LOX-1), thereby inhibiting macrophage accumulation, intimal thickening and atherosclerotic plaque formation in the vascular lumen as well as reducing OS levels in treated arteries as confirmed by 4-hydroxy-2-nonenal (HNE) staining.

Analysis of human PON1 and PON2 gene polymorphisms and their relationship with atherosclerotic disease, CAD and coronary outcomes like MI have shown a significant association in a number of studies in specific populations. Two genetic polymorphisms in *PON1* (Leu55Met and Gln192Arg) and one in *PON2* (Ser311Cys) have been reported to be associated with CAD risk in several case-control studies [60–65], albeit several of these were limited to CAD in patients with type 2 diabetes [60, 61], or were in Japanese subjects [61, 64, 65] and Asian-Indians [62]. For instance, a study of a Japanese population including 431 control subjects, 210 CAD patients, and 235 ischemic stroke patients found that the R192 allele frequency was significantly higher in CAD and ischemic stroke patients than in control subjects and was an independent determinant even when confounding influences of other risk factors were controlled for by multivariate analysis [65]. This finding was not replicated in other populations including Italian, Turkish, and Chinese[63, 66–69].

In a study investigating the association between PON polymorphic variants and the severity of CAD as determined by the number of diseased coronary artery vessels in 711 subjects (589 whites and 122 blacks) from the Women's Ischemia Syndrome Evaluation (WISE) study, those subjects with significant CAD ($\geq$ 50% stenosis) were further classified into groups with one-, two-, or three-vessel disease if any of the three coronary arteries had diameter stenosis $\geq$ 50% [70]. No significant association was found between the PON polymorphisms and stenosis severity in either white or black women. However, when data were stratified by the number of diseased vessels, the frequencies of the PON1 codon 192 Arg/Arg and of the PON2 codon 311 Cys/Cys genotypes were significantly higher in the group with three-vessel disease than in the other groups (those with one-vessel and two-vessel disease).

A number of studies have also reported a significant association of specific PON1 polymorphisms with the risk of MI [71–73]. In a study designed to test whether the PON1-192 polymorphism modulates the MI risk associated with low HDL-C concentrations with 280 MI patients and 396 control subjects, Senti et al. reported a significant decline of PON1 activity levels with advancing age in subjects carrying the low-activity PON1-192 QQ genotype particularly in MI patients [72]. In an analysis of the entire study population, middle-aged and older subjects exhibited MI risks of 1.89 and 2.69 respectively, compared with young subjects. These risks increased to 2.41 and 4.39, respectively, in the older QQ homozygotes in comparison with younger QQ homozygotes, decreased to 1.53 and 2.08, respectively, in QR heterozygotes, and also declined to 1.95 and 0.51 in RR homozygotes who were middle-aged and older, respectively, compared with younger RR carriers. These data indicated that the effect of PON1-192 genotypes on the association of increased age and MI risk was gene-dosage related, with lower PON1 activity levels as a function of age in subjects homozygous for the Q allele and suggested that MI risk increases with advancing age, principally among subjects carrying the low-activity QQ genotype.

Other recent studies have further implicated the PON gene cluster (i.e., including PON1 and PON2) as a susceptibility locus for MI in specific ethnic populations (e.g., Pakistani, Chinese) and suggested that the susceptibility is largely modulated through gene-gene and gene-environment interactions including the involvement of smoking [73, 74]. In addition, in an analysis of 618 CAD subjects, there were more carriers of the PON2 311Cys variation among those who had suffered a MI than among those who had not, and the risk of MI appeared to be influenced by gene-environmental interaction between PON2 Ser311Cys and smoking [75].

Numerous studies have reported that oxLDL is recognized by both the innate and adaptive immune systems of animals and humans. Immune responses to oxLDL including the production of both IgM and IgG autoantibodies are thought to play a key role in the activation and regulation of the inflammatory processes that are featured at different stages in atherogenesis. While there are conflicting findings on whether the immune response to oxidized LDL is predominantly pro- or antiatherogenic in clinical settings in relation to endothelial dysfunction, subclinical atherosclerosis and cardiovascular events, a number of animal studies have indicated that immunization with oxLDL induces antibody formation (both IgG and IgM) with a beneficial role in stemming atherosclerosis development [76].

Increasing evidence indicates that oxLDL plays an important role in endothelial dysfunction. OxLDL induces endothelial injury; inhibits apoptosis, monocyte adhesion, and platelet aggregation; and inhibits endothelial nitric oxide synthase (eNOS) expression/activity, all of which contribute to the atherosclerotic process. OxLDL-induced ROS formation, largely through activation of NADPH oxidase, but also through uncoupling of endothelial NOS and through direct ROS release, also contributes to endothelial dysfunction. Recent evidence suggests that oxLDL also impacts endothelial mitochondrial metabolic and apoptotic function [77], and that endothelial mitochondria may also contribute to the deleterious effects of oxLDL, since mitochondria as a significant source of ROS can increase ROS production in response to lipid oxidation products such as oxLDL [78]. Therefore while enhanced OS is one factor triggering formation of oxLDL, oxLDL itself has been identified as a potent stimulus for vascular ROS formation, potentially causing a vicious circle [79].

Several receptors for oxLDL have been found on endothelial cells. Molecular analysis has resulted in the identification and cloning of the gene for the endothelial lectin-like oxLDL receptor LOX-1 involved in the uptake of oxLDL into endothelial cells [80]. *In vitro* studies have shown that this lectin-like receptor is transcriptionally upregulated by proinflammatory cytokines (e.g., TNF-α), OS, angiotensin II, shear stress and oxLDL itself. The expression of this receptor in concert with oxLDL leads to induction of adhesion molecule expression, activation of nuclear factor-κB (NF-κB) through increased ROS, endothelial apoptosis and decrease of NO release typical of endothelial dysfunction. *In vivo* studies have demonstrated that this receptor is highly expressed in the blood vessels of animals and in humans with hypertension, diabetes mellitus and atherosclerosis. In addition to binding oxLDL, LOX-1 also binds binds apoptotic cells, activated platelets through the interaction with anionic phospholipids and bacteria. Other endothelial scavenger receptors have been identified by expression cloning using modified LDL as a ligand. One characteristic that almost all of these "scavenger receptors" share is the ability to bind with high affinity to a broad spectrum of structurally unrelated ligands. One such protypical receptor includes CD36, a multiple ligand receptor, which binds to oxLDL, thrombospondin, erythrocytes infected with *Plasmodium falciparum*, long-chain fatty acids, and Gram-negative and Gram-positive bacteria [81].

Inflammation and Atherosclerosis

The endothelial dysfunction that arises from injury leads to a series of compensatory responses that can substantially alter the normal homeostatic properties of the endothelium, such as modifying its adhesiveness with respect to leukocytes or platelets, as well as its permeability. The injury also induces the endothelium to form vasoactive molecules, cytokines, and growth factors. If the offending agents are not effectively neutralized or removed, the inflammatory response may continue indefinitely [50]. This inflammatory response stimulates the migration and proliferation of vascular SMCs that become embedded within the area of inflammation to form an intermediate lesion. If these responses continue unabated, they can result in artery wall thickening, which compensates by gradual dilation, so that up to a point, the lumen remains unaltered, leading to vascular remodeling. Monocyte-derived macrophages and specific subtypes of T lymphocytes also largely mediate this response [82].

Continued inflammation results in increased numbers of macrophages and lymphocytes, which both emigrate to and multiply at the lesion. Activation of these cells leads to the release of numerous hydrolytic enzymes, cytokines, chemokines, and growth factors, which further induce damage and can eventually lead to necrosis. The accumulation of mononuclear cells, migration and proliferation of vascular SMCs, and the formation of fibrous tissue promote a further enlargement and restructuring of the lesion, enabling the generation of a fibrous cap that overlies a core of lipid and necrotic tissue. When, at some point, the artery can no longer compensate by dilation, the atherosclerotic lesion may become occlusive compromising blood flow.

LDL modified by oxidation (oxLDL), glycation, aggregation, association with proteoglycans, or incorporation into immune complexes is a important stimulus for injury to the endothelium as described above as well as to underlying smooth muscle. In addition, it is well established that modified lipoproteins interface with monocytes and macrophages, which are also fundamentally implicated in atherogenic pathogenesis. Monocytes evolve into macrophages in the vascular wall. LDL particles entrapped in an artery, often undergo progressive oxidation and are targeted by scavenger receptor on the surfaces of macrophages. LDL internalization leads to the formation of lipid peroxides with the subsequent accumulation of cholesteryl esters, resulting in the formation and activation of foam cells. It has been proposed that the removal and sequestration of modified LDL likely represents an intrinsic, protective role of the macrophage in the inflammatory response to minimize the effects of modified LDL on vascular endothelial cells (ECs) and SMCs. Moreover, oxLDLs stimulate macrophage replication as well as their migration and recruitment into the atherosclerotic lesion in part by upregulating the expression of genes for macrophage colony-stimulating factor (MCSF) [83], and monocyte chemotactic protein (MCP) [84]. *In vitro* studies suggest that after binding to scavenger receptors, modified LDL induces the expression of inflammatory cytokines such as interleukin-1 thereby promoting a vicious circle of inflammation, of lipoprotein modification, and further inflammation in the artery [85]. Continued exposure to MCSF permits macrophages to survive *in vitro* and possibly to multiply within the lesions.

It is noteworthy that both early and later stages in the atherosclerotic development involve the recruitment of inflammatory cells from the circulation and their transendothelial migration, mediated in part by a variety of cellular adhesion molecules, which are expressed in the vascular EC as well as on circulating leukocytes in response to inflammatory stimuli [86]. EC adhesion molecules including selectins, intercellular adhesion molecules, and vascular-cell adhesion molecules serve as receptors for glycoconjugates and integrins present on monocytes and T cells. Molecules associated with the migration of leukocytes across the endothelium act in conjunction with chemoattractant molecules (such as MCP1 generated by the endothelium, SMCs, and monocytes) as well as oxLDL, interleukin-8, platelet-derived growth factor (PDGF), MCSF, and osteopontin to attract monocytes and T cells into the artery. A number of selectins (i.e., P, E and L) and their ligands are involved in the tethering of leukocytes on the vascular wall. Intercellular adhesion molecules (ICAMs) and vascular cell adhesion molecules (VCAM-1), as well as some of the integrins, induce firm adhesion of inflammatory cells at the vascular surface. Interestingly, the expression of specific adhesion molecules (e.g., VCAM-1, ICAM-1 and L-selectin) in ECs has been consistently observed in atherosclerotic plaques, and in some cases has been demonstrated to be regulated by properties of blood flow (e.g., decreased shear stress and increased turbulence) [87]. Several common polymorphisms have been identified in the genes encoding the different adhesion molecules, but their association with CAD has not yet been demonstrated [88].

Several chemokine factors are responsible for the chemotaxis and accumulation of macrophages, lipid-laden monocytes, T lymphocytes and SMCs in fatty streaks. Activation of monocytes and T cells leads to the upregulation of receptors on their surfaces, including molecules that bind selectins, integrins that bind adhesion molecules, and receptors that bind chemoattractant molecules, interactions which profoundly contribute to localizing the lesion and defining the extent of the inflammatory response.

With its array of receptors including Toll-like receptors (TLRs) and scavenger receptors (SRs) that recognize in addition to oxLDL, a broad spectrum of molecular patterns commonly found on pathogens, the macrophage is a principle effector cell in mediating innate immunity which is characteristically antigen- and memory-independent which often constitutes a first line of defense to microbial infection. A list of several ligands and pattern-recognition receptors in macrophages is shown in Table 8.2. Another multi-ligand scavenger receptor present in monocytes/macrophages,

Table 8.2 Ligands for pattern recognition receptor

Ligand	Scavenger receptor (SR)	Toll-like receptor (TLR)
LPS	SR-A	TLR2, TLR4
Lipoteichoic acid	SR-A	TLR2, TLR4
Acetyl-LDL	SR-A, MARCO, SR-B, FEEL	?
Oxidized LDL	SR-A, CD36, SR-PSOX, LOX-1, SR-B	TLR4
AGE	SR-A, CD36, LOX-1, SR-B, FEEL	
Anionic phospholipids	SR-B, CD36,	
HSP60	?	TLR2, TLR4
CpG DNA	?	TLR9
Extra domain A of fibronectin (EDA)		TLR4
Cellular ligands		
Aged/apoptotic cells	LOX-1, SR-A, SR-B, CD36	
Bacteria	LOX-1, SR-A, MARCO, SR-PSOX	TLR2, TLR6, TLR4
Activated platelets	LOX-1, SR-A	

the membrane glycoprotein CD36 binds ligands such as oxLDLs, long-chain fatty acids, collagen, thrombospondin 1, apoptotic cells, anionic phospholipids, and *Plasmodium falciparum*-infected erythrocytes and has been suggested (though not proven) to be a factor in atherosclerosis [89].

A family of mammalian TLRs has recently been identified as a key component of pathogen-associated molecular pattern recognition machinery including the recognition of a large repertoire of microbial pathogens [90]. A variety of bacterial and fungal components are known TLR ligands, including peptidoglycan for TLR2, lipopolysaccharide (LPS) for TLR4, flagellin for TLR5, and unmethylated CpG motifs in bacterial DNA for TLR9 (a cytosolic rather than a plasma-membrane associated TLR). In addition, the binding of the TLRs to oxLDL (but not unmodified LDL) is also accompanied by upregulated TLR4 expression in macrophages *in vitro* [91]. Whereas binding of the recognized particles to SRs leads to endocytosis and lysosomal degradation, engagement of TLR transmits transmembrane signals that activate NF-κB [92], and MAPK pathways [93]. TLR binding induces the expression of a wide variety of genes such as those encoding proteins involved in leukocyte recruitment, ROS production, and phagocytosis. Activation of TLRs can also elicit the production of cytokines that augment local inflammation. Finally, TLR ligation may also directly induce apoptosis [94].

It is noteworthy that ECs also express TLRs and SRs, which upon binding the appropriate ligand, induce the expression of leukocyte adhesion molecules, iNOS2, endothelin, interleukin-1, and other inflammatory molecules. Their activation causes leukocyte recruitment, increased permeability, edema, and other characteristic features of inflammation.

Pathogenic microorganisms such as *Chlamydia pneumoniae*, cytomegalovirus, and *Helicobacter pylori* have been detected with high frequency in atherosclerotic lesions and have been demonstrated to aggravate atherosclerosis in experimental models [95]. However, since neither infection or TLR expression is sufficient to induce atherosclerosis in animal models, these data suggest that the role that microbes and/or TLR signaling play in atherogenesis is unlikely to be causative [96]. However, several lines of evidence suggest the potential involvement of TLR in atherosclerosis. Semiquantitative PCR and immunohistochemical analyses have demonstrated the expression of TLR1, TLR2, and TLR4 was markedly enhanced in human atherosclerotic plaques [97]. While a number of molecular genetic studies have identified several polymorphic variants in the TLR gene with significant association with atherosclerosis [98–100], other studies have not replicated this association [101–103]. Initial studies found that common, missense mutations in TLR4 (i.e., Asp299Gly and Thr399Ile) affecting the extracellular domain of the toll-like receptor 4 receptor were hyposensitive in response to LPS in either homozygous or heterozygous patients [104]. Evidence from a population-based epidemiologic study also found that subjects carrying the Asp299Gly were less susceptible to carotid artery atherosclerosis [99]. Studies have also reported that this TLR4 polymorphism provides protection from carotid and femoral artery atherosclerosis [99, 100] and acute coronary events [105] as well as significantly greater benefit from statin (i.e., pravastatin) therapy [106]. Moreover, several studies are in agreement that specific TLR polymorphic variants are a significant risk factor in coronary restenosis more so than atherosclerosis [102, 104, 107].

In addition to plasma membrane receptors, another type of receptor (present in macrophages as well as in other complicit cell-types), the nuclear receptors have been increasingly recognized as players in atherosclerogenesis. The induction and modulation of both lipid metabolism and inflammatory pathways in activated macrophages by these global regulators of transcription are central to the pathogenesis of atherosclerosis [108]. Nuclear receptors including the peroxisome proliferator-activated receptor gamma (PPAR-γ) and liver X receptors (LXRs) and their ligands mediate the upregulation of expression of genes involved in oxidized lipid uptake (e.g., CD36) and cholesterol efflux in macrophages [109–111]. For instance, a conserved LXR response element was identified by Lafitte et al. in the promoter of the gene for human apoE, a critical macrophage secretory product which plays a protective effect against the development of atherosclerosis, primarily through its ability to promote lipid efflux [109]. Demonstration that the nuclear receptors LXRα and LXRβ and their oxysterol ligands are key regulators of apoE expression in both macrophages and adipose tissues was also confirmed using murine gene knockouts; the ability to regulate apoE expression in adipose tissue and peritoneal macrophages by oxysterols and synthetic ligands was markedly reduced in $LXR\alpha^{-/-}$ or $LXR\beta^{-/-}$ mice and entirely abolished in double knockout strains. Initial studies demonstrated that oxLDL activated macrophage PPAR-γ dependent transcription increased uptake of oxLDL via induced CD36 and that PPAR-γ levels were expressed at high levels in foam cells from atherosclerotic lesions suggesting a potential role in atherogenesis [112, 113]. However, subsequent evidence from the studies of Chawla et al. suggested that the nuclear receptor PPAR-γ orchestrates a complex physiologic response to oxLDL that involves lipoprotein particle uptake into macrophages, processing, and cholesterol removal through induction of the transporter ABCA1 [110]. Ligand activation of PPAR-γ initiated a transcriptional cascade which led to primary induction of LXRα and to the coupled induction of ABCA1 expression resulting in enhanced cholesterol efflux and removal from macrophages. Transplantation of *PPAR-γ* null bone marrow into *LDLR−/−* mice resulted in a significant increase in atherosclerosis, consistent with the hypothesis that the regulation by this nuclear receptor is protective *in vivo*. This was confirmed by studies of Li et al. using LDL-R deficient mice, in which treatment with the PPAR-γ -specific thiazolidenedione (TZD) agonist rosiglitazone strongly inhibited the development of atherosclerosis despite increased CD36 scavenger receptor expression in the arterial wall [114, 115]. Interestingly, agonists of PPAR-β failed to prevent atherosclerotic lesion in this mouse model. Other studies demonstrated that activators of both PPAR-α and PPAR-γ induced ABCA1 gene expression as well as increased apoAI-induced cholesterol efflux from normal macrophages [111].

The nuclear receptors have also been implicated in negatively modulating macrophage inflammatory gene expression [116, 117]. *In vitro* studies demonstrated that LXR ligands inhibit the expression of inflammatory mediators such as inducible nitric oxide synthase (iNOS), cyclooxygenase (COX)-2 and IL-6 in response to bacterial infection or LPS stimulation. *In vivo*, LXR agonists inhibited inflammatory gene expression in the aortas of atherosclerotic mice. Similarly, TZDs inhibit the expression of inflammatory mediators including iNOS, TNF-α and MMP9 as well as gelatinase B and scavenger receptor A genes in macrophages. PPAR-γ inhibits gene expression in part by antagonizing the activities of the transcription factors AP-1, STAT and NF-κB. The mechanism by which the ligand-bound PPAR-γ normally an activator of transcription is converted to a promoter-specific repressor of NF-κB target proinflammory genes that regulate inflammation is not completely understood. However, recent evidence has implicated the ligand-dependent targeting of specific lysine residues on PPAR-γ ligand-binding domain by sumoylation, a post-translational modification by which small ubiquitin-like modifiers (SUMO) are covalently conjugated to a target protein as a potential mechanism. Sumoylation at lysine 365 of PPAR-γ leads to the recruitment and stabilization of the nuclear corepressor (N-CoR) at the promoter sites of proinflammatory genes thereby repressing their transcription [118]. The removal of N-CoR/ histone deacetylase-3 (HDAC3) complexes from gene promoters required for gene activation, a process normally mediated by the ubiquitylation/19S proteosome machinery is impeded by the binding of sumoylated PPAR-γ to these N-CoR/ HDAC3 complexes preventing their dissolution and therefore target genes are maintained in a repressed state through stimulation of the ABCA1 pathway.

The Cap of the Atherosclerotic Lesion and its Rupture

Erosion or uneven thinning and rupture of the atherosclerotic lesion's fibrous cap can lead to MI. This often occurs at the shoulders of the lesion site where macrophages enter, accumulate, and are activated, and where apoptosis may occur [119]. Degradation of the fibrous cap, which is primarily composed of type I and III collagen may result from the increased expression, and activity of metalloproteinases such as collagenases, elastases, and stromelysins. Recent studies have confirmed the presence of both the collagenolytic matrix metalloproteinase MMP-8 protein and its mRNA within unstable carotid atherosclerotic plaques collected from 159 patients undergoing carotid endarterectomy [120]. Cathepsins, and mast cell proteases can also impair the integrity of the fibrous cap by degrading its collagen cap.

Activated T cells may stimulate metalloproteinase production by the macrophages in the lesions, promoting plaque instability. Proinflammatory cytokines can regulate the release of these matrix-degrading proteinases. Moreover, LPS, TNF-α, IL-1, and interferon-γ, all induce tissue-factor (TF) procoagulant gene expression in human ECs. The production of TF procoagulant and other hemostatic factors, is considered to be a principal factor in the thrombosis of the atherosclerotic lesion [121].

Stable advanced lesions usually have uniformly dense fibrous caps. More vulnerable atherosclerotic plaques that might be the site of future acute coronary events tend to have a large lipid core, are rich in TF, with an abundance of inflammatory cells including macrophages and have a thin fibrous cap [121]. Plaque rupture and thrombosis may be responsible for as many as 50% of cases of acute coronary syndromes (ACS) and MI. At autopsy active inflammation is generally evident in the accumulation of macrophages at sites of plaque rupture. In terms of detection, the potentially more dangerous rupture-prone lesions tend to be small and nonocclusive and thus may be difficult to detect by angiography. Since detection of vulnerable plaques (which tend to be multiple) often occurs late in the course of disease after symptoms have presented, much effort has been directed at finding non-invasive imaging modalities including computed tomography (CT) and magnetic resonance imaging (MRI) for early detection to predict plaque vulnerability before irreversible damage has occurred and in defining markers of atherosclerotic disease [122]. Macrophage accumulation may be associated with increased plasma concentrations of both fibrinogen and CRP, two markers of inflammation thought to be early signs of atherosclerosis; other early markers including endothelial dysfunction [123] are discussed in the following section.

Biomarkers

The levels of specific oxidized lipids in plasma and lipoproteins may serve as useful markers of the susceptibility to atherogenesis. The generation of monoclonal antibodies recognizing distinct oxidation-specific epitopes has allowed the development of sensitive and specific assays to measure circulating oxidized LDL. Clinical studies have revealed that circulating oxLDL is associated with preclinical atherosclerosis, coronary and peripheral arterial atherosclerosis, ACS and vulnerable plaques [124]. Another associated marker is the plasma lipoprotein-associated phospholipase A2 (Lp-PLA2), also known as platelet-activating factor acetylhydrolase. Lp-PLA2 is produced by inflammatory cells primarily of myeloid origin and is highly expressed in vulnerable plaques. It is thought that the specific targeting of polar phospholipids in oxidized LDL may be contributory to the formation of downstream intermediates (e.g., lysophosphatidylcholine) that mediate plaque vulnerability by promoting proinflammatory cell phenotype and macrophage death [125]. Furthermore, it is noteworthy that Lp-PLA2 was the first biomarker for predicting stroke risk associated with atherosclerosis and was recently approved by the United States Food and Drug Administration [126].

As noted above, vascular cells and the vascular endothelium are early targets of oxLDL damage disrupting vascular homeostasis as the endothelium provides a host of vasoprotective effects, such as vasodilation, suppression of SMC growth, and inhibition of inflammatory response largely mediated by the production of the endogenous vasodilator NO. Gathering evidence suggests that endothelial dysfunction constitutes an early marker for atherosclerosis and can be detected before structural changes to the vessel wall are apparent on angiography or ultrasound [127].

Gene Expression Profiling and Atherosclerosis

To understand fundamental pathobiological mechanisms in atherogenesis and to develop and target new therapies, information on gene expression patterns (atherogenomics) and protein expression patterns (atheroproteomics) are crucially needed. Unlike the relatively availability of tumor samples for gene expression analysis by the oncologist, access to disease-associated cardiovascular tissues from patients is generally more limited and initially proved to be an impediment to this type of analysis. A large number of profiling studies have been performed in animal models. Csiszar et al [128, 129] using gene expression profiling of rat coronary arteries suggested that aging alters gene expression with a significant shift towards induced proinflammatory, cytokine expression resulting in the upregulation of TNF-α, several interleukin genes (IL-1β, IL-6, and IL-17), IL-6Rα and caspase 9 and the decreased bioavailability of NO, changing vascular cell phenotypes with respect to function, potential inflammation and increased cell death. However, the approach of whole-mount lesions is problematic since arterial tissue is a very heterogeneous collection of cells and localization of expressed transcripts or proteins to certain cell types using *in-situ* hybridization or immunohistochemistry may be a useful adjunct in these studies [130]. The isolation of single cells or small cell populations with the aid of laser microdissection can also be helpful in defining and localizing expression patterns within a atherosclerotic lesion. For instance, Tuomisto et al. used laser microdissection to isolate macrophage-rich shoulder areas from human lesions for profiling gene expression compared to normal intima [131]. Many inflammatory mediators, such as interleukins and their receptors, colony stimulating factor receptors and integrins (i.e., CD11a/CD18 integrins) were upregulated as were calmodulin, NOS, and extracellular superoxide dismutase (EcSOD). Moreover, overexpression of HMG-CoA reductase in macrophage-rich lesion areas may explain some beneficial effects of statins.

Fewer global gene profiling studies have been performed in tissues and cells derived from patients [132–135]. For instance, one recent assessment of the potential of published expression data, compared the data focusing on a CC chemokine gene cluster between 18 murine and human gene expression profiling studies. This analysis concluded that an adequate comparison is mainly hindered by the incompleteness of available data sets, and suggested that further improvement in experimental design, statistical, and bioinformatical analysis are sorely needed as are greater access to data sets [136]. However, several creative approaches to gene profiling in human atherosclerosis have produced interesting findings and this research approach has become substantially more robust. For instance, studies with gene arrays have begun to provide a valuable approach for analysis of atherosclerotic plaque composition and for the identification of candidate markers of plaque progression. In a recent study to identify differences in gene expression between stable and unstable segments of plaque obtained from the same patient, human carotid endarterectomy specimens were analyzed which were segmented and macroscopically classified using a morphological classification system [137]. Using Affymetrix gene chip analysis, two analytical methods were compared, an intraplaque and an interplaque analysis, revealing 170 and 1916 differentially expressed genes, respectively with 115 genes identified from both analyses. The differential expression of eighteen genes not associated previously with plaque instability was found in stable and unstable regions of the same atherosclerotic plaque; genes affected included the metalloproteinase, ADAMDEC1 (approximately 37-fold), retinoic acid receptor responder-1 (approximately 5-fold), and cysteine protease legumain, a potential activator of MMPs and cathepsins (approximately 3-fold). In addition, matrix metalloproteinase-9 (MMP-9), cathepsin B and legumain were also confirmed at the protein level.

Seo et al. examined a collection of human aorta samples containing varying degrees of atherosclerosis in order to identify gene expression patterns predictive of disease state or potential susceptibility [138]. An analysis of minimally compared to severely diseased sections identified a molecular signature comprising a set of 208 genes whose expression patterns provided the power to discriminate and predict disease states in these aorta samples as well as the extent or severity of the lesion. These genes encode proteins previously suspected to play a role in atherosclerosis including *apoE*, osteopontin, and the oxidized LDL receptor 1 (*olr1*) and genes not previously directly associated with atherosclerosis with functions involved in cell cycle regulation and inflammatory response such as *capg, gm2* ganglioside activator protein, matrix metalloproteinase (MMP) 9 (*mmp9*), and chemokine (C-C motif) receptor-like 2 (*ccrl2*). CapG is a key regulatory protein for actin and membrane phospholipids within migrating phagocytes, *gm2* involved in cell proliferation, adhesion, and chemotaxis, MMP vascular remodeling of the extracellular matrix and *ccrl2* encodes a receptor for monocyte chemotactic protein 1 (MCP1) involved in vascular infiltration by monocytes and intimal hyperplasia. In a second analysis comparing gene profiling in proximal and distal sections of the thoracic aorta, a potential surrogate of disease susceptibility, a group of 28 genes were identified that provided the predictive power in the analysis including superoxide dismutase 3 (*sod3*) and protein C receptor (*procr*), previously associated with atherosclerosis. Most of the genes identified were involved with regulation of transcription and signal transduction such as homeobox-containing genes and *gata2*. Homeobox genes, particularly the C class, have been associated with the increased and decreased expression of ICAM-1 while *gata2* is known to mediate VCAM induction in response to thrombin, estrogen, and glucocorticoids.

In another study, a comprehensive analysis of gene expression of coronary atherosclerosis was undertaken using 51 coronary artery segments isolated from the explanted hearts of 22 cardiac transplant patients and subjected to extensive histological grading according to American Heart Association guidelines prior to hybridization analysis of isolated RNA with a customized 22-K oligonucleotide microarray [139]. This study also made novel use of a systems biology/gene ontology approach to examine pathway interactions based on connectivity (determined by information from the published literature), and ranking (as determined by the significance of differentially regulated genes in the network) resulting in the identification of highly connected "nexus" genes that represent potential candidates for therapeutic targeting and follow-up studies. A critical observation emerging from this study indicated that loss of differentiated SMC gene expression is the primary expression signature of disease progression in atherosclerosis.

Another approach has utilized gene expression analysis of specific cell types derived from patients, eliminating some of the difficulties encountered by dealing with heterogenous tissue samples to be discussed in Chapter 13. One tact has been to compare gene expression profiles of primary cultured ECs from human saphenous vein (SVEC), coronary artery (CAEC) or exposed to atherogenic stimuli (including oxLDL, IL-1β or TNF-α) [140]. This study revealed that a different inherent gene expression program in arterial as compared to venous ECs likely underlies differences in atherosclerotic disease susceptibility. Over 285 genes, representing a broad spectrum of atherosclerosis-related pathways including responses to proliferation, oxidoreductase activity, antiinflammatory responses, cell growth, and hemostasis functions were more highly expressed in untreated SVEC compared to untreated CAEC. In addition, treatment of these cell types with oxLDL induced dramatically greater gene expression responses relating to adhesion, proliferation, and apoptosis pathways in CAEC compared with SVEC, while in contrast, IL-1β and TNF-α activated similar gene expression profiles in both CAEC and SVEC.

Several profiling studies have focused on vascular SMCs and their role in atherosclerosis. Profiling analysis of cultured human vascular SMCs using serial analysis of gene expression (SAGE) technology revealed that SMCs treated with an atherogenic stimulus displayed 105 tags induced and 52 tags repressed greater than fivefold [141]. Among the induced set was the gene for the plasminogen activator inhibitor-2 which had not been associated with atherosclerosis before, and was subsequently localized to atherosclerotic lesions. Zhang et al. compared gene expression profiles in cultured normal human medial vascular SMCs and vascular SMCs from primary atherosclerotic plaques or in stent stenosis (ISS) sites [142]. Specific groups of genes were found to be overexpressed in ISS and plaque vascular SMCs, including cell cycle regulatory proteins and cell matrix and contractile proteins in an analysis verified by Northern blot, rt-PCR and *in situ* hybridization analyses. ISS vascular SMCs exhibited a stable gene expression profile reflecting an intimal pattern, intermediate between that found with normal medial and primary plaque vascular SMCs. Jang et al. [143] stimulated vascular SMCs with TNF-α resulting in upregulation of plasminogen activator inhibitor-2, osteoblast-specific factor 2 and cyclin-dependent kinase 3 while the subsequent addition of the antioxidant α-lipoic acid attenuated their expression.

Other studies have found that uptake of aggregated LDL by cultured aortic SMCs as well as exposure of SMCs to the short chain acyl ceramide derivative N hexanoyl D sphingosine (C6 ceramide) upregulated death-associated protein (DAP) kinase, a positive mediator of apoptotic cell death both at the mRNA and protein level [144]. Overexpression of DAP kinase (approximately 5-fold) in atherosclerotic plaques was also found in an analysis of transcript levels of 205 apoptosis-related genes in human carotid endarterectomy specimens as compared to nonatherosclerotic mammary arteries. Studies of Blaschke et al. [145] with microarray profiling of human coronary vascular SMCs treated with CRP revealed that CRP induced caspase-mediated apoptosis in combination with marked upregulation of the transcript for the growth arrest- and DNA damage-inducible gene 153 (GADD153), a gene involved in growth arrest and apoptosis in vascular and nonvascular cells. The CRP-mediated regulation of GADD153 mRNA expression in vascular SMCs was shown to occur primarily at the post-transcriptional level by mRNA stabilization. A functional role for GADD153 in CRP-induced cell death was supported by the demonstration of reduced CRP-induced apoptosis in these cells by small interfering RNA (siRNA) specifically targeted to GADD153, and by the specific localization of GADD153 to apoptotic vascular SMCs in human coronary lesions.

The role of apoptosis and apoptosis-related genes in atherosclerotic lesions is not entirely straightforward. Functional studies have demonstrated that a subset of cells derived from discrete foci within human atherosclerotic lesions (including SMCs) are resistant to antiproliferative and proapoptotic effects of several stimuli including TGF-β1, hydrocortisone and fas ligation compared to cells from the adjacent media [146–148]. Gene expression analysis has shown that TGF-β-resistant cells exhibited selective loss of Type II receptor expression, which could be partially corrected by retroviral transfection of Type II receptor cDNA [146], while hydrocortisone-resistant cells exhibited selective reduction of the glucocorticoid receptor at both the transcript and protein level primarily localized to the fibrous region of the lesion [147]. Microarray profiling of fas-resistant compared to fas-sensitive cells revealed differential expression of a set of genes including STATs, caspase 1, cyclin D1, Bcl-xL, VDAC2, and BAD [148]. Western blot analysis of sensitive and resistant LDC clonal lines corroborated increases in cyclin D1, STAT6, Bcl-xL, and BAD, with decreased expression of caspase 1. One possible explanation for this cell heterogeneity within plaques is that the apoptotic-resistant phenotype may contribute to plaque stability, vascular repair and the slow proliferation of resistant cell subsets, while sensitive cells within the lesion may be involved in plaque rupture and infarction.

Interestingly, an exaggerated neointimal formation developed in response to mechanical injury, a pathologic hallmark of obliterative vascular disease including primary atherosclerosis, has been described in the aging mouse in association with an increased resistance of vascular SMCs to apoptosis in response to nitric oxide and serum starvation [149]. In addition, aging murine vascular SMCs expressed higher levels of PDGFR-α and greater proliferative response (4-fold increase) to PDGF-BB, compared with young vascular SMCs. The mechanism coupling specific transcriptional expression to the similar phenotypes in vascular aging and atherosclerosis needs to be further delineated particularly in the human.

As a tissue surrogate, freshly isolated blood mononuclear cells from patients undergoing carotid endarterectomy due to atherosclerotic stenosis and from matched healthy subjects were profiled. Transcript levels of the Finkel-Biskis-Jenkins osteosarcoma (FOS) gene in circulating monocytes were found to positively correlate with atherosclerosis severity in patients as well as selectively declined with 3-hydroxy-3-methylglutaryl coenzyme A reductase inhibitor (statin) therapy in healthy subjects [150].

Increased insight into the complicity of specific global regulators on human atherosclerosis and/or CAD has been obtained from studies focusing on their specific expression in blood mononuclear cells from patients, correlated with patient data including lipid levels and severity of disease. While expression levels of genes coding for PPARs (α, γ), CD36, and LDLR showed correlation with the severity of coronary atherosclerosis, the expression level of LXRα exhibited a marked negative correlation with the severity of coronary atherosclerosis in subjects with or without hypercholesterolemia suggesting that it may exert a protective effect against the development of CAD [151].

Further studies have also begun to examine how gene profiles may vary in response to diet and specific pharmacological treatments and may be a useful adjunct in tailoring individual therapies [152]. For instance, as we have previously noted statins have various pleiotropic effects on the treatment of atherosclerosis that are not related to their lipid-lowering effects. In oxidized LDL-treated macrophages, gene profiling revealed that statins can attenuate the oxLDL-mediated increase in the expression of the scavenger receptor CD68 and fatty acid binding protein 4 as well as reducing the expression of HDL-binding protein, apolipoprotein E, and matrix metalloproteinase 9 [153]. Statins also affect genes involved in coagulation, vascular constriction and cell growth in a cell-type-specific manner in vascular ECs and SMCs [154]. In cultured human umbilical vein endothelial cells (HUVECs), they induced integrin β4 and thrombomodulin profoundly while in cultured human coronary artery SMCs, statins induced thrombomodulin and urokinase inhibitor, and potently suppressed the cysteine-rich angiogenic inducer 61 and cyclin B. Many genes related to the cell cycle and/or growth were also regulated in HUVECs and SMCs by the statins.

Therapeutic Approaches

While the complex interactions and balance between proinflammatory and anti-inflammatory cellular and molecular elements constitute a significant component in the evolution of the atherosclerotic plaque with a great deal remaining to be learned, these elements also offer potential targets for treatment or stemming disease progression. For instance, several studies have suggested that the reduction of oxidized lipids promoted by the administration of apolipoprotein A-I and apoA-I mimetic peptides may have therapeutic potential [155, 156]. In animals with hypercholesterolemia, antioxidants can reduce the size of the atherosclerotic lesions, and also can reduce the presence of fatty streaks. The latter observation suggests that antioxidants have an anti-inflammatory effect, perhaps by preventing the upregulation of adhesion molecules by monocytes. Antioxidants can also increase the resistance of human LDL to oxidation generated *ex vivo* in proportion to the vitamin

E content of the plasma. Another potential approach that has gained credence in animal studies is the use of antibodies directed against oxLDL using either active (vaccines) or passive (antibodies) immunization. Studies performed in atherosclerosis-prone mice have shown that both peptide-based vaccines and recombinant IgG targeting epitopes in oxidized LDL significantly reduce atherosclerosis [157]. While *in vitro* studies have shown that antioxidants (e.g., β-carotene, vitamin C and vitamin E) can interfere with selected pathomechanisms of atherosclerosis with protective effect and several animal studies have confirmed such a protective effect *in vivo* (especially after administration of high doses of vitamin E), most placebo-controlled randomized clinical studies for primary or secondary atherosclerotic prevention have failed to show a protective effect even after administration of high doses. Only in subsets of patients with high levels of OS or depletion of natural antioxidant defense systems and at high risk for atherosclerosis has a beneficial effect been suggested [158–160].

The use of statin treatment has been shown to provide endothelial stabilization although its mechanisms are not yet clear. The stabilization of endothelial function could result from elevated eNOS activity, reduced ROS production, inhibition of oxLDL action, increased LDL resistance to oxidation, or other undetermined mechanisms [161, 162]. Multiple studies investigating the role of high-dose statin therapy have reinforced the notion that statins have anti-inflammatory and antioxidant properties that go well beyond their lipid-lowering effects [163].

Several lipoprotein-modifying agents have either been recently released, or are still in various phases of development in atherosclerotic intervention. These include agents that reduce LDL-C levels by mechanisms other than HMG-CoA inhibition (such as cholesterol absorption inhibitors, Acyl-CoA cholesterol acyl transferase inhibitors, sterol-regulating binding protein cleavage activating protein ligands, microsomal triglyceride transfer protein inhibitors, LDL receptor activators and farnesoid X receptor antagonists) and agents that raise HDL-C or improve cholesterol efflux (such as CETP inhibitors, retinoid X receptor selective agonists, specific PPAR agonists and estrogen like compounds) [164]. Dissecting the primary mechanism by which these approaches act is often difficult. For instance, it is known that CETP inhibition increases HDL-C and reduces LDL-C levels coincident with beneficial increases in both HDL and LDL particle size [165]. Moreover, CETP inhibition has been recently shown to increase antioxidant enzymes associated with HDL, and is associated with decreased LDL oxidation. This is consistent with CETP lipid transfer activity and its role in reverse cholesterol transport.

Another tactic for intervention employs blocking key aspects of inflammatory pathway including the chemokine receptors involved in leukocyte migration and recruitment from the microcirculation into the inflammatory tissues [166]. For example, blockade of CXC chemokine receptor 2 (CXCR2) implicated in numerous inflammatory disorders substantially reduces leukocyte recruitment, tissue damage and mortality. Selective CXCR2 inhibitors are now being tested in clinical trials [167].

Another viable target for therapy that is being vigorously pursued is the use of high-affinity ligands such as the thiazolidinedione class of drugs to treat atheromatous lesions. It is also noteworthy that PPAR-γ agonism has been found to be an important target in the therapeutic treatment of metabolic syndrome-related conditions [168].

The Role of Altered Immunity in Atherosclerosis in Aging

In 1975, Pierre Grabar proposed that age-associated increase in serum autoantibodies was stimulated by "senescent" epitopes that marked molecules and cells for immune elimination in order to maintain molecular and cellular homeostasis [169]. As we have previously noted, there is considerable evidence that cellular immunity influences the development and progression of atherosclerosis [170]. The concept of protective autoimmunity against atherosclerosis was suggested by an earlier clinical report that post-traumatic splenectomy significantly increased the risk of humans dying from ischemic heart disease [171]. A more recent report indicates that splenectomy also increases atherosclerosis in ApoE-deficient mice and this enhanced development of atherosclerosis could be prevented by transferring syngeneic splenic B cells to splenectomized Apo-E-deficient mice [172]. ApoE-deficient animals are known to have high levels of oxLDL and to have B1 cells that produce anti-oxLDL autoantibodies. These B1 cells are found in the spleen and high titers of IgG autoantibodies to oxLDL developed in splenectomized mice reconstituted with splenic B cells. Such autoantibodies have been shown to inhibit the uptake of oxLDL by macrophages, a key step in atherogenesis, and protect animals from atherosclerosis. The autoantibodies to oxLDL produced by splenic B1 cells express the T15 idiotype and the same unmutated S107 and Vk22 variable genes for the heavy and light chain, respectively, expressed by natural anti-phosphorylcholine (PC) antibodies [173]. Although T15 anti-PC antibodies can be induced by pneumococci and are known to protect mice against pneumococcal infection, their appearance in serum of mice reared in germ-free conditions implies that their development can also be stimulated by non-bacterial determinants. Thus, T15 antibodies recognize not only the PC epitope on pneumococci but also oxLDL and oxidized molecules on the membranes of apoptotic ECs. Even though the immune response to foreign antigens decreases with age, the number of anti-PC antibody forming B cells increases with age, despite the fact that the stimulus for this antibody was thought to be foreign bacteria [174]. However, with the recent recognition that the appearance of anti-PC antibodies occurs in germ-free animals and can be driven by autologous oxidized epitopes on LDL or cell membranes, it suggests that the age-associated increase in anti-PC antibodies may reflect the increase of an autoantibody. However, the genes that code for the anti-PC antibodies are different in young versus old mice. The vast majority of anti-PC antibodies produced in young mice express the T15 idiotype while in old mice only a small minority of anti-PC antibodies expresses the T15 idiotype.9 Thus the impaired production of T-15 idiotype anti-PC antibodies may contribute to the increased susceptibility of old mice to both atherosclerosis and pneumococcal infection. The same amount of anti-PC antibody produced by old mice does not protect naïve young mice from challenge with pneumococci as well as anti-PC antibody from young mice [175]. The age-associated impairment in protection by anti-PC antibody from pneumococcal challenge appears to be due to the lower affinity of the non-T15 compared to T15 anti-PC antibody for the pneumococci. Whether the affinity of non-T15 idiotype antibody is also lower than T15 idiotype antibodies for oxLDL is not known; such a finding might explain an age-associated decline in autoantibody-mediated protection from atherosclerosis.

Acute Coronary Syndrome in the Elderly

Elderly persons and women are generally underrepresented in randomized controlled trials and recent data have suggested that attempts at making cardiovascular trials more inclusive by including the elderly appear to have had limited success [176]. As expected, the prevalence of CAD is very high in elderly patients [177, 178]. Elderly patients with ACS including unstable angina and non-ST segment myocardial infarction (NSTEMI) have a very high prevalence of coronary risk factors [179]. Age ≥75 years constitutes one of the seven prognostic variables in the Thrombolysis In Myocardial Infarction (TIMI) risk score [180]. In general, the management of ACS in the elderly patients should not differ a great deal from that the younger patients in terms of management according to contemporary management guidelines [181, 182].

A prospective study was conducted in 177 consecutive patients aged 70–94 years, hospitalized for ACS [179, 183]. The 177 patients included 91 women and 86 men. Unstable angina was diagnosed in 95 of the 177 (54%) elderly subjects, NSTEMI in 61 (34%) and ST-segment elevation myocardial infarction (STEMI) in 21 (12%). All 177 elderly patients underwent coronary angiography and the coronary anatomy of these elderly subjects is summarized in Table 8.3. Significant obstructive CAD was present in 87%, non-obstructive CAD in 11% and no CAD in 2%. Coronary

Table 8.3 Prevalence and severity of coronary artery disease in elderly subjects hospitalized with acute coronary syndrome*

	Women (n = 91)	Men (n = 86)
Obstructive CAD	73 (80%)	81 (94%)
Nonobstructive CAD	15 (17%)	4 (5%)
No CAD	3 (3%)	1 (1%)
1-vessel CAD	26 (29%)	25 (29%)
2-vessel CAD	23 (25%)	17 (20%)
3-vessel CAD	24 (26%)	39 (45%)
Left Main CAD	2 (2%)	8 (9%)
Left anterior descending or diagonal CAD	53 (58%)	65 (76%)
Left circumflex or obtuse marginal CAD	41 (45%)	53 (62%)
Right CAD	48 (53%)	56 (65%)

**Adapted from Am J Cardiol 2002; 90:1145–1147.*

revascularization was performed in 56% of women, 52% of men, 52% of whites and 64% of African Americans.

Current medical management of STEMI includes intensive antithrombotic therapy, such as clopidogrel, enoxaparin, or unfractionated heparin. The choice of therapy has recently been influenced by the Enoxaparin and Thrombolysis Reperfusion for Acute Myocardial Infarction Treatment (ExTRACT) – Thrombolysis in Myocardial Infarction (TIMI) 25 study [184]. This trial compared enoxaparin versus unfractionated heparin (UFH) as adjunctive therapy for fibrinolysis in STEMI. At 30 days, death or MI was significantly reduced with enoxaparin, as was death, MI, or urgent revascularization; nonfatal MIs were reduced 33% in the enoxaparin group. ExTRACT-TIMI 25 also showed a modest increase in major bleeds associated with enoxaparin (1.4–2.1%) but no increase in intracranial hemorrhages, which occurred in about 0.7% of the patient population. For every 1,000 patients treated with enoxaparin, there would be 28 fewer major cardiovascular events at the cost of four additional major bleeds and no increase in nonfatal intracranial hemorrhage compared to UFH. However, enoxaparin reportedly increases the risk of major bleeding and intracranial hemorrhage in elderly patients (> 75 years of age) [185].

ExTRACT-TIMI 25 devised a specific regimen that adjusted the enoxaparin dosing strategy according to patient age and renal function [186]. For patients younger than 75 years of age, enoxaparin (or matching placebo) was given as a fixed 30 mg IV bolus followed 15 minutes later by a subcutaneous injection of 1.0 mg/kg, with injections administered every 12 hours. For patients at least 75 years of age, the IV bolus was eliminated and the subcutaneous dose was reduced to 0.75 mg/kg every 12 hours. For the first two subcutaneous injections, a maximum of 100 mg (for patients <75 years old) or 75 mg (for those at least 75 years old) was administered. To reduce the risk of bleeding, the IV bolus was omitted for patients who received open-label UFH (at least 4000 U) within 3 hours before randomization. Moreover, for patients with an estimated creatinine clearance of <30 ml/min, the dose was modified to 1.0 mg/kg every 24 hours. The double-blind subcutaneous injections of enoxaparin or matching placebo were to continue until hospital discharge or for a maximum of 8 days (whichever came first). This modified dosing regimen led to a similar reduction in death and MI in the elderly patients compared to younger patients. The number of patients needed to treat to prevent an event was also similar in both groups: 50 patients in the 75 years group versus 67 patients in the group that was 75 years of age or older.

As in the case of STEMI, the elderly are often excluded from clinical trials of non-ST-segment elevation (NSTE)-ACS and are underrepresented in clinical registries. To explore the treatment and outcomes of patients with NSTE-ACS age ≥ 90 years, investigators used data from the CRUSADE registry to study 5,557 patients with NSTE-ACS age ≥ 90 years and compared their baseline characteristics, treatment patterns, and in-hospital outcomes with a cohort age 75–89 years (n = 46,270) [187]. Compared with the younger patients, the older elderly were less likely to be diabetic, smokers, or obese. Among patients without contraindications, the older elderly were less likely to receive glycoprotein IIb/IIIa inhibitors and statins during the first 24 hours and were less likely to undergo cardiac catheterization within 48 hours. The older elderly were also more likely to die (12.0% vs. 7.8%) and experienced more frequent adverse events (26.8% vs. 21.3%) during the hospitalization, differences that persisted after adjustment for baseline patient and hospital characteristics. Increasing adherence to guideline-recommended therapies was associated with both increased bleeding and a graded reduction in risk-adjusted in-hospital mortality across both age groups (Fig. 8.1). These findings therefore underscore the importance of optimizing care patterns for even the oldest patients with NSTE-ACS, while exploring novel approaches to reduce the risk of bleeding in this rapidly expanding patient population.

Myocarditis in the Elderly Population

Myocarditis is an uncommon heart disease. There is general consensus from experimental studies that autoimmune mechanisms follow viral infection, resulting in inflammation and necrosis of the myocardium [188]. In humans, ongoing myocardial inflammation may result in dilated cardiomyopathy (DCM), restrictive cardiomyopathy, or acute left ventricular (LV) failure without dilatation (fulminant myocarditis) [189]. Myocarditis is histologically characterized by both an active inflammatory cellular infiltrate within the myocardium and associated myocyte necrosis (the Dallas pathologic criteria) [190]. Although many clinicians and pathologists consider the Dallas criteria restrictive, this classification has established uniform histologic criteria for diagnosis and has reduced the wide variation in reported rates of this disease. Although the inflammatory infiltrate is lymphocytic in more than 90% of cases, eosinophilic infiltration or giant cell formation may occasionally be seen. The clinical features of myocarditis are quite varied, ranging from asymptomatic electrocardiographic abnormalities observed during viral Coxsackie B outbreaks in the community

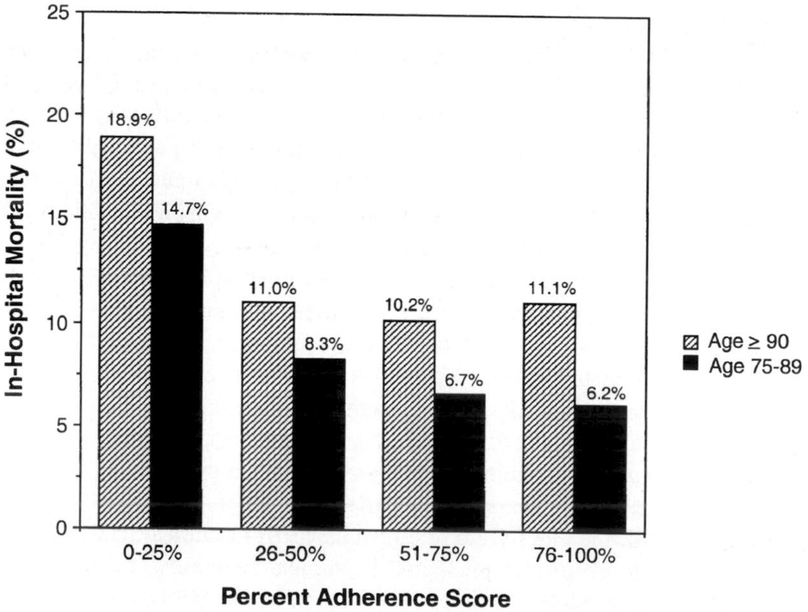

Fig. 8.1 Relationship between in-hospital mortality across each age group with increasing adherence to recommended therapies from the CRUSADE registry
(Adapted from J Am Coll Cardiol 2007;49:1790–7).

to severe DCM with fulminant HF leading to death or need for cardiac replacement therapy [191]. Myocarditis may also cause ventricular dysrhythmias or heart block or mimic acute MI [192]. Both acute and chronic DCM may result from inflammatory heart disease. The histological differentiation of myocarditis from idiopathic DCM remains problematic, because several published series suggest no difference in long-term prognosis, regardless of the presence or absence of myocardial inflammation. Nonetheless, some clinicians believe that myocarditis is a potentially reversible form of cardiomyopathy and continue to perform endomyocardial biopsy searching for its presence. Controversy also continues to surround the best approach to the management of patients considered having myocarditis and thus far controlled trials have failed to demonstrate any significant benefits from immunomodulatory therapy [189].

Recent population-based studies suggest that the proportion of deaths caused by myocarditis appears to be higher in children and younger adults than in older patients. To study the incidence of fatal myocarditis in the general population, one study retrospectively collected all death certificates recording myocarditis as the underlying cause of death in Finland in 1970–1998 [193]. The incidence of myocarditis and its proportion of all deaths were calculated from 141.4 million person-years and 1.35 million deaths. Myocarditis was recorded as the underlying cause of death in 639 cases. The death certificate-based incidence was 0.46 per 100,000 person-years, and it caused 0.47 of 1,000 deaths. The incidence of 0.51 in males was higher than the incidence of 0.42 in females, the odds ratio being 1.34. Importantly, the proportion of deaths caused by myocarditis was highest (up to six of 1,000 deaths) in children and adults aged less than 45 years, when compared to older patients. Because previous histopathologic reanalysis showed that only 32% of cases fulfilled the Dallas criteria, these investigators estimated the incidence of histopathologically certain fatal myocarditis to be 0.15 per 100,000. The death certificate-based incidence of fatal myocarditis was found to be 0.46 per 100,000, and the histopathologically corrected incidence was 0.15 per 100,000.

Hypertension in the Elderly

Hypertension is an increasing clinical and public health problem worldwide [194, 195]. Increasing age is a major risk factor for developing hypertension, and is also a strong confounder of its independent influence on cardiovascular and renal events. This growing group of relatively active and healthy elderly people is at high risk for hypertension, its treatment, and its adverse consequences, including stroke and HF. In the analysis of nearly a million individuals in 61 epidemiological studies followed for an average of 13.3 years, those with blood pressures (BPs) in the highest decile had roughly the same risk of death from either coronary heart disease or stroke as people who were 20 years older, but who had BPs in the lowest decile [196]. In Framingham the Heart Study, the lifetime risk for 55- or 65-year-old men or women to develop hypertension was 90% [197]; among those who survived to ages 65–89 years, systolic BP elevations were found in 87% of the hypertensive men and 93% of the hypertensive women. In an analysis of the Framingham data set, classification of hypertensive people over age 60 years into the appropriate BP stages was done correctly in 99% of the cases using only the systolic BP; diastolic BP was much less useful (at 47%) [198]. These data highlight the great public health importance of systolic BP, particularly among those older than about 53 years. In these older individuals, systolic BP is a much better predictor of hypertensive target-organ damage and future CV and renal events than is diastolic BP [199, 200]. Overall, each 20 mm Hg increase in systolic BP doubles the risk of CV death [201]. Systolic BP is less likely to be controlled than diastolic [202], according to NHANES data from both 1999–2000 and 2001–2002, 65% of those with treated but uncontrolled hypertension in the US are 60 years of age and older [203]. Antihypertensive drug therapy is effective in reducing the risk of CV events across the full age range, including individuals older than 80 years [204, 205].

The public health problem of isolated systolic hypertension has been addressed in part by clinical trials that expressly enrolled individuals with only elevated systolic BP. The first of these was the Systolic Hypertension in the Elderly Program (SHEP), which randomized 4736 people >65 years of age to initial treatment with low-dose chlorthalidone or placebo. The primary end point was fatal or nonfatal stroke, which was 36% lower in those treated with chlorthalidone, despite a 44% prevalence of antihypertensive drug therapy by the end of the study among those assigned to placebo [206]. All subtypes of stroke were equally prevented, and there was evidence that achieving a lower systolic BP (<150 mm Hg) was more effective than leaving the BP higher (<160 mm Hg) [207]. Cardiovascular events were also significantly reduced (by 25%), as well as HF (by 49%) [208]. Placebo-controlled clinical trials involving older patients with isolated systolic hypertension in Europe [209] and China [210] yielded remarkably similar results regarding stroke reduction. A meta-analysis of 15,693 older patients with isolated systolic hypertension in 8 clinical trials against placebo lasting (on average) 3.8 years was published in 2000 [211]. The average age of the patients was 70 years, and the initial BP (174/83 mm Hg) was lowered, on average by 10.4/4.1 mm Hg with active treatment. The investigators concluded that active drug therapy had significant benefits; stroke was reduced by 30%, all cardiovascular events by 26%, MIs by 23%, and all-cause death by 13%. Subgroup analyses of more recent clinical trials including Losartan For Endpoint reduction (LIFE) [212] and the Antihypertensive and Lipid-Lowering Treatment to Prevent Heart Attack Trial (ALLHAT) [213] are consistent with these estimates.

Because no large-scale clinical trial has yet been done in hypertensive people >80 years of age, the best available data come from a meta-analysis of all 1670 hypertensive patients in seven clinical trials that compared active drug therapy versus placebo or no treatment [214]. Octogenarians comprised 13% of the overall population in these trials, averaged 83±3 years of age. Patients had an average BP of 180/84 mm Hg at enrollment and 70% were women. In this meta-analysis, there were 57 strokes and 34 deaths among 874 actively treated patients, compared with 77 strokes and 28 stroke deaths among 796 controls, representing 1 nonfatal stroke prevented for about 100 patients treated each year. In terms of relative risk, active drug therapy significantly reduced strokes by 34%, HF by 39%, and major CV events by 22%. Non-significant differences were also found for coronary events (reduced by 22%), but mortality and cardiovascular death were higher, by 6% and 1%, respectively (Fig. 8.2).

The outcome benefits of drug therapy for hypertension may be different in the elderly when compared to younger subjects. Early clinical trials in hypertension enrolled very few individuals over 80 years of age. An earlier study analyzed 13 trials involving 16,564 elderly persons aged 60 years and older and compared therapeutic benefits of medications (e.g., β-blockers or diuretics) with effects in younger subjects [215]. There were 13 trials involving 16,564 elderly persons (age 60 years and older), 6 of which proved to be high quality. The prevalence of cardiovascular risk factors, CVD and competing comorbid diseases was lower among trial participants than the general population of hypertensive elderly persons. When the six large high-quality trials were combined, trial results showed 43 subjects (95% confidence interval [CI], 31–69) and 61 subjects (95% CI, 39–141) needed to be treated for 5 years to prevent one cerebrovascular event and one coronary heart disease event, respectively. Including the other seven trials did not change the results significantly. Only 18 subjects (95% CI, 14–25) needed to be treated to prevent one cardiovascular event (cerebrovascular or cardiac). Twelve trials in primarily younger and middle-aged adults involved approximately 33,000 persons. For all outcomes except cardiac mortality, two to four times as many of the younger subjects as the older subjects needed to be treated for 5 years to prevent morbid and mortal events. No significant effect on cardiac mortality was seen among younger subjects, while 78 older subjects (95% CI, 50–180) needed to be treated to prevent a fatal cardiac event. Thus, randomized trials suggested that treating healthy older persons with hypertension is highly efficacious. Five-year morbidity and mortality benefits derived from trials are greater for older than younger subjects.

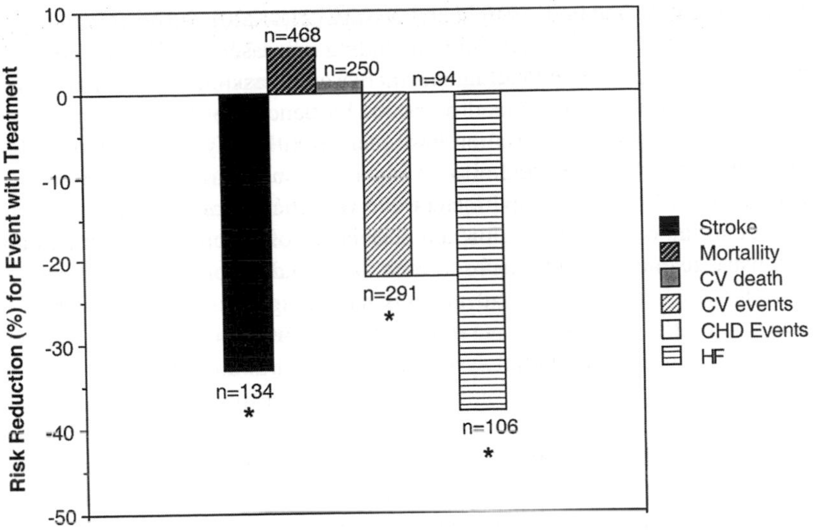

Fig. 8.2 Meta-analysis of 1670 hypertensive subjects >80 years of age from 7 clinical trials
$^*p < 0.05$, CV: Cardiovascular; CHD: Coronary heart disease; HF: Heart failure.

The Hypertension in the Very Elderly Trial (HYVET) is a randomized, double-blind, placebo-controlled trial designed to assess the benefits of treating over 2000 very elderly patients with hypertension [216]. HYVET will compare placebo with a low dose diuretic (indapamide sustained release 1.5 mg daily) and additional angiotensin-converting enzyme (ACE) inhibitor (perindopril) therapy if required. The primary endpoint will be incident fatal and non-fatal stroke during 5 years of follow up. The HYVET pilot trial recruited 1283 patients with systolic and diastolic BPs exceeding 160/95 mm Hg, ≥80 years of age, and randomized them to either a diuretic (usually bendroflumethiazide; n=426), an ACE inhibitor (usually lisinopril; n=431), or placebo (n=426). Mean age was 84 years; and 63% were women. The initial BP was 181/100, but the average follow-up was only 1.1 years. Preliminary results have been presented but not yet published. The results of the meta-analysis by Staessen et al. indicate that the number of deaths and cardiovascular deaths were slightly lower with ACE inhibitor treatment (27 and 22, respectively) than with diuretic treatment (30 and 23) [217]. These data, however, are still very preliminary.

A large body of data has been gathered from 5710 patients ≥ 80 years of age in the INdividual Data ANalysis of Antihypertensive (INDANA) meta-analysis, ALLHAT, and HYVET pilot to provide an initial estimate of the impact of antihypertensive therapy in the elderly, but the results have not been commingled. The results in octogenarians in the last 2 studies have not yet been published, and the number and outcomes are still not in the public domain. When the 2953 patients in the main HYVET trial have completed the follow up, the number will be 5053. Given the current data, it is unlikely that antihypertensive drug treatment will be associated with a significant difference in all-cause mortality among subjects ≥ 80 years of age. Nevertheless, currently available meta-analyses do suggest that antihypertensive drug therapy results in a significant prevention of stroke and HF, 2 events of primary concern to many elderly individuals.

Genetics and Environmental Factors in Essential or Primary Hypertension

A number of family and epidemiological studies support the view that hypertension arises from a complex interplay between genetic and environmental factors including dietary sodium intake, hypertension phenotype. Several studies have recently suggested that blood pressure is governed by multiple genetic loci each with a relatively modest effect [239, 240]. The number of human hypertension loci has recently been proposed to be in the order of tens of genes each with a relatively modest effect on hypertension in the population at large (e.g., relative risk of 1.2–1.5) [241, 242]. In contrast, dramatic progress has been made in our understanding of several forms of secondary hypertension in which a number of single-genes and defined mutations have been implicated.

Conclusion

In this chapter, we surveyed much of the current literature to provide the reader with an overall perspective concerning the pathogenesis and treatment of these chronic cardiovascular diseases in which age has been clearly identified as a risk factor. In doing so, we presented both findings from molecular and clinical studies to attempt to highlight the most critical components and pathways involved. The polygenic nature of both diseases as well as the important contribution of numerous environmental factors has made the precise evaluation of specific component's roles challenging and clearly much remains to be learned in both the realms of gene-gene and gene-environment interactions. Findings with genomics, proteomics and gene expression profiling have continued to reveal critical insights relevant to both the roles of aging, genes and environment in these disorders and will continue to refine our understanding of how diet, exercise and pharmacological intervention can most effectively be applied to treatment and potential reversal of these diseases and should provide impetus for a more personalized approach to medicine. Increasing information in these areas will undoubtedly impact the approaches to treatment and earlier diagnosis allowing the elderly to enjoy their later years with a higher quality of life.

Summary

- With advancing age, a series of structural, architectural and compositional modifications takes place in the vasculature including vessel diameter increase, thickening of intimal and medial layers, increased content of blood-derived leukocytes and "activated" smooth muscle cells (SMCs) in the subendothelial space, accumulation of extracellular matrix (ECM) particularly rich in glycosaminoglycans, with increased collagen content and with progressively disorganized, thinner, and fragmented elastin fibers.
- Animal experiments have demonstrated that aging predisposes the vasculature to advanced atherosclerotic disease and vessel injury and that this predisposition is a function of age-associated changes in the vessel wall itself.
- Compared to vessels from young animals, older ones show a greater reactivity to mechanical injury and to chronic insults.
- Atherosclerosis is a complex disease caused by multiple genetic and environmental factors and gene-environment interactions involving diverse physiological processes and a wide spectrum of cell types and organs even beyond the vasculature.
- Molecular mechanisms of atherosclerosis involve lipid metabolism, inflammatory signaling and thrombosis as well as immunity and oxidative stress (OS). Risk factors involved in these areas such as dyslipidemia and diabetes, pro- and anti-coagulant factors have provided information about genes, which play a significant role in establishing the risk of developing atherosclerosis.
- Over 100 genes have been identified that influence the development of atherosclerotic lesions underlining the complex and polygenic nature of this disorder.
- Rare monogenic forms of atherosclerosis resulting from dyslipidemias have allowed the identification of genes and pathways involved some which play a role as well in more common form(s)

of atherosclerosis, and have clearly demonstrated the effects of endogenously increased LDL on the evolution of atherosclerosis.

- Most studies concur that excess serum LDL in individuals from western countries is related to environmental factors such as diet as compared to changes in HDL, which are primarily genetic.
- Endothelial cell (EC) dysfunction injury is an early event leading to atherosclerosis and is promoted by elevated and modified LDL, hypertension, smoking, diabetes mellitus, elevated plasma homocysteine, infectious microorganisms such as *Chlamydia pneumoniae*, and various combinations of these or other factors,
- Oxidized LDL (oxLDL) is a pivotal factor in the initial endothelial damage by its infiltration into the arterial endothelium, and also involved in recruitment and activation of inflammatory elements including monocytes and macrophages into the atherosclerotic lesion.
- The role of inflammatory and immune pathways and common elements (e.g., TLR, inflammatory genes, CRP) in both longevity and atherosclerosis may provide further insights concerning the relationship between age and atherosclerosis susceptibility.
- A number of markers of inflammation, lipid dysfunction and endothelial dysfunction have become increasingly useful as reliable biomarkers of atherosclerosis.
- Gene expression profiling has begun to provide insights into the elements (and sequence of events) involved in the pathogenesis of atherosclerosis, as well as potential landmarks for diagnosis and therapeutic management, and delineating critical targets for therapeutic intervention.
- Age is an independent and critical factor in the development of essential/primary hypertension, a polygenic disorder with a variety of environmental determinants including diet (especially salt), body mass/obesity.
- A variety of genes involved in arterial remodeling pathways, intracellular signaling and the renin-angiotensin pathways have been identified which have modest effects at best on the development of hypertension and which are often modulated by environmental factors and population-specific indicating the presence of substantial gene-gene (e.g., modifier genes) and gene-environment interactions in defining hypertensive phenotype.
- Hypertension may also cause accelerating aging including endothelial and endothelial progenitor cell (EPC) senescence and increased apoptosis and cell death leading to arterial and cardiac remodeling.

References

1. Lundberg MS, Crow MT. Age-related changes in the signaling and function of vascular smooth muscle cells. Exp Gerontol 1999;34:549–557
2. Bilato C, Crow MT. Atherosclerosis and the vascular biology of aging. Aging (Milano) 1996;8:221–234
3. Pauly RR, Bilato C, Sollott SJ, Monticone R, Kelly PT, Lakatta EG, Crow MT. Role of calcium/calmodulin-dependent protein kinase II in the regulation of vascular smooth muscle cell migration. Circulation 1995;91:1107–1115
4. Lusis AJ. Atherosclerosis. Nature 2000;407:233–241
5. Rader DJ, Cohen J, Hobbs HH. Monogenic hypercholesterolemia: new insights in pathogenesis and treatment. J Clin Invest 2003;111:1795–1803
6. Goldstein JL, Brown MS. Regulation of low-density lipoprotein receptors: implications for pathogenesis and therapy of hypercholesterolemia and atherosclerosis. Circulation 1987;76:504–507
7. Soria LF, Ludwig EH, Clarke HR, Vega GL, Grundy SM, McCarthy BJ. Association between a specific apolipoprotein B mutation and familial defective apolipoprotein B-100. Proc Natl Acad Sci USA 1989;86: 587–591
8. Abifadel M, Varret M, Rabes JP, Allard D, Ouguerram K, Devillers M, Cruaud C, Benjannet S, Wickham L, Erlich D, Derre A, Villeger L, Farnier M, Beucler I, Bruckert E, Chambaz J, Chanu B, Lecerf JM, Luc G, Moulin P, Weissenbach J, Prat A, Krempf M, Junien C, Seidah NG, Boileau C. Mutations in PCSK9 cause autosomal dominant hypercholesterolemia. Nat Genet 2003;34:154–156

9. Soutar AK, Naoumova RP, Traub LM. Genetics, clinical phenotype, and molecular cell biology of autosomal recessive hypercholesterolemia. Arterioscler Thromb Vasc Biol 2003;23:1963–1970
10. Garcia CK, Wilund K, Arca M, Zuliani G, Fellin R, Maioli M, Calandra S, Bertolini S, Cossu F, Grishin N, Barnes R, Cohen JC, Hobbs HH. Autosomal recessive hypercholesterolemia caused by mutations in a putative LDL receptor adaptor protein. Science 2001;292:1394–1398
11. Pullinger CR, Eng C, Salen G, Shefer S, Batta AK, Erickson SK, Verhagen A, Rivera CR, Mulvihill SJ, Malloy MJ, Kane JP. Human cholesterol 7alpha-hydroxylase (CYP7A1) deficiency has a hypercholesterolemic phenotype. J Clin Invest 2002;110:109–117
12. McGill HC Jr, McMahan CA, Kruski AW, Mott GE. Relationship of lipoprotein cholesterol concentrations to experimental atherosclerosis in baboons. Arteriosclerosis 1981;1:3–12
13. Kannel WB, Castelli WP, Gordon T. Cholesterol in the prediction of atherosclerotic disease. New perspectives based on the Framingham study. Ann Intern Med 1979;90:85–91
14. Hoff HF, Bradley WA, Heideman CL, Gaubatz JW, Karagas MD, Gotto AM Jr. Characterization of low density lipoprotein-like particle in the human aorta from grossly normal and atherosclerotic regions. Biochim Biophys Acta 1979;573:361–374
15. Grundy SM. Role of low-density lipoproteins in atherogenesis and development of coronary heart disease. Clin Chem 1995;41:139–146
16. Joossens JV. Mechanisms of hypercholesterolemia and atherosclerosis. Acta Cardiol Suppl 1988;29:63–83
17. Kesaniemi YA, Grundy SM. Increased low density lipoprotein production associated with obesity. Arteriosclerosis 1983;3:170–177
18. Ericsson S, Eriksson M, Vitols S, Einarsson K, Berglund L, Angelin B. Influence of age on the metabolism of plasma low density lipoproteins in healthy males. J Clin Invest 1991;87:591–596
19. Kreisberg RA, Kasim S. Cholesterol metabolism and aging. Am J Med 1987;82:54–60
20. Brooks-Wilson A, Marcil M, Clee SM, Zhang LH, Roomp K, van Dam M, Yu L, Brewer C, Collins JA, Molhuizen HO, Loubser O, Ouelette BF, Fichter K, Ashbourne-Excoffon KJ, Sensen CW, Scherer S, Mott S, Denis M, Martindale D, Frohlich J, Morgan K, Koop B, Pimstone S, Kastelein JJ, Genest J Jr, Hayden MR. Mutations in ABC1 in Tangier disease and familial high-density lipoprotein deficiency. Nat Genet 1999;22: 336–345
21. Bodzioch M, Orso E, Klucken J, Langmann T, Bottcher A, Diederich W, Drobnik W, Barlage S, Buchler C, Porsch-Ozcurumez M, Kaminski WE, Hahmann HW, Oette K, Rothe G, Aslanidis C, Lackner KJ, Schmitz G. The gene encoding ATP-binding cassette transporter 1 is mutated in Tangier disease. Nat Genet 1999;22: 347–351
22. Brousseau ME, Schaefer EJ, Dupuis J, Eustace B, Van Eerdewegh P, Goldkamp AL, Thurston LM, FitzGerald MG, Yasek-McKenna D, O'Neill G, Eberhart GP, Weiffenbach B, Ordovas JM, Freeman MW, Brown RH Jr, Gu JZ. Novel mutations in the gene encoding ATP-binding cassette 1 in four tangier disease kindreds. J Lipid Res 2000;41:433–441
23. Remaley AT, Rust S, Rosier M, Knapper C, Naudin L, Broccardo C, Peterson KM, Koch C, Arnould I, Prades C, Duverger N, Funke H, Assman G, Dinger M, Dean M, Chimini G, Santamarina-Fojo S, Fredrickson DS, Denefle P, Brewer HB Jr. Human ATP-binding cassette transporter 1 (ABC1): genomic organization and identification of the genetic defect in the original Tangier disease kindred. Proc Natl Acad Sci USA 1999;96: 12685–12690
24. Klein HG, Santamarina-Fojo S, Duverger N, Clerc M, Dumon MF, Albers JJ, Marcovina S, Brewer HB Jr. Fish eye syndrome: a molecular defect in the lecithin-cholesterol acyltransferase (LCAT) gene associated with normal alpha-LCAT-specific activity. Implications for classification and prognosis. J Clin Invest 1993;92:479–485
25. Kuivenhoven JA, Stalenhoef AF, Hill JS, Demacker PN, Errami A, Kastelein JJ, Pritchard PH. Two novel molecular defects in the LCAT gene are associated with fish eye disease. Arterioscler Thromb Vasc Biol 1996;16: 294–303
26. Assmann G, Gotto AM Jr. HDL cholesterol and protective factors in atherosclerosis. Circulation 2004;109: III8–III14
27. Caslake MJ, Packard CJ. Lipoprotein-associated phospholipase A2 (platelet-activating factor acetylhydrolase) and cardiovascular disease. Curr Opin Lipidol 2003;14:347–352
28. Wilson PW, Anderson KM, Harris T, Kannel WB, Castelli WP. Determinants of change in total cholesterol and HDL-C with age: the Framingham Study. J Gerontol 1994;49:M252–M257
29. Traissac T, Salzmann M, Rainfray M, Emeriau JP, Bourdel-Marchasson I. [Significance of cholesterol levels in patients 75 years or older]. Presse Med. 2005;34:1525–1532
30. Weverling-Rijnsburger AW, Jonkers IJ, van Exel E, Gussekloo J, Westendorp RG. High-density vs low-density lipoprotein cholesterol as the risk factor for coronary artery disease and stroke in old age. Arch Intern Med 2003;163:1549–1554
31. Barzilai N, Atzmon G, Schechter C, Schaefer EJ, Cupples AL, Lipton R, Cheng S, Shuldiner AR. Unique lipoprotein phenotype and genotype associated with exceptional longevity. JAMA 2003;290:2030–2040

32. Barbagallo CM, Averna MR, Frada G, Noto D, Cavera G, Notarbartolo A. Lipoprotein profile and high-density lipoproteins: subfractions distribution in centenarians. Gerontology 1998;44:106–110
33. Arai Y, Hirose N, Nakazawa S, Yamamura K, Shimizu K, Takayama M, Ebihara Y, Osono Y, Homma S. Lipoprotein metabolism in Japanese centenarians: effects of apolipoprotein E polymorphism and nutritional status. J Am Geriatr Soc 2001;49:1434–1441
34. Middelberg RP, Spector TD, Swaminathan R, Snieder H. Genetic and environmental influences on lipids, lipoproteins, and apolipoproteins: effects of menopause. Arterioscler Thromb Vasc Biol 2002;22:1142–1147
35. Middelberg RP, Martin NG, Whitfield JB. Longitudinal genetic analysis of plasma lipids. Twin Res Hum Genet 2006;9:550–557
36. Inazu A, Brown ML, Hesler CB, Agellon LB, Koizumi J, Takata K, Maruhama Y, Mabuchi H, Tall AR. Increased high-density lipoprotein levels caused by a common cholesteryl-ester transfer protein gene mutation. N Engl J Med 1990;323:1234–1238
37. Yamashita S, Hui DY, Wetterau JR, Sprecher DL, Harmony JA, Sakai N, Matsuzawa Y, Tarui S. Characterization of plasma lipoproteins in patients heterozygous for human plasma cholesteryl ester transfer protein (CETP) deficiency: plasma CETP regulates high-density lipoprotein concentration and composition. Metabolism 1991;40:756–763
38. Hirano K, Yamashita S, Kuga Y, Sakai N, Nozaki S, Kihara S, Arai T, Yanagi K, Takami S, Menju M, Ishigami M, Yoshida Y, Kameda-Takemura K, Hayashi K, Matsuzawa Y. Atherosclerotic disease in marked hyperalphalipoproteinemia. Combined reduction of cholesteryl ester transfer protein and hepatic triglyceride lipase. Arterioscler Thromb Vasc Biol 1995;15:1849–1856
39. de Grooth GJ, Klerkx AH, Stroes ES, Stalenhoef AF, Kastelein JJ, Kuivenhoven JA. A review of CETP and its relation to atherosclerosis. J Lipid Res 2004;45:1967–1974
40. Stein O, Stein Y. Lipid transfer proteins (LTP) and atherosclerosis. Atherosclerosis 2005;178:217–30
41. Arai Y, Hirose N, Yamamura K, Nakazawa S, Shimizu K, Takayama M, Ebihara Y, Homma S, Gondo Y, Masui Y, Inagaki H. Deficiency of choresteryl ester transfer protein and gene polymorphisms of lipoprotein lipase and hepatic lipase are not associated with longevity. J Mol Med 2003;81:102–109
42. Bruce C, Sharp DS, Tall AR. Relationship of HDL and coronary heart disease to a common amino acid polymorphism in the cholesteryl ester transfer protein in men with and without hypertriglyceridemia. J Lipid Res 1998;39:1071–1078
43. Gronholdt ML, Sillesen H, Wiebe BM, Laursen H, Nordestgaard BG. Increased acute phase reactants are associated with levels of lipoproteins and increased carotid plaque volume. Eur J Vasc Endovasc Surg 2001;21: 227–234
44. Strandberg TE, Vanhanen H, Tikkanen MJ. Associations between change in C-reactive protein and serum lipids during statin treatment. Ann Med 2000;32:579–583
45. Arai Y, Hirose N. Aging and HDL metabolism in elderly people more than 100 years old. J Atheroscler Thromb 2004;11:246–252
46. Bruunsgaard H, Skinhoj P, Pedersen AN, Schroll M, Pedersen BK. Ageing, tumour necrosis factor-alpha (TNF-alpha) and atherosclerosis. Clin Exp Immunol 2000;121:255–260
47. Ansell BJ, Watson KE, Weiss RE, Fonarow GC. hsCRP and HDL effects of statins trial (CHEST): rapid effect of statin therapy on C-reactive protein and high-density lipoprotein levels a clinical investigation. Heart Dis 2003;5:2–7
48. Karaca I, Ilkay E, Akbulut M, Yavuzkir M, Pekdemir M, Akbulut H, Arslan N. Atorvastatin affects C-reactive protein levels in patients with coronary artery disease. Curr Med Res Opin 2003;19:187–191
49. Ridker PM, Rifai N, Lowenthal SP. Rapid reduction in C-reactive protein with cerivastatin among 785 patients with primary hypercholesterolemia. Circulation 2001;103:1191–1193
50. Ross R. Atherosclerosis: an inflammatory disease. N Engl J Med 1999;340:115–126
51. Mosinger BJ. Human low-density lipoproteins: oxidative modification and its relation to age, gender, menopausal status and cholesterol concentrations. Eur J Clin Chem Clin Biochem 1997;35:207–214
52. Holvoet P, Harris TB, Tracy RP, Verhamme P, Newman AB, Rubin SM, Simonsick EM, Colbert LH, Kritchevsky SB. Association of high coronary heart disease risk status with circulating oxidized LDL in the well-functioning elderly: findings from the Health, Aging, and Body Composition study. Arterioscler Thromb Vasc Biol 2003;23:1444–1448
53. Nakamura YK, Read MH, Elias JW, Omaye ST. Oxidation of serum low-density lipoprotein (LDL) and antioxidant status in young and elderly humans. Arch Gerontol Geriatr 2006;42:265–276
54. Stulnig TM, Jurgens G, Chen Q, Moll D, Schonitzer D, Jarosch E, Wick G. Properties of low density lipoproteins relevant to oxidative modifications change paradoxically during aging. Atherosclerosis 1996;126:85–94
55. Marathe GK, Prescott SM, Zimmerman GA, McIntyre TM. Oxidized LDL contains inflammatory PAF-like phospholipids. Trends Cardiovasc Med 2001;11:139–142
56. Tokumura A, Sumida T, Toujima M, Kogure K, Fukuzawa K. Platelet-activating factor (PAF)-like oxidized phospholipids: relevance to atherosclerosis. Biofactors 2000;13:29–33

57. Shih DM, Gu L, Xia YR, Navab M, Li WF, Hama S, Castellani LW, Furlong CE, Costa LG, Fogelman AM, Lusis AJ. Mice lacking serum paraoxonase are susceptible to organophosphate toxicity and atherosclerosis. Nature 1998;394:284–287
58. Tward A, Xia YR, Wang XP, Shi YS, Park C, Castellani LW, Lusis AJ, Shih DM. Decreased atherosclerotic lesion formation in human serum paraoxonase transgenic mice. Circulation 2002;106:484–490
59. Miyoshi M, Nakano Y, Sakaguchi T, Ogi H, Oda N, Suenari K, Kiyotani K, Ozono R, Oshima T, Yoshida T, Chayama K. Gene delivery of paraoxonase-1 inhibits neointimal hyperplasia after arterial balloon-injury in rabbits fed a high-fat diet. Hypertens Res 2007;30:85–91
60. Ruiz J, Blanche H, James RW, Garin MC, Vaisse C, Charpentier G, Cohen N, Morabia A, Passa P, Froguel P. Gln-Arg192 polymorphism of paraoxonase and coronary heart disease in type 2 diabetes. Lancet 1995;346: 869–872
61. Odawara M, Tachi Y, Yamashita K. Paraoxonase polymorphism (Gln192-Arg) is associated with coronary heart disease in Japanese noninsulin-dependent diabetes mellitus. J Clin Endocrinol Metab 1997;82:2257–2260
62. Sanghera DK, Aston CE, Saha N, Kamboh MI. DNA polymorphisms in two paraoxonase genes (PON1 and PON2) are associated with the risk of coronary heart disease. Am J Hum Genet 1998;62:36–44
63. Sanghera DK, Saha N, Aston CE, Kamboh MI. Genetic polymorphism of paraoxonase and the risk of coronary heart disease. Arterioscler Thromb Vasc Biol 1997;17:1067–1073
64. Zama T, Murata M, Matsubara Y, Kawano K, Aoki N, Yoshino H, Watanabe G, Ishikawa K, Ikeda Y. A 192Arg variant of the human paraoxonase (*HUMPONA*) gene polymorphism is associated with an increased risk for coronary artery disease in the Japanese. Arterioscler Thromb Vasc Biol 1997;17:3565–3569
65. Imai Y, Morita H, Kurihara H, Sugiyama T, Kato N, Ebihara A, Hamada C, Kurihara Y, Shindo T, Oh-hashi Y, Yazaki Y. Evidence for association between paraoxonase gene polymorphisms and atherosclerotic diseases. Atherosclerosis 2000;149:435–442
66. Aynacioglu AS, Kepekci Y. The human paraoxonase Gln-Argl92 (Q/R) polymorphism in Turkish patients with coronary artery disease. Int J Cardiol 2000;74:33–37
67. Gardemann A, Philipp M, Heÿ K, Katz N, Tillmanns H, Haberbosch W. The paraoxonase Leu-Met54 and Gln-Arg191 gene polymorphisms are not associated with the risk of coronary heart disease. Atherosclerosis 2000;152:421–431
68. Ko YL, Ko YS, Wang SM, Hsu LA, Chang CJ, Chu PH, Cheng NJ, Chen WJ, Chiang CW, Lee YS. The Gln-Arg 191 polymorphism of the human paraoxonase gene is not associated with the risk of coronary artery disease among Chinese in Taiwan. Atherosclerosis 1998;141:259–264
69. Ombres D, Pannitteri G, Montali A, Candeloro A, Seccareccia F, Campagna F, Cantini R, Campa PP, Ricci G, Arca M. The Gln-Arg192 polymorphism of human paraoxonase gene is not associated with coronary artery disease in Italian patients. Arterioscler Thromb Vasc Biol 1998;18:1611–1616
70. Chen Q, Reis SE, Kammerer CM, McNamara DM, Holubkov R, Sharaf BL, Sopko G, Pauly DF, Merz CN, Kamboh MI. WISE Study Group. Association between the severity of angiographic coronary artery disease and paraoxonase gene polymorphisms in the National Heart, Lung, and Blood Institute-sponsored Women's Ischemia Syndrome Evaluation (WISE) study. Am J Hum Genet 2003;72:13–22
71. Tobin MD, Braund PS, Burton PR, Thompson JR, Steeds R, Channer K, Cheng S, Lindpaintner K, Samani NJ. Genotypes and haplotypes predisposing to myocardial infarction: a multilocus case-control study. Eur Heart J 2004;25:459–467
72. Senti M, Tomas M, Vila J, Marrugat J, Elosua R, Sala J, Masia R. Relationship of age-related myocardial infarction risk and Gln/Arg 192 variants of the human paraoxonase1 gene: the REGICOR study. Atherosclerosis 2001;156:443–449
73. Baum L, Ng HK, Woo KS, Tomlinson B, Rainer TH, Chen X, Cheung WS, Chan DK, Thomas GN, Tong CS, Wong KS. Paraoxonase 1 gene Q192R polymorphism affects stroke and myocardial infarction risk. Clin Biochem 2006;39:191–195
74. Saeed M, Perwaiz Iqbal M, Yousuf FA, Perveen S, Shafiq M, Sajid J, Frossard PM. Interactions and associations of paraoxonase gene cluster polymorphisms with myocardial infarction in a Pakistani population. Clin Genet 2007;71:238–244
75. Martinelli N, Girelli D, Olivieri O, Stranieri C, Trabetti E, Pizzolo F, Friso S, Tenuti I, Cheng S, Grow MA, Pignatti PF, Corrocher R. Interaction between smoking and PON2 Ser311Cys polymorphism as a determinant of the risk of myocardial infarction. Eur J Clin Invest 2004;34:14–20
76. Hulthe J. Antibodies to oxidized LDL in atherosclerosis development – clinical and animal studies. Clin Chim Acta 2004;348:1–8
77. Ramachandran A, Levonen AL, Brookes PS, Ceaser E, Shiva S, Barone MC, Darley-Usmar rley-Usmar V. Mitochondria, nitric oxide, and cardiovascular dysfunction. Free Radic Biol Med 2002;33:1465–1474
78. Zmijewski JW, Moellering DR, Le GC, Landar A, Ramachandran A, Darley-Usmar VM. Oxidized LDL induces mitochondrially associated reactive oxygen/nitrogen species formation in endothelial cells. Am J Physiol Heart Circ Physiol 2005;289:H852–H861

79. Galle J, Hansen-Hagge T, Wanner C, Seibold S. Impact of oxidized low density lipoprotein on vascular cells. Atherosclerosis 2006;185:219–226
80. Chen M, Masaki T, Sawamura T. LOX-1, the receptor for oxidized low-density lipoprotein identified from endothelial cells: implications in endothelial dysfunction and atherosclerosis. Pharmacol Ther 2002;95: 89–100
81. Adachi H, Tsujimoto M. Endothelial scavenger receptors. Prog Lipid Res 2006;45:379–404
82. Jonasson L, Holm J, Skalli O, Bondjers G, Hansson GK. Regional accumulations of T cells, macrophages, and smooth muscle cells in the human atherosclerotic plaque. Arteriosclerosis 1986;6:131–138
83. Rajavashisth TB, Andalibi A, Territo MC, Berliner JA, Navab M, Fogelman AM, Lusis AJ. Induction of endothelial cell expression of granulocyte and macrophage colony-stimulating factors by modified low-density lipoproteins. Nature 1990;344:254–257
84. Cushing SD, Berliner JA, Valente AJ, Territo MC, Navab M, Parhami F, Gerrity R, Schwartz CJ, Fogelman AM. Minimally modified low density lipoprotein induces monocyte chemotactic protein 1 in human endothelial cells and smooth muscle cells. Proc Natl Acad Sci USA 1990;87:5134–5138
85. Palkama T. Induction of interleukin-1 production by ligands binding to the scavenger receptor in human monocytes and the THP-1 cell line. Immunology 1991;74:432–438
86. Hwang SJ, Ballantyne CM, Sharrett AR, Smith LC, Davis CE, Gotto AM Jr, Boerwinkle E. Circulating adhesion molecules VCAM-1, ICAM-1, and E-selectin in carotid atherosclerosis and incident coronary heart disease cases: the Atherosclerosis Risk In Communities (ARIC) study. Circulation 1997;96:4219–4225
87. Cunningham KS, Gotlieb AI. The role of shear stress in the pathogenesis of atherosclerosis. Lab Invest 2005;85:9–23
88. Auer J, Weber T, Berent R, Lassnig E, Lamm G, Eber B. Genetic polymorphisms in cytokine and adhesion molecule genes in coronary artery disease. Am J Pharmacogenomics 2003;3:317–328
89. Collot-Teixeira S, Martin J, McDermott-Roe C, Poston R, McGregor JL. CD36 and macrophages in atherosclerosis. Cardiovasc Res 2007 Mar 14
90. Johnson GB, Brunn GJ, Platt JL. Activation of mammalian Toll-like receptors by endogenous agonists. Crit Rev Immunol 2003;23:15–44
91. Xu XH, Shah PK, Faure E, Equils O, Thomas L, Fishbein MC, Luthringer D, Xu XP, Rajavashisth TB, Yano J, Kaul S, Arditi M. Toll-like receptor-4 is expressed by macrophages in murine and human lipid-rich atherosclerotic plaques and upregulated by oxidized LDL. Circulation 2001;104:3103–3108
92. Edfeldt K, Swedenborg J, Hansson GK, Yan ZQ. Expression of toll-like receptors in human atherosclerotic lesions: a possible pathway for plaque activation. Circulation 2002;105:1158–1161
93. Uematsu S, Sato S, Yamamoto M, Hirotani T, Kato H, Takeshita F, Matsuda M, Coban C, Ishii KJ, Kawai T, Takeuchi O, Akira S. Interleukin-1 receptor-associated kinase-1 plays an essential role for Toll-like receptor (TLR)7- and TLR9-mediated interferon-{alpha} induction. J Exp Med 2005;201:15–923
94. Ruckdeschel K, Pfaffinger G, Haase R, Sing A, Weighardt H, Hacker G, Holzmann B, Heesemann J. Signaling of apoptosis through TLRs critically involves toll/IL-1 receptor domain-containing adapter inducing IFN-beta, but not MyD88, in bacteria-infected murine macrophages. J Immunol 2004;173:3320–3328
95. Blessing E, Campbell LA, Rosenfeld ME, Chough N, Kuo CC. Chlamydia pneumoniae infection accelerates hyperlipidemia induced atherosclerotic lesion development in C57BL/6J mice. Atherosclerosis 2001;158:13–17
96. Caligiuri G, Rottenberg M, Nicoletti A, Wigzell H, Hansson GK. Chlamydia pneumoniae infection does not induce or modify atherosclerosis in mice. Circulation 2001;103:2834–2838
97. Edfeldt K, Swedenborg J, Hansson GK, Yan ZQ. Expression of toll-like receptors in human atherosclerotic lesions: a possible pathway for plaque activation. Circulation 2002;105:1158–1161
98. Schwartz DA, Cook DN. Polymorphisms of the Toll-like receptors and human disease. Clin Infect Dis 2005;41:S403–S407
99. Arbour NC, Lorenz E, Schutte BC, Zabner J, Kline JN, Jones M, Frees K, Watt JL, Schwartz DA. TLR4 mutations are associated with endotoxin hyporesponsiveness in humans. Nat. Genet 2000;25:187–191
100. Kiechl S, Lorenz E, Reindl M, Wiedermann CJ, Oberhollenzer F, Bonora E, Willeit J, Schwartz DA. Toll-like receptor 4 polymorphisms and atherogenesis. N Engl J Med 2002;347:185–192
101. Labrum R, Bevan S, Sitzer M, Lorenz M, Markus HS. Toll receptor polymorphisms and carotid artery intima-media thickness. Stroke 2007;38:1179–1184
102. Hamann L, Glaeser C, Hamprecht A, Gross M, Gomma A, Schumann RR. Toll-like receptor (TLR)-9 promotor polymorphisms and atherosclerosis. Clin Chim Acta 2006;364:303–307
103. Norata GD, Garlaschelli K, Ongari M, Raselli S, Grigore L, Benvenuto F, Maggi FM, Catapano AL. Effect of the Toll-like receptor 4 (TLR-4) variants on intima-media thickness and monocyte-derived macrophage response to LPS. J Intern Med 2005;258:21–27
104. Hernesniemi J, Lehtimaki T, Rontu R, Islam MS, Eklund C, Mikkelsson J, Ilveskoski E, Kajander O, Goebeler S, Viiri LE, Hurme M, Karhunen PJ. Toll-like receptor 4 polymorphism is associated with coronary stenosis but not with the occurrence of acute or old myocardial infarctions. Scand J Clin Lab Invest. 2006;66:667–675

149. Vazquez-Padron RI, Lasko D, Li S, Louis L, Pestana IA, Pang M, Liotta C, Fornoni A, Aitouche A, Pham SM. Aging exacerbates neointimal formation, and increases proliferation and reduces susceptibility to apoptosis of vascular smooth muscle cells in mice. J Vasc Surg 2004;40:1199–1207
150. Kang JG, Patino WD, Matoba S, Hwang PM. Genomic analysis of circulating cells: a window into atherosclerosis. Trends Cardiovasc Med 2006;16:163–168
151. Baba MI, Kaul D, Grover A. Importance of blood cellular genomic profile in coronary heart disease. J Biomed Sci 2006;13:17–26
152. Miller DT, Ridker PM, Libby P, Kwiatkowski DJ. Atherosclerosis: the path from genomics to therapeutics. J Am Coll Cardiol 2007;49:1589–1599
153. Llaverias G, Noe V, Penuelas S, Vazquez-Carrera M, Sanchez RM, Laguna JC, Ciudad CJ, Alegret M. Atorvastatin reduces CD68, FABP4, and HBP expression in oxLDL-treated human macrophages. Biochem Biophys Res Commun 2004;318:265–274
154. Morikawa S, Takabe W, Mataki C, Wada Y, Izumi A, Saito Y, Hamakubo T, Kodama T. Global analysis of RNA expression profile in human vascular cells treated with statins. J Atheroscler Thromb 2004;11:62–72
155. Navab M, Ananthramaiah GM, Reddy ST, Van Lenten BJ, Ansell BJ, Fonarow GC, Vahabzadeh K, Hama S, Hough G, Kamranpour N, Berliner JA, Lusis AJ, Fogelman AM. The oxidation hypothesis of atherogenesis: the role of oxidized phospholipids and HDL. J Lipid Res 2004;45:993–1007
156. Navab M, Anantharamaiah GM, Hama S, Garber DW, Chaddha M, Hough G, Lallone R, Fogelman AM. Oral administration of an Apo A-I mimetic Peptide synthesized from D-amino acids dramatically reduces atherosclerosis in mice independent of plasma cholesterol. Circulation 2002;105:290–292
157. Nilsson J, Nordin Fredrikson G, Schiopu A, Shah PK, Jansson B, Carlsson R. Oxidized LDL antibodies in treatment and risk assessment of atherosclerosis and associated cardiovascular disease. Curr Pharm Des 2007;13:1021–1030
158. Robinson I, de Serna DG, Gutierrez A, Schade DS. Vitamin E in humans: an explanation of clinical trial failure. Endocr Pract 2006;12:576–582
159. Williams KJ, Fisher EA. Oxidation, lipoproteins, and atherosclerosis: which is wrong, the antioxidants or the theory? Curr Opin Clin Nutr Metab Care 2005;8:139–146
160. Cherubini A, Vigna GB, Zuliani G, Ruggiero C, Senin U, Fellin R. Role of antioxidants in atherosclerosis: epidemiological and clinical update. Curr Pharm Des 2005;11:2017–2032
161. Li D, Mehta JL. 3-hydroxy-3-methylglutaryl coenzyme a reductase inhibitors protect against oxidized low-density lipoprotein-induced endothelial dysfunction. Endothelium 2003;10:17–21
162. Rosenson RS. Statins in atherosclerosis: lipid-lowering agents with antioxidant capabilities. Atherosclerosis 2004;173:1–12
163. Patel TN, Shishehbor MH, Bhatt DL. A review of high-dose statin therapy: targeting cholesterol and inflammation in atherosclerosis. Eur Heart J 2007;28:664–672
164. Nachimuthu S, Raggi P. Novel agents to manage dyslipidemias and impact atherosclerosis. Cardiovasc Hematol Disord Drug Targets 2006;6:209–217
165. Klerkx AH, El Harchaoui K, van der Steeg WA, Boekholdt SM, Stroes ES, Kastelein JJ, Kuivenhoven JA. Cholesteryl ester transfer protein (CETP) inhibition beyond raising high-density lipoprotein cholesterol levels: pathways by which modulation of CETP activity may alter atherogenesis. Arterioscler Thromb Vasc Biol 2006;26:706–715
166. Kraaijeveld AO, de Jager SC, van Berkel TJ, Biessen EA, Jukema JW. Chemokines and atherosclerotic plaque progression: towards therapeutic targeting? Curr Pharm Des 2007;13:1039–1052
167. Reutershan J. CXCR2–the receptor to hit? Drug News Perspect 2006;19:615–623
168. Campbell IW. The clinical significance of PPAR gamma agonism. Curr Mol Med 2005;5:349–363
169. Grabar P. Hypothesis. Auto-antibodies and immunological theories: an analytical review. Clin Immunol Immunopathol 1975;4:453–466
170. Witztum JL. Splenic immunity and atherosclerosis: a glimpse into a novel paradigm? J Clin Invest 2002;109:721–724
171. Robinette CD, Fraumeni JF Jr. Splenectomy and subsequent mortality in veterans of the 1939–45 war. Lancet 1977;2:127–129
172. Caligiuri G, Nicoletti A, Poirier B, Hansson GK. Protective immunity against atherosclerosis carried by B cells of hypercholesterolemic mice. J Clin Invest 2002;109:745–753
173. Weksler ME, Goodhardt M. Do age-associated changes in 'physiologic' autoantibodies contribute to infection, atherosclerosis, and Alzheimer's disease? Exp Gerontol 2002;37:971–979
174. Riley SC, Froscher BG, Linton PJ, Zharhary D, Marcu K, Klinman NR. Altered VH gene segment utilization in the response to phosphorylcholine by aged mice. J Immunol 1989;143:3798–3805
175. Nicoletti C. Antibody protection in aging: influence of idiotypic repertoire and antibody binding activity to a bacterial antigen. Exp Mol Pathol 1995;62:99–108

176. Lee PY, Alexander KP, Hammill BG, Pasquali SK, Peterson ED. Representation of elderly persons and women in published randomized trials of acute coronary syndromes. JAMA 2001;286:708–713
177. Aronow WS. The older man's heart and heart disease. Med Clin North Am 1999;83:1291–1303
178. Aronow WS, Ahn C, Gutstein H. Prevalence and incidence of cardiovascular disease in 1160 older men and 2464 older women in a long-term health care facility. J Gerontol A Biol Sci Med Sci 2002;57:M45–M46
179. Woodworth S, Nayak D, Aronow WS, Pucillo AL, Koneru S. Comparison of acute coronary syndromes in men versus women > or = 70 years of age. Am J Cardiol 2002;90:1145–1147
180. Antman EM, Cohen M, Bernink PJ, McCabe CH, Horacek T, Papuchis G, Mautner B, Corbalan R, Radley D, Braunwald E. The TIMI risk score for unstable angina/non-ST elevation MI: A method for prognostication and therapeutic decision making. JAMA 2000;284:835–842
181. Smith SC Jr, Feldman TE, Hirshfeld JW Jr, Jacobs AK, Kern MJ, King SB III, Morrison DA, O'neill WW, Schaff HV, Whitlow PL, Williams DO, Antman EM, Smith SC Jr, Adams CD, Anderson JL, Faxon DP, Fuster V, Halperin JL, Hiratzka LF, Hunt SA, Jacobs AK, Nishimura R, Ornato JP, Page RL, Riegel B. ACC/AHA/SCAI 2005 guideline update for percutaneous coronary intervention a report of the American College of Cardiology/American Heart Association Task Force on Practice Guidelines (ACC/AHA/SCAI Writing Committee to Update the 2001 Guidelines for Percutaneous Coronary Intervention). J Am Coll Cardiol 2006;47: e1–121
182. Braunwald E, Antman EM, Beasley JW, Califf RM, Cheitlin MD, Hochman JS, Jones RH, Kereiakes D, Kupersmith J, Levin TN, Pepine CJ, Schaeffer JW, Smith EE III, Steward DE, Theroux P, Alpert JS, Eagle KA, Faxon DP, Fuster V, Gardner TJ, Gregoratos G, Russell RO, Smith SC Jr. ACC/AHA guidelines for the management of patients with unstable angina and non-ST-segment elevation myocardial infarction. A report of the American College of Cardiology/American Heart Association Task Force on Practice Guidelines (Committee on the Management of Patients With Unstable Angina). J Am Coll Cardiol 2000;36:970–1062
183. Woodworth S, Nayak D, Aronow WS, Pucillo AL, Koneru S. Cardiovascular medications taken by patients aged >or=70 years hospitalized for acute coronary syndromes before hospitalization and at hospital discharge. Prev Cardiol 2002;5:173–176
184. Antman EM, Morrow DA, McCabe CH, Murphy SA, Ruda M, Sadowski Z, Budaj A, Lopez-Sendon JL, Guneri S, Jiang F, White HD, Fox KA, Braunwald E. Enoxaparin versus unfractionated heparin with fibrinolysis for ST-elevation myocardial infarction. N Engl J Med 2006;354:1477–1488
185. Wallentin L, Goldstein P, Armstrong PW, Granger CB, Adgey AA, Arntz HR, Bogaerts K, Danays T, Lindahl B, Makijarvi M, Verheugt F, Van de Werf F. Efficacy and safety of tenecteplase in combination with the low-molecular-weight heparin enoxaparin or unfractionated heparin in the prehospital setting: the Assessment of the Safety and Efficacy of a New Thrombolytic Regimen (ASSENT)-3 PLUS randomized trial in acute myocardial infarction. Circulation 2003;108:135–142
186. Antman EM, Morrow DA, McCabe CH, Jiang F, White HD, Fox KA, Sharma D, Chew P, Braunwald E. Enoxaparin versus unfractionated heparin as antithrombin therapy in patients receiving fibrinolysis for ST-elevation myocardial infarction. Design and rationale for the Enoxaparin and Thrombolysis Reperfusion for Acute Myocardial Infarction Treatment-Thrombolysis In Myocardial Infarction study 25 (ExTRACT-TIMI 25). Am Heart J 2005;149:217–226
187. Skolnick AH, Alexander KP, Chen AY, Roe MT, Pollack CV Jr, Ohman EM, Rumsfeld JS, Gibler WB, Peterson ED, Cohen DJ. Characteristics, management, and outcomes of 5,557 patients age > or =90 years with acute coronary syndromes: results from the CRUSADE Initiative. J Am Coll Cardiol 2007;49:1790–1797
188. Chen H, Liu J, Yang M. Corticosteroids for viral myocarditis. Cochrane Database Syst Rev 2006;4:CD004471
189. Heart Failure Society Of America. Myocarditis: Current treatment. J Card Fail 2006;12:e120–e122
190. Aretz HT, Billingham ME, Edwards WD, Factor SM, Fallon JT, Fenoglio JJ Jr, Olsen EG, Schoen FJ. Myocarditis. A histopathologic definition and classification. Am J Cardiovasc Pathol 1987;1:3–14
191. Dec GW Jr, Waldman H, Southern J, Fallon JT, Hutter AM Jr, Palacios I. Viral myocarditis mimicking acute myocardial infarction. J Am Coll Cardiol 1992;20:85–89
192. Dec GW Jr, Palacios IF, Fallon JT, Aretz HT, Mills J, Lee DC, Johnson RA. Active myocarditis in the spectrum of acute dilated cardiomyopathies. Clinical features, histologic correlates, and clinical outcome. N Engl J Med 1985;312:885–890
193. Kyto V, Saraste A, Voipio-Pulkki LM, Saukko P. Incidence of fatal myocarditis: a population-based study in Finland. Am J Epidemiol 2007;165:570–574
194. Elliott WJ. Systemic hypertension. Curr Probl Cardiol 2007;32:201–259
195. Kearney PM, Whelton M, Reynolds K, Muntner P, Whelton PK, He J. Global burden of hypertension: analysis of worldwide data. Lancet 2005;365:217–223
196. Lewington S, Clarke R, Qizilbash N, Peto R, Collins R. Age-specific relevance of usual blood pressure to vascular mortality: a meta-analysis of individual data for one million adults in 61 prospective studies. Lancet 2002;360:1903–1913

197. Vasan RS, Beiser A, Seshadri S, Larson MG, Kannel WB, D'Agostino RB, Levy D. Residual lifetime risk for developing hypertension in middle-aged women and men: the Framingham Heart Study. JAMA 2002;287: 1003–1010
198. Lloyd-Jones DM, Evans JC, Larson MG, O'Donnell CJ, Levy D. Differential impact of systolic and diastolic blood pressure level on JNC-VI staging. Joint National Committee on Prevention, Detection, Evaluation, and Treatment of High Blood Pressure. Hypertension 1999;34:381–385
199. Lewington S, Clarke R, Qizilbash N, Peto R, Collins R. Age-specific relevance of usual blood pressure to vascular mortality: a meta-analysis of individual data for one million adults in 61 prospective studies. Lancet 2002;360:1903–1913
200. Jafar TH, Stark PC, Schmid CH, Landa M, Maschio G, de Jong PE, de Zeeuw D, Shahinfar S, Toto R, Levey AS. Progression of chronic kidney disease: the role of blood pressure control, proteinuria, and angiotensin-converting enzyme inhibition: a patient-level meta-analysis. Ann Intern Med 2003;139:244–252
201. Lewington S, Clarke R, Qizilbash N, Peto R, Collins R. Age-specific relevance of usual blood pressure to vascular mortality: a meta-analysis of individual data for one million adults in 61 prospective studies. Lancet 2002;360:1903–1913
202. Hyman DJ, Pavlik VN. Characteristics of patients with uncontrolled hypertension in the United States. N Engl J Med 2001;345:479–486
203. Hajjar I, Kotchen TA. Trends in prevalence, awareness, treatment, and control of hypertension in the United States, 1988–2000. JAMA 2003;290:199–206
204. Elliott WJ. Management of hypertension in the very elderly patient. Hypertension 2004;44:800–804
205. Gueyffier F, Bulpitt C, Boissel JP, Schron E, Ekbom T, Fagard R, Casiglia E, Kerlikowske K, Coope J. Antihypertensive drugs in very old people: a subgroup meta-analysis of randomised controlled trials. INDANA Group. Lancet 1999;353:793–796
206. Prevention of stroke by antihypertensive drug treatment in older persons with isolated systolic hypertension. Final results of the Systolic Hypertension in the Elderly Program (SHEP). SHEP Cooperative Research Group. JAMA 1991;265:3255–3264
207. Perry HM Jr, Davis BR, Price TR, Applegate WB, Fields WS, Guralnik JM, Kuller L, Pressel S, Stamler J, Probstfield JL. Effect of treating isolated systolic hypertension on the risk of developing various types and subtypes of stroke: the Systolic Hypertension in the Elderly Program (SHEP). JAMA 2000;284:465–471
208. Kostis JB, Davis BR, Cutler J, Grimm RH Jr, Berge KG, Cohen JD, Lacy CR, Perry HM Jr, Blaufox MD, Wassertheil-Smoller S, Black HR, Schron E, Berkson DM, Curb JD, Smith WM, McDonald R, Applegate WB. Prevention of heart failure by antihypertensive drug treatment in older persons with isolated systolic hypertension. SHEP Cooperative Research Group. JAMA 1997;278:212–216
209. Staessen JA, Fagard R, Thijs L, Celis H, Arabidze GG, Birkenhager WH, Bulpitt CJ, de Leeuw PW, Dollery CT, Fletcher AE, Forette F, Leonetti G, Nachev C, O'Brien ET, Rosenfeld J, Rodicio JL, Tuomilehto J, Zanchetti A. Randomised double-blind comparison of placebo and active treatment for older patients with isolated systolic hypertension. The Systolic Hypertension in Europe (Syst-Eur) Trial Investigators. Lancet 1997;350: 757–764
210. Liu L, Wang JG, Gong L, Liu G, Staessen JA. Comparison of active treatment and placebo in older Chinese patients with isolated systolic hypertension. Systolic Hypertension in China (Syst-China) Collaborative Group. J Hypertens 1998;16:1823–1829
211. Staessen JA, Gasowski J, Wang JG, Thijs L, Den HE, Boissel JP, Coope J, Ekbom T, Gueyffier F, Liu L, Kerlikowske K, Pocock S, Fagard RH. Risks of untreated and treated isolated systolic hypertension in the elderly: meta-analysis of outcome trials. Lancet 2000;355:865–872
212. Kjeldsen SE, Dahlof B, Devereux RB, Julius S, Aurup P, Edelman J, Beevers G, de FU, Fyhrquist F, Ibsen H, Kristianson K, Lederballe-Pedersen O, Lindholm LH, Nieminen MS, Omvik P, Oparil S, Snapinn S, Wedel H. Effects of losartan on cardiovascular morbidity and mortality in patients with isolated systolic hypertension and left ventricular hypertrophy: a Losartan Intervention for Endpoint Reduction (LIFE) substudy. JAMA 2002;288:1491–1498
213. Major outcomes in moderately hypercholesterolemic, hypertensive patients randomized to pravastatin vs usual care: The Antihypertensive and Lipid-Lowering Treatment to Prevent Heart Attack Trial (ALLHAT-LLT). JAMA 2002;288:2998–3007
214. Gueyffier F, Bulpitt C, Boissel JP, Schron E, Ekbom T, Fagard R, Casiglia E, Kerlikowske K, Coope J. Antihypertensive drugs in very old people: a subgroup meta-analysis of randomised controlled trials. INDANA Group. Lancet 1999;353:793–796
215. Mulrow CD, Cornell JA, Herrera CR, Kadri A, Farnett L, Aguilar C. Hypertension in the elderly. Implications and generalizability of randomized trials. JAMA 1994;272:1932–1938
216. Bulpitt C, Fletcher A, Beckett N, Coope J, Gil-Extremera B, Forette F, Nachev C, Potter J, Sever P, Staessen J, Swift C, Tuomilehto J. Hypertension in the Very Elderly Trial (HYVET): protocol for the main trial. Drugs Aging 2001;18:151–164

217. Staessen JA, Wang JG, Thijs L. Cardiovascular prevention and blood pressure reduction: a quantitative overview updated until 1 March 2003. J Hypertens 2003;21:1055–1076
218. Snieder H, Harshfield GA, Treiber FA. Heritability of blood pressure and hemodynamics in African- and European-American youth. Hypertension 2003;41:1196–1201
219. Snieder H, Treiber FA. The Georgia Cardiovascular Twin Study. Twin Res 2002;5:497–498
220. Imumorin IG, Dong Y, Zhu H, Poole JC, Harshfield GA, Treiber FA, Snieder H. A gene-environment interaction model of stress-induced hypertension. Cardiovasc Toxicol 2005;5:109–132
221. Truswell AS, Kennelly BM, Hansen JD, Lee RB. Blood pressures of Kung bushmen in Northern Botswana. Am Heart J 1972;84:5–12
222. Poulter NR, Khaw KT, Mugambi M, Peart WS, Rose G, Sever P. Blood pressure patterns in relation to age, weight and urinary electrolytes in three Kenyan communities. Trans R Soc Trop Med Hyg 1985;79:389–392
223. Taddei S, Virdis A, Mattei P, Ghiadoni L, Fasolo CB, Sudano I, Salvetti A. Hypertension causes premature aging of endothelial function in humans. Hypertension 1997;29:736–743
224. Hamet P, Thorin-Trescases N, Moreau P, Dumas P, Tea BS, deBlois D, Kren V, Pravenec M, Kunes J, Sun Y, Tremblay J. Workshop: excess growth and apoptosis: is hypertension a case of accelerated aging of cardiovascular cells? Hypertension 2001;37:760–766
225. Liu JJ, Peng L, Bradley CJ, Zulli A, Shen J, Buxton BF. Increased apoptosis in the heart of genetic hypertension, associated with increased fibroblasts. Cardiovasc Res 2000;45:729–735
226. Imanishi T, Moriwaki C, Hano T, Nishio I. Endothelial progenitor cell senescence is accelerated in both experimental hypertensive rats and patients with essential hypertension. J Hypertens 2005;23:1831–1837
227. Rodriguez-Iturbe B, Sepassi L, Quiroz Y, Ni Z, Wallace DC, Vaziri ND. Association of mitochondrial SOD deficiency with salt-sensitive hypertension and accelerated renal senescence. J Appl Physiol 2007;102:255–260
228. Rao DC, Province MA, Leppert MF, Oberman A, Heiss G, Ellison RC, Arnett DK, Eckfeldt JH, Schwander K, Mockrin SC, Hunt SC. HyperGEN Network. A genome-wide affected sibpair linkage analysis of hypertension: the HyperGEN network. Am J Hypertens 2003;16:148–150
229. Jeunemaitre X, Inoue I, Williams C, Charru A, Tichet J, Powers M, Sharma AM, Gimenez-Roqueplo AP, Hata A, Corvol P, Lalouel JM. Haplotypes of angiotensinogen in essential hypertension. Am J Hum Genet 1997;60:1448–1460
230. Kato N, Sugiyama T, Morita H, Kurihara H, Yamori Y, Yazaki Y. Angiotensinogen gene and essential hypertension in the Japanese: extensive association study and meta-analysis on six reported studies. J Hypertens 1999;17:757–763
231. Inoue I, Nakajima T, Williams CS, Quackenbush J, Puryear R, Powers M, Cheng T, Ludwig EH, Sharma AM, Hata A, Jeunemaitre X, Lalouel JM. A nucleotide substitution in the promoter of human angiotensinogen is associated with essential hypertension and affects basal transcription in vitro. J Clin Invest 1997;99:1786–1797
232. Sethi AA, Nordestgaard BG, Gronholdt ML, Steffensen R, Jensen G, Tybjaerg-Hansen A. Angiotensinogen single nucleotide polymorphisms, elevated blood pressure, and risk of cardiovascular disease. Hypertension 2003;41:1202–1211
233. Zhu X, Chang YP, Yan D, Weder A, Cooper R, Luke A, Kan D, Chakravarti A. Associations between hypertension and genes in the renin-angiotensin system. Hypertension 2003;41:1027–1034
234. Higaki J, Baba S, Katsuya T, Sato N, Ishikawa K, Mannami T, Ogata J, Ogihara T. Deletion allele of angiotensin-converting enzyme gene increases risk of essential hypertension in Japanese men: the Suita Study. Circulation 2000;101:2060–2065
235. Turner ST, Boerwinkle E, Sing CF. Context-dependent associations of the ACE I/D polymorphism with blood pressure. Hypertension 1999;34:773–778
236. Bray MS, Krushkal J, Li L, Ferrell R, Kardia S, Sing CF, Turner ST, Boerwinkle E. Positional genomic analysis identifies the beta(2)-adrenergic receptor gene as a susceptibility locus for human hypertension. Circulation 2000;101:2877–2882
237. Herrmann SM, Nicaud V, Tiret L, Evans A, Kee F, Ruidavets JB, Arveiler D, Luc G, Morrison C, Hoehe MR, Paul M, Cambien F. Polymorphisms of the beta2 -adrenoceptor (ADRB2) gene and essential hypertension: the ECTIM and PEGASE studies. J Hypertens 2002;20:229–235
238. Krushkal J, Xiong M, Ferrell R, Sing CF, Turner ST, Boerwinkle E. Linkage and association of adrenergic and dopamine receptor genes in the distal portion of the long arm of chromosome 5 with systolic blood pressure variation. Hum Mol Genet 1998;7:1379–1383
239. Thiel BA, Chakravarti A, Cooper RS, Luke A, Lewis S, Lynn A, Tiwari H, Schork NJ, Weder AB. A genome-wide linkage analysis investigating the determinants of blood pressure in whites and African Americans. Am J Hypertens 2003;16:151–153
240. Province MA, Kardia SL, Ranade K, Rao DC, Thiel BA, Cooper RS, Risch N, Turner ST, Cox DR, Hunt SC, Weder AB, Boerwinkle E. National Heart, Lung and Blood Institute Family Blood Pressure Program. A meta-analysis of genome-wide linkage scans for hypertension: the National Heart, Lung and Blood Institute Family Blood Pressure Program. Am J Hypertens 2003;16:144–147

241. Koivukoski L, Fisher SA, Kanninen T, Lewis CM, von Wowern F, Hunt S, Kardia SL, Levy D, Perola M, Rankinen T, Rao DC, Rice T, Thiel BA, Melander O. Meta-analysis of genome-wide scans for hypertension and blood pressure in Caucasians shows evidence of susceptibility regions on chromosomes 2 and 3. Hum Mol Genet 2004;13:2325–2332
242. Mein CA, Caulfield MJ, Dobson RJ, Munroe PB. Genetics of essential hypertension. Hum Mol Genet 2004;13:R169–R175

Chapter 9
Metabolic Syndrome, Diabetes and Cardiometabolic Risks in Aging

Overview

Two related chronic disorders metabolic syndrome and diabetes can present with significant microvascular and macrovascular complications including CAD, hypertension and atherosclerosis leading to increased morbidity and mortality in the elderly. While genetic, epigenetic and environmental factors have been shown to underlie the etiology and progression of both these increasingly epidemic disorders, a clear-cut and complete understanding of their precise role in disease pathogenesis still remains undefined. Molecular analysis has begun to identify the generally polygenic elements that constitute susceptibility risk and protective factors in both these disorders. These studies have lead to increased focus on to the role(s) that vascular inflammation, altered transcriptional programming and disturbed intracellular/metabolic signaling play in these disorders, elements that are also markedly impacted upon in the elderly. This approach may lead to facilitate earlier diagnosis of these disorders, improved treatment via more effective drugs and gene and cell-based therapies and eventually to potential prevention or attenuation by gene profiling and appropriate counseling.

Introduction

The metabolic syndrome (MetSyn) is a term used to describe a clustering of metabolic risk factors that have been found to occur in an individual more than by chance alone. This clustering of cardiovascular risk factors has become much more prevalent in the general population and appears to be associated with an increasingly sedentary society and a global epidemic of obesity and diabetes [1]. The following are the components of this syndrome:

- insulin resistance
- central obesity
- atherogenic dyslipidemia
- hypertension

It is now recognized that there are many other conditions and findings associated with this syndrome such as renal disease, elevation in inflammatory markers, and polycystic ovarian syndrome. Moreover, MetSyn is characterized by chronic inflammation and thrombotic disorder contributing to endothelial dysfunction and, subsequently, to accelerated atherosclerosis and coronary artery disease (CAD). Underlying the pathological link of metabolic syndrome to these cardiovascular diseases (CVDs) is the inflammation in the vasculature accompanied by atherogenic dyslipidemia including the combination of hypertriglyceridemia, low levels of high-density lipoprotein cholesterol

J. Marín-García, *Aging and the Heart*,

(HDL-C), and a preponderance of small, dense low-density lipoprotein (LDL) particles, critical components of the syndrome. Furthermore, it has become increasingly recognized that a primary factor by which obesity acts as a central component in the development of MetSyn is the production by adipose cells of bioactive substances that directly influence insulin sensitivity and vascular injury. Given that many of the components of the syndrome are also recognized cardiovascular risk factors, it is not surprising that individuals with MetSyn have up to a five-fold increased risk of developing early atherosclerotic heart disease [2], and hence the term cardiometabolic risks.

The Metabolic Syndrome and the Concept of Cardiometabolic Risks

Although it has just been in the past decade that the concept of a "metabolic syndrome" has been popularized, components of this syndrome have been described for close to a century. Previous names used to describe this condition include Syndrome X [3], insulin resistance syndrome [4], hypertriglyceridemic waist [5] and the deadly quartet [6]. One of the first physicians to describe features of the syndrome was Kylin, who in 1923 described the coexistence of hypertension, diabetes and hyperuricemia, and proposed there was a common mechanism for the development of these conditions. A number of years later, Vague first described an association between upper body adiposity (android phenotype) and the development of diabetes, hypertension, gout and atherosclerosis. In 1988, Reaven hypothesized that insulin resistance was the common etiological factor in this clustering of metabolic disorders and referred to it as Syndrome X [4]. He also pointed out that these patients were at increased risk for the development of atherosclerosis.

In recent years, there have been different criteria proposed for diagnosing an individual with the metabolic syndrome, as illustrated in Table 9.1.

While these definitions all have common elements that include parameters for obesity, hypertension, dyslipidemia and impaired glucose tolerance, there are significant differences between them. The World Health Organization (WHO) was the first group to formally define this syndrome in 1998 [7]. Similar to the European Group for Insulin Resistance (EGIR) definition [8] and the American Academy of Clinical Endocrinologists (AACE) definition [9], the WHO definition mandates that patients must demonstrate evidence of insulin insensitivity to meet their criteria for the MetSyn. Unlike the WHO definition that includes patients with overt diabetes, the latter two definitions do not apply to patients once they develop type-2 diabetes.

Other diagnostic criteria have been proposed that do not mandate insulin insensitivity to be present in order to be diagnosed with the metabolic syndrome, including definitions from the National Cholesterol Education Program Adult Treatment Panel III (NCEP ATP III) [10] and the International Diabetes Federation (IDF). While the NCEP ATP III allows any 3 of 5 diagnostic criteria to be present, the IDF requires the demonstration of central obesity in addition to two other criteria. In addition, the IDF have recommended different waist measurements to define abdominal obesity based on ethnic background. For example, for individuals of European origin, waist circumferences $\geq$ 94 cm in men and $\geq$ 80 cm in women should be used to define abdominal obesity. Asian populations (excluding Japanese) should use waist circumference thresholds $\geq$ 90 cm and $\geq$ 80 cm for men and women respectively. For Japanese, they recommend using a waist circumference $\geq$ 85 cm in men and $\geq$ 90 cm in women respectively.

The American Heart Association (AHA) and the National Heart, Lung and Blood Institute (NHLBI) have published new criteria for the diagnosis of the metabolic syndrome that largely uses the NCEP ATP III definition, with some minor modifications (included in Table 9.1) [11]. The major difference here is a lower threshold for impaired fasting glucose, which corresponds to the AHA criteria for impaired fasting glucose. Therefore, using this definition, patients meet the criteria for the metabolic syndrome if any 3 out the 5 criteria are met. A caveat to this is for individuals

Table 9.1 Criteria used in clinical diagnosis of metabolic syndrome

Clinical measure	WHO 1998	IDF 2005	NCEP ATP III 2003/AHA/NHLBI 2004	AACE 2003	EGIR 1999
Insulin resistance	Any 1 of the following: • Type 2 diabetes (T2D) • Impaired fasting glucose (IFG) • Impaired glucose tolerance (IGT) plus any 2 of the following	None	None	IGT or IFG plus any of the following	Plasma insulin >75th percentile plus any 2 of the following
Body weight	BMI >30 kg/m^2 or waist:hip ratio: >0.9 in men >0.85 in women	Waist circumference- ethnicity specific (plus any 2 of the following)	Waist circumference- ≥102 cm (≥40 ") in men; ≥88 cm (≥35 ") in women;	BMI >25 kg/m2	Waist circumference ≥94 cm in men or ≥80 cm in women
Lipid	TG >150 mg/dl HDL-C <35 mg/dl in men <39 mg/dl in women	TG >150 mg/dl HDL-C <40 mg/dl in men <50 mg/dl in women	TG ≥150 mg/dl HDL-C <40 mg/dl in men <50 mg/dl in women or on drug treatment for elevated TG or HDL-C	TG >150 mg/dl HDL-C <40 mg/dl in men <50 mg/dl in women	TG >150 mg/dl HDL-C <40 mg/dl in men <50 mg/dl in women
Blood Pressure (BP)	≥140 mmHg systolic BP; ≥90 mmHg diastolic BP or on drug treatment for HT	≥130 mmHg systolic BP; ≥85 mmHg diastolic BP	≥130 mmHg systolic BP; ≥85 mmHg diastolic BP or on drug treatment for HT	≥130 mmHg systolic BP; ≥85 mmHg diastolic BP	≥140 mmHg systolic BP; ≥90 mmHg diastolic or on drug treatment for HT
Glucose	Fasting plasma glucose ≥110 mg/dl; IGT, IFG or T2D	Fasting glucose ≥100 mg/dl	≥100 mg/dl or on drug treatment for elevated glucose	IGT or IFG (but not diabetes)	IGT or IFG (but not diabetes)
Other risk factors	Urinary albumin excretion rate 20 µg/min or albumin:creatinine ratio 30 mg/g		Family history of T2D, HT or CVD, polycystic ovary syndrome; Sedentary lifestyle, age, ethnic groups having high risk for T2D or CVD		

TG, triglyceride; HDL-C, high density lipoprotein cholesterol; HT, hypertension; BMI, body mass index;T2D, type 2 diabetes; IFG, impaired fasting glucose; IGT, impaired glucose tolerance.

of Asian descent or with other conditions associated with the metabolic syndrome not included in the standard definition (for example polycystic ovary disease, elevated C-reactive protein > 3 mg/L, fatty liver, elevated total apolipoprotein B). If these individuals have a moderately increased waist circumference (94–101 cm for men, 80–87 cm women) and 2 additional ATP III/AHA criteria, consideration should be made to manage them in the same fashion as people with 3 ATP III/AHA risk factors.

The association of visceral adipose tissue with incident MI in older men and women was evaluated in the Health, Aging and Body Composition Study [12], in which 1,116 men and 1,387 women aged 70–79 years were followed. Analysis of the 71 myocardial infarction (MI) events observed in elderly men revealed no association between incident MI and the adiposity or fat distribution variables. However, for elderly women, visceral adipose tissue was an independent predictor of MI, hazard ratio (HR) 1.67, 95 % confidence interval (CI) 1.28–2.17. No association was found between body mass index or total fat mass and MI events in elderly women. Furthermore, the association of visceral adipose tissue with MI in women was independent of HDL-C, interleukin-6 concentration, hypertension, and diabetes.

While the adverse effects of classical risk factors such as hypercholesterolemia, hypertension and smoking are relatively well understood, increased understanding of the pathophysiology of CVD has revealed new cardiovascular risk factors. Among these, abdominal obesity, low HDL-C, hypertriglyceridemia and the hyperglycemia associated with insulin resistance are all recognized criteria for the diagnosis of MetSyn. However, a range of important novel risk factors or risk markers for CVD is also associated with the metabolic syndrome, although not yet included within its definition. These include chronic, low-grade inflammation, and disturbances in the secretion of bioactive substances from adipocytes ("adipokines") that influence cardiovascular structure and function. Adipokines that are elevated in abdominally obese subjects include pro-inflammatory molecules such as interleukin-6 (IL-6) and tumor necrosis factor-α (TNF-α) which play a critical role in macrophage infiltration in atherosclerosis, reduce insulin sensitivity of adipocytes and can impact the production of other inflammatory mediators including C-reactive protein (CRP) by the liver. In contrast, another adipokine, adiponectin which is reduced in obese individuals particularly with intra-abdominal obesity has a variety of cardioprotective actions including improving insulin sensitivity and glycemic control, and several anti-atherogenic actions such as inhibition of endothelial activation, reduced conversion of macrophages to foam cells, and inhibition of the smooth muscle proliferation and arterial remodeling featured in atherosclerotic plaque development [13].

The cardiometabolic risk factors associated with MetSyn, whether included within its diagnostic criteria or not, do contribute to the progression of atherosclerotic cardiometabolic disease and represent an important clinical entity inadequately addressed by current therapies. Clinicians therefore need to extend routine systematic assessment from cardiovascular risk to cardiometabolic risk—that is, risk for developing CVD and/or diabetes—and increase the understanding of the basic mechanisms that regulate energy balance and metabolic risk factors.

The Effects of CB1 Blockade on Cardiometabolic Risk

The endocannabinoids are endogenous lipids capable of binding to two cannabinoid receptors (CB), CB1 and CB2. These receptors belong to the G protein–coupled superfamily and were discovered during investigation of the mode of action of delta9-tetrahydrocannabinol, an exogenous cannabinoid and an important component of *Cannabis sativa*, which they bind with high affinity [14]. CB1 is widely distributed in the Central Nervous System (CNS) including the hypothalamic nuclei which are involved in the control of energy balance and body weight, as well as in neurons of the mesolimbic system believed to mediate the incentive value of food [14], and is also expressed in peripheral tissues [14]. On the other hand, CB2 is mainly expressed in immune cells and does not appear to play a role in food intake [15]. At around the same time as CB1and CB2 was cloned, CB1 endogenous ligands, named endocannabinoids, were identified and synthesized. The most important are anandamide and 2-arachidonoylglycerol (2-AG) [16]. The discovery of specific receptors and their endogenous ligands therefore support the existence of an endogenous cannabinoid system. Endogenous cannabinoids are lipids synthesized and released from neurons in response to membrane depolarization. Following their release, their rapid inactivation is induced by specific enzymes [17]. Therefore, the endocannabinoid system serves as a general stress-recovery system.

Strong evidence exists that has helped establish the role of CB1 receptors in hunger-induced food intake and energy balance. For example, CB1 activation may restore feeding in satiated animals [18], whereas CB1 receptor blockade decreases the rates of responding to food [19]. Recent data from animal models have provided solid evidence that genetically-induced obesity is accompanied by chronic and intense activation of the endocannabinoid system [20]. Moreover, CB1 is also present in peripheral organs, including adipose tissue and gastrointestinal system, major organs in the regulation of energy metabolism [13, 21]. Indeed, CB1 receptor deficient mice have reduced body weight, fat mass and activation of metabolic processes that are independent of reduced food intake [22]. Furthermore, these CB1 receptor-deficient mice are resistant to diet-induced obesity and the development of what in humans would be regarded as MetSyn [23]. CB1 receptor blockade provides a novel approach to the management of multiple cardiometabolic risk factors by addressing abdominal obesity and directly improving lipid and glucose metabolism and insulin resistance. The discovery of rimonabant [24], the first specific CB1 receptor blocker, made it possible to understand the many facets of the endocannabinoid system and set the stage for the development of novel pharmacotherapeutic approaches to treat obesity.

Clinical Management and Trials with Metabolic Syndrome

The RIO programme enrolled over 6,600 subjects in an investigation of the impact of rimonabant on cardiometabolic risk factors in an overweight/obese population. RIO-North America [25] and RIO-Europe [26] were two-year studies that enrolled patients with body mass index (BMI) >30 kg/m^2, or BMI >27 kg/m^2 with comorbid factors, such as hypertension and dyslipidemia. RIO-Lipids was a one-year study designed to evaluate rimonabant in patients with untreated dyslipidemia [27]. In addition, RIO-Lipids included measurement of additional parameters related to atherosclerotic risk, including adiponectin levels, LDL particle size and density and CRP levels. RIO-Diabetes was a one-year study conducted in overweight/obese patients with type-2 diabetics treated with metformin or sulfonylurea [28]. The design of RIO-North America differed from the other RIO trials, in that a second randomization was included after year one, with patients subsequently randomly allocated to continue their original study therapy or switch to placebo. In this way, this trial evaluated the effects of rimonabant on the change in cardiometabolic factors at one year, the maintenance of these effects in the second year and the impact of discontinuing the drug. All 4 trials in the RIO program utilized a randomized, double-blind, placebo-controlled, parallel group, fixed dose design. A single-blind placebo run-in of four weeks, accompanied by a mild hypocaloric diet (600 kcal/day energy deficit diet) preceded randomization which was maintained. In RIO-Europe and RIO-North America, patients were randomized to receive placebo, rimonabant 5 mg, or rimonabant 20 mg in 1:2:2 ratios. Patients in RIO-Lipids and RIO-Diabetes were also stratified before randomization according to their triglyceride levels and antidiabetic treatment, respectively. Randomization to the three treatment groups in these trials was carried out in a 1:1:1 ratio. Efficacy endpoints included weight change (primary endpoint for RIO-North American and RIO-Europe), waist circumference (WC), a marker of intra-abdominal adiposity, effects on lipids (e.g., HDL-C, triglycerides), glycemic parameters and prevalence of MetSyn as defined by NCEP/ATPIII criteria. Majority of patients were female in RIO-North America and RIO-Europe, while men and women were equally represented in RIO-Lipids and RIO-Diabetes. Close to 90 % included in the 4 studies had abdominal obesity, defined as a WC >102 cm (40") for men and >88 cm (35") in women, i.e. the diagnostic criterion for abdominal obesity by NCEP/ATP III. In addition, in RIO Diabetes the patients had an average glycosylated hemoglobin (HbA1c) of 7.5 % at screening. The presence of multiple cardiometabolic risk factors was common at baseline in participants in the RIO programme [25]. Over half of the populations of RIO-North America, RIO-Europe and RIO Diabetes had elevated lipids at baseline. One quarter and two thirds of the patient populations had hypertension. A high proportion of the overall study population had NCEP/ATPIII defined MetSyn at baseline (from nearly 35 % in RIO North America to nearly 80 % in RIO Diabetes population) indicating the presence of multiple cardiometabolic risk factors.

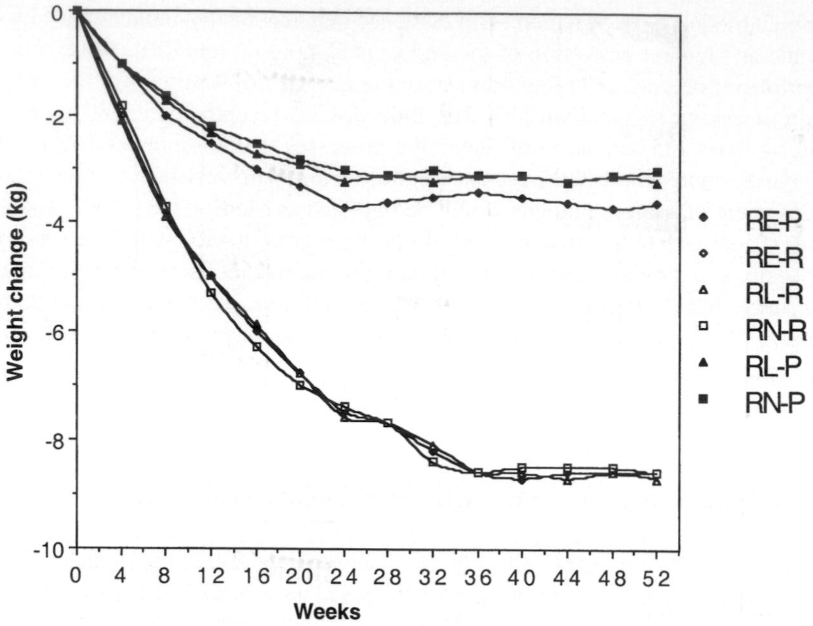

Fig. 9.1 Effect of rimonabant on MetSyn in 3 RIO clinical studies
The graph shows the decline in patients' body weight (in kg) in placebo-treated (P) and in patients treated with 20 mg rimonabant(R) over a 52-week period in 3 independent RIO clinical trials, including the RIO European (RE), the RIO Lipid (RL) and the RIO North American (RN) studies.

Results of RIO-North America, RIO-Europe and RIO-Lipids have been published, [25–27] and the primary results can be summarized as depicted in Figs. 9.1 and 9.2. In obese subjects, CB1 receptor blockade with rimonabant resulted in:

- significant reductions in waist circumference and body weight
- significant improvement in metabolic profile including:
  - increased HDL-C and decreased triglyceride levels
  - improved insulin sensitivity
  - improvement in HbA1c in type-2 diabetes
  - significant decrease in the percent of subjects with MetSyn
- improvement in other metabolic and cardiovascular risk factors including:
  - increased adiponectin
  - decreased CRP
  - improved small dense LDL particles profile

Cardiometabolic Risk Factor in the Elderly

Much less is known regarding cardiometabolic risks or the MetSyn in the elderly as few studies have compared cardiometabolic risks and their impact between the young and the elderly. Conceivably, in general the pathogenesis of the MetSyn in the elderly should be comparable to that in younger subjects although there may be physiological alterations specific to the elderly that render these people more prone to the development of MetSyn while on the other hand the impact of cardiometabolic risks clinical outcome may also be different.

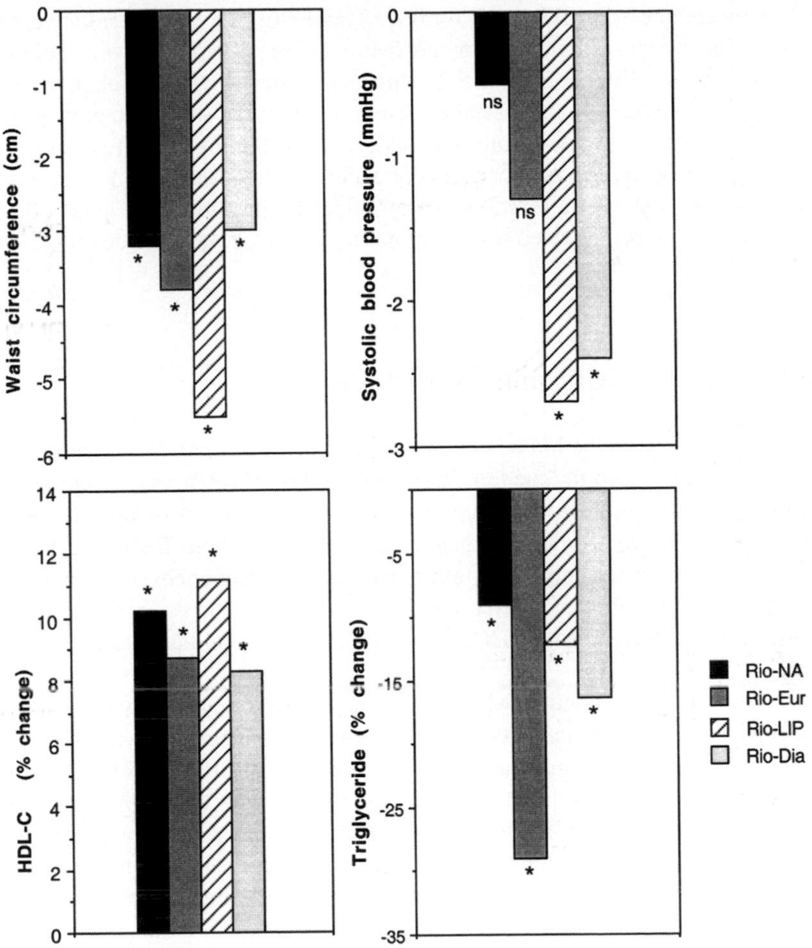

Fig. 9.2 Rimonabant effects on selected MetSyn parameters
Shown are changes in waist circumference (cm), serum HDL-cholesterol level (HDL-C in % change), serum triglyceride level (in % change) and systolic blood pressure (in mm Hg) obtained in 4 different RIO clinical studies as indicated in the legend.
*indicates $p < 0.05$; ns indicates non-significant changes compared to placebo.

Endogenous Sex Hormones and Metabolic Syndrome in the Elderly

Decline of both testicular and adrenal function with aging causes a decrease in androgen concentrations in the male [29]. Evidence from several studies has suggested that sex steroid hormones are related to type-2 diabetes and vascular disease in elderly men [30, 31]. To study the association between endogenous sex hormones and characteristics of the MetSyn, 400 independently living men between 40 and 80 year of age were enrolled in a cross-sectional study in the Netherlands [32]. Serum lipids, glucose, insulin, Total Testosterone (TT), Sex Hormone Binding Globulin (SHBG), estradiol (E2), and dehydroepiandrosterone sulfate (DHEAS) were measured. Bioavailable Testosterone (BT) was calculated using TT and SHBG. Body height, weight, waist-hip circumference, blood pressure, and physical activity were assessed, smoking and alcohol consumption were estimated from self-report and insulin sensitivity was calculated. The MetSyn was defined according to the NCEP ATP III definition. Multiple logistic regression analyses demonstrated an inverse relationship according to 1 standard deviation (SD) increase for circulating TT, BT, SHBG, and DHEAS with MetSyn. Adjusted mean for BT levels for 0, 1, 2, and 3 or more risk factors were 8.5, 8.3, 8.2, and 7.6 nmol/L, respectively. The number of risk factors increased with lower circulating T, SHBG, and DHEAS levels and with higher E2 levels. Exclusion of subjects with prevalent diabetes and CVD did not change the observed estimates. Linear regression analyses showed that higher TT, BT, and SHBG levels were related to higher insulin sensitivity. These findings therefore suggest that higher testosterone and SHBG levels in aging males are independently associated with a higher insulin sensitivity and reduced risk of the MetSyn, independent of insulin levels and body composition measurements, suggesting that reduced sex hormones may play a role in the development of MetSyn in elderly men.

Leptin and Metabolic Syndrome in the Elderly

Since leptin has been shown to be linked to adiposity and insulin resistance in middle-aged individuals, studies have recently been initiated to examine the relationship between leptin and MetSyn in the elderly [33, 34]. A recent study evaluated a potential independent relation between leptin and the components of the MetSyn in 107 women aged 67–78 years with BMI ranging from 18.19 to 36.16 kg/m^2 [33]. In all participants, BMI, waist and hip circumferences, body composition determined by dual energy X-ray absorptiometry, fasting, and 2-hour glucose, lipids, insulin, homeostasis model assessment of insulin resistance (HOMA), systolic (SBP) and diastolic blood pressure (DBP) and leptin levels were measured.

Significant correlation was found between leptin, BMI, waist circumference, fat mass, DBP, SBP, cholesterol, triglycerides, insulin, and HOMA. After adjusting for age and waist circumference, and for age and fat mass, leptin was significantly related to insulin levels, HOMA, and cholesterol. In a stepwise multiple regression analysis using insulin levels or HOMA as dependent variables and age, waist circumference, fat mass, leptin, blood pressure, cholesterol, and triglycerides as independent variables, leptin entered the regression first, waist circumference second, and age third. Their data demonstrate that leptin is related to indices of adiposity in elderly women, and leptin is significantly associated with insulin levels, HOMA, and cholesterol, independent of age, body fat, and fat distribution. Leptin, waist circumference, and age together explained 31 % and 33 % of insulin levels and HOMA variance, respectively, in healthy elderly women.

In a study of 452 Italian men aged 65 and older enrolled in the Invecchiare in Chianti (InCHIANTI) study, levels of a number of hormones including testosterone, SHBG, DHEAS, cortisol and leptin were assessed for their relationship/association with MetSyn [34]. MetSyn as defined by the ATP III criteria was present in roughly 16 % (73 men) and exhibited an inverse association with SHBG and total testosterone levels, and a positive association with leptin (i.e., Log leptin was significantly associated with each component of MetSyn). Other hormones assessed such as cortisol, DHEAS, free and bioavailable testosterone, and IGF-1 were not found to be associated with MetSyn in this cohort of elderly males.

Metabolic Syndrome and Oxidative Stress in the Elderly

Oxidized LDL (oxLDL) has been shown to play an important role in the pathogenesis of atherosclerosis [35]. The generation of oxLDL arising from the oxidation of both lipid and protein components of LDL is primarily attributed to the triggering of inflammatory pathways in several vascular cell types. While obesity and dyslipidemia are particularly strong predictors of levels of oxLDL in middle age individuals [36], a relationship of oxLDL with MetSyn in elderly individuals and consequences with respect to incident CVD events has only recently been addressed. OxLDL was measured in plasma from 3,033 elderly participants in the Health, Aging, and Body Composition study, to determine whether an association exists between MetSyn and oxLDL and to assess the risk for CAD in relation to MetSyn and levels of oxLDL [37]. The presence of MetSyn was associated with higher levels of oxLDL primarily due to a higher fraction of circulating oxLDL, even after adjustment for LDL-C. Compared with those not having MetSyn, individuals with MetSyn had twice the odds of having high oxLDL (> 1.90 mg/dl) after adjusting for age, sex, ethnicity, smoking status and LDL-C. Among those participants who had MetSyn at study entry, incidence of future CAD events were 1.6-fold higher, after adjusting for age, sex, ethnicity, and smoking status. While oxLDL was not an independent predictor of total CAD risk, those individuals with high oxLDL had a significantly greater disposition to MI. Accordingly, MetSyn, a risk factor for CAD, is associated with higher levels of circulating oxLDL that are associated with a greater disposition to atherothrombotic events.

Cardiac Remodeling and Insulin Resistance in the Elderly

An association between MetSyn, particularly the insulin resistance component, and left ventricular hypertrophy (LVH) has been appreciated for some time, albeit primarily in middle-aged men [38, 39]. These associations were examined in a cohort of 475 elderly Swedish men (including 157 hypertensives) over 70 years of age, followed over a 20 year period using echocardiography, oral glucose tolerance test (OGTT), hyperinsulinemic euglycemic clamp, lipid and 24-hour ambulatory blood pressure monitoring [40]. Analysis of the relationship between components of the insulin resistance syndrome and left ventricular geometric parameters indicated that LV relative wall thickness (RWT) was significantly related to clamp insulin sensitivity index, fasting insulin, 32–33 split proinsulin, triglycerides, nonesterified fatty acids, OGTT glucose and insulin levels, waist-to-hip ratio, body mass index, 24-hour blood pressure, and heart rate as shown in Table 9.2. On the other hand, only 24-hour systolic blood pressure (directly), heart rate and OGTT 2-hour insulin

Table 9.2 Relationship between components of insulin resistance syndrome and parameters of left ventricular geometry

	Relative wall thickness		LV mass index	
	r	P	r	P
24-hour SBP	0.22	<0.0001	0.15	0.001
24-hour DBP	0.21	<0.0001	0.09	0.052
24-hour heart rate	0.17	0.0003	−0.14	0.003
Insulin sensitivity index	−0.14	0.002	0.07	0.15
Fasting plasma glucose	0.08	0.08	−0.06	0.22
OGTT 2-hour glucose	0.13	0.005	−0.06	0.20
Fasting immunoreactive insulin	0.05	0.24	20.04	0.35
OGTT 2-hour immunoreactive insulin	0,07	0.10	20.1	0.03
Fasting specific insulin	0.11	0.02	0.009	0.57
Fasting proinsulin	0.07	0.14	0.03	0.47
Fasting 32–33 split proinsulin	0.1	0.03	0.11	0.12
Waist-to-Hip ratio	0.15	0.001	0.02	0.73
Body mass index (BMI)	0.17	0.0002	0.001	0.99
Serum non esterified fatty acids	0.14	0.002	20.08	0.1
Serum triglycerides	0.11	0.01	0.07	0.12
Serum total cholesterol	0.04	0.33	0.02	0.71
LDL cholesterol	0.02	0.61	0.008	0.86
HDL cholesterol	0.02	0.62	−0.03	0.49

(adapted from Sundstrom et al. 2000) [40]
Significance differences of P<0.05 are shown in bold

(both inversely) were significantly related to LV mass index (LVMI). Moreover, neither RWT nor LVMI was significantly related to serum levels of total cholesterol, LDL-C, HDL-C, fasting plasma glucose, immunoreactive insulin, proinsulin, 2-hour immunoreactive insulin level, or the AUC of immunoreactive insulin at the OGTT.

Comparing subjects with various LV geometry (i.e., normal, concentric remodeling and concentric and eccentric hypertrophy) revealed that several components of the insulin resistance syndrome differed significantly between the 4 left ventricular geometric groups. In particular, the values of 24-hour heart rate, waist-to-hip ratio, BMI, and 2-hour OGTT glucose level, were significantly higher and clamp insulin sensitivity index was significantly lower in the concentric remodeling geometry group than in the normal LV geometry group. In addition the 24-hour blood pressure (both SBP and DBP) was significantly higher in the concentric hypertrophy group than in the normal LV geometry group. These data therefore indicate that a number of the components of the MetSyn are related to thick LV walls and concentric remodeling but less so to LV hypertrophy in elderly men.

Cardiometabolic Risk Factors and Cardiovascular Disease in the Elderly

The association between MetSyn components and the prevalence of ischemic heart disease were investigated in a cross-sectional, community-based study of subjects aged 50–89 years (1015 men, 1259 women) [41]. In both sexes, significant positive associations were found between ischemic heart disease as defined by resting electrocardiographic criteria and factors including age, systolic blood pressure, fasting and post-challenge hyperglycemia, total cholesterol/HDL-C ratio, and triglycerides, whereas an inverse association with HDL-C was noted. Using factor analysis performed separately for each sex, three uncorrelated principal components were identified in both men and women, which contribute to the association between MetSyn variables and ischemic heart disease.

These components include a central metabolic factor (comprised by BMI, fasting and nonfasting serum insulin, and dyslipidemia including high serum triglycerides, and low HDL-C), a glucose factor (including both fasting and nonfasting plasma glucose and which was independent of insulin as represented in the metabolic factor), and a blood pressure factor (including both SBP and DBP). In this cross-sectional study, all three factors were significantly and independently associated with ischemic heart disease as was age. Moreover, in a multivariate logistic regression model with age and sex, all three factors were significantly associated with ischemic heart disease as defined by electrocardiogram criteria. These results suggest that in elderly subjects, the metabolic syndrome can increase the risk of ischemic heart disease acting through different risk factors and by multiple mechanisms, and that factor analysis may simplify the complex cluster of inter-related variables, reducing the overall number of factors involved and making them more interpretable, with no significant loss of predictive value

Metabolic Syndrome, Diabetes and Cognitive Decline in the Elderly

In the elderly, the complexity of the elements of the cardiometabolic risks may be of extra concern; namely the potential for cognitive decline [42, 43]. In elderly subjects, elevated glucose levels have not only been linked to the development of retinopathy, neuropathy, and nephropathy, but also to a decline in cognitive abilities [44]. For example, in an analysis of a change in cognitive performance among older adults according to glucose tolerance status it was found that older women with diabetes mellitus had a 4-fold increased risk of a major cognitive decline on a verbal fluency test after 4 years compared with nondiabetic women [45]. In an analysis of data from a 4-year randomized trial of raloxifene among 7,027 osteoporotic postmenopausal women (mean age, 66.3 years), women with diabetes (n = 267) or with impaired fasting glucose (IFG), n = 290, showed an almost two-fold decline in cognitive function compared to women with normal glucose levels [46]. Furthermore, the results of longitudinal studies suggest that diabetes is an independent risk factor for cognitive decline and dementia [47, 48]. In a prospective population-based cohort study among 6,370 elderly subjects, followed for 2 years (on average), diabetes mellitus almost doubled the risk of dementia and Alzheimer disease [48]. Interestingly, patients treated with insulin were at highest risk of dementia.

In addition, recent brain imaging studies using magnetic resonance imaging (MRI) have shown that both lacunar and cortical infarctions were more common and cortical atrophy more pronounced among elderly diabetic patients supporting the notion that the increased risk of cognitive decline and dementia in elderly subjects with diabetes is due to dual pathology, involving both cerebrovascular disease and cortical atrophy [49]. Similar findings of an increased association of type 2 diabetes with markers of brain aging detectable by MRI, including infarcts, lacunes, and white matter hyperintensities as markers of vascular damage and hippocampal atrophy as markers of neurodegeneration were recently reported in a population of older Japanese men (described further below) in the Honolulu-Asia Aging Study [50]. Subjects with type 2 diabetes had a moderately elevated risk for lacunes and hippocampal atrophy and had a two-fold increase in risk for both hippocampal atrophy and lacunes/infarcts compared with those without type 2 diabetes.

Therefore, investigators have found a significant link between the presence of type 2 diabetes or pre-diabetes and an elevated risk for cognitive impairment and dementia in elderly populations. While several studies have demonstrated that older women are particularly targeted, others have shown that elderly males are also significantly affected. Studies with co-twin control method have been shown to improve on traditional case-control approaches by controlling for within-twin pair similarities of genetic and early environmental influences. Cognitive decline was studied over a 12-year period in members of the National Academy of Sciences-National Research Council Twin Registry of World War II male veterans, with respect to potential association of diabetes, hypertension, hypercholesterolemia, and elevated BMI [51]. Difference in cognitive decline within twin pairs discordant for the vascular risk factors were assessed while controlling for baseline differences in education, smoking, and alcohol history. Among twin pairs discordant for diabetes (n = 177), the diabetic twins significantly declined cognitively compared to their nondiabetic co-twins (p = 0.018). Moreover further analyses showed that this was in large part due to greater decline among older men (age 76–84 years). Interestingly, cognitive change was not significantly different between members of pairs discordant for hypertension (n = 326), hypercholesterolemia (n = 282), or elevated BMI. This study based on the analysis of male twin pairs who share similar genetic and early environmental risks for cardiovascular risk factors confirmed that diabetes is associated with greater cognitive decline, particularly among the oldest men.

The Honolulu-Asia Aging Study (HAAS) examined the long-term association between the cardiometabolic syndrome at middle age and the risk of dementia in old age [52]. The HAAS was based on a cohort of Japanese-American men followed since 1965. The original cohort included 8006 Japanese-American men who were born between 1900 and 1919 and were living on the island of Oahu, Hawaii, in 1965. Cardiometabolic risk factors were assessed at baseline when the men were aged 45–68 years. Screening for dementia took place in 1991–1993, when the men ranged in age from 71–93 years. Of the 4678 men who were still alive at that time, 3734 (80 %) participated in the dementia prospective case-finding cohort. Cardiovascular metabolic risk factors were measured at baseline (1965) and included the following: BMI, subscapular skinfold thickness (in millimeters), diastolic and systolic blood pressure, random post-load glucose, random triglycerides, and total cholesterol, and Z scores were calculated for these seven factors. Dementia was diagnosed in 215 men, according to international criteria, and was based on a clinical examination, neuropsychological testing, and an informant interview. The relative risk of dementia was assessed after adjustment for age, education, occupation, alcohol consumption, and cigarette smoking. The z-score sum was higher in demented subjects than in non-demented subjects, indicating a higher risk factor burden; per SD increase in the z-score sum, the risk of dementia was increased by 5 %. The z-score sum was specifically associated with vascular dementia but not with Alzheimer's disease. Findings from the HAAS therefore suggested that the clustering of cardiometabolic risk factors increased the risk of dementia primarily of vascular origin.

To examine the issue of whether the presence of the MetSyn, using NCEP ATP criteria, accelerates the rate of cognitive decline and the emergence of dementia in the elderly and whether this association is mediated by inflammation, Yaffe and colleagues [53] conducted a 5-year prospective observational study that included 2632 elderly subjects (mean age 74 years), 1016 of whom met the criteria for MetSyn [53]. Association of the MetSyn and high inflammation, defined as above median serum level of IL-6 and CRP, was examined with changes in cognition assessed by the Modified Mini-Mental State Examination (3MS) at 3 and 5 years. When compared with those without MetSyn, elderly subjects with MetSyn accompanied by high levels of pro-inflammatory markers manifested a 20 % increased risk for cognitive impairment. Elevated blood levels of IL-6 and CRP supported the significant interaction between the presence of inflammation and MetSyn in the development of cognitive impairment. Subjects with MetSyn and evidence of high inflammation experienced a 66 % increase in risk for cognitive impairment, when compared with subjects without MetSyn. In contrast, the risk for cognitive impairment in subjects with MetSyn and low levels of inflammation was similar to that seen in subjects without MetSyn. These findings support the hypothesis that the MetSyn contributes to cognitive impairment in elders, primarily in individuals with high levels of inflammation.

Several possible mechanisms may explain the association between the MetSyn and cognitive decline including micro- and macro-vascular disease, inflammation, adiposity and insulin resistance [43]. To examine whether markers of inflammation are associated with cognitive decline in well-functioning African-American and white elderly subjects, 3,031 African-American and white men and women (mean age 74 years) enrolled in the Health, Aging, and Body Composition Study were studied [54]. Serum levels of IL-6, CRP and plasma levels of TNF-α were measured at baseline; cognition was assessed with the 3MS examination at baseline and at follow-up. Participants in the highest tertile of IL-6 or CRP performed significantly lower on baseline and follow-up 3MS and declined over the >2 years compared with those in the lowest textiles. After multivariate adjustment, 3MS scores among participants in the highest tertile of IL-6 and CRP were similar at baseline but remained significantly lower at follow-up. Those in the highest inflammatory marker tertile were also more likely to have cognitive decline compared with the lowest tertile for IL-6 and for CRP. It appears that serum markers of inflammation, especially IL-6 and CRP, are prospectively associated with cognitive decline in well-functioning elderly subjects lending further support to the hypothesis that inflammation is contributory to cognitive decline in the elderly. A recent longitudinal study by these investigators with a large cohort of 1624 elderly Latinos has revealed that those subjects with MetSyn at baseline (over 44 % of this cohort) showed a significant decline in cognitive function over a 3 year period [55]. This association was especially pronounced in participants with MetSyn also exhibiting a high serum level of inflammation. Interestingly, individual components of MetSyn were not associated with cognitive decline indicating that a composite measure of MetSyn is a greater risk for cognitive decline than its individual components. If MetSyn is associated with increased risk of developing cognitive impairment, regardless of mechanism, then early identification and treatment of these individuals might offer avenues for disease course modification.

MetSyn interacts with other conventional cardiovascular risk factors. ERIC-HTA was a cross-sectional, multicenter study carried out in primary care, on non-diabetic hypertensive patients aged 55 or older aimed to assess the relationship among MetSyn, target organ damage and established CVD [56]. In 8331 non-diabetic hypertensive patients (3663 men and 4668 women, mean age 67.7 years), the prevalence of MetSyn was 32.6 % (men: 29.0 %; women: 36.8 %). A linear association was observed between a greater number of MetSyn components and a greater prevalence of LVH assessed by electrocardiogram, impaired kidney function and established CVD. In a multivariate model, MetSyn in non-diabetic hypertensive patients was related to a greater prevalence of LVH, impaired kidney function and established CVD, a relationship that persisted after stratifying by gender. Thus, in elderly non-diabetic hypertensives, the presence of MetSyn may be independently related to a greater prevalence of hypertensive target organ damage and established CVD, suggesting a role of MetSyn as a cardiovascular risk marker in hypertension.

Genes Involved in Metabolic Syndrome

Numerous groups are seeking to identify key genes involved as risk factors in MetSyn with many of the common polymorphic genetic variants showing some complicity/association with either the overall syndrome or with some of its central components [57–89], as well as to establish presymptomatic disease biomarkers [90]. Table 9.3 contains information concerning several of the candidate genetic loci which have been examined for significant association with MetSyn and its components.

Insight into the understanding of MetSyn has come from recent studies of familial partial lipodystrophy (FPLD) as a potential model MetSyn. FPLD is a rare monogenic form of insulin resistance, with a gradual evolution and marked recapitulation of key clinical and biochemical features of MetSyn [91]. FPLD can be caused by mutations in either LMNA, encoding nuclear lamin A/C (subtype FPLD2) [92–94], or PPAR-γ (subtype FPLD3), a transcription factor with a key role in adipocyte differentiation and metabolic regulation [95, 96]. Most of the mutations in LMNA associated with FPLD2 are missense mutations localized near the 3′ end of the gene proximal to the DNA-binding domain at the C terminus of the protein suggesting that a probable molecular pathogenic mechanism elicited by these mutations involves their interaction with transcription factors or other DNA-binding elements [97]. Interestingly, mutations in lamin A/C also cause cardiomyopathy and Hutchinson-Gilford progeria syndrome (HGPS). Over a dozen mutations in PPAR-γ have been implicated in FPLD3, some acting by a dominant-negative mechanism, others through haploinsufficiency. Dominant-negative mutations in PPAR-γ leading to MetSyn with severe hyperinsulinemia and early-onset hypertension have also been reported (e.g., proline-467-leucine (P467L) [98]. Moreover, recent studies have described several mutations in the DNA-binding domain of human PPAR-γ that lead to lipodystrophy and severe insulin resistance [99]. These mutant PPAR-γ proteins lack DNA binding and transcriptional activity but can translocate to the nucleus, interact with PPAR-γ coactivators and have been shown to inhibit coexpressed wild-type receptor. Expression of target genes dependent on PPAR-γ was markedly attenuated.

About 50 % of FPLD patients do not have mutations in either LMNA or PPAR-γ suggesting the potential involvement of either unidentified regulatory mutations, novel causative/pathogenic sequences in these genes or undiscovered genetic loci [97].

Given the list of genetic factors that have thus far been implicated from association studies in MetSyn, it is noteworthy that a good proportion are involved in transcription regulation including the previously discussed LMNA, PPARs (α and γ), PGC-1, the forkhead transcription factor FOXC2 and the hepatic nuclear factor-4α (HNF- 4α).

Alterations in the abundance and activity of transcription factors can lead to complex dysregulation of gene expression, which is pivotal in the generation of insulin resistance and its associated clustering of coronary risk factors at the cellular or gene regulatory level. Members of the nuclear hormone receptor superfamily – for example, peroxisome proliferator-activated receptors (PPARs), PGC-1, RXR-α and sterol regulatory element-binding proteins (SREBPs) have all been implicated in both insulin resistance and MetSyn. [100–102] In addition to their regulation by a host of metabolites and nutrients, these transcription factors are also targets of hormones (like insulin and leptin), growth factors, inflammatory signals, and drugs. Extracellular stimuli are coupled to transcription factors by a variety of signaling pathways including the MAP kinase cascades. For instance, SREBPs appear to

Table 9.3 Relationship of gene polymorphisms with respect to insulin resistance and MetSyn

Phenotype	Variants (gene)	Polymorphism	Ref.
Insulin resistance, FPLD	LMNA	1908C/T, R482Q, R133L, H566H	57–59
Body fat/insulin sensitivity; MetSyn	Tyrosine phosphatase 1β (PTPN1)	Pro387Leu haplotypes	60–62
Insulin resistance/premature CHD/obesity MetSyn	β3-adrenoceptor (ADRB3)	Trp64Arg	63–65
Insulin resistance	PPAR-α	Leu162Val	66–67
Increased risk of MetSyn	PPAR-γ	Pro12Ala; 3 SNPs including P2 -689C>T, Pro12 Ala (C/G) and 1431C>T- act together not independently	68–69 70
Improvement in IR after exercise	PPAR-γ	Pro12Ala	71
No significant association with overall MetSyn or with insulin resistance; ↑ BMI with both Ala and T allele	PPAR-γ	Pro12Ala C161T	72
No association with overall MetSyn, IR or BMI but with other MetSyn components (e.g., ↑ WHR and DBP/HT)	PPAR-γ	Pro12Ala	73
No association with MetSyn	PPAR-δ	14 SNPs	74
Insulin resistance/MetSyn	β2-adrenoceptor (ADRB2)	Arg16Gly	75
Association with MetSyn	PGC-1α	Gly482 Ser	76
Not associated with MetSyn but with some MetSyn components (e.g., ↑ WHR and SBP/HT)	PGC-1α	Gly482 Ser	77, 73
Association with Met Syn	Fatty acid binding protein 2 gene (FABP2)	Ala54Thr	78–81
No association with MetSyn in CHD patients	FABP2	Ala54Thr	82
Association with MetSyn	Adiponectin (APM1)	I164T	83
No association with IR or MetSyn	Transcription factor 7-like 2 (TCF7L2)	Two SNPs rs12255372 and rs7903146	84–85
No association with MetSyn	Ghrelin	Leu72Met	86
Association with BMI + MetSyn	FOXC2	−512C>T	87
Association with MetSyn	Hepatic nuclear factor-4α (HNF-4α)	2 haplotypes containing 5 intronic SNPs	88
Association with MetSyn	APOC3	C-482T + T-455C	79,8089

be substrates of MAP kinases and have been proposed to play a contributory role in the development of cellular features belonging to lipid toxicity and MetSyn [100]. Therefore, MetSyn appears to be not only a disease or state of altered glucose tolerance, plasma lipid levels, blood pressure, and body fat distribution, but rather a complex clinical phenomenon of dysregulated gene expression.

In addition, variants of genes encoding protein components of intracellular metabolic signaling pathways including fatty acid binding protein (FABP2), adiponectin, tyrosine phosphatase 1β (PTPN1), apolipoprotein C (ApoC) and β-adrenergic receptor have also been implicated or associated with MetSyn.

These findings have suggested an important approach for the clinical management and treatment of MetSyn [103–105]. Both PPAR-α activators such as the fibric acid class of hypolipidemic drugs and PPAR-γ agonists including antidiabetic thiazolidinediones (TZDs) have proved to be effective for improving MetSyn. PPAR-α agonists, such as the fibrates, correct dyslipidemia, thus decreasing CVD risk while PPAR-γ agonists, such as the glitazones, increase insulin sensitivity and decrease plasma glucose levels in patients with diabetes. Moreover, both PPAR-α and PPAR-γ agonists exert anti-inflammatory activities in liver, adipose and vascular tissues.

Diabetes in the Elderly

Diabetes is one of the most common chronic diseases affecting older persons in the US occurring in 18 % of persons between 65 and 75 years of age and in as many as 40 % in individuals over 80 years of age. Both significant microvascular and macrovascular (including CAD and atherosclerosis) complications arising from this disorder are a common cause of morbidity and mortality in both the elderly and in minority populations [106, 107]. Though type 1 diabetes (T1D) and closely-related autoimmune diabetes (LADA) can occur in the elderly, the most prevalent type in the elderly is non-insulin-dependent type 2 diabetes (T2D).

Genes Associated with Diabetes

The genetic basis for diabetes has been a matter of increasing interest. In several rare forms of diabetes including neonatal diabetes and maturity onset diabetes, a monogenic etiology has been elucidated. As with more common forms of hypertension, the common types of diabetes (type 1 and 2) are polygenic; a large number of genes appear to be involved with extensive modulation by environmental and epigenetic factors. We briefly describe several relatively rare monogenic forms of diabetes, since their genes implicate important mechanisms that appear to be relevant to the more common polygenic forms.

Several studies have identified discrete activating mutations in the *KCNJ11* gene, which encodes the Kir6.2 subunit of the sarcolemmal K_{ATP} channels that prevent its closure in the pancreatic β-cells (and affect insulin secretion) as a primary cause of neonatal diabetes [108–111]. The mutated K_{ATP} channels do not close in the presence of metabolically generated ATP and therefore the β-cell membrane is hyperpolarized and insulin secretion does not occur. The degree of K_{ATP} channel overactivity has been shown to correlate with the severity of the diabetic phenotype. Mutations in channel properties of Kir6.2 that underlie transient neonatal diabetes (I182V) or more severe forms of permanent neonatal diabetes (V59M, Q52R, and I296L) have been identified, which in all cases result in a significant decrease in sensitivity to inhibitory ATP correlating with channel overactivity in intact cells and increasing the K_{ATP} current, which inhibits β-cell electrical activity and insulin secretion.

The targeted ATP-sensitive potassium channel couples membrane excitability to cellular metabolism and is a critical mediator in the process of glucose-stimulated insulin secretion. Importantly, these findings have proven applicable to studies of T2D. A number of K_{ATP} channel polymorphisms have been described and linked to altered insulin secretion indicating that genes encoding this ion channel could be susceptibility markers for T2D and that genetic variants of K_{ATP} channels may underlie altered β-cell electrical activity, and glucose homeostasis, in addition to increased susceptibility to T2D [112]. In particular, the Kir6.2 E23K polymorphism has been linked to increased susceptibility to T2D in Caucasian populations [113]. As with many of the genetic polymorphisms associated with diabetes, this polymorphism has also been associated with weight gain and obesity, both of which constitute major diabetes risk factors. Mechanistically, it has been proposed that the accumulation of long chain fatty acids in the plasma and in pancreatic β-cells in obese and T2D patients elicit an enhanced stimulation of K_{ATP} channels containing subunits encoded by the polymorphic Kir6.2 E23K allele [114].

Moreover, loss-of-function mutations in the genes encoding the two subunits of K_{ATP} channels which reduce K_{ATP} channel activity have been shown to lead to the most common form of congenital hyperinsulinism, resulting in persistent and severe hypoglycemia [115]. Moreover, sulfonylureas, which inhibit K_{ATP} channels, can enhance insulin secretion in type 2 diabetics. This has led to their widespread use in treating patients who were insulin-dependent and provides an important alternative treatment to the use of insulin injections with improved glycemic control.

Another type of monogenic subtype of diabetes, maturity-onset diabetes of the young (MODY) is characterized by an early onset of T2D (usually presenting in children or young adults), including some abnormalities of the β-cell function and an autosomal dominant inheritance with high penetrance [116]. MODY types represent less than 5 % of all cases of T2D. Thus far, mutations in six genes have been described; these different gene mutations are associated with different clinical forms of the disease. For instance, mutation in the *GCK* gene encoding glucokinase, a key regulatory glycolytic enzyme of the β-cell is found in MODY 2 patients. The other mutant *loci* present in MODY 1, 3, 4, 5, 6 respectively, include defects in specific transcription factors including the hepatocyte nuclear factors-1α, -4 α and –1β (HNF-1α, HNF-4α and HNF-1β), the insulin promoter factor-1 (IPF-1) and NeuroD [117–119]. Individuals harboring either of the two most frequently found forms of MODY 2 display a more benign clinical prognosis with an elevated threshold for glucose sensing resulting in mild, regulated hyperglycemia or impaired glucose tolerance with relatively few cardiovascular complications. In contrast, subjects with MODY 3 (with defective HNF-1α) exhibit a much more severe disorder, more typical of T2D and frequently require treatment with sulfonylurea or insulin.

Other monogenic forms of T2D characterized by severe insulin resistance are the result of mutations in genes encoding PPAR-γ (PPARG), Akt (AKT2), and the insulin receptor (INSR) [120–123]. These patients often develop discrete extra-pancreatic phenotypes such as lipid abnormalities or a variety of cystic renal diseases.

Efforts to identify genes responsible for more common, polygenic forms of T1D and T2D diabetes have been less clear-cut than with the monogenic forms of this disorder. Moreover, despite intensive research, there is still no definitive genetic test to diagnose T1D or T2D. Data obtained from both animal and clinical studies have revealed multiple overlaps in the genes implicated in both types of diabetes as well as in the pathogenic pathways including apoptotic remodeling. Notably, both types of diabetes have been shown to be associated with significant damage to mitochondria in pancreatic β-cells, liver and heart [124, 125].

Other genetically influenced traits like obesity and hyperlipidemia are strongly associated with T2D. Interestingly, many of the risk factors implicated in the development of T2D, including weight gain, lack of physical exercise and increasing age, are associated with an impaired mitochondrial function. Furthermore, recent studies have suggested that mitochondrial bioenergetic dysfunction largely underlies the defects in insulin responsiveness found in skeletal muscle and liver responsible for insulin resistance [126], and for defects in glucose-stimulated insulin secretion by pancreatic β-cells responsible for the progression to hyperglycemia [127–130].

In addition, several predisposition loci have significant influence on the susceptibility to T1D. Multifactorial and polygenic T1D is strongly influenced by multiple genes controlling the immune system, within the major histocompatibility complex primarily HLA-DQ and DR [131]. Another well-characterized susceptibility locus is the insulin gene, including the variable nucleotide tandem repeat locus within the regulatory region of the gene. This genetic variation affects the expression of insulin in the thymus and may play a role in the modulation of tolerance to this molecule [132]. Moreover, a significant autoimmune component has been identified in a large subset of T1D cases, with measurable autoantibodies a useful diagnostic and prognostic marker [133]. In addition, polymorphic variants of genes involved in signal transduction including the cytotoxic T lymphocyte-associated molecule 4 (CTLA-4) [134], and the PTPN22 gene encoding the lymphoid protein tyrosine phosphatase (LYP) [135], and in some populations, genomic variations of vitamin D metabolism and target cell action predispose to T1D. There is increasing epidemiological evidence suggesting that vitamin D deficiency in early life increases the incidence of later onset autoimmune diseases, such as T1D, in genetically predisposed individuals, and that high dose vitamin D supplementation can be protective against its development in both animals and humans [136, 137].

In T2D, which accounts for about 85 % of all diabetic patients, the body either produces too little insulin, or does not respond well to it. Forms of T2D tend to have a middle/late age of onset and occur with both impaired insulin secretion and insulin resistance. While this type of diabetes might be predicted to be induced by multiple gene defects specifically involved in insulin action and/or insulin secretion, a rather large variety of other genes have been at least partially implicated in its genesis as shown in Table 9.4 [138–188]. The majority of these genes identified thus far are involved in intracellular and metabolic signaling (e.g., KCNJ11, adiponectin, IRS-1, FABP2, MTP, calpain 10) and with transcription regulation (e.g., HNF-1α, PPAR-γ, LMNA, TCF7L2, TFAP2B) not surprisingly similar (and in a number of cases overlapping) to the previously presented list of genes associated with MetSyn (see Table 9.3). In addition, polymorphic allelic variants of inflammatory cytokines (e.g., IL-6, TNF-α) and of stress-response genes (e.g., MTHFR) have been associated with the increased risk or protection against T2D. In a number of cases, there is strong evidence indicating that the clinical manifestations and course of this disease is fostered by the interaction of environmental and genetic factors, including frequent polymorphisms of many genes, not just one.

Table 9.4 Specific gene polymorphisms and diabetes

Phenotype	Variants (gene)	Polymorphism	Ref
T2D	Interleukin-6 (IL-6)	C-174G, A-598G	138–139
T2D	Methylenetetrahydrofolate reductase (MTHFR)	677C>T	140–141
T2D, T1D	Hepatocyte nuclear factor 1-α (HNF-1α) also known as transcription factor 1 [TCF1]	I27L	142
T2D	Transcription-factor-activating protein 2β (TFAP2B)	Variable # of tandem repeats	143
T2D	PGC-1α	Thr394Thr	144–147
Not associated with T2D	PGC-1α	Gly482Ser	148–150
T2D	TNF-α	G-308 A allele	151–152
T2D	SUR1/Kir6.2/(KCNJ11)	E23K	153
T2D	Calpain 10 (CAPN10)	SNP44/ Thr504Ala, 3 intronic SNPs43,19,63	154–158
T2D	LMNA	1908C/T rs4641	159–160
Not associated with T2D	LMNA	Rs4641 H566H (rs4641)	161–162
T2D	IRS-1	Gly972Arg	163–164
Not associated with T2D	IRS-1	Gly972Arg	165
T2D/CAD	Adiponectin (APM1)	SNP exon 2 (45T/G)	166–168
T2D/CAD	Adiponectin (APM1)	SNP intron 2 (276G/T)	166–167, 169
T2D/CAD	Adiponectin receptor (ADIPOR1)	3 SNPs at 3' end, 3 intronic SNPs	170–171
T2D	FABP2	Ala54Thr	172–175
T2D	PPAR-α	Leu162Val	176–177
Not associated with T2D	PPAR-α	Leu162Val	178
T2D	PPAR-γ	Pro12Ala Ala reduces risk	179–182
Not associated with T2D	PPAR-δ	Several SNPs	74
Lower incidence of T2D	Microsomal triglyceride transfer protein (MTP)	I128T	183
T2D	Transcription factor 7-like 2 (TCF7L2)	Several positive haplotypes and one protective haplotype	84–85, 184–188

Type 2 diabetes: T2D; CAD: Coronary artery disease

These polymorphisms may be localized in the coding or regulatory parts of the genes and are present, although with different frequencies, in both patients as well as healthy individuals. Moreover, some of the polymorphic alleles affect specific clinical presentation more so in the elderly individuals. For instance, elderly individuals carrying the T allele of the TCF7L2 with diabetes tended to have poorer renal function (reduced 24-hour creatinine clearance), and possibly more retinopathy but fewer metabolic syndrome features displaying smaller waist circumference, and lower risk lipid profiles [85]. A large number of pathogenic mechanisms for T2D diabetes have been proposed including increased non-esterified fatty acids, inflammatory cytokines, adipokines, and mitochondrial dysfunction for insulin resistance, and glucotoxicity, lipotoxicity, and amyloid formation for β-cell dysfunction.

Relationship Between Metabolic Syndrome and Diabetes

As suggested by the rather close overlap of predisposing genes, there is a very close relationship between type 2 diabetes and MetSyn. This is further supported by the presence of most of the components of MetSyn in over 75 % of patients classified as prediabetic. According to one perspective championed by Grundy [189], the MetSyn has two underlying primary risk factors insulin resistance and obesity (the latter attributed to the recent remarkable increase in MetSyn incidence); exacerbating factors include physical inactivity, advancing age, endocrine and genetic factors which result in progressive disease which can culminate in several outcomes including atherosclerotic CVD, CVD with type 2 diabetes or type 2 diabetes alone (as shown in Fig. 9.3). The complications of CVDs associated with MetSyn include cardiac dysrhythmias, HF and thrombotic episodes. Diabetic complications that can arise include renal failure, diabetic cardiomyopathy and neuropathy.

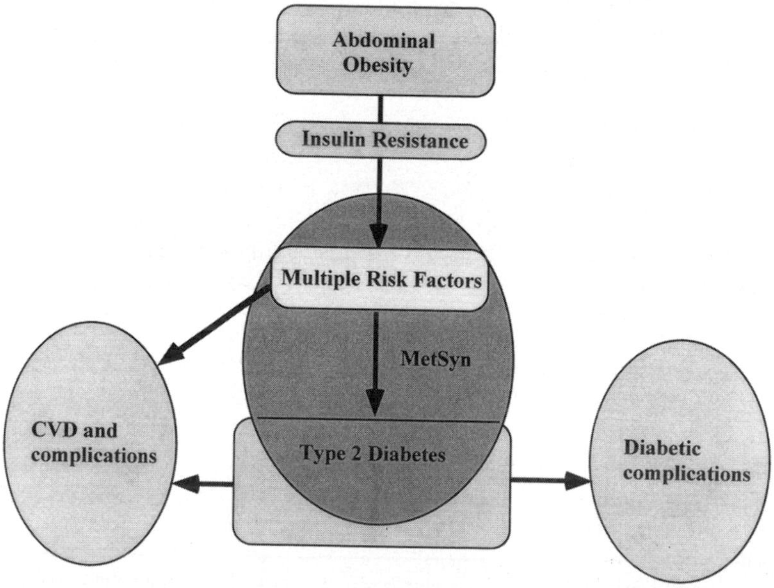

Fig. 9.3 Progression and outcome of metabolic syndrome (MetSyn)
Arising largely from abdominal obesity, MetSyn develops further with multiple added metabolic risk factors and with aging. Many MetSyn subjects develop type 2 diabetes. MetSyn encompasses each stage in the development of risk factors. As the syndrome develops, risks of atherosclerotic cardiovascular disease (CVD) and its complications including increased cardiac dysrhythmia, heart failure and thrombosis. With diabetes, other diabetic complications in addition to CVD develop.

Several studies have demonstrated that when diabetes is not yet present, the risk for progression to type 2 diabetes is greater than five-fold in subjects with MetSyn compared to subjects without the syndrome.

Conclusion

While molecular analysis of factors involved in both MetSyn and diabetes has progressed rapidly in a relatively short period, clearly much remains to be learned about the characterization of these elements and the role that they play in disease pathogenesis. Findings from case-control association studies remain often unclear due to population/individual heterogeneity, often underpowered studies, and differences in both methodological approaches and even clinical end-points leading to frequent conflicting findings. Further studies for both diseases are urgently needed in elderly populations for which there is often limited data; the increased use of gene profiling and increased availability of age, gender and ethnic-based findings on gene expression should also prove useful in further understanding the effects of specific gene variants on the expression of these diseases in elderly individuals.

While this information should eventually provide the clinician with important pharmacogenetic and nutrigenomic tools to improve treatment and disease management at an individualized level, novel strategies for disease prevention and reversal may also be in the cards. In addition to improved drugs, new techniques for gene and cell based therapies may also be employed as suggested by findings in animal models. For instance, recent studies in a rat model of MetSyn caused by leptin insufficiency and abnormal fat accumulation have shown that the single central administration of a recombinant adeno-associated virus vector containing the gene encoding leptin severely depleted fat and ameliorated the major symptoms of MetSyn for extended periods in rodents [190]. In addition, endogenous hematopoietic stem cells have been deployed to regenerate pancreatic β-cells and produce insulin which may be helpful in targeting autoimmune diabetes [191]. Other cell-based approaches include the engineering of extrapancreatic cells (using a patient's somatic cells) to secrete insulin [192]. While some of the techniques may take many years of testing before they can be implemented on a clinical level, other less-invasive approaches including metabolite modulation targeting glucose and fatty acid uptake and utilization pathway components may also be incorporated into treating these disorders [193]. The use of fibrates and PPAR agonists, β-adrenergic blockers and fatty acid oxidation inhibitors in redirecting bioenergetic pathways have also shown promise in treating cardiovascular disorders and diabetes as well as MetSyn [194–198]. Again, the impact of these approaches needs to be further gauged in the elderly.

Summary

- The increasingly prevalent metabolic syndrome (MetSyn) involves the clustering of several phenotypes including hypertension, insulin resistance, atherogenic dyslipidemia and obesity.
- Other conditions and findings associated with this syndrome include renal disease, elevation in inflammatory markers, and polycystic ovarian syndrome.
- MetSyn is also characterized by chronic inflammation and thrombotic disorder contributing to endothelial dysfunction and, subsequently, to accelerated atherosclerosis and coronary artery disease (CAD). Individuals with the metabolic syndrome have up to a five-fold increased risk of developing early atherosclerotic heart disease.
- Underlying the pathological link of MetSyn to these CVDs is the inflammation in the vasculature accompanied by atherogenic dyslipidemia including the combination of hypertriglyceridemia,

low levels of HDL-C, and a preponderance of small, dense low-density lipoprotein (LDL) particles, critical components of the syndrome.

- It has become increasingly recognized that a primary factor by which obesity acts as a central component in the development of MetSyn is the production by adipose cells of bioactive substances (e.g., adipokines) that directly influence insulin sensitivity and vascular injury.
- Blockade of the receptors (e.g., CB1 receptor) of endogenous cannabinoids with agents such as rimonabant provides a novel approach to the management of multiple cardiometabolic risk factors and MetSyn by addressing abdominal obesity and directly improving lipid and glucose metabolism and insulin resistance.
- In the elderly, MetSyn has been shown to be associated with increased cardiac remodeling as well as modulated in part by changes in leptin and endogenous hormones.
- Both MetSyn and diabetes have significant effects on cognitive function and dementia which are particularly evident in the elderly.
- The identification of contributory genes and biomarkers in MetSyn is underway and has begun to allow the identification of the pathways involved in disease onset as well as therapeutic targets. These include transcriptional factors (e.g., LMNA, PPARs, PGC-1, FOXC2 and HNF-4α), lipid pathway factors (e.g., FABP2, APOC3) and metabolic signaling components (β-AR, PTPN1).
- Diabetes affects nearly 20 % of people between 65 and 75 years of age and as many as 40 % over 80 years of age. Though type 1 diabetes (T1D) and closely-related autoimmune diabetes (LADA) can occur in the elderly, the most prevalent type in the elderly is non-insulin-dependent type 2 diabetes (T2D).
- Both type 1 and 2 diabetes are polygenic disorders which involve the interaction of several polymorphic gene variants, which are gradually being identified with environmental risk factors including stressors, neurohormones and dietary factors.
- Gene variants affecting T2D presentation include intracellular and metabolic signaling factors (e.g., KCJN11, adiponectin, IRS-1, FABP2, MTP, calpain 10) transcription regulatory factors (e.g., HNF-1α, PPAR-γ, LMNA, TCF7L2, TFAP2B), inflammatory cytokines (e.g., IL-6, TNF-α) and stress-response genes (e.g. MTHFR).
- Metabolic therapy utilizing fibrates and agonists of PPAR, β-blockers and fatty acid oxidation (FAO) inhibitors to redirecting bioenergetic pathway have also shown promise in treating cardiac dysfunction and diabetes.
- Gene and cell-mediated therapy holds promise in treating diabetes and insulin resistance.

References

1. Zimmet P, Alberti KG, Shaw J. Global and societal implications of the diabetes epidemic. Nature 2001;414: 782–787
2. Vasudevan AR, Ballantyne CM. Cardiometabolic risk assessment: an approach to the prevention of cardiovascular disease and diabetes mellitus. Clin Cornerstone 2005;7:7–16
3. DeFronzo RA, Ferrannini E. Insulin resistance. A multifaceted syndrome responsible for NIDDM, obesity, hypertension, dyslipidemia, and atherosclerotic cardiovascular disease. Diabetes Care 1991;14:173–194
4. Reaven GM. Banting lecture 1988. Role of insulin resistance in human disease. Diabetes 1988;37:1595–1607
5. Lemieux I, Pascot A, Couillard C, Lamarche B, Tchernof A, Almeras N, Bergeron J, Gaudet D, Tremblay G, Prud'homme D, Nadeau A, Despres JP. Hypertriglyceridemic waist: a marker of the atherogenic metabolic triad (hyperinsulinemia; hyperapolipoprotein B; small, dense LDL) in men? Circulation 2000;102:179–184
6. Kaplan NM. The deadly quartet. Upper-body obesity, glucose intolerance, hypertriglyceridemia, and hypertension. Arch Intern Med 1989;149:1514–1520
7. Alberti KG, Zimmet PZ. Definition, diagnosis and classification of diabetes mellitus and its complications. Part 1: diagnosis and classification of diabetes mellitus provisional report of a WHO consultation. Diabet Med 1998;15:539–553
8. Balkau B, Charles MA. Comment on the provisional report from the WHO consultation. European Group for the Study of Insulin Resistance (EGIR). Diabet Med 1999;16:442–443

9. Einhorn D, Reaven GM, Cobin RH, Ford E, Ganda OP, Handelsman Y, Hellman R, Jellinger PS, Kendall D, Krauss RM, Neufeld ND, Petak SM, Rodbard HW, Seibel JA, Smith DA, Wilson PW. American College of Endocrinology position statement on the insulin resistance syndrome. Endocr Pract 2003;9:237–252
10. Third Report of the National Cholesterol Education Program (NCEP) Expert Panel on Detection, Evaluation, and Treatment of High Blood Cholesterol in Adults (Adult Treatment Panel III) final report. Circulation 2002;106:3143–3421
11. Grundy SM, Cleeman JI, Daniels SR, Donato KA, Eckel RH, Franklin BA, Gordon DJ, Krauss RM, Savage PJ, Smith SC Jr, Spertus JA, Costa F. Diagnosis and management of the metabolic syndrome: an American Heart Association/National Heart, Lung, and Blood Institute Scientific Statement. Circulation 2005;112:2735–2752
12. Nicklas BJ, Penninx BW, Cesari M, Kritchevsky SB, Newman AB, Kanaya AM, Pahor M, Jingzhong D, Harris TB. Association of visceral adipose tissue with incident myocardial infarction in older men and women: the Health, Aging and Body Composition Study. Am J Epidemiol 2004;160:741–749
13. Despres JP, Lemieux I. Abdominal obesity and metabolic syndrome. Nature 2006;444:881–887
14. Pagotto U, Vicennati V, Pasquali R. The endocannabinoid system and the treatment of obesity. Ann Med 2005;37:270–275
15. Howlett AC, Barth F, Bonner TI, Cabral G, Casellas P, Devane WA, Felder CC, Herkenham M, Mackie K, Martin BR, Mechoulam R, Pertwee RG. International Union of Pharmacology. XXVII. Classification of cannabinoid receptors. Pharmacol Rev 2002;54:161–202
16. Mechoulam R, Ben-Shabat S, Hanus L, Ligumsky M, Kaminski NE, Schatz AR, Gopher A, Almog S, Martin BR, Compton DR. Identification of an endogenous 2-monoglyceride, present in canine gut, that binds to cannabinoid receptors. Biochem Pharmacol 1995;50:83–90
17. Dinh TP, Carpenter D, Leslie FM, Freund TF, Katona I, Sensi SL, Kathuria S, Piomelli D. Brain monoglyceride lipase participating in endocannabinoid inactivation. Proc Natl Acad Sci USA 2002;99:10819–10824
18. Kirkham TC. Endogenous cannabinoids: a new target in the treatment of obesity. Am J Physiol Regul Integr Comp Physiol 2003;284:R343–R344
19. Freedland CS, Poston JS, Porrino LJ. Effects of SR141716A, a central cannabinoid receptor antagonist, on food-maintained responding. Pharmacol Biochem Behav 2000;67:265–270
20. Di MV, Goparaju SK, Wang L, Liu J, Batkai S, Jarai Z, Fezza F, Miura GI, Palmiter RD, Sugiura T, Kunos G. Leptin-regulated endocannabinoids are involved in maintaining food intake. Nature 2001;410:822–825
21. Kirkham TC. Endogenous cannabinoids: a new target in the treatment of obesity. Am J Physiol Regul Integr Comp Physiol 2003;284:R343–R344
22. Cota D, Marsicano G, Tschop M, Grubler Y, Flachskamm C, Schubert M, Auer D, Yassouridis A, Thone-Reineke C, Ortmann S, Tomassoni F, Cervino C, Nisoli E, Linthorst AC, Pasquali R, Lutz B, Stalla GK, Pagotto U. The endogenous cannabinoid system affects energy balance via central orexigenic drive and peripheral lipogenesis. J Clin Invest 2003;112:423–431
23. Osei-Hyiaman D, DePetrillo M, Pacher P, Liu J, Radaeva S, Batkai S, Harvey-White J, Mackie K, Offertaler L, Wang L, Kunos G. Endocannabinoid activation at hepatic CB1 receptors stimulates fatty acid synthesis and contributes to diet-induced obesity. J Clin Invest 2005;115:1298–1305
24. Rinaldi-Carmona M, Barth F, Heaulme M, Shire D, Calandra B, Congy C, Martinez S, Maruani J, Neliat G, Caput D. SR141716A, a potent and selective antagonist of the brain cannabinoid receptor. FEBS Lett 1994;350:240–244
25. Pi-Sunyer FX, Aronne LJ, Heshmati HM, Devin J, Rosenstock J. Effect of rimonabant, a cannabinoid-1 receptor blocker, on weight and cardiometabolic risk factors in overweight or obese patients: RIO-North America: a randomized controlled trial. JAMA 2006;295:761–775
26. Van Gaal LF, Rissanen AM, Scheen AJ, Ziegler O, Rossner S. Effects of the cannabinoid-1 receptor blocker rimonabant on weight reduction and cardiovascular risk factors in overweight patients: 1-year experience from the RIO-Europe study. Lancet 2005;365:1389–1397
27. Despres JP, Golay A, Sjostrom L. Effects of rimonabant on metabolic risk factors in overweight patients with dyslipidemia. N Engl J Med 2005;353:2121–2134
28. Scheen AJ, Finer N, Hollander P, Jensen MD, Van Gaal LF. RIO-Diabetes Study Group. Efficacy and tolerability of rimonabant in overweight or obese patients with type 2 diabetes: a randomised controlled study. Lancet 2006;368:1660–1672
29. Lamberts SW, van den Beld AW, van der Lely AJ. The endocrinology of aging. Science 1997;278:419–424
30. Kapoor D, Malkin CJ, Channer KS, Jones TH. Androgens, insulin resistance and vascular disease in men. Clin Endocrinol (Oxf) 2005;63:239–250
31. Muller M, van den Beld AW, Bots ML, Grobbee DE, Lamberts SW, van der Schouw YT. Endogenous sex hormones and progression of carotid atherosclerosis in elderly men. Circulation 2004;109:2074–2079
32. Muller M, Grobbee DE, den TI, Lamberts SW, van der Schouw YT. Endogenous sex hormones and metabolic syndrome in aging men. J Clin Endocrinol Metab 2005;90:2618–2623
33. Zamboni M, Zoico E, Fantin F, Panourgia MP, Di FV, Tosoni P, Solerte B, Vettor R, Bosello O. Relation between leptin and the metabolic syndrome in elderly women. J Gerontol A Biol Sci Med Sci 2004;59:396–400

34. Maggio M, Lauretani F, Ceda GP, Bandinelli S, Basaria S, Ble A, Egan J, Paolisso G, Najjar S, Jeffrey Metter E, Valenti G, Guralnik JM, Ferrucci L. Association between hormones and metabolic syndrome in older Italian men. J Am Geriatr Soc 2006;54:1832–1838
35. Goldstein JL, Brown MS. Molecular medicine. The cholesterol quartet. Science 2001;292:1310–1312
36. Holvoet P, Mertens A, Verhamme P, Bogaerts K, Beyens G, Verhaeghe R, Collen D, Muls E, Van de Werf F. Circulating oxidized LDL is a useful marker for identifying patients with coronary artery disease. Arterioscler Thromb Vasc Biol 2001;21:844–848
37. Holvoet P, Kritchevsky SB, Tracy RP, Mertens A, Rubin SM, Butler J, Goodpaster B, Harris TB. The metabolic syndrome, circulating oxidized LDL, and risk of myocardial infarction in well-functioning elderly people in the health, aging, and body composition cohort. Diabetes 2004;53:1068–1073
38. Lind L, Berne C, Lithell H. Prevalence of insulin resistance in essential hypertension. J Hypertens 1995;13:1457–1462
39. Lind L, Andersson PE, Andren B, Hanni A, Lithell HO. Left ventricular hypertrophy in hypertension is associated with the insulin resistance metabolic syndrome. J Hypertens 1995;13:433–438
40. Sundstrom J, Lind L, Nystrom N, Zethelius B, Andren B, Hales CN, Lithell HO. Left ventricular concentric remodeling rather than left ventricular hypertrophy is related to the insulin resistance syndrome in elderly men. Circulation 2000;101:2595–2600
41. Lindblad U, Langer RD, Wingard DL, Thomas RG, Barrett-Connor EL. Metabolic syndrome and ischemic heart disease in elderly men and women. Am J Epidemiol 2001;153:481–489
42. Tangalos EG, Cota D, Fujioka K. Complex cardiometabolic risk factors: impact, assessment, and emerging therapies. J Am Med Dir Assoc 2006;7:1–10
43. Yaffe K. Metabolic syndrome and cognitive decline. Curr Alzheimer Res 2007;4:123–126
44. Morley JE. An overview of diabetes mellitus in older persons. Clin Geriatr Med 1999;15:211–224
45. Kanaya AM, Barrett-Connor E, Gildengorin G, Yaffe K. Change in cognitive function by glucose tolerance status in older adults: a 4-year prospective study of the Rancho Bernardo study cohort. Arch Intern Med 2004;164:1327–1333
46. Yaffe K, Blackwell T, Kanaya AM, Davidowitz N, Barrett-Connor E, Krueger K. Diabetes, impaired fasting glucose, and development of cognitive impairment in older women. Neurology 2004;63:658–663
47. Messier C, Awad N, Gagnon M. The relationships between atherosclerosis, heart disease, type 2 diabetes and dementia. Neurol Res 2004;26:567–572
48. Ott A, Stolk RP, van HF, Pols HA, Hofman A, Breteler MM. Diabetes mellitus and the risk of dementia: the Rotterdam Study. Neurology 1999;53:1937–1942
49. Biessels GJ, Koffeman A, Scheltens P. Diabetes and cognitive impairment. Clinical diagnosis and brain imaging in patients attending a memory clinic. J Neurol 2006;253:477–482
50. Korf ES, White LR, Scheltens P, Launer LJ. Brain aging in very old men with type 2 diabetes: the Honolulu-Asia Aging Study. Diabetes Care 2006;29:2268–2274
51. Xiong GL, Plassman BL, Helms MJ, Steffens DC. Vascular risk factors and cognitive decline among elderly male twins. Neurology 2006;67:1586–1591
52. Kalmijn S, Foley D, White L, Burchfiel CM, Curb JD, Petrovitch H, Ross GW, Havlik RJ, Launer LJ. Metabolic cardiovascular syndrome and risk of dementia in Japanese-American elderly men. The Honolulu-Asia aging study. Arterioscler Thromb Vasc Biol 2000;20:2255–2260
53. Yaffe K, Kanaya A, Lindquist K, Simonsick EM, Harris T, Shorr RI, Tylavsky FA, Newman AB. The metabolic syndrome, inflammation, and risk of cognitive decline. JAMA 2004;292:2237–2242
54. Yaffe K, Lindquist K, Penninx BW, Simonsick EM, Pahor M, Kritchevsky S, Launer L, Kuller L, Rubin S, Harris T. Inflammatory markers and cognition in well-functioning African-American and white elders. Neurology 2003;61:76–80
55. Yaffe K, Haan M, Blackwell T, Cherkasova E, Whitmer RA, West N. Metabolic syndrome and cognitive decline in elderly latinos: findings from the sacramento area latino study of aging study. J Am Geriatr Soc 2007;55: 758–762
56. Navarro J, Redon J, Cea-Calvo L, Lozano JV, Fernandez-Perez C, Bonet A, Gonzalez-Esteban J, Study OB. Metabolic syndrome, organ damage and cardiovascular disease in treated hypertensive patients. The ERIC-HTA study. Blood Press 2007;16:20–27
57. Steinle NI, Kazlauskaite R, Imumorin IG, Hsueh WC, Pollin TI, O'Connell JR, Mitchell BD, Shuldiner AR. Variation in the lamin A/C gene: associations with metabolic syndrome. Arterioscler Thromb Vasc Biol 2004;24:1708–1713
58. Murase Y, Yagi K, Katsuda Y, Asano A, Koizumi J, Mabuchi H. An LMNA variant is associated with dyslipidemia and insulin resistance in the Japanese. Metabolism 2002;51:1017–1021
59. Caux F, Dubosclard E, Lascols O, Buendia B, Chazouilleres O, Cohen A, Courvalin JC, Laroche L, Capeau J, Vigouroux C, Christin-Maitre S. A new clinical condition linked to a novel mutation in lamins A and C with

generalized lipoatrophy, insulin-resistant diabetes, disseminated leukomelanodermic papules, liver steatosis, and cardiomyopathy. J Clin Endocrinol Metab 2003;88:1006–1013

60. Ukkola O, Rankinen T, Lakka T, Leon AS, Skinner JS, Wilmore JH, Rao DC, Kesaniemi YA, Bouchard C. Protein tyrosine phosphatase 1B variant associated with fat distribution and insulin metabolism. Obes Res 2005;13:829–834
61. Spencer-Jones NJ, Wang X, Snieder H, Spector TD, Carter ND, O'Dell SD. Protein tyrosine phosphatase-1B gene PTPN1: selection of tagging single nucleotide polymorphisms and association with body fat, insulin sensitivity, and the metabolic syndrome in a normal female population. Diabetes 2005;54:3296–3304
62. Palmer ND, Bento JL, Mychaleckyj JC, Langefeld CD, Campbell JK, Norris JM, Haffner SM, Bergman RN, Bowden DW. Insulin Resistance Atherosclerosis Study (IRAS) family study. Association of protein tyrosine phosphatase 1B gene polymorphisms with measures of glucose homeostasis in Hispanic Americans: the insulin resistance atherosclerosis study (IRAS) family study. Diabetes 2004;53:3013–3019
63. Manraj M, Francke S, Hebe A, Ramjuttun US, Froguel P. Genetic and environmental nature of the insulin resistance syndrome in Indo-Mauritian subjects with premature coronary heart disease: contribution of beta3-adrenoreceptor gene polymorphism and beta blockers on triglyceride and HDL concentrations. Diabetologia 2001;44:115–122
64. Strazzullo P, Iacone R, Siani A, Cappuccio FP, Russo O, Barba G, Barbato A, D'Elia L, Trevisan M, Farinaro E. Relationship of the Trp64Arg polymorphism of the beta3-adrenoceptor gene to central adiposity and high blood pressure: interaction with age. Cross-sectional and longitudinal findings of the Olivetti Prospective Heart Study. J Hypertens 2001;19:399–406
65. Bracale R, Pasanisi F, Labruna G, Finelli C, Nardelli C, Buono P, Salvatori G, Sacchetti L, Contaldo F, Oriani G. Metabolic syndrome and ADRB3 gene polymorphism in severely obese patients from South Italy. Eur J Clin Nutr 2007
66. Robitaille J, Brouillette C, Houde A, Lemieux S, Perusse L, Tchernof A, Gaudet D, Vohl MC. Association between the PPARalpha-L162V polymorphism and components of the metabolic syndrome. J Hum Genet 2004;49:482–489
67. Tai ES, Collins D, Robins SJ, O'Connor JJ Jr, Bloomfield HE, Ordovas JM, Schaefer EJ, Brousseau ME. The L162V polymorphism at the peroxisome proliferator activated receptor alpha locus modulates the risk of cardiovascular events associated with insulin resistance and diabetes mellitus: the Veterans Affairs HDL Intervention Trial (VA-HIT). Atherosclerosis 2006;187:153–160
68. Frederiksen L, Brodbaek K, Fenger M, Jorgensen T, Borch-Johnsen K, Madsbad S, Urhammer SA. Comment: studies of the Pro12Ala polymorphism of the PPAR-gamma gene in the Danish MONICA cohort: homozygosity of the Ala allele confers a decreased risk of the insulin resistance syndrome. J Clin Endocrinol Metab 2002;87:3989–3992
69. Li S, Chen W, Srinivasan SR, Boerwinkle E, Berenson GS. The Bogalusa Heart Study the peroxisome proliferator-activated receptor-gamma2 gene polymorphism (Pro12Ala) beneficially influences insulin resistance and its tracking from childhood to adulthood: the Bogalusa Heart Study. Diabetes 2003;52: 1265–1269
70. Meirhaeghe A, Cottel D, Amouyel P, Dallongeville J. Association between peroxisome proliferator-activated receptor gamma haplotypes and the metabolic syndrome in French men and women. Diabetes 2005;54: 3043–3048
71. Kahara T, Takamura T, Hayakawa T, Nagai Y, Yamaguchi H, Katsuki T, Katsuki K, Katsuki M, Kobayashi K. PPARgamma gene polymorphism is associated with exercise-mediated changes of insulin resistance in healthy men. Metabolism 2003;52:209–212
72. Rhee EJ, Oh KW, Lee WY, Kim SY, Oh ES, Baek KH, Kang MI, Kim SW. Effects of two common polymorphisms of peroxisome proliferator-activated receptor-gamma gene on metabolic syndrome. Arch Med Res 2006;37:86–94
73. Sookoian S, Garcia SI, Porto PI, Dieuzeide G, Gonzalez CD, Pirola CJ. Peroxisome proliferator-activated receptor gamma and its coactivator-1 alpha may be associated with features of the metabolic syndrome in adolescents. J Mol Endocrinol 2005;35:373–380
74. Grarup N, Albrechtsen A, Ek J, Borch-Johnsen K, Jorgensen T, Schmitz O, Hansen T, Pedersen O. Variation in the peroxisome proliferator-activated receptor delta gene in relation to common metabolic traits in 7,495 middle-aged white people. Diabetologia 2007;50:1201–1208
75. Dallongeville J, Helbecque N, Cottel D, Amouyel P, Meirhaeghe A. The Gly16→Arg16 and Gln27→Glu27 polymorphisms of beta2-adrenergic receptor are associated with metabolic syndrome in men. J Clin Endocrinol Metab 2003;88:4862–4866
76. Vohl MC, Houde A, Lebel S, Hould FS, Marceau P. Effects of the peroxisome proliferator-activated receptor-gamma co-activator-1 Gly482Ser variant on features of the metabolic syndrome. Mol Genet Metab 2005;86:300–306

77. Ambye L, Rasmussen S, Fenger M, Jorgensen T, Borch-Johnsen K, Madsbad S, Urhammer SA. Studies of the Gly482Ser polymorphism of the peroxisome proliferator-activated receptor gamma coactivator 1alpha (PGC-1alpha) gene in Danish subjects with the metabolic syndrome. Diabetes Res Clin Pract 2005;67: 175–179
78. Boullu-Sanchis S, Lepretre F, Hedelin G, Donnet JP, Schaffer P, Froguel P, Pinget M. Type 2 diabetes mellitus: association study of five candidate genes in an Indian population of Guadeloupe, genetic contribution of FABP2 polymorphism. Diabetes Metab 1999;25:150–156
79. Guettier JM, Georgopoulos A, Tsai MY, Radha V, Shanthirani S, Deepa R, Gross M, Rao G, Mohan V. Polymorphisms in the fatty acid-binding protein 2 and apolipoprotein C-III genes are associated with the metabolic syndrome and dyslipidemia in a South Indian population. J Clin Endocrinol Metab 2005;90:1705–1711
80. Pollex RL, Hanley AJ, Zinman B, Harris SB, Khan HM, Hegele RA. Metabolic syndrome in aboriginal Canadians: prevalence and genetic associations. Atherosclerosis 2006;184:121–129
81. Vimaleswaran KS, Radha V, Mohan V. Thr54 allele carriers of the Ala54Thr variant of FABP2 gene have associations with metabolic syndrome and hyper-triglyceridemia in urban South Indians. Metabolism 2006;55: 1222–1226
82. Erkkila AT, Lindi V, Lehto S, Pyorala K, Laakso M, Uusitupa MI. Variation in the fatty acid binding protein 2 gene is not associated with markers of metabolic syndrome in patients with coronary heart disease. Nutr Metab Cardiovasc Dis 2002;12:53–59
83. Ohashi K, Ouchi N, Kihara S, Funahashi T, Nakamura T, Sumitsuji S, Kawamoto T, Matsumoto S, Nagaretani H, Kumada M, Okamoto Y, Nishizawa H, Kishida K, Maeda N, Hiraoka H, Iwashima Y, Ishikawa K, Ohishi M, Katsuya T, Rakugi H, Ogihara T, Matsuzawa Y. Adiponectin I164T mutation is associated with the metabolic syndrome and coronary artery disease. J Am Coll Cardiol 2004;43:1195–1200
84. Marzi C, Huth C, Kolz M, Grallert H, Meisinger C, Wichmann HE, Rathmann W, Herder C, Illig T. Variants of the transcription factor 7-like 2 gene (TCF7L2) are strongly associated with type 2 diabetes but not with the metabolic syndrome in the MONICA/KORA surveys. Horm Metab Res 2007;39:46–52
85. Melzer D, Murray A, Hurst AJ, Weedon MN, Bandinelli S, Corsi AM, Ferrucci L, Paolisso G, Guralnik JM, Frayling TM. Effects of the diabetes linked TCF7L2 polymorphism in a representative older population. BMC Med 2006;4:34
86. Bing C, Ambye L, Fenger M, Jorgensen T, Borch-Johnsen K, Madsbad S, Urhammer SA. Large-scale studies of the Leu72Met polymorphism of the ghrelin gene in relation to the metabolic syndrome and associated quantitative traits. Diabet Med 2005;22:1157–1160
87. Carlsson E, Groop L, Ridderstrale M. Role of the FOXC2 -512C>T polymorphism in type 2 diabetes: possible association with the dysmetabolic syndrome. Int J Obes (Lond) 2005;29:268–274
88. Weissglas-Volkov D, Huertas-Vazquez A, Suviolahti E, Lee J, Plaisier C, Canizales-Quinteros S, Tusie-Luna T, Aguilar-Salinas C, Taskinen MR, Pajukanta P. Common hepatic nuclear factor-4alpha variants are associated with high serum lipid levels and the metabolic syndrome. Diabetes 2006;55:1970–1977
89. Miller M, Rhyne J, Chen H, Beach V, Ericson R, Luthra K, Dwivedi M, Misra A. APOC3 promoter polymorphisms C-482T and T-455C are associated with the metabolic syndrome. Arch Med Res 2007;38:444–451
90. Koh KK, Han SH, Quon MJ. Inflammatory markers and the metabolic syndrome: insights from therapeutic interventions. J Am Coll Cardiol 2005;46:1978–1985
91. Hegele RA. Familial partial lipodystrophy: a monogenic form of the insulin resistance syndrome. Mol Genet Metab 2000;71:539–544
92. Caux F, Dubosclard E, Lascols O, Buendia B, Chazouilleres O, Cohen A, Courvalin JC, Laroche L, Capeau J, Vigouroux C, Christin-Maitre S. A new clinical condition linked to a novel mutation in lamins A and C with generalized lipoatrophy, insulin-resistant diabetes, disseminated leukomelanodermic papules, liver steatosis, and cardiomyopathy. J Clin Endocrinol Metab 2003;88:1006–1013
93. Haque WA, Oral EA, Dietz K, Bowcock AM, Agarwal AK, Garg A. Risk factors for diabetes in familial partial lipodystrophy, Dunnigan variety. Diabetes Care 2003;26:1350–1355
94. Cao H, Hegele RA. Nuclear lamin A/C R482Q mutation in canadian kindreds with Dunnigan-type familial partial lipodystrophy. Hum Mol Genet 2000;9:109–112
95. Hegele RA, Cao H, Frankowski C, Mathews ST, Leff T. PPARG F388L, a transactivation-deficient mutant, in familial partial lipodystrophy. Diabetes 2002;51:3586–3590
96. Hegele RA, Pollex RL. Genetic and physiological insights into the metabolic syndrome. Am J Physiol Regul Integr Comp Physiol 2005;289:R663–R669
97. Hegele RA, Joy TR, Al-Attar S, Rutt BK. Lipodystrophies: windows on adipose biology and metabolism. J Lipid Res. 2007 Mar 20 [Epub ahead of print]
98. Savage DB, Tan GD, Acerini CL, Jebb SA, Agostini M, Gurnell M, Williams RL, Umpleby AM, Thomas EL, Bell JD, Dixon AK, Dunne F, Boiani R, Cinti S, Vidal-Puig A, Karpe F, Chatterjee VK, O'Rahilly S. Human metabolic syndrome resulting from dominant-negative mutations in the nuclear receptor peroxisome proliferator-activated receptor-gamma. Diabetes 2003;52:910–917

99. Agostini M, Schoenmakers E, Mitchell C, Szatmari I, Savage D, Smith A, Rajanayagam O, Semple R, Luan J, Bath L, Zalin A, Labib M, Kumar S, Simpson H, Blom D, Marais D, Schwabe J, Barroso I, Trembath R, Wareham N, Nagy L, Gurnell M, O'Rahilly S, Chatterjee K. Non-DNA binding, dominant-negative, human PPARgamma mutations cause lipodystrophic insulin resistance. Cell Metab 2006;4:303–311
100. Kotzka J, Muller-Wieland D. Sterol regulatory element-binding protein (SREBP)-1: gene regulatory target for insulin resistance? Expert Opin Ther Targets 2004;8:141–149
101. Koo SH, Satoh H, Herzig S, Lee CH, Hedrick S, Kulkarni R, Evans RM, Olefsky J, Montminy M. PGC-1 promotes insulin resistance in liver through PPAR-alpha-dependent induction of TRB-3. Nat Med 2004;10: 530–534
102. Shulman AI, Mangelsdorf DJ. Retinoid x receptor heterodimers in the metabolic syndrome. N Engl J Med 2005;353:604–615
103. Berger JP, Akiyama TE, Meinke PT. PPARs: therapeutic targets for metabolic disease. Trends Pharmacol Sci 2005;26:244–251
104. Han SH, Quon MJ, Koh KK. Beneficial vascular and metabolic effects of peroxisome proliferator-activated receptor-alpha activators. Hypertension 2005;46:1086–1092
105. Chinetti-Gbaguidi G, Fruchart JC, Staels B. Role of the PPAR family of nuclear receptors in the regulation of metabolic and cardiovascular homeostasis: new approaches to therapy. Curr Opin Pharmacol 2005;5:177–183
106. Khan MA, Collins AJ, Keane WF. Diabetes in the elderly population. Adv Ren Replace Ther 2000;7:32–51
107. Kamel HK, Rodriguez-Saldana J, Flaherty JH, Miller DK. Diabetes mellitus among ethnic seniors: contrasts with diabetes in whites. Clin Geriatr Med 1999;15:265–278
108. Koster JC, Permutt MA, Nichols CG. Diabetes and insulin secretion: the ATP-Sensitive K+ Channel (KATP) Connection. Diabetes 2005;54:3065–3072
109. Hattersley AT, Ashcroft FM. Activating mutations in Kir6.2 and neonatal diabetes: new clinical syndromes, new scientific insights, and new therapy. Diabetes 2005;54:2503–2513
110. Gloyn AL, Pearson ER, Antcliff JF, Proks P, Bruining GJ, Slingerland AS, Howard N, Srinivasan S, Silva JM, Molnes J, Edghill EL, Frayling TM, Temple IK, Mackay D, Shield JP, Sumnik Z, van Rhijn A, Wales JK, Clark P, Gorman S, Aisenberg J, Ellard S, Njolstad PR, Ashcroft FM, Hattersley AT. Activating mutations in the gene encoding the ATP-sensitive potassium-channel subunit Kir6.2 and permanent neonatal diabetes. N Engl J Med 2004;350:1838–1849
111. Sperling MA. Neonatal diabetes mellitus: from understudy to center stage. Curr Opin Pediatr 2005;17:512–518
112. Riedel MJ, Steckley DC, Light PE. Current status of the E23K Kir6.2 polymorphism: implications for type-2 diabetes. Hum Genet 2005;116:133–145
113. Gloyn AL, Weedon MN, Owen KR, Turner MJ, Knight BA, Hitman G, Walker M, Levy JC, Sampson M, Halford S, McCarthy MI, Hattersley AT, Frayling TM. Large-scale association studies of variants in genes encoding the pancreatic beta-cell KATP channel subunits Kir6.2 (KCNJ11) and SUR1 (ABCC8) confirm that the KCNJ11 E23K variant is associated with type 2 diabetes. Diabetes 2003;52:568–572
114. Riedel MJ, Boora P, Steckley D, de Vries G, Light PE. Kir6.2 polymorphisms sensitize beta-cell ATP-sensitive potassium channels to activation by acyl CoAs: a possible cellular mechanism for increased susceptibility to type 2 diabetes? Diabetes 2003;52:2630–2635
115. Slingerland AS, Hattersley AT. Mutations in the Kir6.2 subunit of the KATP channel and permanent neonatal diabetes: new insights and new treatment. Ann Med 2005;37:186–195
116. Malecki MT. Genetics of type 2 diabetes mellitus. Diabetes Res Clin Pract 2005;68:S10–S21
117. Gupta RK, Kaestner KH. HNF-4alpha: from MODY to late-onset type 2 diabetes. Trends Mol Med 2004;10:521–524
118. Gloyn AL. Glucokinase (GCK) mutations in hyper- and hypoglycemia: maturity-onset diabetes of the young, permanent neonatal diabetes, and hyperinsulinemia of infancy. Hum Mutat 2003;22:353–362
119. Mitchell SM, Frayling TM. The role of transcription factors in maturity-onset diabetes of the young. Mol Genet Metab 2002;77:35–43
120. George S, Rochford JJ, Wolfrum C, Gray SL, Schinner S, Wilson JC, Soos MA, Murgatroyd PR, Williams RM, Acerini CL, Dunger DB, Barford D, Umpleby AM, Wareham NJ, Davies HA, Schafer AJ, Stoffel M, O'Rahilly S, Barroso I. A family with severe insulin resistance and diabetes due to a mutation in AKT2. Science 2004;304:1325–1328
121. Hone J, Accili D, al-Gazali LI, Lestringant G, Orban T, Taylor SI. Homozygosity for a new mutation (Ile119–>Met) in the insulin receptor gene in five sibs with familial insulin resistance. J Med Genet 1994;31:715–716
122. Kusari J, Takata Y, Hatada E, Freidenberg G, Kolterman O, Olefsky JM. Insulin resistance and diabetes due to different mutations in the tyrosine kinase domain of both insulin receptor gene alleles. J Biol Chem 1991;266:5260–5267
123. Musso C, Cochran E, Moran SA, Skarulis MC, Oral EA, Taylor S, Gorden P. Clinical course of genetic diseases of the insulin receptor (type A and Rabson-Mendenhall syndromes): a 30-year prospective. Medicine 2004;83:209–222

124. Shen X, Zheng S, Thongboonkerd V, Xu M, Pierce WM Jr, Klein JB, Epstein PN. Cardiac mitochondrial damage and biogenesis in a chronic model of type 1 diabetes. Am J Physiol Endocrinol Metab 2004;287:E896–E905
125. Ferreira FM, Seica R, Oliveira PJ, Coxito PM, Moreno AJ, Palmeira CM, Santos MS. Diabetes induces metabolic adaptations in rat liver mitochondria: role of coenzyme Q and cardiolipin contents. Biochim Biophys Acta 2003;1639:113–118
126. Ritov VB, Menshikova EV, He J, Ferrell RE, Goodpaster BH, Kelley DE. Deficiency of subsarcolemmal mitochondria in obesity and type 2 diabetes. Diabetes 2005;54:8–14
127. Petersen KF, Dufour S, Befroy D, Garcia R, Shulman GI. Impaired mitochondrial activity in the insulin-resistant offspring of patients with type 2 diabetes. N Engl J Med 2004;350:664–671
128. Silva JP, Kohler M, Graff C, Oldfors A, Magnuson MA, Berggren PO, Larsson NG. Impaired insulin secretion and beta-cell loss in tissue-specific knockout mice with mitochondrial diabetes. Nat Genet 2000;26:336–340
129. Brownlee M. A radical explanation for glucose-induced beta cell dysfunction. J Clin Invest 2003;112:1788–1790
130. Lowell BB, Shulman GI. Mitochondrial dysfunction and type 2 diabetes. Science 2005;307:384–387
131. Malecki MT. Genetics of type 2 diabetes mellitus. Diabetes Res Clin Pract 2005;68:S10–S21
132. Kelly MA, Mijovic CH, Barnett AH. Genetics of type 1 diabetes. Best Pract Res Clin Endocrinol Metab 2001;15:279–291
133. Achenbach P, Bonifacio E, Ziegler AG. Predicting type 1 diabetes. Curr Diab Rep 2005;5:98–103
134. Kavvoura FK, Ioannidis JP. CTLA-4 gene polymorphisms and susceptibility to type 1 diabetes mellitus: a HuGE Review and meta-analysis. Am J Epidemiol 2005;162:3–16
135. Bottini N, Musumeci L, Alonso A, Rahmouni S, Nika K, Rostamkhani M, MacMurray J, Meloni GF, Lucarelli P, Pellecchia M, Eisenbarth GS, Comings D, Mustelin T. A functional variant of lymphoid tyrosine phosphatase is associated with type I diabetes. Nat Genet 2004;36:337–338
136. Mathieu C, Badenhoop K. Vitamin D and type 1 diabetes mellitus: state of the art. Trends Endocrinol Metab 2005;16:261–266
137. Luong K, Nguyen LT, Nguyen DN. The role of vitamin D in protecting type 1 diabetes mellitus. Diabetes Metab Res Rev 2005;21:338–346
138. Illig T, Bongardt F, Schopfer A, Muller-Scholze S, Rathmann W, Koenig W, Thorand B, Vollmert C, Holle R, Kolb H, Herder C. Kooperative Gesundheitsforschung im Raum Augsburg/Cooperative Research in the Region of Augsburg. Significant association of the interleukin-6 gene polymorphisms C-174G and A-598G with type 2 diabetes. J Clin Endocrinol Metab 2004;89:5053–5058
139. Huth C, Heid IM, Vollmert C, Gieger C, Grallert H, Wolford JK, Langer B, Thorand B, Klopp N, Hamid YH, Pedersen O, Hansen T, Lyssenko V, Groop L, Meisinger C, Doring A, Lowel H, Lieb W, Hengstenberg C, Rathmann W, Martin S, Stephens JW, Ireland H, Mather H, Miller GJ, Stringham HM, Boehnke M, Tuomilehto J, Boeing H, Mohlig M, Spranger J, Pfeiffer A, Wernstedt I, Niklason A, Lopez-Bermejo A, Fernandez-Real JM, Hanson RL, Gallart L, Vendrell J, Tsiavou A, Hatziagelaki E, Humphries SE, Wichmann HE, Herder C, Illig T. IL6 gene promoter polymorphisms and type 2 diabetes: joint analysis of individual participants' data from 21 studies. Diabetes 2006;55:2915–2921
140. Mtiraoui N, Ezzidi I, Chaieb M, Marmouche H, Aouni Z, Chaieb A, Mahjoub T, Vaxillaire M, Almawi WY. MTHFR C677T and A1298C gene polymorphisms and hyperhomocysteinemia as risk factors of diabetic nephropathy in type 2 diabetes patients. Diabetes Res Clin Pract 2007;75:99–106
141. Pollex RL, Mamakeesick M, Zinman B, Harris SB, Hanley AJ, Hegele RA. Methylenetetrahydrofolate reductase polymorphism 677C>T is associated with peripheral arterial disease in type 2 diabetes. Cardiovasc Diabetol 2005;4:17
142. Holmkvist J, Cervin C, Lyssenko V, Winckler W, Anevski D, Cilio C, Almgren P, Berglund G, Nilsson P, Tuomi T, Lindgren CM, Altshuler D, Groop L. Common variants in HNF-1 alpha and risk of type 2 diabetes. Diabetologia 2006;49:2882–2291
143. Maeda S, Tsukada S, Kanazawa A, Sekine A, Tsunoda T, Koya D, Maegawa H, Kashiwagi A, Babazono T, Matsuda M, Tanaka Y, Fujioka T, Hirose H, Eguchi T, Ohno Y, Groves CJ, Hattersley AT, Hitman GA, Walker M, Kaku K, Iwamoto Y, Kawamori R, Kikkawa R, Kamatani N, McCarthy MI, Nakamura Y. Genetic variations in the gene encoding TFAP2B are associated with type 2 diabetes mellitus. J Hum Genet 2005;50:283–292
144. Vimaleswaran KS, Radha V, Ghosh S, Majumder PP, Deepa R, Babu HN, Rao MR, Mohan V. Peroxisome proliferator-activated receptor-gamma co-activator-1alpha (PGC-1alpha) gene polymorphisms and their relationship to Type 2 diabetes in Asian Indians. Diabet Med 2005;22:1516–1521
145. Hara K, Tobe K, Okada T, Kadowaki H, Akanuma Y, Ito C, Kimura S, Kadowaki T. A genetic variation in the PGC-1 gene could confer insulin resistance and susceptibility to Type II diabetes. Diabetologia 2002;45: 740–743
146. Ek J, Andersen G, Urhammer SA, Gaede PH, Drivsholm T, Borch-Johnsen K, Hansen T, Pedersen O. Mutation analysis of peroxisome proliferator-activated receptor-gamma coactivator-1 (PGC-1) and relationships of identified amino acid polymorphisms to Type II diabetes mellitus. Diabetologia 2001;44:2220–2226

147. Andrulionyte L, Zacharova J, Chiasson JL, Laakso M. STOP-NIDDM Study Group. Common polymorphisms of the PPAR-gamma2 (Pro12Ala) and PGC-1alpha (Gly482Ser) genes are associated with the conversion from impaired glucose tolerance to type 2 diabetes in the STOP-NIDDM trial. Diabetologia 2004;47:2176–2284
148. Lacquemant C, Chikri M, Boutin P, Samson C, Froguel P. No association between the G482S polymorphism of the proliferator-activated receptor-gamma coactivator-1 (PGC-1) gene and Type II diabetes in French Caucasians. Diabetologia 2002;45:602–603
149. Nelson TL, Fingerlin TE, Moss L, Barmada MM, Ferrell RE, Norris JM. The Peroxisome Proliferator-activated Receptor Gamma Coactivator-1 Alpha Gene (PGC-1alpha) is Not Associated with Type 2 Diabetes Mellitus or Body Mass Index Among Hispanic and Non Hispanic Whites from Colorado. Exp Clin Endocrinol Diabetes 2007;115:268–275
150. Chen S, Yan W, Huang J, Yang W, Gu D. Peroxisome proliferator-activated receptor-gamma coactivator-1alpha polymorphism is not associated with essential hypertension and type 2 diabetes mellitus in Chinese population. Hypertens Res 2004;27:813–820
151. Nicaud V, Raoux S, Poirier O, Cambien F, O'Reilly DS, Tiret L. The TNF alpha/G-308A polymorphism influences insulin sensitivity in offspring of patients with coronary heart disease: the European Atherosclerosis Research Study II. Atherosclerosis 2002;161:317–325
152. Vendrell J, Fernandez-Real JM, Gutierrez C, Zamora A, Simon I, Bardaji A, Ricart W, Richart C. A polymorphism in the promoter of the tumor necrosis factor-alpha gene (–308) is associated with coronary heart disease in type 2 diabetic patients. Atherosclerosis 2003;167:257–264
153. Florez JC, Burtt N, de Bakker PI, Almgren P, Tuomi T, Holmkvist J, Gaudet D, Hudson TJ, Schaffner SF, Daly MJ, Hirschhorn JN, Groop L, Altshuler D. Haplo-type structure and genotype-phenotype correlations of the sulfonylurea receptor and the islet ATP-sensitive potassium channel gene region. Diabetes 2004;53:13
154. Tsuchiya T, Schwarz PE, Bosque-Plata LD, Geoffrey Hayes M, Dina C, Froguel P, Wayne Towers G, Fischer S, Temelkova-Kurktschiev T, Rietzsch H, Graessler J, Vcelak J, Palyzova D, Selisko T, Bendlova B, Schulze J, Julius U, Hanefeld M, Weedon MN, Evans JC, Frayling TM, Hattersley AT, Orho-Melander M, Groop L, Malecki MT, Hansen T, Pedersen O, Fingerlin TE, Boehnke M, Hanis CL, Cox NJ, Bell GI. Association of the calpain-10 gene with type 2 diabetes in Europeans: results of pooled and meta-analyses. Mol Genet Metab. 2006;89:174–184
155. Evans JC, Frayling TM, Cassell PG, Saker PJ, Hitman GA, Walker M, Levy JC, O'Rahilly S, Rao PV, Bennett AJ, Jones EC, Menzel S, Prestwich P, Simecek N, Wishart M, Dhillon R, Fletcher C, Millward A, Demaine A, Wilkin T, Horikawa Y, Cox NJ, Bell GI, Ellard S, McCarthy MI, Hattersley AT. Studies of association between the gene for calpain-10 and type 2 diabetes mellitus in the United Kingdom. Am J Hum Genet 2001;69: 544–552
156. Horikawa Y, Oda N, Cox NJ, Li X, Orho-Melander M, Hara M, Hinokio Y, Lindner TH, Mashima H, Schwarz PE, del Bosque-Plata L, Horikawa Y, Oda Y, Yoshiuchi I, Colilla S, Polonsky KS, Wei S, Concannon P, Iwasaki N, Schulze J, Baier LJ, Bogardus C, Groop L, Boerwinkle E, Hanis CL, Bell GI. Genetic variation in the gene encoding calpain-10 is associated with type 2 diabetes mellitus. Nat Genet 2000;26:163–175
157. Weedon MN, Schwarz PE, Horikawa Y, Iwasaki N, Illig T, Holle R, Rathmann W, Selisko T, Schulze J, Owen KR, Evans J, Del Bosque-Plata L, Hitman G, Walker M, Levy JC, Sampson M, Bell GI, McCarthy MI, Hattersley AT, Frayling TM. Meta-analysis and a large association study confirm a role for calpain-10 variation in type 2 diabetes susceptibility. Am J Hum Genet 2003;73:1208–1212
158. Iwasaki N, Horikawa Y, Tsuchiya T, Kitamura Y, Nakamura T, Tanizawa Y, Oka Y, Hara K, Kadowaki T, Awata T, Honda M, Yamashita K, Oda N, Yu L, Yamada N, Ogata M, Kamatani N, Iwamoto Y, Del Bosque-Plata L, Hayes MG, Cox NJ, Bell GI. Genetic variants in the calpain-10 gene and the development of type 2 diabetes in the Japanese population. J Hum Genet 2005;50:92–98
159. Liang H, Murase Y, Katuta Y, Asano A, Kobayashi J, Mabuchi H. Association of LMNA 1908C/T polymorphism with cerebral vascular disease and diabetic nephropathy in Japanese men with type 2 diabetes. Clin Endocrinol 2005;63:317–322
160. Wegner L, Andersen G, Sparso T, Grarup N, Glumer C, Borch-Johnsen K, Jorgensen T, Hansen T, Pedersen O. Common variation in LMNA increases susceptibility to type 2 diabetes and associates with elevated fasting glycemia and estimates of body fat and height in the general population: studies of 7,495 Danish whites. Diabetes 2007;56:694–698
161. Mesa JL, Loos RJ, Franks PW, Ong KK, Luan J, O'Rahilly S, Wareham NJ, Barroso I. Lamin A/C polymorphisms, type 2 diabetes, and the metabolic syndrome: case-control and quantitative trait studies. Diabetes 2007;56:884–889
162. Owen KR, Groves CJ, Hanson RL, Knowler WC, Shuldiner AR, Elbein SC, Mitchell BD, Froguel P, Ng MC, Chan JC, Jia W, Deloukas P, Hitman GA, Walker M, Frayling TM, Hattersley AT, Zeggini E, McCarthy MI. Common variation in the LMNA gene (encoding lamin A/C) and type 2 diabetes: association analyses in 9,518 subjects. Diabetes 2007;56:879–883

163. Almind K, Bjørbaek C, Vestergaard H, Hansen T, Echwald S, Pedersen O. Aminoacid polymorphisms of insulin receptor substrate-1 in non-insulin dependent diabetes mellitus. Lancet 1993;342:828–832
164. Jellema A, Zeegers MP, Feskens EJ, Dagnelie PC, Mensink RP. Gly972Arg variant in the insulin receptor substrate-1 gene and association with type 2 diabetes: a metaanalysis of 27 studies. Diabetologia 2003;46: 990–995
165. Florez JC, Sjögren M, Burtt N, Orho-Melander M, Schayer S, Sun M, Almgren P, Lindblad U, Tuomi T, Gaudet D, Hudson TJ, Daly MJ, Ardlie KG, Hirschhorn JN, Altshuler D, Groop L. Association testing in 9,000 people fails to confirm the association of the insulin receptor substrate-1 G972R polymorphism with type 2 diabetes. Diabetes 2004;53:3313–3318
166. Hara K, Boutin P, Mori Y, Tobe K, Dina C, Yasuda K, Yamauchi T, Otabe S, Okada T, Eto K, Kadowaki H, Hagura R, Akanuma Y, Yazaki Y, Nagai R, Taniyama M, Matsubara K, Yoda M, Nakano Y, Tomita M, Kimura S, Ito C, Froguel P, Kadowaki T. Genetic variation in the gene encoding adiponectin is associated with an increased risk of type 2 diabetes in the Japanese population. Diabetes 2002;51:536–540
167. Zacharova J, Chiasson JL, Laakso M. STOP-NIDDM Study Group. The common polymorphisms (single nucleotide polymorphism [SNP] +45 and SNP +276) of the adiponectin gene predict the conversion from impaired glucose tolerance to type 2 diabetes: the STOP-NIDDM trial. Diabetes 2005;54:893–899
168. Lacquemant C, Froguel P, Lobbens S, Izzo P, Dina C, Ruiz J. The adiponectin gene SNP+45 is associated with coronary artery disease in Type 2 (non-insulin-dependent) diabetes mellitus. Diabet Med 2004;21: 776–781
169. Bacci S, Menzaghi C, Ercolino T, Ma X, Rauseo A, Salvemini L, Vigna C, Fanelli R, Di Mario U, Doria A, Trischitta V. The +276 G/T single nucleotide polymorphism of the adiponectin gene is associated with coronary artery disease in type 2 diabetic patients. Diabetes Care 2004;27:2015–2020
170. Soccio T, Zhang YY, Bacci S, Mlynarski W, Placha G, Raggio G, Di Paola R, Marucci A, Johnstone MT, Gervino EV, Abumrad NA, Klein S, Trischitta V, Doria A. Common haplotypes at the adiponectin receptor 1 (ADIPOR1) locus are associated with increased risk of coronary artery disease in type 2 diabetes. Diabetes 2006;55:2763–2770
171. Damcott CM, Ott SH, Pollin TI, Reinhart LJ, Wang J, O'connell JR, Mitchell BD, Shuldiner AR. Genetic variation in adiponectin receptor 1 and adiponectin receptor 2 is associated with type 2 diabetes in the Old Order Amish. Diabetes 2005;54:2245–2250
172. Albala C, Villarroel A, Santos JL, Angel B, Lera L, Liberman C, Sanchez H, Perez-Bravo F. FABP2 Ala54Thr polymorphism and diabetes in Chilean elders. Diabetes Res Clin Pract 2007;77:245–250
173. Canani LH, Capp C, Ng DP, Choo SG, Maia AL, Nabinger GB, Santos K, Crispim D, Roisemberg I, Krolewski AS, Gross JL. The fatty acid-binding protein-2 A54T polymorphism is associated with renal disease in patients with type 2 diabetes. Diabetes 2005;54:3326–3330
174. Li Y, Fisher E, Klapper M, Boeing H, Pfeiffer A, Hampe J, Schreiber S, Burwinkel B, Schrezenmeir J, Doring F. Association between functional FABP2 promoter haplotype and type 2 diabetes. Horm Metab Res 2006;38: 300–337
175. Georgopoulos A, Bloomfield H, Collins D, Brousseau ME, Ordovas JM, O'connor JJ, Robins SJ, Schaefer EJ. Codon 54 polymorphism of the fatty acid binding protein (FABP) 2 gene is associated with increased cardiovascular risk in the dyslipidemic diabetic participants of the veterans affairs HDL intervention trial (VA-HIT). Atherosclerosis 2006 Aug 28; [Epub ahead of print]
176. Tai ES, Collins D, Robins SJ, O'Connor JJ Jr, Bloomfield HE, Ordovas JM, Schaefer EJ, Brousseau ME. The L162V polymorphism at the peroxisome proliferator activated receptor alpha locus modulates the risk of cardiovascular events associated with insulin resistance and diabetes mellitus: the Veterans Affairs HDL Intervention Trial (VA-HIT). Atherosclerosis 2006;187:153–160
177. Flavell DM, Ireland H, Stephens JW, Hawe E, Acharya J, Mather H, Hurel SJ, Humphries SE. Peroxisome proliferator-activated receptor alpha gene variation influences age of onset and progression of type 2 diabetes. Diabetes 2005;54:582–586
178. Sparso T, Hussain MS, Andersen G, Hainerova I, Borch-Johnsen K, Jorgensen T, Hansen T, Pedersen O. Relationships between the functional PPARalpha Leu162Val polymorphism and obesity, type 2 diabetes, dyslipidaemia, and related quantitative traits in studies of 5799 middle-aged white people. Mol Genet Metab 2007;90:205–209
179. Mori H, Ikegami H, Kawaguchi Y, Seino S, Yokoi N, Takeda J, Inoue I, Seino Y, Yasuda K, Hanafusa T, Yamagata K, Awata T, Kadowaki T, Hara K, Yamada N, Gotoda T, Iwasaki N, Iwamoto Y, Sanke T, Nanjo K, Oka Y, Matsutani A, Maeda E, Kasuga M. The Pro12→Ala substitution in PPAR-gamma is associated with resistance to development of diabetes in the general population: possible involvement in impairment of insulin secretion in individuals with type 2 diabetes. Diabetes 2001;50:891–894
180. Doney AS, Fischer B, Leese G, Morris AD, Palmer CN. Cardiovascular risk in type 2 diabetes is associated with variation at the PPARG locus: a Go-DARTS study. Arterioscler Thromb Vasc Biol 2004;24:2403–2407

181. Altshuler D, Hirschhorn JN, Klannemark M, Lindgren CM, Vohl MC, Nemesh J, Lane CR, Schaffner SF, Bolk S, Brewer C, Tuomi T, Gaudet D, Hudson TJ, Daly M, Groop L, Lander ES. The common PPARgamma Pro12Ala polymorphism is associated with decreased risk of type 2 diabetes. Nat Genet 2000;26:76–80
182. Andrulionyte L, Peltola P, Chiasson JL, Laakso M. STOP-NIDDM Study Group. Single nucleotide polymorphisms of PPARD in combination with the Gly482Ser substitution of PGC-1A and the Pro12Ala substitution of PPARG2 predict the conversion from impaired glucose tolerance to type 2 diabetes: the STOP-NIDDM trial. Diabetes 2006;55:2148–2152
183. Rubin D, Helwig U, Pfeuffer M, Schreiber S, Boeing H, Fisher E, Pfeiffer A, Freitag-Wolf S, Foelsch UR, Doering F, Schrezenmeir J. A common functional exon polymorphism in the microsomal triglyceride transfer protein gene is associated with type 2 diabetes, impaired glucose metabolism and insulin levels. J Hum Genet 2006;51:567–574
184. Damcott CM, Pollin TI, Reinhart LJ, Ott SH, Shen H, Silver KD, Mitchell BD, Shuldiner AR. Polymorphisms in the transcription factor 7-like 2 (TCF7L2) gene are associated with type 2 diabetes in the Amish: replication and evidence for a role in both insulin secretion and insulin resistance. Diabetes 2006;55:2654–2659
185. Grant SF, Thorleifsson G, Reynisdottir I, Benediktsson R, Manolescu A, Sainz J, Helgason A, Stefansson H, Emilsson V, Helgadottir A, Styrkarsdottir U, Magnusson KP, Walters GB, Palsdottir E, Jonsdottir T, Gudmundsdottir T, Gylfason A, Saemundsdottir J, Wilensky RL, Reilly MP, Rader DJ, Bagger Y, Christiansen C, Gudnason V, Sigurdsson G, Thorsteinsdottir U, Gulcher JR, Kong A, Stefansson K. Variant of transcription factor 7-like 2 (TCF7L2) gene confers risk of type 2 diabetes. Nat Genet 2006;38:320–323
186. Lehman DM, Hunt KJ, Leach RJ, Hamlington J, Arya R, Abboud HE, Duggirala R, Blangero J, Goring HH, Stern MP. Haplotypes of transcription factor 7-like 2 (TCF7L2) gene and its upstream region are associated with type 2 diabetes and age of onset in Mexican Americans. Diabetes 2007;56:389–393
187. van Vliet-Ostaptchouk JV, Shiri-Sverdlov R, Zhernakova A, Strengman E, van Haeften TW, Hofker MH, Wijmenga C. Association of variants of transcription factor 7-like 2 (TCF7L2) with susceptibility to type 2 diabetes in the Dutch Breda cohort. Diabetologia 2007;50:59–62
188. Duggirala R, Blangero J, Almasy L, Dyer TD, Williams KL, Leach RJ, O'Connell P, Stern MP. Linkage of type 2 diabetes mellitus and of age at onset to a genetic location on chromosome 10q in Mexican Americans. Am J Hum Genet 1999;64:1127–1140
189. Grundy SM. Metabolic syndrome: connecting and reconciling cardiovascular and diabetes worlds. J Am Coll Cardiol 2006;47:1093–1100
190. Kalra SP, Kalra PS. Gene-transfer technology: a preventive neurotherapy to curb obesity, ameliorate metabolic syndrome and extend life expectancy. Trends Pharmacol Sci 2005;26:488–495
191. Shah R, Jindal RM. Reversal of diabetes in the rat by injection of hematopoietic stem cells infected with recombinant adeno-associated virus containing the preproinsulin II gene. Pancreatology 2003;3:422–428
192. Sasaki T, Fujimoto K, Sakai K, Nemoto M, Nakai N, Tajima N. Gene and cell-based therapy for diabetes mellitus: endocrine gene therapeutics. Endocr Pathol 2003;14:141–144
193. Stanley WC. Rationale for a metabolic approach in diabetic coronary patients. Coron Artery Dis 2005;16: S11–S15
194. Chinetti-Gbaguidi G, Fruchart JC, Staels B. Role of the PPAR family of nuclear receptors in the regulation of metabolic and cardiovascular homeostasis: new approaches to therapy. Curr Opin Pharmacol 2005;5:177–183
195. Berger JP, Akiyama TE, Meinke PT. PPARs: therapeutic targets for metabolic disease. Trends Pharmacol Sci 2005;26:244–251
196. Han SH, Quon MJ, Koh KK. Beneficial vascular and metabolic effects of peroxisome proliferator-activated receptor-alpha activators. Hypertension 2005;46:1086–1092
197. Bell DS. Optimizing treatment of diabetes and cardiovascular disease with combined alpha,beta-blockade. Curr Med Res Opin 2005;21:1191–1200
198. Fragasso G, Piatti Md PM, Monti L, Palloshi A, Setola E, Puccetti P, Calori G, Lopaschuk GD, Margonato A. Short- and long-term beneficial effects of trimetazidine in patients with diabetes and ischemic cardiomyopathy. Am Heart J 2003;146:E18

Chapter 10
Gender and Cardiovascular Diseases in Aging

Overview

There are significant sex differences in the incidence and severity of cardiac defects in human although the mechanisms underlying gender-specific differences in regard to CVD in aged human remains poorly understood. A primary difference, that women develop heart disease later in life than man has been largely attributed to the loss of protective female hormones at menopause [1]. However, Hormone Replacement Therapy (HRT) in menopausal women, both asymptomatic and those with known coronary artery disease, have not generated consistent data regarding its potential benefits. Alternatives to HRT are been sought, and Selective Estrogen Receptor Modulators (SERMs) with both estrogen antagonist effects in the breast and agonist effects in the heart that appear to be clinically safe, have recently began to be used. These include raloxifene, tamoxifen, and a third-generation derivative of SERMs, lasofoxifene. Notwithstanding the progress achieved so far, further understanding of the molecular and cellular physiology of these compounds, and their receptors in the heart of postmenopausal women is necessary. In this chapter the effect of gender on the incidence and phenotypic characteristics of CVD in aging will be analyzed, and the potential pathways that men and women seem to follow to achieve longevity will be discussed.

Introduction

Sex steroid hormones and their receptors mostly caused gender differences in cardiovascular (CV) aging. Both transcriptional and non-genomic actions of estrogen and Estrogen Receptors (ER) have been demonstrated to be critical determinants in cardiovascular physiology and disease. While less well studied, evidence concerning the role and importance of testosterone and its receptors (PR and AR) in cardiovascular regulation is only recently emerging. The specific molecular mechanism (s) underlying the gender factor in the incidence and phenotypes of CVD remains poorly understood; however, observations mainly derived from animal models have generated important information on basic issues vital to the understanding of the effect of gender on the heart, such as molecular signaling pathways, genetics, energy metabolism and post-injury repair. On the other hand, translating research data from animal models, mainly rodent, to human regarding the pathogenesis of CVD and the response to different modulatory factors, such as aging and therapies has to be carefully and critically evaluated. From a clinical standpoint, sex differences in morbidity and mortality have been primarily attributed to the earlier perceived protective actions of female hormones as suggested by the increased cardiovascular risk in men and in women after menopause compared to pre-menopausal women [2].

However, clinically and experimentally reported benefits of HRT have been challenged by the negative outcomes in a number of recent large-scale clinical trials including the Heart and

J. Marín-García, *Aging and the Heart*,

Estrogen/Progestin Replacement Study (HERS) and the Women's Health Initiative (WHI) studies [3, 4]. A number of issues need to be resolved to clearly understand why there is sexual dimorphism in regard to CVD in aged human. While not denying the importance of research with animal's models, it is also imperative to generate more investigative studies in human where the molecular and cellular mechanisms, and differences in cardiac phenotypes can be properly addressed.

Gender Effect/Mechanisms on Specific CVDs

Normally there are a number of differences between male and female hearts even in the absence of pathology. For example, cardiac contractility is higher in women than men, in part due to estrogen and ER-mediated changes in the levels and regulation of myocardial calcium-contractility coupling proteins. Furthermore, women tend to maintain better myocardial mass. This is in part related to existing differences in the myocardial expression of glycolytic and mitochondrial metabolic enzymes, and/or to the prosurvival effects mediated by ERs and PI3K–Akt–dependent pathways on cardiomyocytes [5].

Gender-specific differences also exist in cardiac electrophysiology, and in the myocardial response to ischemic insult and heart failure (women are more protected against the former and tend to have better cardiac function and survival in the latter). These differences can become more pronounced with subjects exhibiting cardiac dysfunction and hypertrophy. For example, a recent study found that while the basic mechanical performance of healthy isolated feline myocardium was not significantly different between males and females under normal physiological conditions, under physiological stress sex differences in myocardial function emerged, which may reflect gender-specific differences in intracellular Ca^{2+} regulation in cardiomyocytes [6]. Vascular gender-specific differences include changes in vascular tone and blood pressure, lipoprotein metabolism and lipid accumulation, response to vessel injury, including angiogenesis, hemostasis and thrombosis – processes in which estrogen and ERs play a critical role. However, recent observations suggest that testosterone and ART (androgen replacement therapy) may have a beneficial role as well [1]. The increased vascular contraction observed in males, compared to females, is in large part attributable to the impact of the sex hormones (estrogen, progesterone, and testosterone), albeit the mechanism is not clear [7]. For instance, gender-specific differences in rat aortic contractility appear to be related to estrogen actions on both vascular endothelial (ECs) and smooth muscle cells (SMCs) resulting in altered sensitivity to receptor-mediated stimulation with norepinephrine [8].

Beyond the sex steroids and their receptors, other, genetic, inflammatory and environmental factors may play an important role in determining the gender-specific probability of achieving longevity. Age-related immunoinflammatory factors increase during proinflammation, and the frequency of pro/anti-inflammatory gene variants also shows gender differences. People genetically predisposed to weak inflammatory activity may be at reduced chance of developing Coronary Artery Disease (CAD) and may achieve longer life span if they avoid serious life-threatening infectious disease throughout life [9].

The interaction of pathogens with the individual genotype, may determine the type and intensity of the immune-inflammatory response responsible for both proinflammatory status and CAD. In males more than in females there is an apparent stronger relationship between the genetics of inflammation, successful aging, and the control of CVD. To know these facts is important since females outlive males by approximately 10 %, and as pointed out by Candore et al. understanding the different pathways that men and women seem to follow to achieve longevity, may help us to understand better the basic underlying phenomenon of aging and the search for safe ways to increase male, as well as female, life span [9].

Furthermore, distinctive differences between male and female are well established in animal models, e.g., Spontaneously Hypertensive Rats (SHR). Estrogen seems to preserve the NO-mediated portion of flow/shear stress-induced dilation in female hypertensive rats resulting in a lower maintained wall shear stress in female than in male SHR. This lower wall shear stress may in part contribute to the mechanism by which estrogen lowers systemic blood pressure and incidence of CVDs in women. Moreover, according to Huang et al. in NO-deficient female rats and mice there is an estrogen-dependent, cytochrome P450 (CYP)-mediated dilator responses to shear stress in arterioles [10]. These investigators measured flow-induced dilation in isolated arterioles from N(G)-nitro-L-arginine methyl ester (L-NAME)-treated male and ovariectomized female rats before and after overnight incubation with 17β-estradiol and found that estrogen, via a receptor-dependent, PI3K/Akt-mediated pathway, transcriptionally upregulates CYP activity leading to enhanced arteriolar response to shear stress.

Cell Death

Differences in life span between women and men may also be related to a better preservation of myocardial structure in the female heart with aging; thus, the aging process may have a different impact on the integrity of the myocardium in the two genders. Olivetti et al. in their study on human gender differences and aging reported that the effect of age is different on the myocardial integrity because compared to men, aging was accompanied by less myocyte cell loss, myocyte cellular reactive hypertrophy and myocardial remodeling in women [11]. While subsequent studies by Mallat et al. have not found that aging substantially influences the relative percentage of cardiomyocyte apoptosis in normal human cardiac aging, they did confirm and extend Olivetti' s finding of increased apoptosis in men (3-fold higher than women) and that gender appears to be an important determinant of the occurrence of apoptosis [12]. Moreover, the overall uncertainty concerning the extent of apoptosis in the aging heart may be in part due to the occurrence of other ongoing modes of cell death, which occur in the aging cardiomyocyte (e.g., necrosis, autophagy), commonalities in their signaling pathways with apoptosis and methodological difficulties distinguishing between them (as discussed in Chapter 4) [13–16]. Recent analysis of the effect of age and gender on apoptosis in the human coronary arterial wall revealed that apoptosis is not a key factor in aging of the arterial wall [17].

Since cardiomyocyte apoptosis is in part determined by gender-associated components (e.g., estrogen/ERs), reversal of apoptosis and attenuation of its effects in cardiomyocyte function might be mediated by modulating levels of these components in the cardiomyocyte. In studies of the effect of 17β-estradiol on murine cardiomyocyte apoptosis *in vivo* and *in vitro*, Patten et al. found that physiological E2 replacement reduces cardiomyocyte apoptosis after myocardial infarction (MI) in ovariectomized female mice, and E2 treatment *in vivo* increased activation of the prosurvival kinase, Akt, which preceded the reduction in cardiomyocyte apoptosis at 24 and 72 hours post-MI [5].

Age-Associated CVDs and Gender

Heart Failure (HF)

A number of gender-specific differences in both the etiology and pathophysiology of heart failure (HF) have been reported, underlying differences in the clinical presentation and course of the syndrome. Some of these differences are thought to be linked to sexual dimorphism of myocardial growth processes and myocardial calcium handling, as well as related to myocardial remodeling with age [18]. Moreover, both animal and clinical studies have demonstrated that other cardiovascular conditions including hypertension also play a major role in the etiology of HF. Since the Renin-Angiotensin-Aldosterone System (RAAS) and its effect on hypertensive pathophysiology exhibits sexual dimorphism in the aging rat, modulation of the RAAS by estrogens may be contributory in mediating specific differences between pre- and post-menopausal females and males [19, 20].

Studies in human and animals suggest that estrogen receptors participate in the development of myocardial hypertrophy and HF. Changes in human myocardial estrogen receptor α (ERα) expression, localization, and association with structural proteins have been found in end stage-failing hearts. Mahmoodzadeh et al. reported a 1.8-fold increase in ERα mRNA and protein in end-stage human dilated cardiomyopathy (DCM), as compared with controls [21]. ERα was visualized by confocal immunofluorescence microscopy and localized to the cytoplasm, sarcolemma, intercalated discs and nuclei of cardiomyocytes. Also colocalization of ERα with β-catenin at the intercalated disc in control hearts and immunoprecipitation studies confirmed complex formation of both proteins. On the other hand, ERα/β-catenin colocalization was lost at the intercalated disc in DCM hearts. These findings suggest that ERβ/β-catenin colocalization in the intercalated disc may be of functional relevance and a loss of this association may play a role in HF progression.

In experimental models of alcoholic cardiomyopathy, sexual dimorphism was recently demonstrated by the significant thinning of the ventricular wall and intraventricular septum, with diminished levels of myocardial protein synthesis, in response to chronic alcohol consumption in male but not female rats [22]. The decreased protein synthesis underlying the loss of cardiac mass was associated with limitation of mRNA translation, due to a decline in the phosphorylation and activation of a specific eukaryotic initiation factor (eIF4G) and 4E binding protein (4EBP1), leading to reduced assembly of an active eukaryotic initiation factor (eIF)4G/eIF4E complex and increased formation of inactive 4E binding protein (4EBP1)/eIF4E complex.

Several clinical studies have shown that hypertrophic cardiomyopathy (HCM) has components which exhibit sexual dimorphism. Studies examining gender-specific differences in left ventricular cavity size, contractility and left ventricular outflow tract obstruction (LVOTO) in patients with HCM found that females had higher LV contractility and smaller left ventricular cavity size, which predisposed to LVOTO, whereas neither left ventricular cavity size or contractility were predictive of LVOTO in the HCM of males [23]. Furthermore, these gender-specific differences with regards to increased LV contractility and obstruction accompanied by higher fractional shortening in females became more apparent in older patients [24].

Interestingly, in a study of 122 adult patients with obstructive HCM, female patients had smaller interventricular septum thickness and less frequently systolic anterior movement of the mitral valve, and they were significantly older than male patients (mean age 66.7+/−10.5 versus 54.8+/−12.5 years) [25]. Cross-sectional analysis of a cohort of 239 adult HCM patients (aged 18–91 years) found a modest but statistically significant inverse relation between age and LV wall thickness that was largely gender-specific [26]. Smaller degrees of LV hypertrophy was independently associated with increasing age, and was statistically significant only for women. In a recent large-scale study of 969 HCM patients to assess gender-related differences, women with HCM were significantly under-represented, significantly older, more symptomatic than men, with higher frequency of left ventricular outflow obstruction, and showed higher risk of progression to NYHA functional classes III/IV or death from HF or stroke [27]. Interestingly, risk of sudden death, a potential consequence of HCM, were similar in men and women.

From a clinical standpoint, the relationship of gender to phenotype and severity of CVD variably affects different groups of the population. The Beta-Blocker Evaluation of Survival Trial (BEST) study specifically targeted women in HF, because in previous clinical trials women have been under-represented, and limitation of data in women had impeded a clear understanding of gender-related differences in patients with HF [28].

The BEST study analyzed 2,708 randomized patients with NYHA class III/IV and with a left ventricle ejection fraction (LVEF) $\leq$0.35 in response to bucindolol versus placebo. Women were younger, more likely to be black, had a higher prevalence of non-ischemic etiology, had higher RVEF and LVEF, higher heart rate, greater cardiothoracic ratio, higher prevalence of left bundle branch block, lower prevalence of atrial fibrillation, and lower plasma norepinephrine level. While ischemic etiology and measurements of HF severity were found to be predictors of prognosis in women and men, CAD and LVEF appear to be stronger predictors of prognosis in women. Among non-ischemic patients, women had a significantly better survival rate compared with men. These results support earlier findings of significantly enhanced gender-specific survival of women with advanced, non-ischemic LV dysfunction [29–32].

Although the pathophysiologic mechanisms underlying why CVD is often delayed and less common in women than in men, and their overall survival advantage in HF have not yet been established, the involvement of estrogens, β-adrenergic stimulation, RAAS, and a greater resistance to cardiomyocyte apoptosis in females have been suggested as contributing factors [33]. Anversa and al. have further probed the extent of myocyte cell death in HF and cardiac remodeling as a function of gender [34]. Analysis of a small group of patients of both sexes in HF revealed that the level of myocyte necrosis was 7-fold greater than apoptosis, although overall cell death was 2-fold higher in men than in women. This gender-specific difference in myocyte cell death was primarily due to differential apoptosis, which increased 35-fold in women and 85-fold in men. The lower degree of cell death in women was associated with a longer duration of the cardiomyopathy, a later onset of cardiac decompensation, and a longer interval between HF and transplantation.

On the other hand, Crabbe et al. did not observe gender-based differences in cardiac remodeling among a cohort of 50 patients with idiopathic DCM [35]. However, among 50 patients with ischemic cardiomyopathy, males exhibited significantly greater overall heart weight index, as well as a strong trend toward increased LV mass index paralleled by increased myocyte volume (36 % greater in men than in women) in association with a 14 % increase in resting cell length. These data suggested that gender differences in cardiac remodeling in ischemic cardiomyopathy are mainly related to differences in cellular remodeling and that gender may influence the myocardial responses to ischemic injury. Gender-related differences in the heart susceptibility to ischemia-reperfusion (I/R) injury are well established and play an important role in cardioprotection against I/R injury in females, as we shall discuss shortly [36–38].

It is generally accepted that ischemic heart disease is more prevalent in men than in women. The remodeling of extracellular matrix (ECM) represents an integral structural correlate of HF of ischemic origin, and the proliferation of cardiac fibroblasts is a critical factor in this myocardial remodeling. Cardiac fibroblasts derived from male rats are more susceptible to hypoxia, as gauged by diminished DNA synthesis, whereas fibroblasts from age-matched females are hypoxia-resistant and this resistance is dependent on tyrosine kinase activation [39]. Estrogens, via estrogen-receptor-dependent mechanisms, differentially alter the response of male and female cells to hypoxia. In female cells the combined effect of hypoxia and estrogen led to inhibition of DNA synthesis, whereas in male cells estrogen partially reversed the hypoxia-induced inhibition of DNA synthesis.

Myocardial and ECM remodeling in HF, including ventricular dilatation, also involves matrix metalloproteinase (MMP) activation. An association between increased mast cell density, activation of MMPs, and the initiation of cardiac remodeling by induced volume overload in male rats and dogs has been demonstrated [40, 41]. In addition, chemically induced mast cell degranulation (either by treatment with endothelin-1 or synthetic compound 48/80) resulted in MMP activation, extensive collagen matrix degradation, and LV dilatation within 30 min in the isolated, blood-perfused heart from male and ovariectomized female rats [42]. In contrast, hearts from intact females and estrogen-supplemented ovariectomized females did not show the effects of these compounds on mast cell-mediated MMP activation, ECM degradation and cardiac remodeling, likely reflecting an effect on either mast cell composition or release of its contents, including the proinflammatory cytokine TNF-α [43].

As previously discussed in Chapter 7, HF in both clinical and experimental studies is invariably accompanied by abnormalities in Ca^{2+}-handling that will decrease cardiac contractility, and gender can exert a significant effect on the timing and extent of changes in Ca^{2+} cycling. Dash et al. have studied the potential contributory role of gender to altered SR Ca^{2+} cycling by gauging the levels of SR Ca^{2+}-ATPase (SERCA), phospholamban, and calsequestrin, as well as site-specific phospholamban phosphorylation, in a mixed gender population of failing and donor hearts [44]. In failing hearts, while phospholamban and calsequestrin levels were not altered, SERCA protein levels were significantly reduced and phospholamban phosphorylation (at serine-16 and threonine-17 sites) was attenuated in concert with decreased V_{max} and affinity for SR calcium uptake. Analysis of gender in failing hearts indicated male-specific attenuation of phospholamban phosphorylation at serine-16 and decreased Ca^{2+} affinity. Similarly, transgenic mice containing an overexpressed mutant phospholamban allele which acts as a superinhibitor of SERCA affinity for Ca^{2+} showed extensive Ca^{2+} cycling changes, depressed contractility, LV remodeling and hypertrophy at 3 months, progressing in males to DCM with extensive interstitial tissue fibrosis and death at 6 months [45]. Transgenic females also exhibited ventricular hypertrophy at 3 months but exhibited normal systolic function up to 12 months of age. These results suggest a critical relationship between defective SR Ca^{2+} cycling and cardiac remodeling leading to HF, with a gender-dependent impact on the time course of these alterations.

HF with normal ejection fraction (HF-NEF) is believed to be more common in aging women than in men although the interaction of gender and age is not clear. Increases in vascular (Ea), ventricular systolic (Ees), and ventricular diastolic (Ed) elastance (stiffness) appear to be all contributory to the pathogenesis of HF with preserved ejection fraction (HF-nlEF). According to Regitz-Zagrosek et al. [46] among the major risk factors for HF-NEF including hypertension, aging, obesity, diabetes, and ischemia, hypertension is more frequent in women and is a likely gender-specific component contributing to left ventricular and arterial stiffening, whereas ischemia appears to play a greater role in men. Furthermore, these authors suggest that aging, diabetes and obesity affect myocardial and vascular stiffness differently and can lead to different forms of myocardial hypertrophy in men and women. Gender-specific differences in ventricular diastolic distensibility, in vascular stiffness and ventricular/vascular coupling, in skeletal muscle adaptation to HF, as well as in the perception of symptoms may contribute to a greater rate of HF-NEF in women. A number of molecular mechanisms can contribute to the gender differences in HF-NEF, including differences in Ca^{2+} handling, in the NO signaling pathway, and in natriuretic peptides. In addition, and as we have previously noted, estrogen affects collagen synthesis and degradation and modulates the renin-angiotensin system.

Redfield et al. have hypothesized that ventricular-vascular stiffening may occur with age and be more pronounced in women in the general community [47]. In their study of a cross-sectional sample of 2,042 residents of Olmsted County, Minnesota ($\geq$45 year old) using clinical data, Doppler echocardiography, and blood pressure, they found that while Ea, Ees, and Ed all increased with age in both men and in women, the age-related increase in Ees was more steep in women. When adjusted for age, Ea, Ees, and Ed were more significantly increased in women than in men. Interestingly, these findings were similar in individuals (n=623) without known or suspected CVD suggesting that advancing age and female gender are associated with increases in vascular and ventricular systolic and diastolic stiffness even in the absence of CVD. This combined ventricular-vascular stiffening may contribute to the increased prevalence of HF-nlEF with age particularly in elderly women.

Furthermore, Masoudi et al. [48] have evaluated if women are more likely than men to have HF with preserved Left Ventricular Systolic Function (LVSF) after adjustment for potential confounding factors including age. They carried out a large-scale cross-sectional study using data from retrospective medical chart abstraction of a national sample of Medicare beneficiaries hospitalized with the principal discharge diagnosis of HF in acute-care hospitals in the US between April 1998 and March 1999. Criteria for inclusion in this analysis were age (65 years or older), documentation of LVSF status and corroborated HF diagnosis. Of the 19,710 patients included in the analysis, preserved LVSF was present in 6,700 (35 %), 79 % of whom were women. In contrast, among the 12,956 patients displaying impaired LVSF, only 49 % were women. Patients displaying preserved

LVSF were 1.5 years older than those with impaired LVSF. Even after adjustment for age and other risk factors, a strong association was found between female gender with preserved LVSF, which was consistent in all age groups, and similar in patients with or without CAD, hypertension, pulmonary disease, renal insufficiency, or atrial fibrillation (AF). Therefore in elderly patients with HF, preserved systolic function is primarily a condition of women, independent of important demographic and clinical characteristics.

Dysrhythmias

There are significant gender-based differences on cardiac rhythm and electrophysiology and on the development of dysrhythmias. Mechanisms underlying these differences remain largely undefined but are believed to involve gonadal steroids [49].

Recently, Kelley et al. have reported a large-scale analysis of electrocardiographic findings in a targeted population of the oldest old individuals [50]. Retrospective analysis of electrocardiograms of 888 individuals aged ≥90 years using standard criteria for 128 separate ECG findings revealed that left ventricular enlargement (28 %), first-degree atrioventricular (AV) block (16 %), and AF (15 %) were the most common abnormalities found in this cohort as a whole. Sinus rhythm was observed in 79 % of the population. More Caucasians than African-Americans exhibited AF. While women presented normal ECG findings more frequently than men, more women demonstrated complete right bundle branch block. Thus, in this targeted population of the oldest old, the frequency of certain ECG findings was significantly affected by both gender and race.

Although the precise causes of gender-specific differences in cardiac dysrhythmias are not yet known, sex-specific variations in the electrophysiological structure of the heart and/or hormonal effects on modulating ionic channel function may help to explain some of these differences. It is generally accepted that from puberty on women show a higher basic heart rate as well as a longer QT-interval, shorter QRS duration and lower QRS voltage than men. Women tend to have a higher prevalence of sick sinus syndrome, inappropriate sinus tachycardia, AV nodal reentry tachycardia, idiopathic right ventricular tachycardia (VT), and dysrhythmic events in the long-QT syndrome. Men on the other hand tend to have a higher prevalence of carotid sinus syndrome, supraventricular and reentrant VT due to accessory pathways, Wolff-Parkinson-White syndrome, ventricular fibrillation and sudden death (women suffer only 20 % of sudden cardiac deaths) and the Brugada syndrome.

AF is arguably the most frequent cardiac dysrhythmia encountered, is more prevalent in the elderly and poses a risk factor for stroke and premature death. The presence of AF confers a five-fold increased risk of stroke; a figure that may rise as high as 17 times in the presence of structural heart disease, in particular mitral stenosis. While most investigators have suggested that AF is more prevalent in men [51–53], the absolute numbers of men and women with AF are roughly equal, and the associated morbidity and mortality experienced by women with AF appear to be worse [54].

A large-scale study (the Copenhagen City Study) investigated changes in AF prevalence in a random elderly population (aged 50–89 years) at three time points (8,606 patients examined in 1976–1978, 8,943 patients examined in 1981–1983, and in 6,733 subjects examined in 1991–1994) [55]. This study found a significant increase in age-standardized AF prevalence among men (from 1.4 % in 1976–1978 to 3.3 % in 1991–1994) whereas women showed a non-significant decline in AF prevalence over time in these groups. This data suggest that the prevalence of AF in men more than doubled from the 1970s to the 1990s, while it was unchanged in women. The factors responsible for this remarkable gender-specific increase in AF prevalence have yet to be identified. A subsequent study of cardiovascular events occurring over a 5 year follow-up period with these subjects found that, after adjustment for age and co-morbidity, the effect of AF on the risk of stroke was 4.6-fold greater in women than in men. Similarly, the independent effect of AF on cardiovascular death was 2.5-fold greater in women than in men confirming that AF is a much more pronounced risk factor for stroke and cardiovascular death in women than in men [56].

Until recently the effect of patient gender on recurrence of AF after a successful direct current cardioversion was unknown. Gurevitz et al. have reported that women were more likely than men to have recurrence of AF after successful direct current cardioversion [57]. In their study they found that at presentation, women were older and had a higher prevalence of hypertension and valvular disease and worse mechanical left atrial appendage function compared with men. Furthermore, dysrhythmia recurrence was more prevalent in women. Although there was no difference in mortality, patient gender was a significant predictor of dysrhythmia recurrence. Therefore, when making the decision about cardioversion for AF, gender needs to be taken into account.

Furthermore, AF is predominantly a disease of advancing age whose prevalence rises markedly from approximately 0.1 % at age 40, to 6 % at age 65, and 10 % at age 80 and older. The median age for AF in the general population is 75. It might be expected that as the population ages, the number of individuals developing AF will continue to rise. In addition, data from the Framingham Heart Study suggest that the risk of stroke attributable to AF increases significantly with age, rising from 1.5 % for those aged 50–59 years to 23.5 % for individuals aged 80–89 years. Moreover, as pointed out by Camm without more effective therapeutic interventions, AF-related cardiovascular and cerebrovascular morbidity and mortality will also continue to rise [58].

Strategies considered for AF include prevention of thromboembolism and stroke primarily with anticoagulants and restoration and maintenance of sinus rhythm. Anticoagulation is highly effective in preventing stroke in patients with AF, but the risk of hemorrhage may be increased in older patients. The risks and benefits of antithrombotic therapy need to be carefully weighed in stroke prevention in AF in older individuals, particularly in women. In a recent study of stroke prevention using an oral thrombin inhibitor (the SPORTIF trials), the anticoagulant warfarin, of 3,922 subjects with AF including 2,257 women, warfarin-treated women had a slightly higher rate of major and minor bleeding than men, but gender did not appreciably influence rates of major bleeding arguing in favor of anticoagulation for women with AF [59]. Compared with younger women, the elderly had similar rates of major bleeding but slightly more overall bleeding than younger women, thus arguing for anticoagulation of all age groups. Interestingly, in this study over half the female cohort was >75 years of age, a larger proportion than men. Similarly, in a prospective analysis of data from the large *A*n*T*icoagulation and *R*isk factors *I*n *A*F (ATRIA) study cohort involving 13,559 patients, Wang et al. found warfarin to be at least as effective for women in reducing the risk of thromboembolism and ischemic stroke, if not more so, than in men [60]. Moreover, warfarin therapy did not pose a greater risk of major hemorrhagic complications in women in this study, including intracranial hemorrhage. In addition, women off warfarin exhibited significantly higher annual rates of thromboembolism than did men. These results suggest that warfarin treatment of AF has an overall net benefit that appears to be greater in women compared with men. Nevertheless, more studies are critically needed to confirm both the efficacy and safety of anticoagulant treatment of AF in elderly women.

If AF recurs after one or two cardioversions, a rate control strategy may be a better alternative. Interestingly, markedly symptomatic patients who fail cardioversion may benefit from catheter ablation therapy, which can cure AF and confer cardiovascular functional improvement. However, as Camm noted, ablation therapy may not be appropriate for all AF patients and pharmacological therapies will continue to have an important place in the management of AF.

Gender may also play a critical role in the choice of treatment for AF. As we have noted, women with AF tend to be more symptomatic, and because it is frequently associated to HF the outcome is usually worse. Rienstra et al. using data from RACE (rate control versus electrical cardioversion) including 522 patients (192 females) found that at baseline women had more AF-related complaints and their quality of life was worse than men, but similar cardiovascular morbidity and mortality after a 3 year follow-up [61]. On the other hand, women treated with randomized rhythm control developed more end points, including HF, thromboembolic complications, and adverse effects of antidysrhythmic drugs, compared with rate control randomized female patients and during follow-up, the quality of life in women with either treatment approach remained worse compared to men. Since treatment did not significantly change the quality of life in women, it was suggested that a rate control strategy may be considered in these patients. Interestingly, there is little data concerning characteristics of catheter ablation therapy in treating AF as a function of gender. In a recent study of AF patients undergoing ablation therapy over a seven-year period from 1999 through 2005 it was found that the great majority of patients undergoing this procedure were male suggesting a referral bias against this invasive procedure for women [62].

The incidence of spontaneous complete AV block in elderly men and woman with impaired intra-ventricular conduction was analyzed by Snyder et al. in a group of 144 consecutive patients with symptomatic high grade AV block [63]. After excluding cases secondary to congenital heart disease, acute MI, cardiac surgery or digitalis toxicity, AV conduction in the remaining 71 patients was observed either intermittently during complete heart block (CHB) or in electrocardiograms taken within two years prior to documentation of CHB. The mean age was 69 years, and although the analyzed group was rather small, it is interesting to note that the observed peak incidence was in the seventh decade for 43 men and the eighth decade in 28 women. A retrospective analysis of the medical literature dating from 1941 through 1993 identified 72 cases of torsades de pointes (TdP) associated with acquired complete heart block (and unassociated with QT prolonging drugs) [64]. The female prevalence among these patients with TdP during complete heart block was greater (72 %) than expected suggesting increased susceptibility of females to these events.

Ventricular dysrhythmias are more prevalent in aging men, mainly in association with CAD. In a meta-analysis of 748 patients obtained from reviewing 68 articles, Nakagawa et al. found that males had a marked prevalence of VT originating in the LV septum compared to females whereas tachycardia originating in the right outflow tract was more prevalent in females [65].

On the other hand, TdP tachycardias occur more frequently in women, in conjunction with their higher incidence of acquired and congenital long QT syndrome (LQTS). Furthermore, female gender is an independent risk factor for syncope and sudden death in the congenital LQTS. In this regard, a report by the International Long QT Syndrome Registry [66]. found that during childhood, the risk of cardiac events was shown to be significantly higher in males than in females containing mutant alleles in the KCNQ1 potassium channel gene (LQT1) whereas there was no significant gender-related difference in the risk of cardiac events (e.g., syncope, aborted cardiac arrest, or sudden death) among carriers of mutant alleles of the HERG potassium channel gene (LQT2) or of mutant SCN5A sodium channel gene (LQT3) variants. However, during adulthood, female carriers of either LQT2 or LQT1 had a significantly higher risk of cardiac events than respective males. Therefore, age and gender have different, genotype-specific modulating effects on the probability of cardiac events and electrocardiographic presentation in LQT1 and LQT2 patients.

It is known that a single nucleotide polymorphism (SNP) in the KCNQ1 gene resulting in a G643S alteration at codon 643 is associated with long QT syndrome and with a mild reduction in KCNQ1 current. Recently, the KCNQ1genotype was screened in a cohort of 992 individuals from Japan to determine the incidence of this allele and its association with the QT intervals. Eighty-eight individuals were found to have a heterozygous G643S genotype. Age and gender matched, controls (243) with wild-type alleles were selected and the electrocardiogram parameters in both groups compared including; QT intervals, the peak and the end of the T wave (Tpe) interval, and the Tpe/QT ratio [(these two parameters reflect the transmural dispersion of ventricular repolarization (TDR)]. In G643S carriers, both Tpe and Tpe/QT were significantly longer than in non-carriers, without significant QT prolongation. Although both genders showed a tendency for an increase in QT with aging, both Tpe and Tpe/QT showed a similar significant increase with age in females, which was not observed in males. Therefore, in elderly females, the G643S genotype might represent an independent risk factor for secondary LQTS by causing a greater TDR.

Finally, evidence suggests that the risks of pharmacological therapy for treating AF and various dysrhythmias may in fact be different in men and women and in the elderly. Further controlled studies are necessary to specifically address gender-related solutions for adequate risk stratification and therapy. The unsuspected negative effects of HRT revealed by recent large-scale clinical studies might have been initially predicted by the early finding that estrogen HRT was associated with a higher risk of ischemic stroke in patients with AF [67].

Cardiac Hypertrophy

Cardiac hypertrophy frequently accompanied by cardiac fibrosis, and myocardial dysfunction, are associated with gender-based differences with higher mortality in men. Several studies have demonstrated that elderly female patients (over age 60) with aortic stenosis exhibit better preservation of systolic function and increased LV hypertrophy than males [68, 69]. Sex hormones and their receptors are contributory to these gender-based differences in LV function and structural remodeling/hypertrophy although the mechanism by which they do this is not fully known. *In vitro* studies have shown that estrogen can inhibit hypertrophy in cultured rat cardiomyocytes, preventing angiotensin II (AngII)- or endothelin-1 (ET-1)-induced new protein synthesis, skeletal muscle actin expression, and increased surface area [70]. Moreover, in these cells estrogen induced the MCIP1 gene (an inhibitor of calcineurin activity, via phosphatidylinositol 3-kinase transcriptional, and mRNA stability mechanisms) disabling key signaling components of the hypertrophy program [70]. Long-term administration of 16 α-LE2 (an ERα selective agonist) or 17β-estradiol in ovariectomized, spontaneously hypertensive rats (SHR) efficiently attenuated cardiac hypertrophy and increased cardiac output, LV stroke volume, contractility and cardiac α-myosin heavy chain (α-MHC) expression suggesting that activation of ERα attenuates cardiac hypertrophy, and affects myocardial contractility, and gene expression in ovariectomized SH. Subsequent studies with female SHR rats demonstrated a significant attenuation of the ability of estrogen substitution therapy to reduce LV hypertrophy in senescent (24 mo) compared to adult (4 months old) rats [71]. Furthermore, aging was associated with reduced levels in cardiac ERα and altered estradiol metabolism. Studies with transgenic mice have shown that the estrogen receptor β (ERβ) is also necessary for estrogen's protective effect against LV hypertrophy in females [72]. Androgen and its receptors are linked to the development of hypertrophy in cardiomyocytes [73], and in the LV of males [74, 75], although this linkage is less well defined than is estrogen's protective effect. Gathered observations suggest that androgen modulation of cardiac hypertrophy involved functions provided by angiotensin II type 1A receptor gene (AT1A) and guanyl cyclase A. Recently, study of androgen receptor (AR) knockout transgenic mice found that AR-null male mice displayed a loss of cardiac growth and an impaired response to angiotensin-mediated remodeling [76]. This included diminished concentric hypertrophy and strikingly elevated cardiac fibrosis, with enhanced expression of types I and III collagen and transforming growth factor-β1 genes and with increased Smad2 activation.

The relationship of male sex hormones with aging and cardiac hypertrophy has not been established. Data from a recent study suggest that left ventricular mass in 107 elderly men (over age 50) was positively associated with hypertension but not with levels of hormones, including testosterone (T), estradiol (E2), Sex Hormone Binding Globulin (SHBG) or insulin resistance [77]. For females it may be particularly important to regulate the development of cardiac hypertrophy, since female patients with a similar degree of non-ischemic hypertrophy as males exhibit higher mortality rates [78].

Several clinical studies have identified variants in estrogen receptor genes that impact cardiac hypertrophy. A group of 1,249 unrelated individuals, 547 men and 702 women (mean age 59 years) from the Framingham Heart Study, has been screened for the association of 8 SNPs in the genes for ER α (ESR1) and ER β (ESR2) with 5 LV measures: LV mass (LVM), LV wall thickness (LVWT), LV internal diameter at end-diastole and end-systole, and fractional shortening [79]. While no association was found between the ER polymorphisms tested and LV structure or function in men, women contained two polymorphisms, ESR2 rs1256031 and ESR2 rs1256059, associated with both LVM and LVWT; the association was most pronounced in those women with hypertension, although it was not influenced by variation in blood pressure, plasma lipoprotein levels, or hyperglycemia.

Genetic variation in the TA repeat regulatory region upstream of exon 1 of the ERα gene (ESR1) is associated with left ventricular mass. The mean number of TA repeats (n=18) categorized the subjects into long, short and mixed allele genotypes. Among ninety-two patients (mean age 60.3), subjects with at least one long allele had significant difference in left ventricular mass index compared to individuals with short alleles [80]. Three novel polymorphisms in the ERα promoter were recently identified within a sequence which demonstrated significant promoter activity *in vitro* [81]. In a small healthy population one of these polymorphic variants G>A (−721 E) was associated with LV hypertrophy, after controlling for systolic blood pressure and sex (n=74), contributing to 23 % of interventricular septum (IVS) width variance and 9.4 % of left ventricular mass index variance. Male carriers of the A allele (n=8) in a separate hypertensive cohort, exhibited a 17 % increase in IVS and a 19 % increase in LVMI compared to GG homozygote subjects (n=84).

It is well-established that mutations outside the estrogen pathway such as in sarcomeric proteins can lead to either HCM or DCM, and some of these show gender-specificity in their phenotypic expression. In transgenic mice bearing an α-MHC Arg403Gln missense mutation (α-MHC $^{403/+}$), which display a phenotype characteristic of familial HCM, gender-specific electrophysiologic abnormalities have been identified [82]. While female (α-MHC $^{403/+}$) mice had similar ECG's, cardiac conduction times and refractory periods compared with female wild-type mice, male transgenic mice had distinctive surface ECG and electrophysiologic abnormalities, including prolonged ventricular repolarization and sinus node recovery times, as well as elevated levels of inducible VT. Other studies with this mutant model found that aging played a role in the gender-specific expression of the cardiac phenotype in transgenic mice containing the Arg403Gln mutation [83]. At 4 months of age, both male and female transgenic mice developed LV hypertrophy accompanied by LV diastolic dysfunction, but LV systolic function was normal. At 10 months of age, the females continued to present LV concentric hypertrophy and impaired LV diastolic function without evidence of systolic dysfunction, while males began to display LV dilation, LV diastolic function worsened and systolic performance was impaired mimicking the functional decompensation characteristic of HCM. Both 10-month-old transgenic groups displayed diminished coronary flow.

Another transgenic mouse model of familial HCM, resulting from missense mutation in the cardiac troponin T gene (R92Q), showed gender-specific responses to the induction of cardiac hypertrophy by angiotensin II treatment (males had augmented response) [84]. In addition, female transgenic mice with a truncated allele of troponin T (TnT-trunc) had marked myocardial hypertrophy in response to angiotensin II. Moreover, stimulation with isoproterenol (ISO) and/or phenylephrine (PE) as β and α-adrenergic agonists respectively led to sudden cardiac death in all male but not female mutant animals, which suggests altered adrenergic responsiveness in both these two models of familial HCM.

In a recent clinical study, Stefanelli et al. reported a novel cardiac troponin T mutation (A171S) leading to DCM and sudden cardiac death [85]. In contrast to previously described mutations in troponin T, the A171S mutation resulted in significant gender difference and in the severity of the observed phenotype with adult males, demonstrating a more severe LV dilatation and dysfunction than adult females.

Hypertension

It is well recognized that systolic hypertension, the most common type of hypertension in the elderly is associated with a wide pulse pressure resulting largely from excessive large artery stiffness. Evidence suggests that arterial stiffness increases with age independently of mean blood pressure or the presence of other risk factors, and while the contribution of gender to arterial stiffness and hypertension has been suggested, its precise role is not well defined [86, 87].

Age-related large artery stiffening is more pronounced in women compared with men. Interestingly, prepubertal females had stiffer large arteries and higher pulse pressure than age-matched males while postpubertal females developed more distensible large arteries, suggesting that estrogen modulates a reduction in arterial stiffness. On the other hand, postpubertal males developed stiffer large vessels [88]. That the loss of estrogen with menopause and aging likely contributes to the increased stiffening of the arteries and hypertension in women is also suggested by findings that isolated carotid arteries from ovariectomized (OVX) rats, that underwent 1 year of estrogen treatment, had an significantly increased compliance index, reduced levels of pentosidine (which is a specific marker of glycoxidative damage) and reduced endothelial layer permeability indicating estrogen-mediated attenuation of arterial stiffening, glycoxidative damage, and permeability [89].

Similarly, gender has a significant effect on arterial blood pressure, with premenopausal women having a lower arterial blood pressure than age-matched men that increases significantly in post-menopausal women, and implying a modulating role of ovarian hormones [90]. While the precise mechanism of estrogen's modulation of blood pressure and arterial stiffening are not yet known, several potential related actions of estrogen may be contributory and need further exploration. Estrogen receptors have been identified in vascular endothelium and smooth muscle, and estrogen induces vasodilatation and vascular tone by both ER-dependent and ER-independent mechanisms. Multiple mechanisms are involved in estrogen's vasodilatory effects including increased production of NO, activation of adenylyl cyclase activity with increased synthesis of cyclic AMP, stimulation of the production of adenosine in vascular SMCs, increase in intracellular free calcium concentration in endothelial cells, which could contribute to the increase in endothelial-derived NO, increased synthesis of the vasodilator prostacyclin (by inducing the expression of prostacyclin synthase and cyclooxygenase) and opening of calcium-activated K^+ channels. Moreover, estradiol reduces the synthesis of potent vasoconstrictors such as angiotensin II (Ang II), endothelin-1 and catecholamines.

Estrogen also inhibits the mitogenic effects of multiple factors generated at the site of endothelial injury/dysfunction, which trigger stimulation of hyperplastic and/or hypertrophic growth of vascular SMCs, a critical component underlying the elevated total peripheral resistance characteristic of hypertension. Also estrogen blocks key elements of the extensive vascular remodeling processes that in part mediate hypertension, including attenuating inflammation, modulating signaling factors, i.e., homocysteine, ROS and oxidized lipoproteins, decreased adhesion molecule expression, and altered neointimal formation.

Some of the effects of estrogen are initiated by long-term genomic effects and altered transcriptional programming. Others involve the activation of sex hormone receptors on the plasma membrane of vascular cells triggering rapid non-genomic effects, which stimulate endothelium-dependent vascular relaxation via NO-cGMP, prostacyclin-cAMP, and hyperpolarization pathways; [91] these possible pathways are illustrated in Fig. 10.1. In addition, sex hormones cause endothelium-independent inhibition of vascular smooth muscle contraction, $[Ca^{2+}]_i$ and protein kinase C (PKC). Furthermore, androgens have multiple effects on many of these pathways as well.

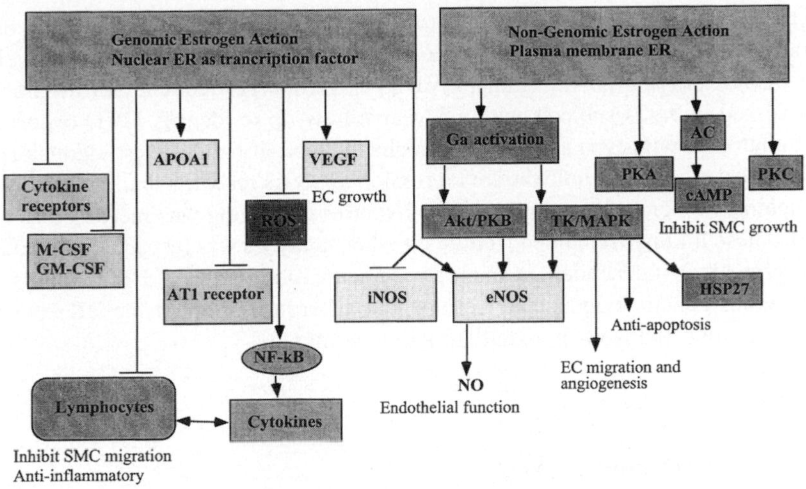

Fig. 10.1 The genomic and post-genomic effects of estrogen on vascular cells
Estrogen can act via nuclear-localized estrogen receptors (ERs) to mediate genomic expression in endothelial (ECs) and smooth muscle cells (SMCs) as well as in lymphocytes to inhibit inflammatory cytokines and their receptors, modulate ROS levels, increase VEGF to enhance EC growth and upregulate eNOS synthesis to increase NO for vasodilatation and improved vascular tone. It also can act more rapidly in a non-genomic pathway via plasma membrane-localized ERs and activating G-proteins (G_a), adenylyl cyclase (AC), PKA, PKC, Akt/PKB, and tyrosine kinases (TK) including MAPK affecting antiapoptotic/prosurvival pathways, elevated EC migration, increased eNOS and NO leading to enhanced endothelial function, and inhibition of SMC migration and growth

These numerous vasorelaxant/vasodilator effects suggest that sex hormone therapy may have a positive vascular effect in natural and surgically induced hypogonadism. Nevertheless, in a number of clinical trials, HRT provided none or minimal benefits in elderly postmenopausal women with hypertension; whether this was due to the type/dose of sex hormone, subject's age or other factors remains unclear.

The potential relationship between estrogen-related gene polymorphisms and blood pressure has been further evaluated recently in a Framingham Heart Study offspring cohort [92]. Untreated cross-sectional and longitudinal analysis of blood pressure was correlated with polymorphic variants in genes encoding the ERα (*ESR1*), ERβ (*ESR2*), aromatase (*CYP19A1*), and nuclear receptor coactivator 1 (*NCOA1*). In men, systolic blood pressure and pulse pressure were significantly associated with two polymorphisms in *ESR1*, while pulse pressure was also associated with variations in *NCOA1* and *CYP19A1*. Polymorphic variants in *ER1, CYP19A1*, and *NCOA1* genes were associated with diastolic blood pressure in women. While the underlying relationship between genes involved in estrogen action and hypertension is presently incompletely understood, these findings suggest estrogen-related genes contribute to gender-specific blood pressure variation. Nevertheless, further studies are warranted to confirm these results.

An increasing number of gene loci (not related to sex hormones) have been shown to contribute to hypertension; a limited subset of these genes has thus far been shown to modulate hypertension in a gender-specific way. An example includes the E65K polymorphism in the β1-subunit of the large-conductance, Ca^{2+}-dependent K^+ (BK) channel, a key element in the control of arterial tone. This channel in vascular SMCs is composed of an ion-conducting α subunit and a regulatory β(1) subunit, and is involved in the coupling of local increases in intracellular Ca^{2+} to augmented channel activity and vascular relaxation. A G352A variant allele in the β(1) gene (KCNMB1) corresponding to an E65K mutation in the channel protein has been identified resulting in a gain-of-function of the channel, and was also found to be associated with a low prevalence of moderate and severe diastolic hypertension [93].

Recently, Senti et al. examined the modulatory effect of sex and age and the association of the E65K polymorphism in KCNMB1 with low prevalence of diastolic hypertension, as well as the protective role of E65K polymorphism against CVD [94]. Genotype frequency of the E65K polymorphism was assessed in 3,924 subjects with a 5-year follow-up to identify CVD occurrence, as was estrogen modulation of wild-type and mutant ion channel activity after heterologous expression and electrophysiological studies. A multivariate regression analysis revealed that the protective effect of the K allele against moderate-to-severe diastolic hypertension aging was increased as a function of increased age. These findings remained significant when analyses was restricted to women but not to men, and this effect was independent of the reported acute modulation of BK channels by estrogen. This study provides genetic evidence concerning the different impact of the BK channel in blood pressure control in men and women, mainly in aging women.

Coronary Artery Disease (CAD)

Many of the effects of sex steroid hormones estrogen on the vascular system presented in the previous discussion of cardiac hypertrophy and hypertension modulate susceptibility and progression of CAD as well. In addition to its vasodilatory effects on the endothelium, inhibition of vascular SMC growth, constriction and attenuation of inflammatory signaling, estrogen significantly improves lipoprotein profiles. With aging, loss of endogenous estrogen contributes to a rapid increase in the incidence of CAD after menopause, and contributes to gender-specific differences in the incidence, pathophysiology and clinical manifestations of the disease. On average, women are 10 years older than men when presenting with CAD, possibly due to delayed diagnosis or presentation. For instance compared with men, women's chest pain is more often associated with abdominal pain, dyspnea, nausea, and fatigue. Gender differences in self-presentation and description of chest pain in part have contributed to underdiagnosis and undertreatment of women with CAD. Moreover, numerous studies have shown that chest pain in women is less likely to be associated with flow-limiting coronary stenoses than chest pain in men. The lack of large obstructive lesions causing artery blockage in women normally detected by coronary angiography may contribute to the discounting of woman's symptoms. Recent findings of the Women's Ischemia Syndrome Evaluation (WISE) Study, a multi-center, long-term investigation sponsored by the National Heart, Lung and Blood Institute suggested that female-specific CAD is more often associated with functional rather than structural abnormalities of the coronary circulation and tends to involve a global pattern of dysfunction in both the large vessels and in the coronary microcirculation, leading to diffuse atherosclerosis [95, 96]. As a corollary, exercise or treadmill stress testing without imaging appears to be insufficient for CAD diagnosis in women whereas functional capacity tests, magnetic resonance spectroscopy and gadolinium cardiac magnetic resonance imaging may identify patients whose chest pain is due to myocardial ischemia without obstructive CAD. Recent innovations in the application of phosphorus-31 nuclear magnetic resonance spectroscopy have provided means for monitoring changes in the myocardial high-energy phosphates, phosphocreatine, and adenosine triphosphate after stress. A transient decrease in myocardial phosphocreatine/adenosine triphosphate ratio during handgrip exercise has been demonstrated [97], indicating a shift toward anaerobic metabolism and myocardial ischemia in 20 % of women with chest pain but normal coronary arteries. Furthermore, emerging evidence implicate microvascular structural damage and abnormalities secondary to aging, hypertension, diabetes, left ventricular hypertrophy are important contributors as well as predictors of CAD outcome in women but not men [98]. Since retinal microvascular structural abnormalities have been linked to past blood pressure, inflammation, and endothelial dysfunction, its assessment enables non-invasive investigation of systemic vascular pathology [98, 99]. Recent studies evaluating risk factors associated with adenosine-related microvascular coronary reactivity in symptomatic women examined for CAD, found that classic atherosclerotic risk factors were not associated with defective coronary microvascular reactivity (to adenosine) in the majority of cases, suggesting that novel gender-specific risk factors need to be identified [100].

The WISE study and others also suggested that chest pain without flow-limiting lesions may be associated with endothelial dysfunction and impaired coronary flow reserve. Furthermore, the finding that women with ischemic heart disease/CAD tend to be older, with more functional disability and a greater susceptibility to morbidity and mortality suggests that gender-specific aging attenuates many estrogen-related potentially beneficial vascular responses, including endothelial progenitor cells (EPCs) and coronary microvascular function, as indicated by the WISE study [98].

Nevertheless, CAD diagnosis in women is generally more difficult than in men because of the lower specificity of symptoms and diagnostic accuracy of non-invasive testing. Wiviott et al. have examined the relationship between gender and the presentation of cardiac biomarkers in patients with unstable angina (UA) and non-ST-segment elevation myocardial infarction (NSTEMI) [101]. Among 1,865 patients with UA/NSTEMI (34 % women), significant gender-specific differences were found in presenting biomarkers. Men were more likely to have elevated creatine kinase-MB and troponins and markers of myocardial necrosis, whereas women were more likely to have elevated C-reactive protein (hs-CRP) and BNP levels. These findings imply that a multimarker approach may be an important adjunct in the initial risk assessment of UA/NSTEMI, and that further research is necessary to determine whether gender-related pathophysiological differences exist in the presentation with acute coronary syndromes.

Recent randomized clinical trials in postmenopausal women have failed to demonstrate that HRT is beneficial for CAD secondary or primary prevention. Interestingly, findings from these randomized studies conflict with numerous observational studies that suggested a significant beneficial effect of estrogen replacement in CAD and these discrepancies are likely related to differences in patient selection, hormone regimen, and most importantly biological effect of hormones in different periods of women's life, particularly in the elderly [102].

Endogenous testosterone (T) in men is correlated positively with HDL-C and negatively with LDL-C, triglycerides, fibrinogen, and plasminogen activator type 1 PAI-1. On the other hand, these relationships are reversed in women [103]. In addition, hypoandrogenemia in men and hyperandrogenemia in women are often confounded by central obesity and insulin resistance making these associations not helpful with respect to deciding if androgens have a direct pro- or antiatherogenic effect. Although a relationship in males of T level with the progression of atherosclerosis, accumulation of visceral adipose tissue, and other risk factors for MI has been reported, neither the level of T nor of estrogen was found to be predictive of coronary events in any of the eight prospective studies that have been carried out. Whereas gender-specific differences in MI incidence tend to support the view that T promotes and/or estrogen prevents MI, it is noteworthy that cross-sectional hormone administration, and prospective studies have suggested that in men T appears to prevent and estrogen promote MI, a so-called estrogen-androgen paradox, meaning that endogenous sex hormones may relate to atherosclerotic CVD, and its risk factors act oppositely in women and men.

In their evaluation of the medical literature (by MEDLINE searches), Wu and von Eckardstein [104] found that the gender difference in CAD could not be explained on the basis of endogenous sex hormone exposure (since none of the epidemiological studies in the literature have showed a positive association between T and CAD in men). In women also, there is not definitive evidence that endogenous T plays a causal or protective role for CAD, although patients with the polycystic ovarian syndrome (PCOS) have shown an adverse risk profile. Furthermore, observational studies on dehydroepiandrosterone (DHEA) do not support the hypothesis that DHEA deficiency is a risk factor for CAD in men or women [104]. Moreover, postmenopausal women treated with either T or DHEA showed no improvement in endothelial vasodilatory function or in modulating endothelin 1 level, as had been suggested by previous animal studies [105].

Besides numerous ethnic and racial differences (which have been described primarily in the prevalence of metabolic syndrome (MetSyn), insulin resistance, type 2 diabetes, and cardiovascular events), increased focus on the importance of family history in CAD development underline the modulatory influence of individual's genotype to vascular disease susceptibility. Several genetic polymorphisms associated with CAD or CAD events have been described in predominantly male populations (which will be discussed more extensively in a later section of this chapter). To understand the interaction between genetic and environmental factors in the incidence of coronary artery spasm (CAS) in Japan. the genotypes for 35 polymorphisms of 29 candidate genes in a large cohort of man and women were analyzed with an allele-specific DNA primer-probe assay [106]. Multivariable logistic regression analysis adjusted for age, body mass index, and the prevalence of smoking, hypertension, diabetes and hypercholesterolemia, demonstrated a significant association with CAS of one polymorphism (242C–>T in the NADH/NADPH oxidase p22 phox gene) in men and two polymorphisms (−1171/5A–>6A in the stromelysin-1 gene and −634C–>G in the interleukin-6 gene) in women. While smoking was found to be the most important risk factor for CAS, the effects of these polymorphic gene variants on CAS were statistically independent of smoking. The NADH/NADPH oxidase p22 phox gene is a susceptibility locus for CAS in men, and the stromelysin-1 and interleukin-6 genes are susceptibility loci in women.

It is widely documented that women have higher hospital mortality rates for acute MI than men, and the difference may be related to the older age and higher prevalence of comorbidities in women [107, 108]. On the other hand it has been suggested that this difference may, at least in part, be related to differences in management with women undergoing less frequently coronary revascularization procedures, such as percutaneous coronary interventions than men [109]. Moreover, in the USA, among the elderly, women have been reported to have lower rates of cardiac catheterization use after an acute MI than men, although it has been suggested that this difference occurred primarily in patients with equivocal indications [110].

As pointed out by Anderson and Pepine gender-specific differences in the outcome of patients with acute MI may be explained in part by biological differences [111]. Conditions found only in women such as early menopause, gestational diabetes, peripartum vascular dissection, preeclampsia and eclampsia, polycystic ovarian syndrome, low-birth-weight children, and hypothalamic hypoestrogenemia suggest gender differences in the pathophysiology of ischemic vascular disease. While many of these conditions occur mainly at a younger age, they carry an increased risk for ischemic heart disease/CAD later in life. Women also tend to have a higher incidence of vascular abnormalities with smooth muscle cell dysfunction such as CAS, and Raynaud's phenomenon as well as higher frequencies of vasculitis (e.g., Takayasu's arteritis, temporal arteritis, rheumatoid vasculitis, lupus vasculitis, polymyalgia rheumatica, etc.) compared with men. In addition to profound gender-specific differences in the vasculature structure, including smaller and less compliant arteries in women (recall the previous discussion of artery stiffening with aging women), functional alterations are clearly involved in the higher risk and more severe CAD-related vascular disease in women.

Increasing evidence suggests that hormone changes/fluctuations impact both the larger vasculature as well as the microvasculature. Estrogen and its loss during aging affect levels of circulating endothelial progenitor cells, which in turn compromises vascular endothelial repair leading to CAD susceptibility.

Smooth muscle dysfunction is also more prevalent in aging women than men, and has been linked to increased CAD. Recent observations have shown that activation of ERα not only reduces the proliferation of vascular SMCs, as previously noted, but also reduces the aortic SMC differentiation [112]. The link between ER activation and vascular health may arise from the influence of the ER activation on SMC phenotype as well as on the ECM production responsible for maintaining a healthy vascular wall. Furthermore, a switch to a dedifferentiated phenotype may contribute to atherosclerotic plaque instability.

There is also a gender-specific response to I/R injury that includes both susceptibility and cardioprotective components. Several components of the cardioprotective signaling pathways have been shown to have gender-specific expression/regulation. Female guinea pig ventricular tissue expresses higher levels of functional cardiac K_{ATP} channels than male due to the higher expression of the SUR2A subunit, which has a significant impact on cardiac response to ischemia-reperfusion challenge [113]. In addition, female gender confers cardioprotection against I/R injury, in part as a function of estrogen's capacity to enhance NO production by endothelial NOS. A gender-specific component in the delayed preconditioning response to isofluorane has been documented in rabbits [114].

McCully et al. have demonstrated that aging is associated with reduced tolerance to ischemia and that the aged (not senescent) female heart has greater susceptibility to ischemia as compared with the aged male heart [115]. These investigators had previously shown that ischemia can be modulated with cardioplegia in the male heart; however, efficacy in the female heart was unknown. Using male and female mature (15–20 weeks) and aged (>32 month) rabbit hearts (n=134) subjected to Langendorff perfusion, it was found that global ischemia significantly decreased postischemic functional recovery and increased infarct size in the mature and aged male and female heart and that the effects of global ischemia were significantly increased in the aged heart as compared with the mature heart. While cardioplegia +/− diazoxide significantly increased postischemic functional recovery and significantly decreased infarct size in mature male and female hearts, these effects were significantly decreased in the aged heart, and particularly in the aged female as compared with the aged male heart. Therefore, postischemic functional recovery and infarct size are affected by age but not by gender. On the other hand, the cardioprotection afforded by cardioplegia is affected by age and gender with a strong age/gender interaction for end-diastolic pressure and infarct size. These data indicate that optimized cardioplegia protocols, are effective in male but not in aged female heart.

Mitochondria play an important role in cardioprotection. When the supply of oxygen becomes limiting as occurs with myocardial ischemia, oxidative phosphorylation (OXPHOS) and mitochondrial electron transport chain (ETC) flux decline. However, hyperthermic stress can protect against myocardial dysfunction after I/R injury [116]. Improved levels of complex I–V activities, heat shock protein expression (i.e., HSP 32, 60, and 72) and ventricular function were reported in heat-stressed hearts. In comparison to untreated reperfused myocardium, in which mitochondria were severely disrupted, the reperfused heat-stressed myocardium exhibited higher respiratory complex activities and mitochondria with intact membranes packed with parallel lamellar cristae. These findings provided evidence that heat-stress-mediated enhancement of mitochondrial energetic capacity is associated with increased tolerance to I/R injury.

Recently, McCully et al. further evaluated the mechanism of cardioprotection provided by cardioplegia as affected by age and gender which as noted above is less effective in the aged female compared with the aged male rabbit heart [117]. They analyzed if these differences are due to age and gender-specific modulation of mitochondrial oxygen consumption and mitochondrial free matrix calcium ($[Ca^{2+}]_{Mito}$) content occurring during early reperfusion in a group of male and female mature (15–20 weeks) and aged (>32 months) subjected to Langendorff perfusion. Interestingly, mitochondrial oxygen consumption was significantly increased in the mature and aged female hearts in all treatment groups. Cardioplegia +/− diazoxide modulated mitochondrial oxygen consumption, but these effects were significantly decreased in the aged heart and in the female heart and cardioplegia (potassium/magnesium) significantly decreased $[Ca^{2+}]_{Mito}$ in aged but not mature hearts. The addition of diazoxide to potassium/magnesium significantly decreased $[Ca^{2+}]_{Mito}$ in mature and aged males (*versus* potassium/magnesium) but not in females. Thus mitochondrial oxygen consumption and $[Ca^{2+}]_{Mito}$ are modulated by age and gender and play an important role in the differences observed between mature and aged male and female response to global ischemia and the cardioprotection afforded by cardioplegia +/− diazoxide.

In women, aging and diabetes increase their susceptibility to myocardial ischemic injury; however, the cellular mechanisms involved are not understood. Desrois et al. have studied the influence of gender on cardiac insulin resistance and ischemic injury in the aging of Goto-Kakizaki (GK) rat, a model of type 2 diabetes [118]. Male and female GK rats had heart/body weight ratios 29 % and 53 % higher, respectively, than their sex-matched controls, with the female GK rat hearts significantly more hypertrophied than the male. Glucose transporter (GLUT) 1 protein levels were the same in all hearts, but GLUT4 protein levels were 28 % lower in all GK rat hearts compared with their sex-matched controls. In isolated, perfused hearts, insulin-stimulated ^{3}H-glucose uptake rates were decreased by 23 % and 40 % in male and female GK rat hearts, respectively, compared with controls, with females showing significantly higher insulin resistance than male GK rat hearts. During low-flow ischemia, glucose uptake was 59 % lower in female, but the same as controls in male GK rat hearts. The recovery of contractile function during reperfusion was 30 % lower in female, but the same as controls in male GK rat hearts. These data suggest that the aging female type 2 diabetic rat heart has increased insulin resistance and greater susceptibility to ischemic injury, than non-diabetic or male type 2 diabetic rat hearts.

Gender and Specific CV Markers

Currently, with our better understanding of the pathophysiology of human CVDs, the development of novel circulating serum and plasma biomarkers is proceeding at an accelerated speed, mainly with the help of new genomic and proteomic technologies. In this section we will describe some of the markers specific of certain CVDs and their gender-specific presentation where present.

Cardiac Troponin (cTn)

cTn, a sensitive indicator of myocardial-cell injury, is the best validated of the new markers in the diagnosis, risk stratification and prognostication of MI, acute coronary syndrome (ACS), and acute myocardial ischemia [119–122]. Because of its sensitivity, detection of elevated cTn levels is common in patients with a large number of acute and chronic CVDs. It is noteworthy, that in a recent study using multiple logistic regression in a Danish population, women >60 years living alone and men >50 years living alone were at especially high risk for ACS. Although they constituted only 5.4 % and 7.7 % respectively of the source population, they accounted for 34.3 % and 62.4 % of ACS patients dying within 30 days [123]. Therefore, age and single living appear to be positively associated with ACS in both sexes.

C-reactive Protein

There are opposing views regarding the variability of CRP levels [124, 125]. Some argue that in the absence of acute illness, including myocardial injury, levels of CRP are stable. Other studies have reported that levels fluctuate and vary by gender and ethnicity [126]. Khera et al. reported that black subjects had higher CRP levels than white subjects, and women had higher CRP levels than men. After adjustment for traditional cardiovascular risk factors, estrogen and statin use, and body mass index, a CRP level >3 mg/l remained more common in white women and black women but not in black men when compared with white men.

In a prospective study of 911 consecutive patients (including 327 women) with typical exertional angina, baseline CRP levels were significantly higher in women than men; however, women had a similar rate of cardiac events (measured over a 3 year follow-up) compared to men. In addition, women on HRT had significantly higher CRP than women not using HRT, and when analyzed as a whole, increased CRP was associated with a higher cardiovascular risk [127]. In addition, as previously noted Wiviott et al. found that among patients with unstable angina, women had increased elevation of CRP and BNP compared to men, who in contrast tended to display elevated levels of CK-MB and troponins [101]. Gender did not change the incidence of ST elevation, TIMI risk scores nor the prognostic value of TACTICS-TIMI 18 markers. However upon using a multimarker approach, a greater proportion of high-risk women were identified suggesting that the use of multimarkers may be more helpful in the initial risk assessment of UA/NSTEMI, mainly in women

Recently, an epidemiological report on the reliability of CRP in the prediction of CAD and global vascular events in the prospective study on pravastatin in the elderly at risk (PROSPER) [128], found that CRP has limited clinical value in CVD risk stratification, or in the predictive response to statin therapy in the elderly. 5,804 cohort members, men and women of 70–82 years of age were studied. Unfortunately, no specific data by gender was provided.

Phospholipase A(2)

It had been hypothesized that lipoprotein-associated phospholipase A2 (Lp-PLA2) level is an independent predictor of cardiovascular risk in hypercholesterolemic men. However, in contrast to data among hyperlipidemic men, a prospective assessment by Blake et al. in a nested case-control study among 28,263 apparently healthy middle-aged women of whether Lp-PLA2 was a predictor of future cardiovascular risk in women revealed that Lp-PLA2 was not a strong predictor of future cardiovascular risk among unselected women [129]. On the other hand, it had been found that both genders have a similar association between the presence of elevated glycated hemoglobin A1c (HbA1c) and CVD and mortality. Khaw et al. have reported that the risk for CVD and total mortality associated with HbA1c concentrations increased continuously in men and women through their sample distribution (4,662 men and 5,570 women of 45–79 years of age) [130]. Interestingly, the relationship was apparent in persons without known diabetes, and most of the events in the sample occurred in persons with moderately elevated HbA1c concentrations. These findings support the need for randomized trials of interventions to reduce HbA1c concentrations in persons without diabetes. However, we agree with the authors that whether HbA1c concentrations and CVD are causally related cannot be concluded from an observational study, and that it will be of further interest to know if this association was stronger with increasing age of the cohort. With this information, interventional studies could be more definitive in determining whether decreasing HbA1c concentrations would reduce CVD.

E-selectin/Atherosclerosis

Atherosclerosis is a complex disease caused by multiple genetic and environmental factors and complex gene-environment interactions as discussed in Chapter 8, The molecular mechanisms of atherosclerosis integrate a complex web of cellular events that is only gradually becoming understandable. These mechanisms involve lipid metabolism, inflammatory signaling and interaction with the complex vascular system involved in thrombosis. The inflammatory signaling involves the recruitment and binding of circulating leukocytes to areas of inflammation within the vascular endothelium, mediated by a diverse array of cellular adhesion molecules. According to Ellsworth et al. a polymorphic variant in the endothelial-leukocyte adhesion molecule 1 (E-selectin) gene has been implicated in early-onset, angiographically defined, severe atherosclerotic disease because it profoundly affects ligand recognition and binding specificity, resulting in a significant increase in cellular adhesion [131].

These investigators evaluated the relationships between the E-selectin S128R polymorphism and coronary artery calcification (CAC), a marker of atherosclerosis in 294 asymptomatic women aged 40–88 years and 314 asymptomatic men aged 30–80 years from the Epidemiology of Coronary Artery Calcification Study. The E-selectin polymorphism was not associated with CAC presence in men of any age or in women over age 50. However, in women 50 years of age or younger, the E-selectin polymorphism was significantly associated with CAC presence after adjustment for age, body mass index, systolic blood pressure, ratio of total cholesterol to HDL-cholesterol, and smoking. The significant association between E-selectin and CAC in women 50 years of age or younger may suggest that the 128R allele is a risk factor for coronary atherosclerosis in younger asymptomatic women, who typically have lower levels of traditional risk factors and reduced adhesion molecule expression due to the presence of higher levels of endogenous hormones.

Lipid Peroxides (LPO)

Using transgenic mice with non-pulsatile circulating human growth hormone (hGH), the gender difference in the effects of chronic exposure to hGH on cardiac risk biomarkers has been investigated by Naraoka et al. [132] Blood plasma was obtained from transgenic and control mice at 8, 12, and 16 weeks of age, and was used for the measurement of hGH and the following cardiac risk biomarkers: total cholesterol, triglyceride, HDL, LDL, non esterified free fatty acids, and lipid peroxides (LPO). Compared to control animals, transgenic males exhibited higher levels of LDL at 8 and 12 weeks of age and higher levels of LPO at every week of age examined, as compared to those of the control males, while transgenic females exhibited somewhat lower levels of LDL and LPO from 8 to 16 weeks of age, as compared to the control females. The relative heart weight in males increased with aging and was significantly higher in the 16-week-old transgenic males compared to those of the control mice. These findings demonstrate that transgenic males exhibit cardiac risk potential caused by chronic exposure to hGH as compared to females and show that the transgenic mouse line is a useful model for the study of gender difference in cardiac disorders caused by hGH.

Mitochondria

Observed gender-specific differences in longevity within a species have been attributed to differences in oxidative stress (OS), and are thought to likely arise from higher female estrogen levels. However, in some species, males live the same or longer despite their lower estrogen values. Recently, Sanz et al. [133] in an analysis of mitochondrial bioenergetics, OS and apoptosis in the B6 (C57Bl/6J) mouse strain found no differences in longevity between males and females in this strain, although estrogen levels were higher in females. They did not find any differences in heart, skeletal muscle and liver mitochondrial oxygen consumption (State 3 and State 4) and ATP content between male and female mice. In addition mitochondrial H_2O_2 generation and OS levels (determined by cytosolic protein carbonyls and 8-hydroxy-2′-deoxyguanosine levels in mtDNA) were similar in both sexes. Furthermore, markers of apoptosis (e.g., caspase-3, caspase-9 and mono- and oligonucleosomes) were not different between male and female mice. The findings are consistent with the Free Radical Theory of Aging (see Chapter 1), by indicating that OS generation independent of estrogen levels determines aging rate.

Resistin

While some investigators have reported that increased serum resistin levels are associated with obesity, visceral fat, insulin resistance, type 2 diabetes and inflammation, others have not found these correlations. The relationship of plasma resistin levels has been examined with markers of MetSyn and atherosclerosis in a large population-based study and related to the presence of obesity, MetSyn, metabolic abnormalities, cardiovascular risk, and progression of intima-media thickness (IMT) [134]. The study group consisting of 1,090 subjects (not taking any medication) was selected from the PLIC study (originally designed to verify the presence of atherosclerotic lesions and progression of IMT in the common carotid artery in the general population). Plasma resistin levels correlated with triglycerides, waist circumference, waist/hip ratio, systolic blood pressure, and ApoAI/ApoB ratio, while they were inversely correlated with HDL and ApoAI levels. Moreover, these findings were gender specific. Plasma resistin levels were significantly higher in women with the MetSyn compared with controls, while no difference was observed in obese subjects. In addition, plasma resistin levels showed a significant correlation with cardiovascular risk.

Adiponectin

Circulating adiponectin derived from fat cells is a marker for insulin sensitivity. Nilsson et al. have recently measured plasma adiponectin levels in 373 men and 514 women of middle age by a time-resolved immunofluorometric assay [135]. The subjects were sampled stratified for degree of insulin sensitivity. In addition, right common carotid artery IMT was assessed by ultrasound. In men, mean IMT was significantly lower with increasing age-adjusted plasma adiponectin levels, while in women no difference in IMT was noted with different adiponectin levels. Hence, plasma adiponectin is a marker of glucose metabolism and obesity and shows an inverse age-adjusted association with carotid ultrasound IMT in men, but not in women. After adjustments for other risk factors this association was attenuated.

Gender-Specific Gene Profiling

While in later chapters we will present a comprehensive discussion of gene profiling in aging using either transcript analysis or proteomic analysis, there have been only limited studies examining these differences in gene programming in aging *vis a vis* gender-specific expression.

In a proteomic investigation of gender-specific differences in gene expression of glycolytic and mitochondrial pathways, Yan et al. have reported a decreased expression of enzymes of glycolysis (e.g., pyruvate kinase, triosephosphate isomerase, α-enolase), glucose oxidation (e.g., pyruvate dehydrogenase E1β -subunit), and the TCA cycle (e.g., 2-oxoglutarate dehydrogenase) in LV samples derived from old males (OM) monkeys, these changes were not observed either in young animals nor in old females (OF) [136]. Gender-specific differences in the reduced expression and function of proteins responsible for mitochondrial ETC and OXPHOS were also only found in hearts from OM monkeys. Moreover, changes in the glycolytic and mitochondrial metabolic pathways in OM monkey hearts were similar to those observed in hearts affected by diabetes or LV dysfunction, suggesting potential involvement in the mechanism of the cardiomyopathy of aging. The finding that OF hearts did not develop these abnormal metabolic changes, may explain the delayed cardiovascular risk observed in OFs.

Gene Polymorphisms in Gender-Specific Age-Related CVDs

An increasing number of gene variants with relatively diverse function have been shown to have significant gender-specific distribution in association with aging-associated CVDs (Table 10.1). Many

Table 10.1 Gender-specific effects of gene variants in aging-associated CVD

Gene	Variant	Phenotype	Refs
APOA5	−1131T>C	Females with C allele had ↑ remnant-like particles and CVD	137
CYP2C9	*3	Hyperlipidemia in females	138
Desmin	Leu370Pro	Males prone to cardiac sudden death	139
ADRB1	Ser49Gly	↑ DBP in females with Gly/Gly	140
ADRA2A	−1297C>G	↑ DBP in females with GG genotype	
ADRB2	Gly16Arg	↑ DBP in men with Arg/Arg	140
AGT	Met235Thr	↑ DBP in men carrying Thr allele	
FYN		Systolic and diastolic BP in women	141
ADRB1	Ser49Gly	Diastolic BP in men	141
QPCT	Arg54Trp	HT in men	141
CYP11B2	−344C>T		
SREBP-2	Gly595Ala	In females, homozygosity for the SREBP-2-595A or for SCAP-796I was associated with ↑ plasma LDL-C	142
SCAP	Ile796Val		
ACADSB	−1187G>C	HT in women	143
COMT	512A>G	HT in men	
eNOS	G894T	↓ BP in black and white females	144
	G10T	↓ BP in white females	
ACE	I/D	↑ BP in males with DD genotype	145
MTHFR	C677T	With TT genotype, ↑ ischemic stroke in women	146
KLOTHO	G-395A	Women carrying A allele had ↑ cardioembolic stroke	147
TGFB1	Pro10Leu	Women with Leu/Leu genotype had ↑ ischemic stroke and SVO	148
Lipoprotein lipase	Asn291Ser	Increased ischemic stroke in women	149

ACADSB: Short/branched chain acyl-CoA dehydrogenase; COMT: Catecholamine-O-methyltransferase; SVO: Small vessel occlusion.

of these identified genetic loci have been discussed in several chapters of this book with regards to be important components of the pathophysiology of specific age-associated CVDs. For instance, APOA5, CYP2 and lipoprotein lipase are important components of lipid metabolism and they clearly impact on atherosclerosis and CVD. Similar relationships pertain to the involvement of gene variants of ACE, eNOS, AGT and adrenergic receptors (ADRs) in blood pressure and hypertension.

Pharmacogenomics and Gender

Variability in the response to cardiovascular drugs fluctuates among patients. While some achieve the desired therapeutic response, others do not. In addition, a subset of patients will experience variable adverse effects ranging from mild to life threatening, and genetics can be an important contributor to this variable drug response.

Pharmacogenomics is a relatively young field focused on unraveling the genetic determinants of variable drug response. A number of gene variants have been identified thus far that have a gender-specific effect on the action of specific drugs used to treat age-associated CVDs (shown in Table 10.2). Clearly, with more intensive research more loci will be uncovered. Importantly, drugs identified in this variable response are commonly used in the treatment of hyperlipidemia (statin) and hypertension (hydrochlorothiazide, atenolol). Genes involved include estrogen receptor, APOE2, MDR1 (suggesting a direct involvement of drug metabolism), ACE, microsomal triglyceride transfer protein (MTP) and preproendothelin-1.

Table 10.2 Gender-associated gene variants and drug response: pharmacogenomics

Drug	Gene variant	Phenotype	Refs
Atorvastatin	*ESR1 Pvu*II(−) *Xba*I(+) haplotype	↑ HDL-C in women not men	150
	APOA1+83	↑ HDL-C in women	
Atorvastatin	MDR1 C3435T	↑ HDL-C in female 3453C carriers	151
Atorvastatin	APOE2 ε 4	↓ LDL-C and ↓ TG in men not women	152
Hydrochlorothiazide	ACE II	↓ SBP and DBP in women	153
	ACE DD	↓ SBP and DBP in men	
Atorvastatin	Microsomal triglyceride transfer protein MTP-493 GT	↓ TG and VLDL in female T carriers	154
Irbesartan or atenolol	Preproendothelin-1 G5665T	↓ SBP response in men carrying TT genotype	155

Current research is largely focused on a limited candidate gene approach, which allows for description of significant genetic associations with variable response, although this approach often does not explain the genetic basis of variable drug response enough to be used effectively in clinical application [156]. Since most drug responses involve a large number of proteins, all of whose genes could have several polymorphisms, it has been argued that a single polymorphism in a single gene would be unlikely to explain a high degree of drug response variability in a consistent fashion, suggesting that a polygenic, or genomic approach might be more informative [156]. Siest et al. [157] in a recent review proposed a comprehensive pharmacogenomic approach in the field of cardiovascular therapy by considering five sources of variability, including the genetics of pharmacokinetics, the genetics of pharmacodynamics (i.e., drug targets), genetics linked to a defined pathology and corresponding drug therapies, the genetics of physiologic regulation, and environmental-genetic interactions. In addition, they illustrated this five-tiered approach by using examples of drugs for CVD treatment in relation to specific genetic polymorphisms.

Presently, with a progressively aging population, the increasing pressure on health-care spending, and the promise of an individualized, safe and effective treatment at lower cost, the public acceptance of pharmacogenomics is apparently high. However, in spite of the great benefits that this new approach may bring, there are a number of hurdles (e.g., ethical, social and legal concerns) to be overcome prior to the successful application of this modality of therapy and building of sufficient shared databases for researchers and clinicians [158]. Undoubtedly, pharmacogenomics has the potential to improve the use of drugs in treating age-associated CVDs through the selection of the most effective drug therapy in an individual, based on their genetic information as well as gender and age. Furthermore, it may take a decade or more before the necessary genetic information will be available for use in making drug therapy decisions, although it is evident that new and important findings in this area will continue to appear, and the experimental approaches will continue to evolve.

Conclusions

Gender-specific changes occur in the heart and vasculature both in aging and in the cardiovascular diseases associated with aging. While information concerning the mechanisms involved in these gender-specific differences is still relatively rudimentary, increasing knowledge concerning both the gender factors themselves (e.g., hormone, receptor), signaling pathways they trigger and cellular targets in both the vasculature [i.e., endothelial cell, smooth muscle cell and stem cells (EPCs)] and in the heart, will enable the identification of viable targets to improved medical therapy for CVDs, including the development of novel effective pharmacological, gene-based and cell-based strategies. Moreover, increasing information about the contribution of specific gene variants to the susceptibility of aging-related CVD, their interaction with other genes as well as with environmental factors, and the modulation of responses to specific drug treatments will be of significant use to the clinical cardiologist treating and managing cardiovascular disorders. Furthermore, given the increased awareness of the role of genetic background, age and assorted risk factors/biomarkers in influencing diagnostic efficacy and therapeutic responses, future clinical trials that fully integrate this information with that of the complex pleiotropic actions of estrogens and progesterone and their analogs will not only provide further insights regarding postmenopausal roles for hormone therapy, but may also prove to be more successful in treating targeted populations.

Summary

- There are a number of differences between male and female hearts even in the absence of pathology. Greater cardiac contractility and improved myocardial mass are found in women.
- Aging is accompanied by less myocyte cell loss, myocyte cellular hypertrophy and myocardial remodeling in women.
- While both necrosis and apoptosis contribute to overall cell death and remodeling in the aging heart, it is not yet clear to what extent each pathway is involved. Several studies have indicated that myocardial apoptosis is markedly increased in aging males compared to females.
- Changes in human myocardial estrogen receptor α (ERα) expression, localization, and association with structural proteins have been found in end stage-failing hearts of patients with dilated cardiomyopathy (DCM).
- Alcoholic cardiomyopathy resulted in male but not in female rats displaying significant ventricular wall and intraventricular septum thinning and decreased levels of myocardial protein synthesis secondary to a decline in the phosphorylation and activation of specific eukaryotic initiation factor (eIF4G) and binding proteins.
- Estrogen, via estrogen-receptor-dependent mechanisms, differentially alters the response of male and female cells to hypoxia. Cardiac fibroblasts derived from male rats are more susceptible to hypoxia as gauged by diminished DNA synthesis, whereas fibroblasts from age-matched females are hypoxia-resistant.
- Increased myocardial and extracellular remodeling in male rats and dogs in response to induced volume overload was accompanied by increased matrix metalloproteinase (MMP) activation and mast cell density.
- In failing hearts abnormal Ca^{2+} cycling in association with male-specific attenuation of phospholamban phosphorylation at serine-16 and decreased Ca^{2+} affinity was found.
- Transgenic mice containing an overexpressed mutant phospholamban allele, which acts as a SERCA superinhibitor, led to progressive DCM with extensive interstitial tissue fibrosis and death at 6 months in males while females exhibited normal systolic function up to 12 months of age.
- Hypertension is more frequent in women and is a likely gender-specific component contributing to left ventricular and arterial stiffening.
- Gender-specific differences in ventricular diastolic distensibility, in vascular stiffness and ventricular/vascular coupling contribute to a greater rate of HF with normal ejection fraction (HF-NEF) in elderly women compared to men.
- The causes of gender-specific differences in the incidence of cardiac dysrhythmias are not yet known, although sex-specific variations in cardiac electrophysiology and/or hormonal effects on modulating ionic channel function are likely contributory factors.
- From puberty on women show a higher basic heart rate than men as well as longer QT interval, shorter QRS duration, and lower QRS voltage.
- Women with long-QT syndrome tend to have a higher prevalence of sick sinus node syndrome, atrioventricular (AV) tachycardia, idiopathic right ventricular tachycardia (VT), and dysrhythmic events.

- Men have a higher prevalence of carotid sinus syndrome, supraventricular and reentrant VT (due to accessory pathways), Wolff-Parkinson-White syndrome, ventricular fibrillation, Brugada syndrome and sudden death.
- Atrial fibrillation (AF) tends to be more prevalent in men but is associated with markedly elevated CVD morbidity (including increased stroke incidence) and mortality in elderly women. Treatment of AF in elderly women with anticoagulants is effective and needs careful consideration.
- *Torsade de pointes* tachycardia occur more frequently in women, in conjunction with the increased incidence of acquired and congenital long-QT Syndrome. Female gender is an independent risk factor for syncope and sudden death in the congenital long QT syndrome.
- Cardiac hypertrophy accompanied by cardiac fibrosis and myocardial dysfunction are often associated with gender-based differences, with higher mortality in men. Elderly female patients with aortic stenosis exhibit better systolic function and increased LV hypertrophy than males.
- Polymorphic variants in genes encoding ERs affect cardiac hypertrophy in women. In rodent models of familial HCM, specific mutations in cardiac troponin T genes have gender-specific phenotypes.
- Striking gender-specific effects on both hypertension and CAD have been reported and are underlined by estrogen's diverse impact on the vasculature (via both genomic and non-genomic mechanisms), including endothelial cell function and growth, on smooth muscle cell migration and proliferation, on the production of eNOS and NO, and on inflammatory events.
- In regard to symptoms and effective diagnosis and treatment of CAD there are significant gender differences.
- The response to ischemia-reperfusion (I/R) injury is gender-specific, including the susceptibility and cardioprotective components (e.g., cardiac K_{ATP} channels and mitochondrial cardioprotective signaling).
- Biomarkers of cardiac and cardiovascular health/disease including cardiac troponin, CRP, phospholipase A2, E-selectin, adiponectin, lipid peroxides and resistin have gender-specific distribution/expression. Gene profiling and proteomic analysis can be used to identify more gender specific biomarkers.
- Polymorphic variants in diverse genes including APOA5, CYP2 and lipoprotein lipase, ACE, eNOS, AGT and adrenergic receptors (ADRs) are associated with gender-specific expression of specific CVD phenotypes including atherosclerosis, hypertension and ischemic stroke.
- Polymorphic variants in genes including the estrogen receptor, APO2, MDR1, ACE, microsomal triglyceride transfer protein (MTP) and preproendothelin-1 have been identified that have a gender-specific effect on the action of specific common drugs (e.g., atorvastatin, hydroclorothiazide) to treat age-associated CVDs.
- Identification of the genetic determinants of variable drug response by pharmacogenetic analysis may prove useful in increasing therapeutic efficacy.

References

1. Mendelsohn ME, Karas RH. Molecular and cellular basis of cardiovascular gender differences. Science 2005;308:1583–1587
2. Babiker FA, De Windt LJ, van Eickels M, Grohe C, Meyer R, Doevendans PA. Estrogenic hormone action in the heart: regulatory network and function. Cardiovasc Res 2002;53:709–719
3. Grady D, Herrington D, Bittner V, Blumenthal R, Davidson M, Hlatky M, Hsia J, Hulley S, Herd A, Khan S, Newby LK, Waters D, Vittinghoff E, Wenger N. Cardiovascular disease outcomes during 6.8 years of hormone therapy: heart and estrogen/progestin replacement study follow-up (HERS II). JAMA 2002;288: 49–57
4. Manson JE, Hsia J, Johnson KC, Rossouw JE, Assaf AR, Lasser NL, Trevisan M, Black HR, Heckbert SR, Detrano R, Strickland OL, Wong ND, Crouse JR, Stein E, Cushman M. Women's health initiative investigators. Estrogen plus progestin and the risk of coronary heart disease. N Engl J Med 2003;349:523–534

5. Patten RD, Pourati I, Aronovitz MJ, Baur J, Celestin F, Chen X, Michael A, Haq S, Nuedling S, Grohe C, Force T, Mendelsohn ME, Karas RH. 17β-estradiol reduces cardiomyocyte apoptosis in vivo and in vitro via activation of phospho-inositide-3 kinase/Akt signaling. Circ Res 2004;95:692–699
6. Petre RE, Quaile MP, Rossman EJ, Ratcliffe SJ, Bailey BA, Houser SR, Margulies KB. Sex-based differences in myocardial contractile reserve. Am J Physiol Regul Integr Comp Physiol 2007;292:R810–R818
7. Denton K, Baylis C. Physiological and molecular mechanisms governing sexual dimorphism of kidney, cardiac, and vascular function. Am J Physiol Regul Integr Comp Physiol 2007;292:R697–R699
8. Paul RJ, Bowman PS, Johnson J, Martin AF. Effects of gender and estrogen on myosin COOH-terminal isoforms and contractility in rat aorta. Am J Physiol Regul Integr Comp Physiol 2007;292:R751–R757
9. Candore G, Balistreri CR, Listi F, Grimaldi MP, Vasto S, Colonna-Romano G, Franceschi C, Lio D, Caselli G, Caruso C. Immunogenetics, gender, and longevity. Ann NY Acad Sci 2006;1089:516–537
10. Huang A, Sun D, Wu Z, Yan C, Carroll MA, Jiang H, Falck JR, Kaley G. Estrogen elicits cytochrome P450 – mediated flow-induced dilation of arterioles in NO deficiency: role of PI3K-Akt phosphorylation in genomic regulation. Circ Res 2004;94:245–252
11. Olivetti G, Giordano G, Corradi D, Melissari M, Lagrasta C, Gambert SR, Anversa P. Gender differences and aging: effects on the human heart. J Am Coll Cardiol 1995;26:1068–1079
12. Mallat Z, Fornes P, Costagliola R, Esposito B, Belmin J, Lecomte D, Tedgui A. Age and gender effects on cardiomyocyte apoptosis in the normal human heart. J Gerontol A Biol Sci Med Sci 2001;56:M719–M723.
13. Bernecker OY, Huq F, Heist EK, Podesser BK, Hajjar RJ. Apoptosis in heart failure and the senescent heart. Cardiovasc Toxicol 2003;3:183–190
14. Goldspink DF, Burniston JG, Tan LB. Cardiomyocyte death and the ageing and failing heart. Exp Physiol 2003;88:447–458
15. Terman A, Gustafsson B, Brunk UT. The lysosomal-mitochondrial axis theory of postmitotic aging and cell death. Chem Biol Interact 2006;163:29–37
16. Powell SR. The ubiquitin-proteasome system in cardiac physiology and pathology. Am J Physiol Heart Circ Physiol 2006;291:H1–H19
17. Boddaert J, Mallat Z, Fornes P, Esposito B, Lecomte D, Verny M, Tedgui A, Belmin J. Age and gender effects on apoptosis in the human coronary arterial wall. Mech Ageing Dev 2005;126:678–684
18. Regitz-Zagrosek V, Lehmkuhl E, Lehmkuhl HB, Hetzer R. Gender aspects in heart failure. Pathophysiology and medical therapy. Arch Mal Coeur Vaiss 2004;97:899–908
19. Radin MJ, Holycross BJ, Sharkey LC, Shiry L, McCune SA. Gender modulates activation of renin-angiotensin and endothelin systems in hypertension and heart failure. J Appl Physiol 2002;92:935–940
20. Yanes LL, Romero DG, Iles JW, Iliescu R, Gomez-Sanchez C, Reckelhoff JF. Sexual dimorphism in the renin-angiotensin system in aging spontaneously hypertensive rats. Am J Physiol Regul Integr Comp Physiol 2006;291:R383–R390
21. Mahmoodzadeh S, Eder S, Nordmeyer J, Ehler E, Huber O, Martus P, Weiske J, Pregla R, Hetzer R, Regitz-Zagrosek V. Estrogen receptor alpha up-regulation and redistribution in human heart failure. FASEB J 2006;20:926–934
22. Vary TC, Kimball SR, Sumner A. Sex-dependent differences in the regulation of myocardial protein synthesis following long-term ethanol consumption. Am J Physiol Regul Integr Comp Physiol 2007;292:R778–R787
23. Dimitrow PP, Czarnecka D, Strojny JA, Kawecka-Jaszcz K, Dubiel JS. Impact of gender on the left ventricular cavity size and contractility in patients with hypertrophic cardiomyopathy. Int J Cardiol 2001;77:43–48
24. Dimitrow PP, Czarnecka D, Kawecka-Jaszcz K, Dubiel JS. The influence of age on gender-specific differences in the left ventricular cavity size and contractility in patients with hypertrophic cardiomyopathy. Int J Cardiol 2003;88:11–16
25. Lin CL, Chiang CW, Shaw CK, Chu PH, Chang CJ, Ko YL. Gender differences in the presentation of adult obstructive hypertrophic cardiomyopathy with resting gradient: a study of 122 patients. Jpn Circ J 1999;63: 859–864
26. Maron BJ, Casey SA, Hurrell DG, Aeppli DM. Relation of left ventricular thickness to age and gender in hypertrophic cardiomyopathy. Am J Cardiol 2003;91:1195–1198
27. Olivotto I, Maron MS, Adabag AS, Casey SA, Vargiu D, Link MS, Udelson JE, Cecchi F, Maron BJ. Gender-related differences in the clinical presentation and outcome of hypertrophic cardiomyopathy. J Am Coll Cardiol. 2005;46:480–487
28. Ghali JK, Krause-Steinrauf HJ, Adams KF, Khan SS, Rosenberg YD, Yancy CW, Young JB, Goldman S, Peberdy MA, Lindenfeld J. Gender differences in advanced heart failure: insights from the BEST study. J Am Coll Cardiol 2003;42:2128–2134
29. Adams KF Jr, Sueta CA, Gheorghiade M, O'Connor CM, Schwartz TA, Koch GG, Uretsky B, Swedberg K, McKenna W, Soler-Soler J, Califf RM. Gender differences in survival in advanced heart failure. Insights from the FIRST study. Circulation 1999;99:1816–1821

30. McKee PA, Castelli WP, McNamara PM, Kannel WB. Natural history of congestive heart failure: the Framingham Study. N Engl J Med 1971;285:1441–1446
31. Ho KKL, Anderson KM, Kannel WB, Grossman W, Levy D. Survival after the onset of congestive heart failure in Framingham Heart Study subjects. Circulation 1993;88:107–115
32. Adams KF, Dunlap SH, Sueta CA, Clarke SW, Patterson JH, Blauwet MB, Jensen LR, Tomasko L, Koch G. Relation between gender, etiology and survival in patients with symptomatic heart failure. J Am Coll Cardiol 1996;28:1781–1788
33. Biondi-Zoccai GG, Baldi A, Biasucci LM, Abbate A. Female gender, myocardial remodeling and cardiac failure: are women protected from increased myocardiocyte apoptosis? Ital Heart J 2004;5:498–504
34. Guerra S, Leri A, Wang X, Finato N, Di Loreto C, Beltrami CA, Kajstura J, Anversa P. Myocyte death in the failing human heart is gender dependent. Circ Res 1999;85:856–866
35. Crabbe DL, Dipla K, Ambati S, Zafeiridis A, Gaughan JP, Houser SR, Margulies KB. Gender differences in post-infarction hypertrophy in end-stage failing hearts. J Am Coll Cardiol 2003;41:300–306
36. Meldrum DR, Wang M, Tsai BM, Kher A, Pitcher JM, Brown JW, Meldrum KK. Intracellular signaling mechanisms of sex hormones in acute myocardial inflammation and injury. Front Biosci 2005;10:1835–1867
37. Bae S, Zhang L. Gender differences in cardioprotection against ischemia/reperfusion injury in adult rat hearts: focus on Akt and protein kinase C signaling. J Pharmacol Exp Ther 2005;315:1125–1135
38. Kuhar P, Lunder M, Drevensek G. The role of gender and sex hormones in ischemic-reperfusion injury in isolated rat hearts. Eur J Pharmacol. 2007 Feb 1
39. Griffin M, Lee HW, Zhao L, Eghbali-Webb M. Gender-related differences in proliferative response of cardiac fibroblasts to hypoxia: effects of estrogen. Mol Cell Biochem 2000;215:21–30
40. Brower GL, Chancey AL, Thanigaraj S, Matsubara BB, Janicki JS. Cause-and-effect relationship between myocardial mast cell number and matrix metalloproteinase activity. Am J Physiol Heart Circ Physiol 2002;283:H518–H525
41. Stewart JA Jr, Wei CC, Brower GL, Rynders PE, Hankes GH, Dillon AR, Lucchesi PA, Janicki JS, Dell'Italia LJ. Cardiac mast cell- and chymase-mediated matrix metalloproteinase activity and left ventricular remodeling in mitral regurgitation in the dog. J Mol Cell Cardiol 2003;35:311–319
42. Chancey AL, Brower GL, Janicki JS. Cardiac mast cell-mediated activation of gelatinase and alteration of ventricular diastolic function. Am J Physiol Heart Circ Physiol 2002;282:H2152–H2158
43. Chancey AL, Gardner JD, Murray DB, Brower GL, Janicki JS. Modulation of cardiac mast cell-mediated extracellular matrix degradation by estrogen. Am J Physiol Heart Circ Physiol 2005;289:H316–H321
44. Dash R, Frank KF, Carr AN, Moravec CS, Kranias EG. Gender influences on sarcoplasmic reticulum Ca2+-handling in failing human myocardium. J Mol Cell Cardiol 2001;33:1345–1353
45. Haghighi K, Schmidt AG, Hoit BD, Brittsan AG, Yatani A, Lester JW, Zhai J, Kimura Y, Dorn GW 2nd, MacLennan DH, Kranias EG. Superinhibition of sarcoplasmic reticulum function by phospholamban induces cardiac contractile failure. J Biol Chem 2001;276:24145–24152
46. Regitz-Zagrosek V, Brokat S, Tschope C. Role of gender in heart failure with normal left ventricular ejection fraction. Prog Cardiovasc Dis 2007;49:241–251
47. Redfield MM, Jacobsen SJ, Borlaug BA, Rodeheffer RJ, Kass DA. Age- and gender-related ventricular-vascular stiffening: a community-based study. Circulation 2005;112:2254–2262
48. Masoudi FA, Havranek EP, Smith G, Fish RH, Steiner JF, Ordin DL, Krumholz HM. Gender, age, and heart failure with preserved left ventricular systolic function. J Am Coll Cardiol 2003;41:217–223
49. Pham TV, Rosen MR. Sex, hormones, and repolarization. Cardiovasc Res 2002;53:740–751
50. Kelley GP, Stellingworth MA, Broyles S, Glancy DL. Electrocardiographic findings in 888 patients > or =90 years of age. Am J Cardiol 2006;98:1512–1514
51. Peters RW, Gold MR. The influence of gender on arrhythmias. Cardiol Rev 2004;12:97–105
52. Larsen JA, Kadish AH. Effects of gender on cardiac arrhythmias. J Cardiovasc Electrophysiol 1998;9:655–664
53. Schulze-Bahr E, Kirchhof P, Eckardt L, Bertrand J, Breithardt G. Gender differences in cardiac arrhythmias. Herz 2005;30:390–400
54. Wolbrette D, Naccarelli G, Curtis A, Lehmann M, Kadish A. Gender differences in arrhythmias. Clin Cardiol 2002;25:49–56
55. Friberg J, Scharling H, Gadsboll N, Jensen GB. Sex-specific increase in the prevalence of atrial fibrillation (The Copenhagen city heart study). Am J Cardiol 2003;92:1419–1423
56. Friberg J, Scharling H, Gadsboll N, Truelsen T, Jensen GB. Copenhagen city heart study. Comparison of the impact of atrial fibrillation on the risk of stroke and cardiovascular death in women versus men (The Copenhagen city heart study). Am J Cardiol 2004;94:889–894
57. Gurevitz OT, Varadachari CJ, Ammash NM, Malouf JF, Rosales AG, Herges RM, Bruce CJ, Somers VK, Hammill SC, Gersh BJ, Friedman PA. The effect of patient sex on recurrence of atrial fibrillation following successful direct current cardioversion. Am Heart J 2006;152:155.e9–13

58. Camm J. Medical management of atrial fibrillation: state of the art. J Cardiovasc Electrophysiol 2006;17 Suppl 2:S2–S6
59. Gomberg-Maitland M, Wenger NK, Feyzi J, Lengyel M, Volgman AS, Petersen P, Frison L, Halperin JL. Anticoagulation in women with non-valvular atrial fibrillation in the stroke prevention using an oral thrombin inhibitor (SPORTIF) trials. Eur Heart J 2006;27:1947–1953
60. Fang MC, Singer DE, Chang Y, Hylek EM, Henault LE, Jensvold NG, Go AS. Gender differences in the risk of ischemic stroke and peripheral embolism in atrial fibrillation: the AnTicoagulation and risk factors in atrial fibrillation (ATRIA) study. Circulation 2005;112:1687–1691
61. Rienstra M, Van Veldhuisen DJ, Hagens VE, Ranchor AV, Veeger NJ, Crijns HJ, Van Gelder IC. RACE investigators. Gender-related differences in rhythm control treatment in persistent atrial fibrillation: data of the rate control versus electrical cardioversion (RACE) study. J Am Coll Cardiol 2005;46:1298–1306
62. Gerstenfeld EP, Callans D, Dixit S, Lin D, Cooper J, Russo AM, Verdino R, Weiner M, Zado E, Marchlinski FE. Characteristics of patients undergoing atrial fibrillation ablation: trends over a seven-year period 1999–2005. J Cardiovasc Electrophysiol 2007;18:23–28
63. Snyder JW, Basta LL, Woolson RF. The relative risk of spontaneous complete atrioventricular block in elderly patients with impaired intra-ventricular conduction. J Electrocardiol 1975;8:95–102
64. Kawasaki R, Machado C, Reinoehl J, Fromm B, Baga JJ, Steinman RT, Lehmann MH. Increased propensity of women to develop torsades de pointes during complete heart block. J Cardiovasc Electrophysiol 1995;6: 1032–1038
65. Nakagawa M, Takahashi N, Nobe S, Ichinose M, Ooie T, Yufu F, Shigematsu S, Hara M, Yonemochi H, Saikawa T. Gender differences in various types of idiopathic ventricular tachycardia. J Cardiovasc Electrophysiol 2002;13:633–638
66. Zareba W, Moss AJ, Locati EH, Lehmann MH, Peterson DR, Hall WJ, Schwartz PJ, Vincent GM, Priori SG, Benhorin J, Towbin JA, Robinson JL, Andrews ML, Napolitano C, Timothy K, Zhang L, Medina A. International long QT syndrome registry. Modulating effects of age and gender on the clinical course of long QT syndrome by genotype. J Am Coll Cardiol 2003;42:103–109
67. Hart RG, Pearce LA, McBride R, Rothbart RM, Asinger RW. Factors associated with ischaemic stroke during aspirin therapy in atrial fibrillation: analysis of 2012 participants in the SPAF I-III clinical trials. The stroke prevention in atrial fibrillation (SPAF) investigators. Stroke 1999;30:1223–1229
68. Aurigemma GP, Silver KH, McLaughlin M, Mauser J, Gaasch WH. Impact of chamber geometry and gender on left ventricular systolic function in patients >60 years of age with aortic stenosis. Am J Cardiol 1994;74: 794–798
69. Carroll JD, Carroll EP, Feldman T, Ward DM, Lang RM, McGaughey D, Karp RB. Sex-associated differences in left ventricular function in aortic stenosis of the elderly. Circulation 1992;86:1099–1107
70. Pedram A, Razandi M, Aitkenhead M, Levin ER. Estrogen inhibits cardiomyocyte hypertrophy in vitro. Antagonism of calcineurin-related hypertrophy through induction of MCIP1. J Biol Chem 2005;280:26339–26348
71. Jazbutyte V, Hu K, Kruchten P, Bey E, Maier SK, Fritzemeier KH, Prelle K, Hegele-Hartung C, Hartmann RW, Neyses L, Ertl G, Pelzer T. Aging reduces the efficacy of estrogen substitution to attenuate cardiac hypertrophy in female spontaneously hypertensive rats. Hypertension 2006;48:579–586
72. Babiker FA, Lips D, Meyer R, Delvaux E, Zandberg P, Janssen B, van Eys G, Grohe C, Doevendans PA. Estrogen receptor beta protects the murine heart against left ventricular hypertrophy. Arterioscler Thromb Vasc Biol 2006;26:1524–1530
73. Marsh JD, Lehmann MH, Ritchie RH, Gwathmey JK, Green GE, Schiebinger RJ. Androgen receptors mediate hypertrophy in cardiac myocytes. Circulation 1998;98:256–261
74. Nahrendorf M, Frantz S, Hu K, von zur Muhlen C, Tomaszewski M, Scheuermann H, Kaiser R, Jazbutyte V, Beer S, Bauer W, Neubauer S, Ertl G, Allolio B, Callies F. Effect of testosterone on post-myocardial infarction remodeling and function. Cardiovasc Res 2003;57:370–378
75. Li Y, Kishimoto I, Saito Y, Harada M, Kuwahara K, Izumi T, Hamanaka I, Takahashi N, Kawakami R, Tanimoto K, Nakagawa Y, Nakanishi M, Adachi Y, Garbers DL, Fukamizu A, Nakao K. Androgen contributes to gender-related cardiac hypertrophy and fibrosis in mice lacking the gene encoding guanylyl cyclase-A. Endocrinology 2004;145:951–958
76. Ikeda Y, Aihara K, Sato T, Akaike M, Yoshizumi M, Suzaki Y, Izawa Y, Fujimura M, Hashizume S, Kato M, Yagi S, Tamaki T, Kawano H, Matsumoto T, Azuma H, Kato S, Matsumoto T. Androgen receptor gene knockout male mice exhibit impaired cardiac growth and exacerbation of angiotensin II-induced cardiac fibrosis. J Biol Chem 2005;280:29661–29666
77. Barud W, Makaruk B, Myslinski W, Palusinski R, Hanzlik J. Hypertension, and not sex hormones or insulin resistance affects left ventricular mass in aging men. Ann Univ Mariae Curie Sklodowska [Med] 2004;59: 232–236
78. Liao Y, Cooper RS, Mensah GA, McGee DL. Left ventricular hypertrophy has a greater impact on survival in women than in men. Circulation 1995;92:805–810

79. Peter I, Shearman AM, Vasan RS, Zucker DR, Schmid CH, Demissie S, Cupples LA, Kuvin JT, Karas RH, Mendelsohn ME, Housman DE, Benjamin EJ. Association of estrogen receptor beta gene polymorphisms with left ventricular mass and wall thickness in women. Am J Hypertens 2005;18:1388–1395
80. Leibowitz D, Dresner-Pollak R, Dvir S, Rokach A, Reznik L, Pollak A. Association of an estrogen receptor-alpha gene polymorphism with left ventricular mass. Blood Press 2006;15:45–50
81. Figtree GA, Kindmark A, Lind L, Grundberg E, Speller B, Robinson BG, Channon KM, Watkins H. Novel estrogen receptor alpha promoter polymorphism increases ventricular hypertrophic response to hypertension. J Steroid Biochem Mol Biol 2007;103:110–118
82. Berul CI, Christe ME, Aronovitz MJ, Maguire CT, Seidman CE, Seidman JG, Mendelsohn ME. Familial hypertrophic cardiomyopathy mice display gender differences in electrophysiological abnormalities. J Interv Card Electrophysiol 1998;2:7–14
83. Olsson MC, Palmer BM, Leinwand LA, Moore RL. Gender and aging in a transgenic mouse model of hypertrophic cardiomyopathy. Am J Physiol Heart Circ Physiol 2001;280:H1136–H1144
84. Maass AH, Ikeda K, Oberdorf-Maass S, Maier SK, Leinwand LA. Hypertrophy, fibrosis, and sudden cardiac death in response to pathological stimuli in mice with mutations in cardiac troponin T. Circulation 2004;110:2102–2109
85. Stefanelli CB, Rosenthal A, Borisov AB, Ensing GJ, Russell MW. Novel troponin T mutation in familial dilated cardiomyopathy with gender-dependant severity. Mol Genet Metab 2004;83:188–196
86. Laurent S, Boutouyrie P, Benetos A. Pathophysiology of hypertension in the elderly. Am J Geriatr Cardiol 2002;11:34–39
87. Breithaupt-Grogler K, Belz GG. Epidemiology of the arterial stiffness. Pathol Biol (Paris) 1999;47:604–613
88. Ahimastos AA, Formosa M, Dart AM, Kingwell BA. Gender differences in large artery stiffness pre- and post puberty. J Clin Endocrinol Metab 2003;88:5375–5380
89. Mullick AE, Walsh BA, Reiser KM, Rutledge JC. Chronic estradiol treatment attenuates stiffening, glycoxidation, and permeability in rat carotid arteries. Am J Physiol Heart Circ Physiol 2001;281:H2204–H2210
90. Dubey RK, Oparil S, Imthurn B, Jackson EK. Sex hormones and hypertension. Cardiovasc Res 2002;53: 688–708
91. Khalil RA. Sex hormones as potential modulators of vascular function in hypertension. Hypertension 2005;46:249–254
92. Peter I, Shearman AM, Zucker DR, Schmid CH, Demissie S, Cupples LA, Larson MG, Vasan RS, D'agostino RB, Karas RH, Mendelsohn ME, Housman DE, Levy D. Variation in estrogen-related genes and cross-sectional and longitudinal blood pressure in the Framingham Heart Study. J Hypertens 2005;23:2193–2200
93. Fernandez-Fernandez JM, Tomas M, Vazquez E, Orio P, Latorre R, Senti M, Marrugat J, Valverde MA. Gain-of-function mutation in the KCNMB1 potassium channel subunit is associated with low prevalence of diastolic hypertension. J Clin Invest 2004;113:1032–1039
94. Senti M, Fernandez-Fernandez JM, Tomas M, Vazquez E, Elosua R, Marrugat J, Valverde MA. Protective effect of the KCNMB1 E65K genetic polymorphism against diastolic hypertension in aging women and its relevance to cardiovascular risk. Circ Res 2005;97:1360–1365
95. Shaw LJ, Bairey Merz CN, Pepine CJ, Reis SE, Bittner V, Kelsey SF, Olson M, Johnson BD, Mankad S, Sharaf BL, Rogers WJ, Wessel TR, Arant CB, Pohost GM, Lerman A, Quyyumi AA, Sopko G. WISE investigators. Insights from the NHLBI-Sponsored Women's Ischemia Syndrome Evaluation (WISE) study: Part I: gender differences in traditional and novel risk factors, symptom evaluation, and gender-optimized diagnostic strategies. J Am Coll Cardiol 2006;47:S4–S20
96. Bairey Merz CN, Shaw LJ, Reis SE, Bittner V, Kelsey SF, Olson M, Johnson BD, Pepine CJ, Mankad S, Sharaf BL, Rogers WJ, Pohost GM, Lerman A, Quyyumi AA, Sopko G. WISE investigators. Insights from the NHLBI-Sponsored Women's Ischemia Syndrome Evaluation (WISE) study: Part II: gender differences in presentation, diagnosis, and outcome with regard to gender-based pathophysiology of atherosclerosis and macrovascular and microvascular coronary disease. J Am Coll Cardiol 2006;47:S21–S29
97. Buchthal SD, den Hollander JA, Merz CN, Rogers WJ, Pepine CJ, Reichek N, Sharaf BL, Reis S, Kelsey SF, Pohost GM. Abnormal myocardial phosphorus-31 nuclear magnetic resonance spectroscopy in women with chest pain but normal coronary angiograms. N Engl J Med 2000;342:829–835
98. Pepine CJ, Kerensky RA, Lambert CR, Smith KM, von Mering GO, Sopko G, Bairey Merz CN. Some thoughts on the vasculopathy of women with ischemic heart disease. J Am Coll Cardiol 2006;47:S30–S35
99. Wong TY, Klein R, Sharrett AR, Duncan BB, Couper DJ, Tielsch JM, Klein BE, Hubbard LD. Retinal arteriolar narrowing and risk of coronary heart disease in men and women the Atherosclerosis risk in communities study. JAMA 2002;287:1153–1159
100. Wessel TR, Arant CB, McGorray SP, Sharaf BL, Reis SE, Kerensky RA, von Mering GO, Smith KM, Pauly DF, Handberg EM, Mankad S, Olson MB, Johnson BD, Merz CN, Sopko G, Pepine CJ. NHLBI Women's Ischemia Syndrome Evaluation (WISE). Coronary microvascular reactivity is only partially predicted by atherosclerosis

risk factors or coronary artery disease in women evaluated for suspected ischemia: results from the NHLBI Women's Ischemia Syndrome Evaluation (WISE). Clin Cardiol 2007;30:69–74
101. Wiviott SD, Cannon CP, Morrow DA, Murphy SA, Gibson CM, McCabe CH, Sabatine MS, Rifai N, Giugliano RP, DiBattiste PM, Demopoulos LA, Antman EM, Braunwald E. Differential expression of cardiac biomarkers by gender in patients with unstable angina/non-ST-elevation myocardial infarction: a TACTICS-TIMI 18 (Treat angina with aggrastat and determine cost of therapy with an invasive or conservative strategy-thrombolysis in myocardial infarction 18) substudy. Circulation 2004;109:580–586
102. Rosano GM, Vitale C, Lello S. Postmenopausal hormone therapy: lessons from observational and randomized studies. Endocrine 2004;24:251–254
103. Phillips GB. Is atherosclerotic cardiovascular disease an endocrinological disorder? The estrogen-androgen paradox. J Clin Endocrinol Metab 2005;90:2708–2711
104. Wu FC, von Eckardstein A. Androgens and coronary artery disease. Endocr Rev 2003;24:183–217
105. Silvestri A, Gambacciani M, Vitale C, Monteleone P, Ciaponi M, Fini M, Genazzani AR, Mercuro G, Rosano GM. Different effect of hormone replacement therapy, DHEAS and tibolone on endothelial function in postmenopausal women with increased cardiovascular risk. Maturitas 2005;50:305–311
106. Murase Y, Yamada Y, Hirashiki A, Ichihara S, Kanda H, Watarai M, Takatsu F, Murohara T, Yokota M. Genetic risk and gene-environment interaction in coronary artery spasm in Japanese men and women. Eur Heart J 2004;25:970–977
107. Vaccarino V, Krumholz HM, Berkman LF, Horwitz RI. Sex differences in mortality after myocardial infarction: is there evidence for an increased risk for women? Circulation 1995;91:1861–1871
108. Kudenchuk PJ, Maynard C, Martin JS, Wirkus M, Weaver WD. Comparison of presentation, treatment, and outcome of acute myocardial infarction in men versus women (the myocardial infarction triage and intervention registry). Am J Cardiol 1996;78:9–14
109. Milcent C, Dormont B, Durand-Zaleski I, Steg PG. Gender differences in hospital mortality and use of percutaneous coronary intervention in acute myocardial infarction: microsimulation analysis of the 1999 nationwide French hospitals database. Circulation 2007;115:833–839
110. Rathore SS, Wang Y, Radford MJ, Ordin DL, Krumholz HM. Sex differences in cardiac catheterization after acute myocardial infarction: the role of procedure appropriateness. Ann Intern Med. 2002;137:487–493
111. Anderson RD, Pepine CJ. Gender differences in the treatment for acute myocardial infarction: bias or biology? Circulation 2007;115:823–826
112. Montague CR, Hunter MG, Gavrilin MA, Phillips GS, Goldschmidt-Clermont PJ, Marsh CB. Activation of estrogen receptor-alpha reduces aortic smooth muscle differentiation. Circ Res 2006;99:477–484
113. Ranki HJ, Budas GR, Crawford RM, Jovanovic A. Gender-specific difference in cardiac ATP-sensitive K(+) channels. J Am Coll Cardiol 2001;38:906–915
114. Wang C, Chiari PC, Weihrauch D, Krolikowski JG, Warltier DC, Kersten JR, Pratt PF Jr, Pagel PS. Gender-specificity of delayed preconditioning by isoflurane in rabbits: potential role of endothelial nitric oxide synthase. Anesth Analg 2006;103:274–280
115. McCully JD, Toyoda Y, Wakiyama H, Rousou AJ, Parker RA, Levitsky S. Age- and gender-related differences in ischemia/reperfusion injury and cardioprotection: effects of diazoxide. Ann Thorac Surg 2006;82:117–123
116. Sammut IA, Jayakumar J, Latif N, Rothery S, Severs NJ, Smolenski RT, Bates TE, Yacoub MH. Heat stress contributes to the enhancement of cardiac mitochondrial complex activity. Am J Pathol 200;158:1821–1831
117. McCully JD, Rousou AJ, Parker RA, Levitsky S. Age- and gender-related differences in mitochondrial oxygen consumption and calcium with cardioplegia and diazoxide. Ann Thorac Surg 2007;83:1102–1109
118. Desrois M, Sidell RJ, Gauguier D, Davey CL, Radda GK, Clarke K. Gender differences in hypertrophy, insulin resistance and ischemic injury in the aging type 2 diabetic rat heart. J Mol Cell Cardiol 2004;37:547–555
119. Alpert JS, Thygesen K, Antman E, Bassand JP. Myocardial infarction redefined—a consensus document of the Joint European Society of Cardiology/American College of Cardiology Committee for the redefinition of myocardial infarction. J Am Coll Cardiol 2000;36:959–969
120. Antman EM, Tanasijevic MJ, Thompson B, Schactman M, McCabe CH, Cannon CP, Fischer GA, Fung AY, Thompson C, Wybenga D. Cardiac-specific troponin I levels to predict the risk of mortality in patients with acute coronary syndromes. N Engl J Med 1996;335:1342–1349
121. Ohman EM, Armstrong PW, Christenson RH, Granger CB, Katus HA, Hamm CW, O'Hanesian MA, Wagner GS, Kleiman NS, Harrell FE Jr, Califf RM, Topol EJ. GUSTO IIA investigators. Cardiac troponin T levels for risk stratification in acute myocardial ischemia. N Engl J Med 1996;335:1333–1341
122. Galvani M, Ottani F, Ferrini D, Ladenson JH, Destro A, Baccos D, Rusticali F, Jaffe AS. Prognostic influence of elevated values of cardiac troponin I in patients with unstable angina. Circulation 1997;95:2053–2059
123. Nielsen KM, Faergeman O, Larsen ML, Foldspang A. Danish singles have a twofold risk of acute coronary syndrome: data from a cohort of 138 290 persons. J Epidemiol Community Health 2006;60:721–728

124. Pearson TA, Mensah GA, Alexander RW, Anderson JL, Cannon RO 3rd, Criqui M, Fadl YY, Fortmann SP, Hong Y, Myers GL, Rifai N, Smith SC Jr, Taubert K, Tracy RP, Vinicor F. Centers for Disease Control and Prevention; American Heart Association. Markers of inflammation and cardiovascular disease: application to clinical and public health practice: a statement for healthcare professionals from the Centers for Disease Control and Prevention and the American Heart Association. Circulation 2003;107:499–511
125. Rifai N, Warnick GR. Quality specifications and the assessment of the biochemical risk of atherosclerosis. Clin Chem Acta 2004;346:55–64
126. Khera A, McGuire DK, Murphy SA, Stanek HG, Das SR, Vongpatanasin W, Wians FH Jr, Grundy SM, de Lemos JA. Race and gender differences in C-reactive protein levels. J Am Coll Cardiol 2005;46:464–469
127. Garcia-Moll X, Zouridakis E, Cole D, Kaski JC. C-reactive protein in patients with chronic stable angina: differences in baseline serum concentration between women and men. Eur Heart J 2000;21:1598–1606
128. Sattar N, Murray HM, McConnachie A, Blauw GJ, Bollen EL, Buckley BM, Cobbe SM, Ford I, Gaw A, Hyland M, Jukema JW, Kamper AM, Macfarlane PW, Murphy MB, Packard CJ, Perry IJ, Stott DJ, Sweeney BJ, Twomey C, Westendorp RG, Shepherd J. PROSPER study group. C-reactive protein and prediction of coronary heart disease and global vascular events in the Prospective study of pravastatin in the elderly at risk (PROSPER). Circulation 2007;115:981–989
129. Blake GJ, Dada N, Fox JC, Manson JE, Ridker PM. A prospective evaluation of lipoprotein-associated phospholipase A(2) levels and the risk of future cardiovascular events in women. J Am Coll Cardiol 2001;38: 1302–1306
130. Khaw KT, Wareham N, Bingham S, Luben R, Welch A, Day N. Association of hemoglobin A1c with cardiovascular disease and mortality in adults: the European prospective investigation into cancer in Norfolk. Ann Intern Med 2004;141:413–420
131. Ellsworth DL, Bielak LF, Turner ST, Sheedy PF 2nd, Boerwinkle E, Peyser PA. Gender- and age-dependent relationships between the E-selectin S128R polymorphism and coronary artery calcification. J Mol Med 2001;79:390–398
132. Naraoka H, Ito K, Suzuki M, Naito K, Tojo H. Analysis of gender difference of cardiac risk biomarkers using hGH-transgenic mice. Exp Anim 2006;55:1–9
133. Sanz A, Hiona A, Kujoth GC, Seo AY, Hofer T, Kouwenhoven E, Kalani R, Prolla TA, Barja G, Leeuwenburgh C. Evaluation of sex differences on mitochondrial bioenergetics and apoptosis in mice. Exp Gerontol 2007;42:173–182
134. Norata GD, Ongari M, Garlaschelli K, Raselli S, Grigore L, Catapano AL. Plasma resistin levels correlate with determinants of the metabolic syndrome. Eur J Endocrinol 2007;156:279–284
135. Nilsson PM, Engstrom G, Hedblad B, Frystyk J, Persson MM, Berglund G, Flyvbjerg A. Plasma adiponectin levels in relation to carotid intima media thickness and markers of insulin resistance. Arterioscler Thromb Vasc Biol 2006;26:2758–2762
136. Yan L, Ge H, Li H, Lieber SC, Natividad F, Resuello RR, Kim SJ, Akeju S, Sun A, Loo K, Peppas AP, Rossi F, Lewandowski ED, Thomas AP, Vatner SF, Vatner DE. Gender-specific proteomic alterations in glycolytic and mitochondrial pathways in aging monkey hearts. J Mol Cell Cardiol 2004;37:921–929
137. Lai CQ, Demissie S, Cupples LA, Zhu Y, Adiconis X, Parnell LD, Corella D, Ordovas JM. Influence of the APOA5 locus on plasma triglyceride, lipoprotein subclasses, and CVD risk in the Framingham Heart Study. J Lipid Res 2004;45:2096–2105
138. Luo CH, Wang A, Zhu RH, Zhang WX, Mo W, Yu BN, Chen GL, Ou-Yang DS, Duan XH, El-Aty AM, Zhou HH. Gender specific association of CYP2C9*3 with hyperlipidaemia in Chinese. Br J Clin Pharmacol 2005;60:629–631
139. Arias M, Pardo J, Blanco-Arias P, Sobrido MJ, Arias S, Dapena D, Carracedo A, Goldfarb LG, Navarro C. Distinct phenotypic features and gender-specific disease manifestations in a Spanish family with desmin L370P mutation. Neuromuscul Disord 2006;16:498–503
140. Rana BK, Insel PA, Payne SH, Abel K, Beutler E, Ziegler MG, Schork NJ, O'Connor DT. Population-based sample reveals gene-gender interactions in blood pressure in White Americans. Hypertension 2007;49:96–106
141. Yamada Y, Ando F, Shimokata H. Association of gene polymorphisms with blood pressure and the prevalence of hypertension in community-dwelling Japanese individuals. Int J Mol Med 2007;19:675–683
142. Durst R, Jansen A, Erez G, Bravdo R, Butbul E, Ben Avi L, Shpitzen S, Lotan C, Leitersdorf E, Defesche J, Friedlander Y, Meiner V, Miserez AR. The discrete and combined effect of SREBP-2 and SCAP isoforms in the control of plasma lipids among familial hypercholesterolaemia patients. Atherosclerosis 2006;189:443–450
143. Kamide K, Kokubo Y, Yang J, Matayoshi T, Inamoto N, Takiuchi S, Horio T, Miwa Y, Yoshii M, Tomoike H, Tanaka C, Banno M, Okuda T, Kawano Y, Miyata T. Association of genetic polymorphisms of ACADSB and COMT with human hypertension. J Hypertens 2007;25:103–110
144. Chen W, Srinivasan SR, Li S, Boerwinkle E, Berenson GS. Gender-specific influence of NO synthase gene on blood pressure since childhood: the Bogalusa Heart Study. Hypertension 2004;44:668–673

145. Stankovic A, Zivkovic M, Alavantic D. Angiotensin I-converting enzyme gene polymorphism in a Serbian population: a gender-specific association with hypertension. Scand J Clin Lab Invest 2002;62:469–475
146. Wu Y, Tomon M, Sumino K. Methylenetetrahydrofolate reductase gene polymorphism and ischemic stroke: sex difference in Japanese. Kobe J Med Sci 2001;47:255–256
147. Kim Y, Kim JH, Nam YJ, Kong M, Kim YJ, Yu KH, Lee BC, Lee C. Klotho is a genetic risk factor for ischemic stroke caused by cardioembolism in Korean females. Neurosci Lett 2006;407:189–194
148. Kim Y, Lee C. The gene encoding transforming growth factor beta 1 confers risk of ischemic stroke and vascular dementia. Stroke 2006;37:2843–2845
149. Ordovas JM. Lipoprotein lipase genetic variation and gender-specific ischemic cerebrovascular disease risk. Nutr Rev 2000;58:315–318
150. Kajinami K, Brousseau ME, Lamon-Fava S, Ordovas JM, Schaefer EJ. Gender-specific effects of estrogen receptor alpha gene haplotype on high-density lipoprotein cholesterol response to ator-vastatin: interaction with apolipoprotein AI gene polymorphism. Atherosclerosis 2005;178:331–338
151. Kajinami K, Brousseau ME, Ordovas JM, Schaefer EJ. Polymorphisms in the multidrug resistance-1 (MDR1) gene influence the response to atorvastatin treatment in a gender-specific manner. Am J Cardiol 2004;93: 1046–1050
152. Pedro-Botet J, Schaefer EJ, Bakker-Arkema RG, Black DM, Stein EM, Corella D, Ordovas JM. Apolipoprotein E genotype affects plasma lipid response to atorvastatin in a gender specific manner. Atherosclerosis 2001;158:183–193
153. Schwartz GL, Turner ST, Chapman AB, Boerwinkle E. Interacting effects of gender and genotype on blood pressure response to hydrochloro-thiazide. Kidney Int 2002;62:1718–1723
154. Garcia-Garcia AB, Gonzalez C, Real JT, Martin de Llano JJ, Gonzalez-Albert V, Civera M, Chaves FJ, Ascaso JF, Carmena R. Influence of microsomal triglyceride transfer protein promoter polymorphism -493 GT on fasting plasma triglyceride values and interaction with treatment response to atorvastatin in subjects with heterozygous familial hypercholesterolaemia. Pharmacogenet Genomics 2005;15:211–218
155. Hallberg P, Karlsson J, Lind L, Michaelsson K, Kurland L, Kahan T, Malmqvist K, Ohman KP, Nystrom F, Liljedahl U, Syvanen AC, Melhus H. Gender-specific association between preproendothelin-1 genotype and reduction of systolic blood pressure during antihypertensive treatment – results from the swedish irbesartan left ventricular hypertrophy investigation versus atenolol (SILVHIA). Clin Cardiol 2004;27:287–290
156. Johnson JA, Cavallari LH. Cardiovascular pharmacogenomics. Exp Physiol 2005;90:283–289
157. Johnson JA. Drug target pharmacogenomics: an overview. Am J Pharmacogenomics 2001;1:271–281
158. Siest G, Jeannesson E, Berrahmoune H, Maumus S, Marteau JB, Mohr S, Visvikis S. Pharmacogenomics and drug response in cardiovascular disorders. Pharmacogenomics 2004;5:779–802

Chapter 11
Cardiac Dysrhythmias and Channelopathies in Aging

Overview

Increasing interaction between clinical cardiologists/gerontologists, molecular biologists and geneticists has facilitated the detection of a number of gene mutations in patients with life-threatening dysrhythmias, particularly mutations in genes encoding most of the proteins forming the ion channels and transporters. On the other hand, there is significant genetic diversity in the channel genes, with allelic heterogeneity spread over the entire gene, often presenting with more than one mutation. Although, genetic heterogeneity represents a tremendous challenge for mutation identification, the availability of new tools, including high-throughput technologies to map the human genome, together with the availability of large databases of single nucleotide polymorphisms (SNPs) and haplotype markers is facilitating the progressive discovery of new mutations and SNPs.

Defects in ion channels (channelopathies) are increasingly found in a large spectrum of human diseases, and in aging. Mutations in genes encoding ion channel proteins, which disrupt channel function, are the most commonly identified cause of channelopathies. Furthermore, mutations in associated proteins, alterations in the expression of ion channels, or changes in the activity of non-mutated channel genes or associated proteins can also produce acquired channelopathies, as they may occur during therapies that affect cellular function. Similarly, defects in the heart rate and rhythm (dysrhythmias) also increase with aging. Compared to young adults a higher incidence of atrial dysrhythmias, including atrial premature beats, atrial fibrillation (AF), atrioventricular block (AV block), and ST-T changes are seen in the elderly with an otherwise normal heart. On the other hand, paroxysmal supraventricular tachycardia (PSVT), ventricular tachycardia (VT) and ventricular blocks in the aging individual are mainly associated with structural cardiac defects. Furthermore, age-related changes also include increased activity of the sympathetic nervous system, which may be an important pathophysiological component in tachydysrhythmias and premature ventricular contractions. In this chapter, the most common channelopathies and dysrhythmias associated with aging will be discussed.

Introduction

Compared to the young a higher incidence of cardiac dysrhythmias occurs in aged patients, and this is true even for elderly patients who are free from structural heart disease. Nevertheless, the majority of cardiac dysrrhythmias in the elderly occur in association with underlying comorbidities,

J. Marín-García, *Aging and the Heart*,

such as hypertension or coronary artery disease (CAD). In addition, aging is a major determinant of heart rate dynamics, which differ between men and women. Women have a higher heart rate and more complex heart rate dynamic regulating heart rhythm and rate (modulated by the nervous system). However, with increasing age there is a decrease of such complexity, and the gender-related differences in neuronal regulation of the heart rate decreases. The mechanisms underlying the gender differences are unclear, although gender differences in neuronal modulation of heart rate could be due to changes in neuronal innervation, amount of cardiac cells or/and changes in ion channel expression (further discussion on the role of gender is presented in Chapter 10).

Significantly, both inherited, and to a lesser degree acquired cardiac dysrhythmias appear to have a genetic basis. For example, changes in channel protein expression, which play a significant role in the cardiomyocyte action potential (AP) and cellular electrical stability may have a significant role in modifying the individual's pharmacological profile by altering the relative expression and contribution of different drug targets. Currently, screening of a significant number of individuals with dysrhythmias has led to the discovery of numerous mutated genes, in particular those encoding subunits of proteins that constitute the cardiac ion channels. In addition, silent mutations and functional DNA polymorphisms have also been found to play a significant role in increasing the susceptibility for these dysrhythmogenic disorders, together with non-genetic or environmental factors such as gender, aging, and the presence of cardiac structural defects.

Sympathetic Nerve System in Aging

With aging, decreased α- and β-AR-mediated contractility contribute to an overall decline in cardiac performance. While impairment in β-AR signaling is well-established in the aging heart, identification of the components of the α1-AR signaling cascade responsible for the aging-associated deficit in α1-AR contractile function, has just begun. These signaling components include protein kinase C (PKC) and associated anchoring proteins receptors for activated C kinase (RACKs). The reperfusion of an isolated mammalian heart with a calcium-containing solution after a brief calcium-free perfusion produces irreversible cell damage (known as the calcium paradox). There is evidence that activation of the α1-AR pathway confers protection against the lethal injury of the Ca^{2+} paradox largely by the PKC-mediated signaling pathways, and this protection is shared by stimuli involved in calcium pre-conditioning [1]. Using 3 month and 24 month old Wistar rats, age-related changes were analyzed with regards to α1-adrenergic stimulation of both cardiomyocyte Ca^{2+} transient and cardiac PKC activity. In a dose-response curve to phenylephrine, the response of Ca^{2+} transient was maximal at 10^{-7} M. While in the young rat this phenylephrine concentration induced a significant increase in Ca^{2+} transient, the aging rat sustained a significant decrease. Moreover, after phenylephrine treatment, a translocation of PKC toward the particulate fraction was observed in young but not in older rats. These results indicate that the negative effect of α1-adrenergic stimulation on cardiomyocyte Ca^{2+} transient observed in old rats may be related to the absence of α1-adrenergic-induced PKC translocation.

Notwithstanding these findings, the effect of aging on the human sympathetic nervous system remains a controversial issue. Since diverse cardiac pathologies, including essential hypertension, CAD, HF and dysrhythmias increase with age, interest in this subject has significantly increased, and the sympathetic nervous system has been proposed as a potential contributory pathophysiological component [2]. However, in an analysis of the role of the sympathetic nervous system in aging and HF, Kaye and Esler [3] found no additive effect of aging in the activation of the sympathetic nervous system in HF, suggesting that other factors such as CAD and myocardial infarction (MI) may impact the increased incidence of HF with aging.

Electrophysiological Studies in Animal Models of Aging

Cardiac electrophysiological studies using a number of animal models have significantly contributed to our knowledge of the changes occurring with aging. For example, using a canine model, electrophysiological changes have been found in the atria with aging including longer duration of the AP, increased negativity of the plateau and reduced L-type Ca^{2+} currents [4]. These changes may provide the basis for the genesis of dysrhythmias and propensity for AF in the aged. Furthermore, histological changes in the atria of old dogs include an increase in fibrous tissue. This heterogeneous atrial interstitial fibrosis is likely contributory to the aging-related increase in atrial conduction slowing, conduction block, and inducible AF seen in older rats [5].

Similarly, using white New Zealand rabbits, Gottwald et al. [6] have reported a higher variability of the activation pattern, increased dispersion of the epicardial potential duration, prolongation of the AV-conduction time and of the duration of epicardial activation signal in old compared to young animals. Moreover, extensive incorporation of fat cells and connective tissue in the ventricular and AV-node tissues, which may explain the prolonged conduction time, and a marked hypertrophy of the ventricular myocytes were found on histological analysis. These findings may explain the enhanced susceptibility to dysrhythmias occurring with increasing age.

Furthermore, Dhein and Hammerath have also reported reduced transversal velocity and enhanced anisotropy but unchanged longitudinal velocity in aged rabbit hearts [7]. Histologically, diffuse deposition of collagen lateral to the fibers and more pronounced expression of connexin43 (Cx43) at lateral cell borders were detected in the ventricles. In addition, the ventricular intercellular coupling transverse to the fiber axis was reduced in aged hearts. Interestingly, these functional age-dependent changes could be mimicked in young rabbit hearts by the gap junction uncoupler palmitoleic acid in a concentration-dependent manner. Complementary to the above findings were increased dispersion, slowed transverse conduction and increased anisotropy, and enhanced Cx43 immunostaining at the lateral cell borders.

The effect of aging on the electrophysiological properties of the left atrium (LA), and in particular on specific LA sites and in ouabain-induced dysrhythmias in rabbits have been evaluated by Wongcharoen et al. [8]. In comparison to the young, the LA in the aging animals had a higher incidence of delayed afterdepolarization with less negative resting membrane potential and smaller maximum upstroke velocity. Aged left atrium posterior walls (LAPWs) had longer AP duration than aged left atrium appendages, and after ouabain treatment the aged LAPWs had a greater shortening of the AP duration. Taken together, aging appears to increase LA regional heterogeneity and LAPW dysrhythmogenesis likely arising from increased atrial fibrosis.

It is worth noting that the use of animal models has been instrumental in providing insight on the correlation of changes in ion channels affecting protein expression with changes in ventricular activity and dysrhythmias. For example, abnormal expression of the *KCNE2* protein has been reported in two different models of cardiac pathology [9]. In the first model, canine myocardial ischemia secondary to coronary microembolizations, the rapid delayed rectifier current (I_{Kr}) density was increased. While the protein level of the ERG (I_{Kr}) pore-forming α subunit was not affected, the auxiliary subunit KCNE2 protein level was markedly reduced. These findings were consistent with effect of heterologously expressed *KCNE2* (also called MiRP1) on ERG, and suggested that KCNE2 may associate with ERG and suppress its current amplitude. In the second model, aging rat ventricle, both the pacemaker current (I_f) density and the KCNE2 protein level were markedly increased, and no significant changes were found in the α-subunit (HCN2). These findings suggest that in the aging ventricle, KCNE2 association with HCN2 can enhance the pacemaker current amplitude. Taken together, these findings show that the KCNE2 protein is differentially expressed in the ventricles under different pathophysiological conditions, such as myocardial ischemia and aging, and this channel protein can play diverse and critical roles in modulating ventricular electrical activity.

Interestingly, Baba et al. [10] have addressed the question if the increases in AF that occur with aging could be related to changes in the intrinsic function of Na^+ currents in cells of the aged atria. They analyzed the RA and LA Na^+ channel protein Na_v 1.5 of aged and adult dogs by immunochemistry, and found that in cells from aged animals Na^+ currents were similar to those measured in adult atria. However, in the aged animals the Na^+ current (I_{Na}) density of the LA cell currents was significantly larger than the RA cell currents. Furthermore, in the aged atrial cells there was no structural remodeling of the fast cardiac Na^+ channel protein Na_v1.5. Therefore, with age there is no change in I_{Na} density in the aging atria, but there are subtle kinetic differences that contribute to some enhancement of use dependence.

The spontaneous activity of pacemaker cells in the sinoatrial (SA) node controls the heart rate under normal physiological conditions, and with age there is an increased incidence of SA node dysfunction with the highest prevalence in the elderly population. Jones et al. [11] using the guinea pig as animal model have investigated whether aging affected the expression of Ca_v 1.2 channels and whether these changes could affect pacemaker activity, in turn leading to age-related SA node degeneration. The SA node region from the right atrium of guinea pigs between birth and 38 months of age, and immunofluorescence studies indicated that Ca_v 1.2 protein was localized around the outer membrane of atrial cells but was absent from the center of the SA node. The area lacking Ca_v1.2 -labeled protein progressively increased from 2.06+/−0.1 mm^2 at 1 month to 18.72+/−2.2 mm^2 at 38 months. In addition, Ca_v1.2 protein expression within the SA node declined during aging as gauged using western blot analysis, and functional assessment showed an increased sensitivity to the L-type Ca^{2+} blocker nifedipine. This study revealed that Ca_v1.2 channel protein decreased concurrently with reduced spontaneous activity of the SA node with increased age, and provided further evidence of the mechanisms underlying the age-related deterioration of the cardiac pacemaker.

Atrial Dysrhythmias

Sinoatrial Node Dysfunction (SND)

With aging a decrease in the sinus node depolarization rate occurs in rats [12], which may be related to a reduction in the accumulation of mRNA encoding β-adrenergic receptors and muscarinic receptors as found in the sinus node region of senescent rat hearts [13]. Increased sensitivity of the senescent rat sinus node to the negative chronotropic effects of adenosine A_1 receptor stimulation has also been reported that may be mediated by an increased density of adenosine A_1 receptors [14, 15]. On the other hand, in human studies aging is associated with a significant decrease in sinus node size and in the volume of sinus cells and a loss of centrally located P cells [16, 17]. Moreover, in human, alterations in sinoatrial channels expression and structural atrial remodeling may occur with aging in association with sinus node disease (SND) and AF. In the absence of structural cardiac defect, it is not clear why SND is silent in some patients and is accompanied with symptoms in others, although this variability may be related to the degree of atrial remodeling. Kistler et al. have reported subclinical SND associated with extensive alterations in the atrial electrical substrate, in otherwise healthy aging indivicuals [18]. We agree with Lamas et al. that the extensive atrial remodeling occurring in aging provides a mechanism not only for SND but also for other atrial dysrhythmias, mainly AF, which may develop in up to 50% of patients with SND [19]. Furthermore, the development of AF may further exacerbate SND, probably related to the high atrial rates [20]. Fortunately, as pointed out by Haqqani and Kalman in a recent editorial [21], at least a partial reversal of this adverse sinus node remodeling may occur after successful catheter ablation of AF [22], or atrial flutter [23].

The forementioned age-dependent loss of the L-type calcium channel in the SA node reported in the guinea pig model likely contributes to aging-associated SND [11]. L-type currents are conducted thru $Ca_v1.2$ channels, integrated by a pore-forming α_1-subunit in association with β- and α2δ-subunits [24]. With aging, $Ca_v1.2$ protein decreased together with a reduction in the spontaneous activity of the SA node, and this decrease in turn increased its susceptibility to L-type calcium channel blockers. Previously, these investigators reported that the progressive loss of connexin-43 expression with aging (in the central and peripheral zones of SA node) resulted in suppressed electrical conductivity in the aged guinea pig node [25]. Therefore, the loss of $Ca_v1.2$ channels together with depletion of Cx43 protein not only will decrease electrical conductivity but also will increase the chances for SA node dysfunction with age as well as the prevalence of dysrhythmias. On the other hand, and in agreement with Haqqani and Kalman [21], it is rather surprising that no changes in collagen content or signs of fibrosis associated with aging were found in this animal SND model. Interestingly, Alings et al. [26] in their comparative study of the age-related SA node structural changes in human and cats have noted that although the relative volume of collagen in human SA node increases from childhood to adulthood, no further increases occur after adulthood. Other investigators have shown that in humans, aging is associated with increasing variability in atrial conduction, which histological analysis revealed to be associated with increasing collagen [27]. Based on these data one can infer that further studies in humans are necessary to settle this issue.

In contrast to the study of Jones et al. [11] that did not evaluate downregulation of the L-type calcium channel in others atrial areas than SA node, downregulation of L-type calcium channel in a canine model of aging atrial cells using cell patch clamp recording techniques has been shown by Dun et al. [28] Under the premise that the ionic basis for the differences in AP contours between normal adult and aged right atrial fibers are unknown, these investigators measured L-type Ca^{2+} currents (I_{CaL}) with either Ca^{2+} or Ba^{2+} (3 mM), and both the transient outward (I_{to}) and sustained potassium currents (I_{sus}) in cells dispersed in normal adult dogs (2–5 years of age) and older dogs (>8 years of age). A significant reduction in peak I_{CaL} (47%) and I_{BaL} (43%) was noted in aged cells; however, these differences in I_{BaL} disappear with maximal β-adrenergic stimulation (isoproterenol, 1 microM). On the other hand, composite I_{to} and I_{sus} densities were significantly increased in the aged versus adult cell group. The decay of I_{to} during a maintained depolarization was slowed in aged cells and I_{to} steady-state inactivation curve was shifted positively in aged cells. Therefore, ionic currents differ in aged versus adult right atrial cells, such that a reduced Ca^{2+} current and augmented outward currents could contribute significantly to the altered AP contour of the aged right atrial cell. Furthermore, adrenergic stimulation appears to restore Ba^{2+} currents in aged cells. Taken together increased TEA sensitive current plays a role in changes of I_{sus} in aged right atrial cells, and the AP contours vary considerably between normal adult and aged right atrial fibers.

Atrioventricular Nodal Reentrant Tachycardia (AVNRT)

AVNRT is the most common regular supraventricular tachycardia in the elderly patients. In patients older than 65 years, AVNRT may lead to severe, sometimes life-threatening symptoms, despite the fact that the tachycardia is not as fast as in younger patients. Radiofrequency (RF) catheter ablation can be performed effectively and safely and should be offered to these patients as first-choice therapy.

In 1998, Kalusche et al. [29] reported in a retrospective analysis of 404 patients who underwent catheter ablation therapy for AVNRT, 85 of which were 65 years old or older. Compared with the younger subgroup, the elderly patients (mean age 70.4 years) more often had organic heart disease (e.g., CAD with or without MI, syncope or presyncope with AVNRT, more hospitalizations and emergency treatments because of their symptoms), although the cycle length of the induced AVNRT was significantly shorter in the younger patient group. Slow pathway ablation was performed in 94% of the young and 82% of the elderly. In 17.5% of the elderly patients versus 6.5% of the young the fast pathway approach was chosen as the first therapy or tried after an unsuccessful approach to the slow pathway. Interestingly, the overall success rate was similar in the young (96.8%) and in the elderly (95.3%) and the recurrence rate was similar in both groups. Therefore, RF catheter ablation is effective and safe and should be offered to these patients as their first-choice therapy.

Recently, Haghjoo et al. [30] also examined the electrophysiological characteristics and results of RF catheter ablation in elderly patients with AVNRT. They compared the electrophysiological characteristics, efficacy, and risks of the RF catheter ablation of the slow pathway in elderly versus young patients with AVNRT. Patients were categorized into two groups; one consisted of patients younger than 65 years ($n = 156$), and another of patients 65 years or older ($n = 112$). As in the previously discussed report by Kalusche et al. [29] elderly patients compared with the younger subgroup, more often had structural heart disease, but there were no statistically significant differences in sex and symptoms during tachycardia. AVNRT cycle length was significantly longer in the older than in the younger group. Among the conduction intervals of tachycardia, only atrio-His (A–H) interval was significantly longer in the older individuals. The ablation fluoroscopy time, RF pulse duration, target temperature, applied energy, and number of RF applications were comparable in both groups. Furthermore, the risk of atrioventricular (AV) block, pericardial effusion, and vascular thrombosis were similar in both groups. They concluded that in the elderly patients, slow pathway ablation is as effective and safe as in younger patients. Therefore, when considering different treatment options, an increased risk of complications or lower efficacy should not be a factor in determining the best therapeutic approach in elderly patients. Also, Meiltz and Zimmermann [31] have examined the efficacy and safety of RF ablation in patients with AVNRT $\geq$ 65 years of age and found that RF ablation of AVNRT was highly effective and safe despite a higher prevalence of structural heart disease and longer A-H intervals at baseline.

Atrial Fibrillation

AF is the most common dysrhythmia seen in the elderly. While AF can develop in the absence of apparent structural changes, it more commonly involves extensive remodeling of the cardiomyocyte electrical properties, extracellular matrix (ECM) and fibrosis, in part mediated by activation of the renin-angiotensin-aldosterone system (RAAS) and induction of proinflammatory pathways. In the aging heart AF can lead to acute HF, without clinically apparent cardiac disease. In the Rotterdam study [32], the prevalence at baseline was assessed in 6,808 participants. Incidence of AF was investigated during a mean follow-up period of 6.9 years in 6,432 persons. The overall prevalence was 5.5%, rising from 0.7% in the age group 55–59 years and to 17.8% in those aged 85 years and above. Also in this prospective study of a European population, the prevalence and incidence were higher in men than in women and the high lifetime risk to develop AF was similar to North American epidemiological data. Recently, similar prevalence has been also reported by Aronow [33] in individuals older than 65 years of age (16% in men and in 13% in women). We agree with this investigator that in the elderly, AF with rapid ventricular rate may precipitate the development of tachycardia-related cardiomyopathy, and that immediate direct-current (DC) cardioversion should be performed in patients with AF and acute MI, AF and chest pain due to myocardial ischemia, hypotension, severe HF, or syncope [34]. In symptomatic life-threatening AF refractory to other drugs, amiodarone can be administrated, as well as anticoagulants since thrombus formation occurred often in elderly individuals. On the other hand, non-drug therapies should be employed in patients with symptomatic AF in whom rapid ventricular rate cannot be slowed by drugs. Finally, paroxysmal AF associated with the tachycardia-bradycardia syndrome should be treated with a permanent pacemaker in combination with drugs. With aging, the atrial myocardium undergoes extensive electrical and structural remodeling both of which may play important roles in the initiation and/or perpetuation of atrial tachydysrhythmias [35]. As noted by Anyukhovsky et al. [4] structurally, the most important change in aged atrial bundles is an enhancement of the fibrous tissue that is interspersed between myocytes. In fact, fibrosis is ubiquitous in the atria of the aging heart and is characterized by excessive accumulation of fibrillar collagen in the extracellular space. Recently, Spach et al. [36] have shown that even in the absence of intrinsic or dynamic electrical heterogeneity, increased microfibrosis can cause a propagation failure in the atria because of a source/sink mismatch and that under the appropriate conditions it can give rise to dysrhythmogenic conduction responses. In experiments conducted on small pieces of old isolated human atrial tissue, Spach et al. observed that an appropriately timed premature stimulus given at the same site where previous stimulation initiated a normal impulse propagation gave rise to extracellular electrograms that were indicative of either: (1) longitudinal propagation in the retrograde direction lateral to the site of stimulus or (2) reentrant activation. To understand the underlying mechanisms, the investigators first experimentally estimated in their preparation the amount of collagenous septa and then used this information to construct a detailed two-dimensional (2D) mathematical model of the atrial syncytium, which was based on a strategy followed earlier for ventricular cells [37]. As pointed out in an editorial comment by Pandit and Jalife [38], by mimicking the experimental stimulus protocol at different sites within the 2D sheet, Spach et al. [36] were able to reproduce/simulate the dysrhythmogenic conduction patterns as recorded in the isolated human atrial tissue. Research into the underlying mechanism suggested that the inward sodium (but not calcium) current was the major determinant of the pattern of propagation and that its interaction with the variable microstructural load (or sink) due to the fibrosis resulted in either microreentry or delayed retrograde conduction lateral to the site of stimulus. These results provide further support to the hypothesis that structural remodeling is a key determinant and by itself can initiate AF, without the need for preexisting repolarization gradients.

AV Conduction in Aging

Aging is frequently associated with progressive AV conduction system disorders affecting the SA node, AV node, and/or the His bundle branch-Purkinje system. Bhat et al. [39] in a study of 1,500 patients over 65 years of age found that AV conduction and intraventricular conduction defects were identified in 30% of patients. As a result, the elderly are prone to develop symptomatic bradydysrhythmias that may require pacemaker implantation. In several animal models, aging is associated with slowing of AV conduction and a blunted response to isoproterenol [6, 40]. This finding may be mediated, at least in part, by a decrease in β-adrenergic receptor density [41]. On the other hand, aging in human in frequently associated with prolonged AV conduction that may be independent of β-adrenergic and parasympathetic effects [42]. With aging the incidence of prolonged PR intervals and first-degree AV block increases in human [43], and this seems to be related to AV node or proximal portion of the His bundle conduction delay [44].

In their study on pacing therapy in the elderly Kusumoto et al. [45] reported that in addition to extracellular changes, apoptosis may play a significant role in the development of AV block with aging since apoptosis appears to be one of the physiologic processes responsible for the normal reduction in AV node size observed from fetus to adulthood. Therefore, inappropriate apoptosis during later adulthood may be a factor in the development of AV block [46]. In cases of isolated AV block there is an increase in fine collagen fibers in and around the AV node and His-Purkinje system [47], and the development of collagen septa leads to cell-to-cell electrical uncoupling and a decrease in conduction velocity particularly in cells that are arranged “side-to-side” [27]. Secondary causes of AV block, such as CAD, annular calcification from valvular disease, infiltrative diseases (amyloidosis, hemochromatosis), and inflammatory diseases (pericarditis, myocarditis, rheumatic heart disease, collagen vascular disease) are more common in the elderly [45].

Initially described as an acquired complete AV block with right (RBBB) or left bundle branch block (LBBB) and widening QRS complexes, hereditary Lenègre/Lev disease has been also associated with mutations in the SCN5A gene (see below). This disease involves fibrosis of the bundle branches of unknown cause and may present with two distinct histological patterns. In Lev's disease, there is progressive loss of myocytes in the proximal bundles, which can result in loss of electrical continuity between the His bundle and the bundle branches [48]. This is often accompanied by calcification of the mitral and aortic valvular annulus, and systemic hypertension appears to accelerate the pathologic process. On the other hand, Lenègre's disease exhibits a more diffuse degenerative process that involves the more distal portions of the bundle branches [49]. Similar to patients with other types of AV conduction block, affected individuals with Lenègre/Lev disease present with syncope, dizziness, and fatigue and often required pacemaker implantation.

In 2002 the guidelines for permanent pacemaker implantation were updated by the ACC/AHA/NASPE (as discussed shortly) and outlined current indications as indicated in the accompanying Tables 11.1–11.3. Nevertheless, since the majority of the recommendations are based on randomized studies and did not specifically address implantation indications in the elderly, they should be used only as a general guide [50].

LQT and Sudden Death

It has been suggested that prolonged QT interval predicts cardiac and all-cause mortality in the elderly. In the Rotterdam study de Bruyne et al. [51] have compared the prognostic value of the QT interval among men and women aged 55 years or older using different formulas to correct for heart rate. They found that in women, the increased risk associated with prolonged QT for cardiac death was more pronounced than in men, and risk estimates did not change after adjustment for potential confounders, including history of MI, hypertension and diabetes mellitus. Therefore, a prolonged heart rate corrected QT (QTc) interval is an independent predictor for cardiac and all-cause mortality in older men and women.

Straus et al. [52] have evaluated the association of prolonged QTc interval and risk of sudden cardiac death in a population of men and women 55 years of age and older. They found that an abnormally prolonged QTc interval (>450 m*s* in men, >470 m*s* in women) was associated with a three-fold increased risk of sudden cardiac death, after adjustment for age, gender, body mass index, hypertension, cholesterol/high-density lipoprotein ratio, diabetes mellitus, MI, HF, and heart rate. In patients with an age below the median of 68 years, the corresponding relative risk was 8.0. Therefore, abnormal QTc prolongation on the electrocardiogram should be viewed as an independent risk factor for sudden cardiac death. On the other hand, an evaluation of the effect of age and gender on QT dispersion has shown that elderly males have significantly greater QT and QTc dispersion than elderly females. In addition, no other gender differences were noted for QT or QTc dispersion in younger individuals. These findings suggest that when evaluating a population of healthy subjects, regardless of age, gender has an impact on QT dispersion but no significant interaction with QTc dispersion. Moreover, evaluating age without examining the data by gender yields no significant differences in QT or QTc dispersion [53].

The modulatory effects of age and gender on the clinical course of long QT syndrome (LQTS) by genotype have been characterized by Zareba et al. [54] The LQTS genotype, QTc duration, and follow-up were determined in 243 cases of LQTS caused by the KCNQ1 potassium channel gene mutations (LQT1), 209 cases of LQTS caused by the HERG potassium channel gene mutations (LQT2), and 81 cases of LQTS caused by the SCN5A sodium channel gene mutation (LQT3) gene carriers. During adulthood, LQT2 females and LQT1 females had a significantly higher risk of cardiac events than respective males. The lethality of cardiac events was highest in LQT3 males and

Table 11.1 Recommendations for permanent pacing in acquired AV block and in chronic Bifascicular and Trifascicular Block

Permanent pacing in acquired AV block in adults	
Class I Evidence and/or general agreement that a given procedure or treatment is useful and effective	3 and advanced 2 AV block at any anatomic level, associated with any one of the following conditions: Bradycardia with symptoms (including HF) presumed to be due to AV block; Dysrhythmias and other medical conditions that require drugs that result in symptomatic bradycardia; Documented periods of asystole ≥ to 3.0 seconds or any escape rate less than 40 beats per minute (bpm) in awake, symptom-free patients; After catheter ablation of the AV junction. There are no trials to assess outcome without pacing, and pacing is virtually always planned in this situation unless the operative procedure is AV junction modification; Postoperative AV block that is not expected to resolve after cardiac surgery; Neuromuscular diseases with AV block, such as myotonic muscular dystrophy, KSS, Erb's dystrophy (limb-girdle), and peroneal muscular atrophy, with or without symptoms, as there may be unpredictable progression of AV conduction disease; 2 AV block regardless of type or site of block, with associated symptomatic bradycardia.
Class II: Conditions with conflicting evidence or divergent opinion about procedure/ treatment efficacy **Class IIa**	Asymptomatic 3 AV block at any anatomic site with average awake ventricular rates of 40 bpm or faster especially if cardiomegaly or LV dysfunction is present; Asymptomatic type II 2 AV block with a narrow QRS. When type II 2 AV block occurs with a wide QRS, pacing becomes a Class I recommendation (see below regarding Pacing for Chronic Bifascicular and Trifascicular Block); Asymptomatic type I 2 AV block at intra- or infra-Hisian. His levels found at electrophysiological study performed for other indications; 1 or 2 AV block with symptoms similar to those of pacemaker syndrome.
Class IIb	Marked first-degree AV block (more than 0.30 seconds) in patients with LV dysfunction and symptoms of congestive HF in whom a shorter AV interval results in hemodynamic improvement, presumably by decreasing left atrial filling pressure; Neuromuscular diseases such as myotonic muscular dystrophy, Kearns-Sayre syndrome, Erb's dystrophy (limb-girdle), and peroneal muscular atrophy with any degree of AV block (including 1 AV block) with/without symptoms, as there may be unpredictable progression of AV conduction disease;
Class III: Evidence of ineffective or harmful treatment	Asymptomatic 1 AV block; Asymptomatic type I 2 AV block at the supra-His (AV node) level or not known to be intra- or infra-Hisian; AV block expected to resolve and/or unlikely to recur (e.g., drug toxicity, Lyme disease, or during hypoxia in sleep apnea syndrome in absence of symptoms).
Permanent pacing in Chronic Bifascicular and Trifascicular Block	
Class I	Intermittent 3 AV block; Type II 2 AV block; Alternating bundle-branch block.
Class IIa	Syncope not demonstrated to be due to AV block when other likely causes have been excluded, specifically ventricular tachycardia (VT); Incidental finding at electrophysiological study of markedly prolonged HV interval (greater than or equal to 100 milliseconds) in asymptomatic patients; Incidental finding at electrophysiological study of pacing-induced infra-His block that is not physiological
Class IIb	Neuromuscular diseases such as myotonic muscular dystrophy, KSS, Erb's dystrophy (limb-girdle), and peroneal muscular atrophy with any degree of fascicular block with or without symptoms, because there may be unpredictable progression of AV conduction.
Class III	Fascicular block without AV block or symptoms; Fascicular block with 1 AV block without symptoms.

Table 11.2 Recommendations for permanent pacing in carotid sinus syndrome and neurocardiogenic syncope, sinus node dysfunction and to terminate and prevent tachycardia

Permanent pacing in hypersensitive sinus syndrome and neurocardiogenic syncope	
Class I	Recurrent syncope caused by carotid sinus stimulation; minimal carotid sinus pressure induces ventricular asystole of more than 3-second duration in the absence of any medication that depresses the sinus node or AV conduction
Class IIa	Recurrent syncope without clear, provocative events and with a hypersensitive cardioinhibitory response; Syncope of unexplained origin when major abnormalities of sinus node function or AV conduction are discovered or provoked in electrophysiological studies. Significantly symptomatic and recurrent neurocardiogenic syncope associated with bradycardia documented spontaneously or at the time of tilt-table testing.
Permanent pacing in sinus node (SN) dysfunction	
Class I	SN dysfunction with documented symptomatic bradycardia, including frequent sinus pauses that produce symptoms. In some patients, bradycardia is iatrogenic and will occur as a consequence of essential long-term drug therapy of a type and dose for which there are no acceptable alternatives; Symptomatic chronotropic incompetence.
Class IIa	SN dysfunction occurring spontaneously or as a result of necessary drug therapy, with heart rate <40 bpm when a clear association between significant symptoms consistent with bradycardia and actual presence of bradycardia has not been documented; Syncope of unexplained origin when major abnormalities of SN function are discovered or provoked in electrophysiological studies.
Class IIb	In minimally symptomatic patients, chronic heart rate <40 bpm while awake.
Class III	SN dysfunction in asymptomatic patients, including those with substantial sinus bradycardia (heart rate <40 bpm) is a consequence of long-term drug treatment; SN dysfunction in patients with symptoms suggestive of bradycardia that are clearly documented as not associated with a slow heart rate; SN dysfunction with symptomatic bradycardia due to nonessential drug therapy.
Permanent pacemakers that automatically detect and pace to terminate tachycardia	
Class I	Symptomatic recurrent supraventricular tachycardia (SVT) reproducibly terminated by pacing after drugs + catheter ablation fail to control dysrhythmia or produce intolerable side effects; Symptomatic recurrent sustained VT as part of an automatic defibrillator system.
Class IIa	Symptomatic recurrent SVT reproducibly terminated by pacing in the unlikely event that catheter ablation and/or drugs fail to control dysrhythmia or produce intolerable side effects.
Class IIb	Recurrent SVT or atrial flutter that is reproducibly terminated by pacing as an alternative to drug therapy or ablation.
Class III	Tachycardias frequently accelerated or converted to fibrillation by pacing; The presence of accessory pathways with the capacity for rapid anterograde conduction whether or not the pathways participate in tachycardia mechanism
Pacing recommendations to prevent tachycardia	
Class I	Sustained pause-dependent VT, with or without prolonged QT, in which the efficacy of pacing is thoroughly documented
Class IIa	High-risk patients with congenital long-QT syndrome.
Class IIb:	AV re-entrant or AV node re-entrant SVT not responsive to medical or ablative therapy; Prevention of symptomatic, drug-refractory, recurrent AF with coexisting SN dysfunction.
Class III	Frequent or complex ventricular ectopic activity without sustained VT in the absence of the LQTS; Torsade de Pointes VT due to reversible causes.

females, and higher in LQT1 and LQT2 males than in LQT1 and LQT2 females. Their conclusion was that age and gender have different, genotype-specific modulating effects on the probability of cardiac events and electrocardiographic presentation in LQT1 and LQT2 patients.

Recently, in an evaluation of the risk factors that influence the clinical course of mutation-confirmed in adult patients with LQTS, the life-threatening cardiac events and protective effect of β-blocker therapy on cardiac events in these patients with known cardiac channel mutations were analyzed by Sauer et al. [55] They found that female gender, QTc interval ≥500 ms, and interim syncopal events were associated with significantly increased risk of life-threatening cardiac events in adulthood. Taken together, the severity of LQTS in adulthood can be risk stratified with information

Table 11.3 Recommendations for permanent pacing in myocardial infarction, hypertrophic and dilated cardiomyopathy

Permanent pacing after the acute phase of myocardial infarction	
Class I	Persistent second-degree AV block in the His-Purkinje system with bilateral bundle-branch block or third-degree AV block within or below the His-Purkinje system after AMI; Transient advanced (second- or third-degree) infranodal AV block and associated bundle-branch block. If the site of block is uncertain, an electrophysiological study may be necessary; Persistent and symptomatic second- or third-degree AV block.
Class IIb	Persistent second- or third-degree AV block at the AV node leve
Class III:	Transient AV block in the absence of intraventricular conduction defects; Transient AV block in the presence of isolated left anterior fascicular block; Acquired left anterior fascicular block in the absence of AV block; Persistent first-degree AV block in the presence of bundle-branch block that is old or age indeterminate.
Pacing recommendations for dilated cardiomyopathy/heart failure (HF)	
Class I	Class I indications for sinus node dysfunction or AV block as previously described.
Class II	Biventricular pacing in medically refractory, symptomatic New York Heart Association (NYHA) class III or IV patients with idiopathic dilated or ischemic cardiomyopathy, prolonged QRS interval (greater than or equal to 130 ms), LV end-diastolic diameter greater than or equal to 55 mm and ejection fraction less than or equal to 35% (In comparison to 1998 guidelines these are new recommendation for biventricular pacing in patients with severe HF following several trials that showed clinical and structural cardiac improvement).
Pacing recommendations for hypertrophic cardiomyopathy	
Class I	Class I indications for sinus node dysfunction or AV block as previously described.
Class IIb	Medically refractory, symptomatic hypertrophic cardiomyopathy with significant resting or provoked LV outflow obstruction.
Class III	Patients who are asymptomatic or medically controlled; Symptomatic patients without evidence of LV outflow obstruction.

regarding genotype, gender, QTc duration, and history of cardiac events. Also, β-blockers effectively reduced but did not eliminate the risk of both syncopal and life-threatening cardiac events in adult patients with mutation-confirmed LQTS. Moreover, the effect of gender and age on ventricular repolarization abnormality have been analyzed in Japanese carriers of a G643S common SNP for the KCNQ1 gene that is known to be associated with secondary LQTS and to cause a mild reduction in KCNQ1 current. Both genders showed a tendency for an increase in QT corrected by Fridericia's formula with aging. Interestingly, in females, both the peak and the end of the T wave (Tpe) interval, and the Tpe/QT ratio were significantly increased with age, which was not observed in males [56].

Besides LQTS and Brugada syndromes, mutations in the SCN5A gene have been also associated with hereditary Lenègre/Lev disease [57]. Initially, Lenègre/Lev disease was described as an acquired complete AV block with right (RBBB) or left bundle branch block (LBBB) and widening QRS complexes, and affected individuals often required pacemaker implantation [48, 58]. The theory mainly accepted is that the disease develops over several decades, affecting the His bundle and its branches. Lenègre and Lev hypothesized that it was a primary degenerative disease or an exaggerated aging process of unknown origin with sclerosis selectively affecting the conducting tissue. In 1995, a first locus was mapped to chromosome 19q13.2–13.3 [59]. In 1999, Schott and associates reported the first mutation in the SCN5A gene that segregated with progressive cardiac conduction defect (PCCD), in an autosomal dominant manner in a large French family, and a second SCN5A mutation which co-segregated in a smaller Dutch family with familial non-progressive conduction defect [57]. Fifteen patients from the French family were clinically and electrocardiographically affected (the mean QRS duration was 135 ±7 ms). RBBB was present in five patients, LBBB in two, left anterior or posterior hemiblock in three and long PR interval (>210 ms) in eight. None of the patients had structural heart disease. Of significance, four patients received a pacemaker implantation because of syncope or complete AV block, and in a number of affected patients the conduction defect increased in severity with age. On the other hand, in the Dutch family the proband presented after birth with an asymptomatic first-degree AV block associated with RBBB. Three brothers were asymptomatic, one of which had RBBB, and the asymptomatic mother had a non-specific conduction defect with a QRS duration of 120 ms. Using markers flanking SCN5A in the French family, these investigators demonstrated segregation of the disease with marker D3S1260 in every affected individual, and analyses with flanking markers of the region confirmed a linkage to the 3p21 locus. Sequencing the entire SCN5A coding region in this family identified a T→C substitution in the highly conserved +2 donor-splicing site of intron 22. This abnormal transcript predicts an in-frame skipping of exon 22 and an impaired gene product lacking the voltage-sensitive domain III S4 segment. Importantly, this mutation was found in all affected members, but not in 100 control chromosomes. In the Dutch family, sequence analysis of the SNC5A gene revealed a deletion of a single nucleotide (G) at position 5,280 resulting in a frame shift and a premature stop codon. This mutation co-segregated with the phenotype in all affected family members. These findings also indicated that with aging there is a progressive increase in cardiac fibrosis, which in association with the SNC5A gene mutation can slow the impulse along the electrical conduction system. In the Dutch family, the mutation conferring a premature stop codon and the presentation of PCCD at birth suggest that as a consequence of the sodium channel mutation a congenital phenotype can arise that may be either progressive or immediate.

Probst et al. [60] have extended the size of the pedigree of Lenègre/Lev disease to 65 potentially affected members, from which 25 individuals were carriers of the IVS.22+2 T→C *SCN5A* mutation. In relation to aging, gene carriers exhibited various types of conduction defects. P-wave, PR, and QRS duration increased progressively with age in gene carriers and in noncarriers. Of significance is that whatever the age, conduction parameters were longer in gene carriers. In addition, they examined *in vitro* the functional consequences of the mutation and found that the *SCN5A* gene induces a progressive alteration in the conduction of the cardiac impulse in the atria as well as the ventricle. The cardiac conduction defect already present in infancy worsened progressively with age, leading to the typical aspect of the idiopathic progressive conduction block as originally described by Lenègre and Lev. They also showed that hereditary Lenègre/Lev disease is caused by a haploinsufficiency mechanism, which in combination with aging leads to progressive defects of the conduction velocity.

Syncope/Tilt Test

Syncope, a common occurrence in the elderly, is often associated with a worse outcome than in adult patients requiring complementary tests, such as tilt-table test (TTT). Besides syncope secondary to AV block or other structural cardiac pathologies (e.g., aortic valve stenosis, obstructive cardiomyopathy, ischemic heart disease, hypertension), syncope in aging is mainly of unknown etiology. It is apparent that the test carries in the elderly a higher risk in comparison to young/adult patients. For example, in an evaluation of the utility of TTT with sublingual nitroglycerin, as a provocative agent, in elderly patients with unexplained syncope, Timoteo et al. [61] concluded that the test helps on the differential diagnosis of the cause of the syncope, and when potentiated by nitroglycerin, it produces a significant increase in positive responses. Furthermore, the test identified a considerable number of patients with an exaggerated response to nitrates. Also, Han et al. [62] assessed the incidence of serious responses occurring during the performance of the TTT in a cohort of 76 elderly individuals, and its prophylactic management. Fifty-one of the 76 patients studied had a positive test, and 23 had significant complications, including cardiac arrest in six cases, marked bradycardia in seven (two associated to 2nd degree AV block and five with AF) and severe hypotension in 10 cases. These findings clearly suggest that although non-invasive, TTT in the elderly may result in serious complications, and to prevent these side effects caution is recommended with patient selection, as well as with close control of isoproterenol infusion and vital signs.

The hemodynamic responses of the elderly to TTT until recently have been lacking. In the study of deCastro and de Nobrega [63], a cohort of elderly patients (n = 165) who sought medical assistance because of recurrent syncope were evaluated. For a period of 18 months they were initially enrolled and submitted to a two-stage, nitroglycerin-potentiated TTT. A subset of these patients who presented with dysautonomic response to TTT performed clinical autonomic tests, and they found that the most frequent cause of syncope during TTT was the dysautonomic pattern (43%), followed by a mixed type of neurocardiogenic syncope (35%). Interestingly, most patients who remained asymptomatic during TTT showed clear abnormal hemodynamic response during examination. Thus, autonomic dysfunction, which can be detected during TTT, is probably an important cause of syncope in the elderly regardless of the occurrence of symptoms during the TTT.

Pacer Therapy in the Elderly

In the previously mentioned 2002 ACC/AHA/NASPE guidelines update for implantation of pacemakers and antidysrhythmia devices, the indications were classified in several categories based on causal factors as indicated in Tables 11.1–11.3 [50]. In addition to these major classes (with the most relevance to elderly patients), for recommendations for permanent pacing in children, adolescents, and patients with congenital heart disease the reader is referred to the 2002 ACC/AHA/NASPE recommendations.

Since the publication of the above recommendations in 2002 the indications for pacemaker therapy in the elderly continue to evolve, and these include use as an adjunct therapy in the advanced stages of HF and in dysrhythmias unresponsive to medical therapy.

Advanced Heart Failure

One of the most recent and interesting applications of pacemaker implantation has been for cardiac resynchronization in advanced HF. As described by Wenger et al. in their review article [64], in the Multisite Stimulation in Cardiomyopathy (MUSTIC) study, patients (mean age, 64 years) with a left ventricular ejection fraction of 35% or less, NYHA class III symptoms, and QRS duration of more than 150 mseconds were randomly assigned to biventricular pacing or inactive pacing. The active pacing group showed a significant improvement in the distance walked in 6 minutes, peak oxygen consumption on exercise testing, and quality of life as measured with the Minnesota Living with Heart Failure questionnaire. Furthermore, biventricular pacing decreased the rate of hospitalizations for HF and resulted in an improvement in NYHA class [65]. These results were reproduced in a larger trial with a very similar design conducted in the US [66]. According to Wenger et al. [64] the benefits of cardiac resynchronization were later expanded to patients with QRS durations of 120–150 msec, and to those with narrow QRS (incomplete left bundle branch block and QRS <120 msec) and echocardiographic evidence of dysynchrony [67, 68].

Previously, several studies have reported the use of left ventricular and biventricular pacing using specialized leads placed in the cardiac veins via the coronary sinus in order to achieve ventricular "resynchronization." In one study [69], temporary biventricular pacing improved cardiac output by 40%. Several multicenter studies have assessed the use of biventricular pacing for advanced HF [70–72]. Two large randomized trials, the COMPANION and the CARE-HF studies unequivocally demonstrated that cardiac resynchronization therapy (CRT) conferred significant mortality and quality-of-life benefits for HF patients [72]. In the COMPANION trial, subjects receiving CRT with a defibrillator (CRT-D) fared better than those who received a device with CRT pacing capability only (CRT-P), albeit both studies found CRT-P reduced risk of death and hospitalization.

Pacemaker Implantation as an Adjunct Therapy for Atrial Fibrillation

Although many elderly patients tolerate AF without medications (because of concomitant AV nodal disease) in others, AF can be associated with rapid ventricular rates that medically are difficult to control. One method for treating the tachycardia associated with AF is to create AV block by applying radiofrequency energy and implanting a pacing system to provide appropriate heart rates. As reported by Fitzpatrick et al. [73] His bundle ablation and pacing may improve the quality of life in the elderly with medically unresponsive AF while reducing health care expenditure [74]. Similarly, pacing therapy may be effective in patients with drug-refractory paroxysmal AF. Delfault et al. [75] studied 30 patients with drug-refractory AF and pacing resulted in increase the temporal symptomatic dysrhythmia-free interval from 9 to 143 days. Indicators of pacemaker therapy are shown in Table 11.4.

Ventricular Dysrhythmias

Premature Ventricular Beats

It is established that aging is associated with an increase in both the prevalence and complexity of premature ventricular beats (PVB). These can be single (uniform or multiform), in couplets, or in short runs of ventricular tachycardia. In the absence of cardiac functional or structural defects, increases in cardiac mortality in these individuals are not apparent. On the other hand, because the risk of developing dysrhythmias increases even with healthy aging, an interesting question is whether high intensity physical activity should be contraindicated in the elderly person. Pigozzi et al. [76] have comparatively evaluated using echocardiogram and EKG monitoring 49 male athletes engaged in various sport disciplines, mean age 62.3+/−2.3 and 24 sedentary or moderately physically active

Table 11.4 Clinical conditions and pacemaker therapy

Clinical condition	Evaluation/therapy
Sinus node dysfunction	
Asymptomatic	Pacing not indicated
Symptomatic	Pacing
AV block	
Asymptomatic	
First degree	Pacing not indicated
Second degree	Pacing not indicated if type 1 second degree AV block with a narrow QRS complex is present; Electrophysiological study should be considered if type 1 second degree AV block and a wide QRS complex are present
	Pacing recommended if type II block is present
Third degree	Pacing
Symptomatic	Pacing regardless of type
Fascicular block	
Asymptomatic	
Bifascicular block	Pacing not indicated
Trifascicular block	Pacing
Syncope/presyncope	
Bifascicular block	Electrophysiological study to assess inducible ventricular dysrhythmias and His-Purkinje conduction

healthy males, mean age 62.9+/−1.7 years as controls. No pathological findings were detected in both experimental groups and the exercise performance was greater in athletes than controls (206.9+/−5.2 *versus* 156.3+/−12 watt, $p < 0.01$). During exercise test, there were no significant difference between-groups in the incidence of ventricular dysrhythmias including multiple PVB polymorphisms, or repetitive PVBs. Interestingly, on EKG monitoring the number of PVBs was significantly greater in controls than athletes, whereas no significant difference were detected in the incidence of discrete ventricular dysrhythmias between athletes and controls. Therefore, in elderly healthy athletes, vigorous training even to competition does not result in a greater incidence of ventricular dysrhythmias, although these investigators suggest caution and preparticipation evaluation is recommended.

Ventricular Tachycardia (VT)

In VT the sinoatrial node does not control the beating of the ventricles. Instead, other areas along the lower electrical pathway take over the pacemaking role. The new signal does not run thru the regular pathway, the heart muscle does not beat normally, and one may feel "skipping beats." This dysrhythmia may cause severe shortness of breath, dizziness, or syncope. VT is frequently present in aging individuals with structural cardiac defects, CAD as well as in those with hypertension. In 1995 Mercando et al. [77] carried out signal-averaged electrocardiography and 24-hour ambulatory electrocardiographic monitoring in 121 elderly patients > 6 months after acute MI and found that all patients had asymptomatic complex ventricular dysrhythmias and a left ventricular ejection fraction ≥ 40%. Rates of sudden, cardiac, and total death were compared between groups with and without nonsustained VT and between normal and abnormal signal-averaged electrocardiographic studies. The prevalence of an abnormal signal-averaged electrocardiographic study was 36%. Thirty-seven percent of the patients had nonsustained VT, and the remaining patients had complex ventricular dysrhythmias other than VT. There were 27 sudden and 48 total cardiac deaths, and 66 deaths from all causes during a mean follow-up period of 30 months. The lower rate of sudden and cardiac death was in the group without nonsustained VT. Although there was a trend toward a lower rate of sudden death in patients with a normal signal-averaged electrocardiogram, there was no statistical difference in the rates of sudden, cardiac or total death between patients with normal or abnormal studies. The negative predictive value of having neither an abnormal signal-averaged electrocardiogram nor nonsustained VT was 94% for sudden death. The authors concluded that in elderly patients with complex ventricular dysrhythmias and ejection fraction ≥40% for at least 6 months after an acute MI, the presence of nonsustained VT predicted a higher rate of sudden and cardiac death; however, signal-averaged electrocardiography alone was not predictive. In a later study by the same group of investigators on the prevalence of VT and complex ventricular dysrhythmias, and their association to new coronary events in old men and women they found similar prevalence in both sexes (16% in males and 15% in women) with CAD, as well as in individual with hypertension, cardiomyopathy and valvular disease [78]. Similarly, no significant difference was noted in those subjects without structural defects or hypertension (3% in men versus 2% in females), nor differences by gender were noted for complex ventricular dysrhythmias. On the other hand, Lampert et al. [79] in their study on gender differences in ventricular dysrhythmia recurrence in patients with CAD and implantable cardioverter-defibrillators found that women were less likely to have VT/ VF, and had fewer VT/VF episodes than men. These findings were strongest in patients with evidence of a stable anatomic VT circuit: those with clinical or electrophysiologically induced VT. It appears that differences in susceptibility to dysrhythmia triggering may underlie the known differences in sudden cardiac death rates between men and women.

Ventricular Fibrillation (VF)

The most serious dysrhythmia is VF, a chaotic heartbeat that may reach 300/minute. Since the heart pumps very little blood to the brain and body, syncope may occur. This dysrhythmia is an emergency requiring immediate action either with CPR and/or electrical shock. Damage to the heart can be minimized if a normal rhythm can be quickly re-established. Approximately 220,000 deaths from heart attacks occur each year in the US, a large number probably caused by VF. Elderly individuals who have a history of CAD or suffer episodes of acute myocardial ischemia are at the highest risk for VF.

It has been reported that VT triggers many episodes of VF, and patients who present with VT or VF are usually grouped together in reports on natural history and treatment. However, there are significant differences in the clinical profiles of these two individual groups, with some studies suggesting differences in their response to therapy. In the Antiarrhythmics Versus Implantable Defibrillators (AVID) trial to determine whether patients who receive an implantable cardioverter-defibrillator (ICD) after VT have dysrhythmias during follow-up, which are different from patients who present with VF, Raitt et al. [80] have suggested that there are important differences in the electrophysiologic characteristics of patients with VT versus those with VF since ventricular dysrhythmias recurrence at follow-up was different in patients who presented with VT than in those who originally presented with VF. More recently, Daubert et al. [81] in their study on the predictive value of ventricular dysrhythmia inducibility for subsequent VT or VF in the Multicenter Automatic Defibrillator Implantation Trial (MADIT) II patients, found inducibility (i.e., sustained monomorphic or polymorphic VT induced with three or fewer extrastimuli or VF induced with two or fewer extrastimuli) was associated with an increased likelihood of VT. The cohort consisted of 720 ICD randomized males, of which 593 (82%) underwent electrophysiological testing. Patients received an ICD whether they were inducible or not. Patients were subcategorized based on monomorphic VT (n = 169, age range 62 ± 12); Polymorphic VT or VF with S2–3 (n = 42, 62 ± 11); VF with S4 (n = 32, age 65 ± 10), and nor VT or VF induced (n = 350, age 64 ± 10). Noninducible MADIT II study subjects using this electrophysiological protocol had a considerable incidence of VT event rate and a higher VF event rate than inducible patients. Therefore, induction of polymorphic VT or VF, even with double extrastimuli, appears less relevant than induction of monomorphic VT. The author's conclusion was that electrophysiological testing using a stimulation protocol up to three extrastimuli at two sites for ruling out subsequent VT or VF events was of a limited predictive value. Although noninducible patients in the MADIT II study population do have a slightly lower risk of the combined dysrhythmic end point of VT or VF, their risk of VF tended to be higher than in inducible patients. In addition they found that postinfarction patients with an ejection fraction of $\leq$0.30, noninducibility at electrophysiological testing did not equate with a low dysrhythmic risk. Finally, based on the collected data this study does not support excluding noninducible patients from ICD therapy.

Dysrhythmogenic Right Ventricular Dysplasia in the Elderly (DRVD)

DVRD is a rare cardiac anomaly occurring mainly in young men. However, isolated cases of DVRD in elderly individual have been reported. Recently, Garcia-Quintana et al. [82] reported a case of a 76 years old man presenting with VT, wide QRS and morphology of left bundle branch block. Cardiac catheterization and echocardiogram revealed dilated and dysfunctional right ventricle. The patient underwent implantation of a cardioverter-defibrillator since while on treatment with amiodarone presented further episodes of VT. Later on, the VT was controlled with sotalol. The authors examined the literature and found five more cases of DRVD in aging individuals (four males, two females) with mean age of 75.8 years, and 4 have presented with VT. Therefore, the diagnosis of

DRVD should be considered in individuals of all ages who present with clinical signs consistent with DRVD and electrocardiographic data consistent with this entity.

Antidysrhythmic Therapy in Aging

With aging, serum drug concentration is prone to increase rapidly and is maintained at high levels for a longer time than desirable because of impaired liver and kidney functions. Therefore efficacy and side effects both occur rapidly and for a long time. In the elderly, the specialized conduction system, including the sinus node and the AV node are often impaired, and antidysrhythmic drugs often induce bradycardia, widening of the QRS duration and LQT interval. The elderly should be treated initially at a lower dosage than adults and should be followed with frequent determinations of serum drug concentration to achieve positive results without serious adverse effect. The promising new fields of pharmacogenetics/pharmacogenomics (discussed later in this chapter) may provide the solution for drug selection and dosage indications particularly in aging.

The use of cardiopulmonary resuscitation in elderly patients in treating dysrhythmias has been increasingly reported. In a recent study, Elshove-Bolk et al. demonstrated in a geriatric hospitalized cohort that resuscitation provided particular benefits in those patients admitted for cardiac ischemia suffering cardiac arrest with VT or VF as a primary dysrhythmia [83].

Channelopathies

Introduction to Channelopathies

Ion channels, particularly K^+ channels and Ca^{2+} channels play pivotal roles in communication between the cell membrane and cytosol. However, with aging these ion channels undergo functional and/or structural alterations, which are not only associated with the development of cellular dysfunction but also contribute to the progression of cellular senescence, defining an age-associated channelopathy. Elucidation of the genetic structure of the molecular components of these channels will lead to the identification of mutational or polymorphic gene variants which mediate the effects of aging, therapeutic treatments or diverse physiological stimuli on channel function.

Calcium and Potassium Currents

Action potential (AP) contours vary considerably between normal adult and aged right atrial fibers. However, the ionic bases for these differences remain unknown. As noted previously, Dun et al. [28] using whole cell patch clamp recording techniques in a canine model have measured L-type Ca^{2+} currents (I_{CaL}) with either Ca^{2+} or Ba^{2+} (3 mM) as the charge carrier, and both the transient outward (I_{to}) and sustained potassium currents (I_{sus}) in cells dispersed from normal adult (2–5 years) and older dogs (>8 years). A significant reduction was found in peak I_{CaL} (47%) and I_{BaL} (43%) in aged cells, yet the differences in I_{BaL} disappeared with maximal β-adrenergic stimulation (isoproterenol, 1 μM). Moreover, composite I_{to} and I_{sus} densities were significantly increased in the aged versus adult cell group. I_{to} decay during maintained depolarization was slowed in aged cells, and I_{to} steady-state inactivation curve was shifted positively in aged cells. Furthermore, composite I_{to} and I_{sus} currents of aged cells were more sensitive to tetraethylammonium chloride (TEA), a specific inhibitor of some types of K^+ currents, and in the presence of TEA (5 mM), I_{to} in aged cells was significantly greater than that in adult cells. Taken together, this interesting study revealed that ionic currents differ in aged versus adult right atrial cells, that reduced Ca^{2+} current and augmented outward currents could contribute significantly to the altered AP contour of the aged right atrial cell, that adrenergic stimulation appears to restore Ba^{2+} currents in aged cells, and that an augmented TEA sensitive current seems to play a role in changes of I_{sus} in aged right atrial cells. Similarly, changes in whole cell K^+ and L-type Ca^{2+} currents in aging rat ventricular myocytes have been studied by Liu et al. [84]. Using whole cell patch-clamp techniques they measured the inward rectifier K^+ current (I_{K1}), the transient outward K^+ current (I_{to}), and the L-type Ca^{2+} channel current ($I_{Ca,L}$) in ventricular myocytes isolated from young adult (6 month) and aged (> 27 month) Fischer 344 rats. Besides an increase in cell size and membrane capacitance, aged myocytes exhibited the same magnitude of peak I_{K1} with a greater slope conductance, while displayed smaller steady-state I_{K1}. In addition, aged myocytes had a greater I_{to} with an increased rate of activation, but the I_{to} inactivation kinetics, steady-state inactivation, and responsiveness to L-phenylephrine, a α1-adrenergic agonist, were unaltered. The magnitude of peak $I_{Ca,L}$ in aged myocytes was decreased and accompanied by a slower inactivation confirming previous findings [85], however the $I_{Ca,L}$ steady-state inactivation was unaltered. AP duration in aged myocytes was prolonged only at 90% of full repolarization (APD_{90}) when compared with the AP duration of young adult myocytes. Taken together, these findings demonstrated aging-associated changes in AP, morphology, in I_{K1}, I_{to}, and $I_{Ca,L}$ of rat ventricular myocytes, which possibly contribute to dysfunction in the aging heart.

Sarcolemmal K_{ATP} Channels in Aging

Opening of sarcolemmal K_{ATP} channels is an important endogenous cardioprotective mechanism, mainly in the aging heart. These channels are abundant in cardiac myocytes where they are essential in coupling the cellular metabolic state with membrane excitability. The opening of sarcolemmal ATP-sensitive K^+ (K_{ATP}) channels occurs during ischemia and protects the heart against injury. Age-dependent changes in the myocardial susceptibility to ischemia have been observed in different species, including humans. Recent research has demonstrated that aging is associated with reduced numbers of sarcolemmal K_{ATP} channels in hearts from females, but not males [86]. This phenomenon seems to be associated with an age-dependent decrease in the concentration of circulating estrogens. Cardiac K_{ATP} channels, gated by cellular metabolism, are formed by association of the inwardly rectifying potassium channel Kir6.2, the potassium conducting and pore-forming subunit, and SUR2A, the ATP-binding cassette protein that serves as the regulatory subunit and member of the ABCC subfamily of ABC proteins [87]. Kir6.2 is the principal site of ATP-induced channel inhibition, while SUR2A regulates K^+ flux through adenine nucleotide binding and catalysis. The findings of Jovanovic et al. have suggested that in the heart basal levels of expression of SUR2A are lower than Kir6.2, albeit stoichiometry of subunits in sarcolemmal K_{ATP} channels is 4:4 [86]. The consequence of this is that SUR2A is a limiting subunit that controls the number of sarcolemmal K_{ATP} channels [88].

Estrogens specifically upregulate SUR2A and, thereby, control the number of sarcolemmal K_{ATP} channels. Ranki et al. [89] found that a decrease in the number of sarcolemmal ATP-sensitive K^+ channels appears to be gender-dependent in aging. Using young and old, male and female guinea-pigs as animal model they studied whether aging changes the expression of cardiac sarcolemmal K_{ATP} channels. RT-PCR conducted with primers specific for K_{ATP} channel subunits, Kir6.2, Kir6.1 and SUR2A subunits using total RNA from ventricular tissue was carried out. Besides whole cell electrophysiology done on ventricular cardiomyocytes, Western blotting using anti-Kir6.2 and anti-SUR2A antibodies, was done on cardiac membrane fraction. No significant age-related changes in levels of Kir6.1 or Kir6.2 mRNAs were detected, although levels of SUR2A transcripts were significantly lower in old than in young females. Interestingly, these findings were not detected in male animals. In both old and young males, pinacidil (100 μM) induced outward currents, and the difference between current density of pinacidil-sensitive component in females, but not males, was statistically significant. Western blotting analysis demonstrated higher levels of Kir6.2 and SUR2A proteins in cardiac membrane fractions from young than old females. These observations suggest that aging in females, but not males, is accompanied by a decrease in the number of cardiac K_{ATP} channels secondary to decreased levels of the SUR2A subunit. Since estrogens specifically upregulate SUR2A and control the number of sarcolemmal K_{ATP} channels, an age-dependent decrease in the concentration of circulating estrogens may underlie a number of the effects of decreasing estrogen levels on the heart and on the plasma membrane [88]. Moreover, age-dependent decrease in the number of sarcolemmal K_{ATP} channels generates a cardiac phenotype more sensitive to ischemia, which again seems to be responsible for decrease in myocardial tolerance to stress that occurs in elderly women.

Calcium Channels

It has been previously mentioned that the Cav1.2 channel protein plays an essential role in the aged-related deterioration of a functioning pacemaker [11]. With age, Cav1.2 channel protein expression decreases, and concurrently there is a reduction in the spontaneous activity of the SA node providing evidence of the significant role that Ca^{2+} channels play in the genesis of dysrhythmias associated with aging. Furthermore, the E65K polymorphism in the β1-subunit of the large-conductance, Ca^{2+}-dependent K^+ (BK) channel, is a key element in the control of arterial tone, and recently has been associated with a low prevalence of diastolic hypertension. Senti et al. have reported on the modulatory effect of sex and age and the association of the E65K channel protein polymorphism with a low prevalence of diastolic hypertension, and the protective role of E65K polymorphism against CVD [90]. The genotype frequency of the E65K polymorphism was evaluated in a study group composed of 3,924 participants 25–74 years of age including 1973 women and 1951 men, and determined its potential effect on subsequent cardiovascular events occurring since inclusion with a five-year follow-up of the cohort. Estrogen modulation of wild-type and mutant ion channel activity was carried out after heterologous expression and electrophysiological studies. Multivariate regression analysis showed that aging upregulates the protective effect of the K allele against moderate-to-severe diastolic hypertension. When analyses were restricted to women the findings remained significant, and this effect was independent of the reported acute modulation of BK channels by estrogen. These observations provide genetic evidence on the different impact of the BK channel in control of blood pressure in men and women, and mainly in aging women. Furthermore, the E65K polymorphism seems to be a major genetic factor in the prevention of myocardial infarction and stroke.

Josephson et al. [91] have also reported changes in the characteristics of the L-type Ca^{2+} channels with aging. They observed that the peak ensemble-averaged single Ca^{2+}channel currents in the aging heart were enhanced compared to those from young adult or adult hearts, which was partially attributed to an apparent increase in the number of active Ca^{2+} channels per patch in aging (1.90+/−0.23) as compared to young adult (1.33+/−0.19) or adult heart (1.50+/−0.2). In addition, an increase in the time constant for inactivation of the ensemble-averaged Ca^{2+} currents in aging was observed compared to young and adult heart. Furthermore, the aging-related changes were also traced to altered single Ca^{2+} channel gating, including the increased probability of being open, and increased availability of single Ca^{2+} currents in aging heart. In contrast, the unitary Ca^{2+} current amplitude was unchanged with aging. Taken together, these findings suggest that the compensatory increase in L-type Ca^{2+} currents occurring with aging may be a consequence of a potential increase in both the number and the activity of individual L-type Ca^{2+} channels. A diagram of the subunit structure of the voltage-gated cardiac L-type Ca^{2+} channel is presented in Fig. 11.1.

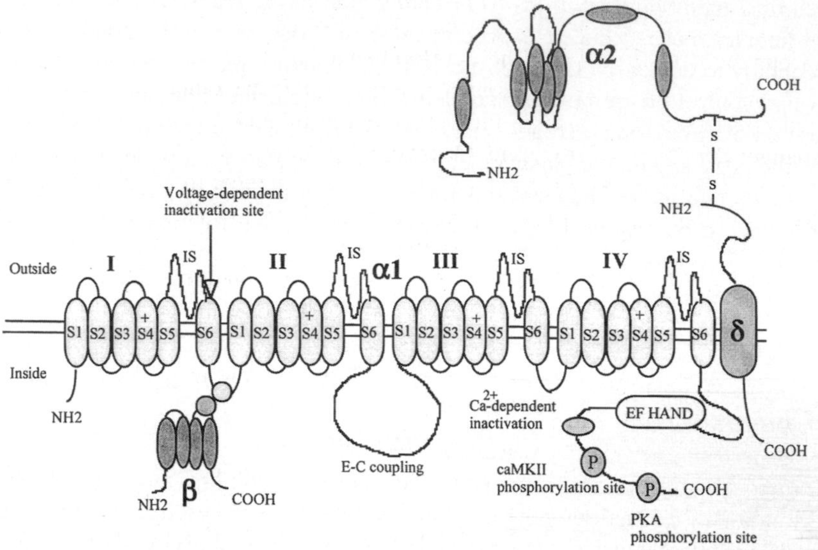

Fig. 11.1 Voltage-Gated Ca^{2+} channel structure
The Ca^{2+} channels are composed of a pore forming α1 subunit, a transmembrane δ subunit covalently linked to an extracellular α2 subunit, and an intracellular β subunit bound to the α1 at the link between domains I and II. The α1 subunit of Ca^{2+} channels is composed of four homologous membrane spanning internal domains, each with six transmembrane helices (S1–S6) and a pore forming loop. S4 segment in each domain serves as a voltage sensor for channel activation, the IS sequence between S5 and S6 in all four domains are involved in ion selectivity and the S6 in domain one contains the voltage-inactivation gate. The loop between domains II-III is involved in excitation-contraction (E-C) coupling. Consensus sites for phosphorylation by cAMP-dependent PKA and by CaMKII have been localized near the C-terminal tail of α1, as have sites for CaM binding (including EF HAND) and Ca^{2+} dependent inactivation as shown. The intracellular β subunit is bound to the α1 subunit at the link between domains I and II. The α2δ complex is derived from a precursor protein that is cleaved to yield separate α2 and δ proteins linked by disulfide bonds.

Connexins

With aging there is an increasing incidence of sinus node dysfunction. The possible mechanisms leading to nodal dysfunction have been evaluated in guinea pigs during their life span (i.e., birth to 38 months). Using immunofluorescence with confocal microscopy, Cx43 protein expression was shown to be present at birth throughout the sinoatrial node and atrial muscle by Jones et al. [25] However, at one month Cx43 protein was not expressed in the center of the SA node, and there was a progressive increase of the area lacking the protein. Throughout the remainder of the animal's life span the area of tissue lacking Cx43 protein progressively increased. That Cx43 protein expression within the SA node was decreasing with age was shown by Western blots; however, the expression of other cardiac connexins, Cx40 and Cx45, did not change with age. Analysis of conduction maps showing propagation of the AP across the SA node, from the initiation point to the crista terminalis, revealed that the AP conduction time taken and conduction distance increased proportionally with age; conversely the conduction velocity decreased with age. It has been shown that aging induces degenerative changes in AP conduction, contributed to by the observed loss of Cx43 protein. Cx43 is a potential therapeutic target for attenuating the age-related deterioration of the cardiac pacemaker.

KCNQ Potassium Channel

Although the incidence and prevalence of cardiovascular pathologies are known to increase with aging, the molecular and genetic basis of these processes has been difficult to decipher, in part because of the lack of suitable model systems. However, some animal models have been very rewarding in our quest to understand the developmental mechanisms of cardiac dysfunction and certain dysrhythmias. For example, *Drosophila melanogaster* has emerged as one of the principal model organisms used for studying the biology of aging in general, and in particular the cardiac functional changes developing with aging. Ocorr et al. [92] have developed specific heart function assays in *Drosophila* and found that the fly's cardiac performance, in a way similar to the human heart, deteriorates with aging by developing a progressive increase in electrical pacing-induced HF as well as in dysrhythmias [92]. According to these investigators, the insulin receptor and associated pathways have a dramatic and heart-autonomous influence on age-related cardiac performance in flies, suggestive of potentially similar mechanisms in regulating cardiac aging in vertebrates. Dysfunction in KCNQ and K_{ATP} ion channels also appears to contribute to the decline in heart performance in the aging flies, in addition to their conserved role in protecting against dysrhythmias. Further studies on *Drosophila* by Ocorr et al. [93] revealed that the aging fly tends to develop an elevated incidence of cardiac dysfunction and dysrhythmias concomitantly associated with a decrease in the expression of the *Drosophila* homolog of human KCNQ1-encoded K^+ channel α-subunits. In humans, this channel is involved in myocardial repolarization, and functional defects in it are associated with increased risk for Torsades de Pointes dysrhythmias and sudden death. On the other hand, and as pointed out by these investigators hearts from young KCNQ1 mutant flies exhibit prolonged contractions and fibrillations reminiscent of Torsades de Pointes dysrhythmias. Interestingly, these mutant flies exhibit markedly increased susceptibility to pacing-induced cardiac dysfunction at young ages, characteristics that are observed only at advanced ages in the wild-type (WT) flies. Furthermore, the fibrillations observed in mutant flies correlate with delayed relaxation of the myocardium, as revealed by increases in the duration of phasic contractions, extracellular field potentials, and in the baseline diastolic tension. The authors noted that their findings suggest that K^+ currents, mediated by a KCNQ channel, contribute to the repolarization reserve of the fly hearts, ensuring normal excitation-contraction coupling and rhythmical contraction. However, since these dysrhythmias, in both WT and KCNQ1 mutants, become worse as flies age, additional factors may be also involved.

Mitochondrial Channels

Mitochondria, the powerhouse of the cells, are considered to be the most important cellular organelles to contribute to aging, mainly because of their role in the production of reactive oxygen species (ROS), in the initiation of apoptotic cell remodeling and in efficient ATP synthesis. Besides their important roles in normal cell functioning, mitochondria participate in many events including calcium signaling, stress responses and regulation of the cell life-death transition, both in necrosis and apoptosis. Defects in mitochondria function are associated with aging including changes in mitochondrial membrane potential (ΔΨm) and the opening of the mitochondrial permeability transition pore (either termed the PT pore or mitoPTP), essential components to the cell life-death transition and the promotion/acceleration of aging [94–100].

The chemiosmotic gradient of protons across the inner mitochondrial membrane is, in large part a result of an ion concentration difference that provides the energy necessary to synthesize ATP by the respiratory chain. Ca^{2+}influx into mitochondria via the Ca^{2+}-uniporter, driven by ΔΨm plays a contributory role in ATP production in response to the increased demands for metabolic energy by the cell. On the other hand, excessive uptake of Ca^{2+} by mitochondria can trigger the mitoPTP opening, which then causes collapse of the $\Delta\Psi m$. As a result, not only will ATP synthesis be further compromised but also a more severe cellular damage will occur.

Importantly, the mitochondrial K_{ATP} (mitoK_{ATP}) channel is involved in ischemic preconditioning (IPC) in heart and brain [95, 100]. Blockage of the K^+ movement through this channel in mitochondria will abolish the endogenous protective effect induced by either multiple brief periods of ischemia or pharmacological treatments, whereas enhancement of mitoK_{ATP} activity by selective K^+ channel openers can protect cells from severe ischemia-reperfusion (I/R) injury. Furthermore, defects in the mitoPTP, Ca^{2+} transporter, and mitoK_{ATP} are involved in the aging processes, including the aging heart [94–100].

Ion Channels/Transporters in Mitochondria

While ion channels have been described in all intracellular membranes, and in particular in the sarcoplasmic membrane (with its fundamental involvement in cellular electrophysiological function), mitochondrial channels are implicated in the maintenance of ion homeostasis, mitochondrial matrix volume, membrane potential, and ATP synthesis. For instance, Ca^{2+} influx into mitochondria through specific uniporters can buffer excessive $Ca^{2+}$when too much Ca^{2+} is loaded in the cytosol, whereas Ca^{2+}efflux, via antiporters, can release extra Ca^{2+}into the cytosol, when an increased requirement for $Ca^{2+}$is signaled [101, 102]. Furthermore, Ca^{2+}influx signaling can directly stimulate ATP production pathways in mitochondria, and other ion transport channels (e.g., potassium, sodium and chloride) participate in the formation of electrochemical gradient across the mitochondrial membranes and generation of a membrane potential. It is evident that this substantially negative membrane potential is essential for ATP synthesis and constitutes a driving force for Ca^{2+}uptake by mitochondria. In addition, mitochondrial transporters for Ca^{2+}, K^+, Cl^+, and Na^+ play important roles in cell growth, death, and functioning under both physiological and pathological states.

Mitochondrial Ca^{2+}-Channels/Transporter

$Ca^{2+}$is taken up by mitochondria by a pump driven by proton-motive force (i.e., $\delta\Psi m$), employing a ruthenium red sensitive-uniporter [103]. Despite extensive attempts to purify the transporter [104–108], the molecular and biochemical identity of the mitochondrial Ca^{2+} uniporter remains undetermined.

With the development of sensitive fluorescent Ca^{2+}indicators and new techniques, including microscope-based photometry and laser confocal microscopy, real time mitochondrial Ca^{2+}uptake in intact cells can be measured. For example, Ca^{2+}transients have been shown in mitochondria of hepatocytes, neurons. skeletal and smooth muscle cells, vascular endothelial cells and beating cardiomyocytes [109–111]. Studies with isolated adult rabbit cardiac myocytes loaded with fluorescent Ca^{2+} indicators demonstrated that mitochondrial Ca^{2+}levels rise and fall during excitation-contraction (E-C) coupling in response to electrical stimulation and isoproterenol [109, 110]. In addition, studies using two-photon microscopy and genetically expressed "chameleon" Ca^{2+} sensors have shown that skeletal muscle mitochondria take up Ca^{2+} during *in vivo* contraction induced by motor nerve stimulation, which is rapidly released during relaxation [111]. These studies have confirmed not only the presence of the uniporter mediating mitochondrial Ca^{2+} influx but have also indicated that the primary (but not exclusive) mechanism of Ca^{2+} efflux involves the mitochondrial Na^+/Ca^{2+} antiporter or Na^+/Ca^{2+} exchanger (mNCX) in exchanging Ca^{2+} for influx of Na^+.

Mitochondrial Ca^{2+} Cycling

Consistently, in both non- and excitable cells, there is Ca^{2+} cycling taking place in respiring mitochondria. Mitochondrial Ca^{2+} cycling plays a very important role in the modulation of oxidative phosphorylation (OXPHOS), namely ATP production, and in the regulation of global cellular Ca^{2+} homeostasis. Calcium is an allosteric activator of several mitochondrial dehydrogenases, including glycerol 3-phosphate dehydrogenase, the pyruvate dehydrogenase multienzyme complex (PDH), α ketoglutarate dehydrogenase (also called 2-oxoglutarate dehydrogenase, OGDH), and NAD-linked isocitrate dehydrogenase (NAD-IDH) [112]. While FAD-glycerol 3-phosphate dehydrogenase is located on the outer surface of the inner mitochondrial membrane, PDH, NAD-IDH and OGDH are located within the matrix. PDH is the rate-limiting enzyme for glucose oxidation, and NAD-IDH and OGDH are important enzymes in the tricarboxylate (TCA) cycle. Therefore, the changes in matrix free Ca^{2+} determined by the Ca^{2+} uniporter and Na^{+}/Ca^{2+} exchanger directly modulate these activities and consequently ATP production. In fact, it has been found that the active uptake of two Ca^{2+} ions yielded the same amount of O_2 uptake as one molecule of ADP, indicating that Ca^{2+} influx signaling could stimulate mitochondrial respiration. Moreover, in cultured cardiomyocytes, increased mitochondrial ATP synthase activity has been demonstrated in response to increased intramitochondrial Ca^{2+}levels [113].

Mitochondrial Ca^{2+} cycling plays a pivotal role in the regulation of intracellular Ca^{2+} homeostasis, in both non- and excitable cells, although only a small amount of Ca^{2+} is taken up by mitochondria [114]. Mitochondrial free Ca^{2+} content is estimated to be $\sim$ 100 nM in unstimulated cells while it increased to 600 nM in stimulated cells. Increased mitochondrial Ca^{2+} levels were found over the course of many contractions in rapid paced cardiac myocytes [115]. In addition, mitochondrial Ca^{2+} content varied with cytosolic Ca^{2+}, which increases upon activation of specific signaling events giving rise to Ca^{2+} transients. In electrically stimulated cardiac myocytes, changes in mitochondrial Ca^{2+}content were detected during each individual contraction cycle; namely, a substantial amount of Ca^{2+} was rapidly taken up during early systole and released during later systole and diastole [116]. Treatment with ruthenium red to block the Ca^{2+} uniporter in neurons immediately following challenge with N-methyl-D-aspartate (NMDA) resulted in a rapid and transient increase in cytosolic Ca^{2+} without a corresponding increase in mitochondrial matrix Ca^{2+}, whereas blocking mitochondrial Ca^{2+} extrusion with a mNCX inhibitor depressed cytosolic Ca^{2+} and prolonged the time for matrix Ca^{2+} level to recover [117]. These findings suggest that mitochondrial Ca^{2+} cycling is significantly involved in intracellular Ca^{2+} handling.

Further support for the view that the mitochondria organelle participates in the regulation of intracellular Ca^{2+} signaling emerged from the recent studies by Cheranov and Jaggar with smooth muscles from cerebral artery which found that pharmacological depolarization of mitochondria reduced Ca^{2+} sparks and waves frequency and increased global intracellular Ca^{2+} concentration, whereas inhibition of mitoPTP caused opposite changes [118]. Although a large amount of Ca^{2+} can be accumulated in mitochondria, the ionic concentration of Ca^{2+} inside the mitochondria may be only slightly affected suggesting that mitochondria might act as Ca^{2+} sinks under conditions of cytosolic Ca^{2+} overload.

Ca^{2+} Transporter in Aging

There is increasing evidence that mitochondrial Ca^{2+} cycling is impaired in aging, by declining Ca^{2+} uptake via Ca^{2+} uniporter, reduced Ca^{2+} retention capacity, a possible decrease in mNCX activity and elevated Ca^{2+} extrusion instead through sensitized mitoPTP opening. For instance, during aging, the calcium compartmentation in synaptosomal mitochondria decreases, and this decline has been associated with a reduction in the activity of the mitochondrial Ca^{2+} uniporter [119]. Moreover, in aging rodent cerebral neurons and synaptosomes, increased cytosolic Ca^{2+} levels have been reported in both basal and depolarization-induced states, likely a consequence of age-modified intracellular Ca^{2+}buffering and extrusion systems rather than a result of increased calcium influx. The recovery rate of cytosolic Ca^{2+} after stimulation is also slowed in aged cells. Altered Ca^{2+} handling in aged neurons, characterized by increased cytosolic Ca^{2+} at rest and slowed recovery after stimulation, is directly correlated with mitochondrial membrane potential and significantly delayed mitochondrial repolarization, which suggest that mitochondrial dysfunction (e.g., reduced mitochondrial Ca^{2+} uptake or Ca^{2+}- mediated bioenergetic activation) may contribute to changes in intracellular Ca^{2+} homeostasis [120]. Similarly, Jahangir et al. [96] reported that Ca^{2+} content in heart mitochondria from senescent rat was significantly reduced compared to adult mitochondria, and suggested that the age-associated decline in mitochondrial Ca^{2+} content could arise from decreased Ca^{2+} uptake, impaired binding capability or enhanced Ca^{2+} extrusion.

Recently, Murchison et al. [121] evaluated the capacity of mitochondria to buffer large Ca^{2+} influxes in forebrain neurons from aged Fischer rats. The amplitude of Ca^{2+} transients induced by high K^+ depolarization was significant less in aged neurons than in young neurons when assessed n the presence of a mitochondrial Ca^{2+} uniporter inhibitor, indicating that aging mitochondria have a significant buffering deficit during larger Ca^{2+} influx through voltage-gated Ca^{2+} channels (VGCCs). This was accompanied by decreased mitochondrial membrane potential as gauged by JC-1 staining. The decreased capacity of buffering Ca^{2+} influx in mitochondria is mainly due to a dysfunctional Ca^{2+} uniporter in the aging neurons. This view is consistent with gathered observations from studies of mitochondria of senescent rat hearts, in which the rate of Ca^{2+} uptake was reduced by about 20% in senescent compared to adult rats [96], and also from studies in aging rat brain synaptosomes [122].

At present, it is unknown whether slower Ca^{2+} uptake by mitochondria is due to a depressed function or a reduced density of Ca^{2+} uniporters. However, it is well-recognized that mitochondrial membrane potential, maintained by electrochemical gradients across the organelle, is a major driving force of Ca^{2+} influx through Ca^{2+} uniporters, and it has also been documented in a variety of cells from different animal species, including human that aged mitochondria exhibit decreased membrane potential, as demonstrated by staining of cells with fluorescent dyes including rhodamine 123, JC-1, tetramethylrhodamine methyl ester (TMRM), chloromethyl-tetramethylrosamine (CMTMR, Mitotracker Orange), and chloromethyl-X rosamine (CMX-Ros) [96–125]. Unfortunately, the changes or differences in fluorescence intensity may not precisely mirror the changes in mitochondrial membrane potential. However, the use of a tetraphenylphosphonium electrode to monitor changes in $\Delta\Psi m$ may avoid many of the problems associated with fluorescent probes [126]. Using a tetraphenylphosphonium-cation sensitive electrode, Kokoszka et al. [127] have measured $\Delta\Psi m$ in mouse liver mitochondria preparations and found a decrease of 10 mV in membrane potential in organelles derived from old mice as compared to young and middle-aged animals. Similarly, analysis of the distribution of labeled tetraphenylphosphonium revealed several distinct subpopulations of hepatocytes from old but not young rats indicating marked heterogeneity in mitochondrial membrane potential in aging [128]. Although 10% of cells from old rats maintained the same $\Delta\Psi m$ (154 mV) as young animals, 65% were depolarized by 60 mV and 25% exhibited dramatic depolarization by more than 80 mV. Using a multichannel system equipped with tetraphenylphosphonium (TTP+)-selective probe and a Ca^{2+}-selective electrode, Jahangir et al. [96] found that senescent cardiac mitochondria displayed both a 15% reduction in membrane potential and a significantly slower rate of mitochondrial Ca^{2+} uptake compared to adult mitochondria. Taken together, it is reasonable to conclude that decreased mitochondrial membrane potential is a prominent feature of aging cells, which is most likely responsible for the reduced mitochondrial Ca^{2+} uptake. However, whether changes in expression or density of the Ca^{2+} uniporter within the mitochondria are the primary cause of aging-mediated decline in mitochondrial Ca^{2+}uptake remains undetermined. Changes in Ca^{2+} affinity and cooperativity of the uniporter have been demonstrated in synaptosomes of senescent rats [119]. The eventual determination of the gene sequence and structure of the mitochondrial Ca^{2+} uniporter should allow further clarification of the age-mediated regulation of its expression and provide further insight into its role in aging-mediated channelopathy.

Reduced Ca^{2+} content in mitochondria with aging may also be associated with increased mitoPTP opening or increased Ca^{2+} extrusion through Ca^{2+}antiporters. Enhanced activation of mitoPTP has been reported in a variety of aged or senescent cells including lymphocytes, neurons, hepatocytes, and cardiac myocytes [94, 125, 129–131]. One measure of mitoPTP activation is its susceptibility to Ca^{2+} load as assessed by mitochondrial Ca^{2+} retention capacity (CRC) in isolated mitochondria [94]. Upon exposure to a sequence of Ca^{2+} pulses, energized mitochondria accumulate Ca^{2+} until a threshold matrix load is reached promoting opening of the mitoPTP, in association with an abrupt release of accumulated $Ca^{2+}$from mitochondria. In addition, Goodell and Cortopassi have reported that mitoPTP rates in response to 20 mM Ca^{2+}were significantly faster in hepatocyte mitochondria from old mice compared to mitochondria from young adult mice [129]. A reduced threshold for calcium-induced, cyclosporin-sensitive calcium release, was demonstrated in isolated brain and liver mitochondria by Mather and Rottenberg [131]. Subsequently, this group reported that the enhanced activation of the mitochondrial permeability transition in T lymphocytes of old mice is likely responsible for the aging-induced attenuation of sustained elevation of cell free calcium (in response to ionomycin) and Ca^{2+} signaling in T lymphocytes [125]. Interestingly, heart mitochondria from 24 month old senescent Fischer 344 rats when challenged with consecutive 15 nmoles Ca^{2+}pulses accumulated Ca^{2+} for 3–4 pulses compared to seven pulses for mitochondria from young adult rat heart [96]. This resulted in nearly a 45% reduction in the overall Ca^{2+} retained in senescent compared to adult mitochondria. Taking into account the 20% reduction in Ca^{2+} uptake, a large amount of Ca^{2+} might "leak" out from aged mitochondria. Furthermore, increased susceptibility of mitoPTP opening to Ca^{2+}, which likely arises from reduced mitochondrial membrane potential may result in enhancement of Na^{+}-independent Ca^{2+} extrusion in aged mitochondria.

Another possibility leading to decreased mitochondrial matrix Ca^{2+} levels may be linked to age-associated changes in mitochondrial NCX activity or expression; altered activity or expression of sarcolemmal NCX has been reported in aging cells [132, 133, 134]. However, it is presently undetermined whether mitochondrial NCX is involved in disturbed Ca^{2+} handling in aging despite its critical role as the major mechanism to extrude mitochondrial Ca^{2+} and in maintaining a certain amount of matrix Ca^{2+} under physiological condition.

It should be noted that reduced mitochondrial Ca^{2+} content may have deleterious effects on mitochondrial function including ATP synthesis because of the involvement of Ca^{2+} in the activation of mitochondrial Ca^{2+}-dependent dehydrogenases, which control substrate oxidative phosphorylation. Several studies have reported that mitochondrial ATP production is decreased in aging albeit in a tissue-specific manner [135–137]. Drew et al. [135, 138] reported that with age, ATP content and production decreased by approximately 50% in isolated rat mitochondria from gastrocnemius muscle, although no effect was noted in the heart, brain or liver. On the other hand, Jahangir et al. [96] reported an aging-associated 58% decrease in ADP-stimulated mitochondrial respiration rate and 23% reduction in ATP production rate in cardiac mitochondria from 24 month old Fischer rats. Recently, an estimated 8% per decade reduction in mitochondrial ATP production rate has been found in aged human skeletal muscle [136]. Therefore, the efficiency of ATP synthesis in aging mitochondria is reduced in some tissues, which is not only associated with reduction in mitochondrial respiratory enzyme complex (i.e., I, II, and IV) activities [137, 139], but also with reduced matrix Ca^{2+}, and the functional depression of mitochondrial Ca^{2+}-dependent dehydrogenases. PDH activity, rate-limiting enzyme for glucose oxidation, was found to be reduced by 40% in brain tissues from patients with autopsy-confirmed Alzheimer's disease (AD) [140], though conflicting results have been obtained from aged animals [141]. Also, NAD-ICD activity was decreased in aged rat brain, skeletal muscle, and heart suggesting defective activity of the TCA cycle in aged mitochondria [142–145]. Furthermore, glycerol-3-phosphate dehydrogenase, an important enzyme that transfers electrons from glycerol-3-phosphate to the mitochondrial ETC was also decreased in aged skeletal muscle [142] and this may have an inhibitory effect on ETC efficiency. Finally, at present it is unknown to what extent reduced matrix Ca^{2+} content influences the TCA cycle and ATP synthesis efficiency in aged mitochondria.

Mitochondrial K^+ Channels

K^+ Uniporter/K_{ATP} Channel

Net K^+ flux across the inner mitochondrial membrane is extremely important for the control of mitochondrial volume. Mitochondrial K^+ uptake is primarily mediated by diffusive leak through a K^+ uniporter driven by the high electrical membrane potential maintained by redox-driven, electrogenic proton ejection and K^+ efflux is regulated by an 82-kDa inner membrane K^+/H^+ antiporter.

Mitochondrial K^+-selective channels were first reported by Inoue et al. who described a K^+ current with a conductance of ~10 pS recorded in fused giant mitoplasts prepared from rat liver using inside-out patch clamp technique [146]. Its activity was further confirmed in studies with liposomes and lipid bilayers reconstituted with proteins partially prepared from the inner membranes of mitochondria [147–149]. This channel (shown in Fig. 11.2) is blocked not only by ATP with a K_i of 0.8 mM but also by a number of inhibitors including antidiabetic sulfonylureas, 5-hydrodecanoic acid (5-HD), MCC-134, as well as plasma membrane K_{ATP} channel blockers 4-aminopyridine (4-AP), glibenclamide, glipizide, glimepiride, and HMR 1098 and is activated by potassium channel openers (KCOs) [150], and reactive free radicals (superoxide anion) [148].

While the sarcolemmal K_{ATP} channels are composed of heteromultimeric complexes of regulatory sulfonylurea receptors (SUR) and potassium inward rectifier (Kir) subunits, the molecular identity of mitoK_{ATP} channels is not yet completely known. Reports from a number of different laboratories suggest that the mitoK_{ATP} channel like the sarcolemmal K_{ATP} channel belongs to the inward rectifier K^+ channel family [149, 151]. Using immunofluorescence and immunogold staining, it has been shown that the pore-forming α-subunits of sarcolemmal K_{ATP} channels, Kir 6.1, are also present in rat skeletal muscle and liver mitochondria [152]. In addition, using immunohistochemistry and *in situ* hybridization this subunit was localized in rat brain mitochondria. Recently, using antibodies and confocal microscopy, Singh et al. [153] found that both Kir 6.1 and Kir 6.2 subunits were localized to mitochondria of rat ventricular myocytes. In brain mitochondria, similar findings were reported as well [154]. On the other hand, the presence of either known sulfonylurea receptors (SUR1 or SUR2 subunits) in the mitochondria appears to be questionable, though it has been suggested that SUR2A-subunit might exist in rat cardiac mitochondria [153]. Furthermore, other components are potentially present in the mitoK_{ATP} channel, which may be responsible for distinguishing its responses from the sarcolemmal K_{ATP} channel [150].

Recent studies have suggested that activation of PKCepsilon leads to an increase in Kir6.2-containing K_{ATP} channels localized in mitochondria [155]. Nevertheless, the lack of agreed upon structure for the mitoK_{ATP} channel including a well-defined pore forming subunit has hampered a more complete understanding of its role and significance in IPC and of its demonstrated cardiprotective role by modulating mitochondrial membrane potential, energy metabolism and apoptosis as discussed below.

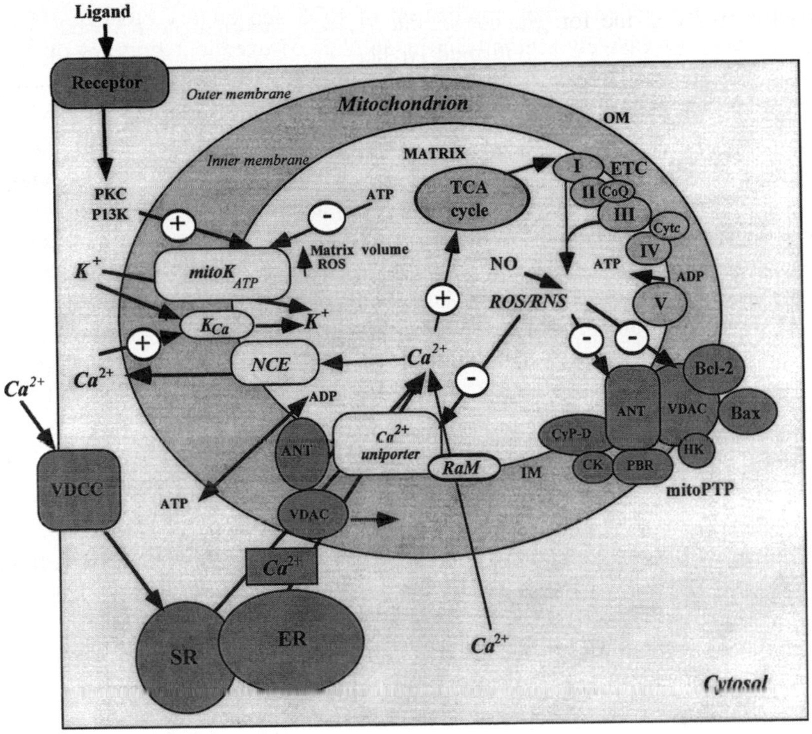

Fig. 11.2 Mitochondrial Ion channels in aging
The opening of mitochondrial K^+ channels (mitoK_{ATP}) in the inner membrane normally triggered by ROS, ATP levels, ligands binding to an assortment of membrane receptors and the involvement of protein kinases (PKC, P13K), which can mediate cytoprotection are affected with aging. In addition to K^+ influx, matrix volume and ROS levels are affected by the opening of these channels. Mitochondrial K^+ influx is also mediated by the K_{Ca} channel, which is activated by Ca^{2+}. Ca^{2+} enters the mitochondria via an aging-regulated uniporter (with VDAC involvement) and by the RaM transporter; increased mitochondrial Ca^{2+} can activate enzymes of the TCA cycle, ETC and complex V as well as modulate the opening of the mitoPTP; Ca^{2+} efflux is primarily managed by the Na^+/Ca^{2+} exchanger (NCE). Ca^{2+} can also enter the mitochondria as can a large number of small metabolites via the mitoPTP opening The major proteins comprising the mitoPTP at contact sites, adjoining the inner (IM) and outer mitochondrial (OM) membranes, including hexokinase (HK), adenine nucleotide translocator (ANT), creatine kinase (CK), cyclophilin-D (CyP-D), porin (VDAC) and the peripheral benzodiazepine receptor (PBR) as well as the VDAC-associated proapoptotic protein (e.g., Bax) and antiapoptotic protein (Bcl-2), whose competition is paramount in apoptotic cell death are also shown. Aging affects VDAC and ANT proteins, mainly by ROS/RNS oxidative damage.

Mitochondrial K_{ATP} Channel in Aging

The biological significance of mitochondrial K_{ATP} channels in cardiac function and cardioprotection has attracted a great deal of attention. Gathered observations indicated that the mitochondrial K_{ATP} channels play a crucial role in endogenous cardioprotection, and K_{ATP} channel openers can prevent myocardial I/R injury in both organ and cell levels. Numerous studies have suggested that the protective effects of ischemic (IPC) and pharmacologic preconditioning (induced by anesthetics, adenosine receptor agonists, PKC activators, opioid agonists, adrenergic receptor agonists, nitric oxide releasers, B_2-bradykinin receptor agonists, M_2-muscarinic receptor agonists, and AT1-receptor antagonists) involve the activation of mitoK_{ATP} channels. The opening of mitoK_{ATP} under conditions of high mitochondrial membrane potential leads to matrix alkalinization and consequently to generation of moderate levels of ROS, which may beneficially trigger the activation of multi-signaling pathways responsible for cardioprotection [156]. This finding is further supported by evidence that application of ROS scavengers blocked IPC. This important finding has been extensively studied and a number of excellent reviews on the subject are available [150, 157–160].

It has been suggested that mitoK_{ATP} opening participates in the regulation of mitochondrial bioenergetics in cardiac myocytes [158, 161–163]. since drug-induced opening of mitoK_{ATP} causes profound uncoupling of mitochondrial oxidative phosphorylation, decreased mitochondrial membrane potential, and a decline in mitochondrial Ca^{2+} uptake [164–166]. Reduced membrane potential has also been observed in liver mitochondria treated with a mitoK_{ATP} opener [167], although diazoxide or pinacidil-induced opening of mitoK_{ATP} channels was found to have little direct effect on mitochondrial bioenergetics or respiration [163]. The uptake of K^+ by the mitoK_{ATP} channels also plays a role in the regulation of mitochondrial steady-state matrix volume. Several studies have suggested that the effects of K_{ATP} channels on mitochondrial bioenergetics may depend on both the work-state of myocytes with a high-work state associated with transient mitochondrial swelling, preservation of intermembrane structure and permeability to adenine nucleotides (i.e., ADP and ATP) as well as in response to ischemic insult [163, 168].

An important issue is whether age-association in alterations in mitoK_{ATP} are involved in mitochondrial defects associated with aging heart, since a significant decline in the density of sarcolemmal K_{ATP} channels (stemming from decreased levels of the SUR2A subunit) has been reported with aging in female guinea pigs as we previously noted [89]. That mitoK_{ATP} channels are impacted in aging has been suggested (albeit indirectly) by observations that aging animals display a reduced myocardial tolerance to I/R injury and an impaired cardioprotection from either IPC [169–171] or anesthetic preconditioning [172, 173]. In addition, other aspects of the preconditioning signaling cascade may be age-sensitive as well.

Lesnefsky et al. [170] have reported that aged rat hearts subjected to I/R exhibited more severe tissue and function damage than adult, suggesting an increased susceptibility to damage in elderly hearts. This phenomenon was thereafter confirmed in different species of animal models and in humans by a number of investigators. In young and adult hearts, an endogenous cardioprotective mechanism can be called into play against lethal challenges when the myocardium or myocytes are preconditioned by a number of sublethal stimuli. This preconditioning mechanism has been found to be insufficient in aged or senescent hearts in experimental animal models [169–175] and in aging humans [176–178].

Since mitoK_{ATP} channel activation is generally considered a contributory effector component in the preconditioning pathway (and may be involved as well in the triggering mechanism of the IPC response, mitoK_{ATP} channel defects may in part lead to ineffective preconditioning in aging hearts [179]. This assumption was tested by studies with isolated Langendorff-perfused hearts from young, middle-aged, and aged Sprague-Dawley rats [175]. One of the intriguing findings was that pretreatment with the mitoK_{ATP} channel opener diazoxide alone failed to produce cardiac protection against I/R in aged rats (age 20 months) although it caused full protection in young adult rats. Furthermore, Lee et al. [176] reported that defective IPC in a cohort of elderly patients could be overcome by the administration of nicorandil, another mitoK_{ATP} channel specific opener, and therefore the aging-mediated decline in IPC effectiveness was attributed to attenuated activation of mitoK_{ATP} channels. Recently the protective effects of mitoK_{ATP} channel opening have been assessed in mature and aged (but not senescent) male and female rabbit hearts against I/R injury [180]. The results of this study demonstrated marked infarct-limiting effects of diazoxide treatment in both mature male and female hearts leading to postischemic functional recovery, whereas benefits of this KCO treatment were more limited in the aged male heart and entirely absent in the aged female heart. These data further suggest that defective function of mitoK_{ATP} channels is more severe in aged female heart.

Although there is evidence that the cardioprotective signaling pathways acting through mitoK_{ATP} channels may be compromised with aging, it is unknown whether aging-attenuated cardiac mitoK_{ATP} channel function is due to changes in their density/number, responsiveness to stress stimuli, or defective communication to downstream effectors (e.g., respiratory ETC). Single channel recordings have shown that the opening and the density of surface sarcolemmal K_{ATP} channels in skeletal muscle were reduced in aging rat [181]. Since mitoK_{ATP} channels likely consist of similar components, pore-forming subunits (Kir 6.1 and Kir 6.2) and regulatory subunits analogous to the sulfonylurea receptor (SUR2), these channels may undergo aging-mediated alterations resembling those in sarcolemmal K_{ATP}. These changes in ion channel function might be regarded as defining an age-associated channelopathy. The modulation of this channel's cardioprotective capacity by diverse signaling ligands (e.g., adenosine and bradykinin) and specific channel openers/closers may be useful in blunting or reversing this aging-mediated channel dysfunction.

The negative effects of mitoK_{ATP} channel defect in aging can also be inferred from its physiological roles in regulating mitochondrial function. The opening of mitoK_{ATP} channels increases K^+ influx leading to increased matrix K^+, and mitochondrial matrix swelling which not only reverses matrix contraction caused by OXPHOS but also may improve fatty acid oxidation, ATP production and help to keep VDAC closed due to space expansion, thereby reducing the rate of ATP hydrolysis [168]. In addition, elevated matrix K^+ results in a small but significant reduction of the mitochondrial membrane potential which reduces the electrogenic driving force for Ca^{2+} uptake through Ca^{2+} uniporter and inhibits mitoPTP opening. Also increased mitochondrial matrix K^+ increases ROS production from ETC [182–185], that activates a wide range of kinases and triggers signaling cascades essential for preconditioning [186–188]. On the other hand, the defect in mitoK_{ATP} channels in aging are likely not so severe and may be masked or compensated by other mechanisms. Probably, the largest influence that aging-altered mitoK_{ATP} channels exert is by increasing the threshold of the myocytes in response to damaging stimuli such that the mitoK_{ATP} channels become less sensitive to stress signals and increased IPC regimens are necessary to promote effective CP in aging animals and humans [175, 176].

Mitochondrial PTP

The mitoPTP was described more than three decades ago following the discovery that energized mitochondria undergo a sudden permeability increase of the inner membrane to solutes of molecular mass up to ~1.5kDa as a result of Ca^{2+} accumulation [101]. The mitoPTP is a regulated pore and also a large-conducting, voltage-dependent, non-selective channel with a diameter of about 3.0 nm. The permeability of this channel can be modulated by factors including anoxia, ROS, and changes in the energetic balance of mitochondria. Although the channel is a complex entity comprised of VDAC at the outer membrane, the adenine nucleotide translocase (ANT) in the inner membrane, and cyclophilin-D (CyP-D) in the mitochondrial matrix [189], (shown in Fig. 11.2), interactions with other proteins including the peripheral benzodiazepine receptor, Bax and Bcl-2 (in the outer membrane), creatine kinase (CK, in the intermembrane space), and hexokinase (HK-1 or II, tethered to VDAC on the cytosolic face of the outer membrane) have also been reported.

Mitochondrial PTP in Aging

Under physiological conditions, the mitochondrial inner membrane is impermeable to almost all metabolites and ions, and the mitoPTP is in a closed conformation, which is essential for normal mitochondrial function. Under some stress conditions such as I/R, oxidative stress (OS), and Ca^{2+} overload, the mitoPTP undergo conformational change, form a non-selective channel, and allow passive diffusion of solutes with molecular masses up to about 1.5 kDa to cross the inner and outer membranes, but do not permit matrix proteins (with masses larger than the mitoPTP exclusion limit) to diffuse through the pore. Therefore, the osmotic force of matrix proteins results in accumulation of water and small molecular solutes increasing matrix volume or matrix swelling. An immediate consequence of mitoPTP opening is the collapse of mitochondrial membrane potential. As a consequence, oxygen consumption is initially increased and ATP produced by glycolysis is hydrolyzed (by the reverse operation of F_0F_1 ATPase leading to ATP depletion) [94, 190, 191]. Severe matrix swelling leads to further rupture of the outer membrane releasing proapoptotic factors like cytochrome *c*, triggering irreversible cell death.

Age-associated increase in mitoPTP opening was first demonstrated in liver [129], and in lymphocyte mitochondria from old mice [130]. Initially, the sensitivity of mitoPTP was assessed by the so-called calcium retention capacity (CRC) [192]. Later, defects in CRC were demonstrated in isolated brain and liver mitochondria from 20 month-old mice [125]. In these studies the age-related dysfunction was attributed to mitoPTP, based on the discovery that *in vitro* CRC and swelling rate of mitochondria from old animals could be restored to control values upon addition of cyclosporin (CsA). Furthermore, increased susceptibility to mitoPTP opening in heart mitochondria has been reported as a reduced CRC in preparations from 24 month-old Fischer 344 rats [96]. In our laboratory, we have found that the opening of mitoPTP, evaluated by mitochondrial swelling, was significantly greater in mitochondria from senescent Fischer 344 rats (30 month-old) than from young adult (Marin–Garcia et al. unpublished data). These data suggest that the mitoPTP complex is susceptible to Ca^{2+} load in the mitochondrial matrix, although this phenomenon has not yet been demonstrated in myocardium *in vivo*; evidence of increased cell death in aged rat heart [193], and skeletal muscle [194], supports the likelihood of mitoPTP opening *in vivo*.

It is not yet clear why the mitochondrial mitoPTP undergoes functional changes during aging. As we have discussed in previous chapters, with aging, there is increased OS in somatic cells, which tends to be more prevalent in those cells rich in mitochondria, such as cardiomyocytes whose mitochondrial respiratory activity is elevated. Increased oxidative damage to proteins by ROS or reactive nitrogen species (RNS) has been broadly implicated in aging, and can be gauged by elevated levels of protein carboxyls and nitrated residues as noted in Chapter 4.

Mitochondria are not only considered the major source but also the targets of ROS during the aging process, and increased mitochondrial ROS formation would be expected to cause mitochondrial protein oxidative damage in the senescent animals [195, 196]. Of particular interest, because of its dual role in mitochondrial bioenergetic metabolism and as a putative component of the mitoPTP, ANT has recently been found to be one of the mitochondrial proteins most susceptible to ROS during aging [197], and this ANT oxidative damage is mostly displayed as carbonylation. Increased ANT carbonyl modification has been found in aged houseflies [197], as well as in aging mammalian species [198]. In addition, ANT contains three redox-sensitive cysteine residues on loops projecting into the matrix compartment. These residues are particularly susceptible to oxidation by sulfenic acid moieties and mixed disulfides if the normally high intramitochondrial glutathione (GSH)/glutathione disulfide (GSSG) ratio is not maintained during periods of OS [199]. Indeed, GSH/GSSG ratio is significantly reduced during aging [200–204]. ANT carbonyl modification is associated with a reduced capability to exchange ADT/ATP across the inner membrane, which may cause the inhibition or uncoupling of OXPHOS and the collapse of $\Delta\Psi m$, turning mitochondrial ATP synthesis into hydrolysis. Moreover, ANT oxidation may also shift from its native state as a gated pore (mediating ADP/ATP exchange) into a non-selective pore, allowing free permeation of small ions and metabolites across the inner membrane.

ANT conformation conversion is affected by cyclophilin-D (CyP-D) in the mitochondrial matrix. CyP-D contains a relatively high proportion of polyunsaturated fatty acids that could be oxidized by ROS to generate highly reactive lipid fragments such as 4-hydroxy-2-nonenal (HNE) and 4-hydroxy-hexenal (HHE). These lipid peroxidation by-products may interact with or modify specific thiol groups on ANT leading to adduct formation, thereby inhibiting ANT activity [205], and also increasing CyP-D binding to ANT [206, 207], thereby destabilizing ANT, and sensitizing mitoPTP to Ca^{2+} [208].

The mitochondrial outer membrane protein VDAC appears also to be particularly targeted in aging. VDAC (originally called porin) serves as a functional channel through which most metabolites entering or leaving the mitochondria pass, and which has been increasingly implicated as a pivotal coordinator in communication between mitochondria and cytosol, by interaction with ANT, CK, and the peripheral benzodiazepine receptor under both physiological and pathological conditions [209, 210]. The conductance of VDAC has been found to be voltage or $\Delta\Psi m$ dependent with marked ion selectivity. Highest conductance occurs at low potential, with preference for anions such as phosphate, chloride, adenosine nucleotides, and other metabolites, while the sub-conductance states occurring at higher positive or negative potential are associated with a shift to small cations and impermeability to ATP and ADP. The closure of VDAC prevents the efficient exchange of ATP and ADP between cytosol and mitochondria. In addition, VDAC contains Ca^{2+} binding sites and participates in the regulation of the mitochondrial Ca^{2+} homeostasis [209, 211]. Moreover, as noted above, VDAC constitutes another mitoPTP component which has been shown to interact directly with proapoptotic stimuli and proteins including Bax resulting in cytochrome *c* permeation through the outer membrane [212–214]. As noted in Chapter 4, tyrosine residues in proteins are particularly vulnerable to oxidative damage and subject to conversion into 3-nitrotyrosine (3-NT) by reactive nitrogen species including NO and peroxynitrite ($ONOO^-$), which are normally produced under physiologic condition and increased with aging. This nitration of tyrosine can compromise the functional and/or structural integrity of target protein [215]. Kanski et al. [216] employing proteomic analysis using 2-D gel electrophoresis combined with nanoelectrospray ionization-tandem mass spectrometry (NSI-MS/MS) revealed that there is an age-dependent nitration of VDAC in mitochondria. Increased VDAC nitration is very likely related to excessive OS in mitochondria since similar changes have been found in diabetic hearts, which exhibit enhanced OS [217]. Importantly, it remains to be determined whether aging-mediated oxidative modification of tyrosine residues directly alters the property of VDAC or sensitize VDAC to its regulators in an *in vivo* model. Cell studies have demonstrated that superoxide anions can induce VDAC-dependent rapid and massive cytochrome *c* release and enhance mitoPTP to Ca^{2+} in permeabilized HepG2 cells [218].

Ca^{2+} is also a key trigger for mitoPTP formation, possibly by binding to the negatively charged cardiolipin head groups on the inner face of the inner membrane, thereby disrupting the stabilizing interactions between cardiolipin and ANT [219]. Since mitochondrial Ca^{2+} content tends to decrease with aging as noted above, the impaired mitochondrial Ca^{2+} handling and reduced threshold of mitoPTP to Ca^{2+} may be critical in further mediating mitoPTP in aging. Moreover, in response to stress such as I/R, heart mitochondrial Ca^{2+} significantly increased with aging (about two-fold greater in senescent animals) indicative of Ca^{2+}overload potentiating mitoPTP opening [97]. Taking these findings together with the evidence of increased lipid peroxidation (e.g., HNE formation, as discussed above) in senescent hearts on reperfusion, it seems that aging hearts are increasingly vulnerable to reperfusion damage brought about by increased mitochondrial Ca^{2+} and OS, the twin triggers for mitoPTP formation. Other factors such as age-dependent increased CK nitration [219, 220], age-dependent decreased hexokinase levels [221, 222], and decreased nucleotide pool [223]. may also facilitate the formation of ANT-VDAC complex, or sensitize mitoPTP promoting permeability transition during the aging.

Pharmacogenetics/Pharmacogenomics in Dysrhythmias/Channelopathies of Aging

Pharmacogenetics and Pharmacogenomics

In the past many marketed drugs, including antidysrhythmics, were withdrawn by the pharmaceutical companies because of the occurrence of prodysrhythmic effects including some with lethal consequences. The related fields of pharmacogenomics and pharmacogenetics appear to have the potential to improve drug development by tailoring drug therapy based mainly on the individual's ability to metabolize drugs which are determined only in part by age, and influenced by disease, environmental factors (e.g., diet), concurrent medications and variant genetic factors specifying the transport, metabolism and targets of the drug. The availability of new pharmacogenetic tests may allow pharmaceutical companies and the physician to identify those individuals who are at risk for severe dysrhythmias.

Genes polymorphisms including SNPs, frequently associated with different types of dysrhythmia phenotypes, may directly affect the heart electrical activity and these gene variants often interact differentially with drug therapy. For example, the voltage-gated potassium channel α subunit KCNE2 protein is expressed in the ventricles, and under different pathophysiological conditions, such as myocardial ischemia and aging, it can play diverse roles in modulating ventricular electrical activity. Careful use of certain drugs with variable interactions with the genetic background may be possible in the future if rapid and affordable genetic screening of defective genes becomes available; nonetheless, this may only apply to the more common polymorphisms predisposing to acquired dysrhythmias, such as T8A and Q9E in *MiRP1* (also known as *KCNE2),* or Y1102 in *SCN5A* (the sodium channel α subunit) [224].

On the other hand, specific DNA polymorphisms may make an individual insensitive to some medications, affecting the overall response to therapy. For example, two variants polymorphisms (P532L and R578K) in the *KCNA5* gene which encodes the α subunit of the I_{Kur} current, both residing in the C-terminus, were found to be resistant to block by quinidine [225]. Furthermore, particular drugs may affect more than just one gene or protein. In a review on the antidysrhythmic potential of the Kv1.5 channel blocker in treating atrial dysrhythmias, Brendel and Peukert noted that these blockers were not selective since they blocked other ion channels [226]. On the other hand, it appears that the additional inhibition of Kv4.3 and K_{ACh} by these compounds may be beneficial in their antidysrhythmic effects, or at least does not affect the atrial selectivity of a Kv1.5 blocker. However, it is worth noting that marked block of I_{K1}, HERG or Na^+ channels may lead to the loss of atrial selectivity thus increasing the risk of lethal ventricular prodysrhythmia.

Since some patients achieve the desired therapeutic response, while others do not, with a subset of patients experiencing variable adverse effects that ranges from mild to life threatening, it is evident that genetics may be an important contributor to this variable drug response. Pharmacogenomics is a field focused on unraveling the genetic determinants of variable drug response. While current research is largely focused on a limited candidate gene approach, which allows for description of significant genetic associations with variable response, it often does not explain the genetic basis of variable drug response enough to be useful clinically [227]. Given that most drug responses involve a large number of proteins, all of whose genes could have several polymorphisms, it seems unlikely that a single polymorphism in a single gene would explain a high degree of drug response variability in a consistent fashion, suggesting that a polygenic, or genomic approach might be more appropriate [228, 229].

Undoubtedly, pharmacogenomics has the potential to improve the use of cardiovascular drugs, particularly in the elderly, through the selection of the most appropriate drug therapy in an individual, based on their genetic information. However, it may take some time before the available genetic information is widely used in making drug therapy decisions, although it is evident that new and important findings in this area will continue to appear, and the experimental approaches will continue to evolve.

Conclusions

The pathophysiology of cardiovascular aging, like aging in any other system in human, is a complex process involving multiple cellular and molecular changes, all part of the multiple phenotypes of aging. For example, aging has significant deleterious effect on the cardiac conduction system,

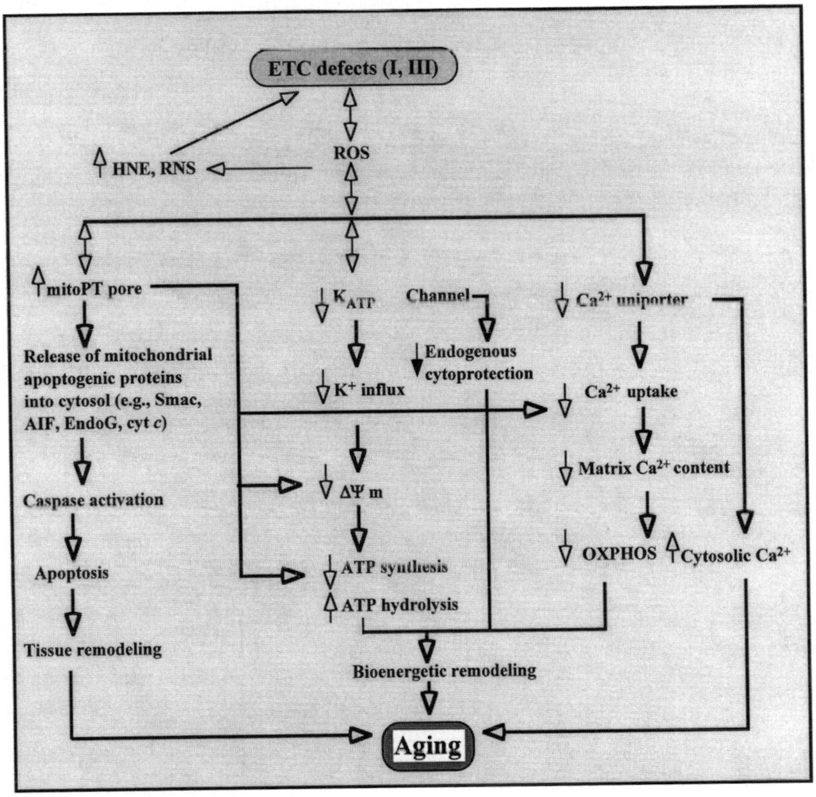

Fig. 11.3 Remodeling resulting from the aging-modulation of mitochondrial ion function
Mitochondrial ETC defects result in electron leak, ROS overproduction followed by formation of reactive nitrogen species (RNS) and lipid peroxidation (e.g., HNE). Increased oxidative stress in turn damages mitochondrial ion channel function. Sensitized mitoPTP causes loss of mitochondrial Ca^{2+}, decreased Ca^{2+} uptake, and reduced $\Delta\Psi_m$, which in turn reduces OXPHOS and ATP synthesis; increased mitoPTP also promotes increased mitochondrial vulnerability to Ca^{2+}loading and the release of apoptogenic factors (e.g., AIF, cyt *c*) from the mitochondria which sets into motion the apoptotic pathway including caspase activation leading to cell death. Mitochondrial K_{ATP} is also targeted in aging resulting in reduced cardiac tolerance to stress and loss of preconditioning cytoprotection; moreover, decreased K^+ influx and electrochemical gradient results in diminished OXPHOS. Reduced Ca^{2+} uniporter activity not only decreases mitochondrial Ca^{2+} uptake, dampening Ca^{2+} stimulatory effects on mitochondrial bioenergetic metabolism but also exaggerates intracellular Ca^{2+} disturbance leading to elevated cytosolic Ca^{2+} levels. Also shown (as indicated by double-headed arrows), is that mitoK_{ATP} and mitoPTP channel modulation can trigger ROS production, which can further target ETC activities, as does increased HNE. HNE: 4-hydroxyl-2-nonal; cyt *c*: cytochrome *c*; AIF: apoptosis inducing factor; $\Delta\Psi_m$: mitochondrial membrane potential. Lighter vertical arrows indicate reduced or increased levels whereas denser arrows denote relationship within a pathway.

and processes leading to sinus node dysfunction and AV block are common in the elderly. Besides advances in pharmacotherapy and pharmacogenomics (see above section), in the last 3–4 decades through technological advances, refined pacing therapies, and advanced algorithms and database resources now provide the physician with a wealth of clinically important information. While adding to the complexity of pacing therapy, these features, if used correctly, can lead to improve the outcomes and quality of life in many patients. Therefore, it is important for cardiologists/physicians involved in care of the elderly to clearly understand pacing therapy and to consider its potential application.

With aging the ion channels undergo functional and/or structural changes that are not only associated with cellular dysfunction but which also may contribute to the progression of cellular senescence and defining the age-associated channelopathy. Of particular interest the mitochondrial ion channels, particularly K^+ channels, Ca^{2+} channels, and megachannel (mitoPTP), play pivotal roles in the communication between mitochondria and cytosol, regulation of intracellular Ca^{2+} homeostasis, mitochondrial bioenergetic, metabolism, and modulation of cell survival and death. However, with aging these ion channels undergo functional and/or structural alterations, which are not only associated with the development of mitochondrial dysfunction but also contribute to the progression of cellular senescence (Fig. 11.3) defining an age-associated channelopathy.

Blockade or reversal of ion channel degeneration may improve not only mitochondrial function but it may also be beneficial in slowing the process of aging. Furthermore, elucidation of the genetic structure of the molecular components of these channels will lead to the identification of mutational or polymorphic gene variants which mediate the effects of aging, therapeutic treatments or diverse physiological stimuli on channel function. Increased awareness that with aging the incidence of dysrhythmias and channelopathies increase may lead to better management and further research interest in the search for the basic molecular mechanisms that underly aging. Furthermore, this will significantly enhance our understanding of the spectrum of aging phenotypes.

Summary

- Defects in the heart rate and rhythm (dysrhythmias) increase with aging.
- Compared to young adults a higher incidence of atrial dysrhythmias, including atrial premature beats, atrial fibrillation (AF), atrioventricular block (AV block), and ST-T changes are present in the elderly with an otherwise normal heart.
- Paroxysmal supraventricular tachycardia (PSVT), ventricular tachycardia (VT) and ventricular blocks in the aging individual are mainly associated with structural cardiac defects. Furthermore, age-related changes also include increased activity of the sympathetic nervous system, which may be an important pathophysiological component in tachydysrhythmias and premature ventricular contractions.
- Screening of a significant number of individuals with dysrhythmias has led to the discovery of numerous mutated genes, in particular those encoding subunits of proteins that constitute the cardiac ion channels.
- Aging does not effect the activation of the sympathetic nervous system occurring in HF, suggesting that other factors such as CAD and MI may impact the increased incidence of HF with aging.
- Cardiac electrophysiological studies using a number of animal models have significantly contributed to our knowledge of the changes occurring with aging.
- The effect of aging on the electrophysiological properties of the left atrium (LA), and in particular on specific LA sites and in ouabain-induced dysrhythmias in rabbits have been recently evaluated.
- LA regional heterogeneity and LAPW dysrhythmogenesis appear to increase with aging.

- Experimental studies in animal models have provided key insights on the correlation of changes in ion channels affecting protein expression, with changes in ventricular activity and dysrhythmias.
- With age there is an increased incidence of SA node dysfunction with the highest prevalence found in the elderly population.
- Extensive atrial remodeling occurring in aging provides a mechanism not only for SND but also for other atrial dysrhythmias, mainly AF, which may develop in up to 50% of patients with SND.
- With aging, $Ca_v1.2$ protein decreased together with a reduction in spontaneous activity of SA node. This decrease in turn increases susceptibility of the node to L-type Ca^{2+} channel blockers.
- The loss of $Ca_v1.2$ channels together with depletion of Cx43 protein not only will decrease electrical conductivity but also will increase the chances for SA node dysfunction with age as well as the prevalence of dysrhythmias.
- Ionic currents differ in aged versus adult right atrial cells, such that a reduced Ca^{2+} current and augmented outward currents could contribute significantly to the altered AP contour of the aged RA cell.
- AVNRT is the most common regular supraventricular tachycardia in the elderly patients.
- In patients older than 65 years, AVN-RT may lead to severe, sometimes life-threatening symptoms, despite the fact that the tachycardia is not as fast as in younger patients.
- AF is the most common dysrhythmia seen in the elderly. It involves extensive remodeling of the cardiomyocyte electrical properties, ECM and fibrosis, and in the aging heart it could lead to acute HF, without clinically apparent cardiac disease.
- Atrial structural remodeling is a key determinant and by itself can initiate AF, without the need for preexisting repolarization gradients.
- Aging is frequently associated with progressive AV conduction system disorders affecting the SA node, AV node, and/or the His bundle branch-Purkinje system.
- The elderly are prone to develop symptomatic bradydysrhythmias that may require pacemaker implantation.
- In addition to extracellular changes, with aging apoptosis may play a significant role in the development of AV block since apoptosis appears to be one of the physiologic processes responsible for the normal reduction in AV node size observed from fetus to adulthood.
- Histological studies from patients who developed isolated AV block demonstrated an increase in fine collagen fibers in and around the AV node and His-Purkinje system.
- Mutations in the SCN5A gene have been associated with hereditary Lenègre/Lev disease initially described as an acquired complete AV block with RBBB or LBBB and widening QRS complexes.
- In women, the increased risk associated with prolonged QT for cardiac death was more pronounced than in men, and risks estimates did not change after adjustment for potential confounders, including history of myocardial infarction, hypertension and diabetes mellitus.
- Abnormal QTc prolongation on the electrocardiogram should be viewed as an independent risk factor for sudden cardiac death.
- Studies on the effect of age and gender on QT dispersion have shown that elderly males have significantly greater QT and QTc dispersion than elderly female.
- Age and gender have different, genotype-specific modulating effects on the probability of cardiac events and electrocardiographic presentation in LQT1 and LQT2 patients.
- Syncope, a common occurrence in the elderly, is often associated with a worse outcome than in adult patients requiring complementary tests, such as tilt-table test (TTT).
- Guidelines update for implantation of pacemakers and antidysrhythmia devices and their indications have been classified in several categories by the ACC/AHA/NASPE in 2002.

- Since the publication of the above recommendations, the indications for pacemaker therapy in the elderly have continued to evolve including as an adjunct therapy in advanced stages of HF and in dysrhythmias unresponsive to medical therapy (e.g., adjunct therapy for AF).
- Aging is associated with an increase in both the prevalence and complexity of PVBs; these can be single (uniform or multiform), in couplets, or in short runs of ventricular tachycardia. In the absence of cardiac functional or structural defects there are not apparent increases in cardiac mortality in these individuals.
- There are important differences in the electrophysiologic characteristics of patients with VT versus those with VF since ventricular dysrhythmias recurrence at follow-up was different in patients who presented with VT than in those who originally presented with VF.
- With aging ion channels undergo functional and/or structural alterations, which are not only associated with the development of cellular dysfunction but also contribute to the progression of cellular senescence, defining an age-associated channelopathy.
- Aging-associated changes in AP, I_{K1}, I_{to}, and $I_{Ca,\,L}$ of rat ventricular myocytes possibly contribute to the cardiac dysfunction of the aging heart.
- Opening of sarcolemmal K_{ATP} channels is an important endogenous cardioprotective mechanism, mainly in the aging heart.
- Aging is associated with a decrease in the number of sarcolemmal K_{ATP} channels in hearts from females, but not males. This phenomenon seems to be associated with an age-dependent decrease in concentration of circulating estrogens.
- Age-dependent decrease in the number of sarcolemmal K_{ATP} channels generates a cardiac phenotype more sensitive to ischemia, which again seems to be responsible for decrease in myocardial tolerance to stress that occurs in elderly women.
- The Cav1.2 channel protein plays an essential role in the aged-related deterioration of a functioning pacemaker. With age its protein expression decreases, and concurrently there is a reduction in the spontaneous activity of the SA node providing evidence of the significant role that Ca^{2+} channels play in the genesis of dysrhythmias associated with aging.
- Aging induces degenerative changes in action potential conduction, contributed to by the loss of Cx43 protein. Interestingly, Cx43 is a potential therapeutic target for quashing the age-related deterioration of the cardiac pacemaker.
- *Drosophila melanogaster* has emerged as one of the principal model organisms used for studying the biology of aging in general, and in particular the cardiac functional changes developing with aging. Dysfunction in KCNQ and K_{ATP} ion channel seems to contribute to the decline in heart performance in aging flies.
- *Drosophila* tends to develop an elevated incidence of cardiac dysfunction and dysrhythmias concomitantly associated with a decrease in the expression of the *Drosophila* homolog of human KCNQ1-encoded K^+ channel α-subunits. In humans, this channel is involved in myocardial repolarization, and functional defects in it are associated with increased risk for Torsades de Pointes dysrhythmias and sudden death.
- Defects in mitochondria function are tightly associated with aging, and these defects include changes in mitochondrial membrane potential ($\Delta\Psi$m) and the opening of the mitochondrial permeability transition pore (mitoPTP), essential components to the cell life-death transition and the promotion/acceleration of aging.
- Mitochondrial Ca^{2+} cycling has been characterized as impaired in aging, by a reduction in Ca^{2+} uptake via Ca^{2+} uniporter, reduced Ca^{2+} retention capacity, a possible decrease in NCX activity, but elevated Ca^{2+} extrusion through sensitized mitoPTP opening.
- During aging, Ca^{2+} compartmentation in synaptosomal mitochondria decreases, and this decline has been associated with a reduction in the activity of mitochondrial Ca^{2+} uniporter.
- Enhanced activation of mitoPTP from a variety of aged or senescent cells including lymphocytes, neurons, hepatocytes, and cardiac myocytes has been reported.

- That mitoK_{ATP} channels participate in the processes of aging has been suggested by observations in aging animals that their heart has a reduced tolerance to I/R injury and experiences diminished overall effectiveness of cardiac IPC.
- Evidence suggests that the cardioprotective signaling pathways acting through mitoK_{ATP} channels are compromised with aging. It is unclear whether aging-attenuated cardiac mitoK_{ATP} channel function is due to changes in its density, responsiveness to stress stimuli, or defective communication to respiratory ETC.
- It is not clear why mitochondrial mitoPTP undergoes functional changes during the aging. With aging, there is increased OS in somatic cells, which tends to be more prevalent in cells rich in mitochondria, such as cardiomyocytes whose mitochondrial respiratory activity is elevated. Increased oxidative damage to proteins by ROS or reactive nitrogen species (RNS) has been implicated in aging, gauged by increased protein carbonyls and nitration.
- Proteomic analysis showed that there is an age-dependent nitration of VDAC in mitochondria. Increased VDAC nitration is very likely related to excessive OS in mitochondria since similar changes have been found in diabetic hearts, which exhibit enhanced OS.
- The related fields of pharmacogenomics and pharmacogenetics appear to have the potential to improve drug development by tailoring drug therapy based mainly on the individual's ability to metabolize drugs which are determined only in part by age, and influenced by disease, environmental factors (e.g., diet), concurrent medications and variant genetic factors specifying the transport, metabolism and targets of the drug.
- Increased awareness that with aging the incidence of dysrhythmias and channelopathies increase may lead to better management and further research interest in the discovery of the molecular mechanisms that underlie aging.

References

1. Montage O, Le Corvoisier P, Guenoun T, Laplace M, Crozatier B. Impaired alpha1-adrenergic responses in aged rat hearts. Fundam Clin Pharmacol 2005;19:331–339
2. Esler M, Kaye D. Sympathetic nervous system activation in essential hypertension, cardiac failure and psychosomatic heart disease. J Cardiovasc Pharmacol 2000;35:S1–S7
3. Kaye D, Esler M. Sympathetic neuronal regulation of the heart in aging and heart failure. Cardiovasc Res 2005;66:256–264
4. Anyukhovsky EP, Sosunov EA, Plotnikov A, Gainullin RZ, Jhang JS, Marboe CC, Rosen MR. Cellular electrophysiologic properties of old canine atria provide a substrate for arrhythmogenesis. Cardiovasc Res 2002;54:462–469
5. Hayashi H, Wang C, Miyauchi Y, Omichi C, Pak HN, Zhou S, Ohara T, Mandel WJ, Lin SF, Fishbein MC, Chen PS, Karagueuzian HS. Aging-related increase to inducible atrial fibrillation in the rat model. J Cardiovasc Electrophysiol 2002;13:801–808
6. Gottwald M, Gottwald E, Dhein S. Age-related electrophysiological and histological changes in rabbit hearts: age-related changes in electrophysiology. Int J Cardiol 1997;62:97–106
7. Dhein S, Hammerath SB. Aspects of the intercellular communication in aged hearts: effects of the gap junction uncoupler palmitoleic acid. Naunyn Schmiedebergs Arch Pharmacol 2001;364:397–408
8. Wongcharoen W, Chen YC, Chen YJ, Lin CI, Chen SA. Effects of aging and ouabain on left atrial arrhythmogenicity. J Cardiovasc Electrophysiol 2007 Mar 6
9. Jiang M, Zhang M, Tang DG, Clemo HF, Liu J, Holwitt D, Kasirajan V, Pond AL, Wettwer E, Tseng GN. KCNE2 protein is expressed in ventricles of different species, and changes in its expression contribute to electrical remodeling in diseased hearts. Circulation 2004;109:1783–1788
10. Baba S, Dun W, Hirose M, Boyden PA. Sodium current function in adult and aged canine atrial cells. Am J Physiol Heart Circ Physiol 2006;291:H756–H761
11. Jones SA, Boyett MR, Lancaster MK. Declining into failure: the age-dependent loss of the L-type calcium channel within the sinoatrial node. Circulation 2007;115:1183–1190
12. Schmidlin O, Bharati S, Lev M, Schwartz JB. Effects of physiological aging on cardiac electrophysiology in perfused Fischer 344 rat hearts. Am J Physiol 1992;262:H97–H105

112. Hansford RG, Zorov D. Role of mitochondrial calcium transport in the control of substrate oxidation. Mol Cell Biochem 1998;184:359–369
113. Das AM, Harris DA. Control of mitochondrial ATP synthase in heart cells: inactive to active transitions caused by beating or positive inotropic agents. Cardiovasc Res 1990;24:411–417
114. Shannon TR, Bers DM. Integrated Ca management in cardiac myocytes. Ann NY Acad Sci 2004;1025:28–38
115. Miyata H, Silverman HS, Sollott SJ, Lakatta EG, Stern MD, Hansford RG. Measurement of mitochondrial free Ca^{2+} concentration in living single rat cardiac myocytes. Am J Physiol 1991;261:H1123–3H1124
116. Isenberg G, Han S, Schiefer A, Wendt-Gallitelli MF. Changes in mitochondrial calcium concentration during the cardiac contraction cycle. Cardiovasc Res 1993;27:1800–1809
117. Wang GJ, Thayer SA. NMDA-induced calcium loads recycle across the mitochondrial inner membrane of hippocampal neurons in culture. J Neurophysiol 2002;87:740–749
118. Cheranov SY, Jaggar JH. Mitochondrial modulation of Ca^{2+} sparks and transient KCa currents in smooth muscle cells of rat cerebral arteries. J Physiol 2004;556:755–771
119. Satrustegui J, Villalba M, Pereira R, Bogonez E, Martinez-Serrano A. Cytosolic and mitochondrial calcium in synaptosomes during aging. Life Sci 1996;59:429–434
120. Xiong J, Verkhratsky A, Toescu EC. Changes in mitochondrial status associated with altered Ca^{2+} homeostasis in aged cerebellar granule neurons in brain slices. J Neurosci 2002;22:10761–10771
121. Murchison D, Zawieja DC, Griffith WH. Reduced mitochondrial buffering of voltage-gated calcium influx in aged rat basal forebrain neurons. Cell Calcium 2004;36:61–67
122. Vitorica J, Satrustegui J. Involvement of mitochondria in the age-dependent decrease in calcium uptake of rat brain synaptosomes. Brain Res 1986;378:36–48
123. Nicholls DG. Mitochondrial membrane potential and aging. Aging Cell 2004;3:35–40
124. Sugrue MM, Wang Y, Rideout HJ, Chalmers-Redman RM, Tatton WG. Reduced mitochondrial membrane potential and altered responsiveness of a mitochondrial membrane megachannel in p53-induced senescence. Biochem Biophys Res Commun 1999;261:123–130
125. Mather MW, Rottenberg H. The inhibition of calcium signaling in T lymphocytes from old mice results from enhanced activation of the mitochondrial permeability transition pore. Mech Ageing Dev 2002;123:707–724
126. Kamo N, Muratsugu M, Hongoh R, Kobatake Y. Membrane potential of mitochondria measured with an electrode sensitive to tetraphenyl phosphonium and relationship between proton electrochemical potential and phosphorylation potential in steady state. J Membr Biol 1979;49:105–121
127. Kokoszka JE, Coskun P, Esposito LA, Wallace DC. Increased mitochondrial oxidative stress in the Sod2 (+/–) mouse results in the age-related decline of mitochondrial function culminating in increased apoptosis. Proc Natl Acad Sci USA 2001;98:2278–2283
128. Hagen TM, Yowe DL, Bartholomew JC, Wehr CM, Do KL, Park JY, Ames BN. Mitochondrial decay in hepatocytes from old rats: membrane potential declines, heterogeneity and oxidants increase. Proc Natl Acad Sci USA 1997;94:3064–3069
129. Goodell S, Cortopassi G. Analysis of oxygen consumption and mitochondrial permeability with age in mice. Mech Ageing Dev 1998;101:245–256
130. Rottenberg H, Wu S. Mitochondrial dysfunction in lymphocytes from old mice: enhanced activation of the permeability transition. Biochem Biophys Res Commun 1997;240:68–74
131. Mather M, Rottenberg H. Aging enhances the activation of the permeability transition pore in mitochondria. Biochem Biophys Res Commun 2000;273:603–608
132. Canzoniero LM, Rossi A, Taglialatela M, Amoroso S, Annunziato L, Di Renzo G. The Na+-Ca^{2+} exchanger activity in cerebrocortical nerve endings is reduc in old compared to young and mature rats when it operates as a Ca^{2+} influx or efflux pathway. Biochim Biophysi Acta 1992;1107:175–178
133. Martinez-Serrano A, Blanco P, Satrustegui J. Calcium binding to the cytosol and calcium extrusion mechanisms in intact synaptosomes and their alterations with aging. J Biol Chem 1992;267:4672–4679
134. Koban MU, Moorman AF, Holtz J, Yacoub MH, Boheler KR. Expressional analysis of the cardiac Na-Ca exchanger in rat development and senescence. Cardiovasc Res 1998;37:405–423
135. Drew B, Phaneuf S, Dirks A, Selman C, Gredilla R, Lezza A, Barja G, Leeuwenburgh C. Effects of aging and caloric restriction on mitochondrial energy production in gastrocnemius muscle and heart. Am J Physiol 2003;284:R474–R480
136. Short KR, Bigelow ML, Kahl J, Singh R, Coenen-Schimke J, Raghavakaimal S, Nair KS. Decline in skeletal muscle mitochondrial function with aging in humans. Proc Natl Acad Sci USA 2005;102:5618–5623
137. Shigenaga MK, Hagen TM, Ames BN. Oxidative damage and mitochondrial decay in aging. Proc Natl Acad Sci USA 1994;19:10771–10778
138. Drew B, Leeuwenburgh C. Method for measuring ATP production in isolated mitochondria: ATP production in brain and liver mitochondria of Fischer-344 rats with age and caloric restriction. Am J Physiol Regul Integr Comp Physiol 2003;285:R1259–R1267

139. Kwong LK, Sohal RS. Age-related changes in activities of mitochondrial electron transport complexes in various tissues of the mouse. Arch Biochem Biophys 2000;373:16–22
140. Bubber P, Haroutunian V, Fisch G, Blass JP, Gibson GE. Mitochondrial abnormalities in Alzheimer brain: mechanistic implications. Ann Neurol 2005;57:695–703
141. Moreau R, Heath SH, Doneanu CE, Harris RA, Hagen TM. Age-related compensatory activation of pyruvate dehydrogenase complex in rat heart. Biochem Biophys Res Commun 2004;325:48–58
142. Piec I, Listrat A, Alliot J, Chambon C, Taylor RG, Bechet D. Differential proteome analysis of aging in rat skeletal muscle. FASEB J 2005;19:1143–1145
143. Kumaran S, Subathra M, Balu M, Panneerselvam C. Supplementation of L-carnitine improves mitochondrial enzymes in heart and skeletal muscle of aged rats. Exp Aging Res 2005;31:55–67
144. Lai JC, Leung TK, Lim L. Activities of the mitochondrial NAD-linked isocitric dehydrogenase in different regions of the rat brain: changes in ageing and the effect of chronic manganese chloride administration. Gerontology 1982;28:81–85
145. Vitorica J, Cano J, Satrustegui J, Machado A. Comparison between develop-mental and senescent changes in enzyme activities linked to energy metabolism in rat heart. Mech Ageing Dev 1981;16:105–116
146. Inoue I, Nagase H, Kishi K, Higuti T. ATP-sensitive K+ channel in the mitochondrial inner membrane. Nature 1991;352:244–247
147. Paucek P, Mironova G, Mahdi F, Beavis AD, Woldegiorgis G, Garlid KD. Reconstitution and partial purification of the glibenclamide-sensitive, ATP-dependent K+ channel from rat liver and beef heart mitochondria. J Biol Chem 1992;267:26062–26069
148. Zhang DX, Chen YF, Campbell WB, Zou AP, Gross GJ, Li PL. Characteristics and superoxide-induced activation of reconstituted myocardial mitochondrial ATP- sensitive potassium channels. Circ Res 2001;89:1177–1183
149. Mironova GD, Negoda AE, Marinov BS, Paucek P, Costa AD, Grigoriev SM, Skarga YY, Garlid KD. Functional distinctions between the mitochondrial ATP-dependent K+ channel (mitoKATP) and its inward rectifier subunit (mitoKIR). J Biol Chem 2004;279:32562–32568
150. Ardehali H, O'Rourke B. Mitochondrial K(ATP) channels in cell survival and death. J Mol Cell Cardiol 2005;39:7–16
151. Yarov-Yarovoy V, Paucek P, Jaburek M, Garlid KD. The nucleotide regulatory sites on the mitochondrial KATP channel face the cytosol. Biochim Biophys Acta 1997;1321:128–136
152. Debska G, Kicinska A, Skalska J, Szewczyk A. Intracellular potassium and chloride channels: an update. Acta Biochim Pol 2001;48:137–144
153. Singh H, Hudman D, Lawrence CL, Rainbow RD, Lodwick D, Norman RI. Distribution of Kir6.0 and SUR2 ATP-sensitive potassium channel subunits in isolated ventricular myocytes. J Mol Cell Cardiol 2003;35:445–459
154. Lacza Z, Snipes JA, Kis B, Szabo C, Grover G, Busija DW. Investigation of the subunit composition and the pharmacology of the mitochondrial ATP-dependent K^+ channel in the brain. Brain Res 2003;994:27–36
155. Garg V, Hu K. Protein kinase c isoform-dependent modulation of ATP-sensitive K+ channels in mitochondrial inner membrane. Am J Physiol Heart Circ Physiol 2006;293:H322–H332
156. Garlid KD, Dos Santos P, Xie ZJ, Costa AD, Paucek P. Mitochondrial potassium transport: the role of the mitochondrial ATP-sensitive K^+ channel in cardiac function and cardioprotection. Biochim Biophys Acta 2003;1606:1–21
157. Otani H. Reactive oxygen species as mediators of signal transduction in ischemic preconditioning. Antioxid Redox Signal 2004;6:449–469
158. Garlid KD, Paucek P. Mitochondrial potassium transport: the K(+) cycle. Biochim Biophys Acta 2003;1606: 23–41
159. Oldenburg O, Cohen MV, Yellon DM, Downey JM. Mitochondrial K(ATP) channels: role in cardioprotection. Cardiovasc Res 2002;55:429–437
160. Wang Y, Haider HK, Ahmad N, Ashraf M. Mechanisms by which K(ATP) channel openers produce acute and delayed cardioprotection. Vascul Pharmacol 2005;42:253–264
161. Rousou AJ, Ericsson M, Federman M, Levitsky S, McCully JD. Opening of mitochondrial KATP channels enhances cardioprotection through the modulation of mitochondrial matrix volume, calcium accumulation, and respiration. Am J Physiol 2004;287:H1967–H1976
162. Costa AD, Quinlan CL, Andrukhiv A, West IC, Jaburek M, Garlid KD. The direct physiological effects of mitoK_{ATP} opening on heart mitochondria. Am J Physiol 2006;290:H406–H415
163. Kowaltowski AJ, Seetharaman S, Paucek P, Garlid KD. Bioenergetic consequences of opening the ATP-sensitive K^+ channel of heart mitochondria. Am J Physiol 2001;280:H649–H657
164. Liu Y, Sato T, Seharaseyon J, Szewczyk A, O'Rourke B, Marban E. Mitochondrial ATP-dependent potassium channels. Viable candidate effectors of ischemic preconditioning. Ann NY Acad Sci 1999;874:27–37
165. Holmuhamedov EL, Wang L, Terzic A. ATP-sensitive K^+ channel openers prevent Ca^{2+} overload in rat cardiac mitochondria. J Physiol 1999;519:347–360

166. Holmuhamedov EL, Jovanovic S, Dzeja PP, Jovanovic A, Terzic A. Mitochondrial ATP-sensitive K^+ channels modulate cardiac mitochondrial function. Am J Physiol 1998;275:H1567–H1576
167. Szewczyk A, Wojcik G, Nalecz MJ. Potassium channel opener, RP 66471, induces membrane depolarization of rat liver mitochondria. Biochem Biophys Res Commun 1995;207:126–132
168. Dos Santos P, Kowaltowski AJ, Laclau MN, Seetharaman S, Paucek P, Boudina S, Thambo JB, Tariosse L, Garlid KD. Mechanisms by which opening the mitochondrial ATP- sensitive K(+) channel protects the ischemic heart. Am J Physiol Heart Circ Physiol 2002;283:H284–H295
169. Fenton RA, Dickson EW, Meyer TE, Dobson JG Jr. Aging reduces the cardioprotective effect of ischemic preconditioning in the rat heart. J Mol Cell Cardiol 2000;32:1371–1375
170. Lesnefsky EJ, Gallo DS, Ye J, Whittingham TS, Lust WD. Aging increases ischemia-reperfusion injury in the isolated, buffer-perfused heart. J Lab Clin Med 1994;124:843–851
171. Przyklenk K, Li G, Simkhovich BZ, Kloner RA. Mechanisms of myocardial ischemic preconditioning are age related: PKC-epsilon does not play a requisite role in old rabbits. J Appl Physiol 2003;95:2563–2569
172. Riess ML, Camara AK, Rhodes SS, McCormick J, Jiang MT, Stowe DF. Increasing heart size and age attenuate anesthetic preconditioning in guinea pig isolated hearts. Anesth Analg 2005;101:1572–1576
173. Sniecinski R, Liu H. Reduced efficacy of volatile anesthetic preconditioning with advanced age in isolated rat myocardium. Anesthesiology 2004;100:589–597
174. Tani M, Honma Y, Hasegawa H, Tamaki K. Direct activation of mitochondrial K(ATP) channels mimics preconditioning but protein kinase C activation is less effective in middle-aged rat hearts. Cardiovasc Res 2001;49: 56–68
175. Schulman D, Latchman DS, Yellon DM. Effect of aging on the ability of preconditioning to protect rat hearts from ischemia-reperfusion injury. Am J Physiol 2001;281:H1630–H1636
176. Lee TM, Su SF, Chou TF, Lee YT, Tsai CH. Loss of preconditioning by attenuated activation of myocardial ATP-sensitive potassium channels in elderly patients undergoing coronary angioplasty. Circulation 2002;105: 334–340
177. Longobardi G, Abete P, Ferrara N, Papa A, Rosiello R, Furgi G, Calabrese C, Cacciatore F, Rengo F. "Warm-up" phenomenon in adult and elderly patients with coronary artery disease: further evidence of the loss of "ischemic preconditioning" in the aging heart. J Gerontol A Biol Sci Med Sci 2000;55:M124–M129
178. Abete P, Ferrara N, Cioppa A, Ferrara P, Bianco S, Calabrese C, Cacciatore F, Longobardi G, Rengo F. Preconditioning does not prevent postischemic dysfunction in aging heart. J Am Coll Cardiol 1996;27:1777–1786
179. McCully JD, Levitsky S. The mitochondrial K(ATP) channel and cardioprotection. Ann Thorac Surg 2003;75:S667–S673
180. McCully JD, Toyoda Y, Wakiyama H, Rousou AJ, Parker RA, Levitsky S. Age- and gender-related differences in ischemia/reperfusion injury and cardioprotection: effects of diazoxide. Ann Thorac Surg 2006;82:117–123
181. Tricarico D, Camerino DC. ATP-sensitive K^+ channels of skeletal muscle fibers from young adult and aged rats: possible involvement of thiol-dependent redox mechanisms in the age-related modifications of their biophysical and pharmacological properties. Mol Pharmacol 1994;46:754–761
182. Krenz M, Oldenburg O, Wimpee H, Cohen MV, Garlid KD, Critz SD, Downey JM, Benoit JN. Opening of ATP-sensitive potassium channels causes generation of free radicals in vascular smooth muscle cells. Basic Res Cardiol 2002;97:365–373
183. Oldenburg O, Yang XM, Krieg T, Garlid KD, Cohen MV, Grover GJ, Downey JM. P1075 opens mitochondrial K_{ATP} channels and generates reactive oxygen species resulting in cardioprotection of rabbit hearts. J Mol Cell Cardiol 2003;35:1035–1042
184. Pain T, Yang XM, Critz SD, Yue Y, Nakano A, Liu GS, Heusch G, Cohen MV, Downey JM. Opening of mitochondrial K_{ATP} channels triggers the preconditioned state by generating free radicals. Circ Res 2000;87: 460–466
185. Carroll R, Gant VA, Yellon DM. Mitochondrial K-$_{ATP}$ channel opening protects a human atrial-derived cell line by a mechanism involving free radical generation. Cardiovasc Res 2001;51:691–700
186. McCubrey JA, Lahair MM, Franklin RA. Reactive oxygen species-induced activation of the MAP kinase signaling pathways. Antioxid Redox Signal 2006;8:1775–1789
187. McCubrey JA, Franklin RA. Reactive oxygen intermediates and signaling through kinase pathways. Antioxid Redox Signal 2006:1745–1748
188. Lahair MM, Howe CJ, Rodriguez-Mora O, McCubrey JA, Franklin RA. Molecular pathways leading to oxidative stress-induced phosphorylation of Akt. Antioxid Redox Signal 2006;8:1749–1756
189. Crompton M. The mitochondrial permeability transition pore and its role in cell death. Biochem J 1999;341: 233–249
190. Weiss JN, Korge P, Honda HM, Ping P. Role of the mitochondrial permeability transition in myocardial disease. Circ Res 2003;93:292–301
191. Halestrap AP, Clarke SJ, Javadov SA. Mitochondrial permeability transition pore opening during myocardial reperfusion – a target for cardioprotection. Cardiovasc Res 2004;61:372–385

192. Ichas F, Jouaville LS, Sidash SS, Mazat JP, Holmuhamedov EL. Mitochondrial calcium spiking: a transduction mechanism based on calcium-induced permeability transition involved in cell calcium signaling. FEBS Lett 1994;348:211–215
193. Kwak HB, Song W, Lawler JM. Exercise training attenuates age-induced elevation in Bax/Bcl-2 ratio, apoptosis, and remodeling in the rat heart. FASEB J 2006;20:791–793
194. Dirks A, Leeuwenburgh C. Apoptosis in skeletal muscle with aging. Am J Physiol 2002;282:R519–R527
195. Lucas DT, Szweda LI. Cardiac reperfusion injury: aging, lipid peroxidation, and mitochondrial dysfunction. Proc Natl Acad Sci USA 1998;95:510–514
196. Sohal RS, Arnold LA, Sohal BH. Age-related changes in antioxidant enzymes and prooxidant generation in tissues of the rat with special referenceto parameters in two insect species. Free Radic Biol Med 1990;9: 495–500
197. Yan LJ, Sohal RS. Mitochondrial adenine nucleotide translocase is modified oxidatively during aging. Proc Natl Acad Sci USA 1998;95:12896–12901
198. Nohl H, Kramer R. Molecular basis of age-dependent changes in the activity of adenine nucleotide translocase. Mech Ageing Dev 1980;4:137–144
199. Hashimoto M, Majima E, Goto S, Shinohara Y, Terada H. Fluctuation of the first loop facing the matrix of the mitochondrial ADP/ATP carrier deduced from intermolecular cross linking of Cys_{56} residues by bifunctional dimaleimides. Biochemistry 1999;38:1050–1056
200. Yokozawa T, Satoh A, Cho EJ. Ginsenoside-Rd attenuates oxidative damage related to aging in senescence-accelerated mice. J Pharm Pharmacol 2004;56:107–113
201. Zhu Y, Carvey PM, Ling Z. Age-related changes in glutathione and glutathione-related enzymes in rat brain. Brain Res 2006;1090:35–44
202. Judge S, Jang YM, Smith A, Hagen T, Leeuwenburgh C. Age-associated increases in oxidative stress and antioxidant enzyme activities in cardiac interfibrillar mitochondria: implications for the mitochondrial theory of aging. FASEB J 2005;19:419–421
203. Suh JH, Heath SH, Hagen TM. Two subpopulations of mitochondria in the aging rat heart display heterogenous levels of oxidative stress. Free Radic Biol Med 2003;35:1064–1072
204. Mo JQ, Hom DG, Andersen JK. Decreases in protective enzymes correlates with increased oxidative damage in the aging mouse brain. Mech Ageing Dev 1995;81:73–82
205. Chen JJ, Bertrand H, Yu BP. Inhibition of adenine nucleotide translocator by lipid peroxidation products. Free Radic Biol Med 1995;19:583–590
206. Pepe S. Effect of dietary polyunsaturated fatty acids on age-related changes in cardiac mitochondrial membranes. Exper Gerontol 2005;40:751–758
207. Kristal BS, Park BK, Yu BP. 4-Hydroxyhexenal is a potent inducer of the mitochondrial permeability transition. J Biol Chem 1996;271:6033–6038
208. Hansford RG, Castro F. Effect of senescence on Ca-ion transport by heart mitochondria. Mech Ageing Dev 1982;19:5–13
209. Shoshan-Barmatz V, Gincel D. The voltage-dependent anion channel: characterization, modulation, and role in mitochondrial function in cell life and death. Cell Biochem Biophys 2003;39:279–292
210. Vyssokikh M, Brdiczka D. The function of complexes between the outer mitochondrial membrane pore (VDAC) and the adenine nucleotide translocase in regulation of energy metabolism and apoptosis. Acta Bochimica Polonica 2003;50:389–404
211. Hajnoczky G, Csordas G, Yi M. Old players in a new role: mitochondria- associated membranes, VDAC, and ryanodine receptors as contributors to calcium signal propagation from endoplasmic reticulum to the mitochondria. Cell Calcium 2002;32:363–377
212. Shoshan-Barmatz V, Israelson A, Brdiczka D, Sheu SS. The voltage-dependent anion channel (VDAC): function in intracellular signalling, cell life and cell death. Curr Pharm Des 2006;12:2249–2270
213. Zaid H, Abu-Hamad S, Israelson A, Nathan I, Shoshan-Barmatz V. The voltage-dependent anion channel-1 modulates apoptotic cell death. Cell Death Differ 2005;12:751–760
214. Cheng EH, Sheiko TV, Fisher JK, Craigen WJ, Korsmeyer SJ. VDAC2 inhibits BAK activation and mitochondrial apoptosis. Science 2003;301:513–517
215. Beckman JS, Koppenol WH. Oxidative damage and tyrosine nitration from peroxynitrite. Chem Res Toxicol 1996;9:836–844
216. Kanski J, Behring A, Pelling J, Schoneich C. Proteomic identification of 3-nitrotyrosine-containing rat cardiac proteins: effects of biological aging. Am J Physiol 2005;288:H371–H381
217. Turko IV, Li L, Aulak KS, Stuehr DJ, Chang JY, Murad F. Protein tyrosine nitration in the mitochondria from diabetic mouse heart. Implications to dysfunctional mitochondria in diabetes. J Biol Chem 2003;278:33972–33977
218. Madesh M, Hajnoczky G. VDAC-dependent permeabilization of the outer mitochondrial membrane by superoxide induces rapid and massive cytochrome c release. J Cell Biol 2001;155:1003–1015

219. Kanski J, Schoneich C. Protein nitration in biological aging: proteomic and tandem mass spectrometric characterization of nitrated sites. Methods Enzymol 2005;396:160–171
220. Pastoris O, Boschi F, Verri M, Baiardi P, Felzani G, Vecchiet J, Dossena M, Catapano M. The effects of aging on enzyme activities and metabolite concentrations in skeletal muscle from sedentary male and female subjects. Exp Gerontol 2000;35:95–104
221. Nehal M, Azam M, Baquer NZ. Changes in the levels of catecholamines, hexokinase and glucose 6-phosphate dehydrogenase in red cell aging. Biochem Int 1990;22:517–522
222. Moorthy K, Yadav UC, Siddiqui MR, Sharma D, Basir SF, Baquer NZ. Effect of estradiol and progesterone treatment on carbohydrate metabolizing enzymes in tissues of aging female rats. Biogerontology 2004;5:249–259
223. Nohl H, Kramer R. Molecular basis of age-dependent changes in the activity of adenine nucleotide translocase. Mech Ageing Dev 1980;4:137–144
224. Roepke TK, Abbott GW. Pharmacogenetics and cardiac ion channels. Vascul Pharmacol 2006;44:90–106
225. Simard C, Drolet B, Yang P, Kim RB, Roden DM. Polymorphism screening in the cardiac K+ channel gene KCNA5. Clin Pharmacol Ther 2005;77:138–144
226. Brendel J, Peukert S. Blockers of the Kv1.5 channel for the treatment of atrial arrhythmias. Curr Med Chem Cardiovasc Hematol Agents 2003;1:273–287
227. Johnson JA, Cavallari LH. Cardiovascular pharmacogenomics. Exp Physiol 2005;90:283–289
228. Johnson JA. Drug target pharmacogenomics: an overview. Am J Pharmacogenomics 2001;1:271–281
229. Mahlknecht U, Voelter-Mahlknecht S. Pharmacogenomics: questions and concerns. Curr Med Res Opin 2005;21:1041–1047

Part V
Genetics

Chapter 12
Genetics of Life Span: Lessons from Model Organisms

Overview

Until the early 1990s, the evidence for genetic components involved in aging and longevity was rather lacking with no actual aging genes formally defined. In this chapter, we will discuss the use of model organisms to identify and functionally characterize genes that affect aging and longevity. In particular, we will focus on data from yeast, *C. elegans*, *Drosophila* and mice that have not only identified, highly conserved genes (most with homologues in human), which can modulate aging and longevity in all species thus far tested, but that also implicate the involvement of larger signaling pathways to which the genetic components identified contribute. Further progress in the identification of upstream and downstream components in these pathways is beginning to provide both illumination of the sequence of intracellular events that are involved in aging/longevity pathways, and delineation of extracellular stimuli and environmental factors and stresses that can modulate their operation. Identification of both the genetic components, their interaction with upstream and downstream components and modulating factors, may be of great significance in the discovery of new targets for aging therapies.

Introduction

The identification of genetic factors involved in determining longevity in relatively simple organisms such as the nematode *C. elegans*, the yeast *Saccharomyces cerevisiae* and the fly *Drosophila melanogaster* derives in large part from their relatively short generation and overall lifetime, the extremely well-defined genetic and cell information available for each of these species and perhaps most importantly, the capacity to use in each extremely powerful and informative molecular techniques of gene targeting and gene transfer. In yeast, gene targeting by homologous recombination, gene overexpression on episomal plasmids and genetic techniques to definine epistatic and gene-product interactions, including yeast 2-hybrid analysis, may allow construction of strains null for specific alleles, correction of specific defects and overall elucidation of the sequence of upstream and downstream pathway components. Similarly, molecular genetic techniques including the use of RNA-mediated interference (RNAi) to target specific gene action in *C. elegans* cells and p-element insertion for targeting gene action in *Drosophila* have been instrumental in identifying specific genetic components, and definition of their role, in pathways of aging. Moreover, mice that have been shown to contain homologues/orthologues of the great majority of the genes identified in the other simpler model organisms (showing the striking conservation of these genes in aging longevity pathways), also offer an unusual well-developed transgenic technology (as described in Chapter 3) with the ability to construct strains with specific null alleles or overexpressed functions. Strains of mice also have been created that model many of the aging phenotypes characteristic of human premature aging and progeria diseases, as well as aging-associated cardiovascular pathologies.

J. Marín-García, *Aging and the Heart*,

Insulin/IGF-1 Pathway in *C. elegans*

Mutations in daf-2, a regulatory gene encoding a insulin/IGF-1 receptor [1] doubled the life span of fertile, active *C. elegans* [2]. Moreover, genetic mosaics that lack the DAF-2 protein in either cell at the two-cell stage, are long-lived suggesting that cells that lack DAF-2 must be able to transmit a signal for longevity to wild-type cells [3]. This life span extension required the activity of a second gene, daf-16 which encodes a forkhead FOXO-related transcription factor (DAF-16). Further observations have showed that the DAF-2 receptor activates a conserved phosphatidylinositol 3-OH kinase (PI3-K) signaling pathway that affects life span, in part by regulating the nuclear localization of the DAF-16 protein [4, 5]. Null mutations in daf-16 suppressed the increased longevity resulting from mutations in daf-2 indicating that lack of DAF-16 bypasses the need for this insulin receptor-like signaling pathway, and also suggests that the principal role of DAF-2 signaling is to antagonize downstream DAF-16 function. Furthermore, human FKHRL1 could partially replace DAF-16 in *C. elegans* which suggests it is a DAF-16 orthologue [5].

Besides DAF-16, the heat shock-transcription factor HSF-1 is also required for daf-2 mutations to extend life span by activating specific longevity genes, including small heat-shock proteins (HSPs) [6, 7]. Overexpresssion of HSF-1 extends worm life span as does stress-activated HSF-1, accompanied by the downstream expression of the small HSPs. Heat shock also promotes DAF-16 nuclear localization, and DAF-16 is required for the expression of small HSPs after heat shock [6, 8].

Longevity of daf-2 mutants and the impact of heat stress on longevity also requires the function of AAK-2, a catalytic subunit of AMP-activated protein kinase [9]. This implied that AAK-2 functions as a sensor that couples life span to metabolic energy levels and insulin-like signals. Moreover, the overexpression of AAK-2 in *C. elegans* increased life span, and the ability of a number of other genes (to be discussed later) to promote longevity (e.g., daf-2, sir-2, clk-1, isp-2) was dependent on AAK-2 function [10].

Mutations in other genes from within the insulin/IGF pathway also lead to enhanced longevity. Mutations in age-1 encoding the catalytic subunit of the PI3 kinase result in longer life [11]. Although it has been suggested that the reduced fecundity noted in age-1 mutant strains might be associated with the increased longevity, recent data have showed that the age-1 mutant, as well as the daf-2 mutant, can extend *C. elegans* life span without leading to a reduction or delay in fecundity [2, 12]. Furthermore, other observations have indicated that the insulin/IGF-1 signaling pathway controls longevity and reproduction independently of one another. Studies with RNAi directed against daf-2 demonstrated that decreased activity of DAF-2 resulting from RNAi treatment, maintained only during early development (in pre-adult worms), resulted in reduced fecundity with no effect on life span; however, reduced DAF-2 expression, resulting from RNAi treatment initiated in adulthood, significantly increased life span without reducing fecundity [13]. Additionally, DAF-18, a homologue of the tumor suppressor PTEN in *C. elegans* regulates both longevity and the formation of the dauer quiescence stage by mediating insulin/IGF-signaling pathway [14].

PTEN encodes a dual-specificity phosphatase that regulates the intracellular levels of phosphatidylinositol 3, 4, 5-trisphosphate (PIP3), generated by AGE-1/PI3-K, by specifically dephosphorylating position 3 on the inositol ring; this suggests that PTEN/DAF-18 antagonizes the DAF-2/AGE-1 pathway. Mutation of daf-18 suppresses life extension and constitutive dauer formation associated with daf-2 or age-1 mutants, and inactivation of daf-18 by RNAi mimics this suppression which suggests a longevity-promoting action of DAF-18/PTEN [14, 15]. Moreover, human PTEN can substitute for DAF-18 and can restore the dauer and longevity phenotypes in worms devoid of DAF-18 [16].

Using a variety of methodologies, it has been possible to identify a large number of genes that are transcriptional targets of DAF-16. A subset of these downstream genes are involved in the modulation of OS, including several antioxidant proteins; other genes are involved in cellular stress signaling (e.g., HSPs), metabolic regulation and fat storage functions [17–20]. Comparative genetics has also been employed to identify 17 genes shared by both *C. elegans* and *Drosophila*, each of which contained a DAF-16/FOXO binding site (TTGTTTAC) within its promoter region [18]. Interestingly, both negatively and positively regulated genes were found to bear conserved DAF-16 binding sites suggesting that DAF-16 can act both as a transcriptional activator and a repressor. The model emerging from these studies is that the insulin/IGF-1 system acts as a longevity module with upstream master regulators (e.g., DAF-2 and DAF-16/FOXO) controlling a wide variety of downstream genes with diverse functions (shown in Fig. 12.1) [21, 22].

It is noteworthy that the DAF-2/DAF-16 downstream longevity genes not only extend life span but also serve to protect the worms from harsh external environmental stresses such as heat, UV and oxidative damage. The stress-resistant phenotype, encompassed by these genes expression, can be effective with metabolic as well as environmental stresses. Beyond regulating adult longevity in *C. elegans*, the insulin/IGF pathway also can trigger entry into a growth-arrested larval state of metabolic quiescence called the dauer state. Progression of a dauer-specific altered morphology, including the development of an impermeable cuticle, and metabolic program (i.e., reduced Krebs [TCA]) cycle and respiratory [ETC] metabolism) in response to harsh environmental stresses, is in part triggered by a downregulation of the insulin/IGF-1 signaling pathway [23].

It has been suggested that the decline in TCA cycle activity and ETC pathways serves as a common element of both the dauer and long-lived phenotypes, resulting in reduced ROS generation [24], although a recent transcript profiling study found decreased levels of ETC and TCA gene expression in dauers but not in daf-2 mutants [25]. Nevertheless, both dauer and long-lived mutants have been shown to utilize alternative sources of metabolic energy (with less ROS generation), including the upregulation of genes involved in the glyoxylate cycle (primarily located in the peroxisomes), as well as gluconeogenesis and trehalose synthesis [25, 26]. Gene transcript profiling by SAGE analysis with dauer larvae has also indicated significant upregulation of anaerobic pathways [27].

While the insulin/IGF-1 pathway can be invoked into triggering the dauer-specific responses to environmental stress, as well as for protection against endogenous stresses that accelerate aging, the responses are not invariably the same (i.e., the long-lived insulin/IGF-1 mutants are not in fact dauers in disguise) [21]. Although some daf-2 mutations (termed class II) can produce dauer-traits in adults, other mutations (class I) do not. Extension of life span in these mutant worms occurs with normal metabolism, reproduction and body morphology [28]. Similarly, mutations that moderately

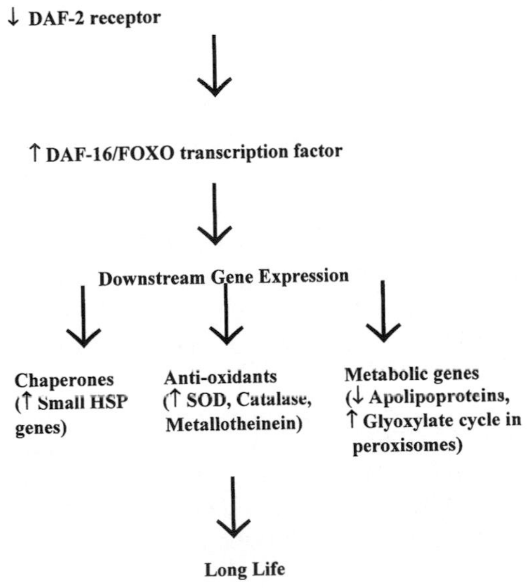

Fig. 12.1 Insulin-IGF-1 signaling regulates longevity in *C. elegans*

increase the activity of DAF-16 result only in life span extension, while more severe mutations result in a constitutive dauer phenotype.

Insulin/IGF Signaling in Other Eucaryotes

In *Drosophila melanogaster* similar to *C. elegans*, when insulin-like signaling is reduced aging is slowed. When the insulin-like receptor (InR) or its receptor substrate (chico) are mutated [29, 30], or when insulin-producing cells are ablated, life expectancy is extended by more than 50%. In both these organisms, the presence of a functional insulin/IGF-signaling pathway accelerates biological aging, and inhibition of this axis extends life span.

Observations with mice and mammalian systems have been rather ambiguous. Using genetic mouse models, e.g., the Ames and Snell dwarf mice, and female mice that are heterozygous for the IGF-1 receptor, Igf1r $^{+/-}$, it was found that a reduction in plasma levels of insulin and/or IGF-1, or reduction in insulin/IGF-1 signaling may be correlated with increased longevity and retarded aging [31]. At least three genes have been identified (Pit1dw, Prop1df, Ghr) in which loss-of-function mutations lead to dwarfism with reduced levels of IGF-1 and insulin, as well as to increased longevity in mice [32–35]. However, animal models with deficiencies in IGF-1 are complicated by the simultaneous alterations in growth hormone or hypopituitarism, which result in multiple endocrine defects and developmental abnormalities. These factors markedly complicate the interpretation of data drawn from dwarf mice in the assessment of the role of IGF-1 in biological aging and life span. On the other hand, loss-of-function mutations in the insulin receptor can result in shortened life span in mice, albeit tissue-specific constructs have provided variable responses.

Brain-specific (NIRKO), liver-specific (LIRKO), and muscle specific insulin receptor knock mice (MIRKO) develop obesity, insulin resistance and impaired glucose regulation and have increased morbidity and shorter life span [36–38]. However, mutations of the insulin receptor in adipose tissue have the opposite effect. Fat-specific insulin receptor knockout mice (FIRKO) have normal food intake, marked decrease in fat mass, lower fasting plasma insulin levels at 2 and 10 months respectively, and live longer [38]. Mice with global mutations of the insulin receptor genes exhibit metabolic derangements at birth, with β-cell failure in days, and death due to diabetes ketoacidosis [39]. Interestingly, mutations of the insulin receptor have been described in humans, causing different degrees of insulin resistance and diabetes and are associated with increased morbidity and mortality due to atherosclerosis, CVD, obesity and diabetes.

Similarly in humans, reduced IGF-1 activity is known to be associated with significant morbidity in adulthood with an increased risk of developing CVD, diabetes, osteoporosis and neurodegenerative diseases. IGF-1 knockout mice (Igf1–/–) show severe intrauterine growth restriction with a birth weight 60% of normal, and a majority die shortly after birth; though, depending on genetic background, some do survive and reach adulthood [40]. Similarly, mice homozygous for the IGF receptor null allele are not viable at birth. However, heterozygous knockout mice for the IGF-1 receptor live 26% longer than the wild type. This increase is gender-specific; females live 33% longer than wild-type females, whereas the male mice have an increase in life span of 16% [35]. The Igf1r (+/–) mice display greater resistance to oxidative stress (OS), a known determinant of aging and no changes in metabolism, physical activity or fertility.

Moreover, information from studies with both human and other mammals clearly indicate a progressive decrease in IGF-1 with age. Restoration of IGF-1 levels in elderly individuals by growth hormone (GH)-replacement therapy have shown to reverse the age-related decline in IGF-1 and have significant health benefits. Gathered observations suggest that an aged phenotype results from anabolic hormone deficiency in which GH and subsequently IGF-1 deficiencies play significant roles.

The contradictions between increased life span, resulting from disruption of the insulin/IGF-1 receptor in nematodes and flies, and the shortened life span and increased aging in mammals with genetic or acquired defects in insulin signaling pathway have been in part explained by the acquisition in mammals of more complicated metabolic pathways over evolution with different receptors for insulin and IGF-1, and distinct pathways and diverse functions in specific tissues of the mammal. In higher organisms, signaling through the insulin/IGF-1 pro-survival pathway is widely recognized to be neuroprotective and cardioprotective as well as important for neuronal and myocyte growth and physiology.

Another interesting wrinkle involving the insulin/IGF-1 signaling with respect to aging/longevity in mice has come from the identification of the Klotho gene, named after the Greek goddess who spun the thread of life. Klotho is an aging suppressor gene which is predominantly expressed in the distal convoluted tubules in the kidney, the parathyroid glands, and the choroid plexus in the brain, all of which interestingly enough are indispensable for the regulation of calcium homeostasis, and which extends life span when overexpressed in mice [41]. Mice carrying a loss-of-function mutation (arising from an insertional mutation at the gene's 5′ end) in the Klotho gene [KL (–/–) mice] also known as the *klotho* mouse, develop aging-like symptoms around 4 weeks after birth and suffer from multiple age-related disorders observed in humans, including osteoporosis, skin atrophy, ectopic calcification, arteriosclerosis, and pulmonary emphysema as well as a shortened life span (usually around 2 months of age) [42]. Klotho deficient mice also display severe hyperphosphatemia (high serum concentrations of phosphates) in association with increased concentrations of 1,25(OH)2D3, the active metabolite of vitamin D, which plays an important role in calcium metabolism [43]. In addition, the *klotho* mouse has reduced blood glucose and insulin levels and exhibits abnormal energy homeostasis manifested by increased glucose tolerance and insulin sensitivity, lower energy reserves (e.g., glycogen and lipid) and reduced body temperature [44]. Moreover, Klotho overexpression induces resistance to insulin and IGF-1 [41].

The Klotho gene encodes a single-pass transmembrane protein whose extracellular domain shares sequence homology with the β-glucosidase enzymes. In addition to its membrane form, the Klotho protein is present in the cytoplasm mostly in association with the endoplasmic reticulum and Golgi apparatus. In addition, the extracellular domain is cleaved and secreted into the blood and cerebrospinal fluid and functions as a circulatory hormone that binds to a cell-surface receptor and inhibits insulin/IGF-1 signaling [45]. Other functions of Klotho associated with its cellular, membrane and secreted forms will undoubtedly surface as discussed below.

Several observations have shown that Klotho can effectively block insulin-mediated glucose uptake, not at the level of insulin receptor-ligand binding, but by disrupting one or more alternative insulin-dependent intracellular signaling pathways including both the suppression of the tyrosine phosphorylation of insulin and IGF-1 receptors leading to their inactivation as well to the repression of already active insulin receptors, which were previously tyrosine phosphorylated by insulin stimulation [41]. This inactivation of insulin/IGF-1 receptors results in reduced activity of IRS proteins and their association with PI3-kinase, thereby inhibiting insulin and IGF-1 signaling.

Klotho protein increases the resistance to OS at the cellular and organismal level, which potentially contributes to its anti-aging properties. Klotho protein activates the FoxO forkhead transcription factors that are negatively regulated by insulin/IGF-1 signaling, thereby inducing expression of manganese superoxide dismutase (MnSOD), thereby facilitating ROS removal and confers OS resistance [46].

A premature aging-like phenotype that is quite similar to that of Klotho-deficient mice has been found in transgenic mice containing knock-out alleles of fibroblast growth factor23 (FGF23), albeit many of the abnormalities in *klotho* mice including arteriosclerosis, skin atrophy and emphysema are not present [47]. Common to both phenotypes, is the development of severe hyperphosphatemia in association with increased concentrations of 1,25(OH)2D3 [48]. As a potential explanation for this overlap in premature-aging and biochemical phenotypes, it has been suggested that Klotho affects the signal-transducing activity of multiple FGFs by binding to their receptors as the cofactor with FGF23; direct binding of Klotho to multiple FGF receptors (FGFRs) has been demonstrated [49]. Moreover, both Klotho and FGF23 functions are required for the negative regulation of the 1-hydroxylase gene, encoding a rate-limiting enzyme involved in active vitamin D synthesis [43]. Therefore, in addition to the OS generated by the insulin/IGF-1 pathway by disruption of Klotho function, Klotho can also contribute to the premature-aging phenotype by virtue of its effect on phosphate and calcium homeostatic regulation, and the hyper-production of the vitamin D metabolite in Klotho-deficient strains. We hesitate to call this a secondary function of Klotho since recent reports have shown that the premature aging phenotype in both the Klotho$^{-/-}$ and Ffg23$^{-/-}$ mice can be dramatically reversed (prolonging knockout-mouse survival to more than 6 months with few observable abnormalities) when fed a vitamin D-deficient diet or by ablation of the 1-hydroxylase gene [50]. Another Ca^{2+} related function of the Klotho protein that has been recently revealed is that it can modify sugar chains (hydrolysizing extracellular N-linked oligosaccharides) and activate the transient receptor potential ion channel TRPV5 through its activity as a β-glucuronidase, preventing the internalization and inactivation of plasma-membrane located Ca^{2+} channels with a net effect of increasing Ca^{2+} reabsorption in the kidney [51]. It remains to be seen whether the effects of the multi-functional Klotho protein on Ca^{2+} and phosphate homeostasis reported in the mouse are as highly-conserved as the insulin/IGF-1 pathway and operative in determining aging/longevity phenotypes in other organisms, including both worms and man.

Tissue-Specific Roles of Insulin/IGF-Signaling

Kenyon et al. have shown that the insulin/IGF-1 pathways involved in aging are tissue-specific, with certain cell-types acting as 'signaling centers" [52]. In particular, activity of the forkhead transcription factor DAF-16 in the intestine, which also serves as the animal's adipose tissue, completely restores the longevity of daf-16^{-} germline-deficient animals therefore affecting DAF-16 activity in other tissues, and substantially increases the life span of daf-16^{-} mutants. In addition, recent data suggest that several tissues in *C. elegans* act as signaling centers to mediate function of the ortholog of the human tumor suppressor gene PTEN, DAF-18 in regulating both dauer formation and life span [53].

The *D. melanogaster* insulin-like receptor mediates the phosphorylation of dFOXO, the equivalent of nematode DAF-16 and mammalian FOXO3a. dFOXO regulates *D. melanogaster* aging when activated in the adult pericerebral fat body [54]. Moreover, increasing FOXO activity in adipose tissue affected the activation of this pathway (i.e., insulin gene expression) in other tissues (i.e., neurons). This is similar to findings with FIRKO mice, which have reduced fat mass, are protected against age-related obesity and resulting metabolic abnormalities, and display an increased life span probably brought about by effects on insulin signaling [38]. This suggests that reduced adiposity, even in the presence of normal or increased food intake, can extend life span, perhaps as a result of the prevention of obesity-related metabolic disorders including type 2 diabetes and atherosclerosis [55].

Metabolic Pathways Involved in Longevity in *C. elegans*

A pivotal link between mitochondrial metabolism and longevity has been pointed out by the demonstration of long-lived strains with a dysfunctional electron transport chain (ETC). The isp-1 mutation is a missense mutation in a nuclear-DNA encoded component of respiratory complex III and results in reduced oxygen consumption, decreased sensitivity to ROS, and increased life span [56].

In addition to mutations that target mitochondrial ETC, gene silencing experiments using RNAi have also shown that downregulated mitochondrial function (e.g., mitochondrial leucyl-tRNA synthetase [lrs-2], ATP synthase) significantly increased life span and stress resistance in *C. elegans* [57, 58], as has treatment with the mitochondrial inhibitor antimycin A [59]. Given the essential role that ETC plays in the production of ATP and the demonstration that complete removal of this capacity often results in extensive cell dysfunction and premature death in most cell-types, the findings in *C. elegans* are somewhat surprising because they revealed that disruption of many of the key components of the normal mitochondrial energy-generating machinery do not result in death, but rather result in adult life span extension.

Four maternal-effect mutations termed the clock mutations were shown to promote life span extension independent of the insulin/IGF-1 pathways affected in dauer formation (i.e., involving DAF-2 and DAF-16) [60]. Amongst these long-lived mutants of *C. elegans*, clk-1, is unable to synthesize ubiquinone, CoQ(9), a cofactor in the mitochondrial respiratory chain. Instead, the mutant accumulates a novel ubiquinone species called demethoxyubiquinone(9) (DMK) and small amounts of rhodoquinone(9) as well as dietary CoQ(8) [61]. The CLK-1 protein is highly conserved among eucaryotes with structurally-related homologues in yeast and human and localizes to mitochondria [62]. Overexpression of CLK-1 activity in wild-type worms shortens life span and increases mitochondrial respiration whereas the clk-1 mutants, associated with life span extension, sustain moderately reduced mitochondrial respiration [61].However, no gross changes in metabolic output, as assessed by oxygen consumption, heat production rates and ATP content were found in clk-1 mutants (nor in any of the other clock-mutant strains), nor was there evidence of cooperatively increased ROS scavenging activity (i.e., catalase and SOD activities) in the clk-1 mutant [63]. Recently, analysis of isolated mitochondria from clk-1 mutants revealed a specific OXPHOS defect resulting from impaired electron transfer from complex I to complex III, whereas individual respiratory complex activities and OXPHOS initiated through complex II were normal [64]. Since both complex I and II use quinone, differential interactions with the quinone pool may be inferred and indicates that a more detailed examination of electron transport may be required beyond measurements of total oxygen consumption and of individual complex evaluation. Nevertheless, the electron transport defect present in the clk-1 mutant appears to relate less to a change in overall metabolic function (since ATP levels appear normal) but may pertain more to altered ROS levels and OS generation by the disabled respiratory complexes.

Silencing of ubiquinone biosynthesis genes including clk-1 in *C. elegans* using RNAi recapitulated the clk-1 mutant phenotype extending life span, lowered ubiquinone levels and reduced superoxide levels [65]. Moreover, withdrawal of coenzyme Q from the diet of wild-type worms extends the adult life span by approximately 60% [66]. The discovery that ROS production is reduced in the clk-1 mutants further supports the oxidative damage theory of aging [67]. Parenthetically, cytoplasmic ROS reduction has also been implicated in germline and vulval developmental delays occurring in clk-1 mutants, calling attention to the importance of ROS as signaling molecules in development [68].

It is also noteworthy that both human and mouse CLK-1 not only show strong structural similiarities but are functionally conserved as well [69, 70]. Transgenic expression of the wild-type mouse clk-1 orthologue into clk-1 *C. elegans* mutants reverted the extended life span of clk-1 mutants to levels comparable to those found in wild-type control [70]. Analysis of the knockout mutation of the mouse orthologue mclk1 indicated that CLK-1 and ubiquinone are necessary for normal mouse development, with mclk1$^{-/-}$ embryos arresting development at midgestation [71, 72]. Embryonic stem (ES) cells and embryos from these knockout strains accumulate a metabolic intermediate, demethoxyubiquinone instead of ubiquinone and exhibit a modest decline in respiratory function and lower ROS levels. Hekimi et al. have demonstrated that ES cells derived from mclk-inactivated embryos tend to be more protected from OS and damage to DNA [73]. Moreover, they also found that mclk1 $^{+/-}$ mice, whose growth and fertility are normal, display a substantial increase in life span in each of three different genetic backgrounds. These observations suggest that the distinct mechanism by which clk-1/mclk1 affects lifespan is evolutionarily conserved from nematodes to mammals.

A methyl viologen (paraquat)-sensitive mutant, mev-1, hypersensitive to oxygen exhibits a markedly shorter life span compared to wildtype *C. elegans* [74]. Furthermore, increasing levels of oxygen concentration exacerbated the aging rate and life span reduction of mev-1 mutants [75]. Strains bearing this mutation accumulate markers of aging (such as fluorescent material resembling lipofuscin and protein carbonyls) faster than the wild-type. Ishii et al. have found that mev-1 is a missense mutation in the SDHC gene encoding the large subunit of the enzyme succinate dehydrogenase cytochrome *b*, a component of respiratory complex II, and the ability of complex II to catalyze electron transport from succinate is compromised in mev-1 worms [76]. This mutation leads to a marked increase in superoxide anion levels, suggesting that endogenous ROS production at a defective complex II leads to the onset of oxygen hypersensitivity and premature aging [77]. Studies employing ultrastructural analysis of mev-1 mutants noted evidence of mitochondrial abnormalities (especially in muscle cells), a loss of mitochondrial membrane potential, and altered and supernumerary apoptotic cells [78]. In addition, mev-1 mutant worms harbor increased levels of nuclear DNA damage as indicated by significantly higher mutation frequencies under hypoxia than in the wild-type strain and suggesting that enhanced mitochondrial OS can be a significant source of genomic instability, which is a landmark of aging [79]. These defects resulting from increased ROS (and aberrant ETC) likely underlie the failure of mev-1 mutants to complete embryonic development under hyperoxia, as well as its reduced life span. It is also noteworthy that treatment of mev-1 mutant strains with coenzyme Q_{10} (CoQ_{10}) both eliminated the life span reduction, reduced superoxide levels and the number of apoptotic cells [80].

The gas-1 mutation was detected initially by its capacity to confer enhanced sensitivities to volatile anesthetics such as isoflurane [81]. Similar to mev-1 mutants, life span of gas-1 mutants are decreased compared to wild-type worms [82]. The gas-1 mutant contains a Arg-> Lys missense mutation in the gene encoding the 49-kDa subunit of the mitochondrial NADH: ubiquinone-oxidoreductase (respiratory complex I). This mutation results in a profound decline in complex I-dependent metabolism in mitochondria, as measured by rates of both OXPHOS, electron transport and increase in complex II-dependent metabolism [83]. Moreover, strains containing suppressors of gas-1 had elevated OXPHOS rates, decreased oxidative damage to mitochondrial proteins and increased life span. Interestingly, in contrast to wild-type strains in which the DAF-16/FOXO transcription factor normally resides in the cytoplasm and only becomes translocated to nuclei upon activating stimuli such as OS, DAF-16 resides and is constitutively expressed in the nuclei of both mev-1 and gas-1 mutants even under normal growth conditions [84]. Treatment of these mutants with the antioxidant CoQ_{10} reversed the nuclear translocation of DAF-16. These findings further implicate the role of OS from mitochondrial perturbations in impacting the insulin/IGF-1 signaling pathway.

While it is well-established that a deficiency of the mitochondrial protein frataxin causes Friedreich ataxia, an autosomal recessive neurological disorder, presumably because of altered iron metabolism and increased mitochondrial ROS production, the precise physiological role of frataxin in mitochondria and its role in aging remain largely undetermined. Studies in patient lymphoblasts have demonstrated decreased activity levels of enzymes containing iron-sulfur clusters including mitochondrial aconitase and succinic dehydrogenase (complex II), reduced heme levels and elevated superoxide levels [85]. Two recent studies have also demonstrated using a transient knockdown model of *C. elegans* frataxin deficiency, that RNA interference applied to the expression of the frataxin homologue (frh-1) significantly altered life span and sensitivity to OS [86, 87]. One study found that reduced frataxin levels increased life span [86], while the second study in contrast reported a decrease in life span, and increased sensitivity to OS [87]. The latter study also demonstrated genetic interaction between frh-1 and mev-1 suggesting a possible role of the *C. elegans* frataxin in the ETC. Moreover, studies with targeted disruption of hepatic frataxin in mice obtained similar results to the latter study including impaired mitochondrial function, increased OS and decreased life span [88].

Despite the large accumulation of mutant genes which impact longevity in *C. elegans*, there is limited information concerning the pathobiology of aging in this organism. In a recent study examining the cell integrity of different tissues in aging animals using ultrastructural analysis and specific cell-type visualization with green fluorescent protein, a striking preservation of the nervous system, even in advanced old age, was reported in contrast to a gradual, progressive deterioration of muscle, resembling human sarcopenia [89]. This study also reported evidence of both stochastic processes as well as contributory genetic factors as significant in *C. elegans* aging, contributing to extensive variability both among same-age animals and between cells of the same type within individuals

Several studies have extended the search for genetic mutations and factors that influence longevity by making use of RNA interference to systematically screen large sets of *C. elegans* genes for gene inactivations that increase life span [90–92]. In screening 5690 genes, Lee et al. reported that genes critical to mitochondrial function stood out as a principal sub-group of genes affecting *C. elegans* life span [90]. While long-lived worms with impaired mitochondria had lower ATP content and oxygen consumption, they exhibited differential responses to free-radical and other stresses suggesting longer life span could not be necessarily attributed to lower free radical production. Another screen found 23 novel genes which increase life span and these fell broadly into 4 classes: genes that influence life span through DAF16/FOXO/insulin/IGF-1, genes that influence mitochondrial respiration, genes that affect the response to dietary or caloric restriction and genes that affect integrin signaling, which are known to influence life span in flies [92]. Using genetic epistasis interaction analysis, nearly all of the novel genes detected could be associated with known aging-regulatory pathways or processes; conversely, mutations in other pathways (except DNA metabolism) were not contributory to life span extension in this study. Interestingly, many genes already known to be involved in aging in *C. elegans* were not identified in this screen suggesting that this selection was under-representing the full spectrum of longevity genes and that more genes remain to be found. Moreover, this selection would not be expected to include functionally redundant genes nor neuronal genes (which interestingly are refractory to RNAi in *C. elegans*). This caveat is important since other types of genetic screens revealed that loss-of-function mutations in several genes important for sensory neuron development can extend life span [93].

Another systematic screening of RNAi selected genes reported 89 novel longevity genes [91]. Over 25% of the genes identifiable by function (17 of 66), were involved in some aspect of metabolism, such as carbohydrate metabolism, alcohol metabolism, citric acid cycle, OXPHOS, and purine metabolism. In addition, this analysis identified genes encoding components of the DAF-2/insulin-like signaling pathway, as well as genes involved in signal transduction, protein turnover, and gene expression. A considerable number of these candidate longevity genes are highly conserved. Genetic interaction analyses with the new longevity genes revealed a subset that acted upstream of the DAF16/FOXO transcription factor or the Sir2.1 protein deacetylase, while others appear to function independently of DAF16/FOXO and Sir2.1, and may define new pathways to regulate life span [94].

SIR/Sirtuins

Using the genetically tractable model organism baker's yeast, *Saccharomyces cerevisiae,* primary genetic determinants of replicative life span in yeast were initially identified from genetic screens of starvation-resistant strains for long-lived mutants. Among these mutants were included members of the SIR (silent information regulator) gene family [95]. Subsequent studies revealed that loss-of-function of SIR2 significantly shortened yeast life span, whereas increased SIR2 gene dosage extended it [96]. A SIR2 orthologue subsequently detected in *C. elegans* was similarly shown to extend life span with increased dosage [97].

Interestingly, SIR2 had been previously identified as a mediator of gene silencing of the mating type loci in yeast [98]. In yeast, transcriptional silencing occurs at a number of chromosomal loci including telomeres, the two mating-type loci (*HML* and *HMR*), and rDNA locus *RDN1*. The establishment of inactive heterochromatin at telomeres, mating-type loci and at the rDNA requires a complex including Sir2. Overexpression of Sir2 increases the extent of silencing at both telomeres and rDNA, suggesting that Sir2 is a limiting component of the silencing apparatus. Evidence strongly suggests that SIR2 mediates its effect on yeast aging primarily through its generation of heterochromatin at the rDNA, and suppression of both the recombination between rDNA repeats and the formation of extra-chromosomal circular forms of rDNA (ERCs) [99]. SIR2's action as a NAD-dependent histone deacetylase (HDAC) mediates this chromatin remodeling effect, and has rendered it the founding member of a large family of NAD-dependent histone deacetylases termed the sirtuins. The sirtuin proteins are conserved from prokaryotes to eucaryotes, and include seven human sirtuin isoforms. The NAD^+ dependence of SIR2 may permit the regulation of its activity through changes in the availability of this co-substrate, allowing the enzyme to sense the bioenergetic and redox states of the cell and set the life span accordingly. Moreover, SIR2 activity can be elevated by genetic and physiological interventions that decrease the levels of NADH, a competitive inhibitor of Sir2 [100].

A critical target of the SIR2 deacetylase activity is the FOXO forkhead transcription factors, shifting FOXO dependent responses away from cell death and towards cell survival contributing to enhanced longevity. In addition to the demonstration by genetic analysis in *C. elegans* that SIR2 acts upstream of DAF-16 in the insulin-like signaling pathway [97], several studies have shown that SIRT1, the mammalian homologue of SIR2, deacetylates FOXO factors (e.g., FOXO 1,3 and/or 4) and modulates their transactivation function [101–103]. The effect on FOXO function lead to the attenuation of FOXO-induced apoptosis and potentiation of FOXO3's ability to induce resistance to OS. Other recently identified SIRT1-regulated transcription factors which operate in aging as well of considerable significance in cardiovascular signaling pathways include peroxisome proliferator-activated receptor γ (PPAR-γ), peroxisome proliferator-activated receptor γ coactivator 1α (PGC-1α), NF-κB, p53, p300 and the cell-cycle and apoptosis regulator E2F1 [104–107].

While an extensive discussion of caloric restriction (CR) in mediating aging and longevity will be forthcoming in a later chapter, it is important to mention here that a link between SIR2 and CR has been suggested by studies in yeast [100], although recent studies have found evidence of life span extension in yeast strains which is SIR-2 independent [108]. Similarly, while some studies supported a role for respiration in adjusting NAD+/NADH ratios affecting SIR2 with CR in yeast [109], more recent observations have shown that CR can occur in yeast in respiration-deficient strains [110]. In nematodes while increased Sir2 can extend life span, a direct link to CR has not been demonstrated.

A direct connection between SIR2 activation and CR has been more convincingly demonstrated in studies with *Drosophila* [111]. This study found that an increase in *Drosophila* Sir2 (dSir2) extends fly life span, whereas a decrease in dSir2 blocks the life span-extending effect of CR. Recent studies have suggested that the mammalian Sir2 orthologue, Sirt1, is required for the induction of at least a phenotypic component of the complex physiological and behavior patterns associated with CR in mice [112]. Moreover, Sirt1 activates a critical tissue-specific component of CR in mammals; i.e., fat mobilization in white adipocytes [113]. Upon food withdrawal, Sirt1 protein binds to and represses PPAR-γ transcriptional activation downregulating genes mediating fat storage. In Sirt1 $^{+/-}$ mice, mobilization of fatty acids from white adipocytes upon fasting is compromised. In 3T3-L1 adipocytes, overexpression of Sirt1 attenuates adipogenesis, and RNAi-mediated silencing of Sirt1 expression enhances it. In addition, upregulation of Sirt1 in differentiated fat cells triggers lipolysis and loss of fat. The involvement of Sirt1 in fat reduction is likely a contributory factor in extending life span.

TOR

Several components (TOR and raptor) of another nutrient sensing pathway have been recently implicated in both life span extension in several model organisms, and as part of the CR pathway in yeast [114]. The target of rapamycin (TOR) encodes a protein kinase that mediates a highly conserved signaling pathway that couples amino acid availability to ribosomal S6 protein kinase activation, translation initiation, and cell growth. In addition, TOR responds to changes in growth factors, amino acids, oxygen tension, and energy status. As with the insulin/IGF-1 pathway, inhibition of the TOR signaling pathway in *Drosophila* extends life span. Overexpression of upstream regulators such as tuberous sclerosis complex genes 1 and 2 (dTsc1, dTsc2), which inhibit TOR expression, or dominant-negative forms of dTOR or dS6K all cause life span extension, dependent on the nutritional status [115]. Similar to findings with the insulin/IGF-1 pathway, modulation of TOR signaling expression in fat tissues is sufficient for life span extension. In *C. elegans,* LET-363/TOR deficiency mediated by targeted RNA interference more than doubles the worm life span [116]. Evidence from genetic analysis suggests an interaction of the insulin/IGF-1 and TOR pathways with nutrient-sensing TOR acting downstream of DAF-16 to regulate protein synthesis. Mutations in the *C. elegans* homologue of the TOR accessory protein, raptor (DAF-15) also extend adult life span and daf-15 transcription is regulated by DAF-16, that in turn is regulated by daf-2 insulin/IGF signaling [117].

Disruption in TOR signaling, as a result of either mutation or targeted pharmacological intervention (e.g., rapamycin treatment), resulted in enhanced chronological life span in yeast (i.e., the time cells in a stationary phase culture remain viable), a potential model for aging of post-mitotic tissues in mammals [118]. Decreased TOR activity also resulted in increased accumulation of storage carbohydrates and enhanced stress resistance. Furthermore, removal of either asparagine or glutamate from the media significantly increased stationary phase survival suggesting that TOR plays a role in starvation-induced stress and CR modulation of life span. In addition, TOR modulates replicative life span in yeast in response to nutrients and modulates CR; CR failed to increase life span in TOR mutants [114].

Another critical aspect of TOR action relevant to aging is its effect on stress response and signaling of mitochondrial dysfunction. The mTOR is mainly localized in the mitochondrial outer membrane (although a cytosolic form has also been reported) [119]. Moreover, mTOR along with accessory proteins such as raptor form a stress-sensing module consisting of mitochondria and mitochondrial outer membrane-associated mTOR, integrate diverse stress signals, including nutrients, cAMP levels, and osmotic stress with cellular responses such as transcription, translation, and autophagy. Mitochondrial bioenergetic function and membrane potential serve as a regulatory intermediate on TOR activity [120, 121]. Raptor (regulatory associated protein of mTOR) binds to p70S6 kinase ($p70^{s6k}$) and 4E-BP1 and is essential for TOR signaling *in vivo* and it appears to serve as an mTOR scaffold protein; binding to mTOR substrates is required for effective mTOR-catalyzed phosphorylation *in vivo* [122].

Interestingly, mTOR pathway plays a significant role in determining both resting oxygen consumption. and oxidative capacity [123]. This conclusion was mainly inferred from the correlation of mTOR/raptor complex formation with overall mitochondrial activity. Following treatment with the mTOR inhibitor rapamycin, disruption of this complex lowered membrane potential, oxygen consumption and ATP synthetic capacity. Furthermore, this inhibition resulted in marked alteration in the mitochondrial phospho-proteome suggesting that TOR phosphorylation of intramitochondrial proteins is part of the mechanism of TOR action.

Modulation of the mitochondrial permeability transition (PT) pore (also located at the junction of the mitochondrial inner and outer membranes) is regulated by the activity of glycogen synthase kinase-3β (GSK-3β), which is under convergent regulation by the protein kinase B/Akt and mTOR/$p70^{s6k}$ pathways [124]. This pathway has been described in cardiomyocytes and implicated in the cardioprotective pathway in response to hypoxic insult. In isolated mouse heart and cardiomyocytes inhibition of TOR signaling with rapamycin confers preconditioning-like protection against ischemia-reperfusion injury [125]. Limiting the opening of the PT pore also likely prevents apoptosis (Fig. 12.2). Furthermore, studies in yeast and animal cells have shown that mTOR serves as part of the mitochondrial retrograde response, a signaling pathway of communication from mitochondria to the nucleus that involves multiple factors that sense mitochondrial dysfunction and transmit signals to effect changes in nuclear gene expression [126, 127].

Other Genetic Factors in Aging Drosophila

Drosophila is another valuable model organism employed to identify genetic determinants of aging and to find genetic variations that can affect aging. Flies are particularly well suited for such studies since they develop to adulthood quickly, have a relatively short life span, their genome has been sequenced and contains extensive homologues in mammals; powerful genetic tools are available to

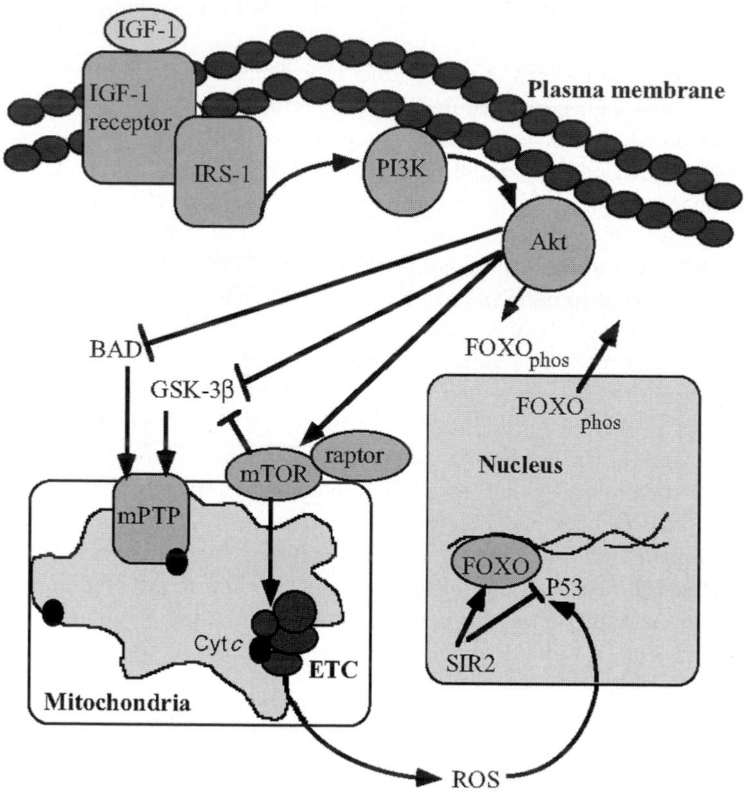

Fig. 12.2 Several signaling pathways, including IGF-1, mTOR and SIR2 interact in aging
Shown is the IGF-1 ligand binding to its cell surface receptor (associated with insulin receptor substrate-1 (IRS-1). Downstream of the receptor, the signal is transmited to the kinases (PI3K and subsequently Akt). The activated Akt inhibits the translocation of the proapoptotic BAD to the mitochondria, stemming mitoPTP (mPTP) and inhibiting apoptosis; similarly, it attenuates glycogen synthase kinase-3β (GSK-3β) activity-reducing mPTP. Akt also activates mTOR signaling part of the mitochondrial retrograde pathway. Akt phosphorylates FOXO, inactivating it, increasing its translocation from the nucleus to the cytosol, reducing its DNA binding and stemming its positive effect on longevity. In contrast, the sirtuin (SIR2) activates FOXO transcriptional activity by reversing its acetylation. Similarly, SIR2 inactivates p53 by deacetylation and attenuates its apoptotic program.

manipulate it [128, 129]. A number of genes involved in the prolongation of life span have been found, further increasing the number of pathways involved in aging response, and noticeable parallels between functional senescence in *Drosophila* and humans have been revealed. In addition, the aging fly heart is an informative model to study the genetics of age-sensitive organ-specific pathology [130]. For instance, as in elderly humans, maximal heart rate is significantly and reproducibly reduced with aging in *Drosophila,* which also manifests an age-associated increase in cardiac dysrhythmias [131].

Besides the previously discussed defects in the insulin/IGF-signaling (e.g., *chico* and *InR*), SIR2 and TOR pathways that promote increased longevity in flies, mutations in other pathways affecting fly aging have also been identified.

Mutations that confer resistance to OS have been noted to display a longevity phenotype. For instance, fly longevity was found to be prolonged by mutations in the Egm gene encoding enigma, a mitochondrial protein with homology to enzymes of the β-oxidation of fatty acids [132]. Complete loss of enigma function affects development and is lethal; low levels engendered by a hypomorphic allele also resulted in premature lethality. Nevertheless, intermediate amounts of the enigma protein present in heterozygous flies, significantly increase life span and tolerance to OS. Egm's extensive sequence homology to ACAD, an enzyme that catalyzes the first of the four reactions that constitute one cycle of the β-oxidation pathway, its mitochondrial localization, and the decreased levels of triglycerides reported in Egm mutant cells, suggest that mutations in β-oxidation metabolism can mediate both life span extension and OS, and appear to characterize a novel longevity pathway.

Mutations in components of several signal transduction pathways have been shown to impact longevity in flies. The evolutionarily conserved Jun N-terminal kinase (JNK) signaling pathway has been shown to be a genetic determinant of aging in *Drosophila*, and acts as a coordinator in the induction of protective genes in response to oxidative challenge with JNK signaling activity, alleviating the toxic effects of ROS [133]. Besides, flies harboring mutations that augment JNK signaling accumulate less oxidative damage and live dramatically longer than wild-type flies. Further analysis of the JNK mediated longevity extension has shown that JNK signaling interfaces and/or overlaps with the insulin/IGF-1 signaling pathway. JNK requires the transcription factor Foxo to extend life span in *Drosophila* [134], and under conditions of low insulin/IGF-1 pathway activity Foxo increases life span. This analysis has also demonstrated that JNK antagonizes insulin/IGF 1 signaling, causing nuclear localization of Foxo and inducing its targets, including growth control and stress defense genes; both JNK and Foxo restrict insulin/IGF-1 activity systemically by repressing ligand expression, particularly in neuroendocrine cells.

That the G-protein signaling system has a potential role in aging has been suggested by the discovery that mutation of a G-protein coupled receptor (GPCR), encoded by *Methuselah,* extends *Drosophila* life span and provides enhanced resistance to various forms of stress, including starvation, high temperature, and dietary paraquat, a free-radical generator [135]. Moreover, mutations in two endogenous peptide ligands of *Methuselah*, designated Stunted A and B result in increased life span and resistance to OS [136].

The observation that long-lived mutants are more resistant to multiple environmental stresses underlies the use of screening cDNA libraries of stressed *versus* unstressed flies by subtractive hybridization to identify stress-regulated genes, which can subsequently be tested for their effect on longevity [137]. Profiling of stress-mediated gene expression identified 13 genes, several already known to be involved in longevity and other genes such as hsp26 and hsp27. Overexpression of either hsp26 or hsp27 extended the fly life span by 30%, and increased stress resistance to multiple stimuli, validating the use of multiple-stress screening to identify new longevity genes. It is noteworthy that both ubiquitous or motorneuron-targeted overexpression of HSP22, a small mitochondrial heat shock protein, significantly increased life span and increased resistance to oxidative damage and thermal stress [138].

Insertional mutations in the INDY gene ("I'm not dead yet"), resulted in a near doubling of the average fly adult life span without a decline in fertility or physical activity [139]. Sequence analysis revealed that Indy is closely related to a mammalian sodium dicarboxylate cotransporter, a membrane protein that transports Krebs cycle intermediates (e.g., dicarboxylates and citrate) through the epithelium of the gut and across the plasma membranes of organs involved in intermediary metabolism and storage.

Given that ROS and OS are a focal point in several aging signaling pathways in *Drosophila*, increasing mitochondrial proton leakage by augmenting mitochondrial uncoupling would appear to be a viable intervention postulated to decrease mitochondrial ROS production, and also a potential site to impact longevity. Introduction of the gene for the human uncoupling protein UCP2 (hUCP2), targeted to the mitochondria of adult fly neurons, resulted in increased state 4 respiration, reduced ROS production and oxidative damage, elevated resistance to the free radical generator paraquat, and an extension in life span without compromising fertility or physical activity [140]. These findings were complemented by an entirely different experimental approach, the addition of the uncoupler 2, 4-dinitrophenol (DNP) to the nutritional mixture of larvae that significantly increased the average life span of the flies without changing their maximal life span [141], although this treatment resulted in poor overall viability.

Caution must be used in inferring that reducing OS in itself can promote fly longevity. Mutant flies overexpressing the mitochondrial adenine nucleotide translocase (ANT) had significantly lower ROS production mainly because they had lower membrane potential, but their life span was not significantly extended compared to wild type [142]. Conversely, the use of CR in flies extended life span but was not correlated with a significant difference in mitochondrial ROS production, compared with controls. In addition, simultaneous overexpression of the antioxidant enzymes MnSOD and catalase, ectopically targeted to the mitochondrial matrix of transgenic *Drosophila* strains resulted in a decrease in mitochondrial H_2O_2 release, enhancement of free methionine content, enhanced resistance to experimental OS (induced by dietary H_2O_2 administration or by exposure to 100% ambient oxygen) and surprisingly, resulted in reduced life span by up to 43% [143]. Furthermore, feeding the SOD mimetic drugs Euk-8 and −134 and the mitochondria-targeted mitoquinone (MitoQ) to both, wild type and SOD-deficient flies also demonstrated that exogenous antioxidants can rescue the pathology associated with compromised defenses to OS, but failed to extend the life span of normal, wild-type animals [144]. In wild-type flies all three drugs showed a dose-dependent increase in toxicity, an effect that was further exacerbated in the presence of the redox-cycling drug paraquat. A potential conclusion from these findings is that mitochondrial ROS/H_2O_2 is essential in normal physiological processes and needed to attain a normal life span. Interestingly, in SOD-deficient flies, antioxidant drugs increased life span and the effects were sex-specific and variable, depending on dosage and the developmental stage when drugs were given.

Presently, increasing attention has been focused on a complex series of phenotypes that promote longevity in *Drosophila* [145, 146]. These phenotypes involve antioxidant upregulation, altered metabolic and mitochondrial energetic regulation (including changes in ETC as well as fatty acid metabolism), mechanisms to stem ROS production, protection against OS and leakage from mitochondria. Critical to the success of a long-lived phenotype, is a finely tuned balance of oxidant and antioxidant, stressor and stress-responder. The identification of genetic factors that can provide protection against stress and affect life span continues to grow, and has provided both insights and several surprises. In *Drosophila*, systematic gain-of-function mutagenesis utilizing GAL4-UAS constructs has permitted the identification of genes that may not be easily detectable by loss-of-function screening approaches. This has been assisted by conditional features of gene "mis"-expression systems especially useful for studying late-stage biological processes, such as those involving adult behavior or life span [147, 148]. This method employed the mis-expression of large gene inserts, incorporated into a vector and containing an upstream activating sequence (UAS), in the presence of a GAL4 transgene induced throughout the adult stage to assess the effects on the aging process.

Of 616 inserts, 23 conferred relatively longer longevity with six related to stress resistance or redox balance (DmGST2, hsp26, nla, and *Drosophila* homologues of mammalian TRX, GILT and POSH), confirming the importance of stress resistance in the extension of longevity. Further experiments with POSH, a scaffold protein containing RING finger and four SH3 domains whose ubiquitous overexpression in adult stage extends fly longevity, showed that its overexpression in neural-specific tissues was sufficient to extend longevity, whereas overexpression during development in non-neural tissues induced apoptosis, largely via activation of the JNK/SAPK pathway [149].

Recently, gathered observations have shown that overexpression of a homologue of apolipoprotein D (ApoD) resulted in increased resistance to hyperoxia and starvation, as well as extension of fly life span under normoxia [145]. Moreover, targeting specific tissues/organs (e.g., neuronal, fat bodies etc.) with specific genes has proved to be highly successful. In addition, the identification of molecular changes, landmarks of longevity and development of biomarkers of aging have presented an alternative to survivorship as a measure of longevity accelerating the potential identification of both genetic and pharmacological interventions that can prolong fly life span [150]. Obviously, it will be of great interest to find if the same series of phenotypic changes and molecular landmarks of longevity can be replicated in human.

Mouse Models of Aging

Previously, we have briefly discussed insulin/IGF-1 signaling in mouse models. In this section, we will present several mouse aging/longevity models that appear to be independent of this pathway.

Mice containing a homozygous deletion of the p66Shc gene have an extended life span (by 30%) and exhibit increased stress resistance [151]. The p66Shc adaptor protein is a cytoplasmic signal transducer involved in the transmission of mitogenic signals from activated receptors to Ras. In addition to mitogenic signaling, p66Shc promotes apoptosis in several cell-types acting in response to a variety of stimuli, and is an indispensable downstream target of the stress-activated tumor suppressor p53 in promoting apoptosis [152]; the absence of p66Shc in null mice correlates with reduced levels of apoptosis in response to H_2O_2 or UV light. Moreover, deletion of p66Shc protects mouse embryo fibroblasts from apoptosis induced by OS, while overexpression of p66Shc in wild-type fibroblasts increases their susceptibility to H_2O_2 [153].

Several recent studies have reported that a fraction of cytosolic p66Shc localizes to the mitochondria [154, 155]. Within the mitochondria, p66Shc complexes with mitochondrial HSP70, a chaperone that acts as an antiapoptotic factor. Dissociation of this inhibitory complex by UV radiation leads to the release of monomeric p66Shc. p66Shc causes apoptosis by modulating ROS-induced mitochondrial damage and by the release of apoptogenic factors. Activated p53 effects a sustained rise in ROS levels implicated in the opening of the mitochondrial PT pore, the release of apoptogenic factors including cytochrome *c*, and the cytosolic assembly of the apoptosome. While expression of p66Shc is required for p53 to increase ROS and induce cytochrome *c* release [152], its role in PT pore modulation remains undetermined. In cells in which p66Shc is absent, the characteristic response to OS (i.e., H_2O_2 treatment) of cytochrome *c* release and reduced membrane potential is blunted indicating that p66Shc, when present, spurs the destruction of mitochondria and the dispersal of cytochrome *c* [154].

Several elegant experiments have shown that p66Shc serves as a redox enzyme in mitochondria resulting in the direct generation of mitochondrial ROS (i.e., H_2O_2) by using reducing equivalents of the mitochondrial ETC, through the oxidation of cytochrome *c* [156]. In support of this mechanism, redox-defective mutants of p66Shc are unable to induce mitochondrial ROS generation and swelling *in vitro* or to mediate mitochondrial apoptosis *in vivo*.

In addition, p66Shc$^{-/-}$ fibroblasts derived from transgenic mouse embryos display abnormal mitochondrial energetics, with reduced oxygen consumption in both coupled and uncoupled states and reduced mitochondrial NADH metabolism [155]. The reduced oxidative capacity observed in p66Shc^{-} cells is counter-balanced by a metabolic switch encompassing augmented aerobic glycolysis and increased lactate production.

Similarly, mouse transgenic models have been informative to support a role of mitochondrial bioenergetic function in aging. Larsson et al. have shown markedly increased apoptosis in cells from embryos containing a homozygous disruption of the mitochondrial transcription factor A gene (TFAM), and increased apoptosis in the hearts from cardiac-specific TFAM knockout animals that also displayed severe myocardial respiratory chain deficiency [157]. These findings have provided direct *in vivo* evidence that respiratory chain deficiency (as a result of reduced mtDNA expression) predisposes cells to apoptosis. However, in *TFAM* knockout mice, no evidence for induction in the expression of enzymes involved in ROS scavenging was found, suggesting that OS is not an important pathophysiological mechanism at least in these animals. As previously noted the critical role of point mutations in mtDNA in aging has been recently highlighted in homozygous knock-in mouse strains that express a proof-reading-deficient version of Polγ, the nuclear-encoded catalytic subunit of mtDNA polymerase [158]. The knock-in mice developed a three-to five-fold increase in the levels of mtDNA point mutations, as well as increased amount of deleted mtDNA. Increased somatic mtDNA mutations were associated with reduced life span and premature onset of aging-related phenotypes, including cardiomegaly, thus, providing further link between mtDNA mutations and aging. Further observations in mtDNA mutator mice unexpectedly did not find significant accumulation of ROS, changes of antioxidant enzymes nor markers of OS; this occurs despite severe respiratory deficiency, which in these strains may be the primary inducer of aging rather than ROS [159].

In longevity studies with higher organisms, there has been limited direct evidence for the role of ROS and OS, pivotal features of the free radical theory of aging. Numerous studies have reported a positive correlation between increased ROS production/oxidative damage and age [160–162], and diverse manipulations that increase life span also diminish the age-related increase in oxidatively damaged molecules [163, 164]. As previously discussed in this chapter, support for ROS involvement in aging has been obtained from studies with different genetically modified *C. elegans* strains. Studies with *Drosophila* in which antioxidant gene expression was modulated have been more equivocal. For instance, overexpression of the cytosolic Cu–ZnSOD (SOD1) in a single cell-type, the adult motoneuron, resulted in increased fly life span of up to 40% [165]. Similarly, CuSOD overexpression extended the mean fly life span up to 48% [166], and MnSOD overexpression up to 37% extension [167], with no additional benefit of overexpressing catalase in the same models. Orr and Sohal have argued that life span extension in the fly model may be limited to short-lived strains with a specific genetic background [168]. Other investigators have been unable to replicate the increase in longevity with overexpression of CuSOD, MnSOD, catalase or thioredoxin reductase in a variety of long-lived recipient strains [169].

Findings in mouse genetic models, in which the expression of different antioxidant enzymes has been altered, have also cast doubt on the centrality of ROS accumulation in determining longevity/aging. Homozygous transgenic mice with a two- to five-fold elevation of Cu-ZnSOD in various tissues showed a slight reduction in life span, whereas hemizygous mice with a 15- to 3-fold increase of Cu-ZnSOD showed no difference compared to nontransgenic littermate controls [170]. Another study has been reported in which overexpression of human Cu–ZnSOD in mice over a 19 month period resulted in neither changes in life span nor neuroprotection [171]. In mice heterozygous for a null mutation of *SOD2* (MnSOD), reduced activity (roughly 50%) of this enzyme is present in most tissues [172]. Increased oxidative damage, including markedly elevated levels of 8-oxo-2-deoxyguanosine (8oxodG) was found in both in nuclear DNA and mtDNA in all examined tissues of *SOD2*$^{+/-}$ mice compared with wild-type mice, as was a marked increase in tumor incidence with aging. However, no difference in either mean or maximal life span was evident, nor was there any significant accumulation of biomarkers of aging, such as cataract formation, immune response, and formation of glycoxidation products carboxymethyl lysine and pentosidine in skin collagen in the life-long MnSOD-deficient strains. Therefore, life-long reduction of MnSOD activity leads to increased levels of oxidative damage to DNA and increased cancer incidence but does not appear to directly affect aging.

Studies in rat heart and liver [173, 174], and in aging human tissues including diaphragm, heart and brain [175–177] have found marked aging-dependent elevation of oxo8-dG levels in mtDNA. In rat heart, increase in mtDNA damage was correlated with mitochondrial respiratory dysfunction, (i.e., reduced levels of complex I and IV activity) [174]. Collectively, these findings have led to the hypothesis that aging-mediated accumulation of oxo8-dG to high levels leads to increased levels of mtDNA mutations, triggering mtDNA instability, reduced rates of mitochondrial protein synthesis, and production of mutant polypeptides that compromise mitochondrial respiration [178].

Nevertheless, a rigorous demonstration of mitochondrial dysfunction secondary to oxo8-dG accumulation in mtDNA is still lacking. One recent study failed to find evidence of mitochondrial respiratory dysfunction even when levels of oxo8-dG are highly elevated [179]. Mice deficient for oxoguanine DNA glycosylase (OGG1), an enzyme responsible for oxo8-dG removal, accumulate oxo8-dG in mtDNA to levels 20-fold higher than in wild-type mice, yet their mitochondria are functionally normal. No significant differences in either coupled or uncoupled respiration rates, ATP synthesis rate or nor maximal activities of complexes I and IV (in liver and heart) were found. Neither was there indication of increased OS in mitochondria from $OGG1^{-/-}$ mice, as gauged by levels of mitochondrial protein carbonyl content. This suggests that the accumulation of oxo8-dG is not sufficient for the onset of mitochondrial respiratory dysfunction. Accordingly, both environmental and genetic factors that might impact on the action of OS are being sought [180].

In addition, mice deficient for both of the major mitochondrial antioxidant enzymes MnSOD and glutathione peroxidase (GPx) ($SOD2^{+/-}/GPX1^{-/-}$) appear phenotypically normal, and can exhibit normal longevity and yet are extremely sensitive to OS [181]. Survival of the $SOD2^{+/-}/GPX1^{-/-}$ mice in response to exogenous stress including whole body γ irradiation or paraquat administration was reduced compared with that of wild-type. Moreover, endogenous OS induced by cardiac ischemia/reperfusion injury promoted increased apoptosis in heart tissue from the double mutant mice, compared to levels of mice deficient in either MnSOD or GPx alone. Therefore, while longevity appears to be unaffected in these strains by modulating antioxidant enzyme levels, aging-associated susceptibility to OS (particularly in specific tissues, including myocardium) is more pronounced with increased ROS levels.

Interestingly, support for the role of ROS and for the free radical theory of aging has recently emerged from the studies of Schriner et al. in which the overexpression of human catalase, normally localized in the peroxisome, when targeted to the mitochondria resulted in a 20% extension of median and maximum life span in two strains of transgenic mice [182]. Older transgenic strains harboring a 50-fold increase in their expression of the antioxidant catalase in cardiac and skeletal muscle mitochondria, exhibited diminished H_2O_2 production, H_2O_2-induced aconitase inactivation and oxidative DNA damage including reduced levels of aging-stimulated mtDNA deletions and oxo8-dG. Moreover, older transgenic animals showed marked reduction in the aging-tissue pathologies found in older control mice; in particular, a delay in the development of cataract formation, arteriosclerosis and cardiac structural changes (e.g., subendocardial interstitial fibrosis, hyaline cytoplasmic change, vacuolization of cytoplasm, variable myocyte fiber size, hypercellularity, collapse of sarcomeres and mineralization). In contrast, targeting human catalase to peroxisomes or nucleus did not significantly extend the life span of transgenic mice. The increase in life span resulting from the upregulation of a single gene involved in boosting antioxidant defenses, and its targeting to the mitochondria, reinforces the notion that mitochondrial ROS and OS play a role in defining life span.

Parenthetically, it is interesting to note that the very long-lived naked mole rat (whose life span of 27 years is over 10-fold longer than its close rodent relatives, rat and mice) exhibits neither an increased level of antioxidant enzymes (such as SOD, catalase and GPx) with age nor does it possess a superior antioxidant armamentarium as compared to its shorter-lived relatives [183]. Moreover, young naked mole-rats surprisingly have high levels of accrued oxidative damage [184].

Models for Premature Aging Syndromes and Progeria

An interesting model for studying human aging is a rare autosomal recessive disorder known as the Werner syndrome (WS), which is characterized by accelerated aging *in vivo* and *in vitro*. Mutations in the WRN gene encoding a RecQ DNA helicase are associated with the development of premature aging in early adulthood including atherosclerosis, which would normally be primarily found in old individuals. The vast majority of WRN mutations produce C-terminal truncations resulting in impaired nuclear localization of the protein and functionally null alleles [185]. Cultured fibroblasts from patients with WS display defects associated with telomere dysfunction, including accelerated telomere erosion and premature senescence. These cells are genetically unstable, characterized by an increased frequency of nonclonal translocations and extensive nuclear DNA deletions and have a markedly reduced growth potential [186]. The WRN protein has been found to co-localize with telomeric factors as well as with a number of proteins involved in DNA metabolism including replication protein A (RPA), proliferating cell nuclear antigen (PCNA), DNA topoisomerase I, DNA polymerase δ and p53, and primarily (although not exclusively) resides in the nucleolus [186, 187]. In addition to its helicase function, WRN has exonuclease activity, and participates in recombination, DNA replication and repair functions as well as acts as a transcriptional activator. A model of WRN and its contribution in aging is shown in Fig. 12.3.

Homologues for the WRN gene have been found in yeast, *Drosophila, C. elegans* and mice and gathered observations in those model systems have proved informative. In yeast, the WRN

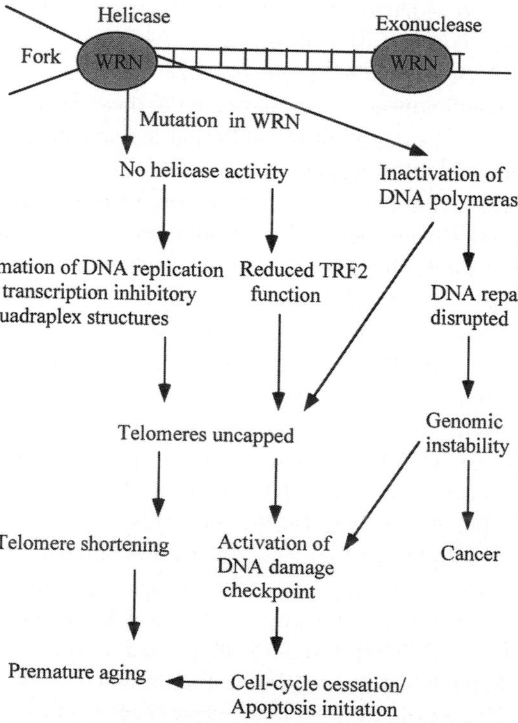

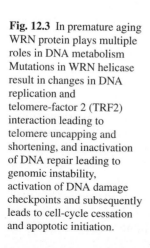

Fig. 12.3 In premature aging WRN protein plays multiple roles in DNA metabolism Mutations in WRN helicase result in changes in DNA replication and telomere-factor 2 (TRF2) interaction leading to telomere uncapping and shortening, and inactivation of DNA repair leading to genomic instability, activation of DNA damage checkpoints and subsequently leads to cell-cycle cessation and apoptotic initiation.

homologue SGS1 is required for genome stability; strains deleted for sgs1 show mitotic hyper-recombination [188]. Mutation of SGS1 caused premature aging in yeast mother cells, on the basis of a shortened life span, and also promoted aging-induced phenotypes of sterility and the relocation of the Sir3 silencing protein from telomeres to the nucleolus [189]. Furthermore, older SGS1-deficient cells displayed enlarged and fragmented nucleoli. Mutations in SGS1 increased the rate of accumulating gross chromosomal rearrangements including translocations and deletions containing extended regions of imperfect homology at their breakpoints [190]. In the absence of telomerase activity, sgs1 mutants show defective telomere metabolism with a higher rate of telomere erosion, and display increased rates of growth arrest in the G_2/M phase of the yeast cell cycle [191, 192].

Recent observations suggest that *C. elegans* may be a useful model for studying the premature aging associated with WS. A *C. elegans* WRN protein homologue (WRN-1) has been immunolocalized to the nuclei of germ cells, embryonic cells, and other cells of larval and adult worms [193]. Interestingly, RNA interference studies have shown that inhibition of WRN-1 expression caused a variety of developmental defects with accompanying signs of premature aging, such as earlier accumulation of lipofuscin, increased tissue deterioration in the head as well as altered life span. WRN-1 deficient worms also exhibited abnormal DNA replication (accelerated S phase) and responses to DNA damage, consistent with roles of the WRN protein in both DNA replication and repair, and its contribution to the aging process.

In studies with the murine homologue of WRN, deletion mutations within the coding sequence were generated in both ES cells and animals [194]. Although they exhibit reduced embryonic survival, homozygous WS mice appear normal during their first year of life. Homozygous WS ES cells display a higher mutation rate and are significantly more sensitive to topoisomerase inhibitors (e.g., camptothecin) than are wild-type ES cells. Furthermore, mouse embryo fibroblasts derived from homozygous WS embryos show premature loss of proliferative capacity recapitulating the phenotype of cultured fibroblasts from WS patients. However, in transgenic mice harboring a mutation that eliminates expression of the C-terminus of the helicase domain of the WRN protein (analogous to the most prevalent type of human WRN mutation), there was no overt sign of premature aging or of altered life span [195]. Given the indicated importance of telomere events as a locus of WRN action in both patient fibroblast and yeast studies, the different phenotypic responses to WRN mutation in mice, compared to human, might be attributed to longer telomeres and a more prevalent telomerase, which are known to be present in mice. Employing mice containing a telomerase (TERC-) mutation (to shorten the telomeres) and WRN-null mutations, strains were eventually generated (several generations were required for the telomere loss) that recapitulated many of the features of the WS phenotype including cataract development, graying hair, alopecia, osteoporosis, type II diabetes and slow wound healing [196, 197]. These strains also developed cancers such as lymphomas and soft-tissue sarcomas, that typically strike Werner syndrome patients but are rare in the general population. Moreover, this mouse model also showed accelerated replicative senescence and accumulation of DNA-damage foci in cultured cells. The pathology in these mouse strains was also accompanied by enhanced telomere dysfunction, including end-to-end chromosome fusions and loss of telomere repeat DNA [198]. These data suggest that the delayed manifestation of the complex aging phenotypes associated with WRN deficiency are precipitated by the exhaustion of telomere reserves in mice as indicated by telomere shortening. This notion is strongly supported by recent findings of physical and functional interactions between WRN and TRF2, a telomeric repeat binding factor essential for proper telomeric structure, [199, 200] and between WRN and telomeric DNA [201].

Another mouse model of WS in which part of the helicase domain of the murine WRN homologue was deleted has shown critical aspects of cardiovascular aging pathology. Homozygous mutant mice developed severe cardiac interstitial fibrosis in addition to tumors, displayed features of aortic stenosis, abnormal increases in visceral fat deposition and fasting blood triglyceride and cholesterol levels followed by insulin resistance and high blood glucose levels [202], more so in adult female than males. Prior to the development of cardiac fibrosis, adult mice showed higher levels of ROS in serum and heart tissue followed in time by an increase in cardiac oxidative DNA damage. The increase in cardiac DNA damage can be easily anticipated since the WRN helicase plays a pivotal role in DNA repair and it has been shown, using targeted RNAi in primary human fibroblasts, to protect nonproliferating cells from oxidative DNA damage [203]. Furthermore, in a recent study, Bohr et al. have shown that in contrast to normal diploid fibroblast, WS diploid fibroblasts continue to proliferate after extensive H_2O_2-induced DNA damage and accumulate oxidative DNA lesions further suggesting a specific role for wild-type WRN in the detection and/or processing of oxidative DNA lesions [204]. WRN directly interacts with poly(ADP-ribose) polymerase 1 (PARP-1), a nuclear enzyme that protects the genome by responding to DNA damage and facilitating DNA repair, and theWRN/PARP-1 complex is involved in the cellular response to OS and alkylating agents, in particular base excision DNA repair [205].

The source of increased generation of cardiac ROS and OS in the WRN-helicase deficient mice is not clear, although it may in part originate from damage to mitochondrial respiration secondary to increased DNA damage. Evidence of increased levels of leukocyte 8-hydroxy-2′-deoxyguanosine and glutathione from whole blood have recently been reported in WS patients compared to controls [206]. Interestingly, in a double mutant mouse strain containing mutations in both PARP-1 and WRN, *in vivo* analyses revealed increased apoptosis and developmental defects in embryos, as well as major increase in intracellular phosphorylation and oxidative DNA damage in adult tissues [207]. Gene expression profiling of cultured cells from these double mutants showed major misregulation of genes involved in apoptosis, cell cycle control, embryonic development, metabolism and signal transduction. Notably, these mice exhibited a progressive increase in OS with age.

Conclusion

It should be evident from the foregoing discussion that the use of this rather diverse group of organisms has provided significant information about the genes and signaling pathways in aging and life span determination. The strikingly conservation of genes and pathways involved in aging has provided further insights into the insulin/IGF-1 and metabolic/OS contribution to aging and life span extension, and imply numerous interactions between key components of these pathways that may allow the identification of promising targets for reversing aging phenotypes and enhancing longevity. The development of new screening modalities will undoubtedly define new genes and further define relationships between the critical subcellular events underlying aging phenotype. Interestingly, while many of these models have confirmed the negative role of ROS in aging, there is also some evidence that ROS may provide important beneficial signaling in aging pathways. Furthermore, the use of these models to recapitulate both phenotypic aspects of aging-associated diseases (including premature aging syndromes and progeria), and to work out key molecular events underlying these phenotypes, underline the relevance of these models in the understanding of human aging in addition to defining tissue-specific changes with the aging processes.

Summary

- The identification of genetic factors involved in determining longevity in relatively simple organisms such as the nematode *C.elegans*, the yeast *Saccharomyces cerivisiae* and the fly *Drosophila melanogaster* derives in large part from their relatively short generation and overall lifetime, the extremely well-defined genetics available for each of these species and most importantly, the capacity to use extremely powerful and informative molecular techniques of gene targeting and gene transfer.

- In *C.elegans,* the insulin/IGF-1 system acts as a longevity module with upstream master regulators (e.g., DAF-2 and DAF-16/FOXO) controlling a wide variety of downstream genes with diverse functions including chaperones, antioxidants and metabolic genes.
- Homologues of the *C.elegans* genes involved in insulin/IGF-1 are directly implicated in *Drosophila* aging. Other genes (i.e., Klotho) involved in that pathway have been also described in murine and human aging.
- Genes involved in mitochondrial bioenergetic functioning and in orchestrating OS responses have been implicated in *C. elegans* and *Drosophila* longevity.
- Highly conserved sirtuin proteins (e.g., SIR2) originally described in yeast as a critical determinant of longevity have also been found in *C.elegans*, *Drosophila*, mice and man, and are thought to contribute significantly to aspects of aging in most of these species.
- Among their many regulatory roles, sirtuins are involved in chromatin remodeling, and interface with the insulin/IGF-1 pathway, regulate in a variety of cell-types critical metabolic functions including fat metabolism. In several species, sirtuins appear to modulate many of the responses to caloric restriction (CR).
- The several components of the highly conserved TOR pathway (e.g., TOR and its accessory protein raptor) comprise another nutrient sensing pathway that recently has been implicated in extension of the life span of several model organisms, and also as part of the CR pathway in yeast. TOR responds to changes in growth factors, amino acids, oxygen tension/stress, energy status, integrates stress/starvation responses, mitochondrial bioenergetic function and protein synthetic capacity.
- In mice p66Shc function has been shown to be an important determinant of life span and increased stress resistance.
- The p66Shc adaptor protein is a cytoplasmic signal transducer involved in the transmission of mitogenic signals from activated receptors to Ras; within mitochondria p66Shc induces apoptosis by modulating ROS-induced mitochondrial damage and release apoptogenic factors acting in response to a variety of stimuli as well as directly inducing the generation of ROS through the oxidation of cytochrome *c*.
- Mouse transgenic models have been very important in defining the relationships between increased tissue-specific apoptosis and respiratory damage, with mitochondrial-targeted dysfunction (e.g., TFAM knock-outs), increased apoptosis and cardiac dysfunction, with premature aging phenotype in mice, with increased mtDNA mutations (e.g., DNA polymerase γ mutator strains), and increased longevity and reduced aging-associated tissue dysfunction in transgenic strains harboring mitochondrial-targeted antioxidant (e.g., catalase).
- Several human premature aging and progeriod syndromes have been shown to have well-conserved components (e.g., WRN helicase protein) which affect DNA repair, mitotic instability and DNA damage in model systems including yeast, *Drosophila, C. elegans* and mice. These model systems have also provided further insights on the broad role of WRN in aging-associated DNA damage and the function of a broad array of DNA-associated proteins involved in repair, transcription and replication.

References

1. Kimura KD, Tissenbaum HA, Liu Y, Ruvkun G. DAF-2, an insulin receptor-like gene that regulates longevity and diapause in Caenorhabditis elegans. Science 1997;277:942–946
2. Kenyon C, Chang J, Gensch E, Rudner A, Tabtiang R. A C. elegans mutant that lives twice as long as wild type. Nature 1993;366:461–464

3. Apfeld J, Kenyon C. Cell nonautonomy of C. elegans daf-2 function in the regulation of diapause and life span. Cell 1998;95:199–210
4. Lin K, Dorman JB, Rodan A, Kenyon C. daf-16: an HNF-3/forkhead family member that can function to double the life-span of Caenorhabditis elegans. Science 1997;278:1319–1322
5. Lee RY, Hench J, Ruvkun G. Regulation of C. elegans DAF-16 and its human ortholog FKHRL1 by the daf-2 insulin-like signaling pathway. Curr Biol 2001;11:1950–1957
6. Hsu AL, Murphy CT, Kenyon C. Regulation of aging and age-related disease by DAF-16 and heat-shock factor. Science 2003;300:1142–1145
7. Morley JF, Morimoto RI. Regulation of longevity in Caenorhabditis elegans by heat shock factor and molecular chaperones. Mol Biol Cell 2004;15:657–664
8. Lin K, Hsin H, Libina N, Kenyon C. Regulation of the Caenorhabditis elegans longevity protein DAF-16 by insulin/IGF-1 and germline signaling. Nat Genet 2001;28:139–145
9. Apfeld J, O'Connor G, McDonagh T, DiStefano PS, Curtis R. The AMP-activated protein kinase AAK-2 links energy levels and insulin-like signals to lifespan in C. elegans. Genes Dev 2004;18:3004–3009
10. Curtis R, O'Connor G, DiStefano PS. Aging networks in Caenorhabditis elegans: AMP-activated protein kinase (aak-2) links multiple aging and metabolism pathways. Aging Cell 2006;5:119–126
11. Dorman JB, Albinder B, Shroyer T, Kenyon C. The age-1 and daf-2 genes function in a common pathway to control the lifespan of Caenorhabditis elegans. Genetics 1995;141:1399–1406
12. Johnson TE, Tedesco PM, Lithgow GJ. Comparing mutants, selective breeding, and transgenics in the dissection of aging processes of Caenorhabditis elegans. Genetica 1993;91:65–77
13. Dillin A, Crawford DK, Kenyon C. Timing requirements for insulin/IGF-1 signaling in C. elegans. Science 2002;298:830–834
14. Rouault JP, Kuwabara PE, Sinilnikova OM, Duret L, Thierry-Mieg D, Billaud M. Regulation of dauer larva development in Caenorhabditis elegans by daf-18, a homologue of the tumour suppressor PTEN. Curr Biol 1999;9:329–332
15. Mihaylova VT, Borland CZ, Manjarrez L, Stern MJ, Sun H. The PTEN tumor suppressor homolog in Caenorhabditis elegans regulates longevity and dauer formation in an insulin receptor-like signaling pathway. Proc Natl Acad Sci USA 1999;96:7427–7432
16. Solari F, Bourbon-Piffaut A, Masse I, Payrastre B, Chan AM, Billaud M. The human tumour suppressor PTEN regulates longevity and dauer formation in Caenorhabditis elegans. Oncogene 2005;24:20–27
17. McElwee J, Bubb K, Thomas JH. Transcriptional outputs of the Caenorhabditis elegans forkhead protein DAF-16. Aging Cell 2003;2:111–121
18. Lee SS, Kennedy S, Tolonen AC, Ruvkun G. DAF-16 target genes that control C. elegans life-span and metabolism. Science 2003;300:644–647
19. Murphy CT, McCarroll SA, Bargmann CI, Fraser A, Kamath RS, Ahringer J, Li H, Kenyon C. Genes that act downstream of DAF-16 to influence the lifespan of Caenorhabditis elegans. Nature 2003;424:277–283
20. Walker GA, Lithgow GJ. Lifespan extension in C. elegans by a molecular chaperone dependent upon insulin-like signals. Aging Cell 2003;2:131–139
21. Kenyon C. The plasticity of aging: insights from long-lived mutants. Cell 2005;120:449–460
22. Murphy CT, McCarroll SA, Bargmann CI, Fraser A, Kamath RS, Ahringer J, Li H, Kenyon C. Genes that act downstream of DAF-16 to influence the lifespan of Caenorhabditis elegans. Nature 2003;424:277–283
23. Rea S, Johnson TE. A metabolic model for life span determination in Caenorhabditis elegans. Dev Cell 2003;5:197–203
24. Balaban RS, Nemoto S, Finkel T. Mitochondria, oxidants, and aging. Cell 2005;120:483–495
25. McElwee JJ, Schuster E, Blanc E, Thornton J, Gems D. Diapause-associated metabolic traits reiterated in long-lived daf-2 mutants in the nematode Caenorhabditis elegans. Mech Ageing Dev 2006;127:458–472
26. Wadsworth WG, Riddle DL. Developmental regulation of energy metabolism in Caenorhabditis elegans. Dev Biol 1989;132:167–173
27. Holt SJ, Riddle DL. SAGE surveys C. elegans carbohydrate metabolism: evidence for an anaerobic shift in the long-lived dauer larva. Mech Ageing Dev 2003;124:779–800
28. Gems D, Sutton AJ, Sundermeyer ML, Albert PS, King KV, Edgley ML, Larsen PL, Riddle DL. Two pleiotropic classes of daf-2 mutation affect larval arrest, adult behavior, reproduction and longevity in Caenorhabditis elegans. Genetics 1998;150:129–155
29. Tatar M, Kopelman A, Epstein D, Tu MP, Yin CM, Garofalo RS. A mutant *Drosophila* insulin receptor homolog that extends life-span and impairs neuroendocrine function. Science 2001;292:107–110
30. Clancy DJ, Gems D, Harshman LG, Oldham S, Stocker H, Hafen E, Leevers SJ, Partridge L. Extension of life-span by loss of CHICO, a Drosophila insulin receptor substrate protein. Science 2001;292: 104–106
31. Richardson A, Liu F, Adamo ML, Van Remmen H, Nelson JF. The role of insulin and insulin-like growth factor-I in mammalian ageing. Best Pract Res Clin Endocrinol Metab 2004;18:393–406

32. Hsieh CC, DeFord JH, Flurkey K, Harrison DE, Papaconstantinou J. Effects of the Pit1 mutation on the insulin signaling pathway: implications on the longevity of the long-lived Snell dwarf mouse. Mech Ageing Dev 2002;123:1245–1255
33. Flurkey K, Papaconstantinou J, Miller RA, Harrison DE. Lifespan extension and delayed immune and collagen aging in mutant mice with defects in growth hormone production. Proc Natl Acad Sci USA 2001;98:6736–6741
34. Coschigano KT, Clemmons D, Bellush LL, Kopchick JJ. Assessment of growth parameters and life span of GHR/BP gene-disrupted mice. Endocrinology 2000;141:2608–2613
35. Holzenberger M, Dupont J, Ducos B, Leneuve P, Geloen A, Even PC, Cervera P, Le Bouc Y. IGF-1 receptor regulates lifespan and resistance to oxidative stress in mice. Nature 2003;421:125–126
36. Bruning JC, Michael MD, Winnay JN, Hayashi T, Horsch D, Accili D, Goodyear LJ, Kahn CR. A muscle-specific insulin receptor knockout exhibits features of the metabolic syndrome of NIDDM without altering glucose tolerance. Mol Cell 1998;2:559–569
37. Bruning JC, Gautam D, Burks DJ, Gillette J, Schubert M, Orban PC, Klein R, Krone W, Muller-Wieland D, Kahn CR. Role of brain insulin receptor in control of body weight and reproduction. Science 2000;289:2122–2125
38. Bluher M, Kahn BB, Kahn CR. Extended longevity in mice lacking the insulin receptor in adipose tissue. Science 2003;299:572–574
39. Accili D, Drago J, Lee EJ, Johnson MD, Cool MH, Salvatore P, Asico LD, Jose PA, Taylor SI, Westphal H. Early neonatal death in mice homozygous for a null allele of the insulin receptor gene. Nat Genet 1996;12:106–109
40. Liu JP, Baker J, Perkins AS, Robertson EJ, Efstratiadis A. Mice carrying null mutations of the genes encoding insulin-like growth factor I (Igf-1) and type 1 IGF receptor (Igf1r). Cell 1993;75:59–72
41. Kurosu H, Yamamoto M, Clark JD, Pastor JV, Nandi A, Gurnani P, McGuinness OP, Chikuda H, Yamaguchi M, Kawaguchi H, Shimomura I, Takayama Y, Herz J, Kahn CR, Rosenblatt KP, Kuro-o M. Suppression of aging in mice by the hormone Klotho. Science 2005;309:1829–1833
42. Kuro-o M, Matsumura Y, Aizawa H, Kawaguchi H, Suga T, Utsugi T, Ohyama Y, Kurabayashi M, Kaname T, Kume E, Iwasaki H, Iida A, Shiraki-Iida T, Nishikawa S, Nagai R, Nabeshima YI. Mutation of the mouse klotho gene leads to a syndrome resembling ageing. Nature 1997;390:45–51
43. Nabeshima Y. Toward a better understanding of Klotho. Sci Aging Knowledge Environ 2006;2006:pe11
44. Mori K, Yahata K, Mukoyama M, Suganami T, Makino H, Nagae T, Masuzaki H, Ogawa Y, Sugawara A, Nabeshima Y, Nakao K. Disruption of klotho gene causes an abnormal energy homeostasis in mice. Biochem Biophys Res Commun 2000;278:665–667
45. Bartke A. Long-lived Klotho mice: new insights into the roles of IGF-1 and insulin in aging. Trends Endocrinol Metab 2006;17:33–35
46. Yamamoto M, Clark JD, Pastor JV, Gurnani P, Nandi A, Kurosu H, Miyoshi M, Ogawa Y, Castrillon DH, Rosenblatt KP, Kuro-o M. Regulation of oxidative stress by the anti-aging hormone klotho. J Biol Chem 2005;280:38029–38034
47. Shimada T, Kakitani M, Yamazaki Y, Hasegawa H, Takeuchi Y, Fujita T, Fukumoto S, Tomizuka K, Yamashita T. Targeted ablation of Fgf23 demonstrates an essential physiological role of FGF23 in phosphate and vitamin D metabolism. J Clin Invest 2004;113:561–568
48. Razzaque MS, Sitara D, Taguchi T, St-Arnaud R, Lanske B. Premature aging-like phenotype in fibroblast growth factor 23 null mice is a vitamin D-mediated process. FASEB J 2006;20:720–722
49. Kurosu H, Ogawa Y, Miyoshi M, Yamamoto M, Nandi A, Rosenblatt KP, Baum MG, Schiavi S, Hu MC, Moe OW, Kuro-o M. Regulation of fibroblast growth factor-23 signaling by klotho. J Biol Chem 2006;281:6120–6123
50. Tsujikawa H, Kurotaki Y, Fujimori T, Fukuda K, Nabeshima Y. Klotho, a gene related to a syndrome resembling human premature aging, functions in a negative regulatory circuit of vitamin D endocrine system. Mol Endocrinol 2003;17:2393–2403
51. Chang Q, Hoefs S, van der Kemp AW, Topala CN, Bindels RJ, Hoenderop JG. The beta-glucuronidase klotho hydrolyzes and activates the TRPV5 channel. Science 2005;310:490–493
52. Libina N, Berman JR, Kenyon C. Tissue-specific activities of C. elegans DAF-16 in the regulation of lifespan. Cell 2003;115:489–502
53. Masse I, Molin L, Billaud M, Solari F. Lifespan and dauer regulation by tissue-specific activities of Caenorhabditis elegans DAF-18. Dev Biol 2005;286:91–101
54. Hwangbo DS, Gershman B, Tu MP, Palmer M, Tatar M. Drosophila dFOXO controls lifespan and regulates insulin signalling in brain and fat body. Nature 2004;429:562–566
55. Kloting N, Bluher M. Extended longevity and insulin signaling in adipose tissue. Exp Gerontol 2005;40:878–883
56. Feng J, Bussiere F, Hekimi S. Mitochondrial electron transport is a key determinant of life span in Caenorhabditis elegans. Dev Cell 2001;1:633–644
57. Dillin A, Hsu AL, Arantes-Oliveira N, Lehrer-Graiwer J, Hsin H, Fraser AG, Kamath RS, Ahringer J, Kenyon C. Rates of behavior and aging specified by mitochondrial function during development. Science 2002;298:2398–2401

58. Lee SS, Lee RY, Fraser AG, Kamath RS, Ahringer J, Ruvkun G. A systematic RNAi screen identifies a critical role for mitochondria in C. elegans longevity. Nat Genet 2003;33:40–48
59. Anson RM, Hansford RG. Mitochondrial influence on aging rate in Caenorhabditis elegans. Aging Cell 2004;3:29–34
60. Lakowski B, Hekimi S. Determination of life-span in Caenorhabditis elegans by four clock genes. Science 1996;272:1010–1013
61. Felkai S, Ewbank JJ, Lemieux J, Labbe JC, Brown GG, Hekimi S. CLK-1 controls respiration, behavior and aging in the nematode Caenorhabditis elegans. EMBO J 1999;18:1783–1792
62. Ewbank JJ, Barnes TM, Lakowski B, Lussier M, Bussey H, Hekimi S. Structural and functional conservation of the Caenorhabditis elegans timing gene clk-1. Science 1997;275:980–983
63. Braeckman BP, Houthoofd K, Brys K, Lenaerts I, De Vreese A, Van Eygen S, Raes H, Vanfleteren JR. No reduction of energy metabolism in Clk mutants. Mech Ageing Dev 2002;123:1447–1456
64. Kayser EB, Sedensky MM, Morgan PG, Hoppel CL. Mitochondrial oxidative phosphory-lation is defective in the long-lived mutant clk-1. J Biol Chem 2004;279:54479–54486
65. Asencio C, Rodriguez-Aguilera JC, Ruiz-Ferrer M, Vela J, Navas P. Silencing of ubiquinone biosynthesis genes extends life span in Caenorhabditis elegans. FASEB J 2003;17:1135–1137
66. Larsen PL, Clarke CF. Extension of life-span in Caenorhabditis elegans by a diet lacking coenzyme Q. Science 2002;295:120–123
67. Rodriguez-Aguilera JC, Gavilan A, Asencio C, Navas P. The role of ubiquinone in Caenorhabditis elegans longevity. Ageing Res Rev 2005;4:41–53
68. Shibata Y, Branicky R, Landaverde IO, Hekimi S. Redox regulation of germline and vulval development in Caenorhabditis elegans. Science 2003;302:1779–1782
69. Vajo Z, King LM, Jonassen T, Wilkin DJ, Ho N, Munnich A, Clarke CF, Francomano CA. Conservation of the Caenorhabditis elegans timing gene clk-1 from yeast to human: a gene required for ubiquinone biosynthesis with potential implications for aging. Mamm Genome 1999;10:1000–1004
70. Takahashi M, Asaumi S, Honda S, Suzuki Y, Nakai D, Kuroyanagi H, Shimizu T, Honda Y, Shirasawa T. Mouse coq7/clk-1 orthologue rescued slowed rhythmic behavior and extended life span of clk-1 longevity mutant in Caenorhabditis elegans. Biochem Biophys Res Commun 2001;286:534–540
71. Nakai D, Shimizu T, Nojiri H, Uchiyama S, Koike H, Takahashi M, Hirokawa K, Shirasawa T. coq7/clk-1 regulates mitochondrial respiration and the generation of reactive oxygen species via coenzyme Q. Aging Cell 2004;3:273–281
72. Levavasseur F, Miyadera H, Sirois J, Tremblay ML, Kita K, Shoubridge E, Hekimi S. Ubiquinone is necessary for mouse embryonic development but is not essential for mitochondrial respiration. J Biol Chem 2001;276:46160–46164
73. Liu X, Jiang N, Hughes B, Bigras E, Shoubridge E, Hekimi S. Evolutionary conservation of the clk-1-dependent mechanism of longevity: loss of mclk1 increases cellular fitness and lifespan in mice. Genes Dev 2005;19:2424–2434
74. Ishii N, Takahashi K, Tomita S, Keino T, Honda S, Yoshino K, Suzuki K. A methyl viologen-sensitive mutant of the nematode Caenorhabditis elegans. Mutat Res 1990;237:165–171
75. Honda S, Ishii N, Suzuki K, Matsuo M. Oxygen-dependent perturbation of life span and aging rate in the nematode. J Gerontol 1993;48:B57–B61
76. Ishii N, Fujii M, Hartman PS, Tsuda M, Yasuda K, Senoo-Matsuda N, Yanase S, Ayusawa D, Suzuki K. A mutation in succinate dehydrogenase cytochrome b causes oxidative stress and ageing in nematodes. Nature 1998;394:694–697
77. Senoo-Matsuda N, Yasuda K, Tsuda M, Ohkubo T, Yoshimura S, Nakazawa H, Hartman PS, Ishii N. A defect in the cytochrome b large subunit in complex II causes both superoxide anion overproduction and abnormal energy metabolism in Caenorhabditis elegans. J Biol Chem 2001;276:41553–41558
78. Senoo-Matsuda N, Hartman PS, Akatsuka A, Yoshimura S, Ishii N. A complex II defect affects mitochondrial structure, leading to ced-3- and ced-4-dependent apoptosis and aging. J Biol Chem 2003;278:22031–22036
79. Hartman P, Ponder R, Lo HH, Ishii N. Mitochondrial oxidative stress can lead to nuclear hypermutability. Mech Ageing Dev 2004;125:417–420
80. Ishii N, Senoo-Matsuda N, Miyake K, Yasuda K, Ishii T, Hartman PS, Furukawa S. Coenzyme Q10 can prolong C. elegans lifespan by lowering oxidative stress. Mech Ageing Dev 2004;125:41–46
81. Kayser EB, Morgan PG, Sedensky MM. GAS-1: a mitochondrial protein controls sensitivity to volatile anesthetics in the nematode Caenorhabditis elegans. Anesthesiology 1999;90:545–554
82. Kayser EB, Sedensky MM, Morgan PG. The effects of complex I function and oxidative damage on lifespan and anesthetic sensitivity in Caenorhabditis elegans. Mech Ageing Dev 2004;125:455–464
83. Kayser EB, Morgan PG, Hoppel CL, Sedensky MM. Mitochondrial expression and function of GAS-1 in Caenorhabditis elegans. J Biol Chem 2001;276:20551–20558

84. Kondo M, Senoo-Matsuda N, Yanase S, Ishii T, Hartman PS, Ishii N. Effect of oxidative stress on translocation of DAF-16 in oxygen-sensitive mutants, mev-1 and gas-1 of Caenorhabditis elegans. Mech Ageing Dev 2005;126:637–641
85. Napoli E, Taroni F, Cortopassi GA. Frataxin, iron-sulfur clusters, heme, ROS, and aging. Antioxid Redox Signal 2006;8:506–516
86. Ventura N, Rea S, Henderson ST, Condo I, Johnson TE, Testi R. Reduced expression of frataxin extends the lifespan of Caenorhabditis elegans. Aging Cell 2005;4:109–112
87. Vazquez-Manrique RP, Gonzalez-Cabo P, Ros S, Aziz H, Baylis HA, Palau F. Reduction of Caenorhabditis elegans frataxin increases sensitivity to oxidative stress, reduces life-span, and causes lethality in a mitochondrial complex II mutant. FASEB J 2006; 20:172–174
88. Thierbach R, Schulz TJ, Isken F, Voigt A, Mietzner B, Drewes G, von Kleist-Retzow JC, Wiesner RJ, Magnuson MA, Puccio H, Pfeiffer AF, Steinberg P, Ristow M. Targeted disruption of hepatic frataxin expression causes impaired mitochondrial function, decreased life span and tumor growth in mice. Hum Mol Genet 2005;14:3857–3864
89. Herndon LA, Schmeissner PJ, Dudaronek JM, Brown PA, Listner KM, Sakano Y, Paupard MC, Hall DH, Driscoll M. Stochastic and genetic factors influence tissue-specific decline in ageing C. elegans. Nature 2002;419:808–814
90. Lee SS, Lee RY, Fraser AG, Kamath RS, Ahringer J, Ruvkun G. A systematic RNAi screen identifies a critical role for mitochondria in C. elegans longevity. Nat Genet 2003;33:40–48
91. Hamilton B, Dong Y, Shindo M, Liu W, Odell I, Ruvkun G, Lee SS. A systematic RNAi screen for longevity genes in C. elegans. Genes Dev 2005;19:1544–1555
92. Hansen M, Hsu AL, Dillin A, Kenyon C. New genes tied to endocrine, metabolic, and dietary regulation of lifespan from a Caenorhabditis elegans genomic RNAi screen. PLoS Genet 2005;1:119–128
93. Apfeld J, Kenyon C. Regulation of lifespan by sensory perception in Caenorhabditis elegans. Nature 1999;402:804–809
94. Hekimi S, Lakowski B, Barnes TM, Ewbank JJ. Molecular genetics of life span in C. elegans: how much does it teach us? Trends Genet 1998;14:14–20
95. Kennedy BK, Austriaco NR Jr, Zhang J, Guarente L. Mutation in the silencing gene SIR4 can delay aging in S. cerevisiae. Cell 1995;80:485–496
96. Kaeberlein M, McVey M, Guarente L. The SIR2/3/4 complex and SIR2 alone promote longevity in Saccharomyces cerevisiae by two different mechanisms. Genes Dev 1999;13:2570–2580
97. Tissenbaum HA, Guarente L. Increased dosage of a sir-2 gene extends lifespan in Caenorhabditis elegans. Nature 2001;410:227–230
98. Rine J, Herskowitz I. Four genes responsible for a position effect on expression from HML and HMR in Saccharomyces cerevisiae. Genetics 1987;116:9–22
99. Sinclair DA, Guarente L. Extrachromosomal rDNA circles – a cause of aging in yeast. Cell 1997;91:1033–1042
100. Lin SJ, Ford E, Haigis M, Liszt G, Guarente L. Calorie restriction extends yeast life span by lowering the level of NADH. Genes Dev 2004;18:12–16
101. Motta MC, Divecha N, Lemieux M, Kamel C, Chen D, Gu W, Bultsma Y, McBurney M, Guarente L. Mammalian SIRT1 represses forkhead transcription factors. Cell 2004;116:551–563
102. Brunet A, Sweeney LB, Sturgill JF, Chua KF, Greer PL, Lin Y, Tran H, Ross SE, Mostoslavsky R, Cohen HY, Hu LS, Cheng HL, Jedrychowski MP, Gygi SP, Sinclair DA, Alt FW, Greenberg ME. Stress-dependent regulation of FOXO transcription factors by the SIRT1 deacetylase. Science 2004;303:2011–2015
103. Daitoku H, Hatta M, Matsuzaki H, Aratani S, Ohshima T, Miyagishi M, Nakajima T, Fukamizu A. Silent information regulator 2 potentiates Foxo1-mediated transcription through its deacetylase activity. Proc Natl Acad Sci USA 2004;101:10042–10047
104. Wang C, Chen L, Hou X, Li Z, Kabra N, Ma Y, Nemoto S, Finkel T, Gu W, Cress WD, Chen J. Interactions between E2F1 and SirT1 regulate apoptotic response to DNA damage. Nat Cell Biol 2006;8:1025–1031
105. Nemoto S, Fergusson MM, Finkel T. SIRT1 functionally interacts with the metabolic regulator and transcriptional coactivator PGC-1{alpha}. J Biol Chem 005;280:16456–16460
106. Bouras T, Fu M, Sauve AA, Wang F, Quong AA, Perkins ND, Hay RT, Gu W, Pestell RG. SIRT1 deacetylation and repression of p300 involves lysine residues 1020/1024 within the cell cycle regulatory domain 1. J Biol Chem 2005;280:10264–10276
107. Yang T, Fu M, Pestell R, Sauve AA. SIRT1 and endocrine signaling. Trends Endocrinol Metab 2006;17:186–911
108. Kaeberlein M, Kirkland KT, Fields S, Kennedy BK. Sir2-independent life span extension by calorie restriction in yeast. PLoS Biol 2004;2:E296
109. Lin SJ, Kaeberlein M, Andalis AA, Sturtz LA, Defossez PA, Culotta VC, Fink GR, Guarente L. Calorie restriction extends Saccharomyces cerevisiae lifespan by increasing respiration. Nature 2002;8;418: 344–348

110. Kaeberlein M, Hu D, Kerr EO, Tsuchiya M, Westman EA, Dang N, Fields S, Kennedy BK. Increased life span due to calorie restriction in respiratory-deficient yeast. PLoS Genet 2005;1:e69
111. Rogina B, Helfand SL. Sir2 mediates longevity in the fly through a pathway related to calorie restriction. Proc Natl Acad Sci USA 2004;101:15998–16003
112. Chen D, Steele AD, Lindquist S, Guarente L. Increase in activity during calorie restriction requires Sirt1. Science 2005;310:1641
113. Picard F, Kurtev M, Chung N, Topark-Ngarm A, Senawong T, Machado De Oliveira R, Leid M, McBurney MW, Guarente L. Sirt1 promotes fat mobilization in white adipocytes by repressing PPAR-gamma. Nature 2004;429:771–776
114. Kaeberlein M, Powers RW 3rd, Steffen KK, Westman EA, Hu D, Dang N, Kerr EO, Kirkland KT, Fields S, Kennedy BK. Regulation of yeast replicative life span by TOR and Sch9 in response to nutrients. Science 2005;310:1193–1196
115. Kapahi P, Zid BM, Harper T, Koslover D, Sapin V, Benzer S. Regulation of lifespan in Drosophila by modulation of genes in the TOR signaling pathway. Curr Biol 2004;14:885–890
116. Vellai T, Takacs-Vellai K, Zhang Y, Kovacs AL, Orosz L, Muller F. Genetics: influence of TOR kinase on lifespan in C. elegans. Nature 2003;426:620
117. Jia K, Chen D, Riddle DL. The TOR pathway interacts with the insulin signaling pathway to regulate C. elegans larval development, metabolism and life span. Development 2004;131:3897–3906
118. Powers RW 3rd, Kaeberlein M, Caldwell SD, Kennedy BK, Fields S. Extension of chronological life span in yeast by decreased TOR pathway signaling. Genes Dev 2006;20:174–184
119. Desai BN, Myers BR, Schreiber SL. FKBP12-rapamycin-associated protein associates with mitochondria and senses osmotic stress via mitochondrial dysfunction. Proc Natl Acad Sci USA 2002;99:4319–4324
120. Kim DH, Sarbassov DD, Ali SM, King JE, Latek RR, Erdjument-Bromage H, Tempst P, Sabatini DM. mTOR interacts with raptor to form a nutrient-sensitive complex that signals to the cell growth machinery. Cell 2002;110:163–175
121. Tokunaga C, Yoshino K, Yonezawa K. mTOR integrates amino acid- and energy-sensing pathways. Biochem Biophys Res Commun 2004;313:443–446
122. Nojima H, Tokunaga C, Eguchi S, Oshiro N, Hidayat S, Yoshino K, Hara K, Tanaka N, Avruch J, Yonezawa K. The mammalian target of rapamycin (mTOR) partner, raptor, binds the mTOR substrates p70 S6 kinase and 4E-BP1 through their TOR signaling (TOS) motif. J Biol Chem 2003;278:15461–15464
123. Schieke SM, Phillips D, McCoy JP Jr, Aponte AM, Shen RF, Balaban RS, Finkel T. The mammalian target of rapamycin (mTOR) pathway regulates mitochondrial oxygen consumption and oxidative capacity. J Biol Chem 2006;281:27643–27652
124. Juhaszova M, Zorov DB, Kim SH, Pepe S, Fu Q, Fishbein KW, Ziman BD, Wang S, Ytrehus K, Antos CL, Olson EN, Sollott SJ. Glycogen synthase kinase-3beta mediates convergence of protection signaling to inhibit the mitochondrial permeability transition pore. J Clin Invest 2004;113:1535–1549
125. Khan S, Salloum F, Das A, Xi L, Vetrovec GW, Kukreja RC. Rapamycin confers preconditioning-like protection against ischemia-reperfusion injury in isolated mouse heart and cardiomyocytes. J Mol Cell Cardiol 2006;41:256–264
126. Liu Z, Butow RA. Mitochondrial retrograde signaling. Annu Rev Genet 2006;40:159–185
127. Butow RA, Avadhani NG. Mitochondrial signaling: the retrograde response. Mol Cell 2004;14:1–15
128. Grotewiel MS, Martin I, Bhandari P, Cook-Wiens E. Functional senescence in Drosophila melanogaster. Ageing Res Rev 2005;4:372–397
129. Ballard JW. Drosophila simulans as a novel model for studying mitochondrial metabolism and aging. Exp Gerontol 2005;40:763–773
130. Wessells RJ, Fitzgerald E, Cypser JR, Tatar M, Bodmer R. Insulin regulation of heart function in aging fruit flies. Nat Genet 2004;36:1275–1281
131. Paternostro G, Vignola C, Bartsch DU, Omens JH, McCulloch AD, Reed JC. Age-associated cardiac dysfunction in Drosophila melanogaster. Circ Res 2001;88:1053–1058
132. Mourikis P, Hurlbut GD, Artavanis-Tsakonas S. Enigma, a mitochondrial protein affecting lifespan and oxidative stress response in Drosophila. Proc Natl Acad Sci USA 2006;103:1307–1312
133. Wang MC, Bohmann D, Jasper H. JNK signaling confers tolerance to oxidative stress and extends lifespan in Drosophila. Dev Cell 2003;5:811–816
134. Wang MC, Bohmann D, Jasper H. JNK extends life span and limits growth by antago-nizing cellular and organism-wide responses to insulin signaling. Cell 2005;121:115–125
135. Lin YJ, Seroude L, Benzer S. Extended life-span and stress resistance in the Drosophila mutant methuselah. Science 1998;282:943–946
136. Cvejic S, Zhu Z, Felice SJ, Berman Y, Huang XY. The endogenous ligand Stunted of the GPCR Methuselah extends lifespan in Drosophila. Nat Cell Biol 2004;6:540–546

137. Wang HD, Kazemi-Esfarjani P, Benzer S. Multiple stress analysis for isolation of Drosophila longevity genes. Proc Natl Acad Sci USA 2004;101:12610–12615
138. Morrow G, Samson M, Michaud S, Tanguay RM. Overexpression of the small mitochondrial Hsp22 extends Drosophila life span and increases resistance to oxidative stress. FASEB J 2004;18:598–599
139. Rogina B, Reenan RA, Nilsen SP, Helfand SL. Extended life-span conferred by cotransporter gene mutations in Drosophila. Science 2000;290:2137–2140
140. Fridell YW, Sanchez-Blanco A, Silvia BA, Helfand SL. Targeted expression of the human uncoupling protein 2 (hUCP2) to adult neurons extends life span in the fly. Cell Metab 2005;1:145–152
141. Padalko VI. Uncoupler of oxidative phosphorylation prolongs the lifespan of Drosophila. Biochemistry (Mosc) 2005;70:986–989
142. Miwa S, Riyahi K, Partridge L, Brand MD. Lack of correlation between mitochondrial reactive oxygen species production and life span in Drosophila. Ann N Y Acad Sci 2004;1019:388–391
143. Bayne AC, Mockett RJ, Orr WC, Sohal RS. Enhanced catabolism of mitochondrial superoxide/hydrogen peroxide and aging in transgenic Drosophila. Biochem J 2005;391:277–284
144. Magwere T, West M, Riyahi K, Murphy MP, Smith RA, Partridge L. The effects of exogenous antioxidants on lifespan and oxidative stress resistance in Drosophila melanogaster. Mech Ageing Dev 2006;127:356–370
145. Walker DW, Muffat J, Rundel C, Benzer S. Overexpression of a Drosophila homolog of apolipoprotein d leads to increased stress resistance and extended lifespan. Curr Biol 2006;16:674–679
146. Arking R, Buck S, Hwangbo DS, Lane M. Metabolic alterations and shifts in energy allocations are corequisites for the expression of extended longevity genes in Drosophila. Ann N Y Acad Sci 2002;959:251–262
147. Aigaki T, Ohsako T, Toba G, Seong K, Matsuo T. The gene search system: its application to functional genomics in Drosophila melanogaster. J Neurogenet 2001;15:169–178
148. Seong KH, Ogashiwa T, Matsuo T, Fuyama Y, Aigaki T. Application of the gene search system to screen for longevity genes in Drosophila. Biogerontology 2001;2:209–217
149. Aigaki T, Seong KH, Matsuo T. Longevity determination genes in Drosophila melanogaster. Mech Ageing Dev 2002;123:1531–1541
150. Bauer JH, Goupil S, Garber GB, Helfand SL. An accelerated assay for the identification of lifespan-extending interventions in Drosophila melanogaster. Proc Natl Acad Sci USA 2004;101:12980–12985
151. Migliaccio E, Giorgio M, Mele S, Pelicci G, Reboldi P, Pandolfi PP, Lanfrancone L, Pelicci PG. The p66shc adaptor protein controls oxidative stress response and life span in mammals. Nature 1999;402: 309–313
152. Trinei M, Giorgio M, Cicalese A, Barozzi S, Ventura A, Migliaccio E, Milia E, Padura IM, Raker VA, Maccarana M, Petronilli V, Minucci S, Bernardi P, Lanfrancone L, Pelicci PG. A p53–p66Shc signalling pathway controls intracellular redox status, levels of oxidation-damaged DNA and oxidative stress-induced apoptosis. Oncogene 2002;21:3872–3878
153. Migliaccio E, Mele S, Salcini AE, Pelicci G, Lai KM, Superti-Furga G, Pawson T, Di Fiore PP, Lanfrancone L, Pelicci PG. Opposite effects of the p52shc/p46shc and p66shc splicing isoforms on the EGF receptor-MAP kinase-fos signalling pathway. EMBO J 1997;16:706–716
154. Orsini F, Migliaccio E, Moroni M, Contursi C, Raker VA, Piccini D, Martin-Padura I, Pelliccia G, Trinei M, Bono M, Puri C, Tacchetti C, Ferrini M, Mannucci R, Nicoletti I, Lanfrancone L, Giorgio M, Pelicci PG. The life span determinant p66Shc localizes to mitochondria where it associates with mitochondrial heat shock protein 70 and regulates trans-membrane potential. J Biol Chem 2004;279:25689–25695
155. Nemoto S, Finkel T. Redox regulation of forkhead proteins through a p66shc-dependent signaling pathway. Science 2002;295:2450–2452
156. Giorgio M, Migliaccio E, Orsini F, Paolucci D, Moroni M, Contursi C, Pelliccia G, Luzi L, Minucci S, Marcaccio M, Pinton P, Rizzuto R, Bernardi P, Paolucci F, Pelicci PG. Electron transfer between cytochrome c and p66Shc generates reactive oxygen species that trigger mitochondrial apoptosis. Cell 2005;122:221–233
157. Wang J, Silva JP, Gustafsson CM, Rustin P, Larsson NG. Increased in vivo apoptosis in cells lacking mitochondrial DNA gene expression. Proc Natl Acad Sci USA 2001;98:4038–4043
158. Trifunovic A, Wredenberg A, Falkenberg M, Spelbrink JN, Rovio AT, Bruder CE, Bohlooly-Y M, Gidlof S, Oldfors A, Wibom R, Tornell J, Jacobs HT, Larsson NG. Premature ageing in mice expressing defective mitochondrial DNA polymerase. Nature 2004;429:417–423
159. Trifunovic A, Hansson A, Wredenberg A, Rovio AT, Dufour E, Khvorostov I, Spelbrink JN, Wibom R, Jacobs HT, Larsson NG. Somatic mtDNA mutations cause aging phenotypes without affecting reactive oxygen species production. Proc Natl Acad Sci USA 2005;102:17993–17998
160. Ku HH, Brunk UT, Sohal RS. Relationship between mitochondrial superoxide and hydrogen peroxide production and longevity of mammalian species. Free Radic Biol Med 1993;15:621–627
161. Sohal RS, Toy PL, Allen RG. Relationship between life expectancy, endogenous antioxidants and products of oxygen free radical reactions in the housefly, Musca domestica. Mech Ageing Dev 1986;36:71–77

162. Munkres K, Rana RS. Antioxidants prolong life span and inhibit the senescence-dependent accumulation of fluorescent pigment (lipofuscin) in clones, of Podospora anserina. Mech Ageing Dev 1978;7:407–415
163. Orr WC, Sohal RS. Extension of life-span by overexpression of superoxide dismutase and catalase in Drosophila melanogaster. Science 1994;263:1128–1130
164. Melov S, Ravenscroft J, Malik S, Gill MS, Walker DW, Clayton PE, Wallace DC, Malfroy B, Doctrow SR, Lithgow GJ. Extension of life-span with superoxide dismutase/catalase mimetics. Science 2000;289:
1567–1569
165. Parkes TL, Elia AJ, Dickinson D, Hilliker AJ, Phillips JP, Boulianne G. Extension of Drosophila lifespan by overexpression of human SOD1 in motorneurons. Nat Genet 1998;19:171–174
166. Sun J, Tower J. FLP recombinase-mediated induction of Cu/Zn-superoxide dismutase transgene expression can extend the life span of adult Drosophila melanogaster flies. Mol Cell Biol 1999;19:216–228
167. Sun J, Folk D, Bradley TJ, Tower J. Induced overexpression of mitochondrial Mn-superoxide dismutase extends the life span of adult Drosophila melanogaster. Genetics 2002;161:661–672
168. Orr WC, Sohal RS. Does overexpression of Cu, Zn-SOD extend life span in Drosophila melanogaster? Exp Gerontol 2003;38:227–230
169. Orr WC, Mockett RJ, Benes JJ, Sohal RS. Effects of overexpression of copper-zinc and manganese superoxide dismutases, catalase, and thioredoxin reductase genes on longevity in Drosophila melanogaster. J Biol Chem 2003;278:26418–26422
170. Huang TT, Carlson EJ, Gillespie AM, Shi Y, Epstein CJ. Ubiquitous overexpression of CuZn superoxide dismutase does not extend life span in mice. J Gerontol A Biol Sci Med Sci 2000;55:B5–B9
171. Gallagher IM, Jenner P, Glover V, Clow A. CuZn-superoxide dismutase transgenic mice: no effect on longevity, locomotor activity and 3H-mazindol and 3H-spiperone binding over 19 months. Neurosci Lett 2000;289:221–223
172. Van Remmen H, Ikeno Y, Hamilton M, Pahlavani M, Wolf N, Thorpe SR, Alderson NL, Baynes JW, Epstein CJ, Huang TT, Nelson J, Strong R, Richardson A. Life-long reduction in MnSOD activity results in increased DNA damage and higher incidence of cancer but does not accelerate aging. Physiol Genomics 2003;16:29–37
173. Richter C, Park JW, Ames BN. Normal oxidative damage to mitochondrial and nuclear DNA is extensive. Proc Natl Acad Sci USA 1988;85:6465–6467
174. Takasawa M, Hayakawa M, Sugiyama S, Hattori K, Ito T, Ozawa T. Age-associated damage in mitochondrial function in rat hearts. Exp Gerontol 1993;28:269–280
175. Hayakawa M, Torii K, Sugiyama S, Tanaka M, Ozawa T. Age-associated accumulation of 8-hydroxydeoxyguanosine in mitochondrial DNA of human diaphragm. Biochem Biophys Res Commun 1991;179:1023–1029
176. Hayakawa M, Hattori K, Sugiyama S, Ozawa T. Age-associated oxygen damage and mutations in mitochondrial DNA in human hearts. Biochem Biophys Res Commun 1992;189:979–985
177. Mecocci P, MacGarvey U, Kaufman AE, Koontz D, Shoffner JM, Wallace DC, Beal MF. Oxidative damage to mitochondrial DNA shows marked age-dependent increases in human brain. Ann Neurol 1993;34:609–616
178. Richter C. Oxidative damage to mitochondrial DNA and its relationship to ageing. Int J Biochem Cell Biol 1995;27:647–653
179. Stuart JA, Bourque BM, de Souza-Pinto NC, Bohr VA. No evidence of mitochondrial respiratory dysfunction in OGG1-null mice deficient in removal of 8-oxodeoxyguanine from mitochondrial DNA. Free Radic Biol Med 2005;38:737–745
180. Huang TT, Carlson EJ, Kozy HM, Mantha S, Goodman SI, Ursell PC, Epstein CJ. Genetic modification of prenatal lethality and dilated cardiomyopathy in Mn superoxide dismutase mutant mice. Free Radic Biol Med 2001;31:1101–1110
181. Van Remmen H, Qi W, Sabia M, Freeman G, Estlack L, Yang H, Mao Guo Z, Huang TT, Strong R, Lee S, Epstein CJ, Richardson A. Multiple deficiencies in antioxidant enzymes in mice result in a compound increase in sensitivity to oxidative stress. Free Radic Biol Med 2004;36:1625–1634
182. Schriner SE, Linford NJ, Martin GM, Treuting P, Ogburn CE, Emond M, Coskun PE, Ladiges W, Wolf N, Van Remmen H, Wallace DC, Rabinovitch PS. Extension of murine life span by overexpression of catalase targeted to mitochondria. Science 2005;308:1909–1911
183. Andziak B, O'Connor TP, Buffenstein R. Antioxidants do not explain the disparate longevity between mice and the longest-living rodent, the naked mole-rat. Mech Ageing Dev 2005;126:1206–1212
184. Buffenstein R. The naked mole-rat: a new long-living model for human aging research. J Gerontol A Biol Sci Med Sci 2005;60:1369–1377
185. Yu CE, Oshima J, Wijsman EM, Nakura J, Miki T, Piussan C, Matthews S, Fu YH, Mulligan J, Martin GM, Schellenberg GD. Mutations in the consensus helicase domains of the Werner syndrome gene. Werner's Syndrome Collaborative Group. Am J Hum Genet 1997;60:330–341

186. Shen J, Loeb LA. Unwinding the molecular basis of the Werner syndrome. Mech Ageing Dev 2001;122:921–944
187. Szekely AM, Chen YH, Zhang C, Oshima J, Weissman SM. Werner protein recruits DNA polymerase delta to the nucleolus. Proc Natl Acad Sci USA 2000;97:11365–11370
188. Watt PM, Hickson ID, Borts RH, Louis EJ. SGS1, a homologue of the Bloom's and Werner's syndrome genes, is required for maintenance of genome stability in Saccharomyces cerevisiae. Genetics 1996;144:935–945
189. Sinclair DA, Mills K, Guarente L. Accelerated aging and nucleolar fragmentation in yeast sgs1 mutants. Science 1997;277:1313–1316
190. Myung K, Datta A, Chen C, Kolodner RD. SGS1, the Saccharomyces cerevisiae homologue of BLM and WRN, suppresses genome instability and homologous recombination. Nat Genet 2001;27:113–116
191. Johnson FB, Marciniak RA, McVey M, Stewart SA, Hahn WC, Guarente L. The Saccharomyces cerevisiae WRN homolog Sgs1p participates in telomere maintenance in cells lacking telomerase. EMBO J 2001;20:905–913
192. Cohen H, Sinclair DA. Recombination-mediated lengthening of terminal telomeric repeats requires the Sgs1 DNA helicase. Proc Natl Acad Sci USA 2001;98:3174–3179
193. Lee SJ, Yook JS, Han SM, Koo HS. A Werner syndrome protein homolog affects C. elegans development, growth rate, life span and sensitivity to DNA damage by acting at a DNA damage checkpoint. Development 2004;131:2565–2575
194. Lebel M, Leder P. A deletion within the murine Werner syndrome helicase induces sensitivity to inhibitors of topoisomerase and loss of cellular proliferative capacity. Proc Natl Acad Sci USA 1998;95:13097–13102
195. Lombard DB, Beard C, Johnson B, Marciniak RA, Dausman J, Bronson R, Buhlmann JE, Lipman R, Curry R, Sharpe A, Jaenisch R, Guarente L. Mutations in the WRN gene in mice accelerate mortality in a p53-null background. Mol Cell Biol 2000;20:3286–3291
196. Chang S. A mouse model of Werner Syndrome: what can it tell us about aging and cancer? Int J Biochem Cell Biol 2005;37:991–999
197. Chang S, Multani AS, Cabrera NG, Naylor ML, Laud P, Lombard D, Pathak S, Guarente L, DePinho RA. Essential role of limiting telomeres in the pathogenesis of Werner syndrome. Nat Genet 2004;36:877–882
198. Du X, Shen J, Kugan N, Furth EE, Lombard DB, Cheung C, Pak S, Luo G, Pignolo RJ, DePinho RA, Guarente L, Johnson FB. Telomere shortening exposes functions for the mouse Werner and Bloom syndrome genes. Mol Cell Biol 2004;24:8437–8446
199. Opresko PL, von Kobbe C, Laine JP, Harrigan J, Hickson ID, Bohr VA. Telomere-binding protein TRF2 binds to and stimulates the Werner and Bloom syndrome helicases. J Biol Chem 2002;277:41110–41119
200. Machwe A, Xiao L, Orren DK. TRF2 recruits the Werner syndrome (WRN) exonuclease for processing of telomeric DNA. Oncogene 2004;23:149–156
201. Opresko PL, Otterlei M, Graakjaer J, Bruheim P, Dawut L, Kolvraa S, May A, Seidman MM, Bohr VA. The Werner syndrome helicase and exonuclease cooperate to resolve telomeric D loops in a manner regulated by TRF1 and TRF2. Mol Cell 2004;14:763–774
202. Massip L, Garand C, Turaga RV, Deschenes F, Thorin E, Lebel M. Increased insulin, triglycerides, reactive oxygen species, and cardiac fibrosis in mice with a mutation in the helicase domain of the Werner syndrome gene homologue. Exp Gerontol 2006;41:157–168
203. Szekely AM, Bleichert F, Numann A, Van Komen S, Manasanch E, Ben Nasr A, Canaan A, Weissman SM. Werner protein protects nonproliferating cells from oxidative DNA damage. Mol Cell Biol 2005;25:10492–10506
204. Von Kobbe C, May A, Grandori C, Bohr VA. Werner syndrome cells escape hydrogen peroxide-induced cell proliferation arrest. FASEB J 2004;18:1970–1972
205. von Kobbe C, Harrigan JA, May A, Opresko PL, Dawut L, Cheng WH, Bohr VA. Central role for the Werner syndrome protein/poly(ADP-ribose) polymerase 1 complex in the poly(ADP-ribosyl)ation pathway after DNA damage. Mol Cell Biol 2003;23:8601–8613
206. Pagano G, Zatterale A, Degan P, d'Ischia M, Kelly FJ, Pallardo FV, Kodama S. Multiple involvement of oxidative stress in Werner syndrome phenotype. Biogerontology 2005;6:233–243
207. Deschenes F, Massip L, Garand C, Lebel M. In vivo misregulation of genes involved in apoptosis, development and oxidative stress in mice lacking both functional Werner syndrome protein and poly(ADP-ribose) polymerase-1. Hum Mol Genet 2005;14:3293–3308

Chapter 13
Profiling the Aging Cardiovascular System: Transcriptional, Proteomic, SNPs, Gene Mapping and Epigenetics Analysis

Overview

Transcriptional and proteomic analysis of cardiovascular genes involved in aging and in age-associated diseases and reported findings in animal models, cells models and human will be discussed in this chapter. Furthermore, mapping of aging-susceptibility genes in human studies, analysis of mutations and genetic polymorphic variants (including SNPs) in candidate genes and their relationship with longevity and the phenotype of aging will be addressed together with the most recent evidence that epigenetics, including DNA methylation and chromatin remodeling, may contribute to the aging phenotype of cardiovascular cells.

Introduction

A primary tool for understanding the cellular and organ-specific changes occurring in aging is the analysis of gene expression. Furthermore, age-associated changes in heart structure and function, both in the normal and in the diseased state and even with specific aging interventions such as caloric restriction, are associated with altered patterns of gene expression with characteristic profiles for specific gene. The most common approach to examine quantitative and qualitative changes in gene expression is to gauge relative changes in the abundance of gene transcripts. Until recently, most of the changes in transcript abundance were identified one gene at a time, but new and more global techniques including microarray profiling have permitted rapid, large-scale expression profiling. With this approach, simultaneous evaluation of the expression of diverse as well as related genes may be achieved; in some cases elaborating a molecular signature that can uncover commonalities in regulation that might not have been suspected otherwise, and also providing a unique opportunity to identify aging biomarkers in specific cell-types, tissues or organs. A second approach to evaluate gene expression and define novel aging biomarkers uses proteomic analysis. In addition to gene expression analysis, this technique can be adapted to assess both qualitatively and quantitatively post-translational modifications in proteins that may accumulate with aging and senescence.

The use of linkage-analysis and case-association analysis to define genetic determinants in aging has identified thus far a limited number of genes that impact longevity. However, new observations using SNP polymorphisms and assessment of epigenetic factors in association with age appear to promise new progress in the study of longevity and function. These represent nascent areas of great interest and potential in defining the molecular subcontext of aging.

J. Marín-García, *Aging and the Heart,*

Transcriptional Gene Profiling

In Chapter 3 we have examined the methodology of transcriptome profiling (primarily by microarray analysis) and discussed its application to tissues and cell-types of several animal models as well as noting several limitations with this approach. In this chapter we will explore in greater depth the data collected with this technique and their potential significance.

Normal Aging Studies

Lee et al. in their study focusing on gene expression profiles in hearts of 30 month-old compared with 5 month-old B6C3F1male mice, found with aging significant modulation of gene expression with over 10% of myocardial transcripts significantly changed [1]. Consistent with previous findings that the aging heart undergoes extracellular matrix (ECM) protein deposition, fibrosis and cardiomyocyte hypertrophy, genes that exhibited increased age-mediated expression included myocardial structural genes involved in ECM components, collagen deposition, cell adhesion, and cell growth. Significant upregulation was found for troponin T1, the gap junction protein connexin 43, intercellular adhesion molecule 2, integrin-α6, actin-α 2 and a variety of collagens. Downregulated expression was found with genes involved in protein synthesis (including numerous translation initiation and elongation factors) and in genes associated with fatty acid oxidation (FAO), metabolism and transport including carnitine palmitoyltransferase I (*Cpt1*), carnitine acetyltransferase, mitochondrial carnitine/acylcarnitine translocase and carnitine palmitoyltransferase II (*Cpt2*). These findings, in concert with increased expression of genes involved in carbohydrate metabolism, in particular glycolysis and glucose uptake (increased phosphofructokinase [PFK] and *GLUT4*) and downregulation of the glycolytic inhibitor *PDK4*, which phosphorylates mitochondrial pyruvate dehydrogenase and inhibits its activity, suggested an aging-induced shift in myocardial energy metabolism.

Later on this group of investigators reported that genes involved in myocardial inflammatory and stress responses are affected (primarily upregulated) in the aging sedentary mouse, suggesting that the aging heart experiences oxidative stress (OS) leading to a pro-inflammatory state [2]. Upregulation was found in the genes of the mitochondrial electron transport chain (ETC) such as cytochrome *c* oxidase subunits COX Va and COX VIa, although genes for the uncoupling protein (UCP3) and mitochondrial F1-F0 ATP synthase were downregulated. Decreased expression of genes involved in fatty acid metabolism, such as methylacyl-CoA racemase, involved in peroxisomal FAO, and heart fatty-acid binding protein (HFABP), which functions as a vehicle of cytosolic fatty acid transport, was found. This is in agreement with previous observation of impaired cardiac FAO oxidation with aging. As we shall discuss in more depth in a later chapter, a high proportion of the aging-mediated transcriptional changes were reversed or at least partially attenuated in older animals subjected to intensive exercise training.

Widespread alterations in gene expression in aging mouse heart have been also recently documented in 309 genes (from 26–28 month old mice), with roughly 50% of them upregulated [3]. Interestingly, this study also revealed that re-programming of myocardial gene expression appears somewhat modest compared to transcriptome changes in the liver (over 1819 transcripts) and hypothalamus (1085 transcripts), with only 9 transcripts shared between each type of tissue (including the RIKEN cDNA 1500005K14 gene encoding cfm, and Amylase I). Of the remaining 300 genes altered in the aging heart, 91 genes also changed expression in either liver or hypothalamus. Grouping of the aging-affected myocardial genes by functional category showed a striking upregulation of immune system-related and stress-response genes, and significant downregulation of macromolecule biosynthesis as well as ion transport, particularly metal ion transport. Interestingly, significant changes in myocardial FAO gene expression were not found unlike in the liver.

Presumably the discrepancies between different studies arise from use of different strains and/or the variability in the experimental animal ages.

The enzymes participating in FAO (which takes place both in the peroxisome and in the mitochondria) are largely regulated at the transcriptional level by the global nuclear regulators including the fatty acid activated-peroxisomal proliferating activating receptor (PPAR) and its coactivator (PGC-1). Compared with 4 month-old sedentary rats, 23 month old sedentary rats exhibited lower myocardial expression of PPAR-α, which was significantly higher in exercise-trained aged rats, compared with sedentary aged rats. Moreover, Ietmitsu et al. found that in association with changes in myocardial PPAR-α mRNA and protein levels, PPAR-α DNA binding to the transcriptional regulatory elements on PPAR-α target genes encoding FAO metabolic enzymes is altered in the aging heart, resulting in lower mRNA expression and enzyme activity of 3-hydroxyacyl CoA dehydrogenase (*HAD*) and carnitine palmitoyltransferase-I (*CPT1*) [4]. On the other hand, Lemoine et al. reported no significant changes in relative transcript levels of nuclear transcriptional regulators, including PPAR-α, PPAR-β, PPAR-γ or PGC-1 (or of Sirt1, a histone-modifying enzyme that interacts with PGC-1) in very old Fischer 344 rats (35 months) [5].

In contrast to the extensive "reprogramming" of the myocardial transcriptome revealed by the aforementioned observations, Bodyak et al., in their gene profiling analysis of isolated ventricular cardiomyocytes of aging mice compared to cardiomyocytes from young mice [6], have identified a more limited subset of gene transcripts that accumulated at significantly different levels with age. The age-affected genes included decreased transcript levels of several stress response proteins including heat shock proteins (e.g., HSP70 and HSP25) and heme oxygenase (HO-1 also known as HSP32), decreased levels of mitochondrial DNA (mtDNA) encoded-ETC transcripts (e.g., cytochrome *b*, COX3), mitochondrial creatine kinase (Mi-CK), decreased transcript levels of proteins involved in contraction (e.g., dystrophin, tropomyosin, troponin I, α-MHC, skeletal actin, connexin43 and sarcoplasmic reticulum Ca^{2+}-ATPase (SERCA2), and more uniquely, reduced mRNA levels of several transcription factors (e.g., Nkx2.5, GATA-4, c-jun, JunB). Interestingly, other investigators have also suggested that only a relatively small cohort (approximately 2%) of expressed genes show significant changes in their levels of expression during aging [7]. Differential display of gene expression during aging of the rat brain, heart and liver, revealed that levels of c-fos, a component of the AP-1 transcription factor were downregulated with age. This is consistent with previous data showing that reduced level of fos expression and of fos inducibility in rat hearts occurred with age [8]. In addition, this study revealed a significant increase in mitochondrial RNA during aging of the heart, in contrast to the findings of Bodyak et al. [6]

Mitochondrial gene expression in the aging heart has long been a contentious issue. Whereas some investigators have reported a decline in the levels of mtDNA-encoded transcripts in senescent rat heart [9–11], others have found either no significant changes[5, 12] or increased levels of mtDNA-encoded mRNAs [7]. No changes in activity or transcript level of the mitochondrial transcription factor mtTFA (also termed TFAM), implicated in mtDNA replication and transcription, were detected in the aging rat and mouse heart compared to age-related increases reported in liver and brain [13, 14], and in human skeletal muscle from aged subjects [15]. On the other hand, global nuclear regulators of mitochondrial transcription such as the nuclear respiratory factors NRF-1 and NRF-2 were found to be upregulated in the aging heart [5], as they have in skeletal muscle [15]. From these observations it is evident that further research in this area is needed to elucidate the role of nuclear regulatory factors and nuclear-encoded enzymes (Table 13.1) which regulate mitochondrial biogenesis and mtDNA transcription, in the aging heart.

These gene profiling data have shown in some cases striking differences in comparison to Lee's et al. findings and suggest that a large subset of age-associated changes in myocardial transcript abundance may in fact be associated with non-cardiomyocytes, strain differences or abnormal transcript abundance that may be related to the isolation procedures used and not necessarily to aging. Furthermore, altered gene expression in specific cell sub-populations (e.g., myocytes), including

Table 13.1 Nuclear-encoded factors involve in the regulation of myocardial mitochondrial biogenesis and mtDNA transcription

Factor	Function	Principle target
PPAR-α	Global transcription factor	FAO genes
PGC-1	Transcription factor/coactivator	FAO genes NRF-1,NRF-2, mtTFA
NRF-1	Transcription factor	Nuclear ETC genes
NRF-2	Transcription factor	Nuclear ETC genes
MtTFA (TFAM)	Mitochondrial transcription factor, mtDNA replication and maintenance	MtDNA-encoded ETC genes
TR	Thyroid hormone receptor, transcription factor	MtDNA and nuclear ETC genes
ANT	Adenine nucleotide translocator, PT pore component, DNA maintenance,	MtDNA
DNA polymerase γ	mtDNA replication and repair	MtDNA
TWINKLE	mtDNA replication and repair, heliease	MtDNA

changes in less-abundant transcription factors, might be obscured by transcript levels in neighboring cells (e.g., cardiac fibroblasts). Moreover, the disparity found in connection with mitochondrial RNA levels in the aging heart compared to isolated cardiomyocytes, might be explained in part by increased levels of mitochondrial RNA in other cell-types such as fibroblasts and vascular endothelial cells (ECs). Expression levels of ND3, ND2, ATPase6 and 16S rRNA have been reported to be elevated in senescent ECs and fibroblasts [16]. This highlights the necessity of taking into account biological diversity when performing studies of aging, and that heart transcriptome (as well as proteomic) analyses are complicated by factors such as tissue and cellular heterogeneity, genetic variability, disease state and pharmacological intervention [17].

Another complicating factor that contributes to gene expression variation to be considered in transcript analysis is the element of circadian regulation in which gene expression may follow a temporal or diurnal rhythm. A number of critical physiological events including fatty acid responsiveness in isolated adult rat cardiomyocytes, changes in blood pressure, heart rate, and cardiac output, diurnal variations in metabolic flux and contractile function have been primarily attributed to both extracardiac (e.g., neurohumoral factors) and intracardiac (i.e., circadian clock) influences and their complex interplay [18–21]. The intracellular circadian clock is largely transcriptionally based, and functions to allow the cell to perceive the time of day, thereby enabling preparation for anticipated environmental stimuli [20]. In adult rat cardiomyocytes, two metabolic genes whose expression, both *in vivo* and *in vitro*, has been identified as undergoing significant circadian oscillation, are pyruvate dehydrogenase kinase4 (*pdk4*) and uncoupling protein 3 (*ucp3*), both genes regulated by PPAR-α. Storch et al. have reported that 8–10% of the myocardial genes assessed had circadian expression patterns suggesting that temporal expression can be a critical variable in microarray/gene profiling studies [22]. There is also evidence that the temporal pattern of circadian rhythms and the transcriptional events that underlie them may also be profoundly altered in aging [23–25].

Age-associated Myocardial Transcription Responses to Oxidative and Ischemic Stress

One of the surprising findings in the study of Lee et al. was the apparent absence of aging-mediated changes in transcriptional profile for OS genes. To further investigate the age-modulated transcriptional response to OS in the heart, the cardiac gene expression profiles of young (5 months old), middle-aged (15 months old), and old (25 months old) C57BL/6 mice were subjected to a single intraperitoneal injection of the ROS generator paraquat (50 mg/kg) [26]. A total of 55 transcripts were found to be paraquat-responsive for all age groups. Genes commonly induced in all age groups include those associated with stress, inflammatory, immune, and growth factor responses. Paraquat treatment induced several genes previously known to mediate stress responses, including metallothioneins 1 and 2, GADD45, p21, and sestrin. In addition, the induction of several genes appears to be associated with a protective metabolic stress response in the heart including Bcl-XL, an antiapoptotic protein that allows cells to maintain oxidative metabolism during cellular stress by a continuous transport of metabolites across the outer mitochondrial membrane, and 5′ nucleotidase, an enzyme that controls the production of adenosine in the heart through the dephosphorylation of AMP. Interestingly, only young mice displayed a significant increase in expression of all three isoforms of GADD45, a DNA damage-responsive gene. Several immediate early response genes (IEGs), including *zfp36*, *btg2*, *cyr61*, *nr4a1*, *ptpn16* and *atf3*, induced by paraquat were considerably higher in the younger animals. Many of these IEGs exhibit age-related alterations in expression and have been shown to be dependent on mitogen-activated protein kinase kinase (MAPKK) signaling for expression. Aging was also associated with impairment in the induction of several stress response genes, including MAP3K6, and JunB. These data are, in great part, in agreement with earlier findings showing that reduced levels of expression of the IEGs *c-fos* and *c-jun* in aged rat hearts follow hemodynamic stress [27]. It is noteworthy that lower constitutive levels of several antioxidant genes have been found in the aged heart, including glutathione peroxidase (GPx4), peroxiredoxin 1, peroxiredoxin 2, peroxiredoxin 5, and both the cytosolic and mitochondrial superoxide dismutases, Sod1, and Sod2 which suggest that with aging the ability of the heart to cope with OS decreases.

The differential transcriptional response of the aging heart to ischemia-reperfusion (I/R) was evaluated in normoxic and post-ischemic murine hearts from young (2-4 months) and aged (16–18 months) mice. RNA was extracted from isolated hearts subjected to either normoxic perfusion or 20 min of global normothermic ischemia and 60 min of reperfusion and analyzed by cDNA microarray analysis and quantitative RT-PCR [28]. Aged normoxic hearts exhibited upregulation of genes involved in cell death (e.g., *Bnip*, *Casp*12, *Fgf*12, *Myc*, *Pdcd7*), transporter activity (e.g., oxygen transport) and metabolism (primarily fatty acid metabolism: *Aacs*, *Acsl*5, *Elovl*6, *Fasn* and *Lpd*). Most of the downregulated transcripts in aged normoxic hearts were involved in transcription (including transcription cofactor activities), and cell communication such as G-protein coupled receptor (GPCR) and bone morphogenetic protein (BMP) signaling components, with significant changes in components of MAPK, WNT, JAK-STAT and TGF-β signaling pathways. Significantly modified transcriptional response was found in association with the greater degree of ischemic stress-mediated contractile impairment and cellular damage in aged as compared to young hearts with selective changes in Ca^{2+}, WNT, and NOTCH signaling pathways in aged hearts. Despite a number of common responses to ischemia in both young and aged hearts (i.e., induction of stress/defense response, heat shock protein and protein folding factors such as *Brca2*,*Dnaja*1, *Dnajb*1, *Dnajb*9, *Hsp*105, *Txnip*), aging selectively modified ischemic transcriptional responses. Genes uniquely induced by ischemia in aged hearts include the kruppel-like transcription factors (Klf4 and Klf6), involved in regulating growth proliferation, *ID1, ID2* and *ID3* that are triggers of cardiac apoptosis, and inhibitors of DNA binding and of bHLH transcription factors, protective molecular chaperones that regulate apoptosis/survival pathways (e.g., *Hspd*1 also HSP60, *Hspca*), BCL2-associated athanogene 3 (Bag3) and the tissue inhibitor of matrix metalloproteinases, TIMP4. Nearly 25% of the identified downregulated transcripts possessed binding properties, including protein and nucleic acid binding. Genes involved in modulating apoptosis (e.g., *Hspd*1, *Bag*3, *Hspca*, *Lnk*, *Dnm*2), hypertrophy and remodeling (e.g., *Timp*4, *Il6st*, *Dscr*1, *Plaur*), and angiogenesis (e.g., *Klf*4, *Klf*6, *Wt*1, *F*11*r*, *Plaur*) are altered in the aging ischemic heart.

IEGs are thought to trigger "adaptive" responses to stress/ischemia resulted in selective induction of *Ier*5 and selective repression of *Cebpg*, *Nr*1*d*2, *Atf*3, and *Atf*4 in aged hearts. With some exceptions, a general picture of repressed IEG expression emerges in older hearts, consistent with impaired adaptation to stress. On the other hand, young ischemic hearts displayed modified expression of four genes involved in Toll-like receptor, WNT and TGF-β signaling (*Jun*, *Atm*,

Nfkb1, *Apc*). Jun is upregulated (albeit not in the aging ischemic heart), whereas the other genes are downregulated.

At the conclusion of this discussion, a few remarks are pertinent: (1) Aging is associated with shifts in cardiovascular gene expression consistent with the phenotypic features of older hearts. (2) Reduced tolerance with age may be related to modification of signaling (particularly WNT and TGF-β). (3) Shifts in expression of immediate early genes, and genes important in control of cell death/survival, angiogenesis and cardiac remodeling likely contribute to the aging phenotype. (4) This phenotype is characterized by dysregulation of apoptosis with increased cardiomyocyte loss, reduced vascularity and vasodilator reserve, and abnormal remodeling responses

CR in Heart and Skeletal Muscle

Lee et al. had also examined the effects of caloric restriction (CR) dietary regimen on transcript profiles, initiated in middle-age in a second cohort of aging animals, and identified an altered transcriptional pattern (compared to the untreated aging animals) that was rather broad-based (over 20% of profiled genes showed significant changes), with more than 75% of the changes associated with myocardial aging, being either completely or partially reversed. The CR-mediated myocardial transcriptome changes included the suppression of the structural gene transcription (e.g., collagen and ECM proteins), downregulation of DNA-inducible transcripts (presumably indicative of less endogenous DNA damage) and proapoptotic factors, and upregulation of DNA repair and antiapoptotic factors, consistent with CR mediating a reduction of aging-induced endogenous damage. In addition, CR mediated a reversal of a number of age-induced transcript changes leading to upregulated glycolysis and downregulated FAO; CR also completely prevented both age-related downregulation of the glycolytic inhibitor *PDK4* and PFK upregulation, and partially restored FAO gene expression consistent with CR modulating the age-induced myocardial metabolic shift, as shown in Fig. 13.1 [29]. Further microarray-based observations on the effects on long-term CR on cardiac gene expression also detected a pattern of altered murine gene expression consistent with reduced myocardial remodeling and fibrosis, enhanced contractility and energy production, via FAO [30]. An 8-week regimen of CR reproduces nearly 20% of the genomic effects of long-term CR in heart, compared to 75% in liver, suggesting that the genomic effects of CR may be established more rapidly in mitotic (i.e., liver) than in post-mitotic (i.e., heart) tissues. Nevertheless, rapid reversal of the aging phenotype by CR appears possible in both tissue-types. Molecular and histochemical analysis revealed that both types of CR reduced myocardial natriuretic peptide precursor type B, collagen expression and reduced perivascular collagen deposition. Moreover, the presence of smaller cardiomyocytes in the left ventricle of long-term CR mice, suggests reduced age-related cell death.

Not unexpectedly, microarray gene profiling analysis of murine and monkey skeletal muscle transcripts revealed a number of striking tissue-specific differences with regards to aging, as well as sharing some commonalities with the myocardial/cardiomyocyte profiles [30, 31]. A reduced proportion of genes appear to be affected overall in murine skeletal muscle aging as compared to heart; roughly 2% of 6347 genes surveyed by microarray analysis displayed a greater than twofold increase or decrease in expression levels as a function of age. A large percentage (nearly 20%) of the aging-associated upregulated genes in gastrocnemius muscle in 30 month old mice are involved in the induction of stress response including heat shock response genes (e.g., Hsp71 and Hsp27), OS-inducible genes (e.g., HIC-5, a transcriptional factor induced by oxidative damage), DNA damage-inducible genes (e.g., GADD45) and the mitochondrial creatine kinase. Genes involved in energy metabolism were downregulated with aging, including genes associated with mitochondrial function and turnover (e.g., mitochondrial lon protease, ATP synthase A subunit, NADP transhydrogenase) as were genes associated with glycogen metabolism and glycolysis (e.g., α-enolase, phosphoprotein

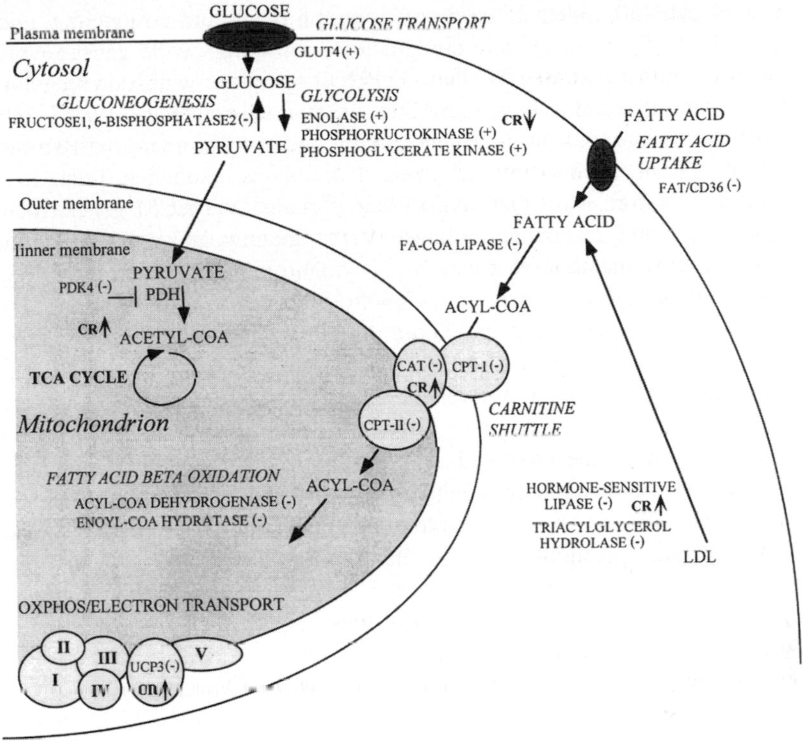

Fig. 13.1 Profiling of murine myocardial genes during normal aging and during caloric restriction
Specific metabolic genes affected either by upregulation (+) or downregulation (−) in the aging heart are shown, including genes involved in plasma membrane glucose and fatty acid transport (e.g., GLUT4, FAT/CD36), cytosolic gluconeogenesis, fatty acid metabolism and glycolysis (e.g., fructose 1,6 -bisphosphatase 2, enolase, fatty acyl CoA-lipase, hormone sensitive lipase, phosphofructokinase). Also shown are genes involved in mitochondrial-based metabolic processes including carnitine transport (e.g., CPT-1, CAT, CPT-II), fatty acid oxidation (e.g., Acyl CoA dehydrogenase), pyruvate oxidation (e.g., PDK4), OXPHOS and electron transport/coupling (e.g., UCP3). Changes in gene expression with caloric restriction (CR) are shown with arrows.

phosphatase, glucose 6-phosphate isomerase), the latter in marked contrast with their upregulation in heart. Also significantly downregulated were genes involved in macromolecular synthesis including squalene synthase, stearoyl-CoA desaturase, EF1-γ and the chaperone HSP70, and a concerted decrease in the expression of genes involved in protein turnover. A significant number of downregulated genes such as the 20*S* proteasome subunit, the 26*S* proteasome component TBP1, ubiquitin-thiolesterase, and the ubiquitin-specific protease UNP, are involved in the ubiquitin-proteasome pathway of protein turnover.

Using a parallel group of animals subjected to CR, comparison of 30 month old control and CR mice revealed that aging-related changes in gene expression profiles were significantly attenuated by CR, with 29% completely prevented by CR and 34% partially suppressed. Moreover, CR induced a metabolic reprogramming characterized by a transcriptional shift toward energy metabolism, increased biosynthesis, and protein turnover by both attenuating several key aging-mediated changes (e.g., G-6-P isomerase, EF-1-γ, 26*S* proteasome component TBP1) as well as by induction/repression of other genes. For instance, CR enhanced expression of transketolase, PPAR-γ and PPAR-α, pyruvate kinase and fatty acid synthase and downregulated inducible genes involved in metabolic detoxification, DNA repair, and the response to OS.

In a similar profiling analysis with vastus lateralis skeletal muscle derived from Rhesus monkeys, genes involved in OS responses (e.g., NF-κB, metallothionein 1B, HSP70), detoxification (e.g., several isoforms of cytP450, aldehyde oxidase), neuronal death and remodeling, and DNA repair (e.g., p21, uracil-DNA glycosylase) were upregulated with aging, while genes involved in energy metabolism, such as mitochondrial ETC and OXPHOS function, were downregulated, including sarcomeric mitochondrial creatine kinase, NADH: ubiquinone reductase, ATP synthase-α and- γ subunits, succinate dehydrogenase iron-protein subunit and cytochrome *c* oxidase subunits IV and VIa [32]. Onset of CR in the middle-aged group of monkeys resulted in induction of structural genes (e.g., desmin, laminin, actin and myosin heavy chain) and ECM genes, including several collagens (collagen I 1 and 2 subunits, collagen VII 2 subunit, and collagen III 1 subunit) and downregulation of energy metabolism genes (e.g., cytochrome *c*1, cytochrome *c* oxidase subunit VII, cytochrome *c* subunit IV, sarcomeric mitochondrial creatine kinase, several ATP synthase subunits, and ubiquinol:cytochrome *c* reductase core protein II) suggesting that CR monkeys may be in a hypometabolic state associated with reduced activity of the mitochondrial ETC. However, in contrast to the significant reversal of age-related alterations at the transcriptional level in murine skeletal muscle by CR, which include energy metabolism reprogramming, increased macromolecular biosynthesis and turnover, and reduced oxidative induced damage, no beneficial effects of CR were observed in aging rhesus monkey skeletal muscle. The observed differences between murine and *Rhesus* gene expression may be attributable to potential problems with the timing of CR initiation or differential species-specificity regarding the CR mechanism.

Transcriptome Profiling in Age-associated Cardiac Diseases

Global gene profiling analysis has also proven to be informative in documenting gene expression patterns associated with diverse aging-associated cardiac pathologies including cardiac hypertrophy [33], myocardial ischemia [34], dilated cardiomyopathy [33], coronary artery disease [35], atrial fibrillation[36] and heart failure (HF)[37] in tissues and cells from both animal models and human subjects. Nevertheless, gene profiling studies with diseased human heart from either fresh or frozen biopsied samples or transplant tissue contain mixed cell populations, are obtained from patients of different ages, ethnicities and gender making it exceedingly difficult to determine to what extent gene products are responsive to age and not to other sources of biological variation.

An interesting study employing microarray analysis to examine gene expression profiles in failing and non-failing human myocardium identified 162 candidate "HF-responsive" gene products and demonstrated that the majority of changes in abundance were subject to diverse biological inputs [38]. When modeled to take into account the three variables of HF, gender and age, only 5 of these transcripts were linked to HF irrespective of sex or age (e.g., lumican and CCAAT-enhancer binding protein), 15 transcripts demonstrated HF-associated changes in expression, which varied by sex (e.g., calponin 1 and natriuretic peptide precursor A), and 10 transcripts demonstrated complex interactions, involving HF, sex and age while only one of the transcripts, methionine tRNA synthetase demonstrated a HF response that varied only as a function of age. Analysis of candidate gene expression in non-failing myocardium revealed that metallothionein 1L (Mt1l), a protein implicated in cell defense, whose abundance increases with age regardless of normalization, is truly age-responsive and independent of the hypertensive status [17].

This analytical approach has also been revealing in establishing expression profiles of genes involved (or altered) in aging-associated neointimal formation, apoptotic progression and proinflammatory events in vascular cells [39, 40]. Expression analysis by cDNA-based microarray of cytokines, chemokines, and their receptors in isolated coronary arteries of young (3 months old) and aged (25 months old) male Fischer 344 rats showed that TNF-α (3.3-fold), interleukin-1β (IL1β) (3-fold), IL-6 (2.9-fold), IL-6Rα (2.8-fold) and IL-17 (6.1-fold) genes were significantly increased in older compared to young arteries suggesting that a proinflammatory shift in the profile of vascular cytokine expression may contribute to the aging induced phenotypic changes in coronary arteries [40]. Further studies using both microarray and real-time PCR indicated increased expression of proapoptotic caspase 9 as well as TNF-α and TNF-β in aged coronary arteries in parallel with a 5-fold increase in apoptotic ECs as gauged by DNA fragmentation and TUNEL analysis [39]. Interestingly, expression of TNFR1, TNFα-converting enzyme (TACE), Bcl-2, Bcl-X(L), Bid, Bax, caspase 8, and caspase 3 were unchanged

Neointimal formation, a pathologic hallmark of several obliterative vascular diseases, including atherosclerosis, post-stent restenosis, and allograft vasculopathy is more exaggerated in aging rats after arterial injury than in their younger counterparts. Exaggerated neotimal formation in response to mechanical injury has also been more recently reported in aging mice in concert with increased vascular smooth muscle cell (SMC) proliferation and reduced apoptosis [41]. Analysis of angiogenesis-related gene expression in vascular SMCs harvested from aging and young adult mice subjected to wire injury of the carotid artery showed increased expression of PDGFR-α (11.4-fold), restin (10.6-fold), Nos3 (8.6-fold), Fgfr4 (10.2-fold), and Erb2 (6.8-fold) in aging compared with young vascular SMCs. In contrast, expression of Fgf4 (0.25-fold), Fgfr3 (0.11-fold), and cadherin 5 (0.46-fold) were lower in aging. Age-dependent increases in PDGFR-α likely contribute to increased vascular SMC proliferation. This was further supported by a significant increase in overall proliferative growth in aging vascular SMCs in the presence of 10 ng/mL of the PDGFR-α ligand and mitogen PDGF-BB, findings which suggest an important role for the PDGF/PDGFR pathway in the exaggerated neointimal formation associated with aging.

Proteomic Analysis

As with transcriptome analysis, proteomic analysis also provides an opportunity to evaluate gene expression in aging tissues in a global fashion. This approach allows the assessment of gene expression at the protein level, as well as possible identification of novel cardiovascular and cardiac-specific biomarkers of aging. Primarily, two methods have been employed in proteomic research, the complete proteomic screening in which the entire proteome (i.e., all proteins) are characterized, and a more limited proteomic analysis that is either targeted to specific candidate proteins or limited to specific classes of proteins, or sub-proteomes. A critical review of the literature reveals that only a few studies of complete myocardial proteomics in aging at the global level have been published.

One alternative method has been to focus on proteomes contained within specific subcellular organelles such as mitochondria. In Chapter 3 we presented several methodologies for separation and high-yield preparation of subcellular organelles such as mitochondria, Golgi bodies and endoplasmic reticulum that are usually further analyzed by 2D gel electrophoresis, digitized imaging of 2D gel electrophoresis, and mass spectrometry [42, 43]. Other methods of subfractionation of enzymatic complexes have been utilized including the use of blue-native PAGE electrophoresis (BN-PAGE), which allows the separation of large macromolecular complexes with both membrane and soluble components preserving protein-protein interactions. This technique can be used to separate membrane and other functional protein complexes as intact, enzymatically active complexes in the first dimension that may be followed by a second-dimension separation by Tricine–SDS-PAGE, to allow the separation of complexes into their component subunits, and can be combined with MALDI-PMF (matrix-assisted laser desorption ionization peptide mass fingerprinting) for protein identification. Studies with BN-PAGE have been useful in the analysis of all of the individual subunits of the five ETC/OXPHOS respiratory complexes of the mitochondria from human heart [44]. Moreover, BN-PAGE has recently been employed to compare and quantitatively assess (and isolate) the five OXPHOS complexes from solubilized mitochondria of five different rat organs including kidney, liver, heart, skeletal muscle, and brain [45], and to identify "an OXPHOS interactome" of over

100 non-redundant soluble and membrane-embedded non-OXPHOS proteins comprised of constituents of known mitochondrial protein complexes, several novel proteins, and proteins primarily not localized in mitochondria (e.g., glycolytic enzymes). Data obtained from these partial mitochondrial proteome maps of various rat tissues can serve as a database for elucidating age-dependent changes, including alterations in protein-protein interactions as well as in post-translational modifications [46].

Another method of protein analysis, particularly relevant to aging studies,involves the proteomic evaluation of specific post-translational modifications (e.g., phosphorylation or oxidative changes). This methodology has been greatly facilitated by the availability of specific antibodies to phosphorylated residues (e.g., phosphoserine or phosphotyrosine), protein carbonyls or nitrotyrosine. For instance, Kanski et al. have identified cardiac proteins which undergo nitration as a consequence of biological aging in aging Fischer 344/Brown Norway F1 rats using separation by 1- and 2-D gel electrophoresis, and subsequent immunoblot analysis using an anti-nitrotyrosine antibody with further identification by nanoelectrospray ionization-tandem mass spectrometry (NSI-MS/MS) [47]. Both soluble homogenate and solubilized mitochondrial proteins were analyzed and protein profiles from whole hearts of young (5 months old) and old (26 months old) animals compared. Among the 48 nitrated proteins identified in this study were proteins responsible for energy production and metabolism including glycolysis, the tricarboxylic acid (TCA) cycle, or β-oxidation of fatty acids. Affected proteins include α-enolase, α-aldolase, aconitase, methylmalonate semialdehyde dehydrogenase, 3-ketoacyl-CoA thiolase, acetyl-CoA acetyltransferase, GAPDH, malate dehydrogenase (MDH), creatine kinase, electron-transfer flavoprotein (ETF), manganese-superoxide dismutase (MnSOD), F1-ATPase (ATP synthase), and the voltage-dependent anion channel (VDAC), as well as proteins involved in the structural integrity of the cells (e.g., desmin). Since mitochondrial proteins have been reported to be especially sensitive to NO-dependent modification under conditions of acute OS during inflammatory processes or I/R [48, 49], it is not entirely surprising that many of the proteins undergoing 3-NT accumulation are mitochondrial-localized including aconitase (containing a redox-sensitive iron-sulfur cluster), ETF, a critical electron acceptor for several dehydrogenases involved in the transfer of electrons to the main mitochondrial respiratory chain, the TCA cycle enzyme MDH, the FAO enzymes acetyl-CoA acetyltransferase and 3-ketoacyl-CoA thiolase, the mitochondrial-based free radical scavenger MnSOD, ATP synthase, and the outer membrane protein VDAC. Nitration of VDAC and aconitase has also been demonstrated in hearts of diabetic mouse models [50].

There is conclusive evidence of increased levels of protein carbonyl accumulation in aged hearts [51–54], and indications that this accumulation can be reversed by long-term CR (in rodents) [51, 55, 56]. Interestingly, short-term CR has the opposite effect resulting in a significant increase in cardiac protein carbonyl content with aging [57]. At present, there is little information as to which specific cardiac proteins are targeted by protein carbonylation in aging; and conflicting data exist as to whether mitochondrial proteins are selectively targeted [10, 53]. Although a variety of proteomic methods have been employed to identify specific protein carbonyl content in aging liver and brain [58–60], these methods have not yet been applied to the aging heart.

Another critical post-transcriptional protein modification that occurs during aging with significant cardiovascular relevance is glycation (which has been comprehensively discussed in Chapters 3 and 4). This process, which involves the addition of reducing sugars to specific proteins by non-enzymatic reaction can be reversible, although glycated proteins subject to further oxidation can form Advanced Glycation End-products (AGEs) that are irreversible. These modified proteins are frequently heterogeneous and accumulate in the circulatory system and various tissues including the heart [61]. Collagen, elastin and basement membrane are among the proteins most vulnerable to AGE formation presumably because of their long-life and slow rate of turnover. The accumulation of interstitial collagen (found in both the diabetic and in the aging heart), and the development of increasing glucose-cross-links by AGE have been proposed as the primary basis for the increased myocardial stiffness and consequently, diastolic dysfunction in the aging heart. Further support for a pivotal role of AGE in myocardial stiffening has been provided by the discovery that regimens that specifically inhibit AGE formation such as diet restriction [62], and treatment with aminoguanidine [63], effectively prevent the pathological stiffening process associated with diabetes and aging.

Levels of cardiac AGEs determined by AGE-ELISA, evaluated in young (2 months) and aged (24–26 month) mice were approximately 2.5-fold higher in aged hearts than young ones. A group of proteins with a molecular range between 50 and 75 kDa with pI of 4–7 was distinctively modified in the aged heart [64].

An important modulator of AGE and its effect in the myocardium bears particular mention: an integral membrane protein receptor for AGE (RAGE). Interaction of this receptor with diverse AGE has also been reported to lead to the production of pro-inflammatory cytokines and formation of free radicals. By immunohistochemistry, the RAGE antigen was identified in cultured bovine endothelium, vascular smooth muscle, monocyte-derived macrophages, bovine cardiac and neonatal rat cardiac myocytes, diverse neuronal tissues/cell-types and in the expanded intima of human atherosclerotic plaques [65].

A role of RAGE in mediating AGE in I/R has been identified by the demonstration that RAGE (and its ligands) are upregulated in the ischemic heart, and by the striking protection from myocardial I/R injury exhibited by RAGE-null mice [66]. Moreover, RAGE activation is probably associated with increases in inducible nitric oxide synthase expression and levels of nitric oxide, cyclic guanosine monophosphate (cGMP), nitrotyrosine and decreased myocardial energy metabolism; myocardial ATP levels are restored in RAGE-null mice. Upregulation of the RAGE protein (detected by Western blot) has also been reported in the atria of senescent and adult patients, and was associated with reduced heart function [67]. A comprehensive proteomic analysis of the specific proteins targeted by the RAGE/AGE pathway in the aging heart is needed.

Cell Proteomics in Aging

In contrast to the complex tissue and cellular heterogeneity that comprises the heart, cell culture systems are attractive models for proteomic analysis because they may provide more highly defined systems with much lower inherent variability between samples. However, cells maintained in culture (particularly adult cardiomyocytes) while maintaining their protein synthestic capacity [68], may display alterations in their pattern of protein expression significantly distinct from their profile *in vivo* [69]. Nevertheless, the adult cardiac myocyte in culture can remain a highly differentiated cell maintaining many of its previous *in vivo* characteristics [70–72] dependent on the use of low-serum or no serum media and modification of culture growth substrate (e.g., agarose or laminin-coated and not plastic plates or suspension culture). Relatively few proteomic investigations of isolated adult cardiac myocytes have been published, and none, that we are aware, with aging.

Proteomic analysis has been carried out with ECs undergoing replicative senescence, as discussed in Chapters 3 and 5. Since the aging of ECs and vascular SMCs may play a significant role in the pathophysiology of age-related vascular diseases, including atherosclerosis, proteomic analysis may reveal potential mediators of susceptibility to these disorders as well as the triggering elements of replicative senescence. Using *in vitro* cultured human umbilical vein endothelial cells (HUVECs) as an experimental model for replicative senescence, Kamino et al. have identified by 2-D electrophoresis (2-DE), 3 upregulated proteins and 5 downregulated proteins in senescent HUVECs compared to young HUVECs [73]. Among the upregulated proteins in senescent HUVECs was cathepsin B, a protease participating in both intracellular proteolysis and ECM remodeling. Proteomic analysis of 3 isolates of HUVECS derived from 3 umbilical cords has been also recently employed [74]. After HUVEC replicative senescence, lysates were subjected to 2-DE and despite the variability of the three independent isolations, a common set of proteins that showed senescence-dependent expression patterns was identified. Thirty-five proteins were found with LC-Fourier transform MS with significant association to the senescent phenotype. The functional classifications comprised by this protein subset suggest that EC replicative senescence is accompanied by changes in a number of diverse biological pathways. These include increased cellular stress (e.g., upregulation of HSP27, the NUAM subunit of respiratory complex I, transferrin (TRFE) and the glutathione-s-transferease omega), protein biosynthesis (e.g., downregulation of EFI5a and nucleophosmin (NPM)) and reduction in DNA repair and maintenance (e.g., downregulation of KU80 and RFA2) with both nuclear integrity affected (e.g., downregulation of the nuclear-envelope protein, lamin B) and altered cytoskeletal structure (e.g., upregulated α-actinin, annexin V, moesin and downregulated microtubule binding proteins).

A major hallmark of HUVEC *in vitro* senescence is the increased frequency of apoptotic cell death. Recent observations have shown that the onset of HUVEC senescence is accompanied by a striking upregulation of extracellular proteins, including interleukin-8 (over 50-fold increase), VEGI, and the IGF-binding proteins 3 and 5 [75]. These extracellular proteins modulate the apoptotic response of human cells, and in the case of interleukin-8, are linked to the establishment of atherosclerotic lesions.

Proteomic analysis has been used to compare normal and senescent HUVECs with HUVECs transformed (and immortalized) with ectopic expression of the catalytic subunit of telomerase hTERT [76]. While ectopic hTERT expression appears to lead to a stable, proliferating cell line (with a growth rate similar to early passage HUVECs) with many characteristics of differentiation, the protein expression profile was significantly different than that of normal early passage and senescent HUVEC cells. For example, the marked 5-fold reduction in levels of cytokeratin 7 in senescent HUVEC, which by destabilization of the cytoskeleton may contribute to the observed enlarged and flattened morphology of these cells, was not seen in the transformed HUVEC cells. Moreover, glutathione *S*-transferase, which has been described as marker for enhanced OS, is nearly 2-fold upregulated in senescent HUVECs but not in TERT-transformed HUVECs. This study also identified several protein changes specific to the senescent HUVEC phenotype and a role in atherosclerosis worthy of note. ICAM-1 basal expression level was increased in senescent HUVECs promoting the recruitment of monocytes to the artery wall, an early step in the development of atherosclerosis. CHST3, an enzyme which catalyzes the sulfation of chondroitin sulfate and keratan sulfate, both belonging to the ECM, is increased by 3-fold in senescent HUVECs; this is consistent with the noted changes in the composition and structure of the ECM during the progression of atherosclerosis. Also upregulated (by 5-fold) in senescent HUVECs was calumenin, an EF-HAND low affinity calcium binding protein, which has been identified in atherosclerotic lesions, while absent in normal vasculature; it is also associated with the immunological defense system and amyloid formation.

Using cultured human dermal microvascular ECs and 2-DE proteomic mapping, the effects of various treatments (e.g., kinetin, epigallocatechin-3-gallate, all-trans-retinoic acid, and selenium) on cell senescence have been assessed and a search for the aging-related proteins initiated [77]. These treatments resulted in 68 qualitative changes and 172 quantitative changes, of which 46 could be identified. Alteration in expression of proteins associated with cell cycle and cytoskeleton including moesin, rho guanosine-5′-diphosphate-dissociation inhibitor, and actin has been found and confirmed by both immunoblotting and confocal laser microscopy.

Proteomic analysis using 2-DE of vascular SMCs cultured from aorta of newborn (4 day old) and aging (18 months old) Wistar rats found 10 proteins that were increased in the SMCs of older animals; sequence analysis of one of these proteins (expressed only in old SMCs) identified it as cellular retinol-binding protein (CRPB) [78].

Genetics of Aging

In Chapter 12, we have described a number of animal and cell models of aging that have provided multiple and informative tools (e.g., genes, pathways), and even paradigms, with which one can study human aging. In this section, we survey 3 nascent areas of human aging analysis that are currently being developed.

Mapping of Genes Involved in Aging

Genome Wide Scans

In humans, exceptional longevity accompanied by good cardiovascular health has a genetic component that is suggested by identification of rare families showing clustering for this phenotype [79]. Twin studies have revealed that for individuals living to approximately 100 years, approximately 25% of the variation in life span is caused by genetic differences [80]. Such genetic components are likely to influence basic mechanisms of aging, which in turn broadly influence susceptibility to age-related illnesses.

An increased survival advantage may arise in individuals both lacking genetic variations that predispose to disease, and having variations that confer disease resistance (longevity enabling genes). Further molecular genetic studies may allow the discovery of both longevity-enabling genes as well as genes associated with an increased propensity to develop specific diseases. Given the marked improvement in the human haplotype map, large-scale linkage studies of long-lived families will likely be undertaken in the near future to assist in the quest to define genetic determinants of longevity and basic aging [81].

To identify the genes contributing to a cardiovascular-healthy aging phenotype in humans, a 10 centimorgan (cM) genome screen has been performed in 95 pairs of male fraternal twins, concordant for healthy aging [82]. Individuals meeting these criteria were defined as those attaining the age of 70 free of cardiovascular disease (coronary surgery, diabetes, heart attack, and stroke) as well as prostate cancer. Six chromosomal regions were identified with logarithm of odds (LOD) scores greater than 1.2 ($p < 0.01$). A locus on the long arm of chromosome 4 at marker D4S1564 produced a LOD score of 1.67 suggesting an association with better physical aging and/or longevity. This was the same marker previously linked to extreme longevity segregating as an autosomal dominant trait in a study of 143 centenarians and their long-lived siblings [83].

The microsatellite D4S1564 interval spans 12 million bp that contains approximately 50 putative genes. To identify the specific gene and gene variants impacting life span, a haplotype-based fine-mapping study of the interval was performed using densely spaced informative SNP markers [84]. The resulting genetic association study identified a haplotype marker within the microsomal triglyceride transfer protein (MTP) as a modifier of human life span within some individuals of specific backgrounds with evidence of moderate stratification. The genetic variant of MTP associated with longevity involves a 2 SNP haplotype including both a *MTP* promoter mutation (−493G) and with the major Q95 allele of *MTP*. The minor allele MTP95H is a semiconservative mutation in exon 3 of *MTP* Q95H (glutamine to histidine at amino acid 95) and represents a risk allele. Other groups have found genetic associations between MTP and several phenotypes including lipoprotein profiles, insulin resistance, fat distribution, and most of these studies focused on the −493G/T marker [85]. Interestingly, a significant association between specific variants of the MTP gene in a Caucasian population of centenarians (from the US) was found, but this association was not replicated in either French or German study populations [86]. The microsomal triglyceride transfer protein has been identified as the rate-limiting step in lipoprotein synthesis and may affect longevity by subtly modulating this pathway and affecting lipid profiles; other data suggest that this gene may also affect susceptibility to insulin resistance and obesity.

SNP Analysis in Aging and Aging Associated Disease Susceptibility

Studies of the frequencies of different alleles in young adults and aged individuals have implicated several genes, such as ApoE and ACE, in longevity. However, such association studies are fraught with difficulty, can easily give rise to spurious and unreproducible results through unsuspected population subdivision; an approach making use of genetic relationships among relatives often is desirable.

Lipoproteins (APOE)

Absence of DNA polymorphisms predisposing to age-associated diseases may be one way to achieve exceptional old age. The marked decreased frequency of the apolipoprotein (apo) E4 allele among centenarians exemplifies such a mechanism [87]. This finding is consistent with the strong association of APOE4 with hypercholesteremia, ischemic heart disease, age-related cognitive decline and Alzheimer's disease. Conversely, the E2 allele has been associated with longevity in French centenarians and their siblings [88]. In a study of nonagenarian subjects from Belfast where there is a high intrinsic incidence of cardiovascular disease, the E4 allele was reduced in the nonagenarian group, the E3 unchanged and E2 frequency was increased suggesting that longevity is negatively associated with the E4 allele and may be associated with E2 [89].

In a case-control study featuring Ashkenazi Jews, individuals with exceptional longevity and their offspring were found to have significantly larger high-density lipoprotein (HDL) and low-density lipoprotein (LDL) particle size [90]. In addition, these subjects have a lower prevalence of hypertension, cardiovascular disease, and the metabolic syndrome in association with increased homozygosity for the 405V variant in cholesteryl ester transfer protein (CETP), which is involved in the regulation of lipoprotein and its particle sizes. Lipoprotein particle sizes may be heritable and able to promote healthy aging.

A more recent longitudinal study examining 11 common polymorphisms in 224 older ($\geq$75 years) Jerusalem residents of Ashkenazi ethnicity compared to a group of 441 younger subjects (mean age, 22 years) found that variants in apoE, MHTFR, SOD2, IGF2, ApaI, and factor VII are risk factors for a single outcome, survival to 75 years, in this population [91]. This is consistent with the view that deleterious genes can significantly affect aging and predisposition to early-life pathology and disease, including those that confer risk for developing vascular disease in the heart, brain, or peripheral vessels (e.g., APOE, methyltetrahydrofolate-reductase (MTFHR), and mutation at factor VII genes). A polymorphism in MTHFR, caused by the C677T point mutation, leads to increased thermolability of the enzyme with reduced enzyme activity and has been associated with longevity [92], and in selective populations, vascular defects such as stroke [93]. Further longitudinal candidate-gene association studies will likely provide potential future progress in this area.

A recent study conducted in a relatively homogeneous population (making stratification effects less likely) of US Ashkenazi Jewish centenarians, their offspring, and Ashkenazi controls found that the −641C allele in the APOC3 promoter is present at a significant higher frequency in centenarians and their offspring (20–25%), compared to controls (10%) [94]. This genotype was also associated with lower APOC3 serum levels, a favorable profile for lipoproteins, reduction in cardiovascular risk factors, including hypertension and decreased insulin sensitivity, as well as with enhanced survival.

ACE

Variants in the gene encoding angiotensin I-converting enzyme (ACE) are biologically plausible candidates for longevity. The cleavage of angiotensin I by ACE produces the octapeptide angiotensin II, which is a potent vasoconstrictor, and polymorphisms in ACE have been reported to be involved in cardiovascular diseases, including ischemic disease and myocardial infarction. One human ACE polymorphism is caused by an Alu element insertion resulting in three genotypes (Alu+/+, Alu+/−, Alu−/−, or ACE-II, ACE-ID, and ACE-DD, respectively), with ACE-II displaying lower ACE activity.

The ACE genotype may be associated with longevity. Increased frequency of homozygosity for the ACE-D allele in a German population of octogenarians has been found [95], which was further supported in a longitudinal study;[96] however, this could not be confirmed in two large studies of centenarians and younger controls [88, 97]. In addition, there is evidence from numerous studies that differential ethnic and geographic distribution of specific ACE alleles may underlie or modulate the age-related findings.

To clarify the functional role of the ACE polymorphism, its direct effect on cell survival has been recently assessed [98]. ACE-II human ECs had lower angiotensin-II levels and 20-fold increased viability after slow starvation compared to EC cells with the ACE-DD genotype. Moreover, only ACE-II cells expressed the pluripotent/stem cell-maintenance factors nanog, numb, and klotho. ACE inhibition by captopril in ACE-DD cells mimicked the ACE-II genotype. These results provide the first evidence of a functional role for a naturally occurring polymorphism, having broad implications in human biology, longevity, and disease.

KLOTHO

Longevity may also be affected by variants in the human homologues of the aging suppressor gene Klotho (KLOTHO), which extends life span when overexpressed in mice. As we have previously noted in Chapter 12, mice carrying a loss-of-function mutation in the Klotho gene develop aging-like symptoms around 4 weeks after birth and suffer from multiple age-related disorders similar to those observed in humans, including osteoporosis, skin atrophy, ectopic calcification, arteriosclerosis, and pulmonary emphysema, as well as manifest a shortened life span (usually around 2 months of age). A functional variant of KLOTHO (termed "KL-VS"), which harbors two amino acid substitutions (F352V and C370S) in complete linkage disequilibrium is associated with reduced human longevity (in a carefully selected population of homogenous Bohemian Czechs) when in homozygosity [99]. In a subsequent study of 525 Ashkenazi Jews composed of 216 probands (age $\geq$ 95 years) and 309 unrelated individuals (ages 51–94) genotyped for the KL-VS allele, a heterozygous advantage for longevity was observed for individuals $\geq$ 79 years of age [100]. Furthermore, both decreased HDL and higher systolic blood pressure (SBP) are associated with the homozygous KL-VS genotype whereas the heterozygous individuals had a reduced incidence of stroke, lower SBP and increased longevity.

Studies with gene variants in human homologues of another pivotal aging-pathway gene, previously identified in mouse studies (p66Shc) and discussed in Chapter 12, have suggested that p66Shc may be another aging-determinant factor in human longevity. In two independent cohorts of respectively, 730 and 563 subjects aged 85 and over, when tested for association of the only known non-synonymous polymorphism, Met(410)Val in p66SHC with longevity, an increasing valine allele frequency was associated with increased age at death and lower mortality rate [101]

Epigenetics

Epigenetics can be defined as the study of heritable changes in gene expression non-related to changes in the sequence of DNA. A number of processes are involved in epigenetics including chemical modifications to DNA or to proteins closely interacting with DNA (e.g., histones), as well as RNA. Moreover, epigenetic influences can be disrupted during aging, as well as by environmental factors including toxins and diet.

DNA Methylation

Genomic methylation, which influences many cellular processes such as gene expression and chromatin organization, generally declines with cellular senescence although some genes paradoxically undergo hypermethylation during cellular aging and immortalization. Epigenetic modification of CpG islands in promoter regions is an important regulatory mechanism of gene expression in eukaryotic cells. Hypermethylation of CpG islands may silence a gene, whereas hypomethylation of previously methylated CpG islands may facilitate gene expression. The pattern of methylation is cell-type-specific and established during development of the organisms. Limited findings in a changed CpG island methylation pattern have been found in a number of aging cardiovascular cells [102, 103], and more extensively in cancer. Aging-mediated changes in the levels of methylated cytosines may promote chromosomal instability and rearrangements, which can increase the risk of neoplasia

Lopatina et al. [104] have found evidence that overall methylating activity by DNA methyltransferases (Dnmts), and in particular the maintenance of methylation activity of the Dnmt1 isozyme is greatly decreased during cellular senescence in aging WI-38 fibroblasts. In contrast, in immortalized WI-38 cells, DNA methylating activity was similar to that of normal young cells. Interestingly, 2 other Dnmt activities are upregulated in both senescence and immortalized cells. Reduced genome-wide methylation in aging cells may be attributable to attenuated Dnmt1 activity whereas sporadic hypermethylation in aging and immortalized cells may be linked to increased *de novo* methylation by Dnmts other than the maintenance methyltransferase.

The majority of DNA methylation screening protocols generally utilize methylation-sensitive endonuclease digestion or bisulfite treatment of the template followed by subsequent PCR amplification of a specific sequence (usually assessed with a single DNA gene sequence at a time). A new more global approach combines methylation-sensitive enzyme digestion with the comparative genomic hybridization technique to develop an array-based method to screen the entire genome for changes of methylation patterns [105].

Chromatin Modifications

In addition to DNA methylation, post-translational changes (e.g., methylation, acetylation) to the histone proteins comprising the chromatin scaffold enveloping the chromosomal DNA orchestrate DNA organization and gene expression. Histone-modifying enzymes including methylases, acetylases and deacetylases are recruited to ensure that a receptive DNA region is either accessible for transcription or that DNA is targeted for silencing. Active regions of chromatin tend to have unmethylated DNA and have high levels of acetylated histones, whereas inactive regions of chromatin contain methylated DNA and deacetylated histones. Thus, an epigenetic "tag" is placed on targeted DNA, marking it with a special status that specifically activates or silences genes.

The histone deacetylases (HDACs) are enzymes that are able to deacetylate lysine side chains in histones as well as in specific non-histone proteins leading to altered states of conformation and activity [106, 107]. Of the 3 classes of human histone deacetylases, class I and II are zinc-dependent amidohydrolases and class III enzymes depend in their catalysis on NAD^+. Due to the homology to the yeast HDAC Sir2p, the NAD^+-dependent deacetylases are also termed sirtuins with seven members (Sirt1-7) presently known in humans. As discussed in Chapter 12, sirtuins have been implicated in the regulation of molecular mechanisms of aging with overexpression of sirtuin enzymatic activity resulting in an increase of life span in the yeast *S. cerevisiae* and in *C. elegans*. Sirtuins have been proposed to act as sensors for glucose uptake that respond to the levels of NAD^+ but other complex ways of action have been suggested as well. Sirtuin regulation of the highly conserved insulin-IGF-1 signaling pathway has been observed for *C. elegans* and mammals, indicating a role for sirtuins in the modulation of cell and organism adaptation to nutritional intake. In addition, the human sirtuin SIRT1 regulates a number of transcription factors that modulate endocrine signaling, including PPAR-γ, PGC-1α, forkhead-box transcription factors and p53.

Studies with the human sirtuin 3 (SIRT3) gene, which belongs to the evolutionary conserved family of sirtuin 2 (SIR2) proteins that control life span in the forementioned model organisms, found that a G477T variant of SIRT3 was associated with human longevity [108]. Males harboring the TT genotype increased survival in the elderly, while the GT genotype was associated with decreased survival.

Another variation in the human SIRT3 gene has been related to human longevity and arises as a result of a VNTR polymorphism (72-bp repeat core) localized to intron 5 [109]. Varied SIRT3 alleles differ both for the number of repeats and for presence/absence of potential regulatory sites. The VNTR region also has an allele-specific enhancer activity. In the analysis of allele frequencies as a function of age in a sample of 945 individuals (20–106 years), the allele completely lacking enhancer activity was found to be virtually absent in males older than 90 years suggesting that underexpression of a human sirtuin gene may be detrimental for longevity.

Numerous environmental factors as well as physiological (e.g., ROS) and pharmacological stimuli may impact epigenetic regulation of gene expression in aging. Among the many agents that have recently been assigned a potential role in epigenetic activation are plant-derived polyphenols, such as resveratrol, found in grapes and red wine, which some evidence suggest act via activation of sirtuins in cells [110]. Moreover, sirtuins may be impacted by metabolic factors and by CR albeit the mechanism remains largely undefined. Furthermore, recent observations indicate that environmental factors and diet can perturb the way genes are controlled by DNA methylation and covalent histone modifications. Clearly, further research on the link between environment and epigenetics in relationship to aging may result in potential therapeutic options, which could be used to reverse some of aging's detrimental consequences. Some of these will be described in Chapter 15.

Conclusion

Studies involving transcriptome analysis of aging tissues have begun to provide an overall picture of which genes are upregulated and which are downregulated. This can provide a "snapshot" or molecular signature of aging that depicts some general programming changes in overall gene expression, dependent on sampling time and tissue. This type of analysis has begun to facilitate the identification of biomarkers that are not only associated with aging phenotypic changes but also can be reversed with interventions such as CR. These investigations have also unveiled a classical pattern of heterogeneity in genotypic expression that seems to characterize aging post-mitotic tissues such as the heart. This heterogeneity arises from the multiple cell-types comprising these tissues that is even more evident in cell-to-cell studies of single cardiomyocytes. The use of proteomic analysis in aging studies has thus far been more limited. The most informative proteomic studies with respect to aging have targeted either specific groups of proteins, either organelle-specific (e.g., mitochondrial), functional (e.g., metabolic) or modified (e.g., nitrated proteins) rather than using global snapshots of the whole proteomic "enchilada".

In reference to the genetic analysis of human aging, despite the problems posed by the pronounced heterogeneity in genotypes, and difficult-to-control environmental factors, practical problems in conducting longitudinal studies and frequent methodological inconsistencies in sampling and assessing phenotypes, a number of genes and gene variants that contribute to aging and to aging-related diseases have been and continue to be identified. Furthermore, the molecular analysis of progeria and premature aging has not only revealed genes involved in the onset of these aging phenotypes and identified commonalities of gene expression profiles shared with normal aging, but also has begun to unveil the epigenetic mechanisms that can be disrupted during aging, including chromatin remodeling and DNA modifications.

Summary

- Gene expression profiling has been conducted in studies of the aging heart in mouse and rat tissues, primarily using microarray analysis.
- In mouse heart, increased age-mediated expression of myocardial structural genes involved in extracellular matrix (ECM) components, collagen deposition, cell adhesion, and cell growth has been found, consistent with findings that the aging heart undergoes ECM protein deposition, fibrosis and cardiomyocyte hypertrophy.
- Downregulated expression of genes involved in protein synthesis, including numerous translation initiation and elongation factors, and in genes associated with fatty acid transport and metabolism has been found.
- Genes involved in myocardial inflammatory and stress responses are primarily upregulated in the aging sedentary mouse, suggesting that the aging heart experiences oxidative stress (OS) leading to a pro-inflammatory state.
- Age-mediated re-programming of mouse heart gene expression was less extensive compared to transcriptome changes in other organs (e.g., liver) and found little overlap in the expression profiles of different aging tissues.
- A limited subset of gene transcripts that accumulated at significantly different levels with age has been found in the gene profiling analysis of isolated ventricular cardiomyocytes of aging mice compared to young mice.
- Biological diversity is necessary to be taking into account when performing studies of aging. Transcriptome (and proteomic) analysis of heart tissue is complicated and limited by factors such as tissue and cellular heterogeneity, genetic variability, disease state and pharmacological intervention.
- Interventions such as caloric restriction (CR) and exercise have significant impact on gene profiles in aging mice with a large proportion of aging-associated transcript changes being either completely or partially reversed.
- Global gene profiling analysis has proven to be informative in diverse aging associated cardiac pathologies including cardiac hypertrophy, myocardial ischemia, dilated cardiomyopathy, coronary artery disease, atrial fibrillation and heart failure.
- In tissues and cells of both animal models and human subjects gene profiling has also been revealing in establishing profiles of genes involved (or altered) in aging-associated neotimal formation, apoptotic progression and proinflammatory events in vascular cells.
- Proteomic analysis allows the assessment of gene expression at the protein level, as well as the identification of novel vascular and cardiac-specific biomarkers of aging.

- Most informative proteomic studies have eschewed a complete proteomic approach in which the entire proteome is characterized, and rather have utilized a more focused proteomic analysis targeted to specific candidate proteins by function, or limited to specific classes of proteins, or sub-proteomes of specific organelles (e.g., mitochondria or lysosomes) or containing specific protein-modifications (e.g., nitration).
- Cell culture systems are attractive models for proteomic analysis since they provide more highly defined systems with much lower inherent variability between samples than with aging tissues.
- Proteomic investigations have been carried out with endothelial cells (ECs) and vascular smooth muscle cells (SMCs) undergoing replicative senescence and have been informative in showing the potential mediators of susceptibility to atherosclerosis, as well as to the triggering elements of replicative senescence.
- Genome-wide screening in some defined populations (e.g., centenarians and their families) and SNP polymorphic variant analysis in case-association studies have allowed the identification of several genes associated with human aging.
- Genes involved in lipoprotein metabolisms (APOE), signaling, inflammation and immune-regulation have been clearly associated with differences in longevity, as well as in the susceptibility to aging-associated diseases.
- Molecular genetic analysis has begun to reveal the mechanism of significant epigenetic contributions to the expression of the aging phenotype, including DNA methylation and chromatin remodeling, primarily through modifications of chromatin proteins including histones.

References

1. Lee CK, Allison DB, Brand J, Weindruch R, Prolla TA. Transcriptional profiles associated with aging and middle age-onset caloric restriction in mouse hearts. Proc Natl Acad Sci USA 2002;99:14988–14993
2. Bronikowski AM, Carter PA, Morgan TJ, Garland T Jr, Ung N, Pugh TD, Weindruch R, Prolla TA. Lifelong voluntary exercise in the mouse prevents age-related alterations in gene expression in the heart. Physiol Genomics 2003;12:129–138
3. Fu C, Hickey M, Morrison M, McCarter R, Han ES. Tissue specific and non specific changes in gene expression by aging and by early stage CR. Mech Ageing Dev 2006;127:905–916
4. Iemitsu M, Miyauchi T, Maeda S, Tanabe T, Takanashi M, Irukayama-Tomobe Y, Sakai S, Ohmori H, Matsuda M, Yamaguchi I. Aging-induced decrease in the PPAR-alpha level in hearts is improved by exercise training. Am J Physiol Heart Circ Physiol 2002;283:H1750-H760
5. LeMoine CM, McClelland GB, Lyons CN, Mathieu-Costello O, Moyes CD. Control of mitochondrial gene expression in the aging rat myocardium. Biochem Cell Biol 2006;84:191–198
6. Bodyak N, Kang PM, Hiromura M, Sulijoadikusumo I, Horikoshi N, Khrapko K, Usheva A. Gene expression profiling of the aging mouse cardiac myocytes. Nucleic Acids Res 2002;30:3788–3794
7. Goyns MH, Charlton MA, Dunford JE, Lavery WL, Merry BJ, Salehi M, Simoes DC. Differential display analysis of gene expression indicates that age-related changes are restricted to a small cohort of genes. Mech Ageing Dev 1998;101:73–90
8. Shida M, Isoyama S. Effects of age on c-fos and c-myc gene expression in response to hemodynamic stress in isolated, perfused rat hearts. J Mol Cell Cardiol 1993;25:1025–1035
9. Gadaleta MN, Petruzzella V, Renis M, Fracasso F, Cantatore P. Reduced transcription of mitochondrial DNA in the senescent rat. Tissue dependence and effect of L-carnitine. Eur J Biochem 1990;187:501–506
10. Andreu AL, Arbos MA, Perez-Martos A, Lopez-Perez MJ, Asin J, Lopez N, Montoya J, Schwartz S. Reduced mitochondrial DNA transcription in senescent rat heart. Biochem Biophys Res Commun 1998;252:577–581
11. Hudson EK, Tsuchiya N, Hansford RG. Age-associated changes in mitochondrial mRNA expression and translation in the Wistar rat heart. Mech Ageing Dev 1998;103:179–193
12. Barazzoni R, Short KR, Nair KS. Effects of aging on mitochondrial DNA copy number and cytochrome c oxidase gene expression in rat skeletal muscle, liver, and heart. J Biol Chem 2000;275:3343–3347
13. Dinardo MM, Musicco C, Fracasso F, Milella F, Gadaleta MN, Gadaleta G, Cantatore P. Acetylation and level of mitochondrial transcription factor A in several organs of young and old rats. Biochem Biophys Res Commun 2003;301:187–191

14. Masuyama M, Iida R, Takatsuka H, Yasuda T, Matsuki T. Quantitative change in mitochondrial DNA content in various mouse tissues during aging. Biochim Biophys Acta 2005;1723:302–308
15. Lezza AM, Pesce V, Cormio A, Fracasso F, Vecchiet J, Felzani G, Cantatore P, Gadaleta MN. Increased expression of mitochondrial transcription factor A and nuclear respiratory factor-1 in skeletal muscle from aged human subjects. FEBS Lett 2001;501:74–78
16. Kumazaki T, Sakano T, Yoshida T, Hamada K, Sumida H, Teranishi Y, Nishiyama M, Mitsui Y. Enhanced expression of mitochondrial genes in senescent endothelial cells and fibroblasts. Mech Ageing Dev 1998;101:91–99
17. Volkova M, Garg R, Dick S, Boheler KR. Aging-associated changes in cardiac gene expression. Cardiovasc Res 2005;66:194–204
18. Young ME, Razeghi P, Cedars AM, Guthrie PH, Taegtmeyer H. Intrinsic diurnal variations in cardiac metabolism and contractile function. Circ Res 2001;89:1199–1208
19. Young ME. Circadian rhythms in cardiac gene expression. Curr Hypertens Rep 2003;5:445–453
20. Durgan DJ, Trexler NA, Egbejimi O, McElfresh TA, Suk HY, Petterson LE, Shaw CA, Hardin PE, Bray MS, Chandler MP, Chow CW, Young ME. The circadian clock within the cardiomyocyte is essential for responsiveness of the heart to fatty acids. J Biol Chem 2006;281:24254–24269
21. Young ME. The circadian clock within the heart: potential influence on myocardial gene expression, metabolism, and function. Am J Physiol Heart Circ Physiol 2006;290:H1–H16
22. Storch KF, Lipan O, Leykin I, Viswanathan N, Davis FC, Wong WH, Weitz CJ. Extensive and divergent circadian gene expression in liver and heart. Nature 2002;417:78–83
23. Duffy PH, Feuers RJ. Biomarkers of aging: changes in circadian rhythms related to the modulation of metabolic output. Biomed Environ Sci 1991;4:182–191
24. Claustrat F, Fournier I, Geelen G, Brun J, Corman B, Claustrat B. Aging and circadian clock gene expression in peripheral tissues in rats. Pathol Biol (Paris) 2005;53:257–260
25. Kunieda T, Minamino T, Katsuno T, Tateno K, Nishi J, Miyauchi H, Orimo M, Okada S, Komuro I. Cellular senescence impairs circadian expression of clock genes in vitro and in vivo. Circ Res 2006;98:532–539
26. Edwards MG, Sarkar D, Klopp R, Morrow JD, Weindruch R, Prolla TA. Age-related impairment of the transcriptional responses to oxidative stress in the mouse heart. Physiol Genomics 2003;13:119–127
27. Takahashi T, Schunkert H, Isoyama S, Wei JY, Nadal-Ginard B, Grossman W, Izumo S. Age-related differences in the expression of proto-oncogene and contractile protein genes in response to pressure overload in the rat myocardium. J Clin Invest 1992;89:939–946
28. Ashton KJ, Willems L, Holmgren K, Ferreira L, Headrick JP. Age-associated shifts in cardiac gene transcription and transcriptional responses to ischemic stress. Exp Gerontol 2006;41:189–204
29. Park SK, Prolla TA. Gene expression profiling studies of aging in cardiac and skeletal muscles. Cardiovasc Res 2005;66:205–212
30. Dhahbi JM, Tsuchiya T, Kim HJ, Mote PL, Spindler SR. Gene expression and physiologic responses of the heart to the initiation and withdrawal of caloric restriction. J Gerontol A Biol Sci Med Sci 2006;61:218–231
31. Lee CK, Klopp RG, Weindruch R, Prolla TA. Gene expression profile of aging and its retardation by caloric restriction. Science 1999:285:1390–1393
32. Kayo T, Allison DB, Weindruch R, Prolla TA. Influences of aging and caloric restriction on the transcriptional profile of skeletal muscle from rhesus monkeys. Proc Natl Acad Sci USA 2001;98:5093–5098
33. Hwang JJ, Allen PD, Tseng GC, Lam CW, Fananapazir L, Dzau VJ, Liew CC. Microarray gene expression profiles in dilated and hypertrophic cardiomyopathic end-stage heart failure. Physiol Genomics 2002;10: 31–44
34. Stanton LW, Garrard LJ, Damm D, Garrick BL, Lam A, Kapoun AM, Zheng Q, Protter AA, Schreiner GF, White RT. Altered patterns of gene expression in response to myocardial infarction. Circ Res 2000:86:939–945
35. Archacki SR, Angheloiu G, Tian XL, Tan FL, DiPaola N, Shen GQ, Moravec C, Ellis S, Topol EJ, Wang Q. Identification of new genes differentially expressed in coronary artery disease by expression profiling. Physiol Genomics 2003;15:65–74
36. Kim YH, Lim do S, Lee JH, Shim WJ, Ro YM, Park GH, Becker KG, Cho-Chung YS, Kim MK. Gene expression profiling of oxidative stress on atrial fibrillation in humans. Exp Mol Med 2003;35:336–349
37. Ueno S, Ohki R, Hashimoto T, Takizawa T, Takeuchi K, Yamashita Y, Ota J, Choi YL, Wada T, Koinuma K, Yamamoto K, Ikeda U, Shimada K, Mano H. DNA microarray analysis of in vivo progression mechanism of heart failure. Biochem Biophys Res Commun 2003;307:771–777
38. Boheler KR, Volkova M, Morrell C, Garg R, Zhu Y, Margulies K, Seymour AM, Lakatta EG. Sex- and age-dependent human transcriptome variability: implications for chronic heart failure. Proc Natl Acad Sci USA 2003;100:2754–2759
39. Csiszar A, Ungvari Z, Koller A, Edwards JG, Kaley G. Proinflammatory phenotype of coronary arteries promotes endothelial apoptosis in aging. Physiol Genomics 2004;17:21–30

40. Csiszar A, Ungvari Z, Koller A, Edwards JG, Kaley G. Aging-induced proinflammatory shift in cytokine expression profile in coronary arteries. FASEB J 2003;17:1183–1185
41. Vazquez-Padron RI, Lasko D, Li S, Louis L, Pestana IA, Pang M, Liotta C, Fornoni A, Aitouche A, Pham SM. Aging exacerbates neointimal formation, and increases proliferation and reduces susceptibility to apoptosis of vascular smooth muscle cells in mice. J Vasc Surg 2004;40:1199–1207
42. Kiri AN, Tran HC, Drahos KL, Lan W, McRorie DK, Horn MJ. Proteomic changes in bovine heart mitochondria with age: using a novel technique for organelle separation and enrichment. J Biomol Tech 2005;16:371–379
43. Drahos KL, Tran HC, Kiri AN, Lan W, McRorie DK, Horn MJ. Comparison of Golgi apparatus and endoplasmic reticulum proteins from livers of juvenile and aged rats using a novel technique for separation and enrichment of organelles. J Biomol Tech 2005;16:347–355
44. Devreese B, Vanrobaeys F, Smet J, Van Beeumen J, Van Coster R. Mass spectrometric identification of mitochondrial oxidative phosphorylation subunits separated by two-dimensional blue-native polyacrylamide gel electrophoresis. Electrophoresis 2002;23:2525–2533
45. Reifschneider NH, Goto S, Nakamoto H, Takahashi R, Sugawa M, Dencher NA, Krause F. Defining the mitochondrial proteomes from five rat organs in a physiologically significant context using 2D blue-native/SDS-PAGE. J Proteome Res 2006;5:1117–1132
46. Dencher NA, Goto S, Reifschneider NH, Sugawa M, Krause F. Unraveling age-dependent variation of the mitochondrial proteome. Ann N Y Acad Sci 2006;1067:116–119
47. Kanski J, Behring A, Pelling J, Schoneich C. Proteomic identification of 3-nitrotyrosine-containing rat cardiac proteins: effects of biological aging. Am J Physiol Heart Circ Physiol 2005;288:H371–H381
48. Aulak KS, Koeck T, Crabb JW, Stuehr DJ. Dynamics of protein nitration in cells and mitochondria. Am J Physiol Heart Circ Physiol 2004;286:H30–H38
49. Elfering SI, Haynes VL, Traaseth NJ, Ettl A, Giulivi C. Aspects, mechanism, and biological relevance of mitochondrial protein nitration sustained by mitochondrial nitric oxide synthase. Am J Physiol Heart Circ Physiol 2004;286:H22–H29
50. Turko IV, Li L, Aulak KS, Stuehr DJ, Chang JY, Murad F. Protein tyrosine nitration in the mitochondria from diabetic mouse heart. Implications to dysfunctional mitochondria in diabetes. J Biol Chem 2003;278: 33973–3977
51. Sohal RS, Ku HH, Agarwal S, Forster MJ, Lal H. Oxidative damage, mitochondrial oxidant generation and antioxidant defenses during aging and in response to food restriction in the mouse. Mech Ageing Dev 1994;74:121–133
52. Bejma J, Ramires P, Ji LL. Free radical generation and oxidative stress with ageing and exercise: differential effects in the myocardium and liver. Acta Physiol Scand 2000;169:343–351
53. Davies SM, Poljak A, Duncan MW, Smythe GA, Murphy MP. Measurements of protein carbonyls, ortho- and meta-tyrosine and oxidative phosphorylation complex activity in mitochondria from young and old rats. Free Radic Biol Med 2001;31:181–190
54. Cocco T, Sgobbo P, Clemente M, Lopriore B, Grattagliano I, Di Paola M, Villani G. Tissue-specific changes of mitochondrial functions in aged rats: effect of a long-term dietary treatment with N-acetylcysteine. Free Radic Biol Med 2005;38:796–805
55. Colotti C, Cavallini G, Vitale RL, Donati A, Maltinti M, Del Ry S, Bergamini E, Giannessi D. Effects of aging and anti-aging caloric restrictions on carbonyl and heat shock protein levels and expression. Biogerontology 2005;6:397–406
56. Forster MJ, Sohal BH, Sohal RS. Reversible effects of long-term caloric restriction on protein oxidative damage. J Gerontol A Biol Sci Med Sci 2000;55:B522–B529
57. Judge S, Judge A, Grune T, Leeuwenburgh C. Short-term CR decreases cardiac mitochondrial oxidant production but increases carbonyl content. Am J Physiol Regul Integr Comp Physiol 2004;286:R254–R259
58. Opii WO, Joshi G, Head E, Milgram NW, Muggenburg BA, Klein JB, Pierce WM, Cotman CW, Butterfield DA. Proteomic identification of brain proteins in the canine model of human aging following a long-term treatment with antioxidants and a program of behavioral enrichment: Relevance to Alzheimer's disease. Neurobiol Aging 2006 Oct 19
59. Nabeshi H, Oikawa S, Inoue S, Nishino K, Kawanishi S. Proteomic analysis for protein carbonyl as an indicator of oxidative damage in senescence-accelerated mice. Free Radic Res 2006;40:1173–1181
60. Chaudhuri AR, de Waal EM, Pierce A, Van Remmen H, Ward WF, Richardson A. Detection of protein carbonyls in aging liver tissue: a fluorescence-based proteomic approach. Mech Ageing Dev 2006;127:849–861
61. Brownlee M. Advanced protein glycosylation in diabetes and aging. Annu Rev Med 1995:46; 223–234
62. Reiser KM. Influence of age and long-term dietary restriction on enzymatically mediated crosslinks and nonenzymatic glycation of collagen in mice. J Gerontol 1994;49:B71–B79
63. Norton GR, Candy G, Woodiwiss AJ. Aminoguanidine prevents the decreased myocardial compliance produced by streptozotocin-induced diabetes mellitus in rats. Circulation 1996;93:1905–1912

64. Li SY, Du M, Dolence EK, Fang CX, Mayer GE, Ceylan-Isik AF, LaCour KH, Yang X, Wilbert CJ, Sreejayan N, Ren J. Aging induces cardiac diastolic dysfunction, oxidative stress, accumulation of advanced glycation endproducts and protein modification. Aging Cell 2005;4:57–64
65. Brett J, Schmidt AM, Yan SD, Zou YS, Weidman E, Pinsky D, Nowygrod R, Neeper M, Przysiecki C, Shaw A, Migheli A, Stern D. Survey of the distribution of a newly characterized receptor for advanced glycation end products in tissues. Am J Pathol 1993;143:1699–1712
66. Bucciarelli LG, Kaneko M, Ananthakrishnan R, Harja E, Lee LK, Hwang YC, Lerner S, Bakr S, Li Q, Lu Y, Song F, Qu W, Gomez T, Zou YS, Yan SF, Schmidt AM, Ramasamy R. Receptor for advanced-glycation end products: key modulator of myocardial ischemic injury. Circulation 2006;113:1226–1234
67. Simm A, Casselmann C, Schubert A, Hofmann S, Reimann A, Silber RE. Age associated changes of AGE-receptor expression: RAGE upregulation is associated with human heart dysfunction. Exp Gerontol 2004;39:407–413
68. Clark WA, Rudnick SJ, Simpson DG, LaPres JJ, Decker RS. Cultured adult cardiac myocytes maintain protein synthetic capacity of intact adult hearts. Am J Physiol 1993;264:H573–H582
69. Nag AC, Cheng M. Biochemical evidence for cellular dedifferentiation in adult rat cardiac muscle cells in culture: expression of myosin isozymes. Biochem Biophys Res Commun 1986;137:855–862
70. Bugaisky LB, Zak R. Differentiation of adult rat cardiac myocytes in cell culture. Circ Res 1989;64:493–500
71. He Q, Cahill CJ, Spiro MJ. Suspension culture of differentiated rat heart myocytes on non-adhesive surfaces. J Mol Cell Cardiol 1996;28:1177–1186
72. Bird SD, Doevendans PA, van Rooijen MA, Brutel de la Riviere A, Hassink RJ, Passier R, Mummery CL. The human adult cardiomyocyte phenotype. Cardiovasc Res 2003;58:423–434
73. Kamino H, Hiratsuka M, Toda T, Nishigaki R, Osaki M, Ito H, Inoue T, Oshimura M. Searching for genes involved in arteriosclerosis: proteomic analysis of cultured human umbilical vein endothelial cells undergoing replicative senescence. Cell Struct Funct 2003;28:495–503
74. Eman MR, Regan-Klapisz E, Pinkse MW, Koop IM, Haverkamp J, Heck AJ, Verkleij AJ, Post JA. Protein expression dynamics during replicative senescence of endothelial cells studied by 2-D difference in-gel electrophoresis. Electrophoresis 2006;27:1669–1682
75. Hampel B, Fortschegger K, Ressler S, Chang MW, Unterluggauer H, Breitwieser A, Sommergruber W, Fitzky B, Lepperdinger G, Jansen-Durr P, Voglauer R, Grillari J. Increased expression of extracellular proteins as a hallmark of human endothelial cell in vitro senescence. Exp Gerontol 2006;41:474–481
76. Chang MW, Grillari J, Mayrhofer C, Fortschegger K, Allmaier G, Marzban G, Katinger H, Voglauer R. Comparison of early passage, senescent and hTERT immortalized endothelial cells. Exp Cell Res 2005;309: 121–136
77. Lee JH, Chung KY, Bang D, Lee KH. Searching for aging-related proteins in human dermal microvascular endothelial cells treated with anti-aging agents. Proteomics 2006;6:1351–1361
78. Cremona O, Muda M, Appel RD, Frutiger S, Hughes GJ, Hochstrasser DF, Geinoz A, Gabbiani G. Differential protein expression in aortic smooth muscle cells cultured from newborn and aged rats. Exp Cell Res 1995;217:280–287
79. Perls T, Shea-Drinkwater M, Bowen-Flynn J, Ridge SB, Kang S, Joyce E, Daly M, Brewster SJ, Kunkel L, Puca AA. Exceptional familial clustering for extreme longevity in humans. J Am Geriatr Soc 2000;48: 1483–1485
80. Herskind AM, McGue M, Holm NV, Sorensen TI, Harvald B, Vaupel JW. The heritability of human longevity: a population-based study of 2872 Danish twin pairs born 1870–1900. Hum Genet 1996;97:319–323
81. Christensen K, Johnson TE, Vaupel JW. The quest for genetic determinants of human longevity: challenges and insights. Nat Rev Genet 2006;7:436–448
82. Reed T, Dick DM, Uniacke SK, Foroud T, Nichols WC. Genome-wide scan for a healthy aging phenotype provides support for a locus near D4S1564 promoting healthy aging. J Gerontol A Biol Sci Med Sci 2004;59: 227–232
83. Puca AA, Daly MJ, Brewster SJ, Matise TC, Barrett J, Shea-Drinkwater M, Kang S, Joyce E, Nicoli J, Benson E, Kunkel LM, Perls T. A genome-wide scan for linkage to human exceptional longevity identifies a locus on chromosome 4. Proc Natl Acad Sci USA 2001;98:10505–10508
84. Geesaman BJ, Benson E, Brewster SJ, Kunkel LM, Blanche H, Thomas G, Perls TT, Daly MJ, Puca AA. Haplotype-based identification of a microsomal transfer protein marker associated with the human lifespan. Proc Natl Acad Sci USA 2003;100:14115–14120
85. Juo SH, Han Z, Smith JD, Colangelo L, Liu K. Common polymorphism in promoter of microsomal triglyceride transfer protein gene influences cholesterol, ApoB, and triglyceride levels in young african american men: results from the coronary artery risk development in young adults (CARDIA) study. Arterioscler Thromb Vasc Biol 2000;20:1316–1322

86. Nebel A, Croucher PJ, Stiegeler R, Nikolaus S, Krawczak M, Schreiber S. No association between microsomal triglyceride transfer protein (MTP) haplotype and longevity in humans. Proc Natl Acad Sci USA 2005;102:7906–7909
87. Schachter F, Faure-Delanef L, Guenot F, Rouger H, Froguel P, Lesueur-Ginot L, Cohen D. Genetic associations with human longevity at the APOE and ACE loci. Nat Genet 1994;6:29–32
88. Blanche H, Cabanne L, Sahbatou M, Thomas G. A study of French centenarians: are ACE and APOE associated with longevity? C R Acad Sci III 2001;324:129–135
89. Rea IM, Mc Dowell I, McMaster D, Smye M, Stout R, Evans A. MONICA group (Belfast). Monitoring of Cardiovascular trends study group. Apolipoprotein E alleles in nonagenarian subjects in the Belfast Elderly Longitudinal Free-living Ageing Study (BELFAST). Mech Ageing Dev 2001;122:1367–1372
90. Barzilai N, Atzmon G, Schechter C, Schaefer EJ, Cupples AL, Lipton R, Cheng S, Shuldiner AR. Unique lipoprotein phenotype and genotype associated with exceptional longevity. JAMA 2003;290:2030–2040
91. Stessman J, Maaravi Y, Hammerman-Rozenberg R, Cohen A, Nemanov L, Gritsenko I, Gruberman N, Ebstein RP. Candidate genes associated with ageing and life expectancy in the Jerusalem longitudinal study. Mech Ageing Dev 2005;126:333–339
92. Todesco L, Angst C, Litynski P, Loehrer F, Fowler B, Haefeli WE. Methylenetetrahydrofolate reductase polymorphism, plasma homocysteine and age. Eur J Clin Invest 1999;29:1003–1009
93. Kohara K, Fujisawa M, Ando F, Tabara Y, Niino N, Miki T, Shimokata H. NILS-LSA Study. MTHFR gene polymorphism as a risk factor for silent brain infarcts and white matter lesions in the Japanese general population: the NILS-LSA Study. Stroke 2003;34:1130–1135
94. Atzmon G, Rincon M, Schechter CB, Shuldiner AR, Lipton RB, Bergman A, Barzilai N. Lipoprotein genotype and conserved pathway for exceptional longevity in humans. PLoS Biol 2006;4:e113
95. Luft FC. Bad genes, good people, association, linkage, longevity and the prevention of cardiovascular disease. Clin Exp Pharmacol Physiol 1999;26:576–579
96. Frederiksen H, Gaist D, Bathum L, Andersen K, McGue M, Vaupel JW, Christensen K. Angiotensin I-converting enzyme (ACE) gene polymorphism in relation to physical performance, cognition and survival-a follow-up study of elderly Danish twins. Ann Epidemiol 2003;13:57–65
97. Bladbjerg EM, Andersen-Ranberg K, de Maat MP, Kristensen SR, Jeune B, Gram J, Jespersen J. Longevity is independent of common variations in genes associated with cardiovascular risk. Thromb Haemost 1999;82:1100–1105
98. Hamdi HK, Castellon R. A genetic variant of ACE increases cell survival: a new paradigm for biology and disease. Biochem Biophys Res Commun 2004;318:187–191
99. Arking DE, Krebsova A, Macek M Sr, Macek M Jr, Arking A, Mian IS, Fried L, Hamosh A, Dey S, McIntosh I, Dietz HC. Association of human aging with a functional variant of klotho. Proc Natl Acad Sci USA 2002;99:856–861
100. Arking DE, Atzmon G, Arking A, Barzilai N, Dietz HC. Association between a functional variant of the KLOTHO gene and high-density lipoprotein cholesterol, blood pressure, stroke, and longevity. Circ Res 2005;96:412–418
101. Mooijaart SP, van Heemst D, Schreuder J, van Gerwen S, Beekman M, Brandt BW, Eline Slagboom P, Westendorp RG. 'Long Life' Study Group. Variation in the SHC1 gene and longevity in humans. Exp Gerontol 2004;39:263–268
102. Post WS, Goldschmidt-Clermont PJ, Wilhide CC, Heldman AW, Sussman MS, Ouyang P, Milliken EE, Issa JP. Methylation of the estrogen receptor gene is associated with aging and atherosclerosis in the cardiovascular system. Cardiovasc Res 1999;43:985–991
103. Kim J, Kim JY, Song KS, Lee YH, Seo JS, Jelinek J, Goldschmidt-Clermont PJ, Issa JP. Epigenetic changes in estrogen receptor beta gene in atherosclerotic cardiovascular tissues and in-vitro vascular senescence. Biochim Biophys Acta 2007;1772:72–80
104. Lopatina N, Haskell JF, Andrews LG, Poole JC, Saldanha S, Tollefsbol T. Differential maintenance and de novo methylating activity by three DNA methyltransferases in aging and immortalized fibroblasts. J Cell Biochem 2002;84:324–334
105. Lopatina N, Haskell JF, Andrews LG, Poole JC, Saldanha S, Tollefsbol T. Differential maintenance and de novo methylating activity by three DNA methyltransferases in aging and immortalized fibroblasts. J Cell Biochem 2002;84:324–334
106. Trapp J, Jung M. The role of NAD+ dependent histone deacetylases (sirtuins) in ageing. Curr Drug Targets 2006;7:1553–1560
107. Longo VD, Kennedy BK. Sirtuins in aging and age-related disease. Cell 2006;126:257–268
108. Rose G, Dato S, Altomare K, Bellizzi D, Garasto S, Greco V, Passarino G, Feraco E, Mari V, Barbi C, BonaFe M, Franceschi C, Tan Q, Boiko S, Yashin AI, De Benedictis G. Variability of the SIRT3 gene, human silent information regulator Sir2 homologue, and survivorship in the elderly. Exp Gerontol 2003;38:1065–1070

109. Bellizzi D, Rose G, Cavalcante P, Covello G, Dato S, De Rango F, Greco V, Maggiolini M, Feraco E, Mari V, Franceschi C, Passarino G, De Benedictis G. A novel VNTR enhancer within the SIRT3 gene, a human homologue of SIR2, is associated with survival at oldest ages. Genomics 2005;85:258–263
110. Haigis MC, Guarente LP. Mammalian sirtuins – emerging roles in physiology, aging, and calorie restriction. Genes Dev 2006;20:2913–2921

Part VI
Therapies

Chapter 14
Translational Research: Gene, Pharmacogenomics and Cell-Based Therapy in the Aging Heart

Overview

Cellular hallmarks of cardiac aging include a progressive accumulation of molecular damage in nucleic acids, proteins and lipids. A primary cause of age-related accumulation of this molecular damage resides in the inefficiency and failure of maintenance, repair and turnover pathways resulting in structural myocardial remodeling and dysfunction. Increasing focus in molecular gerontology has been directed at understanding the genetic and epigenetic regulation of myocardial survival and maintenance mechanisms at the levels of transcription, post-transcriptional processing, post-translational modifications, and interactions among various gene products [1]. In this chapter, we will discuss several potential translational targets for modulating either aging or some of its more pathogenic cardiovascular manifestations. A number of these therapeutic targets have shown some evidence of success in early testing stages, whereas others await to be tested. In addition, we review several approaches that have shown some success with preclinical models including specific gene and cell-based therapy, chemotherapeutic and metabolic modulation, including intervention by free radical scavengers and other molecules.

Introduction

As we have already pointed out, there are a considerable number of events occurring in aging contributing to both the increased levels of cardiac and cardiovascular dysfunction, which appear to occur with normal aging, and the enhanced susceptibility of the aged to age-related diseases.

The use of targeted therapies (primarily at the preclinical level), mainly performed with either animal models or with isolated cells, will be presented in this chapter organized broadly in categories (with some overlap) of targeted organelles/events that are widely considered to be the primary contributors to the aging pathology and phenotype; a number of these show considerable promise in reversing specific aspects of aging. The order that these specific subjects are presented in the text is not necessarily the order of significance in which they are involved in the aging process, nor in the success of the therapies employed. These targeted events include: (1) Cell death and remodeling with both apoptosis and necrosis as targeted events; (2) Initiation of pro-survival/proliferative cell signaling pathways; (3) Modulation of cardioprotective pathways; (4) Attenuation of oxidative stress (OS) and reduction of ROS levels and effects; (5) Treating or reversing mitochondrial dysfunction and structural defects, including mtDNA damage; (6) Removing "biological garbage" (targeting lysosomes, proteasomes and other approaches for enhancing recycling of cellular components); (7) Targeting the nucleus to reverse DNA damage and genomic instability, attenuate transcriptional programming involved in cell and tissue senescence and restore programming associated with proliferative growth, and restoration of telomere function; and (8) Restoring sarcomere contractile function

J. Marín-García, *Aging and the Heart*,

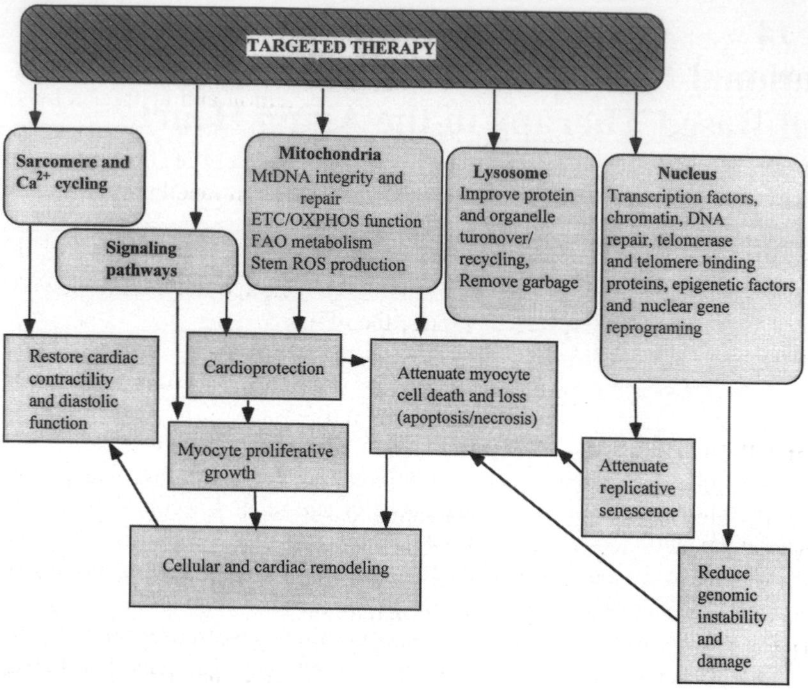

Fig. 14.1 Targeted therapies in cardiac aging
This diagram shows the effects of targeting specific organelles/events associated with aging including sarcomeric/calcium cycling, cytosolic signaling pathways, mitochondria, lysosomes and nuclei. Phenotypic consequences of these therapies including attenuated cell death, increased growth, attenuated replicative senescence, genomic instability and increased contractility are shown in the bottom tier.

by modulation of calcium cycling pathways and enzymes. A brief flow-chart detailing the categories of targeted therapy in aging treatment and how these targeted categories may inter-connect with each other is outlined in Fig. 14.1.

Primary Targets in Reversing Cardiovascular and Cardiac Aging Damage

Attenuating Cell-Death and Remodeling

As discussed in Chapter 3, there is evidence that suggest a significant relationship between cell-death and CVD, particularly ischemic heart disease and congestive heart failure (HF), the most common heart diseases in the elderly. This has provided the rationale for research directed to the treatment and possible prevention of apoptosis, which may provide a means of decreasing the incidence of HF as well as a strategy to increase the survival of endothelial and smooth muscle cells (SMCs) in aging [2]. Interestingly, human endothelial cells from the umbilical vein (HUVECs) tend to acquire a proapoptotic phenotype when reaching senescence, which likely results from ROS-induced damage and associated signaling. This susceptibility to apoptosis in endothelial cells (ECs) is in striking contrast with the replicative senescence exhibited by diploid human fibroblasts at the end of their life span in which growth-arrested cells are resistant to various apoptotic stimuli [3].

A number of critical steps in the apoptotic pathway have been identified as viable targets vis-à-vis apoptotic induction and have stimulated the development of efficient apoptosis-modulating drugs. Interestingly, much of the information on these pathways and their modulators has come from recent studies of several forms of cancer which involve the inactivation of the apoptotic process, thus enabling the cancer cells to continue to proliferate. For instance, compounds directly targeting the mitochondria to trigger mitochondrial membrane permeabilization and apoptosis may be useful as efficient cytotoxic drugs to treat hematological malignancies [4]. These include positively charged α-helical peptides, which are attracted to and disrupt the negatively charged mitochondrial membrane, thus inducing mammalian cell apoptosis when targeted intracellularly, inhibition of Bcl-2 and related antiapoptotic proteins, including antisense oligonucleotides (e.g., Genasense, currently tested in phase III trials), small molecules that mimic the BH3 dimerization domain of these proteins and kinase inhibitors [5]. While the reverse strategy (i.e., apoptotic inhibition) is more likely to be beneficial in age-related targeted therapies, the effectiveness of such apoptotic-modulatory approaches have proved highly informative.

Mitochondrial membrane permeabilization at the mitochondrial PT pore and at the outer membrane (MOMP) has been demonstrated to be a central rate-limiting and critical early step of numerous models of cell death in response to a variety of intracellular and extracellular stimuli. Opening of the PT pore causes massive swelling of mitochondria, and rupture of the outer membrane. Both MOMP and the PT pore are thought to be upstream of caspase activation, are in part under the regulatory control of the Bcl-2 family and contribute to the release of multiple proapoptogenic proteins (e.g., cytochrome *c*, Smac/DIABLO, endonuclease G (Endo G), apoptosis-inducing factor (AIF), and HtrA2/Omi) from the mitochondrial intermembrane space into the cytosol.

Numerous molecular and pharmacological studies have suggested that the adenine nucleotide translocator (ANT), an integral PT pore component could be a therapeutic target [6]. ANT is a bi functional mitochondrial protein, mediating the exchange of cytosolic ADP and mitochondrial ATP, and contributing to cell death via its capacity to become a lethal pore. Both ANT functions are under the control of both the pro- and antiapoptotic factors of the Bax/Bcl-2 family, as well as of a diverse assortment of agents (e.g., proteins, lipids, ions, pro-oxidants or chemotherapeutic agents) that can directly modulate the pore-forming activity of ANT. Other components of the PT pore are the voltage-dependent anion channel (VDAC), cyclophilin-D (Cyp-D: a mitochondrial peptidyl prolyl-cis, *trans*-isomerase) and the mitochondrial peripheral-type benzodiazepine receptors (PBRs). Recent studies performed with mice lacking Cyp-D have suggested that Cyp-D is essential for the PT pore to occur and that the Cyp-D-dependent PT pore appears to be more critical in necrotic as compared to apoptotic cell death and plays a crucial role in ischemia/reperfusion (I/R) injury [7, 8]. Cyp-D is targeted by the immunosuppressant cyclosporin A (CsA), which has been shown to be cytoprotective in many cellular and animal models. Mitochondrial pore opening is inhibited by CsA analogues with the same affinity as they inhibit the peptidyl-prolyl cis–trans isomerase activity of CyP-D [9]. There is strong interest in designing Cyp-D ligands without immunosuppressant properties, which would have the potential of being useful therapeutic agents in a variety of disease states [10].

Another potential target is the outer membrane PT pore component, VDAC/porin. Recent observations have shown that the antiapoptotic proteins Bcl-2 and Bcl-XL block the PT pore by direct inhibition of VDAC activity. There is also evidence suggesting that direct Bcl-2 blockage of VDAC homodimerization determines its gating capacity to cytochrome *c* and represents a novel mechanism for inhibition of apoptosis [11].

Another putative component of the PT pore, highly abundant in cardiovascular cells (e.g., endothelium, the striated cardiac muscle, the vascular smooth muscles as well as circulating cells), is the peripheral-type benzodiazepine receptors (PBRs), whose role in cell death is less clear. A large array of synthetic ligands is available with affinity for PBR including both proapoptotic (FGIN-1-27) and antiapoptotic (SSR180575) effects, suggesting that PBR may represent a promising therapeutic target [12].

While it has become evident that not all apoptotic stimuli trigger PT pore opening, several studies have suggested that stimuli, such as calcium overload, OS, or I/R injury, can mediate cytochrome *c* release directly through the PT pore. Recently, peptides have been employed to target PT pore function and modulate apoptotic and/or necrotic induction [13]. Moreover, experiments with tissue-targeted Bcl-2 overexpression (to be further discussed in a later section of this chapter) have shown attenuation of apoptosis and cardiac dysfunction in an animal model of cardiomyopathy [14]. Using strategies that combine co-immunoprecipitation, proteomics, and functional tests with proteoliposomes, a number of the intra/inter-PT pore protein interactions have been characterized leading to a finer elucidation of the process of mitochondrial membrane permeabilization [15]. This type of approach may also identify other interacting factors and regulators of PT pore function in cell death.

Since myocardial I/R injury involves both apoptotic and necrotic cell death, specifically targeting only apoptosis may not be adequate in entirely stemming myocardial injury. Recent studies in Langendorff-perfused rabbit hearts subjected to global ischemia showed that the contribution of necrosis to infarct size is significantly greater than that of apoptosis, and that treatment with irreversible caspase-3, -8, and -9 inhibitors reduced apoptosis in early reperfusion, but this protection does not result in improved immediate postischemic functional recovery i.e., left ventricular peak developed pressure (LVPDP) and systolic shortening (SS) [16].

Initiating Pro-Survival Pathways

An alternative strategy for reversing cell death progression involves the regulated activation of anti-apoptotic, prosurvival pathways. Studies with IGF-1 have shown that overexpression of this growth factor as well as activation of components of the downstream Akt/PI3K/PKB signaling pathway can have a marked antiapoptotic effect on cells *in vitro* and *in vivo*. In addition to its effectiveness in preventing cardiac apoptosis and promoting survival of cardiomyocytes, IGF-1 overexpression confers extensive cardioprotection in both mouse and rat heart after myocardial infarction (MI) and I/R injury [17–21]. While the precise mechanism by which the IGF-1/PI3K pathway inhibits apoptosis has not yet been fully defined, considerable evidence indicates that both IGF-1 and PI3-kinase (PI3K) inhibit apoptosis by maintaining high levels of the antiapoptotic protein Bcl-2, largely by activation of the transcription factor cAMP response element-binding protein (CREB) [22–24] and by increasing the phosphorylation of the proapoptotic factor Bad [25]. Moreover, studies with IGF-1 overexpressing mice have shown that IGF-1 mediates many of the effects of growth hormone (GH) on cardiovascular structure and function, and that IGF-1 can promote cardiomyocyte hyperplasia and hypertrophy, improve contractility and inhibit apoptosis [21].

Gene products implicated in growth arrest and senescence, such as p27Kip1, p53, p16INK4a, and p19ARF while present in myocytes of young wild-type mice were significantly increased with age [26]. Levels of these proteins were markedly attenuated in transgenic mice containing overexpressed IGF-1. In wild-type aging mice, telomerase activity was diminished; reduced nuclear levels of both telomerase and phospho-Akt resulted in marked telomere shortening and uncapping, and a subpopulation of myocytes (identified as cardiac stem cells) was targeted by senescence and death. In contrast, in IGF-1 transgenic aging mice, telomerase activity and Akt phosphorylation were elevated paralleled by delayed cellular aging and death. Furthermore, in mice with the IGF-1 transgene, the cardiac stem cell population was able to regenerate preventing ventricular dysfunction.

Targeted treatment with exogenous IGF-1 can retard or reverse specific age-related changes in cardiovascular structure and function. In a study assessing the effect of cardiac overexpression of IGF-1 on cardiomyocyte contractile function conducted in young (3 months) and old (26–28 months) mice, the introduction of a IGF-1 transgene had a beneficial effect on aging-associated cardiomyocyte contractile dysfunction, which could be mimicked by short-term treatment *in vitro* with recombinant IGF-1 (500 nM) [27]. Interestingly, increased advanced glycation endproducts (AGE) and protein carbonyl levels, normally found in aged mice, were present and not affected by IGF-1 treatment whereas aging-mediated reduction in SERCA2 expression and activity were reversed. This suggests that the IGF-1 benefit to contractility may be related to improved Ca^{2+} uptake. Recent, data collected in our laboratory showed that IGF-1 also can reverse the mitochondrial dysfunction that occurs with ischemic injury in isolated rat cardiomyocytes.

A similar antiapoptotic, cardioprotective effect versus acute I/R injury has been reported with other growth factors including the cytokine and hepatocyte growth factor (HGF). Gathered observations have shown that post-MI treatment with either the HGF gene or protein attenuates chronic cardiac remodeling and dysfunction in both rat and mouse models [28]. Moreover, HGF can confer cytoprotection versus apoptosis (as well as enhance the repair of DNA strand breaks) by signaling through PI3K/Akt and by up-regulating expression of the anti-apoptotic protein Bcl-XL [29].

Growth hormone (GH) has been found to reverse many of the deficits in cardiovascular function in aged animals and humans [30]. Long-term GH replacement in 30 month old Fischer 344 rats preserved diastolic function and attenuated left ventricular remodeling associated with normal aging. These changes were accompanied by reduced cardiac angiotensin II (Ang II), attenuation in cardiac collagen and restoration of IGF-1 levels [31]. This may be in part due to stimulation of IGF-1 expression, which is under GH regulation. Moreover, administration of GH to aged rats provided protection against postischemic ventricular dysfunction [32].

Modulation of Cardioprotection Pathways as a Potential Strategy

As previously noted, in animal models a variety of treatments have been shown to provide protection to myocardium against ischemic injury. For instance, in ischemic preconditioning (IPC) a single or multiple brief periods of ischemia can protect the heart against a more prolonged ischemic insult. This robust form of cardioprotection has been widely documented in animal models as well as in cardiomyocytes *in vitro*, and appears to occur in humans in response to balloon angioplasty and angina [33–35]. IPC has been shown to have an acute and a delayed cardioprotective phase, both involving the activation within the myocyte of specific triggering pathways including mediating signals, transducing components and end-effectors [36–39]. Treatment with a variety of chemicals can substitute for IPC, generating cardioprotective responses that share aspects of the IPC model involving a variety of cell signaling pathways (many in common with IPC) that appear to converge on several cardiomyocyte end-effectors. This *pharmacological preconditioning* includes the targeted use of volatile anesthetics, potassium channel openers, nitric oxide donors and modulators of some of the downstream components including erythropoietin, statins, insulin, glucagon-like peptide 1 and pyruvate (see Table 14.1). In addition, application of some of these stimuli (either a brief regimen of I/R or the use of pharmacological agents) at the time of reperfusion can also trigger what is termed a *post-conditioning* cardioprotective pathway that involves many of the same components involved in ischemic/anesthetic preconditioning pathways [40, 41].

These complex signaling cardioprotective pathways, which contain many shared elements, are comprised of components including ligand stimuli or triggers (e.g., adenosine, bradykinin), cell-surface receptors, sarcolemmal and mitochondrial ion channels (e.g., K_{ATP} channels), protein kinases (e.g., PI3K, tyrosine kinases, PKC-ε) and a variety of cellular effectors, including the PT pore. A central substrate for cardioprotection resides in the mitochondria providing critical signals (and potential therapeutic targets) at discrete stages within these cardioprotective pathways including ROS generation, calcium flux, bioenergetic function and metabolic uncoupling as well as the regulation of pivotal early events in the apoptotic pathway [36–39].

The cardioprotective potentials of IPC and post-conditioning have been difficult to realize in clinical practice as they necessitate highly invasive interventions, applied either before the onset of

Table 14.1 Pharmacological approaches to cardioprotection

Class	Specific drug/chemical
Potassium channel openers	Nicorandil Diazoxide Pinacidil Cromakalin
Potassium channel blockers	Glibenclamide 5-HD
Inhibitors of mitochondrial PT pore	Cyclosporin A
Receptor-mediated signaling pathways/ligands	Adenosine Opioids Bradykinin Acetylcholine Endothelin PKC-TIP
Sphingolipid/ceramide signaling	Ceramide Sphingosine Chelerythrine (Pan-PKC inhibitors)
Mitochondrial-generated ROS and lipid peroxidation	Idebenone FCCP DNP Coenzyme Q Quercetin Carvedilol
Other pharmacological agents	Erythropoietin (EPO) Statin (avorstatin) Glucose-insulin-potassium (GIK) Insulin Nitroglycerin Pyruvate Glucagon-like peptide Sidenafil Monophosphoryl lipid A

the ischemic insult, which is difficult to predict, or during reperfusion. Therefore, pharmacological preconditioning at the time of myocardial reperfusion may eventually have greater applicability.

Unfortunately, at present there is only limited data from preclinical studies concerning the use of cardioprotective approaches in the elderly; most studies have been conducted with young and healthy animals. Limited preclinical observations have indicated that there is a reduced cardioprotective efficacy of volatile anesthetic preconditioning with advanced age in rat. Furthermore, other experimental studies performed in rodents using infarct size and hemodynamic measures to assess cardioprotection, found that IPC effects are diminished or abolished in the old heart [42, 43]. Interestingly, studies in aging rabbits and sheep have generally found that IPC reduces the infarct size [44, 45].

Abete et al. have reported that the cardioprotective effect of angina before acute MI in adults was significantly reduced in the elderly population [46]. Lee et al. have demonstrated that a loss of the effectiveness of preconditioning in elderly patients undergoing coronary angioplasty was likely secondary to an attenuated activation of the myocardial K_{ATP} channels [47]. Interestingly, the impaired preconditioning responsiveness in the elderly could be reversed by administration of the potassium channel opener (KCO) nicorandil or by a prolonged ischemic period (lengthened to 180 seconds). Other investigators found that IPC had no beneficial effect on the postischemic functional recovery of senescent human myocardium [48], and no differences were found in the expression of cardioprotective proteins such as HSP70, PKC-δ and Bcl-2/-xL in elderly patients, however other critical proteins were not examined [49].

One rationale for this loss of cardioprotective response may be related to the observed age-related alterations in the expression and activation of proteins key to the cardioprotective process. Reduced levels of these critical cardioprotective proteins include nitric oxide synthase (NOS), a central player in the delayed preconditioning response, the sodium-hydrogen exchanger (NHE), the mitogen-activated protein (MAP) kinases, c-Jun N-terminal Kinase (JNK), extracellular signal-regulated kinase (ERK), and p38 [50].

Consistent with age-related changes in the cast of cardioprotective players, several studies have suggested that preconditioning cardioprotective responses do occur in aging albeit with pronounced changes in the transducing elements. Moreover, senescent myocardium is more sensitive to ischemia compared to young adult myocardium which suggests that the protective pathways existing in adult myocardium are modified or impaired by aging [51]. For instance, data obtained from adult cohorts have implicated activation/translocation of specific isoforms of protein kinase C (e.g., PKC-ε as an important cellular mediator of myocardial infarct size reduction with IPC). However, in older rabbits, IPC-induced cardioprotection was maintained despite treatment with either a PKC-ε translocation inhibitor peptide (PKC-ε-TIP) inhibitor or the pan-PKC inhibitor chelerythrine suggesting that IPC in the aging rabbit was not associated with activation/translocation of PKC-ε [52]. Recent studies conducted with 24–26 month old Fischer 344 × Brown Norway hybrid (F344 × BN) rats showed that treatment with the adenosine A1/A(2a) agonist AMP579 resulted in a 50% greater infarct size reduction in aged compared to adult rats suggesting that adenosine A1 and A(2a) receptor-mediated effects are not only diminished in normal aged myocardium, but rather that aged hearts exhibit increased adenosine agonist-induced infarct reduction [53]. This confirmed earlier findings that adenosine-enhanced IPC provides enhanced cardioprotection in the senescent rabbit heart [54], albeit in contrast with several other studies (as reviewed by Willems et al.) [55]. Interestingly, transcription analysis of murine adenosine receptor transcription demonstrated selective modulation of receptor isotypes with age-related reduction in some subtypes (e.g., Adora3), enhanced induction (e.g., Adora3) and others unchanged, although significantly declining during ischemia (e.g., Adora1) [56]. Other investigators have suggested that there are significant age-mediated changes in adenosine-receptor mediated cardioprotection which occur at the level of receptor coupling, generation of protective "signal" (adenosine formation), and/or at sites within signaling cascades triggered, albeit the molecular basis remains unclear [55]. Studies with overexpression of adenosine receptors have shown that overexpression of adenosine receptor subtypes in aged mice bolsters adenosinergic cardioprotection and restores ischemic tolerance to levels found in young myocardium [57].

Given the broad array of animal models used, the different preconditioning regimens, age of subjects and disparate end-points used to gauge successful preconditioning/cardioprotection, it is not entirely surprising that a number of studies have also challenged the view of an aging-diminished cardioprotective response in studies with aging mice, rats and humans [58–61]. Clearly, more well-designed, large-scale studies to be conducted with both older animal models as well as with clinical subjects will be critical in defining and refining effective cardioprotection in the elderly. In addition to the growing list of pharmacological agents that can be used in providing cardioprotection, a therapeutic cocktail of several factors may provide enhanced cardioprotection as found with combined growth factor treatment [platelet-derived growth factor-AB (PDGF-AB), vascular endothelial growth factor and angiopoictin-2] in the reversal of senescent dysfunction in aging Fischer rats [62]. While new drugs/pharmacological agents will likely be developed that can target downstream events (e.g., end-effectors) in the cardioprotective pathway bypassing any upstream age-related signaling defects (e.g., receptors and kinase transducers), extreme caution will have to be taken in their use to ensure their specificity of action and that they do not interfere with endogenous protection-signaling, diminishing the protective response already altered by "physiological" aging [63]. For instance, the use of antioxidants and ROS-scavengers to prevent deleterious ROS-accumulation can interfere with ROS signaling (which plays an obligatory role as a trigger of pre- or post-conditioning) and can attenuate cardioprotection.

Attenuating the Generation of OS and Reducing ROS

As noted in previous chapters, there is a large body of evidence implicating ROS in many of the deleterious effects of cardiovascular aging. As such, there has been an intensive effort to employ agents that can stem ROS accumulation and reverse cardiac/cardiovascular dysfunction and restore a more youthful phenotype. The primary strategies have aimed at bolstering the capability of the cells to neutralize or detoxify ROS. The tactic of attenuating ROS production is a more difficult proposition since ROS is produced as a by-product of normal bioenergetic metabolism. A third approach, which will be discussed in a later section, involves reversing ROS-mediated damage.

Bolstering myocardial antioxidant responses has been a primary tactic. Adenoviral-mediated gene transfer of extracellular superoxide dismutase (EcSOD) restored the relaxation of aorta in response to acetylcholine which was impaired in 29–31 months old Fischer rats with an associated reduction in superoxide levels [64]. Previous studies have shown that intravenous injection of adenoviral vectors expressing EcSOD in rats with HF (due to coronary artery ligation) similarly led to reduced levels of superoxide and improved relaxation in the aorta and mesenteric artery in response to acetylcholine and ADP [65]. Moreover, this study demonstrated that the heparin-binding domain (HBD) of EcSOD, by which EcSOD binds to cells, is required for protective effects of EcSOD against endothelial dysfunction in HF. In addition, introduction and overexpression of CuSOD in targeted cells can enhance intracellular generation of H_2O_2, which can significantly stimulate VEGF production and potentially impact angiogenesis [66].

Cardiac-targeted adenoviral-mediated gene transfer of SOD has been shown to be effective with MnSOD in reducing I/R injury in rats [67], and in attenuating contractile dysfunction after I/R in mice [68]. Adenoviral mediated gene transfer of EcSOD in rabbits to increase systemic levels of EcSOD was shown to provide protection against MI generated by a 30 min coronary occlusion with a reduction of infarct size of 25% [69]. Interestingly, relatively similar findings were obtained with gene transfer and overexpression of a chaperone, the heat shock protein HSP70 [70].

Adenoviral-mediated transfer of catalase in the mouse myocardium was sufficient to prevent the stunning associated with 15 min of ischemia followed by reperfusion [71], as well as effective in attenuating contractile dysfunction after I/R [68]. Moreover, transgenic mice containing a catalase gene localized in cardiac mitochondria showed reduction in aging cardiac pathology, significant reduction in oxidative damage, reduced H_2O_2 production and H_2O_2-mediated damage as well as significantly increasing life span [72], findings that are among the strongest pieces of evidence supporting primary roles of ROS and mitochondria in aging.

Heme oxygenase is another antioxidant enzyme that has been successfully delivered using viral-mediated gene transfer to the myocardium to relieve ischemic injury [73, 74]. Using a recombinant adeno-associated virus (rAAV) as a vector for direct delivery of the human heme oxygenase-1 (HO-1) gene into the rat myocardium, 8 weeks before acute coronary artery ligation, achieved a significant reduction in MI. Reduction in infarct size was accompanied by decreased myocardial lipid peroxidation, proapoptotic Bax and proinflammatory interleukin-1β protein abundance, in parallel with increased Bcl-2 protein level suggesting that the HO-1 transgene exerts its cardioprotective effects in part by reducing OS, associated inflammation and apoptotic cell death [75]. Recent studies have demonstrated that this construct had a considerable impact on postinfarction changes, markedly reducing fibrosis and ventricular remodeling as well as restoring LV function and chamber dimensions [76].

HO-1 may provide long term cardioprotection against repeated, chronic forms of ischemic insult [74]. Since myocardial gene therapy as a targeted intervention against acute cardiac insults (e.g., myocardial ischemia) may have limited efficacy because an extensive period of time is needed for transgene introduction, transcription, translation, and processing of the transgene product, it may be more efficacious to employ a prophylactic or preemptive use of gene therapy to mount a protective response to potential adverse cardiac events. To implement this approach, a cardioprotective vigilant plasmid vector was developed for cardiac-specific expression, and hypoxia-regulatable expression of therapeutic transgenes [77], which provided an oxygen biosensor (i.e., the oxygen-dependent degradation, ODD, domain derived from HIF-1α) fused to the GAL4 transactivator protein under the control of the MLC-2v promoter, located on a sensor plasmid vector. Under hypoxic conditions, the GAL4-ODD protein, which is produced in myocytes, binds and activates the expression of HO-1 equipped with a GAL4 upstream activating sequence site located on a second (effector) plasmid [78]. Rapid and robust cardiac-specific HO-1 transgene expression has been reported with this vector system in transfected cardiomyocytes (H9C2 cells) upon exposure to low oxygen. In a mouse model of MI, transfection with a similar vigilant vector containing HO-1 resulted in marked HO-1 gene upregulation in response to ischemia, significant reduction of apoptosis in the infarct area, and improved cardiac function [79]. Pachori et al. have reported another preemptive strategy using AAV vectors containing human HO-1 and driven by an erythropoietin gene-derived HRE sequence [74]. Administration of this construct into the rat heart prevented the I/R injury induced by MI 8 weeks later. Ischemia resulted in approximately a 50-fold induction in human HO-1 over endogenous rat HO-1. In addition, there was an immediate and sustainable increase in total HO-1 protein levels in human HO-1-transduced animals after 1 hour of ischemia.

Whether this approach of regulatable gene therapy, dependent on the activity of endogenous transcription factors, may present limitations related to a potential disturbance in the expression of endogenous genes remains to be seen [80]. Clearly, long-term preclinical studies will be warranted to test these concerns prior to clinical application.

Considerable evidence supports the concept that overexpression or upregulation of heme oxygenase may be used to provide vascular protection in the aging individual through its antioxidant, antiapoptotic and anti-inflammatory effects [81]. Absence of HO-1 has been suggested to exacerbate atherosclerosis because overexpression of HO-1 in several animal models has been shown to prevent the development of atherosclerosis [82–84].

The role of the antioxidant metallothionein (MT) in aging has been examined in mice containing a cardiac-specific metallothionein transgene [85]. MT-containing mice exhibited a longer life span. Moreover, aging-induced changes in myocyte contractile function, OS (e.g., increased superoxide generation) and related protein biomarkers (cytochrome *c* release, p47phox expression and reduced aconitase activity) were attenuated by MT, and MT-containing myocytes were more resistant to apoptosis. In a follow-up study, Fang et al. have reported that MT-mice displayed a parallel attenuation in both age-related cardiac contractile dysfunction (e.g., prolonged TR[90] and intracellular Ca^{2+} decay) and aberrant insulin signaling (e.g., reduced Akt expression and insulin-stimulated Akt phosphorylation, elevated PTP1B expression and diminished basal insulin receptor tyrosine phosphorylation) [86]. These data suggest that an enhanced antioxidant defense is beneficial for aging-induced cardiac contractile dysfunction and alteration in insulin signaling.

It is well-established that detoxification of mitochondrial ROS is regulated by induction of the SOD2 gene, which encodes the mitochondrial-localized manganese-dependent superoxide dismutase (MnSOD); however, the mechanisms by which mitochondrial OS activates cellular signaling pathways leading to induction of nuclear genes have only recently been unveiled. Storz et al. have recently demonstrated that mitochondrial ROS activates a signal relay pathway in which the serine/threonine protein kinase D (PKD), acting as a mitochondrial sensor of OS, activates the NF-κB transcription factor leading to induction of SOD2 [87]. PKD is localized to the mitochondria in cells exposed to both exogenous and mitochondrial ROS, where it is phosphorylated and activated.

Subsequently, PKD likely dissociates from mitochondria in an activated state and phosphorylates substrates such as those which participate in NF-κB activation, although how this occurs is not known. *SOD2* promoter activation was shown to be dependent on PKD since RNAi-mediated silencing of PKD blunted *SOD2* induction. This conclusion is supported by findings with cells containing constitutively active PKD alleles which also increased *SOD2* reporter activity and MnSOD protein expression [88]. This study identified an important and missing link to targeting aging effects and age-related diseases, which have been linked to mitochondrial dysfunction.

As previously discussed, caloric restriction (CR) decreases mitochondrial ROS generation and oxidative damage to mtDNA and mitochondrial proteins, and increases maximum longevity, although the mechanisms responsible for this remain unknown. Recent observations have suggested that protein restriction and more specifically methionine restriction also produce similar changes independent of energy restriction [89]. Male rats subjected to methionine restriction (MetR) exhibit markedly decreased mitochondrial ROS production, mtDNA oxidative damage, and levels of markers of protein oxidation measured in heart and liver mitochondria [90]. Furthermore, the concentration of respiratory complexes I and IV also decreases in MetR. The decrease in mitochondrial ROS generation (derived from complexes I and III in liver and complex I in heart) appears to be due to increase efficiency of the respiratory chain to avoid electron leak to oxygen. Moreover, in addition to a role in lowering the rate of mitochondrial ROS generation, lowering of methionine levels by MetR also appears to decrease the sensitivity of proteins to oxidative damage, which may further contribute to control of vertebrate longevity.

Directly Targeting Mitochondrial Dysfunction and Structural Defects

As previously noted, mitochondria play a critical role in the cardiac pathology associated with age as well as in the generation of ROS that potentially initiates, accompanies and amplifies the effects of aging on the cardiovascular system, and in particular in the heart. Some of these effects from mitochondria appear to stem from the mitochondrial involvement in cell-death signaling and its role as ROS producer. In Chapter 4, we have also described the significant aging-related effects on cardiac mitochondrial bioenergetic function at the levels of the respiratory chain, the membrane potential and fatty acid beta-oxidation, which is further exacerbated by the toxic effects of ROS on mitochondrial protein, lipid structure and mitochondrial DNA integrity.

The role of mitochondrial DNA mutations in aging has more recently taken center stage after the striking findings in transgenic mouse strains containing increasing mtDNA mutation levels (so called mutator strains). These mouse strains have markedly reduced longevity and also display many of the manifestations seen in premature aging phenotypes in humans such as reduced life span, weight loss, hair loss, curvature of the spine, loss of bone mass, decrease in red blood cells and testicular atrophy [91–93]. While the mitochondrial bioenergetic phenotype was effected in one of these constructs (as was the propensity towards apoptosis) surprisingly, the levels of mitochondrial ROS or of ROS-associated damage were not significant. It is noteworthy that these transgenic strains were constructed by the introduction of a nuclear-DNA encoded error-prone DNA polymerase γ into these mice. Interestingly, a transgenic mouse strain containing a cardiac-specific overexpression of the error-prone DNA polymerase also accumulated point mutations and deletions in mtDNA, but did not show evidence of OXPHOS impairment, increased OS or antioxidant responses; these mice developed dilated cardiomyopathy within 4 weeks of age associated with a wave of myocyte apoptosis [94]. Therefore, the mechanism of how these mutant mitochondrial genomes may contribute to the premature aging phenotypes remains uncertain.

One approach to correcting mtDNA defects is by supplementing mtDNA repair systems. Several studies have reported that using gene therapy DNA repair enzymes can be introduced into the mitochondria. Mitochondria contain several endogenous enzymes (all nuclear encoded) to remove oxidative alterations from mtDNA, largely resulting from ROS production. Several human DNA glycosylases: UNG (uracil DNA glycosylase), OGG1, hMYH (the human homologue of *Escherichia coli* MutY, which excises mispaired adenine opposite 8-oxoguanine) and hNTH1 (the human homologue of *E. coli* endonuclease III) have been localized to mitochondria [95]. The OGG1 enzyme acts on oxidized purines such as 7,8-dihydro-8-oxoguanine (8-oxoG), a highly mutagenic oxidative lesion whose levels in mtDNA significantly increases with age [96]; an age-associated increase in this enzyme has been reported in both rat liver and heart mitochondria indicating induction of this 8-oxo-dG-specific repair pathway with age [97]. hOGG1, a human homologue of the *E coli mutM* DNA glycosylase/AP lyase encodes four isoforms from distinct transcripts generated by alternative splicing, three of which are targeted to mitochondria. Using a vector containing a mitochondrial transport sequence located upstream of the hOGG1 cDNA sequence, transfection of Hela cells resulted in enhancing the repair of mtDNA oxidative damage and increasing the capacity for cells to survive and continue to divide after an oxidative insult (i.e., treatment with increasing dosage of menadione) [98]. Furthermore, the physiological role of the transfected hOGG1 gene when placed under the control of a tetracycline-regulated promoter has also been investigated [99]. Transfected cells that conditionally expressed OGG1 in the absence of the tetracycline analogue doxycycline, and targeted this recombinant protein to mitochondria, were generated and displayed an eight-fold increase in the amount of a functional OGG1 protein in mitochondria. These cells were more proficient at repairing oxidative damage in a synthetic oligonucleotide substrate containing 8-oxoguanine, as well as in their own mtDNA with menadione-induced oxidative damage, this increased repair capacity was shown to lead to increased cellular survival following OS. Experiments in which either a wild-type or R229Q mutant hOGG1 were transfected in Hela cells, and targeted to either the mitochondria or nucleus, demonstrated that overexpression of wild-type hOGG1 resulted in increased cellular survival when compared to vector or mutant overexpression of hOGG1 [100]. In contrast, mitochondrially-targeted mutant hOGG1 resulted in increased cell death compared to nuclear targeted mutant hOGG1 upon exposure of cells to oxidative damage. Moreover, mutant hOGG1 in the mitochondria resulted in reduced mitochondrial DNA integrity (as gauged by real-time quantitative PCR) when compared to the wild-type suggesting that deficiencies in hOGG1, especially in the mitochondria, may lead to reduced mtDNA integrity and consequently result in decreased cell viability. Similar constructs have been used to introduce endonuclease III and endonuclease VIII in the mitochondria to enhance the repair of pyramidine oxidative lesions in mtDNA, leading to increased cellular resistance to OS [101]. Comparable results have been reported in cultured oligodendrocytes with transfected hOGG1 and they have been shown to stem menadione-induced apoptosis, reducing the release of cytochrome *c* from the intermitochondrial space and caspase 9 activation [102]. However, to the best of our knowledge these experiments have not yet been carried out specifically with aging cells or in cardiomyocytes or with animal models *in vivo*.

The transfection and subsequent expression of full-length mtDNA in mammalian mitochondria has not yet been successfully accomplished. As a result, and in contrast to gene therapy for chromosomal DNA defects, mitochondrial gene therapy remains a field that is still in its infancy and attempts towards gene therapy of the mitochondrial genome have been rare. One approach to surmount this limitation has deployed the delivery of DNA into mitochondria in conjunction with a conjugated peptide containing a mitochondrial leader sequence (MLS) recognized by the mitochondrial translocase/protein import apparatus; small peptide nucleic acids (PNAs) attached to oligonucleotide have been delivered to the mitochondria in this way. Efficient delivery of these constructs into the mitochondrial matrix has been achieved with the use of cationic liposomes [103, 104], and, even more effectively, with cationic polyethylenimine [105]. Using this approach, a mitochondrial-specific delivery system has been recently developed using DQAsomes, liposome-like vesicles formed in aqueous medium from a dicationic amphiphile called *dequalinium* [106]. These DQAsomes can also bind and carry DNA (as well as drugs), are able to transfect cells with a high efficiency, and selectively accumulate in the mitochondrial organelle releasing their load. Moreover, in addition to PNA-oligonucleotides, MLS peptide conjugated with plasmid DNAs can be incorporated and condensed within the DQAsomes and exclusively delivered to the mitochondrial compartment [107, 108], albeit these experiments have not yet directly demonstrated the mitochondrial-specific expression of a transgene delivered to mitochondria by these vesicles.

Another approach to correcting mtDNA defects involves expression of the mitochondrial gene of interest in the nucleus with subsequent targeting of the gene product to the mitochondria, via the mitochondrial translocase/import apparatus. This approach also termed allotopic expression has been carried out with mammalian cells in culture with only a few mitochondrial structural genes (i.e., ATPase6, ND4) [109–111]. However, this approach has not been reported with tRNA, or rRNA molecules nor is it feasible with the important non-coding regulatory D-loop region, genetic loci which have been shown to bear many of the most deleterious, pathogenic and common mutations in mtDNA. In addition, competition or toxic effects due to the endogenous mitochondrial product are a concern and gene replacement methods are not evident.

Several convergent lines of evidence have suggested that mitochondrial complementation can occur in mice and human cells [112–114], and that mitochondria can share information with each other through fission and fusion processes. Early studies suggested that exogenous mitochondria added to cells could be incorporated as transforming elements, with chloramphenicol-sensitive mammalian cells acquiring a resistant phenotype from isolated mitochondria from a chloramphenicol-resistant cell line, presumably via mitochondrial endocytosis [115]. With data obtained from cell fusion studies, Enriquez et al. have suggested that inter-mitochondrial complementation between mammalian mitochondria carrying two different non-allelic mtDNA mutations, indicating a capacity of mitochondria to fuse and mix their contents, was a relativity rare event although this capacity may become activated in some developmental or physiological situations, and may be very much dependent on the nuclear genetic background which regulates the mitochondrial fusion/fission machinery [116, 117].

Strong evidence for the presence of extensive *in vivo* inter-mitochondrial complementation was shown in transgenic mice carrying an exogenously-introduced mutant mtDNA with a deletion of 4,696 bp (mtDNA4696) [113]. In all tissues examined containing the mtDNA4696 deletion, Nakada et al. found mitochondria with normal COX activity (preventing those mice from expressing disease phenotypes) until the deletion accumulated to high levels. They also found no evidence of the coexistence of COX-positive and -negative mitochondria within single cells indicative of the occurrence of *in vivo* inter-mitochondrial complementation by the exchange of mitochondrial contents between exogenously introduced mitochondria with mtDNA4696 and host mitochondria with normal mtDNA. An important implication from these studies relates to the possibility that transcomplementation (via gene therapy) may rescue human somatic cells and tissues from aging-dependent mtDNA mutations and dysfunction [118].

Another related recent study has further documented mammalian mitochondrial transfer *in vitro* from skin fibroblast or adult stem cells (i.e., human mesenchymal stem cells) co-cultured with respiratory-deficient A549 p° cells (p° are cells that lack mtDNA). This active transfer of mitochondria from one cell-type to another, resulted in rescued mitochondrial function (gauged by increased ATP levels, ETC function and mitochondrial membrane potential and restored translation of mtDNA-encoded proteins) and diminished ROS levels in the recipient A549 p° cells [119]. While cell fusion was excluded in this study, the mechanism of mitochondrial transfer (which may involve vesicular transfer) remains undetermined thus far. Furthermore, it is not clear whether all mitochondria were transferred or whether the recipient cell incorporated isolated mitochondrial components such as the mtDNA. The utility of this finding in rescuing cells from aging-damage mitochondria by transfer of normally functioning mitochondria from wild-type cells (an approach that most likely will be implemented *ex vivo*) remains to be tested in other cell types including cardiomyocytes.

Significantly, new prospects appear to be available for the targeting and reversing of mtDNA damage in aging [120]. Moreover, therapies aimed at other targets of aging-induced mitochondrial damage are also being developed. This includes therapies to enhance the repair of oxidatively damaged mitochondrial proteins [121], indirect strategies aimed at remedying the age-mediated decline in fatty acid beta oxidation function by upregulating the global regulator PPAR-α with exercise training [122], or atorvastatin treatment [123], and non-specific treatments with agents known to have a beneficial effect on mitochondrial bioenergetic metabolism including creatine, coenzyme Q_{10}, Gingko biloba, nicotinamide, riboflavin, carnitine, lipoic acid, pyruvate and dichloroacetate [124]. In addition, the selective delivery to the mitochondria of a variety of compounds (e.g., antiapoptotic drugs, antioxidants, and proton uncouplers) could be used as an alternative strategy in the treatment of age-mediated mitochondrial dysfunction. For instance, the previously mentioned DQAsome can also deliver drugs that trigger apoptosis to mitochondria and inhibit carcinoma growth in mice. For instance, a synthetic ubiquinone analog (termed *mitoQ*) containing the addition of a lipophilic triphenylphosphate cation has been selectively targeted to the mitochondrial compartment [125]. These positively charged lipophilic molecules can rapidly permeate the mitochondrial lipid bilayers and accumulate at high levels within negatively charged energized mitochondria [126]. Significant doses of these bioactive compounds can be orally administered to mice over long periods of time and accumulate within most organs, including the heart and brain. Interestingly, the incorporation of mitoQ within mitochondria has been shown to prevent apoptotic cell death and caspase activation induced by H_2O_2 (in isolated Jurkat cells) and can function as a potent antioxidant, preventing lipid peroxidation and protecting mitochondria from oxidative damage. In addition, feeding mitoQ to rats significantly decreased heart dysfunction, cell death, and mitochondrial damage after I/R injury [127].

There is evidence that this approach of targeting bioactive molecules to mitochondria can be adapted to other neutral bioactive molecules, offering a potential vehicle for testing mitochondrial-specific therapies of aging. For instance, synthetic peptide, cell-permeable antioxidants containing dimethyltyrosine, concentrate in mitochondria by over 1,000-fold, can reduce intracellular ROS and cell death in a cell model. In ischemic hearts, these peptides were shown to potently improve contractile force in an *ex vivo* model [128]. In addition, the successful incorporation of another modified antioxidant, a synthetic analog of vitamin E (MitoVitE) into the mitochondrial matrix has been shown to significantly reduce mitochondrial lipid peroxidation and protein damage and can accumulate after oral administration at therapeutic concentrations within the cardiac tissue [129]. This type of approach critically needs to be further tested in aging animal models and may have enormous clinical benefit. Moreover, this approach of targeted-organelle delivery of drugs can be adapted to other organelles which as we shall shortly see can also contribute to the aging phenotype.

Removing "Biological Garbage" (Targeting Lysosomes, Proteasomes and Other Approaches for Enhancing Catabolic Remediation)

In Chapter 4, we discussed the cellular requirement for the removal of worn-out and defective macromolecules and organelles and their degradation by proteases including calcium-dependent neutral proteases (calpains), multicatalytic proteinase complexes (proteasomes) and by lysosomes using autophagy. Since the proteasome has been implicated in both general protein turnover and the removal of oxidized protein, its fate during aging has been of increasing interest, with the evidence indicating that impaired proteasome function occurs with age in different cellular systems, particularly in nondividing (post-mitotic) cells [130]. Marked decrease in the activity of both the proteasomal system and the lysosomal proteases was reported during the senescence of nondividing fibroblasts, with the peptidyl-glutamyl-hydrolyzing activity of the proteasome particularly inhibited.

This decline in proteolytic capacity was accompanied by increased accumulation of oxidized proteins [131]. Other studies have found that severe OS causes extensive protein oxidation, directly generating protein fragments, cross-linked and aggregated proteins, that become progressively resistant to proteolytic digestion, and which can bind to the 20S proteasome acting as irreversible inhibitors [132]. The progressive inhibition of the proteasome by binding to increasing levels of oxidized and cross-linked protein aggregates appears both during aging and in many age-related diseases/disorders [133].

Previously we have discussed the sequence of events and specific proteins involved (e.g., atg proteins) in autophagosome formation and the contribution of a variety of signaling pathways in its regulation, including pathways involving insulin signaling, phosphatidylinositol 3-kinases and the protein kinase mTOR. In addition, chaperone-mediated autophagy is responsible for the degradation of specific proteins and is activated by OS [134]. Gathered observations have shown that autophagy is a critical adaptive response to damage ranging from OS and starvation to survival when either extracellular or intracellular nutrients are limited. In animal models, autophagy also appears to be upregulated in aging-associated myocardial diseases including myocardial ischemia, and in association with elevated cardiomyocte cell death in the hamster model of cardiomyopathy. In the latter model, granulocyte colony-stimulating factor (G-CSF) treatment improved survival among 30-week-old hamsters, restored ventricular function and remodeling, increased cardiomyocyte size, and reduced myocardial fibrosis followed by a dramatic reduction in autophagy [135]. In contrast, there is considerable evidence that aging is accompanied by a marked decline in autophagic function, particularly in post-mitotic cells. Abnormal autophagic degradation of damaged macromolecules and organelles, termed biological "garbage", is also considered an important contributor to aging and the death of post-mitotic cells, including cardiomyocytes. This reduction in autophagy is due in part to the inappropriate distribution of lysosomal enzymes [136]. Also contributory to this autophagic dysfunction is the marked increase in levels of oxidatively damaged mitochondria and peroxisomes, cytosolic proteins and increasingly undigestable macromolecules (due to cross-linking), such as the intralysosomal undegradable pigment lipofuscin (Fig. 14.2).

Since autophagy is a primary defense against the accumulation of damaged organelles such as mitochondria and peroxisomes, its dysfunction may be a critical determinant of cell longevity. Experiments with genetically modified mice support the hypothesis that an age-related decrease in macroautophagy may promote accumulation of damaged mitochondria [137]. Furthermore, autophagy of mitochondria, peroxisomes, and possibly other organelles can be selective and non-random, underlined by the term mitophagy, with targeted degradation of defective mitochondria resulting in delaying the accumulation of somatic mutations of mtDNA with aging [138]. Recent observations suggest that rat mtDNA containing 8-OHdG accumulate in a small pool of mitochondria with increasing age; the intraperitoneal administration of the antilipolytic agent [3, 5-dimethylpyrazole (DMP)] rescued older cells from the accumulation of 8-OHdG in the mtDNA in less than 6 hours but did not impact the overall level of cytochrome *c* oxidase activity suggesting the targeting of defective mitochondria [139].

Interventions including caloric restriction, decrease of insulin-like signaling and chronic administration of anti-lipolytic drugs which decrease glucose and insulin levels, stimulate autophagy and may provide antiaging effects [140, 141]. Interestingly, administration of the antibiotic rapamycin, a mTOR inhibitor, to various eukaryotic cells (e.g., yeast and *C. elegans*) results in physiological changes that mimic nutrient starvation, activate autophagy and modulate longevity [142].

To eliminate one of the causes of the aging-associated autophagic dysfunction, the accumulation of undegradable compounds such as lipofuscin, a radically different approach has been recently proposed [143, 144]. This involves augmenting the natural catabolic machinery with hydrolytic microbial enzymes, "xenohydrolases", which can degrade molecules that our natural machinery cannot. The delivery systems envisioned for such enzymes include direct enzyme introduction to lysosomes via targeted endocytosis (a technique successfully used to introduce therapeutic quantities of specific enzymes to treat lysosomal storage diseases, including Gaucher and Fabry disease). Other

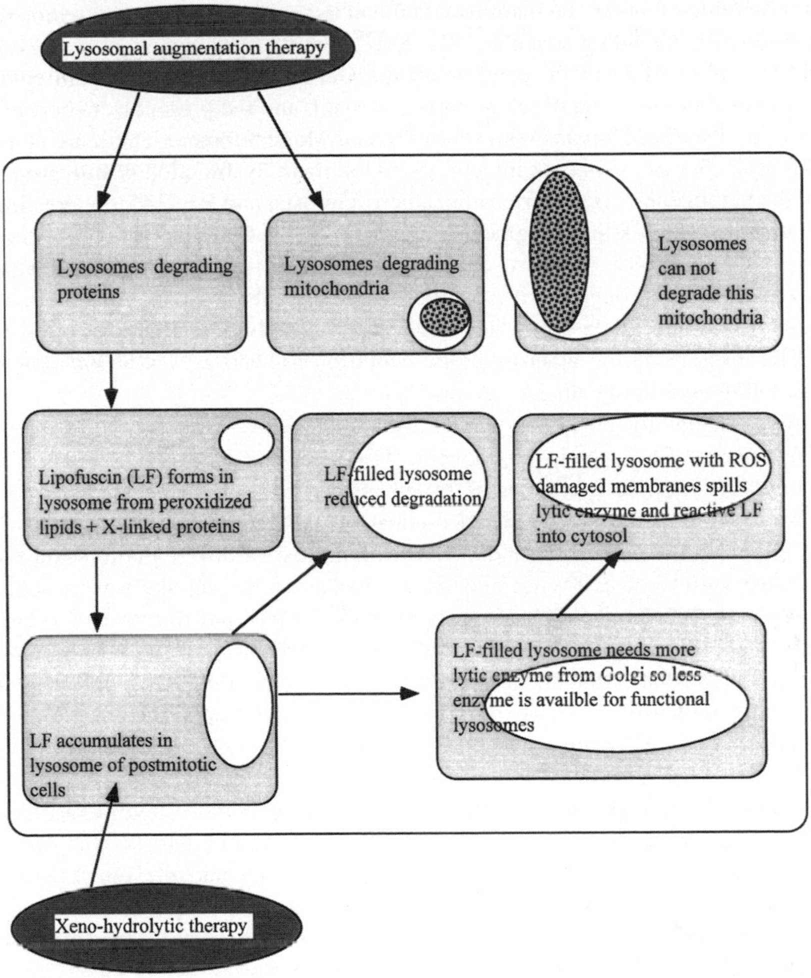

Fig. 14.2 Lysosome in aging. Potential sites for therapy
Shown is the accumulation in some lysosomes of lipofuscin which can reduce overall recycling and even in some cases cause cytosolic leakage of reactive lipofuscin and lytic enzymes triggering injury. Also shown are the degradation of damaged mitochondria and the potential inactivation of lysosomal function by increasingly large, oxidatively damaged mitochondria. Sites amenable to therapeutic interventions are also indicated.

delivery approaches involve gene therapy targeting to the lysosome by: (1) Incorporating signals on the therapeutic protein specifying the addition of mannose 6-phosphate residues; (2) Using specific motifs present for vesicular transport; and (3) By chaperone-mediated autophagy effected by the presence of specific pentapeptide motif, "KFERQ" in association with the cytosolic chaperone HSP 70 that recognizes the targeting signal, the lysosomal membrane protein type 2a, LAMP-2a, which acts as a receptor and a lysosomal luminal variant of HSP 70 that is required for substrate translocation across the lysosomal membrane.

Targeting the Nucleus

In Chapter 3, we have examined evidence that telomerase and telomere binding proteins play a major role in cellular senescence and aging in general. Since telomerase is virtually absent or only transiently active in normal somatic cells throughout postnatal life, telomere length gradually decreases as a function of age in the majority of human tissues. Age-dependent telomere shortening in most somatic cells, including vascular ECs, SMCs, and cardiomyocytes, is thought to impair cellular function and viability of the aged organism. Gathered observations from epidemiological and genetic studies point to a role of telomerase repression and the presence of short telomeres in a broad spectrum of diseases. Humans with shorter than average telomere length are at increased risk of dying from heart disease, stroke, or infection; and telomere dysfunction is emerging as an important factor in the pathogenesis of hypertension, atherosclerosis, and HF [145]. Interestingly, analysis of discrete human coronary arterial segments obtained from heart transplant recipients showed that hTERT was expressed in 88% of atherosclerotic tissues, at a five-fold higher frequency compared with controls and with a strong positive correlation with levels of telomerase bioactivity and the severity of atherosclerotic grade [146], and suggest a marked upregulation of telomerase and its catalytic hTERT protein during atherosclerotic evolution as well as a role for telomerase in the vascular remodeling underlying atherosclerosis.

Therapeutic strategies for enhancing telomerase activity have been primarily directed to components of telomerase (the protein component, TERT, or the RNA component, TERC). Activation of telomerase may be useful in the treatment of diseases associated with telomere loss. Telomerase transduced cells have extended replicative capacities, increased resistance to stress, improved functional activities *in vitro* and *in vivo* with no loss of differentiation capacity or growth control in a large variety of cell-types and tissues including human skeletal muscle [147, 148], human osteoblasts [149], human ECs (from both large vessels and microvessels) [150] and cardiac myocytes [151]. Forced expression of TERT in cardiac muscle in mice was sufficient to rescue telomerase activity and telomere length. Interestingly, the transduced ventricle was initially hypercellular, with increased myocyte density and DNA synthesis, whereas by 12 weeks, cell cycling attenuated and myocyte enlargement (hypertrophy) was noted without fibrosis or impaired function [151].

Reintroduction of one copy of the TERC gene in late generation telomerase-deficient mice (Terc-/-), which have short telomeres and show severe proliferative defects, was sufficient to critically elongate short telomeres, rescue chromosomal instability and prevent severe proliferative defects [152]. These findings suggest that the reintroduction of telomerase activity is a potential model in the treatment of age-related diseases triggered by telomerase exhaustion, or premature aging syndromes accompanied by marked telomere shortening.

Cells subjected to sub-lethal doses of stress such as irradiation or oxidative damage enter a state that closely resembles replicative senescence. The responses of human fibroblasts with and without overexpression of hTERT, when subjected to stress induced by UV, gamma-radiation or OS (e.g., H_2O_2 exposure), were similar suggesting that stress-induced senescence is not triggered by telomere shortening/loss. However, fibroblasts with hTERT were more resistant to stress-induced apoptosis and necrosis [153]. On the other hand, several observations have suggested that OS is a primary determinant of telomere shortening, whereas antioxidants decelerate telomere loss, and that telomeres are extremely sensitive sensors for genomic oxidative damage [154]. The loss of telomerase activity and increase in ROS observed in aging cells was recapitulated in cells exposed to H_2O_2 and resulted in nuclear export of TERT into the cytosol accompanied by increased level of mtDNA damage; these changes preceded the onset of replicative senescence [155]. Incubation of these cells with the antioxidant N-acetylcysteine reduced intracellular ROS formation and prevented mtDNA damage, and significantly delayed the nuclear export of TERT protein, loss in overall TERT activity, and the onset of replicative senescence. Thus, modulation of telomerase activity and control of telomeric length together with the attenuation of ROS formation, may represent important therapeutic tools in regenerative medicine and in the prevention of aging [156].

A further link between OS and telomere function/senescence has been demonstrated in endothelial progenitor cells (EPCs) in which Ang II-mediated OS (gauged by increased levels of peroxynitrite formation and of gp91phox expression) accelerated the onset of EPC senescence with significantly diminished telomerase activity [157]; these effects were attenuated by treatment with 17β-estradiol (E2) [158].

Genomic Instability

One of the features of cellular aging that is less well-understood is genomic instability, whose analysis has been best characterized in studies with premature and accelerated aging (progeria) syndromes. Premature aging syndromes often result from mutations in nuclear proteins involved in the maintenance of genomic integrity. For instance in Hutchinson-Gilford Progeria Syndrome (HGPS), genetic defects in the nuclear envelope protein prelamin A or in the FACE-1 metalloprotease (also termed Zmspte24) involved in prelamin A proteolytic maturation, cause the accumulation of an abnormal form of the lamin A protein and the subsequent disruption of the nuclear envelope integrity. This disruption leads to marked alterations in chromatin organization, genomic instability, transcriptional programming changes, and the activation of a p53-linked signaling pathway, resulting in progeroid phenotypes in mice and humans. Evidence of genetic instability in the Zmpste24-deficient mouse has been demonstrated with embryonic fibroblasts from these mice exhibiting increased DNA damage and chromosome aberrations and are more sensitive to DNA-damaging agents [159]. Moreover, bone marrow cells derived from Zmpste24-/- mice display increased aneuploidy, and the mice are more sensitive to DNA-damaging agents. Lowering prelamin A levels results in a complete recovery of Zmpste24-deficient mice from the accelerated aging process, while downregulation of p53 results in a modest but significant improvement in the premature aging phenotype [160]. Furthermore, the Zmpste24-deficient mice have been used to test different therapeutic approaches to attenuate accelerated aging, including some based on drugs currently available.

Mutations that lead to accumulation of a lipid-modified (farnesylated) form of prelamin A disrupt the critical nuclear scaffolding function of this protein, leading to misshapen nuclei and progeria. Treatment with farnesyltransferase inhibitors (FTIs) can be employed to reverse this cellular abnormality; Zmpste24-deficient mice, treated with FTI exhibited improved body weight, grip strength, bone integrity and survival at 20 weeks of age [161].

Another mutation associated with HGPS, a spontaneous point mutation in lamin A (LMNA) activates an aberrant cryptic splice site in LMNA pre-mRNA, leading to the synthesis of a truncated lamin A protein and concomitant reduction in wild-type lamin A. This cellular disease phenotype is reversible in cells derived from individuals with this mutation [162]. The mutant LMNA mRNA and lamin A protein can be efficiently eliminated by correction of the aberrant splicing, event using a modified oligonucleotide targeted to the activated cryptic splice site. With this splicing correction, HGPS fibroblasts assume normal nuclear morphology, the aberrant nuclear distribution and cellular levels of lamina-associated proteins are rescued, defects in heterochromatin-specific histone modifications are corrected and proper expression of several misregulated genes is reestablished. Interestingly, introduction of wild-type lamin A protein did not rescue the cellular disease manifestations.

Progeria cells bearing the G608G LMNA mutation are characterized by accumulation of a mutated lamin A precursor (progerin), nuclear dysmorphism, chromatin disorganization, heterochromatin loss and transcript redistribution. Combined treatment with mevinolin (a farnesyl inhibitor) and the histone deacetylase inhibitor trichostatin A (targeting chromatin arrangement) dramatically lowered progerin levels, leading to the rescue of heterochromatin organization and reorganization of transcripts in HGPS fibroblasts [163].

Epigenetic chromatin alterations have been reported in premature aging/progeroid syndromes. In the cells derived from female HGPS patients, levels of methylated histones in the inactive X chromosome (Xi) and of an enzyme required for histone methylation of Xi are sharply lower [164].

The effects of chromatin modification on genomic instability have also been underscored in mice null for the histone H2AX [165]. The histone variant H2AX is primarily associated with maintaining genomic integrity by contributing to the repair of double-strand DNA breaks introduced by radiation or chemical damage or by recombination processes.

A role of OS in these epigenetic processes may also be envisioned. Supplementation with the antioxidant coenzyme Q together with a PUFA-rich diet was protective against age-related double strand breaks, and increased rat life span [166].

One key aspect driving aging appears to be DNA damage. Previously, we described several syndromes of premature aging in which defective DNA repair was central to their etiology. Defects in one of the proteins that act in nucleotide excision repair pathway (i.e., XPD) result in three distinct autosomal recessive syndromes: Xeroderma pigmentosum (XP), Cockayne syndrome (CS) and Trichothiodystrophy (TTD). In the human disorder trichothiodystrophy (TTD) a mutation is found in XPD encoding a DNA helicase, which functions in both DNA repair and transcription; TTD mice display many symptoms of premature aging, including osteoporosis and kyphosis, osteosclerosis, early greying, cachexia, infertility, and reduced life span recapitulating the human syndrome. Even greater accelerated aging is found in TTD mice which contain a second mutation affecting DNA repair and exhibit an elevated cellular sensitivity to oxidative DNA damage. The unrepaired DNA damage likely compromises transcription, which can lead to enhance apoptosis [167]. Correction of these cells' DNA repair defects by transducing the complementing wild-type gene, is one potential strategy to help these patients. Using an adenoviral vector carrying the XPD gene, complete correction of SV40-transformed primary skin fibroblasts obtained from XP, TTD and CS patients was reported [168]. Earlier studies utilizing a retroviral based vector gene transfer of a variety of human DNA repair proteins (XPA, XPB, XPC and XPD) corrected the respective DNA repair defects in fibroblasts obtained from specific patient complementation groups (e.g., A, B, C and D) [169, 170].

Attack at the Level of Transcription

In Chapter 13, it was noted that aging is accompanied by significant changes in the transcriptional programme of the cells. Thus, it is not unexpected that the introduction of specific transcriptional factors (primarily by gene therapy) might be a useful therapeutic approach to attenuate specific pathological manifestations of aging. Suggested examples of this methodology include global transcriptional regulators governing lipid metabolism, fat mobilization and mitochondrial function (e.g., PGC-1, PPAR-γ and PPAR-α) [171–175]. Furthermore, the mammalian SIR2 orthologue, Sirt1 binds to and represses genes controlled by the global regulator PPAR-γ including genes that mediate fat storage and contribute to the mammalian caloric restriction program in reference to regulation of fat mobilization in adipocytes [176]. SirT1 is also part of a regulatory loop that limits the production of IGF binding protein (IGFBP1), thereby modulating IGF signaling in mice and the FoxO transcription factor, that is downstream of the IGF signaling pathway [177]. SIRT1 also binds and deacetylates p53, and can repress p53-mediated transactivation. When overexpressed in primary mouse embryo fibroblasts (MEFs), SIRT1 antagonizes the induced acetylation of p53 and rescues induced premature cellular senescence [178].

Gene transfer and overexpression of an engineered VEGF-activating zinc finger protein transcription factor have been successful in improving angiogenesis in aging mice, blood flow and limb salvage [179]. In addition, numerous observations have suggested a beneficial role of testosterone and selective androgen receptor modulators, primarily in men with numerous anabolic effects such as increasing muscle mass and strength, induction of muscle fiber hypertrophy and increased satellite cell number [180].

Targeting the Sarcomere and SR

In preclinical studies, gene therapy approaches have been successful in the restoration of diastolic function in senescent heart. Using a catheter based delivery of an adenoviral construct, transduction of rat myocardium *in vivo* with a SERCA gene was achieved in both young and senescent rats [181]. Two days after infection, parameters of systolic and diastolic function were measured in open-chest rats. Overexpression did not significantly affect left ventricular systolic pressure but did increase dP/dt in the senescent heart. Moreover, SERCA2a overexpression restored the left ventricular time constant of isovolumic relaxation and dP/dt to adult levels and markedly improved rate-dependent contractility and diastolic function in senescent hearts.

Parvalbumin acts as a Ca^{2+} sink and enhances relaxation in skeletal muscle; overexpression of parvalbumin in myocardium increased cardiac relaxation both *in vitro* and *in vivo*. Gene transfer of parvalbumin as an adenoviral construct was conducted with two different rat models of aging: the Fischer 344 (F344) and the Fischer 344 × Brown Norway F1 hybrid (F344 × BN) [182]. *In vivo* overexpression of parvalbumin in both models had no effect on systolic parameters but reduced left ventricular diastolic pressure and the time course of pressure decline. These results suggested that gene therapy of parvalbumin could address the impaired Ca^{2+} homeostasis and diastolic dysfunction without increase in energy expenditure. Other studies have reached the same conclusion [183, 184].

Conclusion and New Horizons

A number of the therapeutic modalities and targeted approaches discussed above represent in fact new discoveries; some of the discoveries have been not repeated by other investigators either because the experimental conditions were different or because the recipients were not the same, and some are even untested at the preclinical stage. Most of the approaches discussed in this chapter have used either pharmacological treatments or gene therapy. Particular promise (from our point of view) may be accorded to the novel finding of transfer of mitochondria (and its phenotype) from one cell to another [119], but this needs further substantiation from other investigators, in other cell-types, and careful consideration of how it could be used in diminishing ROS as well as replacing defective mitochondria in a clinically adaptable fashion. An increasing number of investigators are using gene transfer in preclinical studies as an effective treatment plan. However, before serious considerations of their clinical application, the safety, efficacy and long-term consequences of the vectors and genes used in aging individuals, as well as the mode of gene delivery (e.g., catheter, direct injection, liposome/intracellular carrier, retroperfusion or after *ex vivo* modification) must be assessed.

As noted in Chapter 3, there is increasing interest in the use of cell transplantation with fetal cardiomyocytes, skeletal myoblasts, embryonic or adult stem cells to provide factors such as angiogenic factors or cytokines, to impact cell growth, to overcome myocyte loss (in ischemia/reperfusion), to restore contractile function and to provide cardioprotective signaling.

In some cases these types of cells (e.g., adult stem cells such as bone marrow and myoblasts) can be easily derived from the individual circumventing immune rejection issues and can be produced in culture in rather large number. Some transplanted cell-types may be good for a short-term benefit (e.g., myoblasts), albeit the long-term stability of the phenotype of any of the cell-types considered for transplant, and their responses to the cardiac milieu (particularly in the older and often diseased human heart) are not yet known. Other transplanted cells can serve as platforms for the delivery of recombinant products; an approach increasingly used for effective delivery. Unfortunately, the precise cellular mechanism(s) of action responsible for the beneficial cardiovascular effects reported with the use of stem cell-transplants remain poorly defined. Although this field is still in its infancy, with further experimentation and clinical trials, definition of stem cell markers, elucidation of their regenerative plasticity and stability, and the mechanisms of action within the cardiac milieu will be established. Subsequently, this methodology may evolve into potential therapies for aging, including the myocardial dysfunction of the elderly.

Summary

- Aging-targeted therapies have been performed primarily at the preclinical level with either animal models or isolated cells targeting organelles/events that are considered to be primary contributors to the aging pathology and phenotype.
- Attenuation of cell-loss and cell death (either apoptotic or necrotic) is a potential strategy to treat heart failure (HF) and myocardial ischemic damage. It may also be a viable strategy to increase survival of endothelial and smooth muscle cells (SMCs) in the elderly.
- Endothelial cells (ECs) are particularly susceptible to apoptosis when reaching senescence. These likely results from reactive oxygen species (ROS)-induced damage and associated signaling.
- A key target in stemming cell death are sites on the mitochondrial inner and outer membrane, the mitochondrial PT pore and the MOMP, which control mitochondrial permeability, integrity and function, the release of specific apoptogenic proteins and are early steps in both apoptosis and necrosis.
- The ANT. VDAC, CyP-D and PBR proteins (all components of the MPT pore) are particularly good targets to regulate cell death, as are the use of antiapoptotic Bcl-2 family factors.
- Activation of pro-survival signaling pathways also attenuate cell death progression. IGF-1 and downstream components of its signaling pathway (e.g., PI3K and Akt) are effective in activating growth pathways and reducing apoptosis in aging cardiovascular cells.
- Other growth factors such as GH and HGF have shown similar benefits.
- Cardioprotective signaling pathways can blunt the effects of ischemia on the heart. These can be triggered by brief episodes of ischemia followed by reperfusion prior to a longer ischemic insult termed ischemic preconditioning, IPC), and by pharmacological stimuli and anesthetics which can mimic the effects of IPC. They can also be applied at the time of reperfusion (i.e., postconditioning) with similar benefits.
- These complex signaling cardioprotective pathways contain many shared components including ligand stimuli or triggers (e.g., adenosine, bradykinin), cell-surface receptors, sarcolemmal and mitochondrial ion channels (e.g., K_{ATP} channels), protein kinases (e.g., PI3K, tyrosine kinases, PKC-ε) and a variety of cellular effectors (including the PT pore).
- Central substrates for cardioprotection reside in the mitochondria including ROS generation, calcium flux, bioenergetic function, and metabolic uncoupling.
- Cardioprotection has been reported in a variety of animal models; it can occur in humans (and may occur with angina) albeit its benefits in the elderly have not been clearly established.
- A primary strategy of aging therapy has been to bolster the capability of the cells to neutralize or detoxify ROS as reported with the transfer and overexpression of superoxide dismutase, catalase, heme oxygenase and metallotheinein.
- Mitochondrial damage including mtDNA oxidative damage can be directly targeted using transfer/overexpression of DNA repair enzymes.
- Direct mitochondrial gene therapy with full-length mtDNA is not yet possible; however, introduction of small sequences conjugated with peptides (PNAs) or using synthetic liposome-like vesicles (DQAsomes) is possible although functional studies are limited. Allotopic expression of two mitochondrial structural genes (ATP6, ND4) has been achieved.

- Recent evidence of direct mitochondrial transfer and complementation experiments suggests new possible modes of mitochondrial replacement and therapy.
- Synthetic liposome-like vesicles can be adapted to deliver a variety of compound to mitochondria (e.g., antiapoptotic drugs, antioxidants, and proton uncouplers).
- Defects in lysosomal function may impact the recycling of worn-out proteins, damaged organelles and amplify the effects of aging, including apoptosis.
- Targeting lysosomal dysfunction may invoke the novel use of xeno-hydrolytic enzymes from bacterial and fungal cells as catabolic remediators.
- A number of nuclear processes can be targeted that will affect both the onset of cellular senescence and the gene damage/genomic instability associated with aging. Moreover, these events are ROS-sensitive.
- Overexpression of telomerase and DNA repair proteins and their nuclear localization can reverse nuclear-based defects in aging (particularly in premature aging syndromes). Aging-associated epigenetic alterations in DNA and chromatin also may be reversed. Overexpression of specific transcription factors can impact the overall programming of the aging phenotype.
- Overexpression of calcium cycling proteins (e.g., SERCA, parvalbumin) can reverse diastolic dysfunction and restore contractility in the aging heart.

References

1. Ratta SI, Clark BF. Understanding and modulating ageing. IUBMB Life 2005;57:297–304
2. Duque G. Apoptosis in cardiovascular aging research: future directions. Am J Geriatr Cardiol 2000;9:263–264
3. Hampel B, Malisan F, Niederegger H, Testi R, Jansen-Durr P. Differential regulation of apoptotic cell death in senescent human cells. Exp Gerontol 2004;39:1713–1721
4. Solary E, Bettaieb A, Dubrez-Daloz L, Corcos L. Mitochondria as a target for inducing death of malignant hematopoietic cells. Leuk Lymphoma 2003;44:563–574
5. Vieira HL, Boya P, Cohen I, El Hamel C, Haouzi D, Druillenec S, Belzacq AS, Brenner C, Roques B, Kroemer G. Cell permeable BH3-peptides overcome the cytoprotective effect of Bcl-2 and Bcl-X(L). Oncogene 2002;21:1963–1977
6. Tsujimoto Y, Nakagawa T, Shimizu S. Mitochondrial membrane permeability transition and cell death. Biochim Biophys Acta 2006;1757:1297–1300
7. Baines CP, Kaiser RA, Purcell NH, Blair NS, Osinska H, Hambleton MA, Brunskill EW, Sayen MR, Gottlieb RA, Dorn GW, Robbins J, Molkentin JD. Loss of cyclophilin D reveals a critical role for mitochondrial permeability transition in cell death. Nature 2005;434:658–662
8. Nakagawa T, Shimizu S, Watanabe T, Yamaguchi O, Otsu K, Yamagata H, Inohara H, Kubo T, Tsujimoto Y. Cyclophilin D-dependent mitochondrial permeability transition regulates some necrotic but not apoptotic cell death. Nature 2005;434:652–658
9. Halestrap AP, McStay GP, Clarke SJ. The permeability transition pore complex: another view. Biochimie 2002;84:153–166
10. Waldmeier PC, Zimmermann K, Qian T, Tintelnot-Blomley M, Lemasters JJ. Cyclophilin D as a drug target. Curr Med Chem 2003;10:1485–1506
11. Zheng Y, Shi Y, Tian C, Jiang C, Jin H, Chen J, Almasan A, Tang H, Chen Q. Essential role of the voltage-dependent anion channel (VDAC) in mitochondrial permeability transition pore opening and cytochrome c release induced by arsenic trioxide. Oncogene 2004;23:1239–1247
12. Veenman L, Gavish M. The peripheral-type benzodiazepine receptor and the cardiovascular system. Implications for drug development. Pharmacol Ther 2006;110:503–524
13. Deniaud A, Hoebeke J, Briand JP, Muller S, Jacotot E, Brenner C. Peptido-targeting of the mitochondrial transition pore complex for therapeutic apoptosis induction. Curr Pharm Des 2006;12:4501–4511
14. Weisleder N, Taffet GE, Capetanaki Y. Bcl-2 overexpression corrects mitochondrial defects and ameliorates inherited desmin null cardiomyopathy. Proc Natl Acad Sci USA 2004;101:769–774
15. Verrier F, Mignotte B, Jan G, Brenner C. Study of PTPC composition during apoptosis for identification of viral protein target. Ann NY Acad Sci 2003;1010:126–142
16. McCully JD, Wakiyama H, Hsieh YJ, Jones M, Levitsky S. Differential contribution of necrosis and apoptosis in myocardial ischemia-reperfusion injury. Am J Physiol Heart Circ Physiol 2004;286:H1923–H1935

17. Yamamura T, Otani H, Nakao Y, Hattori R, Osako M, Imamura H. IGF-I differentially regulates Bcl-xL and Bax and confers myocardial protection in the rat heart. Am J Physiol Heart Circ Physiol 2001;280:H1191–H1200
18. Li Q, Li B, Wang X, Leri A, Jana KP, Liu Y, Kajstura J, Baserga R, Anversa P. Overexpression of insulin-like growth factor-1 in mice protects from myocyte death after infarction, attenuating ventricular dilation, wall stress, and cardiac hypertrophy. J Clin Invest 1997;100:1991–1999
19. Yamashita K, Kajstura J, Discher DJ, Wasserlauf BJ, Bishopric NH, Anversa P, Webster KA. Reperfusion-activated Akt kinase prevents apoptosis in transgenic mouse hearts overexpressing insulin-like growth factor-1. Circ Res 2001;88:609–614
20. Fujio Y, Nguyen T, Wencker D, Kitsis RN, Walsh K. Akt promotes survival of cardiomyocytes in vitro and protects against ischemia-reperfusion injury in mouse heart. Circulation 2000:101:660–667
21. Ren J, Samson WK, Sowers JR. Insulin-like growth factor I as a cardiac hormone: physiological and pathophysiological implications in heart disease. J Mol Cell Cardiol 1999;31:2049–2061
22. Burgess W, Liu Q, Zhou J, Tang Q, Ozawa A, VanHoy R, Arkins S, Dantzer R, Kelley KW. The immune-endocrine loop during aging: role of growth hormone and insulin-like growth factor-I. Neuroimmunomodulation 1999;6:56–68
23. Pugazhenth S, Nesterova A, Sable C, Heidenreich KA, Boxer LM, Heasley LE, Reusch JE. Akt/protein kinase B up-regulates Bcl-2 expression through cAMP-response element-binding protein. J Biol Chem 2000;275: 10761–10766
24. Mehrhof FB, Muller FU, Bergmann MW, Li P, Wang Y, Schmitz W, Dietz R, von Harsdorf R. In cardiomyocyte hypoxia, insulin-like growth factor-I-induced antiapoptotic signaling requires phosphatidylinositol-3-OH-kinase-dependent and mitogen-activated protein kinase-dependent activation of the transcription factor cAMP response element-binding protein. Circulation 2001;104:2088–2094
25. Fernandez M, Sanchez-Franco F, Palacios N, Sanchez I, Fernandez C, Cacicedo L. IGF-I inhibits apoptosis through the activation of the phosphatidylinositol 3-kinase/Akt pathway in pituitary cells. J Mol Endocrinol 2004;33:155–163
26. Torella D, Rota M, Nurzynska D, Musso E, Monsen A, Shiraishi I, Zias E, Walsh K, Rosenzweig A, Sussman MA, Urbanek K, Nadal-Ginard B, Kajstura J, Anversa P, Leri A. Cardiac stem cell and myocyte aging, heart failure, and insulin-like growth factor-1 overexpression. Circ Res 2004;94:514–524
27. Li Q, Wu S, Li SY, Lopez FL, Du M, Kajstura J, Anversa P, Ren J. Cardiac specific overexpression of insulin-like growth factor-1 (IGF-1) attenuates aging-associated cardiac diastolic contractile dysfunction and protein damage. Am J Physiol Heart Circ Physiol 2007;292:H1398–H1403
28. Jin H, Wyss JM, Yang R, Schwall R. The therapeutic potential of hepatocyte growth factor for myocardial infarction and heart failure. Curr Pharm Des 2004;10:2525–2533
29. Fan S, Ma YX, Wang JA, Yuan RQ, Meng Q, Cao Y, Laterra JJ, Goldberg ID, Rosen EM. The cytokine hepatocyte growth factor/scatter factor inhibits apoptosis and enhances DNA repair by a common mechanism involving signaling through phosphatidyl inositol 3' kinase. Oncogene 2000;19:2212–2223
30. Khan AS, Sane DC, Wannenburg T, Sonntag WE. Growth hormone, insulin-like growth factor-1 and the aging cardiovascular system. Cardiovasc Res 2002;54:25–35
31. Groban L, Pailes NA, Bennett CD, Carter CS, Chappell MC, Kitzman DW, Sonntag WE. Growth hormone replacement attenuates diastolic dysfunction and cardiac angiotensin II expression in senescent rats. J Gerontol A Biol Sci Med Sci 2006;61:28–35
32. Rossoni G, De Gennaro Colonna V, Bernareggi M, Polvani GL, Muller EE, Berti F. Protectant activity of hexarelin or growth hormone against postischemic ventricular dysfunction in hearts from aged rats. J Cardiovasc Pharmacol 1998;32:260–265
33. Murry CE, Jennings RB, Reimer KA. Preconditioning with ischemia: a delay of lethal cell injury in ischemic myocardium. Circulation 1986;74:1124–1136
34. Riksen NP, Smits P, Rongen GA. Ischaemic preconditioning: from molecular characterisation to clinical application – part I. Neth J Med 2004;62:353–363
35. Murry CE, Jennings RB, Reimer KA. Preconditioning with ischemia: a delay of lethal cell injury in ischemic myocardium. Circulation 1986;74:1124–1136
36. Bolli R. The late phase of preconditioning. Circ Res 2000:87:972–983
37. Yellon DM, Downey JM. Preconditioning the myocardium: from cellular physiology to clinical cardiology. Physiol Rev 2003;83:1113–1151
38. Cohen MV, Baines CP, Downey JM. Ischemic preconditioning: from adenosine receptor of KATP channel. Annu Rev Physiol 2000;62:79–109
39. Murphy E. Primary and secondary signaling pathways in early preconditioning that converge on the mitochondria to produce cardioprotection. Circ Res 2004;94:7–16
40. Vinten-Johansen J, Zhao ZQ, Zatta AJ, Kin H, Halkos ME, Kerendi F. Postconditioning – A new link in nature's armor against myocardial ischemia-reperfusion injury. Basic Res Cardiol 2005;100:295–310

41. Hausenloy DJ, Tsang A, Yellon DM. The reperfusion injury salvage kinase pathway: a common target for both ischemic preconditioning and postconditioning. Trends Cardiovasc Med 2005:15:69–75
42. Fenton RA, Dickson EW, Meyer TE, Dobson JG Jr. Aging reduces the cardioprotective effect of ischemic preconditioning in the rat heart. J Mol Cell Cardiol 2003;32:1371–1375
43. Abete P, Ferrara N, Cioppa A, Ferrara P, Bianco S, Calabrese C, Cacciatore F, Longobardi G, Rengo F. Preconditioning does not prevent postischemic dysfunction in aging heart. J Am Coll Cardiol 1996;7:1777–1786
44. Przyklenk K, Li G, Whittaker P. No loss in the in vivo efficacy of ischemic preconditioning in middle-aged and old rabbits. J Am Coll Cardiol 2001;38:1741–1747
45. Burns PG, Krunkenkamp IB, Calderone CA, Kirvaitis RJ, Gaudette GR, Levitsky S. Is the preconditioning response conserved in senescent myocardium? Ann Thorac Surg 1996;61:925–929
46. Abete P, Ferrara N, Cacciatore F, Madrid A, Bianco S, Calabrese C, Napoli C, Scognamiglio P, Bollella O, Cioppa A, Longobardi G, Rengo F. Angina-induced protection against myocardial infarction in adult and elderly patients: a loss of preconditioning mechanism in the aging heart? J Am Coll Cardiol 1997;30:947–954
47. Lee TM, Su SF, Chou TF, Lee YT, Tsai CH. Loss of preconditioning by attenuated activation of myocardial ATP-sensitive potassium channels in elderly patients undergoing coronary angioplasty. Circulation 2002;105: 334–340
48. Bartling B, Friedrich I, Silber RE, Simm A. Ischemic preconditioning is not cardioprotective in senescent human myocardium. Ann Thorac Surg 2003;76:105–111
49. Bartling B, Hilgefort C, Friedrich I, Silber RE, Simm A. Cardioprotective determinants are conserved in aged human myocardium after ischemic preconditioning. FEBS Lett 2003;555:539–544
50. Taylor RP, Starnes JW. Age, cell signalling and cardioprotection. Acta Physiol Scand 2003;178:107–116
51. Lakatta EG, Yin FC. Myocardial aging: functional alterations and related cellular mechanisms. Am J Physiol 1992;242:H927–H941
52. Przyklenk K, Li G, Simkhovich BZ, Kloner RA. Mechanisms of myocardial ischemic preconditioning are age related: PKC-epsilon does not play a requisite role in old rabbits. J Appl Physiol 2003;95:2563–2569
53. Kristo G, Yoshimura Y, Keith BJ, Mentzer RM Jr, Lasley RD. Aged rat myocardium exhibits normal adenosine receptor-mediated bradycardia and coronary vasodilation but increased adenosine agonist-mediated cardioprotection. J Gerontol A Biol Sci Med Sci 2005;60:1399–1404
54. McCully JD, Uematsu M, Parker RA, Levitsky S. Adenosine-enhanced ischemic preconditioning provides enhanced cardioprotection in the aged heart. Ann Thorac Surg 1998;66:2037–2043
55. Willems L, Ashton KJ, Headrick JP. Adenosine-mediated cardioprotection in the aging myocardium. Cardiovasc Res 2005;66:245–255
56. Ashton KJ, Nilsson U, Willems L, Holmgren K, Headrick JP. Effects of aging and ischemia on adenosine receptor transcription in mouse myocardium. Biochem Biophys Res Commun 2003;312:367–372
57. Headrick JP, Willems L, Ashton KJ, Holmgren K, Peart J, Matherne GP. Ischaemic tolerance in aged mouse myocardium: the role of adenosine and effects of A1 adenosine receptor overexpression. J Physiol 2003;549:823–833
58. Shinmura K, Nagai M, Tamaki K, Bolli R. Gender and aging do not impair opioid-induced late preconditioning in rats. Basic Res Cardiol 2004;99:46–55
59. Loubani M, Ghosh S, Galinanes M. The aging human myocardium: tolerance to ischemia and responsiveness to ischemic preconditioning. J Thorac Cardiovasc Surg 2003;126:143–147
60. Peart JN, Gross GJ. Chronic exposure to morphine produces a marked cardioprotective phenotype in aged mouse hearts. Exp Gerontol 2004;39:1021–1026
61. Sniecinski R, Liu H. Reduced efficacy of volatile anesthetic preconditioning with advanced age in isolated rat myocardium. Anesthesiology 2004;100:589–597
62. Zheng J, Chin A, Duignan I, Won KH, Hong MK, Edelberg JM. Growth factor-mediated reversal of senescent dysfunction of ischemia-induced cardioprotection. Am J Physiol Heart Circ Physiol 2006;290:H525–H530
63. Juhaszova M, Rabuel C, Zorov DB, Lakatta EG, Sollott SJ. Protection in the aged heart: preventing the heartbreak of old age? Cardiovasc Res 2005;66:233–244
64. Brown KA, Chu Y, Lund DD, Heistad DD, Faraci FM. Gene transfer of extracellular superoxide dismutase protects against vascular dysfunction with aging. Am J Physiol Heart Circ Physiol 2006;290:H2600–H2605
65. Iida S, Chu Y, Francis J, Weiss RM, Gunnett CA, Faraci FM, Heistad DD. Gene transfer of extracellular superoxide dismutase improves endothelial function in rats with heart failure. Am J Physiol Heart Circ Physiol 2005;289:H525–H532
66. Grzenkowicz-Wydra J, Cisowski J, Nakonieczna J, Zarebski A, Udilova N, Nohl H, Jozkowicz A, Podhajska A, Dulak J. Gene transfer of CuZn superoxide dismutase enhances the synthesis of vascular endothelial growth factor. Mol Cell Biochem 2004;264:169–181
67. Abunasra HJ, Smolenski RT, Morrison K, Yap J, Sheppard MN, O'Brien T, Suzuki K, Jayakumar J, Yacoub MH. Efficacy of adenoviral gene transfer with manganese superoxide dismutase and endothelial nitric oxide synthase in reducing ischemia and reperfusion injury. Eur J Cardiothorac Surg 2001;20:153–158

68. Woo YJ, Zhang JC, Vijayasarathy C, Zwacka RM, Englehardt JF, Gardner TJ, Sweeney HL. Recombinant adenovirus-mediated cardiac gene transfer of superoxide dismutase and catalase attenuates postischemic contractile dysfunction. Circulation 1998;98:II255–II260
69. Li Q, Bolli R, Qiu Y, Tang XL, Guo Y, French BA. Gene therapy with extracellular superoxide dismutase protects conscious rabbits against myocardial infarction. Circulation 2001;103:1893–1898
70. Okubo S, Wildner O, Shah MR, Chelliah JC, Hess ML, Kukreja RC. Gene transfer of heat-shock protein 70 reduces infarct size in vivo after ischemia/reperfusion in the rabbit heart. Circulation 2001;103:877–881
71. Zhu HL, Stewart AS, Taylor MD, Vijayasarathy C, Gardner TJ, Sweeney HL. Blocking free radical production via adenoviral gene transfer decreases cardiac ischemia-reperfusion injury. Mol Ther 2000;2:470–475
72. Schriner SE, Linford NJ, Martin GM, Treuting P, Ogburn CE, Emond M, Coskun PE, Ladiges W, Wolf N, Van Remmen H, Wallace DC, Rabinovitch PS. Extension of murine life span by overexpression of catalase targeted to mitochondria. Science 2005;308:1909–1911
73. Abraham NG. Therapeutic applications of human heme oxygenase gene transfer and gene therapy. Curr Pharm Des 2003;9:2513–2524
74. Pachori AS, Melo LG, Zhang L, Solomon SD, Dzau VJ. Chronic recurrent myocardial ischemic injury is significantly attenuated by pre-emptive adeno-associated virus heme oxygenase-1 gene delivery. J Am Coll Cardiol 2006;47:635–643
75. Melo LG, Agrawal R, Zhang L, Rezvani M, Mangi AA, Ehsan A, Griese DP, Dell'Acqua G, Mann MJ, Oyama J, Yet SF, Layne MD, Perrella MA, Dzau VJ. Gene therapy strategy for long-term myocardial protection using adeno-associated virus-mediated delivery of heme oxygenase gene. Circulation 2002;105:602–607
76. Liu X, Pachori AS, Ward CA, Davis JP, Gnecchi M, Kong D, Zhang L, Murduck J, Yet SF, Perrella MA, Pratt RE, Dzau VJ, Melo LG. Heme oxygenase-1 (HO-1) inhibits postmyocardial infarct remodeling and restores ventricular function. FASEB J 2006;20:207–216
77. Tang YL, Qian K, Zhang YC, Shen L, Phillips MI. A vigilant, hypoxia-regulated heme oxygenase-1 gene vector in the heart limits cardiac injury after ischemia-reperfusion in vivo. J Cardiovasc Pharmacol Ther 2005;10: 251–263
78. Tang Y, Schmitt-Ott K, Qian K, Kagiyama S, Phillips MI. Vigilant vectors: adeno-associated virus with a biosensor to switch on amplified therapeutic genes in specific tissues in life-threatening diseases. Methods 2002;28:259–266
79. Tang YL, Tang Y, Zhang YC, Qian K, Shen L, Phillips MI. Protection from ischemic heart injury by a vigilant heme oxygenase-1 plasmid system. Hypertension 2004;43:746–751
80. Dulak J, Zagorska A, Wegiel B, Loboda A, Jozkowicz A. New strategies for cardiovascular gene therapy: regulatable pre-emptive expression of pro-angiogenic and antioxidant genes. Cell Biochem Biophys 2006;44:31–42
81. Kruger AL, Peterson SJ, Schwartzman ML, Fusco H, McClung JA, Weiss M, Shenouda S, Goodman AI, Goligorsky MS, Kappas A, Abraham NG. Up-regulation of heme oxygenase provides vascular protection in an animal model of diabetes through its antioxidant and antiapoptotic effects. J Pharmacol Exp Ther 2006;319:1144–1152
82. Juan SH, Lee TS, Tseng KW, Liou JY, Shyue SK, Wu KK, Chau LY. Adenovirus-mediated heme oxygenase-1 gene transfer inhibits the development of atherosclerosis in apolipoprotein E-deficient mice. Circulation 2001;104:1519–1525
83. Hoekstra KA, Godin DV, Cheng KM. Protective role of heme oxygenase in the blood vessel wall during atherogenesis. Biochem Cell Biol 2004;82:351–359
84. Bouche D, Chauveau C, Roussel JC, Mathieu P, Braudeau C, Tesson L, Soulillou JP, Iyer S, Buelow R, Anegon I. Inhibition of graft arteriosclerosis development in rat aortas following heme oxygenase-1 gene transfer. Transpl Immunol 2002;9:235–238
85. Yang X, Doser TA, Fang CX, Nunn JM, Janardhanan R, Zhu M, Sreejayan N, Quinn MT, Ren J. Metallothionein prolongs survival and antagonizes senescence-associated cardiomyocyte diastolic dysfunction: role of oxidative stress. FASEB J 2006;20:1024–1026
86. Fang CX, Doser TA, Yang X, Sreejayan N, Ren J. Metallothionein antagonizes aging-induced cardiac contractile dysfunction: role of PTP1B, insulin receptor tyrosine phosphorylation and Akt. Aging Cell 2006;5:177–185
87. Storz P. Mitochondrial ROS-radical detoxification, mediated by protein kinase D. Trends Cell Biol 2007;17: 13–18
88. Storz P, Doppler H, Toker A. Protein kinase D mediates mitochondrion-to-nucleus signaling and detoxification from mitochondrial reactive oxygen species. Mol Cell Biol 2005;25:8520–8530
89. Sanz A, Caro P, Barja G. Protein restriction without strong caloric restriction decreases mitochondrial oxygen radical production and oxidative DNA damage in rat liver. J Bioenerg Biomembr 2004;36:545–552
90. Sanz A, Caro P, Ayala V, Portero-Otin M, Pamplona R, Barja G. Methionine restriction decreases mitochondrial oxygen radical generation and leak as well as oxidative damage to mitochondrial DNA and proteins. FASEB J 2006;20:1064–1073
91. Kujoth GC, Hiona A, Pugh TD, Someya S, Panzer K, Wohlgemuth SE, Hofer T, Seo AY, Sullivan R, Jobling WA, Morrow JD, Van Remmen H, Sedivy JM, Yamasoba T, Tanokura M, Weindruch R, Leeuwenburgh C, Prolla TA.

Mitochondrial DNA mutations, oxidative stress, and apoptosis in mammalian aging. Science 2005;309: 481–484
92. Trifunovic A, Hansson A, Wredenberg A, Rovio AT, Dufour E, Khvorostov I, Spelbrink JN, Wibom R, Jacobs HT, Larsson NG. Somatic mtDNA mutations cause aging phenotypes without affecting reactive oxygen species production. Proc Natl Acad Sci USA 2005;102:17993–17998
93. Trifunovic A, Wredenberg A, Falkenberg M, Spelbrink JN, Rovio AT, Bruder CE, Bohlooly Y-M, Gidlof S, Oldfors A, Wibom R, Tornell J, Jacobs HT, Larsson NG. Premature ageing in mice expressing defective mitochondrial DNA polymerase. Nature 2004;429:417–423
94. Zhang D, Mott JL, Farrar P, Ryerse JS, Chang SW, Stevens M, Denniger G, Zassenhaus HP. Mitochondrial DNA mutations activate the mitochondrial apoptotic pathway and cause dilated cardiomyopathy. Cardiovasc Res 2003;57:147–157
95. Takao M, Aburatani H, Kobayashi K, Yasui A. Mitochondrial targeting of human DNA glycosylases for repair of oxidative DNA damage. Nucleic Acids Res 1998;26:2917–2922
96. Hudson EK, Hogue BA, Souza-Pinto NC, Croteau DL, Anson RM, Bohr VA, Hansford RG. Age-associated change in mitochondrial DNA damage. Free Radic Res 1998;29:573–579
97. Souza-Pinto NC, Croteau DL, Hudson EK, Hansford RG, Bohr VA. Age-associated increase in 8-oxo-deoxyguanosine glycosylase/AP lyase activity in rat mitochondria. Nucleic Acids Res 1999;27:1935–1942
98. Dobson AW, Xu Y, Kelley MR, LeDoux SP, Wilson GL. Enhanced mitochondrial DNA repair and cellular survival after oxidative stress by targeting the human 8-oxoguanine glycosylase repair enzyme to mitochondria. J Biol Chem 2000;275:37518–37523
99. Rachek LI, Grishko VI, Musiyenko SI, Kelley MR, LeDoux SP, Wilson GL. Conditional targeting of the DNA repair enzyme hOGG1 into mitochondria. J Biol Chem 2002;277:44932–44937
100. Chatterjee A, Mambo E, Zhang Y, Deweese T, Sidransky D. Targeting of mutant hogg1 in mammalian mitochondria and nucleus: effect on cellular survival upon oxidative stress. BMC Cancer 2006;6:235
101. Rachek LI, Grishko VI, Alexeyev MF, Pastukh VV, LeDoux SP, Wilson GL. Endonuclease III and endonuclease VIII conditionally targeted into mitochondria enhance mitochondrial DNA repair and cell survival following oxidative stress. Nucleic Acids Res 2004;32:3240–3247
102. Druzhyna NM, Hollensworth SB, Kelley MR, Wilson GL, Ledoux SP. Targeting human 8-oxoguanine glycosylase to mitochondria of oligodendrocytes protects against menadione-induced oxidative stress. Glia 2003;42:370–378
103. Muratovska A, Lightowlers RN, Taylor RW, Turnbull DM, Smith RA, Wilce JA, Martin SW, Murphy MP. Targeting peptide nucleic acid (PNA) oligomers to mitochondria within cells by conjugation to lipophilic cations: Implications for mitochondrial DNA replication, expression and disease. Nucleic Acids Res 2001;29: 1852–1863
104. Geromel V, Cao A, Briane D, Vassy J, Rotig A, Rustin P, Coudert R, Rigaut JP, Munnich A, Taillandier E. Mitochondria transfection by oligonucleotides containing a signal peptide and vectorized by cationic liposomes. Antisense Nucleic Acid Drug Dev 200;11:175–180
105. Flierl A, Jackson C, Cottrell B, Murdock D, Seibel P, Wallace DC. Targeted delivery of DNA to the mitochondrial compartment via import sequence-conjugated peptide nucleic acid. Mol Ther 2003;7:550–557
106. Weissig V, Lasch J, Erdos G, Meyer HW, Rowe TC, Hughes J. DQAsomes: a novel potential drug and gene delivery system made from Dequalinium. Pharm Res 1998;15:334–337
107. D'Souza GG, Boddapati SV, Weissig V. Mitochondrial leader sequence – plasmid DNA conjugates delivered into mammalian cells by DQAsomes co-localize with mitochondria. Mitochondrion 2005;5:352–358
108. D'Souza GG, Rammohan R, Cheng SM, Torchilin VP, Weissig V. DQAsome-mediated delivery of plasmid DNA toward mitochondria in living cells. J Control Release 2003;92:189–197
109. Guy J, Qi X, Pallotti F, Schon EA, Manfredi G, Carelli V, Martinuzzi A, Hauswirth WW, Lewin AS. Rescue of a mitochondrial deficiency causing leber hereditary optic neuropathy. Ann Neurol 2002;52:534–542
110. Zullo SJ, Parks WT, Chloupkova M, Wei B, Weiner H, Fenton WA, Eisenstadt JM, Merril CR. Stable transformation of CHO Cells and human NARP cybrids confers oligomycin resistance (oli(r)) following transfer of a mitochondrial DNA-encoded oli(r) ATPase6 gene to the nuclear genome: a model system for mtDNA gene therapy. Rejuvenation Res 2005;8:18–28
111. Manfredi G, Fu J, Ojaimi J, Sadlock JE, Kwong JQ, Guy J, Schon EA. Rescue of a deficiency in ATP synthesis by transfer of MTATP6, a mitochondrial DNA-encoded gene, to the nucleus. Nat Genet 2002;30:394–399
112. Ono T, Isobe K, Nakada K, Hayashi J. Human cells are protected from mitochondrial dysfunction by complementation of DNA products in fused mitochondria. Nat Genet 2001;28:272–275
113. Nakada K, Inoue K, Ono T, Isobe K, Ogura A, Goto YI, Nonaka I, Hayashi JI. Inter-mitochondrial complementation: mitochondria-specific system preventing mice from expression of disease phenotypes by mutant mtDNA. Nat Med 2001;7:934–940
114. Khan SM, Smigrodzki RM, Swerdlow R. Cell and animal models of mtDNA biology: progress and prospects. Am J Physiol Cell Physiol 2007;292:C658–C669

115. Clark MA, Shay JW. Mitochondrial transformation of mammalian cells. Nature 1982;295:605–607
116. Enriquez JA, Cabezas-Herrera J, Bayona-Bafaluy MP, Attardi G. Very rare complementation between mitochondria carrying different mitochondrial DNA mutations points to intrinsic genetic autonomy of the organelles in cultured human cells. J Biol Chem 2000;275:11207–11215
117. Attardi G, Enriquez JA, Cabezas-Herrera J. Inter-mitochondrial complementation of mtDNA mutations and nuclear context. Nat Genet 2002;30:360
118. Sato A, Nakada K, Hayashi J. Mitochondrial dynamics and aging: mitochondrial interaction preventing individuals from expression of respiratory deficiency caused by mutant mtDNA. Biochim Biophys Acta 2006;1763: 473–481
119. Spees JL, Olson SD, Whitney MJ, Prockop DJ. Mitochondrial transfer between cells can rescue aerobic respiration. Proc Natl Acad Sci USA 2006;103:1283–1288
120. Khrapko K. Mitochondrial DNA gene therapy: a gene therapy for aging? Rejuvenation Res 2005;8:6–8
121. Hansel A, Kuschel L, Hehl S, Lemke C, Agricola HJ, Hoshi T, Heinemann SH. Mitochondrial targeting of the human peptide methionine sulfoxide reductase (MSRA), an enzyme involved in the repair of oxidized proteins. FASEB J 2002;16:911–913
122. Iemitsu M, Miyauchi T, Maeda S, Tanabe T, Takanashi M, Irukayama-Tomobe Y, Sakai S, Ohmori H, Matsuda M, Yamaguchi I. Aging-induced decrease in the PPAR-alpha level in hearts is improved by exercise training. Am J Physiol Heart Circ Physiol 2002;283:H1750–H1760
123. Sanguino E, Roglans N, Alegret M, Sanchez RM, Vazquez-Carrera M, Laguna JC. Atorvastatin reverses age-related reduction in rat hepatic PPARalpha and HNF-4. Br J Pharmacol 2005;145:853–861
124. Tarnopolsky MA, Beal MF. Potential for creatine and other therapies targeting cellular energy dysfunction in neurological disorders. Ann Neurol 2001;49:561–574
125. Kelso GF, Porteous CM, Coulter CV, Hughes G, Porteous WK, Ledgerwood EC, Smith RA, Murphy MP. Selective targeting of a redox-active ubiquinone to mitochondria within cells: antioxidant and antiapoptotic properties. J Biol Chem 2001;276:4588–4596
126. Smith RA, Porteous CM, Gane AM, Murphy MP. Delivery of bioactive molecules to mitochondria in vivo. Proc Natl Acad Sci USA 2003;100:5407–5412
127. Adlam VJ, Harrison JC, Porteous CM, James AM, Smith RA, Murphy MP, Sammut IA. Targeting an antioxidant to mitochondria decreases cardiac ischemia-reperfusion injury. FASEB J 2005;19:1088–1095
128. Zhao K, Zhao GM, Wu D, Soong Y, Birk AV, Schiller PW, Szeto HH. Cell-permeable peptide antioxidants targeted to inner mitochondrial membrane inhibit mitochondrial swelling, oxidative cell death and reperfusion injury. J Biol Chem 2004;279:34682–34690
129. Torchilin VP. Recent approaches to intracellular delivery of drugs and DNA and organelle targeting. Annu Rev Biomed Eng 2006;8:343–375
130. Farout L, Friguet B. Proteasome function in aging and oxidative stress: implications in protein maintenance failure. Antioxid Redox Signal 2006;8:205–216
131. Grune T, Merker K, Jung T, Sitte N, Davies KJ. Protein oxidation and degradation during postmitotic senescence. Free Radic Biol Med 2005;39:1208–1215
132. Davies KJ. Degradation of oxidized proteins by the 20S proteasome. Biochimie 2001;83:301–310
133. Davies KJ, Shringarpure R. Preferential degradation of oxidized proteins by the 20S proteasome may be inhibited in aging and in inflammatory neuromuscular diseases. Neurology 2006;66:S93–S96
134. Kaushik S, Cuervo AM. Autophagy as a cell-repair mechanism: activation of chaperone-mediated autophagy during oxidative stress. Mol Aspects Med 2006;27:444–454
135. Miyata S, Takemura G, Kawase Y, Li Y, Okada H, Maruyama R, Ushikoshi H, Esaki M, Kanamori H, Li L, Misao Y, Tezuka A, Toyo-Oka T, Minatoguchi S, Fujiwara T, Fujiwara H. Autophagic cardiomyocyte death in cardiomyopathic hamsters and its prevention by granulocyte colony-stimulating factor. Am J Pathol 2006;168:386–397
136. Brunk UT, Terman A. The mitochondrial-lysosomal axis theory of aging: accumulation of damaged mitochondria as a result of imperfect autophagocytosis. Eur J Biochem 2002;269:1996–2002
137. Komatsu M, Waguri S, Ueno T, Iwata J, Murata S, Tanida I, Ezaki J, Mizushima N, Ohsumi Y, Uchiyama Y, Kominami E, Tanaka K, Chiba T. Impairment of starvation-induced and constitutive autophagy in Atg7-deficient mice. J Cell Biol 2005;169:425–434
138. Lemasters JJ. Selective mitochondrial autophagy, or mitophagy, as a targeted defense against oxidative stress, mitochondrial dysfunction, and aging. Rejuvenation Res 2005;8:3–5
139. Cavallini G, Donati A, Taddei M, Bergamini E. Evidence for selective mitochondrial autophagy and failure in aging. Autophagy 2007;3:26–27
140. Donati A. The involvement of macroautophagy in aging and anti-aging interventions. Mol Aspects Med 2006;27:455–470
141. Bergamini E, Cavallini G, Donati A, Gori Z. The anti-ageing effects of caloric restriction may involve stimulation of macroautophagy and lysosomal degradation, and can be intensified pharmacologically. Biomed Pharmacother 2003;57:203–208

142. Abeliovich H, Zhang C, Dunn WA Jr, Shokat KM, Klionsky DJ. Chemical genetic analysis of Apg1 reveals a non-kinase role in the induction of autophagy. Mol Biol Cell 2003;14:477–490

143. de Grey AD, Alvarez PJ, Brady RO, Cuervo AM, Jerome WG, McCarty PL, Nixon RA, Rittmann BE, Sparrow JR. Medical bioremediation: prospects for the application of microbial catabolic diversity to aging and several major age-related diseases. Ageing Res Rev 2005;4:315–338

144. de Grey AD. Bioremediation meets biomedicine: therapeutic translation of microbial catabolism to the lysosome. Trends Biotechnol 2002;20:452–455

145. Serrano AL, Andres V. Telomeres and cardiovascular disease: does size matter? Circ Res 2004;94: 575–584

146. Liu SC, Wang SS, Wu MZ, Wu DC, Yu FJ, Chen WJ, Chiang FT, Yu MF. Activation of telomerase and expression of human telomerase reverse transcriptase in coronary atherosclerosis. Cardiovasc Pathol 2005;14: 232–240

147. Wootton M, Steeghs K, Watt D, Munro J, Gordon K, Ireland H, Morrison V, Behan W, Parkinson EK. Telomerase alone extends the replicative life span of human skeletal muscle cells without compromising genomic stability. Hum Gene Ther 2003;14:1473–1487

148. Di Donna S, Mamchaoui K, Cooper RN, Seigneurin-Venin S, Tremblay J, Butler-Browne GS, Mouly V. Telomerase can extend the proliferative capacity of human myoblasts, but does not lead to their immortalization. Mol Cancer Res 2003;1:643–653

149. Yudoh K, Matsuno H, Nakazawa F, Katayama R, Kimura T. Reconstituting telomerase activity using the telomerase catalytic subunit prevents the telomere shorting and replicative senescence in human osteoblasts. J Bone Miner Res 2001;16:1453–1464

150. Yang J, Chang E, Cherry AM, Bangs CD, Oei Y, Bodnar A, Bronstein A, Chiu CP, Herron GS. Human endothelial cell life extension by telomerase expression. J Biol Chem 1999;274:26141–26148

151. Oh H, Taffet GE, Youker KA, Entman ML, Overbeek PA, Michael LH, Schneider MD. Telomerase reverse transcriptase promotes cardiac muscle cell proliferation, hypertrophy, and survival. Proc Natl Acad Sci USA 2001;98:10308–10313

152. Samper E, Flores JM, Blasco MA. Restoration of telomerase activity rescues chromosomal instability and premature aging in Terc-/- mice with short telomeres. EMBO Rep 2001;2:800–807

153. Gorbunova V, Seluanov A, Pereira-Smith OM. Expression of human telomerase (hTERT) does not prevent stress-induced senescence in normal human fibroblasts but protects the cells from stress-induced apoptosis and necrosis. J Biol Chem 2002;277:38540–38549

154. von Zglinicki T. Oxidative stress shortens telomeres. Trends Biochem Sci 2002;27:339–344

155. Haendeler J, Hoffmann J, Diehl JF, Vasa M, Spyridopoulos I, Zeiher AM, Dimmeler S. Antioxidants inhibit nuclear export of telomerase reverse transcriptase and delay replicative senescence of endothelial cells. Circ Res 2004;94:768–775

156. Harley CB. Telomerase therapeutics for degenerative diseases. Curr Mol Med 2005;5:205–211

157. Imanishi T, Hano T, Nishio I. Angiotensin II accelerates endothelial progenitor cell senescence through induction of oxidative stress. J Hypertens 2005;23:97–104

158. Imanishi T, Hano T, Nishio I. Estrogen reduces endothelial progenitor cell senescence through augmentation of telomerase activity. J Hypertens 2005;23:1699–1706

159. Liu B, Wang J, Chan KM, Tjia WM, Deng W, Guan X, Huang JD, Li KM, Chau PY, Chen DJ, Pei D, Pendas AM, Cadinanos J, Lopez-Otin C, Tse HF, Hutchison C, Chen J, Cao Y, Cheah KS, Tryggvason K, Zhou Z. Genomic instability in laminopathy-based premature aging. Nat Med 2005;11:780–785

160. Cadinanos J, Varela I, Lopez-Otin C, Freije JM. From immature lamin to premature aging: molecular pathways and therapeutic opportunities. Cell Cycle 2005;4:1732–1735

161. Fong LG, Frost D, Meta M, Qiao X, Yang SH, Coffinier C, Young SG. A protein farnesyltransferase inhibitor ameliorates disease in a mouse model of progeria. Science 2006;311:1621–1623

162. Scaffidi P, Misteli T. Reversal of the cellular phenotype in the premature aging disease hutchinson-gilford progeria syndrome. Nat Med 2005;11:440–445

163. Columbaro M, Capanni C, Mattioli E, Novelli G, Parnaik VK, Squarzoni S, Maraldi NM, Lattanzi G. Rescue of heterochromatin organization in hutchinson-gilford progeria by drug treatment. Cell Mol Life Sci 2005;62:2669–2678

164. Shumaker DK, Dechat T, Kohlmaier A, Adam SA, Bozovsky MR, Erdos MR, Eriksson M, Goldman AE, Khuon S, Collins FS, Jenuwein T, Goldman RD. Mutant nuclear lamin A leads to progressive alterations of epigenetic control in premature aging. Proc Natl Acad Sci USA 2006;103:8703–8708

165. Celeste A, Petersen S, Romanienko PJ, Fernandez-Capetillo O, Chen HT, Sedelnikova OA, Reina-San-Martin B, Coppola V, Meffre E, Difilippantonio MJ, Redon C, Pilch DR, Olaru A, Eckhaus M, Camerini-Otero RD, Tessarollo L, Livak F, Manova K, Bonner WM, Nussenzweig MC, Nussenzweig A. Genomic instability in mice lacking histone H2AX. Science 2002;296:922–927

166. Quiles JL, Ochoa JJ, Huertas JR, Mataix J. Coenzyme Q supplementation protects from age-related DNA double-strand breaks and increases lifespan in rats fed on. Exp Gerontol 2004;39:189–194

167. de Boer J, Andressoo JO, de Wit J, Huijmans J, Beems RB, van Steeg H, Weeda G, van der Horst GT, van Leeuwen W, Themmen AP, Meradji M, Hoeijmakers JH. Premature aging in mice deficient in DNA repair and transcription. Science 2002;296:1276–1279
168. Armelini MG, Muotri AR, Marchetto MC, de Lima-Bessa KM, Sarasin A, Menck CF. Restoring DNA repair capacity of cells from three distinct diseases by XPD gene-recombinant adenovirus. Cancer Gene Ther 2005;12:389–396
169. Zeng L, Quilliet X, Chevallier-Lagente O, Eveno E, Sarasin A. Mezzina Retrovirus-mediated gene transfer corrects DNA repair defect of xeroderma pigmentosum cells of complementation groups A, B and C. Gene Ther 1997;4:1077–1084
170. Carreau M, Quilliet X, Eveno E, Salvetti A, Danos O, Heard JM, Mezzina M, Sarasin A. Functional retroviral vector for gene therapy of xeroderma pigmentosum group D patients. Hum Gene Ther 1995;6:1307–1315
171. Erol A. PPARalpha activators may be good candidates as antiaging agents. Med Hypotheses 2005;65:35–38
172. Pineda Torra I, Gervois P, Staels B. Peroxisome proliferator-activated receptor alpha in metabolic disease, inflammation, atherosclerosis and aging. Curr Opin Lipidol 1999;10:151–159
173. Melloul D, Stoffel M. Regulation of transcriptional coactivator PGC-1alpha. Sci Aging Knowledge Environ 2004;2004:pe9
174. Rodgers JT, Lerin C, Haas W, Gygi SP, Spiegelman BM, Puigserver P. Nutrient control of glucose homeostasis through a complex of PGC-1alpha and SIRT1. Nature 2005;434:113–118
175. Ling C, Poulsen P, Carlsson E, Ridderstrale M, Almgren P, Wojtaszewski J, Beck-Nielsen H, Groop L, Vaag A. Multiple environmental and genetic factors influence skeletal muscle PGC-1alpha and PGC-1beta gene expression in twins. J Clin Invest 2004;114:1518–1526
176. Picard F, Kurtev M, Chung N, Topark-Ngarm A, Senawong T, Machado De Oliveira R, Leid M, McBurney MW, Guarente L. Sirt1 promotes fat mobilization in white adipocytes by repressing PPAR-gamma. Nature 2004;429:771–776
177. Lemieux ME, Yang X, Jardine K, He X, Jacobsen KX, Staines WA, Harper ME, McBurney MW. The Sirt1 deacetylase modulates the insulin-like growth factor signaling pathway in mammals. Mech Ageing Dev 2005;126:1097–1105
178. Langley E, Pearson M, Faretta M, Bauer UM, Frye RA, Minucci S, Pelicci PG, Kouzarides T. Human SIR2 deacetylates p53 and antagonizes PML/p53-induced cellular senescence. EMBO J 2002;21:2383–2396
179. Yu J, Lei L, Liang Y, Hinh L, Hickey RP, Huang Y, Liu D, Yeh JL, Rebar E, Case C, Spratt K, Sessa WC, Giordano FJ. An engineered VEGF-activating zinc finger protein transcription factor improves blood flow and limb salvage in advanced-age mice. FASEB J 2006;20:479–481
180. Bhasin S, Calof OM, Storer TW, Lee ML, Mazer NA, Jasuja R, Montori VM, Gao W, Dalton JT. Drug insight: testosterone and selective androgen receptor modulators as anabolic therapies for chronic illness and aging. Nat Clin Pract Endocrinol Metab 2006;2:146–159
181. Schmidt U, del Monte F, Miyamoto MI, Matsui T, Gwathmey JK, Rosenzweig A, Hajjar RJ. Restoration of diastolic function in senescent rat hearts through adenoviral gene transfer of sarcoplasmic reticulum Ca(2+)-ATPase. Circulation 2000;101:790–796
182. Schmidt U, Zhu X, Lebeche D, Huq F, Guerrero JL, Hajjar RJ. In vivo gene transfer of parvalbumin improves diastolic function in aged rat hearts. Cardiovasc Res 2005;66:318–323
183. Michele DE, Szatkowski ML, Albayya FP, Metzger JM. Parvalbumin gene delivery improves diastolic function in the aged myocardium in vivo. Mol Ther 2004;10:399–403
184. Huq F, Lebeche D, Iyer V, Liao R, Hajjar RJ. Gene transfer of parvalbumin improves diastolic dysfunction in senescent myocytes. Circulation 2004;109:2780–2785

Chapter 15
Nutrition and Exercise in Cardiovascular Aging: Metabolic and Pharmacological Interventions

Overview

Caloric restriction (CR) without malnutrition is the most reproducible experimental manipulation that increases the mean and maximum life span of laboratory rodents. Data from a diverse group of organisms including yeast, worms, flies and mammals have shown that CR is an active, highly conserved stress response that likely evolved to increase an organism's chance of surviving adversity. Moreover, evidence suggests that CR significantly reduces the age-mediated morbidity and mortality associated with the cardiovascular system [1].

In this chapter, we will review current evidence that dietary interventions and exercise training, essentially parameters that are under lifestyle control, can impact both overall aging and more particularly cardiac and cardiovascular (CV) aging. While the great majority of this evidence derives from a variety of animal models, there is also some indication from studies of human subjects that these interventions may operate in humans as well, although some indications of species-specific effects (in particular with CR) have also been recently noted. We will further examine available information concerning the molecular and cellular basis underlying the effectiveness of these interventions and we will also discuss the development, and use of CR mimetics in a clinical setting, and potential application of these interventions in stemming aging.

Introduction

CR with adequate nutrition has been found to dramatically extend the maximum life span of a wide spectrum of laboratory organisms. It is important to note that victims of starvation and malnutrition do not experience the life-extending benefits of CR and that adequate nutrition (i.e., vitamins, minerals, essential amino acids and essential fatty acids in adequate quantity) is a prerequisite for CR diets to extend life span. In addition to its effects on longevity, CR markedly reduces the functional decline associated with aging maintaining most physiological functions at levels resembling those found in younger rather than older adults. CR also retards the development of age-related diseases, such as cardiomyopathy, diabetes, hypertension-related diseases, as well as neoplastic processes.

Rats, mice and hamsters experience maximum life span extension from a diet that contains 40–60% of the calories (but all of the required nutrients) consumed from normal diets. When long-term CR is begun just before puberty the mean life span is increased up to 65% and the maximum life span up to 50%. However, many beneficial effects of CR can be observed not only when initiated at a young age, but also in adulthood.

Insofar as CR seems to slow aging in rodents and many other short-lived species, long-term studies of CR on monkeys are presently being conducted to establish if CR also slows aging in primates. Although many of these studies will take years to obtain full longevity data, there are

J. Marín-García, *Aging and the Heart*,

early indications that rhesus monkeys (*Macaca mulatta*) subjected to CR will similarly show a wide spectrum of benefits, including lower body weight, body fat, blood glucose and thus are at lower risk for developing diabetes [2], as well as CR-induced attenuation of aging-associated changes in plasma triglycerides [3], melatonin [4], oxidative damage [5], and glucose tolerance [6]. Furthermore, two of the most robust biomarkers of CR detected in rodents, reduced body temperature and plasma insulin also were found in rhesus monkeys on CR. In addition, CR slows the rate of decline in serum adrenal steroid dehydroepiandrosterone sulfate (DHEAS) with CR monkeys exhibiting more youthful levels. Since DHEAS declines with age in both monkeys and humans, the potential relevance of these findings to human subjects are further underscored by the findings that male human subjects with elevated serum DHEAS levels exhibited greater survival in the Baltimore Longitudinal Study of Aging, and also had reduced body temperature and plasma insulin. [7]. Whether the benefits of CR seen in rodents apply to humans is to be more fully discussed in a later section.

Caloric Restriction (CR)

Overview of CR in Comparative Models

It has been known for over 70 years that restricting the food intake of laboratory rats can extend their mean and maximum life span. Life extension has been observed over the years in a large spectrum of other species, including mice, hamsters, dogs, fish, invertebrate animals, and yeast albeit it is not yet clear whether this kind of life extension can be mediated in primates and humans.

The mechanisms underlying CR's effects on life span remain unclear although several observations support attenuation of oxidative damage and alteration in growth hormone/insulin/IGF signaling in specific tissues. Many of the signaling pathways affected by CR are shared by a vast array of organisms suggesting that the genes involved in these pathways are in fact highly conserved. This has been confirmed by the discovery of mutations in homologous genes affecting growth hormone/insulin/IGF signaling and OS responses in species ranging from worms and yeast to mice and man, which have been shown to increase the life span of model organisms. Signaling and stress responses have been integrated into the hormetic hypothesis that proposes that low-intensity stressors, such as CR, activate ancient hormetic defense mechanisms in organisms ranging from yeast to mammals, protecting them against a variety of afflictions and, when long-term, delaying the senescent processes [8, 9]. Thus, evolution has allowed a way that the aging program can be abated in times of stress (e.g., CR).

Tissue-Specific and Cardiovascular-Specific Transcriptional and Proteomic Profiling of CR

CR in Heart and Skeletal Muscle

As previously discussed, the gene expression programs of several tissues (i.e., heart, and skeletal muscle) from animals subjected to CR have been profiled.

Microarray studies of the effects on long-term CR on cardiac gene expression revealed a pattern of altered murine gene expression consistent with reduced myocardial remodeling and fibrosis, and enhanced contractility and energy production via FAO [10]. An altered transcriptional pattern (compared to the untreated aging animals) was identified which was rather broad-based (over 20% of profiled genes showed significant changes) with over 75% of the changes associated with myocardial aging being either completely or partially reversed. The CR-mediated myocardial transcriptome changes included the suppression of structural genes transcription (e.g., collagen and ECM proteins), downregulation of DNA-inducible transcripts (presumably indicative of less endogenous DNA damage), proapoptotic factors and upregulation of DNA repair and antiapoptotic factors consistent with CR mediating a reduction of aging-induced endogenous damage. In addition, CR mediated a reversal of a number of age-induced transcript changes leading to upregulated glycolysis and downregulated FAO; CR completely prevented both the age-related downregulation of the glycolytic inhibitor *PDK4* and PFK upregulation, and partially restored FAO gene expression consistent with CR preventing the age-induced myocardial metabolic shift [11, 12].

Using microarray analysis of gastrocnemius muscle of male C57BL/6 mice, Lee et al. found, that aging results in a gene expression pattern indicative of marked stress response and lower expression of metabolic and biosynthetic genes. In CR treated mice, these aging-mediated changes in transcript expression were completely or partially prevented and suggested that CR retards the aging process in murine skeletal muscle by causing a metabolic shift toward increased protein turnover and decreased macromolecular damage [13, 14].

Comparison of 30 month old control and a parallel group of age-matched mice subjected to CR revealed that aging-related changes in muscle gene expression profiles were significantly attenuated by CR, with 29% of altered transcripts completely prevented and 34% partially suppressed by CR. Moreover, CR induced a metabolic reprogramming characterized by a transcriptional shift toward energy metabolism, increased biosynthesis, and protein turnover by both attenuating several key aging-mediated changes (e.g., G-6-P isomerase, EF-1-γ, 26*S* proteasome component TBP1) as well as by induction/repression of other genes. For instance, CR enhanced expression of transketolase, PPAR-γ and PPAR-α, pyruvate kinase and fatty acid synthase and downregulated inducible genes involved in metabolic detoxification, DNA repair, and response to OS.

In contrast to the significant reversal of age-related alterations in murine skeletal muscle by CR, including energy metabolism reprogramming, increased macromolecular biosynthesis and turnover, and reduced oxidative induced damage, beneficial aspects of CR at the transcriptional level in aging rhesus monkey skeletal muscle were not observed suggesting potential problems with timing of CR initiation or differential species-specificity regarding the CR mechanism [15].

Specific Pathways Affected

Oxidative Stress and ROS

While CR affects a number of parameters of aging, a highly consistent critical target for its effects is the mitochondria, in which it has shown to reverse the age-related ROS production and to reduce oxidative and mtDNA damage in a tissue-specific fashion.

Gathered observations, largely in rat and mice, have shown a lower mitochondrial free radical generation rate in a variety of tissues (including liver, heart, skeletal muscle and brain) in caloric-restricted animals compared with *ad libitum* (AL) fed animals [16, 17]. In skeletal muscle, the rate of superoxide anion radical generation by submitochondrial particles significantly increased with age in AL-fed mice, whereas in caloric-restricted mice there was no age-associated increase in superoxide anion radical generation [18]. In rat heart, Gredilla et al. [19] demonstrated that H_2O_2 production in mitochondria respiring with complex I-linked substrate pyruvate/malate was increased with age, but not in aging rats under a long-term CR regimen (1 year); however, no significant difference was found in AL and CR tissues in the mitochondrial free radical leak when the complex II-linked substrate succinate was used. Moreover, mitochondrial oxygen consumption with any substrate was not affected with diet in either CR or AL animals. These results suggest that the decrease in mitochondrial ROS production in restricted animals primarily occurs at complex I and is not due to a diminution in mitochondrial oxygen consumption, but rather to a reduction of the complex I ROS generator that decreases its percentage of free radical leak. One year of CR in rats has been shown to reduce liver mitochondrial hydrogen peroxide production from Complex I by 47% [20]. Comparison of different tissue responses to CR-mediated reduction in ROS production is not entirely clear-cut. For instance, in one study senescent brain from CR-mice exhibited a two-fold reduction in superoxide levels compared to old AL mice, whereas reduction in superoxide levels in heart was only 30% [17]. However, in rat, H_2O_2 levels declined with CR treatment by 24% in brain compared to 45% in heart [19, 21, 22]. Interestingly, quantitative reduction in mtDNA oxidative damage (and not nuclear DNA oxidative damage) was strikingly similar to that found for mitochondrial free radical generation (this will be further addressed below). This CR-mediated reduction in mtDNA damage is prevalent in a variety of tissues (e.g., heart, liver, skeletal muscle). In regard to reduction in the mitochondrial rate of free radical generation and the oxidative damage to mtDNA in the rat heart and liver, later observations indicated less clear-cut benefits of either short-term (6 week) or medium-term CR regimen [22]. Similar experiments showed no effect of medium term CR on mitochondrial free radical generation in either kidney or skeletal muscle [23]. Furthermore, Sanz et al. have demonstrated that a 1 year CR regimen started late in life can improve oxidative stress-related parameters. After CR initiation at 24 months of age, the rate of mitochondrial H_2O_2 production significantly decreased (by 24%) and oxidative damage to mtDNA (by 23%) in the brain, below the level of both old and young AL-fed animals rats [21].

Mitochondria Function and Biogenesis

The role that CR may play in mitochondrial physiology is complex; this has been confirmed by several reports indicating that not all mitochondrial dysfunction associated with aging is reversed by CR. For instance, Lambert et al. reported that in isolated mitochondria from liver, heart, brain and kidney of male Brown Norway rats (fully fed and CR) there was no significant effect of CR on state 4 respiration rate [24]. Experiments focusing on the effects of lifelong CR on rat skeletal muscle mitochondria have shown that an aging-mediated decline in ATP content and production (over 50%), which may be a contributory factor in sarcopenia, was not affected by a CR regimen whereas CR significantly reduced both mtDNA damage and ROS (i.e., H_2O_2) production [25]. On the other hand, Hepple et al. have shown that aging-mediated decline in skeletal muscle citrate synthase and respiratory I-IV enzyme activities (in 35 month old rats) were reversed by long-term CR [26]. Subsequent observations by these investigators in skeletal muscle of CR versus AL animals indicated that a factor in CR's prevention of the age-related decline in mitochondrial oxidative capacity was a slower decline with aging in the gene expression of the global mitochondrial biogenesis factor peroxisome proliferation-activated receptor coactivator (PGC-1α), suggesting that overall mitochondrial biogenesis is better maintained with aging in CR animals [27, 28].

Using a novel *in vitro* CR approach, Lopez et al. have demonstrated in a more direct manner that CR stimulates the proliferation of mitochondria through a PGC-1α signaling pathway [29]. This approach features incubation of HeLa cells, FaO cells, and primary hepatocytes in the presence of serum from rats submitted to long-term CR (40% for 6–12 month) compared with cells incubated with serum from age-matched, AL-fed rats. Fluorimetric analysis showed a significant decrease in ROS production and a decline in mitochondrial membrane potential ($\Delta\ \psi$m) in CR cells (analogous to the decreased ROS levels found with CR *in vivo*, as previously noted) when compared with cells grown in AL serum. Bioenergetic analysis revealed that an equivalent amount of ATP was produced in CR-treated cells relative to cells treated with AL serum with significantly lower oxygen consumption and reduced ROS production (i.e., higher overall bioenergetic efficiency). Increased mitochondrial mass (indicated by Mitotracker green staining), increased immunohistochemical staining of

COX subunits, cytochrome *c*, cardiolipin and citrate synthase activity confirmed findings observed by electron microscopy, that the number of mitochondria were significantly elevated in CR cells. This also suggested that the CR-mediated mitochondrial biogenesis and enhanced bioenergetic efficiency involved PGC-1α signaling mediated in part by PGC-1-dependent nuclear respiratory factors (NRFs). Both NRF-1 and NRF-2 transcripts were significantly increased in CR serum-treated cells compared with AL serum-treated cells; disrupted expression of PGC-1 by using RNAi caused attenuation in decreased oxygen consumption in CR serum-treated cells.

Further support for the role of elevated mitochondrial biogenesis in CR has been recently provided by Nisoli et al. who demonstrated that both short-term (3 month) and long-term (12 month) CR in male mice resulted in increased mitochondrial biogenesis, increased oxygen consumption and ATP production, and enhanced expression of sirtuin 1, both preceded by induced endothelial nitric oxide synthase (eNOS) expression and 3′,5′-cyclic guanosine monophosphate formation (shown in Fig. 15.1) While these CR-mediated mitochondrial changes were primarily documented in white adipose tissue, similar findings were obtained in brain, liver and heart [30]. On the other hand, in contrast to the marked effects of CR on free radical production, experiments with rat liver [31], heart [32], and mouse skeletal muscle [18] and kidney [33] have failed to show any clear-cut overall pattern of CR-related changes in antioxidant defenses, ruling out antioxidants as determinants of the lower oxidative damage observed in CR animals.

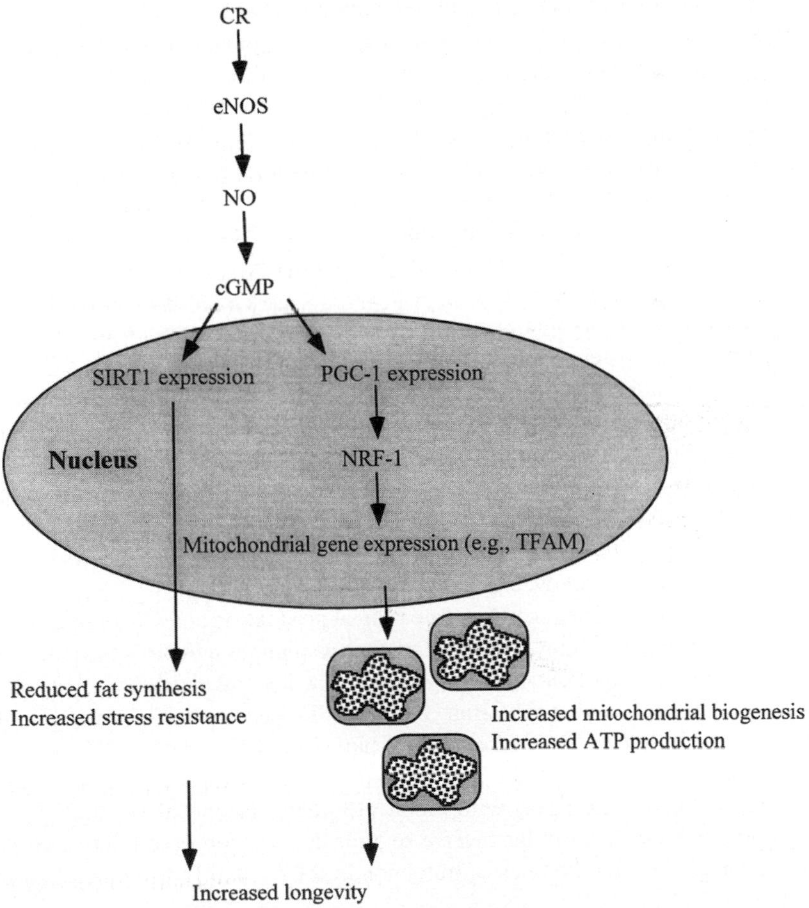

Fig. 15.1 Role of CR in mitochondrial biogenesis. Elevated SIRT1 expression is mediated by NO

MtDNA Damage and Repair

Observations from various tissues and different species revealed that the relative amount of oxidative base damage found in mtDNA was increased compared to nuclear DNA damage. Various base modifications, particularly 8-hydroxydeoxyguanosine (8OHdG) were detected, which can lead to subsequent point mutations because of mispairing. In the liver of 6 month old rats the extent of oxidative damage in mtDNA, gauged by levels of 8-oxodG, is 16 times greater than to nuclear DNA [34]. Similarly, Zastawny et al. found in pig liver significantly increased levels of oxidative base modifications in mtDNA compared to nuclear DNA [35].

There is strong evidence that oxidative DNA damage accumulates with age in rat mitochondrial DNA, an indication that mitochondria are primary targets for a heavy load of oxidative DNA damage. While mitochondria have a base excision repair (BER) process responsible for the removal of most endogenous damage including alkylation damage, depurination reactions and oxidative damage, it remains unclear how much of the age-associated mtDNA damage accumulation is secondary to an aging-mediated decline in DNA repair. Several studies have demonstrated that the accumulation of DNA damage cannot be completely explained by an attenuation of DNA repair since the mitochondrial incision of 8-oxoG increases with age in rodents [36, 37]; however, several observations have shown evidence of declining DNA repair capacity (in both nuclear and mitochondria BER). The import of selective mitochondrial DNA glycosylases (including uracil glycosylase and OGG) into the mitochondrial matrix, necessary for mtDNA base excision repair, is compromised in aging human fibroblasts and defective in aging mice [38]. This would effectively lower the intramitochondrial activity of the enzyme, despite apparently unchanged protein levels. A significant age-dependent decrease in incision activities of three glycosylases (oxoguanine DNA glycosylase, OGG1, uracil DNA glycosylase, UDG and the endonuclease III homologue, NTH1) in the mitochondria of all brain regions has been reported and suggests that decreased efficiency of mitochondrial BER-glycosylases may be insufficient to repair increased mtDNA oxidative damage, and is contributory to the normal aging process [39].

Although CR does not reduce oxidative damage (8-oxodG) to rat liver nuclear DNA and only reduces oxidative damage to mouse liver nuclear DNA by 19%, it completely eliminates mtDNA damage in both the rat and mouse [40, 41]. In mice, CR also significantly reduced the accumulation of mtDNA rearrangements that occurs with aging in post-mitotic tissues, particularly in the brain [42]. The highly-consistent decrease observed in mtDNA damage with CR is not due to a general upregulation of mitochondrial BER in either heart or brain; this is in apparent contrast with nuclear BER pathways that are significantly increased with CR [43]. These findings suggest that the lower mtDNA damage or enhanced mitochondrial genomic stability with CR is primarily due to its effect on decreased ROS production and decreased mtDNA lesion formation, rather than its effect on repair. An alternative explanation is that CR may stimulate macroautophagy (as occurs in response to anti-lipolytic treatment with subsequent removal of 8-OHdG damaged mtDNA) rescuing older cells; this is an interesting but unproven hypothesis [44].

While there is little information regarding free radical production and CR in primates and human, it is noteworthy that studies with long-lived species such as pigeons and birds have demonstrated that oxidative damage to DNA (in particular mtDNA) tends to be lower than in short-lived mammals [45], consistent with the low rate of mitochondrial oxygen radical generation observed in all long-lived species investigated [46]. In fact, an inverse relationship of longevity with mtDNA oxidative damage in the heart and brain has been reported in mammalian species, comparing the relatively short-lived rodents (3–4 year maximum life span) with rabbit (13 year), sheep (20 year), pig (27 year), cow (30 year) and horse (46 year); a similar inverse relationship was observed between maximum life span in mammalian species and the rates of mitochondrial $O^{2\cdot-}$ and H_2O_2 generation in the kidney and the heart [47].

Genomic Instability

Generalized damage to nuclear DNA with aging has been previously discussed in Chapter 4. Mutations in DNA accumulate during the aging of somatic tissues, as well as in cultured fibroblasts during replicative senescence. A contributory factor to the accumulation of genomic damage in aging is a decline in DNA repair. Cabelof et al. found a decline in the repair capacity of the BER pathway in multiple tissues (e.g., brain, liver, spleen and testes) of the 24 month old mouse (compared to tissues of 4 month old mouse) concomitant with 3–5 fold increases in spontaneous and chemically-induced mutation frequency [48]. The age-mediated reduction in repair capacity correlated with decreased levels of DNA polymerase β (β-pol) enzymatic activity, protein and mRNA. Other investigators have observed a lack of inducibility (in response to oxidative damage) of both β-pol, a rate-limiting enzyme in the BER pathway and AP endonuclease (APE) in aging murine tissues [49].

In the previous section of this chapter we have discussed that CR promotes enhanced genomic stability by induction of the BER pathway in the nucleus [43]. While this observation showed increased nuclear BER activity in tissues of CR mice (e.g., kidney, liver), no significant differences were found in activities of nuclear DNA glycosylases (OGG1, UDG, NTH1) or APE. In other experiments, CR completely reversed the age-related decline in BER capacity in all tissues tested (brain, liver, spleen and testes) providing aged, CR animals with the BER phenotype of young, AL-fed animals. This CR-induced reversal of the aged BER phenotype was accompanied by a reversal in the age-related decline in β-pol activity, protein and mRNA levels in all analyzed tissues [48].

In addition to oxidative base damage directed repair, age-related decline in DNA double-strand break (DSB) repair in unstimulated human lymphocytes has been reported [50]. An important element of the DSB recognition and repair pathways is the DNA-dependent protein kinase (DNA-PK), which consists of two components, a catalytic subunit (DNA-PKcs) and a Ku autoantigen (Ku) that is a DNA-binding protein, consisting of Ku70 and Ku80 heterodimeric regulatory components. CR prevented age-associated modulation of Ku70/80 in a tissue-specific manner. CR attenuated decreasing Ku expression and its activity in old aged rat kidney and lung but did not prevent severely impaired Ku expression and activity in the testis and had no effect at all on liver Ku expression [51].

IGF/Growth Hormone/SIR Involvement

In Chapter 12, we have described evidence from a variety of model systems of aging and longevity, ranging from the yeast and *C. elegans* to flies and mice, that IGF and GH signaling pathways are determinant factors of aging and longevity and also play a role (not yet by any means entirely defined) in cardiovascular aging.

The decrease in tissue function that is observed in aging animals has been linked to a decline in rates of protein synthesis, which may be caused, in part, by reduced secretion of growth hormone (GH) and insulin-like growth factor 1 (IGF-1). AL-fed male Brown Norway rats displayed age-related decreases in plasma IGF-1, IGF binding protein (IGF-BP) and in the rates of protein synthesis of the heart (36%) and liver (38%), and maintained a relatively constant density of type 1 IGF receptor in all tissues with age [52]. In contrast, while CR rats exhibited plasma IGF-1 and IGF-BP concentrations lower than the AL-fed animals, rates of protein synthesis increased by 70 and 30% in heart and diaphragm in association with 60–100% increases in type 1IGF receptor densities, when compared with AL fed animals. Moderate CR induces adaptive endocrine changes, including an increase in growth hormone secretory dynamics and a decline in plasma levels of IGF-1 that serve to maintain blood levels of glucose [53]. These alterations are thought to decrease the stimulus for cellular replication, resulting in a decline in pathologies and increased life span in these animals.

Hypopituitary mutant Ames dwarf mice and growth-hormone-resistant (growth hormone receptor knockout, GHR-KO) mice have reduced plasma levels of IGF-1 and insulin, enhanced insulin sensitivity and a remarkably increased life span; strikingly similar to the phenotypic characteristics of normal animals subjected to CR. Interestingly, hepatic Akt phosphorylation was reduced in both CR and GHR-KO mice, the forkhead box (Foxo1) transcription factor was additively increased by both CR and GHR-KO at the mRNA level, and protein levels of the deacetylase sirtuin 1 (SIRT1) were elevated implying a major role for the Akt/Foxo1 pathway in both the CR and GH/IGF axis regulation of longevity in rodents [54]. Interestingly, CR leads to further increases in insulin sensitivity and longevity in Ames dwarf strains but not in GHR-KO mice, suggesting that distinct but overlapping pathways may be involved in these modified aging phenotypes [55]. While the transcript levels of IR, IRS1, IRS2, GLUT4 and IGF-1 were reduced by CR in skeletal muscle in both normal and GHR-KO mice [56, 57], CR increased the cardiac expression of IR, IRS1, IGF-1, IGF-1R and GLUT4 in normal mice and IRS1, GLUT4, PPAR-α and PPAR-β/δ in GHR-KO animals. Elevated levels of hepatic PPAR-γ and PPAR-α mRNAs and proteins, found in long-lived GHR-KO mice as compared to normal mice, may underlie the enhanced insulin sensitivity of GHR-KO mice while CR may increase insulin sensitivity through a different mechanism.

CR reverses age-dependent decreases in the global regulatory factors PPAR-α, PGC-1α, and their regulated genes albeit differentially in a tissue-specific manner [58]. For instance, CR blunts the age-mediated decline in the PPAR family nuclear protein, mRNA level, and DNA binding activity in rat kidney [59], but not in murine skeletal muscle [60]. Long-term CR rats were associated with increased expression of the transcription factor mRNAs in the liver for PPAR-α, γ and δ but decreased expression for the sterol regulatory element binding protein (SREBP-1c) resulting in a concerted modulation in the expression of key transcription target genes involved in fatty acid oxidation [61]. Moreover, the notion that some effects of CR are mediated by PPAR-α has received support by the recent demonstration of significant overlaps between the CR transcript profile in wild-type mice liver and the profiles altered by agonists of lipid-activated PPAR-α, and related nuclear receptors, including liver X receptor, and their obligate heterodimer partner, retinoid X receptor [62]. The overlapping genes included those involved in CVD (lipid metabolism and inflammation) and cancer (cell fate). Moreover, CR protection was lost in PPAR-α -null mice due to inadequate tissue repair.

In yeast, worms and flies, the SIR2 gene has been implicated in mediating the life-extending effects of calorie restriction [63]. There is evidence that the expression of mammalian SIR2 homologue (SIRT1) is induced in many tissues (including brain, liver, visceral fat pads and kidney) of CR rats and likely plays a role in this pathway [64]. Moreover, human cells treated with serum from these CR animals exhibited increased SIRT1 expression and recapitulated key *in vivo* proliferative and phenotypic features of CR including the induction of characteristic stress-response genes and the attenuation of stress-induced apoptosis. Interestingly, cells treated with CR serum supplemented with insulin or IGF-1, displayed reduced SIRT1 expression and no phenotypic effects.

The mammalian SIRT1 (sirtuin 1), activates a critical component of CR in mammals regulating fat mobilization in white adipose tissue [65]. Upon food withdrawal, SIRT1 protein binds to and represses genes controlled by the transcriptional regulator PPAR-γ, including genes mediating fat storage. SIRT1 represses PPAR-γ by docking with its cofactors NCoR (nuclear receptor co-repressor) and SMRT (silencing mediator of retinoid and thyroid hormone receptors). The repression of PPAR-γ by SIRT1 is also evident in adipocytes, where overexpression of SIRT1 attenuates adipogenesis [65]. In differentiated fat cells, upregulation of SIRT1 triggers lipolysis and loss of fat.

A number of other cellular homeostatic and signaling pathways are directly affected by SIRT1 (depicted in Fig. 15.2). For instance, SIRT1is a regulatory factor in the gluconeogenic/glycolytic pathways in liver in response to fasting signals through the transcriptional coactivator PGC-1α [66]. Induction of the SIRT1 protein in liver during fasting is triggered by pyruvate as a result of a nutrient signaling response. Upon induction, SIRT1 interacts with and deacetylates PGC-1α at

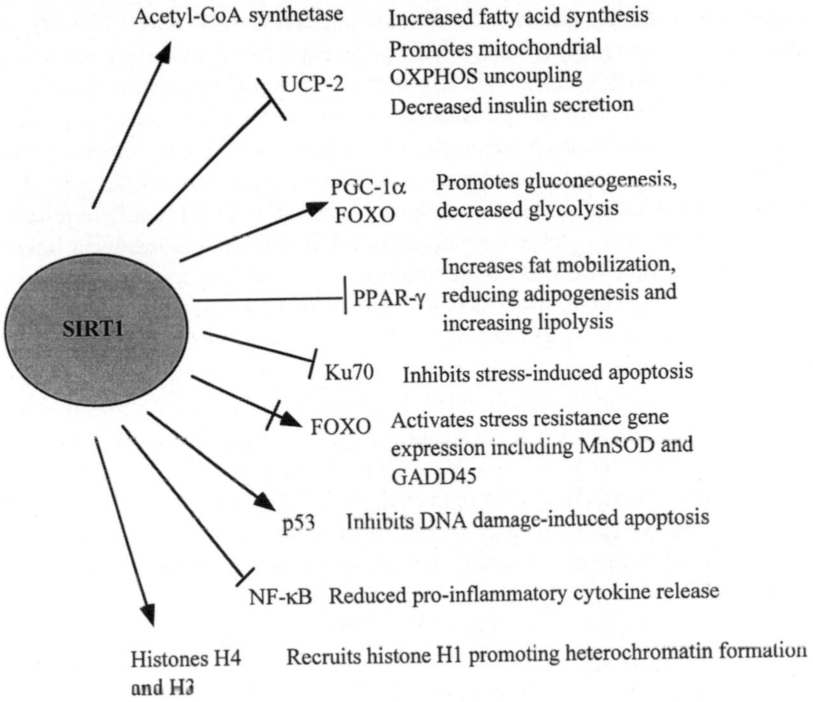

Fig. 15.2 SIRT1 has multiple effects on metabolic and stress signaling components

specific lysine residues in a NAD^+-dependent manner leading to PGC-1α-mediated induction of gluconeogenic genes and hepatic glucose output; it is noteworthy that SIRT1's promotion of hepatic glucose production is opposite to its function in pancreatic β-cells, where it promotes insulin secretion, thus leading to glucose utilization by peripheral tissues. In addition, SIRT1 modulates the effects of PGC-1α repression of glycolytic genes in response to fasting and pyruvate. Sirtuins including SIRT1 also have recently been shown to mediate another relevant metabolic effect, the deacylation and activation of mammalian acetyl-CoA synthetases, which can lead to increased fatty acid synthesis and regulated intracellular acetyl-CoA levels [67]. In addition to SIRT1's critical role in regulating the activities of the nuclear receptor PPAR-γ and PGC-1α, influencing differentiation of muscle cells, adipogenesis, fat storage in white adipose tissue and hepatic metabolism (as discussed above), SIRT1 has other effects on homeostasis and metabolism. Recent observations using either SIRT1-overexpressing (BESTO) mice [68], or SIRT1−/− mice [69], revealed that SIRT1 positively regulates glucose-stimulated insulin secretion in pancreatic β-cells. Moreover, SIRT1 was found to repress transcription of the mitochondrial uncoupling protein UCP-2 gene, which normally acts to uncouple mitochondrial respiration from ATP production, reducing the proton gradient across the mitochondrial membrane and leading to decreased ATP, required for the secretion of insulin. By suppressing the expression of UCP-2 and reducing UCP-2 function in pancreatic β cells, SIRT1 promotes more efficient energy generation and enhances insulin secretion. However, it is not yet known whether SIRT1 regulates insulin secretion during CR or plays any role in pathologies associated with impaired insulin secretion.

SIRT1 function has multiple effects on the regulation of glucose homeostasis through its role in insulin secretion and by its contribution to survival in the context of pancreatic cells and in gluconeogenesis in the liver. Thus, targeting or modulating the activity of SIRT1 and possibly other sirtuins may prove useful in the treatment of diabetes, where aberrant glucose homeostasis and β-cell dysfunction are key manifestations of the disease.

SIRT1 deacetylates a large number of substrates, including p53, Ku70, NF-κB, and forkhead proteins to affect stress resistance in cells, which may relate to the observed stress resistance conferred by CR [64, 70–72]. SIRT1 deacetylates several transcription factors involved in the regulation of cell cycle progression and apoptosis consistent with a role in the fundamental processes underlying cancer. For instance, SIRT1 deacetylates the tumor suppressor p53 to inhibit its transcriptional activity, resulting in reduced apoptosis in response to various genotoxic stimuli [71, 73].

SIRT1 regulates and inactivates the transcription factor NF-κB[72] that is required for the transcription of growth factors and cytokines involved in inflammation and has been linked to diseases such as Type 2 diabetes and cancer. By its regulation of several forkhead family transcription factors, including FOXO1, FOXO3a, and FOXO4, SIRT1 likely enhances the expression of FOXO target genes involved in stress responses and cell cycle arrest such as MnSOD, GADD45 and p27 [70, 74], and suppresses transcription of some insulin response element (IRS)-driven genes (e.g., IGFBP1) [75]. Furthermore, SIRT1 mediates deacetylation of the DNA repair factor Ku70 preserving its association with the proapoptotic protein Bax and preventing the translocation of Bax to mitochondria to initiate apoptosis [76]. SIRT1 also has been shown to have effects on epigenetic alterations of chromatin, which have been implicated in cancer regulation, and are thought to have an impact on genomic stability and aging. SIRT1 deacetylates specific lysine residues (K26) on histone H1 and promotes heterochromatin formation through spreading of hypomethylated lysine residues (K79) on histone H3 [77].

Experimental evidence suggests that SIRT1 has a protective role against neuronal and cardiac damage. Alcendor et al. have shown that sirtuin inhibition, by either nicotinamide or sirtinol in isolated neonatal rat cardiomyocytes resulted in cell death in a p53-dependent manner [78]. They also demonstrated that SIRT1 overexpression caused an increase in cardiomyocyte size and protected cells from apoptosis following serum starvation. In addition, these investigators found that SIRT1 levels were markedly increased in a canine model of heart failure (HF), due to aortic banding and pacing, possibly as a result of failed prevention of cell death.

At least six other sirtuins have been reported in mammalian cells including human. While substantial information is available concerning their subcellular localization (3 have been localized to mitochondria) and regulation, their precise role in aging and in CR has not yet been determined [79]. However, gathered observations have shown that SIRT6 is a nuclear, chromatin-associated protein that promotes resistance to DNA damage and suppresses genomic instability in mouse cells, in association with a role in base excision repair. Mostoslavsky et al. have recently shown that SIRT6 loss in mice leads to premature aging as SIRT6-deficient mice at 2–3 weeks of age develop lymphopenia, loss of subcutaneous fat, decreased bone density, and severe metabolic defects and eventually die at about 4 weeks [80]. In addition, mouse embryonic fibroblasts (MEFs) lacking SIRT6 show impaired proliferation and enhanced sensitivity to DNA-damaging agents, and MEFs derived from SIRT6 null strains exhibit genomic instability in the form of chromosomal translocations, fragments, gaps, and detached centromeres, but maintain normal cell cycle checkpoints, end-joining, and double-strand break DNA repair.

Vascular Inflammation

Studies of vascular aging have shown that aging Fischer rats have elevated levels of prostaglandin E2 (PGE2), PGI2, thromboxane A2 (TXA2) and increased gene expression of several prostanoid synthase enzymes [81]. CR was found to attenuate the age-related prostanoid changes by suppressing inflammatory activities. Activity of myeloperoxidase (MPO), a heme protein existing in neutrophil and monocyte, which has been implicated in various stages of inflammation in concert with the production of a variety of potent oxidants, increased during aging in AL rat kidney, but was significantly attenuated by CR [82]. Furthermore, the amount of dityrosine, a stable MPO-oxidation end product increased in old AL, but not in old CR rats. These findings suggest that increased MPO activity with aging may participate in the increased recruitment of inflammatory cells contributing to protein oxidation accumulation in the aging process, and can be attenuated by CR anti-inflammatory action. Moreover, studies with CR in 24 month-old Fischer rats showed older AL-fed rats exhibited increased levels of vascular adhesion proteins (aortic P-selectin and vascular adhesion molecule-1, VCAM-1) compared to older CR-fed rats [83]. These elevations were also closely related to activation of redox-sensitive NIK/IKK/IκB/nuclear factor-κB pathway brought on by OS. Other observations have established that the serum levels of a number of soluble adhesion molecules, including E-selectin, P-selectin, VCAM-1, and intercellular adhesion molecule 1 (ICAM-1) are significantly increased during aging in AL rats, but effectively blunted in the CR rats [84]. This upregulation of adhesive factors was found to coincide with increased ROS/RNS and superoxide-generating xanthine oxidase levels in serum during aging, and was suppressed by CR.

Examination of the aorta of aging rats fed either AL or CR diets revealed other significant alterations of age-related changes with CR. Compared with aged AL-fed rats, CR-fed animals showed less pronounced age-dependent alterations such as collagen accumulation and elastic fiber degradation, with aortic elastic fibers displaying lower content of LDL, decorin and elastase and higher HDL [85]. These findings suggest that CR likely impacts the aging process of the arterial wall in rats, delaying the appearance of age-related degenerative features, such as structural alterations of cells and matrix and modified interactions of elastin with other extracellular matrix molecules.

Dissection of the CR Process: Which Aspect of the Diet Does the Signaling (Evidence Favoring Protein Restriction Versus Carbohydrate/Lipid)

Several investigators have attempted to delineate whether a single-class of nutrients in the caloric restricted diet might be responsible for some of the aforementioned effects on aging and cardiovascular function. Barja et al. have recently focused on the role of protein and methionine restriction. To investigate the role of dietary proteins, the ingestion of proteins in Wistar rats was decreased by 40%, below that of controls, while other dietary components were ingested at the same level as in AL-fed animals [86]. After seven weeks of this protein restricted (PR) diet, the liver showed 30–40% decreases in mitochondrial production of reactive ROS and in oxidative damage to nuclear and mitochondrial DNA, strikingly similar to data previously obtained after 40% CR in the liver of Wistar rats. These findings suggest that part of the decrease in aging rate induced by CR can be due to decreased intake of proteins acting through reduction in mitochondrial ROS production and oxidative DNA damage. Similar studies in which dietary lipids were restricted by 40% with protein and carbohydrates levels maintained, or in which carbohydrate levels were restricted by 40% without changing the intake level of the other dietary components, found neither changes to liver mitochondrial H_2O_2 production nor hepatic oxidative mtDNA or nuclear DNA damage in lipid-restricted or carbohydrate-restricted animals [87, 88]. Interestingly, methionine may be the key dietary component responsible for the decrease in mitochondrial ROS generation and OS in both PR and CR. Methionine restriction profoundly decreases ROS production, decreases mtDNA oxidative damage, lowers membrane unsaturation, decreases markers of protein oxidation measured in rat heart and liver mitochondria and activity levels of respiratory complexes I and IV [89]. Moreover, methionine restriction also increases maximum longevity in rats [90, 91], and recent observations indicate that methionine levels in tissue negatively correlate with maximum longevity in mammals and bird [92]. Significantly, restricting only the intake of dietary proteins or methionine to nullify aging-mediated OS may represent a more feasible option than CR for adult individuals.

Interestingly, reduction in glucose also may contribute to enhanced longevity as shown directly in yeast [93]. Whether as a diminished component of diet or not, dietary restriction tends to reduce blood glucose levels, reduces cell glycation damage (by reducing exposure to glucose) and delays the development of glucose-induced glycolytic capacity [94], and therefore may mediate many of the cumulative toxic effects of glucose associated with age-related pathologies such as diabetes, cataract, Alzheimer's, atherosclerosis and Parkinson's, as well as physiological aging [95].While there is no direct evidence that CR's effect on glycation plays a major role in its anti-aging action, recent observations have also shown that high caloric intake, based on saturated fat, promotes Alzheimer disease type β-amyloidosis, and conversely dietary restriction based on reduced carbohydrate intake is able to prevent it in a mouse model [96, 97].

Development of CR Mimetics

An alternative way to apply the potential benefits of CR to enhance human cardiovascular health and longevity is to identify and test agents that may mimic critical actions of CR. Several important outcomes of CR including the reduction of oxidative metabolic stress, alterations of the stress signaling response and improved glucoregulation (i.e., lowering circulating glucose and insulin concentrations or to increase insulin sensitivity) have provided a number of candidate targets for CR mimetic action [98]. Several compounds have been identified that mimic CR effects by targeting metabolic and stress response pathways affected by CR, but without actually restricting caloric intake. For example, agents that inhibit glycolysis (2-deoxyglucose 2DG), and enhance insulin action (metformin) have been assessed as CR mimetics [99]. 2DG is a synthetic glucose analog that inhibits the glycolytic enzyme phosphohexose isomerase that upon injection into rodents suppresses tumor growth, decreases insulin and body temperature and increases glucocorticoids, all of which parallel CR [100]. However, chronic administration of 2DG enlarges the heart and increases the chance of congestive HF, making it unlikely to extend animal life span.

Other areas providing potential targets include intermediary metabolism, response to infection, and source of dietary fat. The intriguing relationship between the effects of nuclear receptors which act as specific global transcriptional regulators (e.g., PPAR-α, PPAR-γ and PGC-1) on genes involved in glucose and lipid metabolism, bioenergetics, stress signaling and inflammation and their overlap with CR activated genes suggests that agonists of these nuclear receptors might elicit the same gene expression profiles and metabolic actions as CR [62].

Given that CR affects short-lived organisms including worms, flies and yeast, an attractive approach is to screen for molecules that increase life span in these models or that can activate molecules believed to be associated with CR (e.g., sirtuins).

Resveratrol Studies

A class of polyphenolic molecules produced by plants in response to stress including resveratrol, butein, and piceatannol activates the human sirtuin SIRT1 activity both *in vitro* and *in vivo* [101]. The compound with the greatest stimulatory activity was resveratrol, a polyphenol found in red wine, which activates the SIR2 sirtuin from yeast, increases DNA stability and mimics the effects of CR by extending life span of specific yeast strains. Resveratrol can activate sirtuins from metazoans such as *C. elegans* and *Drosophila melanogaster*, can extend their life span (albeit modestly) without reducing fecundity [102], as well as significantly affect life span and delay the onset of age-related dysfunction in a short-lived fish (*Nothobranchius furzeri*) [103]. Interestingly, despite its potent effect on aging, the activation of sirtuins by resveratrol is presently a subject of some controversy [104, 105], and its known interaction with other proteins including mitochondrial ATP synthase, mitochondrial complex III, fatty-acid synthase, protein kinase C, p53, MEK1, TNF-α, NF-κB and AMP kinase may be important in mediating its *in vivo* effects.

Bauer et al. have recently showed that mice fed a diet akin to coconut cream pie for every meal exhibited a dramatic increase in survival and health when their food was supplemented with resveratrol [106]. Compared with animals fed a more standard diet, mice fed a high-calorie (60% from fat) diet without resveratrol had a shorter life span, displayed obesity, insulin resistance and heart disease. These investigators found that although resveratrol did not prevent obesity, it did prevent obesity-associated disease (in one strain of mouse), and conferred a nearly normal life span on these mice. Furthermore, it simulated a number of the physiological effects of CR including increased insulin sensitivity, reduced IGF-1 levels, increased AMP-activated protein kinase (AMPK) and PGC-1 activity, increased mitochondrial number, and improved motor function. However, many of the plant derived sirtuin activators like resveratrol have poor stability and relatively low potency as SIRT1 activators; synthetically improved derivatives are currently being designed and tested for their effects on life span in the yeast model system [107]. A flow chart of the signaling pathways involved in the activation of CR by mimetics is shown in Fig. 15.3.

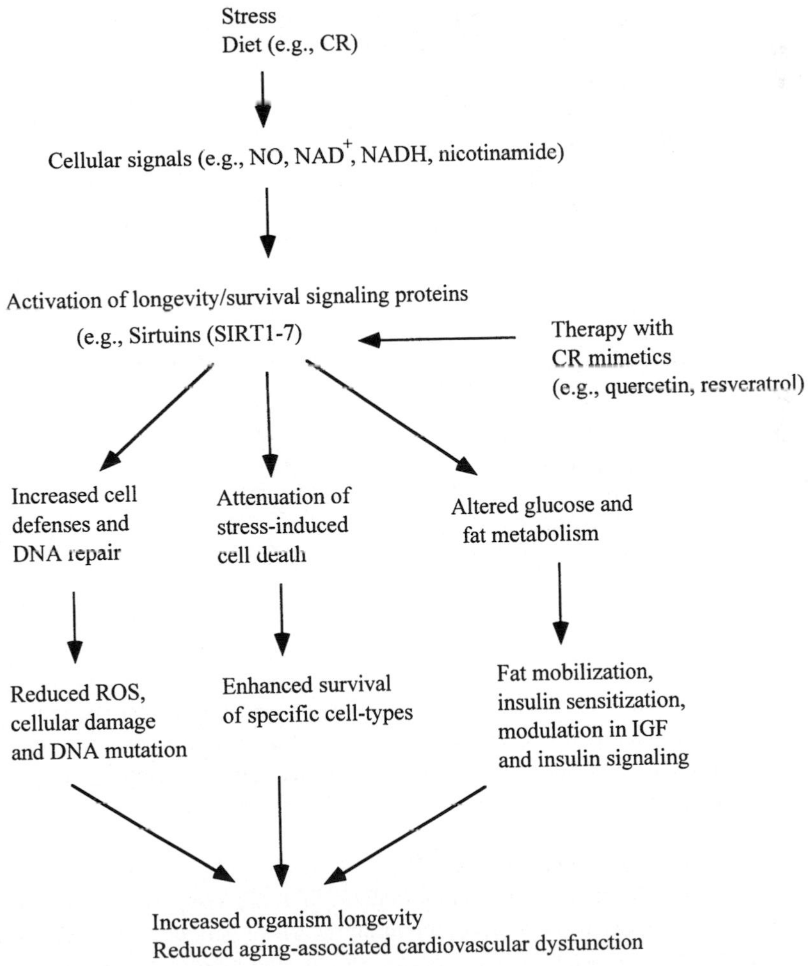

Fig. 15.3 The overall effect of CR and mimetics on aging and signaling pathways shown as a flow chart

Conclusions

Whether CR will offer similar benefits to humans remain unclear. Arguments from an evolutionary point of view have suggested that the large increases in life span resulting from CR observed in rodents such as mice and rats, species with early sexual maturity, narrow reproductive span and large litter size, will not be likely in humans, a species with late sexual maturity, broad reproductive span, small litter size and an entirely different metabolic stability [108, 109]. Moreover, there are some indications of species-specificity in CR responsivity with recent observations that CR decreases the life span of the housefly, *Musca domestica*, and fails to extend the life span of at least one mouse strain [110]. Despite the lack of information on the benefits, potential side-effects and pitfalls of long term CR in humans, research on short-term CR or "weight loss" programs suggest beneficial outcomes in parameters of cardiovascular disease [111]. Furthermore, clinical application of alternative CR mimetics need the unqualified development of more potent, less toxic (safer) well-tested compounds.

New Directions

Pharmacological Reversal of Aging

A complete discussion of pharmacological treatment of aging and its many associated diseases is beyond the perview of this book. In this section we will focus on the use of therapies with pharmacological supplements primarily targeting cardiovascular diseases in aging.

A pharmacological compound, acetylcarnitine (ALCAR) has therapeutic potential for several aging-associated cardiovascular and neurodegenerative disorders, and current evidence suggests that it may play a critical role as a modulator of cellular stress response [112]. Supplements of acetyl-l-carnitine and (R)-α-lipoic acid have been used to improve myocardial bioenergetics and decrease the OS associated with aging while reversing the mitochondrial dysfunction found in the aging heart [113]. A number of tissues from old rats fed with acetyl-l-carnitine showed a reversal of the age-related decline in carnitine levels and improved mitochondrial fatty acid β-oxidation. Lesnefsky et al. have shown that pretreatment with acetylcarnitine in the aged rat following ischemia significantly reduced the heart injury. Indices of mitochondrial function (i.e., overall oxidative phosphorylation rate and respiratory activities of complexes III and IV) were restored to young adult levels as was myocardial contractile recovery during reperfusion [114]. By itself, ALCAR supplementation does not appear to reverse the age-related decline in the cardiac antioxidant status and may not improve the indices of OS [113]. Lipoic acid, a potent thiol antioxidant appears to increase low molecular weight antioxidant status and thereby decreases age-associated oxidative insult, and can reverse an aging-mediated glutathione redox deficit in post-mitotic tissues [115]. Gathered observations have documented the beneficial aspects of acetylcarnitine treatment in combination with lipoic acid in aged rats with a restoration of mitochondrial function, lower oxidant, neuron RNA oxidation and mutagenic aldehydes levels, improved glutathione redox function and increases in rat ambulatory activity and cognition [116, 117]; in addition significant effects on lipid metabolism have been shown. Supplementation of acetyl-l-carnitine for 3 months significantly increased tissue carnitine levels (e.g., heart and brain), decreased all lipoprotein fractions and consequently the levels of triacylglycerol and cholesterol in aged rats [118].

Furthermore, the lipophilic antioxidant and mitochondrial redox coupler coenzyme Q_{10} may have the potential to improve energy production in the aging heart mitochondria by bypassing defective components in the respiratory chain, as well as by reducing the effects of OS. Data from rats and human suggest that coenzyme Q_{10} protects the aging heart against stress [119].

According to the popular media, it would appear that the use of antioxidants to slow/stop aging-related cardiac defects is a well-established fact. However, so far, there is a lack of rigorously obtained evidence supporting this conclusion. In addition, concerns have been raised how much of these antioxidant agents should be administered without jeopardizing the ROS "protector side" role in the heart signaling pathways. Furthermore, Sohal et al. have recently reappraised the role of coenzyme Q as a potential aging-reversal supplement and found no significant effect of coenzyme Q supplementation on murine life span, proxidant generation (e.g., superoxide), protein oxidative damage, or on mitochondrial activities in multiple tissues during aging [120].

The development of myocardial and large vessel stiffness with aging underlies the development of diastolic HF and isolated systolic hypertension. As we have previously discussed, formation of advanced glycation endproducts (AGE), a result of nonenzymatic reaction between glucose and proteins, leads to collagen cross-linking in the myocardium and arterial wall and has been implicated in age-related increase in cardiovascular stiffness and cardiac dysfunction [121]. Several observations indicated that treatment with aminoguanidine (AG), an inhibitor of protein cross-linking, retards age-related decline in the elastic properties of the left ventricle and arteries. Previously, it was found that AG supplementation in both aged Fischer and Sprague-Dawley rats prevented significant increases in the AGE content in aged cardiac, aortic and renal tissues, as well as the marked age-linked vasodilatory impairment in response to acetylcholine and nitroglycerine and the age-related cardiac hypertrophy evident in both strains [122]. Cormon et al. have shown that AG treatment could significantly reduce cardiac hypertrophy as well as arterial stiffness (gauged by prevention of age-related increases in aortic impedance and decreases in carotid distensibility) in 30 month-old rats with no changes in elastin and collagen content [123].

Moreau et al. found in 28 month-old Fischer 344 rats that the levels of Nε-carboxymethyl lysine (CML) content in serum, aorta, and heart proteins was double that found in 4 month-old rats [124]. AG administration (by addition to drinking water) to old rats for 3 months from the age of 25 months lowered CML content by 15, 44, and 28% in serum, aorta, and heart, respectively. In addition, AG can have beneficial effects on the left ventricular-arterial coupling in aged Fischer 344 rats [125], as well as on aortic stiffness [126], mediating significant improvements in aging-diminished arterial and ventricular function. Other AGE cross-link breakers have been shown to have significant effects by reducing age-related left ventricular stiffness and improving cardiac function [127].

Role of Exercise

Exercise has been shown to improve the mean longevity but does not appear to affect the maximal longevity. Cumulative data have shown that exercise training provides beneficial cardiovascular effects in both animal models and human subjects. In addition to numerous hemodynamic effects, there is clear evidence that exercise training participates in tissue remodeling as well as in improving energetic aspects of muscle function, which has been shown to provide benefits in both animal models and patients with HF [128]. In this section we will survey the beneficial effects of exercise as well as examine the most likely molecular and cellular mechanisms by which exercise exerts them.

Gene Profiling

Several investigators have utilized gene profiling of aging subjects to examine the global effects on tissue-specific gene expression in response to exercise. Research on the effects of exercise training on myocardial gene expression has been performed largely in animals, including a large variety of models and conditions such as pacing-induced HF in dogs [129], rats with myocardial infarction [130], pathological cardiac hypertrophy and apoptosis in SHR rats [131]. Moreover, myocardial gene profiling of exercised-trained aging rat showed a reversal of the aging-induced downregulation of cardiac VEGF angiogenic signaling cascade, thereby contributing to the exercise training-induced improvement of angiogenesis and capillary density in the heart [132].

Bronokowski et al. have carried out a comprehensive study on myocardial gene expression in relation to exercise training and aging. They found that exercise training attenuated or reduced many of the gene expression changes that normally occur in the aging heart, including genes involved in inflammatory response, stress response, signal transduction, and energy metabolism [133].

Other investigators have also performed gene expression profiling in skeletal muscle from exercise-trained aging animal models [134] and human subjects [135]. Following exercise training one study found increased expression of VEGF in skeletal muscle of patients with HF [136]. Furthermore, enhanced antioxidant expression (specifically Cu/Zn SOD and GPx) in the skeletal muscle vasculature followed exercise training in patients with chronic HF [137]. Another interesting finding was that skeletal muscle from older men (62–75 year-old) exhibited an altered gene expression profile in response to resistance exercise training compared to younger men, suggesting a variable response at the transcriptional level [138].

Specific Pathways Affected

Ischemia/Reperfusion/Apoptosis/Remodeling

Endurance exercise provides cardioprotection against I/R-induced cell death in aged Fischer 344 rats, primarily by reducing I/R-induced myocardial apoptosis. The mechanisms for this exercise-induced cardioprotection against I/R-induced apoptosis may be mediated by improved myocardial antioxidant capacity and the prevention of calpain and caspase-3 activation [139]. Compared to sedentary animals, French et al. found that exercise training prevented the I/R-induced rise in calpain activity and improved cardiac work in working heart derived from adult male rats [140]. The pharmacological inhibition of calpain activity also resulted in cardioprotection against I/R injury. This exercise-induced protection against I/R-induced calpain activation was not due to abnormal myocardial protein levels of calpain or calpastatin. Interestingly, exercise training was associated with increased levels of myocardial MnSOD, catalase and a reduction in OS. Other studies have also found that exercise training attenuates age-induced increases in remodeling, apoptosis, and Bax/Bcl-2 ratio in rat left ventricle [141]. In addition, exercise training also prevented the I/R-induced degradation of SERCA2a, apparently by increases in endogenous antioxidants.

Exercise intolerance has long been recognized as an important symptom of HF, but it also may develop in aged individuals without cardiac pathology. A number of non-specific factors such as skeletal muscle dysfunction (likely secondary to mitochondrial bioenergetics defects), ventilatory abnormalities, and endothelial dysfunction, individually or in association, may contribute to limitation in exercise capacity. A pivotal contributing factor for skeletal muscle catabolism (e.g., elevated cytokine expression) can be found in both normal, healthy aging, and in patients with HF [142]. This similar spectrum of aging and HF-associated changes in the skeletal muscle may underlie the more severe clinical presentation of the HF syndrome among elderly patients. A decline in maximal aerobic capacity and the ability to sustain submaximal exercise with advancing age was demonstrated in 27 month-old Fischer 344 × Brown Norway rats [143]. Using the same animal model, the effect of aging on muscle blood-flow with similar degrees of myocardial infarct-induced LV dysfunction, was evaluated [144]. A significant age-related redistribution of blood-flow from the highly oxidative to the highly glycolytic muscles of the hind limb was reported during exercise in old rats.

Mitochondrial Function and Stress Responses

The beneficial effects of moderate exercise on overall cardiac physiology and metabolism are well established. Experimental studies have also indicated that mitochondrial function and stress responses are affected by exercise. Fischer rats engaged in long-term voluntary wheel running exhibited significantly reduced H_2O_2 production from both mitochondrial subpopulations (subsarcolemmal [SSM] and interfibrillar [IFM]), and increased daily energy expenditure compared with sedentary controls. Additionally, MnSOD activity was significantly lowered in SSM and IFM from wheel runners, which may reflect a reduction in mitochondrial superoxide production [145].

Moderate exercise in a treadmill increased the life span of male and female mice (aged from 28 to 78 weeks) [146]. In addition, moderate exercise decreased the aging-associated ROS accumulation and ROS-mediated damage (e.g., oxidative damage to proteins and lipids) in a number of tissues including the heart, in part, by lessening the decrease in antioxidant enzymes (e.g., SOD and catalase) and preventing the decline in respiratory complex I and IV activities.

Myocardial Signaling

A number of myocardial signaling pathways are affected by exercise training. For instance, Korzick et al. have assessed cardiac contractility (dP/dt) in Langendorff-perfused hearts isolated from 5 month adult and 24 month-old Wistar rats, following maximal α1-AR stimulation with phenylephrine [147]. They found that the subcellular translocation of PKCα and PKCε, in response to α1-AR stimulation, is disrupted in the aging myocardium. Moreover, an age-related reduction in the levels of PKC-anchoring proteins (e.g., RACK1 and RACK2), which might contribute to impaired PKC translocation and defective α1-AR contraction in the aged rat heart, was found. Subsequently, this group of investigators determined in adult and aged rat whether age-related defects in α1-AR contraction could be reversed by chronic exercise training (treadmill) [148]. They found that the age-related decrease in α1-AR contractility in the rat heart can be partially reversed by exercise, suggesting that alterations in PKC levels underlie, at least in part, exercise training-induced improvements in α1-AR contraction.

As we have previously noted, an age-associated reduction in cardiovascular β-adrenergic (β-AR) responsiveness has been documented in aging Fischer 344 rats that corresponds with alterations in post-receptor adrenergic signaling rather than with a decrease in LV β-AR receptor number [149]. Interestingly, chronic exercise partially attenuated these changes through alterations in post-receptor elements of cardiac signal transduction.

Exercise training also improves the aging-induced downregulation of myocardial PPAR-α mediated signaling pathway, and contributes to an amelioration in fatty acid metabolic enzyme activity in rats [150]. Similar findings of exercise training induction of lipid metabolism gene expression have been reported in skeletal muscle in both animal models and humans [151, 152].

Calcium handling is a primary target of exercise training [129, 140]. Recent observations have demonstrated that aging-related downregulation of MHC and SERCA expression, mediated by myocardial thyroid hormone (TH)-receptor (TR) signaling-induced transcriptional control, can be reversed with exercise [153]. While the expression of the myocardial TRs (TRα1 and TRβ1) is significantly lower in sedentary aged rats than in young rats, their expression is significantly higher in exercise-trained aged rats than in sedentary aged rats. Furthermore, the activity of TR DNA binding to the thyroid hormone response element (TRE) transcriptional regulatory region in the α-MHC and SERCA genes and the subsequent myocardial expression of α-MHC and SERCA (both mRNA and protein) were upregulated with exercise training in the aging heart, in association with changes in the myocardial TR protein levels. In addition, plasma 3,3'-triiodothyronine (T3) and TH levels, which decrease in aging, are increased with exercise training [154]. The reversal of aging-induced downregulation of myocardial TR signaling-mediated transcription of MHC and SERCA genes by exercise training, appears to be related to the cardiac functional improvement observed in exercise-trained aged hearts.

Another critical signaling pathway that appears to be affected in exercise training is the heat shock response. The induction of myocardial heat shock proteins (HSPs) is an important contributory factor to cardioprotection against an I/R insult provided by endurance exercise in both young and old animals [155]. Elevated HSP expression, mediated by endurance exercise, appears to be more essential to the cardioprotective mechanism than increased levels of antioxidants [156]. Other observations have shown a significant age-related decrease in HSP70 production in rat heart and liver following chronic exercise [157].

Vasodilatation/Endothelial-Dependent Effects

In addition to the heart, endothelial function deteriorates with aging in human, and exercise training appears to improve the function of vascular endothelial cells. Regular aerobic-endurance exercise has been found to reduce plasma ET-1 concentration and to increase NO production in previously sedentary older women, with beneficial effects on the cardiovascular system, i.e., prevention of progression of hypertension and/or atherosclerosis by endogenous ET-1 and the potent vasodilatory effects of NO [158, 159]. In addition, regular aerobic exercise may prevent the age-associated loss in endothelium-dependent vasodilatation and restore the levels in sedentary middle aged and older healthy men. This has been proposed to be a potential mechanism by which aerobic exercise lowers the risk of CVD in this population [160]. Furthermore, endothelial release of tissue-type plasminogen activator (tPA), a primary regulator of fibrinolysis and part of the overall endogenous defense mechanism against thrombosis, declines with age in sedentary men, and regular aerobic exercise may not only prevent it, but could also reverse the age-related loss in endothelial fibrinolytic function [161]. In adults with obesity associated with increased risk of atherothrombosis, significant endothelial fibrinolytic dysfunction may be present but regular aerobic exercise can increase the capacity of the endothelium to release tPA [162].

Clinical Applications of Exercise

Collected evidence thus far strongly suggests that moderate exercise may provide a wealth of increased cardioprotective signaling to the aging heart, enhanced bioenergetic, metabolic and calcium cycling changes that can improve remodeling and may provide beneficial angiogenic and endothelial factors to the vasculature. Moreover, exercise training is an important adjuvant therapy with well-documented beneficial effects on exercise tolerance, skeletal muscle function, endothelial function, and respiration and can be useful in treating HF [163]. Is there a downside to this picture? Since strenuous exercise can increase muscle oxygen flux and elicit intracellular events leading to increased ROS and oxidative injury, the question arises as to whether exercise would be advisable to the aged population given their increased susceptibility to muscle injury, inflammation and diminished repair. In spite of these risks, there is evidence that the elderly who are physically active benefit from exercise-induced adaptation in cellular antioxidant defense systems. Improved muscle mechanics, strength, and endurance make them less vulnerable to acute injury and chronic inflammation [164]. Clearly, further studies are needed that may identify genetic, biochemical and epigenetic factors that may increase the beneficial effects and effectiveness of exercise as well as susceptibility factors that might accentuate its deleterious effects.

Summary

- Caloric restriction (CR) increases the life span of a number of organisms and mammals. This represents the most robust intervention to significantly affect both mean and maximum life span as well as aging of the cardiovascular system and is mostly well characterized in rodents. While aspects of this are clearly conserved, there is increasing evidence that there are species-specific aspects to CR.
- Studies that have not yet been completed in monkeys suggest that CR may also be operative in monkeys. It remains to be determined if CR works in humans.
- Animals maintained on a CR diet have a significant reduction in the extension of mtDNA damage and OS. This is largely affected by decrease in ROS production and mediated by increased antioxidant effect.
- The effects on both longevity and reduction of OS are accomplished by highly conserved cellular pathways, involved in metabolic and stress response, and impact both nuclear and mitochondrial components.
- Global gene expression studies have been performed primarily in rodent models of CR and show distinctive profiles in cardiovascular tissues and in skeletal muscle.
- In addition to mitochondrial biogergetics, other critical cellular homeostatic mechanisms are affected by CR including calcium cycling, apoptosis, cardioprotective signaling, nuclear DNA repair pathways, IGF signaling, glucose metabolism and inflammation pathways.
- The highly conserved mammalian sirtuins, in particular SIRT1, a deacetylase have been implicated in the mediation of CR-induced changes in tissue-specific metabolic gene expression and signaling (via changing PPAR-α and PGC-1 levels), insulin and glucose homeostasis, effects on inflammation (via NF-κB), effects on DNA repair proteins, and apoptotic regulators (e.g., p53).
- CR also can stimulate NO production, which can activate SIRT1 expression and increase mitochondrial biogenesis.
- Mimetics to CR are being developed and tested. The plant phenol resveratrol has thus far been the most robust agent capable of mimicking CR action in prolonging life span in some model organisms. Recent studies indicate that resveratrol may function in preserving cardiovascular function in animals fed high lipid diets.
- Agonists of nuclear receptors (e.g., PPARs and PGC-1) have shown strong potential as CR mimetics.
- Protein and methionine restriction has similar effects to CR in relieving OS and mtDNA damage, can also enhance longevity in animal models and may be a critical aspect of CR.
- Pharmacological supplements, including acetylcarnitine in combination with lipoic acid, which target combined mitochondrial bioenergetic dysfunction and OS, have shown benefits in both aging-mediated vascular and cardiac dysfunction. Studies with antioxidant supplementation alone (e.g., coenzyme Q) have shown conflicting results.
- Targeting glycation using cross-linking breakers such as aminoguanidine reduces aging-mediated vascular and aortic stiffening and left ventricular diastolic dysfunction.
- Exercise can increase the mean life span in a variety of model systems. Multiple benefits to the aging cardiovascular system, both heart and vasculature, are apparent in both animal models and aging humans.

- Gene profiling has played a useful role in the identification of signaling pathways, which are involved in exercise-mediated benefits to cardiovascular function.
- Exercise-mediated changes include stress signaling, mitochondrial function, calcium cycling and apoptotic pathways with the involvement of altered expression levels of global regulators, including PPARs and thyroid hormone receptors.

References

1. Dhahbi JM, Tsuchiya T, Kim HJ, Mote PL, Spindler SR. Gene expression and physiologic responses of the heart to the initiation and withdrawal of caloric restriction. J Gerontol A Biol Sci Med Sci 2006;61:218–31
2. Mattison JA, Roth GS, Lane MA, Ingram DK. Dietary restriction in aging nonhuman primates. Interdiscip Top Gerontol 2007;35:137–158
3. Verdery RB, Ingram DK, Roth GS, Lane MA. Caloric restriction increases HDL2 levels in rhesus monkeys (Macaca mulatta). Am J Physiol 1997;273:E714–E719
4. Roth GS, Lesnikov V, Lesnikov M, Ingram DK, Lane MA. Dietary caloric restriction prevents the age-related decline in plasma melatonin levels of rhesus monkeys. J Clin Endocrinol Metab 2001;86:3292–3295
5. Zainal TA, Oberley TD, Allison DB, Szweda LI, Weindruch R. Caloric restriction of rhesus monkeys lowers oxidative damage in skeletal muscle. FASEB J 2000;14:1825–1836
6. Lane MA, Ball SS, Ingram DK, Cutler RG, Engel J, Read V, Roth GS. Diet restriction in rhesus monkeys lowers fasting and glucose-stimulated glucoregulatory end points. Am J Physiol 1995;268:E941–E948
7. Roth GS, Lane MA, Ingram DK, Mattison JA, Elahi D, Tobin JD, Muller D, Metter EJ. Biomarkers of caloric restriction may predict longevity in humans. Science 2002;297:811
8. Masoro EJ. Subfield history: caloric restriction, slowing aging, and extending life. Sci Aging Knowledge Environ 2003;2003:RE2
9. Masoro EJ. Overview of caloric restriction and ageing. Mech Ageing Dev 2005;126:913–922
10. Lee CK, Allison DB, Brand J, Weindruch R, Prolla TA. Transcriptional profiles associated with aging and middle age-onset caloric restriction in mouse hearts. Proc Natl Acad Sci USA 2002;99:14988–14993
11. Park SK, Prolla TA. Gene expression profiling studies of aging in cardiac and skeletal muscles. Cardiovasc Res 2005;66:205–212
12. Park SK, Prolla TA. Lessons learned from gene expression profile studies of aging and caloric restriction. Ageing Res Rev 2005;4:55–65
13. Lee CK, Pugh TD, Klopp RG, Edwards J, Allison DB, Weindruch R, Prolla TA. The impact of alpha-lipoic acid, coenzyme Q10 and caloric restriction on life span and gene expression patterns in mice. Free Radic Biol Med 2004;36:1043–1057
14. Weindruch R, Kayo T, Lee CK, Prolla TA. Microarray profiling of gene expression in aging and its alteration by caloric restriction in mice. J Nutr 2001;131:918S–923S
15. Cefalu WT, Wang ZQ, Bell-Farrow AD, Collins J, Morgan T, Wagner JD. Caloric restriction and cardiovascular aging in cynomolgus monkeys (*Macaca fascicularis*): metabolic, physiologic, and atherosclerotic measures from a 4-year intervention trial. J Gerontol A Biol Sci Med Sci 2004;59:1007–1014
16. Barja G. Aging in vertebrates, and the effect of caloric restriction: a mitochondrial free radical production-DNA damage mechanism? Biol Rev 2004;79:235–251
17. Sohal RS, Weindruch R. Oxidative stress, caloric restriction, and aging. Science 1996;273:59–63
18. Lass A, Sohal BH, Weindruch R, Forster MJ, Sohal RS. Caloric restriction prevents age-associated accrual of oxidative damage to mouse skeletal muscle mitochondria. Free Radic Biol Med 1998;25:1089–1097
19. Gredilla R, Sanz A, Lopez-Torres M, Barja G. Caloric restriction decreases mitochondrial free radical generation at complex I and lowers oxidative damage to mitochondrial DNA in the rat heart. FASEB J 2001;15:1589–1591
20. Lopez-Torres M, Gredilla R, Sanz A, Barja G. Influence of aging and long-term caloric restriction on oxygen radical generation and oxidative DNA damage in rat liver mitochondria. Free Radic Biol Med 2002;32:882–889
21. Sanz A, Caro P, Ibanez J, Gomez J, Gredilla R, Barja G. Dietary restriction at old age lowers mitochondrial oxygen radical production and leak at complex I and oxidative DNA damage in rat brain. J Bioenerg Biomembr 2005;37:83–90
22. Gredilla R, Lopez-Torres M, Barja G. Effect of time of restriction on the decrease in mitochondrial H_2O_2 production and oxidative DNA damage in the heart of food-restricted rats. Microsc Res Tech 2002;59: 273–277
23. Gredilla R, Phaneuf S, Selman C, Kendaiah S, Leeuwenburgh C, Barja G. Short-term caloric restriction and sites of oxygen radical generation in kidney and skeletal muscle mitochondria. Ann NY Acad Sci 2004;1019: 333–342

24. Lambert AJ, Wang B, Yardley J, Edwards J, Merry BJ. The effect of aging and caloric restriction on mitochondrial protein density and oxygen consumption. Exp Gerontol 2004;39:289–295
25. Drew B, Phaneuf S, Dirks A, Selman C, Gredilla R, Lezza A, Barja G, Leeuwenburgh C. Effects of aging and caloric restriction on mitochondrial energy production in gastrocnemius muscle and heart. Am J Physiol Regul Integr Comp Physiol 2003;284:R474–R480
26. Hepple RT, Baker DJ, Kaczor JJ, Krause DJ. Long-term caloric restriction abrogates the age-related decline in skeletal muscle aerobic function. FASEB J 2005;19:1320–1332
27. Baker DJ, Betik AC, Krause DJ, Hepple RT. No decline in skeletal muscle oxidative capacity with aging in long-term calorically restricted rats: effects are independent of mitochondrial DNA integrity. J Gerontol A Biol Sci Med Sci 2006;61:675–684
28. Hepple RT, Baker DJ, McConkey M, Murynka T, Norris R. Caloric restriction protects mitochondrial function with aging in skeletal and cardiac muscles. Rejuvenation Res 2006;9:219–222
29. Lopez-Lluch G, Hunt N, Jones B, Zhu M, Jamieson H, Hilmer S, Cascajo MV, Allard J, Ingram DK, Navas P, de Cabo R. Calorie restriction induces mitochondrial biogenesis and bioenergetic efficiency. Proc Natl Acad Sci USA 2006;103:1768–1773
30. Nisoli E, Tonello C, Cardile A, Cozzi V, Bracale R, Tedesco L, Falcone S, Valerio A, Cantoni O, Clementi E, Moncada S, Carruba MO. Calorie restriction promotes mitochondrial biogenesis by inducing the expression of eNOS. Science 2005;310:314–317
31. Leon TI, Lim BO, Yu BP, Lim Y, Jeon EJ, Park DK. Effect of dietary restriction on age-related increase of liver susceptibility to peroxidation in rats. Lipids 2001;36:589–593
32. Judge S, Judge A, Grune T, Leeuwenburgh C. Short-term CR decreases cardiac mitochondrial oxidant production but increases carbonyl content. Am J Physiol Regul Integr Comp Physiol 2004;286:R254–R259
33. Sohal RS, Ku HH, Agarwal S, Forster MJ, Lal H. Oxidative damage, mitochondrial oxidant generation and antioxidant defenses during aging and in response to food restriction in the mouse. Mech Ageing Dev 1994;74:121–133
34. Richter C, Park JW, Ames BN. Normal oxidative damage to mitochondrial and nuclear DNA is extensive. Proc Natl Acad Sci USA 1988;85:6465–6467
35. Zastawny TH, Dabrowska M, Jaskolski T, Klimarczyk M, Kulinski L, Koszela A, Szczesniewicz M, Sliwinska M, Witkowski P, Olinski R. Comparison of oxidative base damage in mitochondrial and nuclear DNA. Free Radic Biol Med 1998;24:722–725
36. Dianov GL, Souza-Pinto N, Nyaga SG, Thybo T, Stevnsner T, Bohr VA. Base excision repair in nuclear and mitochondrial DNA. Prog Nucleic Acid Res Mol Biol 2001;68:285–297
37. Bohr VA. Repair of oxidative DNA damage in nuclear and mitochondrial DNA, and some changes with aging in mammalian cells. Free Radic Biol Med 2002;32:804–812
38. Szczesny B, Hazra TK, Papaconstantinou J, Mitra S, Boldogh I. Age-dependent deficiency in import of mitochondrial DNA glycosylases required for repair of oxidatively damaged bases. Proc Natl Acad Sci USA 2003;100:10670–10675
39. Imam SZ, Karahalil B, Hogue BA, Souza-Pinto NC, Bohr VA. Mitochondrial and nuclear DNA-repair capacity of various brain regions in mouse is altered in an age-dependent manner. Neurobiol Aging 2006;27:1129–1136
40. Hamilton ML, Van Remmen H, Drake JA, Yang H, Guo ZM, Kewitt K, Walter CA, Richardson A. Does oxidative damage to DNA increase with age? Proc Natl Acad Sci USA 2001;98:10469–10474
41. Hamilton ML, Guo Z, Fuller CD, Van Remmen H, Ward WF, Austad SN, Troyer DA, Thompson I, Richardson A. A reliable assessment of 8-oxo-2-deoxyguanosine levels in nuclear and mitochondrial DNA using the sodium iodide method to isolate DNA. Nucleic Acids Res 2001;29:2117–2126
42. Melov S, Hinerfeld D, Esposito L, Wallace DC. Multi-organ characterization of mitochondrial genomic rearrangements in ad libitum and caloric restricted mice show striking somatic mitochondrial DNA rearrangements with age. Nucl Acids Res 1997;25:974–982
43. Stuart JA, Karahalil B, Hogue BA, Souza-Pinto NC, Bohr VA. Mitochondrial and nuclear DNA base excision repair are affected differently by caloric restriction. FASEB J 2004;18:595–597
44. Donati A, Taddei M, Cavallini G, Bergamini E. Stimulation of macroautophagy can rescue older cells from 8-OHdG mtDNA accumulation: a safe and easy way to meet goals in the SENS agenda. Rejuvenation Res 2006;9:408–412
45. Herrero A, Barja G. 8-oxo-deoxyguanosine levels in heart and brain mitochondrial and nuclear DNA of two mammals and three birds in relation to their different rates of aging. Aging (Milano) 1999;11:294–300
46. Barja G, Herrero A. Oxidative damage to mitochondrial DNA is inversely related to maximum life span in the heart and brain of mammals. FASEB J 2000;14:312–318
47. Ku H H, Brunk UT, Sohal RS. Relationship between mitochondrial superoxide and hydrogen peroxide production and longevity of mammalian species. Free Rad Biol Med 1993;15:621–627

48. Cabelof DC, Yanamadala S, Raffoul JJ, Guo Z, Soofi A, Heydari AR. Caloric restriction promotes genomic stability by induction of base excision repair and reversal of its age-related decline. DNA Repair (Amst) 2003;2: 295–307
49. Cabelof DC, Raffoul JJ, Ge Y, Van Remmen H, Matherly LH, Heydari AR. Age-related loss of the DNA repair response following exposure to oxidative stress. J Gerontol A Biol Sci Med Sci 2006;61:427–434
50. Mayer PJ, Lange CS, Bradley MO, Nichols WW. Gender differences in age-related decline in DNA double-strand break damage and repair in lymphocytes. Ann Hum Biol 1991;18:405–415
51. Um JH, Kim SJ, Kim DW, Ha MY, Jang JH, Kim DW, Chung BS, Kang CD, Kim SH. Tissue-specific changes of DNA repair protein Ku and mtHSP70 in aging rats and their retardation by caloric restriction. Mech Ageing Dev 2003;124:967–975
52. D'Costa AP, Lenham JE, Ingram RL, Sonntag WE. Moderate caloric restriction increases type 1 IGF receptors and protein synthesis in aging rats. Mech Ageing Dev 1993;71:59–71
53. Sonntag WE, Lynch CD, Cefalu WT, Ingram RL, Bennett SA, Thornton PL, Khan AS. Pleiotropic effects of growth hormone and insulin-like growth factor (IGF)-1 on biological aging: inferences from moderate caloric-restricted animals. J Gerontol A Biol Sci Med Sci 1999;54:B521–B538
54. Bartke A, Masternak MM, Al-Regaiey KA, Bonkowski MS. Effects of dietary restriction on the expression of insulin-signaling-related genes in long-lived mutant mice. Interdiscip Top Gerontol 2007;35:69–82
55. Al-Regaiey KA, Masternak MM, Bonkowski M, Sun L, Bartke A. Long-lived growth hormone receptor knockout mice: interaction of reduced insulin-like growth factor i/insulin signaling and caloric restriction. Endocrinology 2005;146:851–860
56. Masternak MM, Al-Regaiey KA, Del Rosario Lim MM, Jimenez-Ortega V, Panici JA, Bonkowski MS, Bartke A. Effects of caloric restriction on insulin pathway gene expression in the skeletal muscle and liver of normal and long-lived GHR-KO mice. Exp Gerontol 2005;40:679–684
57. Masternak MM, Al-Regaiey KA, Del Rosario Lim MM, Jimenez-Ortega V, Panici JA, Bonkowski MS, Kopchick JJ, Wang Z, Bartke A. Caloric restriction and growth hormone receptor knockout: effects on expression of genes involved in insulin action in the heart. Exp Gerontol 2006;41:417–429
58. Corton JC, Brown-Borg HM. Peroxisome proliferator-activated receptor gamma coactivator 1 in caloric restriction and other models of longevity. J Gerontol A Biol Sci Med Sci 2005;60:1494–1509
59. Sung B, Park S, Yu BP, Chung HY. Modulation of PPAR in aging, inflammation, and calorie restriction. J Gerontol A Biol Sci Med Sci 2004;59:997–1006
60. Masternak MM, Al-Regaiey KA, Del Rosario Lim MM, Jimenez-Ortega V, Panici JA, Bonkowski MS, Kopchick JJ, Bartke A. Effects of caloric restriction and growth hormone resistance on the expression level of peroxisome proliferator-activated receptors superfamily in liver of normal and long-lived growth hormone receptor/binding protein knockout mice. J Gerontol A Biol Sci Med Sci 2005;60:1394–1398
61. Zhu M, Miura J, Lu LX, Bernier M, DeCabo R, Lane MA, Roth GS, Ingram DK. Circulating adiponectin levels increase in rats on caloric restriction: the potential for insulin sensitization. Exp Gerontol 2004;39:1049–1059
62. Corton JC, Apte U, Anderson SP, Limaye P, Yoon L, Latendresse J, Dunn C, Everitt JI, Voss KA, Swanson C, Kimbrough C, Wong JS, Gill SS, Chandraratna RA, Kwak MK, Kensler TW, Stulnig TM, Steffensen KR, Gustafsson JA, Mehendale HM. Mimetics of caloric restriction include agonists of lipid-activated nuclear receptors. J Biol Chem 2004;279:46204–46212
63. Guarente L, Picard F. Calorie restriction – the SIR2 connection. Cell 2005;120:473–482
64. Cohen HY, Miller C, Bitterman KJ, Wall NR, Hekking B, Kessler B, Howitz KT, Gorospe M, de Cabo R, Sinclair DA. Calorie restriction promotes mammalian cell survival by inducing the SIRT1 deacetylase. Science 2004;305:390–392
65. Picard F, Kurtev M, Chung N, Topark-Ngarm A, Senawong T, Machado De Oliveira R, Leid M, McBurney MW, Guarente L. Sirt1 promotes fat mobilization in white adipocytes by repressing PPAR-gamma. Nature 2004;429:771–776
66. Rodgers JT, Lerin C, Haas W, Gygi SP, Spiegelman BM, Puigserver P. Nutrient control of glucose homeostasis through a complex of PGC-1alpha and SIRT1. Nature 2005;434:113–118
67. Hallows WC, Lee S, Denu JM. Sirtuins deacetylate and activate mammalian acetyl-CoA synthetases. Proc Natl Acad Sci USA 2006;103:10230–10235
68. Moynihan KA, Grimm AA, Plueger MM, Bernal-Mizrachi E, Ford E, Cras-Meneur C, Permutt MA, Imai S. Increased dosage of mammalian Sir2 in pancreatic β cells enhances glucose-stimulated insulin secretion in mice. Cell Metab 2005;2:105–117
69. Bordone L, Motta MC, Picard F, Robinson A, Jhala US, Apfeld J, McDonagh T, Lemieux M, McBurney M, Szilvasi A. Sirt1 regulates insulin secretion by repressing UCP2 in pancreatic ÿ cells. PLoS Biol 2006;4:31
70. Brunet A, Sweeney LB, Sturgill JF, Chua KF, Greer PL, Lin Y, Tran H, Ross SE, Mostoslavsky R, Cohen HY. Stress-dependent regulation of FOXO transcription factors by the SIRT1 deacetylase. Science 2004;303: 2011–2015

71. Luo J, Nikolaev AY, Imai S, Chen D, Su F, Shiloh A, Guarente L, Gu W. Negative control of p53 by Sir2 promotes cell survival under stress. Cell 2001;107:137–148
72. Yeung F, Hoberg JE, Ramsey CS, Keller MD, Jones DR, Frye RA, Mayo MW. Modulation of NF-κB-dependent transcription and cell survival by the SIRT1 deacetylase. EMBO J 2004;23:2369–2380
73. Vaziri H, Dessain SK, Ng Eaton E, Imai SI, Frye RA, Pandita TK, Guarente L, Weinberg RA. hSIR2(SIRT1) functions as an NAD-dependent p53 deacetylase. Cell 2001;107:149–159
74. Daitoku H, Hatta M, Matsuzaki H, Aratani S, Ohshima T, Miyagishi M, Nakajima T, Fukamizu A. Silent information regulator 2 potentiates Foxo1-mediated transcription through its deacetylase activity. Proc Natl Acad Sci USA 2004;101:10042–10047
75. Motta MC, Divecha N, Lemieux M, Kamel C, Chen D, Gu W, Bultsma Y, McBurney M, Guarente L. Mammalian SIRT1 represses forkhead transcription factors. Cell 2004;116:551–563
76. Cohen HY, Lavu S, Bitterman KJ, Hekking B, Imahiyerobo TA, Miller C, Frye R, Ploegh H, Kessler BM, Sinclair DA. Acetylation of the C terminus of Ku70 by CBP and PCAF controls Bax-mediated apoptosis. Mol Cell 2004;13:627–638
77. Vaquero A, Scher M, Lee D, Erdjument-Bromage H, Tempst P, Reinberg D. Human SirT1 interacts with histone H1 and promotes formation of facultative heterochromatin. Mol Cell 2004;16:93–105
78. Alcendor RR, Kirshenbaum LA, Imai S, Vatner SF, Sadoshima J. Silent information regulator 2alpha, a longevity factor and class III histone deacetylase, is an essential endogenous apoptosis inhibitor in cardiac myocytes. Circ Res 2004;95:971–980
79. Michishita E, Park JY, Burneskis JM, Barrett JC, Horikawa I. Evolutionarily conserved and nonconserved cellular localizations and functions of human SIRT proteins. Mol Biol Cell 2005;16:4623–4635
80. Mostoslavsky R, Chua KF, Lombard DB, Pang WW, Fischer MR, Gellon L, Liu P, Mostoslavsky G, Franco S, Murphy MM, Mills KD, Patel P, Hsu JT, Hong AL, Ford E, Cheng HL, Kennedy C, Nunez N, Bronson R, Frendewey D, Auerbach W, Valenzuela D, Karow M, Hottiger MO, Hursting S, Barrett JC, Guarente L, Mulligan R, Demple B, Yancopoulos GD, Alt FW. Genomic instability and aging-like phenotype in the absence of mammalian SIRT6. Cell 2006;124:315–329
81. Kim JW, Zou Y, Yoon S, Lee JH, Kim YK, Yu BP, Chung HY. Vascular aging: molecular modulation of the prostanoid cascade by calorie restriction. J Gerontol A Biol Sci Med Sci 2004;59:B876–B885
82. Son TG, Zou Y, Yu BP, Lee J, Chung HY. Aging effect on myeloperoxidase in rat kidney and its modulation by calorie restriction. Free Radic Res 2005;39:283–289
83. Zou Y, Yoon S, Jung KJ, Kim CH, Son TG, Kim MS, Kim YJ, Lee J, Yu BP, Chung HY. Upregulation of aortic adhesion molecules during aging. J Gerontol A Biol Sci Med Sci 2006;61:232–244
84. Zou Y, Jung KJ, Kim JW, Yu BP, Chung HY. Alteration of soluble adhesion molecules during aging and their modulation by calorie restriction. FASEB J 2004;18:320–322
85. Fornieri C, Taparelli F, Quaglino D Jr, Contri MB, Davidson JM, Algeri S, Ronchetti IP. The effect of caloric restriction on the aortic tissue of aging rats. Connect Tissue Res 1999;40:131–143
86. Sanz A, Caro P, Barja G. Protein restriction without strong caloric restriction decreases mitochondrial oxygen radical production and oxidative DNA damage in rat liver. J Bioenerg Biomembr 2004;36:545–552
87. Sanz A, Caro P, Sanchez JG, Barja G. Effect of lipid restriction on mitochondrial free radical production and oxidative DNA damage. Ann NY Acad Sci 2006;1067:200–209
88. Sanz A, Gomez J, Caro P, Barja G. Carbohydrate restriction does not change mitochondrial free radical generation and oxidative DNA damage. J Bioenerg Biomembr 2006;38:327–333
89. Sanz A, Caro P, Ayala V, Portero-Otin M, Pamplona R, Barja G. Methionine restriction decreases mitochondrial oxygen radical generation and leak as well as oxidative damage to mitochondrial DNA and proteins. FASEB J 2006;20:1064–1073
90. Richie JP Jr, Leutzinger Y, Parthasarathy S, Malloy V, Orentreich N, Zimmerman JA. Methionine restriction increases blood glutathione and longevity in F344 rats. FASEB J 1994;8:1302–1307
91. Orentreich N, Matias JR, DeFelice A, Zimmerman JA. Low methionine ingestion by rats extends life span. J Nutr 1993;123:269–274
92. Pamplona R, Barja G. Mitochondrial oxidative stress, aging and caloric restriction: the protein and methionine connection. Biochim Biophys Acta 2006;1757:496–508
93. Jiang JC, Jaruga E, Repnevskaya MV, Jazwinski SM. An intervention resembling caloric restriction prolongs life span and retards aging in yeast. FASEB J 2000;14:2135–2137
94. Mobbs CV, Mastaitis JW, Zhang M, Isoda F, Cheng H, Yen K. Secrets of the lac operon. Glucose hysteresis as a mechanism in dietary restriction, aging and disease. Interdiscip Top Gerontol 2007;35:39–68
95. Suji G, Sivakami S. Glucose, glycation and aging. Biogerontology 2004;5:365–373
96. Pasinetti GM, Zhao Z, Qin W, Ho L, Shrishailam Y, Macgrogan D, Ressmann W, Humala N, Liu X, Romero C, Stetka B, Chen L, Ksiezak-Reding H, Wang J. Caloric intake and Alzheimer's disease. Experimental approaches and therapeutic implications. Interdiscip Top Gerontol 2007;35:159–175

97. Wang J, Ho L, Qin W, Rocher AB, Seror I, Humala N, Maniar K, Dolios G, Wang R, Hof PR, Pasinetti GM. Caloric restriction attenuates beta-amyloid neuropathology in a mouse model of Alzheimer's disease. FASEB J 2005;19:659–661
98. Weindruch R, Keenan KP, Carney JM, Fernandes G, Feuers RJ, Floyd RA, Halter JB, Ramsey JJ, Richardson A, Roth GS, Spindler SR. Caloric restriction mimetics: metabolic interventions. J Gerontol A Biol Sci Med Sci 2001;56:20–33
99. Ingram DK, Zhu M, Mamczarz J, Zou S, Lane MA, Roth GS, deCabo R. Calorie restriction mimetics: an emerging research field. Aging Cell 2006;5:97–108
100. Ingram DK, Anson RM, de Cabo R, Mamczarz J, Zhu M, Mattison J, Lane MA, Roth GS. Development of calorie restriction mimetics as a prolongevity strategy. Ann NY Acad Sci 2004;1019:412–423
101. Howitz KT, Bitterman KJ, Cohen HY, Lamming DW, Lavu S, Wood JG, Zipkin RE, Chung P, Kisielewski A, Zhang LL, Scherer B, Sinclair DA. Small molecule activators of sirtuins extend Saccharomyces cerevisiae life span. Nature 2003;425:191–196
102. Wood JG, Rogina B, Lavu S, Howitz K, Helfand SL, Tatar M, Sinclair D. Sirtuin activators mimic caloric restriction and delay ageing in metazoans. Nature 2004;430:686–689
103. Valenzano DR, Terzibasi E, Genade T, Cattaneo A, Domenici L, Cellerino A. Resveratrol prolongs life span and retards the onset of age-related markers in a short-lived vertebrate. Curr Biol 2006;16:296–300
104. Kaeberlein M, McDonagh T, Heltweg B, Hixon J, Westman EA, Caldwell SD, Napper A, Curtis R, DiStefano PS, Fields S, Bedalov A, Kennedy BK. Substrate-specific activation of sirtuins by resveratrol. J Biol Chem 2005;280:17038–17045
105. Borra MT, Smith BC, Denu JM. Mechanism of human SIRT1 activation by resveratrol. J Biol Chem 2005;280:17187–17195
106. Baur JA, Pearson KJ, Price NL, Jamieson HA, Lerin C, Kalra A, Prabhu VV, Allard JS, Lopez-Lluch G, Lewis K, Pistell PJ, Poosala S, Becker KG, Boss O, Gwinn D, Wang M, Ramaswamy S, Fishbein KW, Spencer RG, Lakatta EG, Le Couteur D, Shaw RJ, Navas P, Puigserver P, Ingram DK, de Cabo R, Sinclair DA. Resveratrol improves health and survival of mice on a high-calorie diet. Nature 2006;444:337–342
107. Yang H, Baur JA, Chen A, Miller C, Sinclair DA. Design and synthesis of compounds that extend yeast replicative life span. Aging Cell 2007;6:35–43
108. Demetrius L. Caloric restriction, metabolic rate, and entropy. J Gerontol A Biol Sci Med Sci 2004;59: B902–B915
109. Demetrius L. Aging in mouse and human systems: a comparative study. Ann NY Acad Sci 2006;1067:66–82
110. Mockett RJ, Cooper TM, Orr WC, Sohal RS. Effects of caloric restriction are species-specific. Biogerontology 2006;7:157–160
111. Dirks AJ, Leeuwenburgh C. Caloric restriction in humans: potential pitfalls and health concerns. Mech Ageing Dev 2006;127:1–7
112. Calabrese V, Giuffrida Stella AM, Calvani M, Butterfield DA. Acetylcarnitine and cellular stress response: roles in nutritional redox homeostasis and regulation of longevity genes. J Nutr Biochem 2006;17:73–88
113. Hagen TM, Moreau R, Suh JH, Visioli F. Mitochondrial decay in the aging rat heart: evidence for improvement by dietary supplementation with acetyl-L-cartinine and/or lipoic acid. Ann NY Acad Sci 2002;959: 491–507
114. Lesnefsky EJ, He D, Moghaddas S, Hoppel CL. Reversal of mitochondrial defects before ischemia protects the aged heart. FASEB J 2006;20:1543–1545
115. Suh JH, Wang H, Liu RM, Liu J, Hagen TM. (R)-alpha-lipoic acid reverses the age-related loss in GSH redox status in post-mitotic tissues: evidence for increased cysteine requirement for GSH synthesis. Arch Biochem Biophys 2004;423:126–135
116. Kumaran S, Savitha S, Anusuya Devi M, Panneerselvam C. L-carnitine and DL-alpha-lipoic acid reverse the age-related deficit in glutathione redox state in skeletal muscle and heart tissues. Mech Ageing Dev 2004;125:507–512
117. Ames BN, Liu J. Delaying the mitochondrial decay of aging with acetylcarnitine. Ann NY Acad Sci 2004;1033:108–116
118. Tanaka Y, Sasaki R, Fukui F, Waki H, Kawabata T, Okazaki M, Hasegawa K, Ando S. Acetyl-L-carnitine supplementation restores decreased tissue carnitine levels and impaired lipid metabolism in aged rats. J Lipid Res 2004;45:729–735
119. Rosenfeldt FL, Pepe S, Linnane A, Nagley P, Rowland M, Ou R, Marasco S, Lyon W, Esmore D. Coenzyme Q10 protects the aging heart against stress: studies in rats, human tissues, and patients. Ann NY Acad Sci 2002;959:355–359
120. Sohal RS, Kamzalov S, Sumien N, Ferguson M, Rebrin I, Heinrich KR, Forster MJ. Effect of coenzyme Q10 intake on endogenous coenzyme Q content, mitochondrial electron transport chain, antioxidative defenses, and life span of mice. Free Radic Biol Med 2006;40:480–487

121. Aronson D. Pharmacological prevention of cardiovascular aging – targeting the Maillard reaction. Br J Pharmacol 2004;142:1055–1058
122. Li YM, Steffes M, Donnelly T, Liu C, Fuh H, Basgen J, Bucala R, Vlassara H. Prevention of cardiovascular and renal pathology of aging by the advanced glycation inhibitor aminoguanidine. Proc Natl Acad Sci USA 1996;93:3902–3907
123. Corman B, Duriez M, Poitevin P, Heudes D, Bruneval P, Tedgui A, Levy BI. Aminoguanidine prevents age-related arterial stiffening and cardiac hypertrophy. Proc Natl Acad Sci USA 1998;95:1301–1306
124. Moreau R, Nguyen BT, Doneanu CE, Hagen TM. Reversal by aminoguanidine of the age-related increase in glycoxidation and lipoxidation in the cardiovascular system of Fischer 344 rats. Biochem Pharmacol 2005;69: 29–40
125. Chang KC, Hsu KL, Chou TF, Lo HM, Tseng YZ. Aminoguanidine prevents age-related deterioration in left ventricular-arterial coupling in Fisher 344 rats. Br J Pharmacol 2004;142:1099–1104
126. Chang KC, Hsu KL, Peng YI, Lee FC, Tseng YZ. Aminoguanidine prevents age-related aortic stiffening in Fisher 344 rats: aortic impedance analysis. Br J Pharmacol 2003;140:107–114
127. Asif M, Egan J, Vasan S, Jyothirmayi GN, Masurekar MR, Lopez S, Williams C, Torres RL, Wagle D, Ulrich P, Cerami A, Brines M, Regan TJ. An advanced glycation endproduct cross-link breaker can reverse age-related increases in myocardial stiffness. Proc Natl Acad Sci USA 2000;97:2809–2813
128. Ventura-Clapier R, Mettauer B, Bigard X. Beneficial effects of endurance training on cardiac and skeletal muscle energy metabolism in heart failure. Cardiovasc Res 2007;73:10–18
129. Lu L, Mei DF, Gu AG, Wang S, Lentzner B, Gutstein DE, Zwas D, Homma S, Yi GH, Wang J. Exercise training normalizes altered calcium-handling proteins during development of heart failure. J Appl Physiol 2002;92:1524–1530
130. Orenstein TL, Parker TG, Butany JW, Goodman JM, Dawood F, Wen WH, Wee L, Martino T, McLaughlin PR, Liu PP. Favorable left ventricular remodeling following large myocardial infarction by exercise training. Effect on ventricular morphology and gene expression. J Clin Invest 1995;96:858–866
131. Lee YI, Cho JY, Kim MH, Kim KB, Lee DJ, Lee KS. Effects of exercise training on pathological cardiac hypertrophy related gene expression and apoptosis. Eur J Appl Physiol 2006;97:216–224
132. Iemitsu M, Maeda S, Jesmin S, Otsuki T, Miyauchi T. Exercise training improves aging-induced down-regulation of VEGF angiogenic signaling cascade in hearts. Am J Physiol Heart Circ Physiol 2006;291: H1290–H1298
133. Bronikowski AM, Carter PA, Morgan TJ, Garland T Jr, Ung N, Pugh TD, Weindruch R, Prolla TA. Lifelong voluntary exercise in the mouse prevents age-related alterations in gene expression in the heart. Physiol Genomics 2003;12:129–138
134. Suzuki J. L-arginine supplementation causes additional effects on exercise-induced angiogenesis and VEGF expression in the heart and hind-leg muscles of middle-aged rats. J Physiol Sci 2006;56:39–44
135. Short KR, Vittone JL, Bigelow ML, Proctor DN, Coenen-Schimke JM, Rys P, Nair KS. Changes in myosin heavy chain mRNA and protein expression in human skeletal muscle with age and endurance exercise training. J Appl Physiol 2005;99:95–102
136. Gustafsson T, Bodin K, Sylven C, Gordon A, Tyni-Lenne R, Jansson E. Increased expression of VEGF following exercise training in patients with heart failure. Eur J Clin Invest 2001;31:362–366
137. Ennezat PV, Malendowicz SL, Testa M, Colombo PC, Cohen-Solal A, Evans T, LeJemtel TH. Physical training in patients with chronic heart failure enhances the expression of genes encoding antioxidative enzymes. J Am Coll Cardiol 2001;38:194–198
138. Jozsi AC, Dupont-Versteegden EE, Taylor-Jones JM, Evans WJ, Trappe TA, Campbell WW, Peterson CA. Aged human muscle demonstrates an altered gene expression profile consistent with an impaired response to exercise. Mech Ageing Dev 2000;120:45–56
139. Quindry J, French J, Hamilton K, Lee Y, Mehta JL, Powers S. Exercise training provides cardioprotection against ischemia-reperfusion induced apoptosis in young and old animals. Exp Gerontol 2005;40:416–425
140. French JP, Quindry JC, Falk DJ, Staib JL, Lee Y, Wang KK, Powers SK. Ischemia-reperfusion induced calpain activation and SERCA2a degradation are attenuated by exercise training and calpain inhibition. Am J Physiol Heart Circ Physiol 2006;290:H128–H136
141. Kwak HB, Song W, Lawler JM. Exercise training attenuates age-induced elevation in Bax/Bcl-2 ratio, apoptosis, and remodeling in the rat heart. FASEB J 2006;20:791–793
142. Gielen S, Adams V, Niebauer J, Schuler G, Hambrecht R. Aging and heart failure – similar syndromes of exercise intolerance? Implications for exercise-based interventions. Heart Fail Monit 2005;4:130–136
143. Musch TI, Eklund KE, Hageman KS, Poole DC. Altered regional blood flow responses to submaximal exercise in older rats. J Appl Physiol 2004;96:81–88
144. Eklund KE, Hageman KS, Poole DC, Musch TI. Impact of aging on muscle blood flow in chronic heart failure. J Appl Physiol 2005;99:505–514

145. Judge S, Jang YM, Smith A, Selman C, Phillips T, Speakman JR, Hagen T, Leeuwenburgh C. Exercise by lifelong voluntary wheel running reduces subsarcolemmal and interfibrillar mitochondrial hydrogen peroxide production in the heart. Am J Physiol Regul Integr Comp Physiol 2005;289:R1564–R1572
146. Navarro A, Gomez C, Lopez-Cepero JM, Boveris M. Beneficial effects of moderate exercise on mice aging: survival, behavior, oxidative stress and mitochondrial electron transfer. Am J Physiol Regul Integr Comp Physiol 2004;286:R505–R511
147. Korzick DH, Holiman DA, Boluyt MO, Laughlin MH, Lakatta EG. Diminished alpha1-adrenergic-mediated contraction and translocation of PKC in senescent rat heart. Am J Physiol Heart Circ Physiol 2001;281: H581–H589
148. Korzick DH, Hunter JC, McDowell MK, Delp MD, Tickerhoof MM, Carson LD. Chronic exercise improves myocardial inotropic reserve capacity through alpha1-adrenergic and protein kinase C-dependent effects in senescent rats. J Gerontol A Biol Sci Med Sci 2004;59:1089–1098
149. Roth DA, White CD, Podolin DA, Mazzeo RS. Alterations in myocardial signal transduction due to aging and chronic dynamic exercise. J Appl Physiol 1998;84:177–184
150. Iemitsu M, Miyauchi T, Maeda S, Tanabe T, Takanashi M, Irukayama-Tomobe Y, Sakai S, Ohmori H, Matsuda M, Yamaguchi I. Aging-induced decrease in the PPAR-alpha level in hearts is improved by exercise training. Am J Physiol Heart Circ Physiol 2002;283:H1750–H1760
151. Tunstall RJ, Mehan KA, Wadley GD, Collier GR, Bonen A, Hargreaves M, Cameron-Smith D. Exercise training increases lipid metabolism gene expression in human skeletal muscle. Am J Physiol Endocrinol Metab 2002;283:E66–E72
152. Koves TR, Li P, An J, Akimoto T, Slentz D, Ilkayeva O, Dohm GL, Yan Z, Newgard CB, Muoio DM. Peroxisome proliferator-activated receptor-gamma co-activator 1alpha-mediated metabolic remodeling of skeletal myocytes mimics exercise training and reverses lipid-induced mitochondrial inefficiency. J Biol Chem 2005;280: 33588–33598
153. Iemitsu M, Miyauchi T, Maeda S, Tanabe T, Takanashi M, Matsuda M, Yamaguchi I. Exercise training improves cardiac function-related gene levels through thyroid hormone receptor signaling in aged rats. Am J Physiol Heart Circ Physiol 2004;286:H1696–H1705
154. Tang F. Effect of sex and age on serum aldosterone and thyroid hormones in the laboratory rat. Horm Metab Res 1985;17:507–509
155. Powers SK, Quindry J, Hamilton K. Aging, exercise, and cardioprotection. Ann NY Acad Sci 2004;1019: 462–470
156. Lennon SL, Quindry JC, Hamilton KL, French JP, Hughes J, Mehta JL, Powers SK. Elevated MnSOD is not required for exercise-induced cardioprotection against myocardial stunning. Am J Physiol Heart Circ Physiol 2004;287:H975–H980
157. Starnes JW, Choilawala AM, Taylor RP, Nelson MJ, Delp MD. Myocardial heat shock protein 70 expression in young and old rats after identical exercise programs. J Gerontol A Biol Sci Med Sci 2005;60:963–969
158. Maeda S, Tanabe T, Miyauchi T, Otsuki T, Sugawara J, Iemitsu M, Kuno S, Ajisaka R, Yamaguchi I, Matsuda M. Aerobic exercise training reduce plasma endothelin-1 concentration in older women. J Appl Physiol 2003;95:336–341
159. Maeda S, Tanabe T, Otsuki T, Sugawara J, Iemitsu M, Miyauchi T, Kuno S, Ajisaka R, Matsuda M. Moderate regular exercise increases basal production of nitric oxide in elderly women. Hypertens Res 2004;27:947–953
160. DeSouza CA, Shapiro LF, Clevenger CM, Dinenno FA, Monahan KD, Tanaka H, Seals DR. Regular aerobic exercise prevents and restores age-related declines in endothelium-dependent vasodilation in healthy men. Circulation 2000;102:1351–1357
161. Smith DT, Hoetzer GL, Greiner JJ, Stauffer BL, DeSouza CA. Effects of ageing and regular aerobic exercise on endothelial fibrinolytic capacity in humans. J Physiol 2003;546:289–298
162. DeSouza CA, Van Guilder GP, Greiner JJ, Smith DT, Hoetzer GL, Stauffer BL. Basal endothelial nitric oxide release is preserved in overweight and obese adults. Obes Res 2005;13:1303–1306
163. Gielen S, Adams V, Niebauer J, Schuler G, Hambrecht R. Aging and heart failure – similar syndromes of exercise intolerance? Implications for exercise-based interventions. Heart Fail Monit 2005;4:130–136
164. Ji LL. Exercise at old age: does it increase or alleviate oxidative stress? Ann NY Acad Sci 2001;928:236–247

Part VII
The Future of Aging Research

Chapter 16
Aging and the Frontier Ahead

Overview

The role of molecular genetics in the analysis of aging has just begun to provide major insights to our understanding of the mechanisms of aging, both as to its highly conserved aspects as well as those that may be more specific to human subjects. In this chapter, we will discuss the applicability of results with non-human models of aging, reprising some of the major findings implicating specific genes as well as previewing possible ways to make further inroads in human clinical studies and the genetic analysis of aging. We will also present an overview of the continuing search for aging biomarkers including a review of the current armamentarium of cellular/molecular biomarkers and a discussion on the use of genomic, gene profiling, proteomic and nutrigenomic approaches towards identifying and validating novel biomarkers, as well as elucidating gene-environment interactions in the expression of the aging phenotype. The use of an integrative system biology approach, which has been discussed by several aging scientists, is also appraised. In addition, we will briefly survey the use of highly targeted methods to reverse and/or retard aging, which have shown promise in preclinical models, both animal and cell-based studies that may have application in the future.

Introduction

At this juncture it should be apparent to the reader that an important crossroad in aging research has been reached. Animal studies have begun to provide provocative results revealing some of the genes involved in determining longevity as well as several genes involved in aging-related diseases, particularly cardiovascular disorders. Moreover, these observations have shown that numerous pathways involved in intracellular signaling, genomic damage and expression and responses to oxidative stress (OS) appear to contribute to aging in a seemingly multifactorial fashion. Critiques have been leveled at the strains used in these studies, arguing that inbred and shorter-life span models likely do not reflect the events occurring in human aging. Similar criticism has been also directed at the role of replicative senescence, which emerged from numerous studies with *in vitro* cells and its relevance to aging tissues *in vivo* underlined by the fact that there is no clear evidence that cellular senescence *in vivo* limits animal life span. Nevertheless, the pathways identified in these studies have been increasingly implicated in aging-associated cardiovascular disease (CVD) and also appear to contribute to aging. Despite the lack of a clearly identifiable cause or single theory of aging, a formidable body of evidence suggests that highly conserved genes and pathways are involved in aging (with other important links yet to be identified). The crossroads ahead include how we go from here to identify genes and pathways involved in human aging and define their overlap in aging-related diseases, how to integrate both clinical and molecular/cellular information with a non-reductive systematic approach, and how to devise further targeted experiments to test the role

J. Marín-García, *Aging and the Heart*,

of the identified determinants and ultimately to apply this information to reverse/repair aging CV dysfunction.

Molecular genetic studies with human aging and aging-related diseases have been somewhat limited with major insights arising from focusing on centenarians, data from individuals with premature aging syndromes and on case-association studies. As with many gene-association studies in humans, different populations appear to demonstrate different phenotypic expression, which provide further support for the multifactorial components of aging and for the likely interaction of specific genes with modifying elements that might include other genes, environmental and epigenetic factors. Interestingly, while these studies have revealed novel gene-associations with human aging including identification of novel immune/inflammatory genes, they have also found considerable overlap with elements identified in animal studies, including elements involved in mitochondrial function, chromatin remodeling and cell growth responses. This will be further discussed later as are new approaches to potentially improve association analysis, novel genetic loci and identification of biomarkers of aging and aging-associated diseases including gene expression, proteomic and metabolomic analysis.

The use of a systems biology approach may be important in integrating the diverse and often unwieldy wealth of data generated by the varied approaches and different population analysis in human aging and disease, and in finding the proper context to place molecular and cellular information. This approach involves the integration of clinical and physiological findings with molecular/cellular data as discussed below.

Current evidence, mostly emerging from animal studies, suggests that both longevity and aging dysfunction can be altered/delayed, and in some cases reversed. Although already discussed in previous chapters, promising methodologies including gene therapy to target contractile and signaling dysfunction, pharmacological approaches to target defective lysosomal and mitochondrial function, amelioration of oxidative and glycation damage and emphasis on less invasive modifications of lifestyle including CR, other nutritional concerns and exercise will be summarized in this chapter. In addition, we will examine the potential use of stem cell transplantation and/or activation in mediating cell repair in aging, particularly in reference to the heart, as well as ongoing and potential application of these approaches to human aging and aging-diseases taking note about some of the present controversies concerning these approaches.

New Focus on Genetic Analysis in Aging Research

Animal Models: Can Simpler Models Suffice?

Despite the obvious reservations that one might have in regard to comparing human and the various model systems available (ranging from yeast, *C. elegans*, *Drosophila* to mice), including their shorter life, selection for high fecundity and enormous physiological differences, over the last ten to twenty years intense research efforts have provided the striking finding that many genes substantially modulate aging. In model organisms such as yeast [1], *C. elegans* [2], *Drosophila* [3], and mice [4, 5] many genes have been identified that play a role in the response to stresses (including OS), to caloric restriction, chromatin remodeling and insulin-signaling pathway [6–10]. As previously discussed, mice with experimentally induced mutations or spontaneous genetic alterations have provided supportive evidence of the contribution of intracellular signaling (e.g., Klotho) and mitochondrial bioenergetic pathways (e.g., DNA polymeraseγ/mtDNA mutations) in the mechanism of aging. While the role of these genes and defects in human aging have not yet been fully ascertained, these findings are useful as a basis for further research. For instance, to examine the link between variation in gene expression patterns in specific cell-types (e.g., hematopoietic stem cells) and organs (e.g., brain) and longevity one recently developed method employed a combined genetic and genomic analysis of large families of fully genotyped recombinant inbred mice [11].

In recapitulating aging-associated cardiac diseases and age-related cardiac deterioration, the *Drosophila* model, surprisingly is evocative of the aging human heart; with aging fruit flies exhibiting a progressive increase in electrical pacing-induced HF as well as an increased prevalence of heart rhythm disorders [12, 13]. This model of aging-associated cardiac disease is highly attractive because of *Drosophila*'s simple, well-defined and manipulatable genetics that can be applied to track complex traits defined by polygenic variants. These studies also revealed that reducing insulin receptor (InR) or Target Of Rapamycin (TOR) signaling dramatically lowered the risk of pacing-induced HF in the old flies; and provided support that an age-dependent increase in dysrhythmicity correlated with an age-related decrease in myocardial transcript levels of the single *Drosophila* KCNQ-type K^+ channel and K_{ATP} channel (*dSUR*l) genes. Furthermore, deletion mutants of the *Drosophila* KCNQ gene and cardiac dSUR knockdown exhibit increased pacing-induced HF. Similarly, mutations in human *KCNQ* genes, encoding the pore-forming subunits underlying I_{ks} current, cause type 1 long QT syndrome (LQT1) and associated ventricular dysrhythmias, similar to the heart dysfunction seen in vertebrates with abnormal K_{ATP} channels. In addition, missense and a frameshift mutations in ABCC9 that encodes the regulatory human SUR2A subunit, resulting in structural abnormalities of the K_{ATP} channel and impaired ATP-dependent channel gating, have been found in two independent families with middle age onset dilated cardiomyopathy (DCM) [14]. Therefore, data from this model suggest that reduced *dSUR*-function and resulting K_{ATP} channel insufficiency contribute to an increased risk of HF with age, and may be an indicator of cardiac aging also (although this needs to be further evaluated in aging humans).

On the other hand, mice mutants that show accelerated aging (and a shorter life span) generally display some of the phenotypes observed in older human subjects and occasionally develop phenotypes that are not observed during aging (e.g., the development of phenotypes in the mitochondrial DNA polymerase γ mutator strains, which are not seen in normal mouse aging) and have not been shown to completely recapitulate normal aging, which supports the concept that aging involves more than just genetic inputs. Even more interesting might be the loss-of-function mutations in the genetic models that lead to increased life span, implying that normal gene function can limit life span. It is noteworthy, that these loss-of-function mutations appear to act on the mechanism(s) of aging in a way that might be eventually mimicked by drugs (recapitulating the effects of the mutant gene) [15]. Nevertheless, because of its potential side effects it is unlikely that gene therapy will be used in humans in the near future. Drugs that target products of a mutant gene, whose alterations might affect the rate of aging, might be an important test for the assessment of the relatedness of human and animal models (in regard to aging mechanisms), and might provide a myriad of potential benefits (to be discussed later in this chapter).

Advances in Human Genotyping and Gene Analysis

Longevity and Frailty Genes

It should be stated at the outset that many genes that are associated with human life span are not "longevity genes" per se. For example, mutations in the tumor suppressor genes BRCA-1 and BRCA-2, which increase mortality associated with breast and ovarian cancer are rare among long-lived women [16]. Conversely, genes that reduce the risk of atherosclerosis may be more common in centenarians; two such genes have been identified. The first involves a mutation in the cholesteryl ester transfer protein (CETP) gene that leads to larger-sized lipoproteins and diminished prevalence of CVD [17]. Individuals with exceptional longevity and their offspring have significantly larger

HDL and LDL particle sizes together with significantly lower prevalence of hypertension, CVD, metabolic syndrome, and increased homozygosity for the I405V variant in CETP. The second gene involves variants in the microsomal transfer protein (MTP) – the rate-limiting step in lipoprotein synthesis [18].

Furthermore, several other genes involved in lipoprotein metabolism, affecting both longevity and overall cardiovascular health, have been described. Common variants of APOE have been among the most consistent gene variants associated with longevity. Three isoforms, APOE2, APOE3 and APOE4, encoded by different alleles interact differently with specific lipoprotein receptors that affect circulating levels of cholesterols. *APOE4* has repeatedly been associated with a moderately increased risk of both CVD and Alzheimer disease, whereas *APOE2* is protective. Differences in the APOE frequency between age groups are consistent with APOE4 prevalence nearly half the frequency levels found in young adults. Nevertheless, the overall gain in longevity in individuals carrying the APOE2 genes, albeit highly consistent, is relatively modest; it has been proposed to represent a frailty rather than a longevity determinant [19]. Evidence that common *APOE* variants can impact life span originally elicited a strong search effort to find other common variants with clear-cut association; however, this has not been realized. One possible explanation is that no single gene variant has been identified with aging, suggesting that the genetic architecture of life span is a complex phenotypic trait that likely involves many rare gene variants with small effects that together with environmental factors significantly contribute to slow the progress in this area. This has been reinforced by the great diversity in the findings from centenarian populations.

Interestingly, compared to a control group of Ashkenazi, a group of Ashkenazi Jewish centenarians (n = 213) and their offspring (n = 216), showed homozygosity for the apolipoprotein C-3 (APOC3) -641C allele that has been reported to be more prevalent and is associated with a favorable lipoprotein profile and cardiovascular health, including lower prevalence of hypertension, greater insulin sensitivity and longevity [20].

Therefore while these genes appear to have moderate effects on longevity, their effect appears primarily on the modulation of susceptibility for disease rather than on modulation of the overall aging process. Other genes with demonstrated effects on frailty in older individuals include genes involved in inflammatory pathways such as IL-6 [21]. In contrast, longevity genes are posited to delay the onset, or reduce the rate, of aging (or both) [22], perhaps by slowing cellular senescence, improving repair mechanisms, or increasing resistance to stresses such as infection and injury. Nevertheless, both frailty and longevity determinants both contribute to the increased cardiovascular health with enhanced longevity observed in some individuals. For instance, offspring of centenarians compared to age-matched controls have markedly reduced incidence of diabetes, hypertension and ischemic heart disease [23], suggesting that inheritance from their long-lived parent of longevity and/or frailty gene(s) can provide protection against these infirmities and confirm that low cardiovascular disease susceptibility is a factor in becoming a centenarian.

Methods of Genetic Analysis

Large-scale and carefully designed studies will be essential for progress in genetic studies of human longevity. For instance, in Europe large-scale international collaborations have recently been initiated (e.g., the Genetics of Healthy Ageing [GEHA] project and GenomEUtwin) [24], and in the US (the Long Life Family Study) and the National Institute on Aging-supported Longevity Consortium studies to identify genetic and non-genetic factors of importance for exceptional longevity are underway. These collaborative efforts should facilitate the collection of relatively large samples of long-lived individuals (their siblings and offspring) and may include, beyond longevity, intermediate phenotypes such as cardiovascular risk factors in their offspring.

Linkage analysis of longevity involving genome-wide scans has occasionally proved useful. For instance, Puca et al. [25] have scanned the whole genome using 308 individuals belonging to 137 sibships with exceptional longevity and identified a region on chromosome 4 that is significantly linked to human longevity, using either parametric or nonparametric analysis. Subsequent fine mapping of the 12 million bp chromosomal region identified, containing approximately 50 putative genes, using a haplotype-based association-study design implicated the microsomal transfer protein (MTP) gene in a US caucasian population; although attempts to replicate this association in other study populations (e.g., French, German) have not been successful [18]. Linkage analysis studies are often hampered by a lack of available multi-generational DNA from long-lived individuals, and by the requirement of extremely (and unrealistically) large sample sizes to identify genetic regions that are involved in complex multifactorial phenotypes, such as life span. These problems may be contributory to the primarily discordant findings in the limited linkage studies thus far conducted. Use of expanded haplotype multi-locus analysis and rapidly evolving high-throughput genotyping techniques (such as high density SNP analysis) may harbor new promise for this research endeavor. Moreover, publicly available databases of human haplotype maps (HAPMAP) should also prove useful in the identification of novel genetic loci not previously thought to play a role in aging.

Another type of genetic analysis, usually conducted with unrelated individuals, is the candidate-gene association studies test for statistical associations between one or more genetic polymorphisms in order to identify genetic determinants of longevity/survival by comparing the genotypes at specific loci of long-lived individuals (e.g., centenarians) with those of younger cohorts [27, 28, 29]. In contrast to linkage analysis, gene variants with small effects can be detected. These case-control association studies are limited by the specific biological knowledge required to nominate plausible candidate genes. Furthermore, cases and controls are often born several generations apart; this age-mismatching represents a lack of appropriate control groups, and can lead to faulty interpretation since cohort-specific characteristics may reflect change in population structure over time or different gene-environment interactions across generations and can confound comparisons between centenarians and younger cohorts. Moreover, since very few people will become centenarians, the overall relevance of the phenotype to ordinary older people remains unclear. It is noteworthy that most genetic associations with longevity have not been replicated. Inadequate sample size is also a possible reason for lack of replication; to enlarge the sample size use of post hoc meta analyses has been recommended. These might ensure quality inclusion criteria with carefully matched large samples having sufficient statistical power, to detect the relatively small risks presented by most known variants with well-chosen genetic markers, adequate standards in genotyping, analysis and interpretation.

While the most common association study designs in aging research have been either case-control or cross-sectional format, longitudinal population studies are also possible [30]. Studies of large cohorts of elderly people who are followed longitudinally, although logistically challenging, have proved highly useful for longevity research. For instance, the Danish 1905 cohort assessed in 1998 comprised 3,600 individuals still alive of whom 2,262 participated in a survey that included an interview, physical and cognitive tests, and collection of biological material for molecular genetic analysis [31, 32].

Since chronological age is not necessarily an accurate indicator of the aging process, it is important to emphasize that longevity itself may not be the phenotype of interest, and rather the quality of life in older age together with active life expectancy and duration of disability-free aging should be considered.

Biological age estimates the functional status of an individual in reference to his or her chronological peers on the basis of how well he or she functions in comparison with others of the same chronological age; this may serve as an indicator of an individual's general health status, remaining healthy life span, and active life expectancy. Defining and validating the biomarkers that constitute the measure of biological age is a priority for gerontologists, and this has led several researchers to expand their focus beyond the centenarian to studies beginning in middle-age, in an effort to identify alleles linked to aging in one or more physiological systems [33].

Mitochondrial DNA and Aging

Previously, we have presented evidence from both animal models and human studies (including studies of the heart) that primary somatic or acquired mtDNA damage, including large-scale deletions and point mutations, accumulate in aging. Several observations in elderly humans from a defined ethnic population have shown that specific mitochondrial genotypes are significantly present or absent in the oldest old. For instance, in a Italian population, a C–T mutation found at position 150 of the mtDNA D-loop control region was found to be over-represented in centenarians in comparison to young and old people [34]. This mutation has been suggested to change the origin of replication of the mtDNA heavy strand at position 149, substituting for that at position 151, and represents a rather unique example of a beneficial mtDNA mutation; in general, mtDNA alteration has been thought to be deleterious. Furthermore, this mutation has been found to be an inherited polymorphism in some cases, and may also arise as a result of somatic mutation later in life. It is interesting to note that the C150T mutation has been found associated with longevity in three additional populations, Irish, Finnish and Japanese [35, 36]. Since age-related mutations in the mtDNA D-loop region usually exhibit tissue specificity, it is notable that the C150T mutation has been found so far in three different cell types, i.e., peripheral blood lymphocytes, granulocytes and fibroblasts, and may be linked to immunosenescence, an important marker of morbidity and mortality in the elderly [37].

Previously, Wallace et al. [38] have found that human mtDNA can be characterized by a series of inherited point mutations that define a haplotype, and that these display a region-specific distribution. In a burgeoning research field, the number of mtDNA haplotypes and sub-haplotypes has constantly been increasing. One of these haplotypes (haplotype J) most commonly present in European Caucasians, was found to be over-represented in long-living males and male centenarians in a North Italian cohort suggesting a potential role for this mtDNA variant in the longevity of this group, with gender having also a role in its phenotypic expression [39]. The over-representation of haplogroup J in nonagenarians and centenarians was also independently found in Irish and Finnish elderly populations [36, 41], but not replicated in southern Italians [41]. Collectively, these results support the idea that the effect of mtDNA inherited variants on longevity is geographically/population dependent.

An unexpected but intriguing finding emerging from several studies [42, 43] is that the same mitochondrial haplotype J associated with increased longevity has been also associated with increased prevalence of mitochondrial-based disease, including Leber hereditary optic neuropathy (LHON), a disorder most commonly resulting from pathogenic mtDNA point mutations affecting genes encoding complex I (NADH: ubiquinone oxidoreductase) subunits. Similarly, haplotype J has been reported to contribute to optic neuritis in multiple sclerosis patients [44].

Rose et al. [45] using further sequence analysis (of both the D-loop and mtDNA coding regions) in centenarians have found mutations known to promote mitochondrial cytopathies (e.g., 3010). Since these mutations tend to reduce OXPHOS function, efficiency and coupling, it has been suggested that such mutations would tend to reduce mitochondrial ROS stress and decrease apoptosis [37]. A more elaborate explanation has been offered by Wallace [46]. He proposed that lineage J mtDNAs harbor specific "uncoupling mtDNA variants" that reduce mitochondrial ATP output in favor of heat production exacerbating the partial ATP defect generated by the pathogenic mtDNA mutations. For instance, two polymorphic variants in cyt *b* associated with haplotype J include 15257A and 14798C, altering well-conserved amino acids D171N and F18L respectively. The 15257 variant alters the outer coenzyme Q binding site of complex III, which contacts the Rieske iron-sulfur protein, while the 14798 site alters the inner coenzyme Q binding site of complex III. Since both Qo and Qi binding sites are essential for complex III proton pumping, the np 14798 and 15257 variants are both likely to have disconnected the electron flow through complex III with proton pumping. It is estimated that these variants effectively reduce the coupling efficiency of mitochondrial OXPHOS by nearly one third and increase heat generation. It has been also proposed that these variants in individuals from European climates are cold-adaptive.

Individuals with uncoupled mitochondria would burn calories more rapidly to generate both the required ATP plus increased heat. Increased uncoupling would tend to reduce mitochondrial ROS production, diminish mitochondrial OS and would reduce the activation of the mitochondrial PT pore, thus preserving cells and protecting against cell loss that may lead to neurological and visceral tissue degeneration and aging. On the other hand, the cold-adapted mtDNA uncoupling mutations generate less ATP per calorie consumed and uncoupled mitochondria would be more prone to clinical problems resulting from energy insufficiency, such as LHON.

In an analysis of a population of Japanese centenarians (another longevity-associated mitochondrial genotype), a C→A variant at nucleotide 5178 of mtDNA, was identified at a significantly higher frequency. This variant results in a Leu-to-Met substitution within the mitochondrial NADH dehydrogenase subunit 2 (NADH2) gene [47, 48] The population-specificity of this association was underlined by subsequent molecular studies with an older population from Yunnan province in China, which failed to replicate this association [49]. Subsequent studies have suggested that the Mt5178A variant may promote resistance to adult-onset diseases. Takagi et al. found that the frequency of the Mt5178A genotype was significantly higher in controls than in subjects with myocardial infarction (MI) [50]. Similarly, Mukae et al. [51] noted that the allelic frequency of 5178C was significantly higher in a group of Japanese subjects with acute MI than in a control group. This difference was more pronounced in younger patients. Furthermore, in an analysis of 257 Japanese patients with type 2 diabetes (181 men and 89 women) and 254 control subjects without diabetes, the 5178C genotype was observed more frequently in patients with type 2 diabetes than in control subjects [52]. Interestingly, the mean age at onset of diabetes was significantly lower in patients with mt5178C. Patients with a maternal history of diabetes carried the mt5178C allele more frequently than did patients without a maternal history of diabetes. While another study with a similar Japanese population failed to replicate this association, the mt5178A was reported to have an antiatherogenic effect in type 2 diabetic individuals, as gauged by significantly smaller mean intima-media thickness (IMT) at six sites in the bilateral carotid arteries in the mt5178A group than in the mt5178C group [53]. In addition, upon multiple regression and discriminate analysis, the mt5178 type was significantly correlated with both the mean IMT and the presence of plaque. Kokaze et al. have reported that the mt5178C variant is significantly associated with increased diastolic blood pressure (in Japanese women), increased blood pressure in response to alcohol and intraocular pressure (in Japanese men) [54, 55]. These results suggest that the mt5178A variant is protective against a range of adult-onset diseases in Japanese subjects and this effect may explain, at least in part, its contribution to longevity in that population. Interestingly, besides the forementioned Chinese study [49], we are not aware of any similar study in other non-Japanese population analyzing the effects of age-associated diseases or longevity with this remarkable allele.

Cellular Models

The cell is another widely used model of aging that may be either of human or animal origin. Since the early findings of Hayflick that human fibroblasts grown in culture exhibited a finite proliferative capacity (50-doublings) [56], gathered observations have characterized replicative senescence and have unearthed the rather complex signaling pathway that underlies this program [57]. Triggering of the senescence pathway (found in other cell-types besides fibroblast) can come from a variety of stimuli including OS and can also be mediated by either DNA or telomere damage [58, 59]. In concert with the replicative senescence programme a distinct set of cell biomarkers develops, including β-galactosidase, alterations of some of the proteins involved in the replicative senescence pathway including telomerase, telomere attrition and increased DNA damage (e.g., double strand breaks) in various cell types [60–64]. Recent studies with *in vivo* tissues have not been able to demonstrate a consistent aging-mediated increase in replicative senescence and have challenged its relevance and role in aging [65–68]. These observations suggested that the altered (oxygen-rich) harsh conditions of the *in vitro* culturing are likely responsible for the triggering of the senescence program, which is primarily operative as an anti-cancer strategy. Nevertheless, a role for replicative senescence in aging-associated atherosclerosis in endothelial and vascular smooth muscle cells has been suggested [69, 70]. Furthermore, some aging cell-types, in particular a wide array of stem cells (e.g., embryonic [ESCs], adult cardiac [CSCs], satellite stem cells, hematopoietic [HSCs]) have been shown to be more susceptible to replicative senescence with the concomitant appearance of senescent biomarkers such as telomere attrition [71–73]. For instance, in myocardial aging, CSCs are characterized by telomere dysfunction with alterations in telomeric binding proteins and accompanied by increased expression of p14ARF, p16INK4a, phospho-Ser-15-p53, and p53; p14ARF inhibits p53 degradation, and p16INK4a inhibits cdk4 and cdk6, blocking cells at the G_0-G_1 boundary [74]. The resultant decline of cell proliferation likely has striking effect on aging tissue to replenish/repair itself, a subject to which we will return later on in this chapter.

Search for Biomarkers of Human Aging

At a relatively recent workshop (circa 2004) leading biologists and clinicians interested in aging defined a biomarker of aging as a trait having three criteria [75].

1. The biomarker should predict physiological, cognitive and behavioral function in an age-coherent way, and do so better than chronological age.
2. It should predict remaining longevity at an age at which 90% of the population is still alive (or years of remaining functionality for the clinician), and do so for most of the specific illnesses that afflict the species under study.
3. Its measurement should not alter life expectancy or outcomes of subsequent tests of other age-sensitive parameters (i.e., be minimally invasive as well as accessible/affordable).

A continuing debate among clinicians and scientists has concerned the distinction between processes of aging, which can be identified and studied independently of age-related disease. While it is well-recognized that there are age-related risk factors for disease, and that these may overlap with risk factors for aging, there is no consensus on whether diseases to which older persons are vulnerable should be considered merely a byproduct of aging, or represent an essential component of the aging process. On the other hand, there is general agreement that biomarkers of aging represent a measure by which one could assess how long and how well physiological functions can be maintained with increasing age; with potential to inform the development of interventions that increase life expectancy and/or enhance function in aging populations.

Recently, it has been noted that despite intensive research effort in the search for aging biomarkers with these features, little progress has been achieved and arguably these criteria might in fact be more stringent than necessary [76].

A variety of data could be employed as a panel of potential functional biomarkers of aging, ranging from anthropometric markers (e.g., body mass index, body composition, bone density), functional challenge tests (e.g., glucose tolerance test), biochemical/physiological tests (e.g., HDL-cholesterol and other apolipoproteins, glycosylated hemoglobin, homocysteine), as well as genomic and proteomic data [75].

Consistent with the view of aging as an accumulation of macromolecular and cellular alterations resulting in degeneration and dysfunction, the assessment of damage, primarily resulting from OS, has proved to be useful as an aging biomarker in animal and clinical studies. Recently, after evaluation of several oxidative biomarkers including lipid peroxidation (LPO) products, protein oxidation products, antioxidative enzymes, minerals, vitamins, glutathione, flavonoids, bilirubin and uric acid in a clinical setting it has been suggested that no single marker is sufficient by itself but rather a set of markers should be used to determine the oxidation status of the individual, which should include markers for LPO, protein oxidation, the total antioxidative status as well as one for DNA damage [77].

Similarly, a profiling technique to assess the "Oxidative Stress Profiles (JaICA-Genox OSP)" of individuals and laboratory test animals has been developed as a joint effort by Japan Institute for the Control of Aging (JaICA) and Genox [78]. The JaICA-Genox OSP is comprised of nearly 45 different assays gauging the levels of oxidative damage in lipids and nucleic acids, and the antioxidant defenses in the serum. In addition, several biomarkers for CVD risk are also measured, and assays to measure specific age- and sex-related hormones in serum and urine, and trace elements in serum, urine, and drinking water are also analyzed.

Employing an impressive array of analytical techniques, including immunoblot analysis, microsequencing, immunohistochemistry, HPLC, and GC-MS and HPLC-MS/MS several investigators have suggested that a number of modalities to detect oxidative damage to amino acids (e.g., nitrosylation, accumulation of protein carbonyls and dityrosine residues) may be useful aging biomarkers [79-81]. Several post-translational modifications (such as tyrosine oxidation) are also more prevalent in age-associated diseases including Alzheimer disease and atherosclerosis. However, the specificity of protein damage in aging as well as the correlation between structural defect and protein function remains rather undefined. Activities of several proteins with critical cellular function, which appear to be specifically targeted by OS in aging include the bioenergetic enzymes –*cis*-aconistase, adenine nucleotide translocase (ANT) and the poly adenosine diphosphate-ribose polymerase (PARP), an essential factor for DNA repair (previously discussed in greater depth in Chapter 4) [82–84]. In mice, Navarro has reported that several mitochondrial enzyme activities, including mitochondrial nitric oxide synthase (mtNOS), NADH dehydrogenase (complex I) and cytochrome *c* oxidase (complex IV), behaved as markers of brain aging with the decline in enzyme activities (in concert with increased protein carbonyl levels) correlating with diminished neurological function [85]. Furthermore, this study also showed that a delay in both mitochondrial enzymatic and neurological dysfunction significantly increased mice life span (arising from regimens of exercise and antioxidant supplementation).

Disparities have been observed between intracellular and extracellular proteins with regards to age-associated oxidation. With age the concentration of oxidative markers has been found to increase more in extracellular proteins than in intracellular proteins, which may be in part explained by significant differences in turnover between extracellular (hours to days) and intracellular proteins (minutes to hours) [86].

Another type of post-translational protein damage that can serve as an aging biomarker is the age pigment, lipofuscin. The age-related increase of age pigments was initially demonstrated by Strehler et al. [87] in human myocardium, and by Reichel et al. [88] in rodent brain. The origin of this pigment is thought to stem from cross-linked protein oxidation products, with the involvement of free radicals in the formation of fluorescent oxidized/cross-linked aggregates [89]. Observations on the effects of pro-oxidants and antioxidants on lipofuscin accumulation in cultured rat cardiac myocytes and human glial cells have indicated that pro-oxidants accelerate while antioxidants retard the rate of lipofuscin accumulation [90]. The accumulation of these non-degradable protein aggregates leads to the inhibition of proteasome-mediated degradative pathways, particularly in post-mitotic cells [91].

Another marker of aging is the cross-linked protein resulting from the nonenzymatic Maillard reaction, involving oxidative reactions of carbohydrate and lipid substrates, [92] and acting as an amplifier of reactive oxygen damage generating AGE or glycation elements, also termed Nε Carboxymethyl lysine (CML) [93]. The oxidative formation of CML from glycated proteins was reduced by lipoic acid, aminoguanidine, superoxide dismutase, catalase, and particularly vitamin E and desferrioxamine. Among the numerous organs, which accumulate CML in an age-associated manner, glycated proteins were particularly localized in the arterial wall and in the elastic membrane, as well as within atherosclerotic plaques and in foam cells. These glycated proteins (e.g., the relatively long-lived and abundant collagen molecule is frequently targeted) contribute to increased arterial stiffness, altered extracellular matrix and affect repair of vascular damage and dermal wound healing. Moreover, the properties of collagen as a supporting framework structure and as a controlling factor in cell matrix interactions are compromised. These events are accelerated in metabolic diseases such as diabetes, end-stage renal disease, neurodegenerative diseases such as Alzheimer's disease (AD) and amyotrophic lateral sclerosis (ALS), which have in common with physiological aging the accumulation of various glycation products and cross-links. Also, a linkage of AGE to endothelial cell dysfunction has been observed mediated by specific receptors to AGE (RAGE). AGE-binding to its receptor induces expression of cell adhesion molecules, tissue factor, cytokines such as IL-6, and monocyte chemoattractant protein-1 and stimulation of NADPH oxidase leading to further ROS generation [94].

DNA damage/modifications may also be an important aging biomarker although data available from human are limited. For instance, the detection of 8-hydroxyguanine (8OHdG), an accepted biomarker of OS, in both nuclear and mtDNA was initially proposed as an aging biomarker in rodents [95, 96]. Subsequent observations have found that the levels of mtDNA damage were greatly overestimated [97]. These later findings have been confirmed by other investigators [98], albeit it remains unclear how good an indicator of aging 8OHdG is. Interestingly, measurement of 8OHdG in urine to assess "whole-body" oxidative DNA damage has been used, and significant increase in urinary 8OHdG in elderly men (mean 72 year) versus younger men (mean 22 year) has been reported [99]. However, urinary 8OHdG is a partial measure of damage to guanine residues in DNA as well as to its nucleotide precursor pool, (it can arise from degradation of oxidized dGTP), thus 8OHdG concentrations may not truly reflect rates of oxidative damage to DNA [100].

While there is strong evidence that somatic mtDNA mutations and deletions do accumulate with aging in specific tissues (particularly the heart) in both animals and human [101, 102], their use as a biomarker has been somewhat limited by doubts concerning the mechanism by which these mutations arise, as well as their functional significance in organ function. For instance, accumulation of acquired mtDNA mutations to functionally relevant levels in aged tissues are primarily a consequence of clonal expansions of single founder molecules and not of ongoing stochastic mutational events. Recent observations have also suggested that epigenetic remodeling of DNA occurs in human aging, with older individuals displaying higher levels of promoter hypermethylation compared to younger ones [103]. While techniques initially used for measuring DNA methylation primarily focused on one specific DNA sequence at a time, novel improved techniques that allow a global examination of the whole genome for methylation changes using an array-based method, are emerging and this will increase our understanding of the full extent of DNA methylation in aging [104].

Dolichol is a polyprenol compound broadly distributed in membranes generally tucked between the two leaflets of the lipid bilayer, very close to the tail of phospholipid fatty acids. While no definitive catabolic pathway for this molecule has yet been defined, dolichol may act as a radical scavenger of peroxidized lipids belonging to the cell membranes [105]. Dolichol levels increase dramatically with increasing age. Parentini et al. [106] have recently proposed that dolichol fulfills the criteria for an aging-specific biomarker since: (1) Dolichol levels increase with age in all tissues across several mammalian species, including humans and are not altered by several age-dependent diseases in the same direction as that aging; (2) Dolichol accumulation is not secondary to metabolic changes of aging and is significantly altered by factors that modulate the aging rate, such as caloric restriction and physical exercise; and (3) Reliable changes in tissue dolichol levels are seen in relatively short intervals of time compared to over a life span, and levels can be analyzed on a small amount of tissue without causing death of the animal.

There is significant evidence of an association between human aging and a pro-inflammatory state in which several inflammatory cytokines, including interleukin-6 (IL-6), tumor necrosis factor α (TNF-α) and interleukin-1β (IL-1β) exhibit increased expression. At the same time, aging is associated with a decrease in serum testosterone (T) levels, which appears to be correlated with the increase in inflammatory cytokines [107]. This inverse relationship has been further corroborated in *in vitro* studies indicating that T downregulates the IL-6 gene through androgen receptors [108], and that induction of hypogonadism in older men was followed by a significant increase in IL-6, soluble IL-6 receptor (sIL-6r), and TNF-α [109]. On the other hand, T replacement in both young and old hypogonadal men reduces inflammatory markers leading to decreased levels of TNF-α and IL-1β without significant changes in IL-6 [110]. Collectively, these inflammatory factors may contribute to chronic diseases such as sarcopenia, osteoporosis, and arthritis, and are among the most powerful biomarkers and predictors of frailty and mortality in the elderly [111]. It is well-established that many problems common to older adults including anorexia, lethargy, anemia and the catabolism of muscle can be induced by IL-6. In the "Invecchiare in Chianti" (InCHIANTI) study, a prospective population-based study of 1,020 participants aged 65 years and older living in the Chianti area of Italy older people, inflammation, measured as high levels of IL-6, CRP, and IL-1RA, was significantly associated with poor physical performance and muscle strength in the elderly [112]. Moreover, in studies of adults < 65 years, IL-6, and TNF-α levels have been shown to predict coronary disease and cardiovascular mortality [113]. On the other hand, observations on elderly participants show that CRP and fibrinogen may not be as useful as other markers such as IL-6 and TNF-α, suggesting that a combined evaluation of several biomarkers may increase the specificity of the definition of inflammation. Cesari et al. have combined IL-6, CRP and TNF-α into a single measure by identifying participants having all three markers (in the respective highest tertile), which led to a stronger prediction of CAD events compared to the single strongest individual predictor IL-6 [114].

Over the last decade, considerable attention has focused on the anabolic steroid dehydroepiandrosterone (DHEA) and its prohormome DHEA sulphate (DHEAS) as biomarkers of aging. When human development is completed and adulthood is reached, adrenal gland generated DHEA and DHEAS levels start to decline so that by 80 years of age, peak DHEAS concentrations are only 10–20% of those in young adults. Lane et al. have reported that male and female rhesus monkeys exhibited a steady, age-related decline in serum DHEAS, similar to that observed in humans [115]. These observations provide further evidence that DHEA/DHEAS are aging biomarkers and showed that CR significantly retarded the postmaturational decline in serum DHEAS levels. Furthermore, in the gray mouse lemur, a short living primate (longevity 10–13 years), the DHEAS level was about 30–40% of its adult value with age over 6 years, a stepwise pattern most closely resembling the human pattern and consistent with DHEAS being a biomarker of aging [116].

Epidemiological studies have demonstrated an inverse relationship between plasma DHEA(S) levels in men and age-related illnesses, including cardiovascular and metabolic diseases, immune disorders, malignancies, and neurological dysfunction [117]. Gathered observations have shown that lower plasma DHEAS levels, as an independent risk factor, can be contributory to chronic HF and is a marker of poor prognosis [118, 119, 120]. Moreover, in a random sample prospective study of 1,709 men aged 40–70 years, low serum DHEAS was reported to be an independent risk factor of ischemic heart disease [121]. Although the majority of prospective studies have shown no significant association, others studies investigating the relationship between serum DHEA and DHEAS levels and CAD in men have been rather discordant [122]. From the clinical observations gathered thus far, there is no significant supporting data to use DHEA supplementation (as a replacement therapy) to treat healthy elderly individuals; however, several clinical trials are underway [123].

There is significant evidence that inflammation is implicated in all phases of the atherosclerotic pathogeneic process, from plaque formation to the progression, and ultimately the thrombotic complications of atherosclerosis [124]. The composition of the atherosclerotic plaque, is now recognized as a key feature in determining plaque vulnerability, and hence the risk of acute coronary ischemic events. Arising from the increasing focus on the role of inflammation in atherogenesis, questions have been raised as to whether circulating levels of inflammatory biomarkers can be used to identify those at risk for future cardiovascular events. It is also noteworthy that the Werner syndrome (WS), featuring premature aging, presents with inflammatory diseases such as atherosclerosis and type II diabetes and is accompanied by the presence of high plasma levels of inflammatory cytokines. Fibroblasts derived from individuals with WS have activated a major molecular pathway involved in inflammation suggesting that WS is an example of "inflamm-aging", with many of the phenotypic manifestations potentially resulting from an increased inflammatory state [125].

The hemostatic system has age-dependent components and there are indications that the elderly display a biological picture of a prethrombotic state. In a study of 80 healthy subjects with age ranging between 20 and 94 years, Cadroy et al. [126] have found that three thrombotic markers, i.e., the plasma concentration of prothrombin fragments 1 + 2 (F 1 + 2), thrombin-antithrombin III complexes (TAT) and fibrin degradation fragments D-dimers (D-D) were positively correlated with age with mean plasma levels of each marker two- to five-fold higher in subjects with age greater than or equal to 60 as compared to those less than 60 years.

Interestingly, in a random sample of 1,727 community-dwelling elderly persons (72 years or older) from five rural and urban counties in North Carolina, as part of the Established Populations for the Epidemiologic Studies of the Elderly (Duke University), D-dimer levels increased with increasing age and functional disability and were dramatically higher in blacks (nearly four times more likely to have an extreme value of D-dimer than whites); blacks had an average level that was nearly 40% higher than whites in an analysis of the continuous version of the outcome [127]. The racial effect persisted even after controlling for smoking and factors known to be related to thrombosis and was not mediated by social factors.

Although advanced age, as previously noted, is often associated with elevated IL-6 levels (suggesting that a pro-inflammatory state exists in the elderly that may be an important stimulus for thrombus formation), and can be associated with a dramatic increase in the incidence of venous and arterial thrombotic events, many elderly people do not experience clinical thrombotic events [128]. The identification of modifying elements (both genetic and environmental), which may heighten thrombotic risks in the elderly, is clearly warranted. For instance, obesity may represent such a risk factor since adipose tissue is an important source of inflammatory cytokines and plasminogen activator inhibitor-1 (PAI-1).

Several factors, which are known to play a critical role in cellular senescence, also may constitute aging biomarkers. For instance, the tumor suppressor products of the INK4a/ARF locus–p16INK4a (more simply p16) and ARF – attenuate cell proliferative growth at the senescence stage by exerting their effects on the retinoblastoma (Rb) protein- and p53-mediated responsive pathways. Importantly, these proteins have been linked to the induction of cell cycle arrest in response to DNA damage [129, 130]. Both of these cell cycle inhibitors are upregulated in nearly all tissues examined during aging in rodent [131]. Moreover, the age-associated increase in expression of p16 and ARF was attenuated in the kidney, ovary, and heart by CR.

Telomere attrition is another proposed senescence-associated aging biomarker. Telomere shortening has been successfully associated with cellular senescence and irreversible cell cycle arrest and is implicated in tumorigenesis and cancer [62]. As such telomere length is an indicator of replicative history, and of the cumulative history of OS. In addition, during aging telomeres in many human cell-types shorten *in vivo* as well, suggesting that telomere length could be a biomarker of aging (as an indicator of functional age), and of age-related morbidity. This telomere-associated senescence might be targeted to stem cells in specific tissues, in which replication potential is crucial to function, contributing to age-related functional attenuation in this tissue or alternatively cause systemic effects [132]. However, beyond the available correlative evidence and with nagging questions surrounding the role and impact of cellular senescence on aging, as previously discussed, more definitive proofs are needed linking telomere attrition to aging. Interestingly, recent studies in the nonhuman primate, *Macaca fascicularis* replicated findings similar to those obtained in humans of age-associated telomere-attrition in proliferating tissues including lung, pancreas, skin and thyroid, with significant telomerase activity in spleen, thymus, digestive tract, and gonads, suggesting that factors that modify telomere attrition and aging in humans may also be operative in the macaque model [133].

Gene expression profiling may also be used to identify a pattern of genes (a molecular signature) that serves as biomarker of relevant clinical parameters of CVD (e.g., disease presence, progression or response to therapy) [134]. While not as easy or convenient to perform as the screening of circulating biomarkers, the deployment of gene/transcriptome profiling targeted to specific tissues or cell populations can often provide important information unavailable with other approaches, as well as augmenting the growing list of significant (and novel) biomarkers. Numerous relevant data concerning which pathways (e.g., inflammatory and OS-associated functions) appear to be most significantly affected and take-home lessons (including limitations and biases of this analytical approach) have emerged from the use of gene expression profiling in specific tissues (including heart and skeletal muscle) in rat and mouse models of aging and premature aging [135–137]. Furthermore, the tissue-specific profiling patterns and gene-expression biomarkers have also been gainfully examined under conditions in which aging animals were subjected to stresses (oxidative or ischemic) [138, 139] or subjected to CR or treated with pharmacological mimetics to CR [135, 140, 141]. Mice fed with supplements including creatine displayed significantly increased mean life span (10%), with reduced levels of ROS and lower accumulation of the lipofuscin; expression profiling revealed an upregulation of genes implicated in neuronal growth, neuroprotection, and learning [142].

Furthermore, both major and minor nutrients can affect the specific expression of genes related to aging and inflammation (identifiable by gene profiling), and chemically diverse micronutrients such as polyphenols and tocopherols may exert their effects through modulating the expression of functionally related genes [143]. Thus, novel and diverse transcriptional targets of nutrients operative in aging may be identified using functional genomics (potential biomarkers) as well as bringing insight to the molecular mechanisms involved in the modulation of aging by nutrients [144]. Another closely related way that nutrients can impact the genome (and gene expression) is by directly altering the genome (impacting DNA repair) or by chromatin remodeling, which controls specific transcription through epigenetic-mediated changes in gene expression [145]. Later in this chapter we shall return to the subject of nutrigenomics.

Comprehensive gene profiling in human muscle from healthy young (21–27 years old) and older men (67–75 years old) revealed that expression of numerous genes involved with stress responses, hormone/cytokine/growth factor signaling, control of the cell cycle and apoptosis, and transcriptional regulation were affected by aging. In older muscle, genes encoding proteins involved in energy metabolism and mitochondrial protein synthesis were downregulated while genes encoding metallothioneins, high-mobility-group proteins, heterogeneous nuclear ribonucleoproteins and other RNA binding/processing proteins, and components of the ubiquitin-proteasome proteolytic pathway were upregulated [146]. Moreover, more kinds of transcripts were detected in older muscle, suggesting dedifferentiation, an increased number of splice variants, or increased cellular heterogeneity. Interestingly, a careful profiling analysis of the non-failing human heart also found that metallothionein 1L (Mt1l), a protein implicated in cell defense, increased with age regardless of normalization and independent of the hypertensive status [147]. As metallothionein is involved in cytoprotection against various forms of oxidative injury, its increased abundance in humans with aging may be reflective of oxidative repair mechanisms activated and it may represent an important aging biomarker.

A more recent transcriptome profiling study of human muscle identified a molecular profile for aging consisting of 250 age-regulated genes, which correlated with chronological age as well as with a measure of physiological age and shared a common signature for aging with previously obtained profiles of the kidney and the brain [148]. The common aging signature contained four age-upregulated pathways (affecting genes in the extracellular matrix, involved in cell growth, encoding factors involved in complement activation, and ribosome components) and two age-downregulated pathways (affecting genes involved in chloride transport and encoding subunits of the mitochondrial electron transport chain). Comparison of the human genomic profiling pattern with mouse and fly patterns, revealed a decline in electron transport chain pathway expression with age in all three organisms, suggesting that this may be a common transcriptional biomarker for aging across species.

Transcriptional profiling of the human frontal cortex from individuals ranging from 26 to 106 years of age could define a set of genes known to play critical roles in synaptic plasticity, vesicular transport and mitochondrial function, with reduced expression after age 40 and also identified upregulated genes involved in stress response, antioxidant and DNA repair [149]. Interestingly, promoters of genes with reduced expression in the aged cortex exhibited marked increases in DNA damage *in vivo* and in cultured human neurons subjected to OS; these promoters were selectively damaged and displayed reduced base-excision DNA repair. This suggests that DNA damage may reduce the expression of selectively vulnerable genes involved in learning, memory and neuronal survival, initiating a program of brain aging that starts early in adult life.

Gene profiling studies with premature aging syndromes have also provided important insights into normal human aging [150]. Altered transcription as a result of mutations in DNA metabolism enzymes appear to be fundamentally involved in the pathology of a number of the progeroid disorders including WS, CS and HGPS, albeit the proposed role of altered transcription relative to the mechanism of normal aging is thus far less clear [151]. Nevertheless, Kyng et al. have demonstrated that there is a strikingly similar pattern of gene expression changes in primary human fibroblast cells derived from old donors and in cells derived from patients with Werner syndrome as compared to cells from young donors suggesting a presence of common cellular aging mechanisms in old and progeria [152]. The similarity in genes affected indicated that this was a programmatic shift in gene expression and unlikely a result of stochastic damage. Further studies found a similar expression profile in fibroblasts from WS patients or aged subjects upon stress-induction known to promote DNA damage (i.e., gamma- and UV-irradiation) [153]. Profiled fibroblasts from patients with HGPS compared to normal age-matched controls revealed significant changes in expression of transcription factors and extracellular matrix proteins, many of which are known to function in the tissues severely affected in HGPS including the identification of a large number of genes implicated in atherosclerosis [154].

Moreover, developing proteomic techniques may be useful in confirming and identifying novel biomarkers of aging [155]. For example, using mass spectrometry (MS) technology (specifically SPE-LC-MS/MS), a methodology widely used in the precise quantitative determination of small molecules such as drugs, drug metabolites and hormones, multiple small peptides generated (by proteolytic digestion) from larger plasma proteins can be rapidly detected with high sensitivity and accurately quantitated (compared to other proteomic techniques such as electrophoresis which tend to show great variability in quantitative assessment). In addition, assay technologies with higher sensitivity and a greater dynamic range can also be applied to preselected or pre-fractionated groups of candidate proteins compared to current proteomic analysis. Simultaneous profiling analysis of multiple independent disease-related circulating biomarker proteins and their peptides, considered in the aggregate, should prove less prone to the influence of heterogenous genetic factors and disease processes, as well as environmental "noise" that might impact on the level of a single marker protein giving a better fingerprint with aging or an aging-associated disease. In this regard, multiple biomarkers, considered as a composite, may provide better prediction of a disease state than single markers (e.g., in the assessment of inflammation with a panel of weak acute phase reactants compared to a single marker such as CRP or serum amyloid A). In addition, the relative risk of CAD might be better predicted (by CRP and LDL-cholesterol) together than by either marker alone [156].

Given the more extensive targeting of mitochondrial proteins by oxidative damage, described in several studies, there has been increasing efforts to develop techniques to enrich and to assess both qualitatively and quantitatively the mitochondrial proteome in relation to age-mediated modifications as well as changes in specific peptide abundance, composition, structure, and activity

[157–162]. Because a significant part of the mitochondrial proteome is membrane-associated and functions as oligomeric protein complexes, techniques are being developed to detect and identify both membranous and soluble mitochondrial proteins under conditions preserving protein-protein interactions. The isolation of large supercomplexes (both OXPHOS and nonOXPHOS) from mitochondria by blue-native (BN)-PAGE and subsequent analysis by 2D SDS-PAGE, and MS peptide mass fingerprinting in different tissues has allowed the quantitative analysis of tissue-diverse mitochondrial proteomes [163]. In addition, this proteomic analysis has permitted the identification of over 200 distinct non-OXPHOS proteins and numerous non-mitochondrial proteins that interact with these complexes defining a mitochondrial protein interactome and enlarging the potential sets of markers available. Recent observations suggested that consistent changes in the stoichiometry of the various OXPHOS complexes occurs in aging [162]. Moreover, as previously noted, the proteomic detection of specific post-translational modifications including the addition of 3-nitrotyrosine to specific proteins can be used as a marker of aging [81]. Another age-mediated oxidative modification involves the formation of ROS-induced N-formyl-kynurenine from oxidized tryptophans in certain cardiac mitochondrial proteins, including multiple aconitase isoforms, are resolvable using 2D-PAGE with high resolution IEF in the first dimension [164]. These oxidatively-modified aconitase isoforms might serve as component of a protein biomarker signature of cardiac aging.

Systems Biology: Improved Networking-Enlarging the Perspective

Translation of the wealth of reductionist details about molecules, genes, biochemical pathways, cells and tissues into a real understanding of how these systems function and are perturbed in age and age-mediated disease, remains a primary challenge of the gerontologist. There is increasing acceptance that a more complete understanding of the overall mechanism of aging and the role of genes in fostering its complex phenotypes, particularly with respect to the heart and cardiovascular health will require integrating the large comprehensive and ever-growing information concerning genomic, proteomic, biochemical, anatomical and physiological data in aging individuals [165]. With the important insight that age-related alterations tend to progress in a system-wide fashion, increased emphasis is placed on the overall cellular networks involved in gene regulation, metabolic and growth pathways and protein-protein interaction rather than focusing on single genes and proteins. A primary and attractive feature of systems biology is it's model-building by integrating data incorporating unconnected observations and theories to test *via* simulation and allow the generation and refinement of hypothesis concerning aging. Several *in silico* models are being developed with the primary goal of establishing mechanistic models and algorithms of gene regulatory, metabolic, signaling or DNA repair pathways to recapitulate the dynamics and properties of networks in aging [166, 167].

Interestingly, much pertinent information is already broadly available both in published literature and in online databases that can be searched and retrieved. Moreover, this could eventually lead to simulated modeling of aging cardiac function (or dysfunction) at the genetic, molecular and physiological levels, which can allow predictions about potential interventions to be made. Some investigators have proposed that such simulated modeling would also highlight the gaps in our knowledge of the aging process and elicit new perspectives in how to fill them [168]. The construction of these models, in addition to the array of data discussed above, requires an extensive and sophisticated mathematical and computer algorithmic treatment [165]; its undertaking is clearly a multidisciplinary approach involving mathematics, computer skills, molecular and cell biology, genetics, physiology and anatomy.

In general, system-modeling approaches can be divided into bottom-up and top-down. In top-down mode, the system as a whole is deconstructed into its component parts (i.e., functional groups such as a tissues and cells) and links. The bottoms-up approach tends to be more "reductionist" focusing on the gene and proteins and the pathways they define. Interestingly, as Kriete et al.

have pointed out, there is presently limited quantitative data regarding higher levels of biological organization depicting cells, their arrangements in tissues and supply networks to optimize nutrient distribution and thereby regulate metabolism, in contrast to the expanding wealth of information relating to bottoms-up modeling (i.e., derived from molecular studies) [169]. However, defining and integrating both approaches appears to be important for successful modeling as models built from bottom-up data alone appear to have limited capacity for examining the effect of perturbations on cells as a whole, and even more so, on modeling multicellular entities or organisms.

A top-down model of aging will examine interactions between body mass, metabolism and life span defining a hierarchical branching network; a central premise involves the effect of age on the distribution of life-sustaining nutrition over several orders of scale, providing a consistent supply for all cells to drive metabolism and biosynthetic reactions [170]. These interactions defined in part by so called scaling laws and in part by environmental influences dictating demands for thermoregulation and ATP production can impact many aspects of cellular structure, function and viability. For instance, they can predict turnover rates in mitochondrial respiratory complexes, which in turn can lead to ROS generation that has been linked to life span regulation (see Chapters 2 and 12). The bottom-up focus in aging has tended to concentrate on the identification of gene regulation, chromatin functional remodeling (e.g., telomere function), intracellular signaling, protein and DNA repair networks. It is noteworthy that these aging-models have had to recognize and address the dual-sided features of ROS, both as a participant in the stochastic mechanisms involved in the cell (and DNA) as well as a critical signaling molecule in executing programmed transcriptional responses dealing with cell survival, and also cytoprotective strategies highlighting the increased awareness of both the stochastic and the programmatic aspects of aging. From a physiome perspective, it is apparent that aging can affect all levels of the network in an interconnected and multidirectional fashion, suggesting several feedback loops between the genomic, organelle, cellular and organ level (Fig. 16.1).

While a central component of several aging hypotheses encompasses the free radical theory of aging, which suggests that aging results from the accumulation of unrepaired somatic defects built into aging models, so has the recognition that multiple mechanisms of aging operate in parallel [171]. Distribution processes becomes increasingly dissipative creating entropy and energy-damaging molecules (such as ROS), altering proteins and genes and disturbing a multitude of essential cellular programs such as mitochondrial function. Energy dissipation and damage have been related to the average cellular metabolic rate, increasing with mass/organism size. Age-associated entropy in multiple cellular pathways is also noted with evidence of structural alteration at the cellular and multicellular levels, switches to apoptotic or senescence pathways, impaired intracellular signaling, DNA damage and altered gene expression profiles. Oxidative damage to DNA and increased mutation levels (including mtDNA) may be particularly deleterious dramatically impacting transcription programming and regulation [149], telomere shortening in non-replicating cells such as brain neurons and cardiomyocytes [59], increasing cell death [172], and targeting stem cell populations leading to a profound loss of tissue regenerative capacity [73].

These age-mediated changes also impact the homogeneity and efficiency of the tissue (i.e., increasing cellular heterogeneity), augmented cellular atrophy and hypertrophy as well as altering supplying networks. For instance, significant alterations in the arterial supply network that includes greater vascular stiffness, thickening and dysfunction, contribute to abnormal cardiovascular functioning; moreover, these changes, can impact the vasculature age-associated signaling cascades such as the onset of inflammatory signaling, potentially giving rise to adverse outcomes including neuropathologies. These models also can embrace information concerning the adaptiveness of the aging systems in responding to age-related deterioration, including the ability to foster antioxidant neutralization of ROS, built-in reserves to function and recruitment of the available maintenance/repair systems.

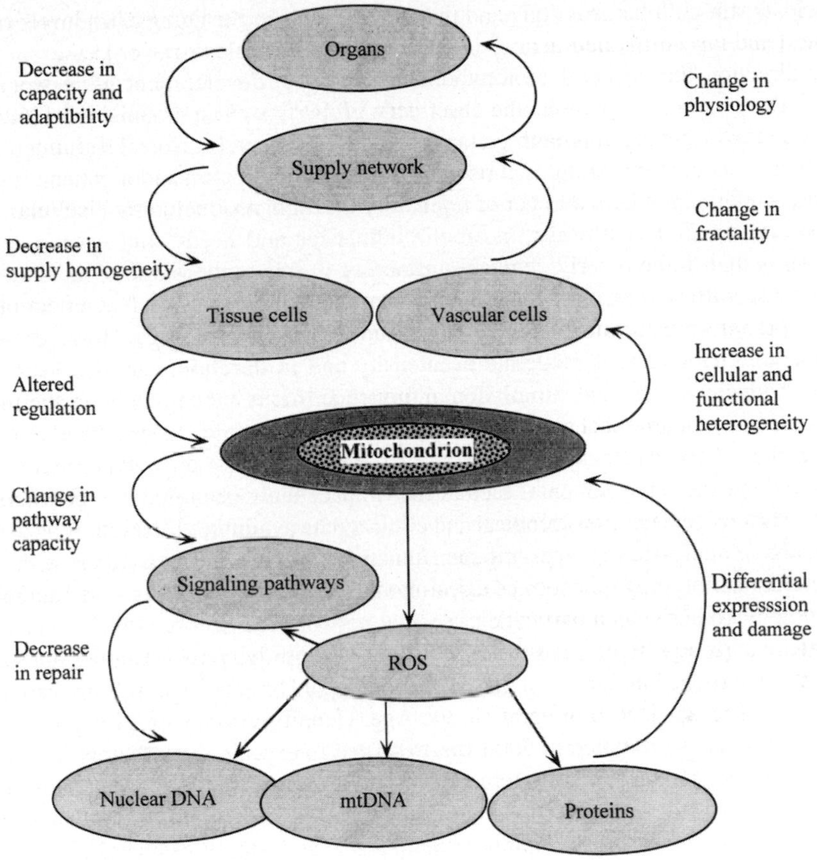

Fig. 16.1 System biology. Top-down and bottom-up analysis of the phenome

It is important to keep in mind that these models underscore that much critical post-genomic data remains to be obtained, including the identification of gene-environmental factor and protein-protein interactions, which appear to underlie many phenotypic changes and signaling events in the aging cell. It is increasingly clear that a number of critical biomolecular modifications and interactions, revealed by proteomic information (including oxidative changes such as nitrosylation and glycation), will be useful for unraveling metabolic and signaling pathways operating in the aging cell, in particular in response to disease and injury. Further identification of functional interactions between signaling pathways and genetic networks will also be of key interest as they may provide insight into regulation of the coordinated expression of functional groups of genes, with a few key pathways switching between alternative cell fates. The integration of molecular, clinical and physiological data into testable aging models should also greatly benefit from information available in online databases, mining of comparative genomics, proteomic and DNA microarray data, and knowledge environments [173–175]. Recent studies have suggested that phenotypic changes on the tissue-structural and physiological level can be effectively used as statistical covariants to enrich the gene expression analysis [176]. This will enable a profiling of genes that likely would have been overlooked by conventional gene expression analyses strategies.

Also underlying these models is the important recognition that the aging cardiovascular system is dynamic and is more than just electrical circuitry or mechanical pumps, and they have the ability to grow, remodel and adapt in response to changing environments partly determined by genes and partly by their physical environment [177]. Such a systems approach may in the near future further elucidate sub-cellular cross-talk and metabolic events in the aging cardiomyocyte, including mitochondrial and lysosomal interactions in concert with organelle turnover [178].

Another direction that systems biology is offering is the development of phenome studies of aging [165]. The phenome represents the observable properties of an organism that have developed under the continued influences of both genome and environmental factors The homeostatic control of these properties necessary for optimal function at the cellular, organ and organism levels is highly complex and is maintained by a number of regulatory mechanisms including neuroendocrine loops, neural networks, signaling pathways, metabolic influences and needs, and genetic switches. One view of aging is that in the elderly, dynamic instability in this homeostatic regulation, particularly when challenged with severe or chronic stress, can lead to progressive loss of normal function, failure of adaptation to environmental challenges and increased pathology. However, such stresses or environmental challenges, if moderate in intensity and in duration, can also lead to beneficial changes; this happens under mild stimulation or *hormesis* that is capable of enhancing DNA repair, immune competence, neuronal activity, vigilance, memory, resistance to stress and longevity [179]. The identification of the particular relationship of human genotype-phenotype, including both the genes involved and the environmental factors that impact their phenotypic expression, requires a large input of various genetic, physiological and clinical data available as databases as well as sophisticated algorithmic analysis encompassing the Human Phenome project. To assist with this analysis high-throughput phenotyping, phenomics research tools involving the use of computation and informatics technology, to derive genome wide molecular networks of genotype-phenotype or phenomic associations, are currently being developed [180]. This integrative post-genomics approach has just begun to be applied to the interaction of genes, phenotype and environment in aging in general and in aging-associated diseases [181]. In addition, the Age, Gene/Environment Susceptibility-Reykjavik Study (AGES-Reykjavik) initiated in 2002 was designed to examine risk factors, including genetic susceptibility and gene/environment interaction, in relation to disease and disability in an elderly human population from Iceland [182]. This phenomics study was multidisciplinary, with detailed phenotypes related to the cardiovascular, neuro-cognitive and musculoskeletal function, as well as to body composition and metabolic regulation. In addition, it detailed in this cohort relevant late-life quantitative traits, subclinical indicators of disease, and medical diagnoses identified using a variety of biomarkers, imaging, and other physiologic indicators. The use of this approach with a relatively genetically homogeneous older population can also facilitate the identification of genetic factors that contribute to healthy aging, as well as the chronic ailing conditions common in the elderly.

Reversing Aging and/or Dysfunction of Age-Associated Diseases

Both, retarding aging and extending longevity (with increased healthy aging) may be possible. However, the majority of the studies supporting this concept have been performed either with cells or in model organisms (very different physiologically from humans), thus the relevance of these observations to human aging has remained quite controversial. On the other hand, the findings that many of the genes and pathways affected are highly conserved and that perturbations in these genes and pathways appear to occur in many species, including in some human subjects, suggest that the findings from model systems about particular targeted pathways should be more seriously considered in regard to human aging. The famous theoretician Aubrey de Grey in collaboration with a group of scientists has proposed that a major long-term research focus directed towards reverse human aging should be undertaken and termed Strategies for Engineering Negligible Senescence (SENS) [183–186]. The reader is referred to his interesting website (www.degrey.org), which is a combination of his stimulating blogs, occasional rants and links to relevant publications supporting his premises. The SENS program has been strongly criticized by a large segment of the aging-science community in part for the aggressive and media-circus-associated manner in which these provocative ideas have been proposed, the questionable feasibility of many of the radical aspects of the SENS plans [187], and by the less-than-rigorous science and often over-exaggerated claims that often characterize its approach. Unfortunately, both sides of this controversy have utilized name-calling and invective to characterize the others position and have largely been unable to produce a meaningful productive debate on anti-aging approaches (at least in public dialogue). Nevertheless, while many of the SENS ideas and approaches are challenging and unlikely to be ever realized, most of the pathways pinpointed as worth targeting using bioengineering strategies are in fact widely viewed as credible targets to reverse and/or to retard aging. In this section we will review the primary targeted pathways so far examined and in several instances a call for attention to some of the proposals.

Targeting Cellular Atrophy and Depletion in Aging

Cell loss in aging is particularly critical in the cardiovascular system and in the brain. Extensive cell depletion in this areas is often accompanied by significant tissue remodeling in which the lost cells are replaced either by hypertrophic cells, by fibrous acellular deposits or not replaced leaving the tissue to shrink (i.e., mostly evident in skeletal muscle). As previously noted (see Chapters 3 and 4) cell death arising from several routes (e.g., apoptosis, necrosis and autophagy) occurs during aging. Moreover, evidence obtained from several animal models has suggested a mechanistic role for cardiac myocyte apoptosis in the development of DCM [188] and in the onset of HF [189], although the overall role of cell loss in human aging remains controversial.

The therapeutic targeting of apoptotic pathway elements has potential in the treatment of HF. For example, systemic administration of the broad-spectrum caspase inhibitor acetyl-Tyr-Val-Ala-Asp chloromethylketone significantly decreased apoptosis in infarcted regions of the myocardium, with subsequent reduction in infarct size in rabbit hearts during experimentally induced ischemia and reperfusion [190]. Caspase inhibition using pharmacological inhibitors or genetic approaches can be protective against ischemic injury to various organs including brain, heart and kidney [191]. Similarly, overexpression of a human Bcl-2 transgene in a mouse model of ischemia and reperfusion caused substantial reduction in apoptotic cells and infarct size and improvement in cardiac function [192]. In a rat model of HF, direct intramyocardial injection of adenovirus vector containing the gene for hepatocyte growth factor (HGF) 3 weeks post-MI resulted in increased expression of HGF and Bcl-2 proteins, in enhanced angiogenesis, reduced apoptosis, greater preservation of ventricular geometry, and cardiac contractile function [193]. In addition, to directly targeting cell death events, there is also evidence that activating components of pro-survival pathways in the myocardium, including IL-6-related cytokines, calcineurin, and IGF-1/PI3K/Akt signaling pathways can also provide antiapoptotic effects. However, the long-term consequences of inhibiting apoptosis must be carefully considered before its incorporation into potential therapies. Apoptotic cell death is a key element in maintaining immune homeostasis and preventing the emergence of lymphomas, or the development of autoimmunity, and therefore chronic systemic inhibition of apoptosis could have significant deleterious effects on organs other than the heart. Moreover, inhibition of apoptosis may also result in activation of other modes of cell death, such as necrosis that could have more deleterious effects on neighboring cells and a worse outcome, or might result in unwanted proliferative growth. In fact, many of the chemotherapeutic treatments directed against cancer cell growth target apoptosis.

Information concerning the effects of modulating apoptosis or cell depletion in aging is presently limited. It has been suggested that in the process of endothelial cell (EC) aging, laminar flow in the blood vessel and shear stress, which normally provide a potent endogenous protective force against endothelial cell apoptosis (primarily by increasing eNOS expression leading to increasing NO bioavailability), fails to induce eNOS and NO availability leading to increased EC apoptosis [193].

As we previously noted the targeted deletion of p66shc in mice causes increased longevity and p66shc, a redox enzyme directly involved in mitochondrial ROS production, is a critical promoter of apoptosis in several cell-types. Deletion of p66shc also reduces systemic and tissue OS, vascular cell apoptosis, and early atherogenesis in mice fed a high-fat diet [194], and by reducing OS effects protection against diabetic glomerulopathy [195]. Moreover, in a mouse model of insulin-dependent diabetes, ablation of the p66shc gene prevents ROS generation, telomere-shortening-associated senescence and apoptosis of the cardiac progenitor cells interfering with the acquisition of the heart senescent phenotype and the development of HF with diabetes [196].

A signaling route was recently demonstrated by which protein kinase C-β (PKC-β), activated by oxidative conditions in the cell, induces p66Shc phosphorylation and triggered mitochondrial accumulation of the p66Shc protein after it is recognized by the prolyl isomerase Pin1 causing downstream alteration of mitochondrial Ca^{2+} responses and structure; hence inducing apoptosis [197] may provide a viable target of pharmacological approaches to inhibit aging. Regulation of Shc isoforms in receptor-dependent pathways leading to cardiac hypertrophy and HF transition revealed that p66Shc expression is induced by a Gαq agonist. Furthermore, p66Shc has been identified as a candidate for a hypertrophy-induced mediator of cardiomyocyte apoptosis and HF suggesting that p66Shc represents an attractive novel molecular target for HF therapy [198].

Aging-associated apoptosis can also be targeted by lifestyle modifications such as CR and endurance exercise training. Observations with CR in mice have documented a decline in the myocardial cellular redox balance, that is critical with apoptosis [199]. The thioredoxin system, which is a necessary contributory factor to enhanced susceptibility to apoptotic stimuli in aging myocardium, has a transcriptional profile which can be reversed by CR. Rohrbach et al. [200] recently reported that mitochondrial thioredoxin reductase (TrxR2) is markedly decreased in aging skeletal and cardiac muscle and renormalized after CR, while the cytosolic thioredoxin reductase isoform remained unchanged. Experiments with RNAi have demonstrated that reduction of TrxR2 in myoblasts, under exposure to ceramide or TNF-α resulted in marked enhancement of nucleosomal DNA cleavage, caspase 9 activation, and mitochondrial ROS release, together with reduced cell viability. Furthermore, recent observations have shown that 12 weeks of exercise training provided significant protection against loss of cardiac myocytes in the aging rat heart attenuating age-induced increases in remodeling, apoptosis, and Bax/Bcl-2 ratio in the left ventricle. Moreover, exercise training in the aging rat reduced caspase-9 levels and Bax/Bcl-2 ratio by lowering Bax protein expression, while increasing Bcl-2 levels [201].

Stem Cells as both Primary Targets of Aging and a Potential Treatment Plan

Stem cells, which play a role in regenerative function, are particularly susceptible to aging-mediated loss and senescence programs. In the heart, a small pool of cardiac-specific stem (CSCs) and progenitor cells have been shown to be particularly sensitive to different forms of stress and in response can acquire a senescent, dysfunctional phenotype. This is particularly evident in the aging heart. Histological examination of cardiac tissue from older patients with signs of CVD has shown that c-kit+ resident CSCs undergo apoptosis and express the cyclin-dependent kinase p16INK4a [73]. In mice, CSC apoptosis was more prevalent in older animals, and CSC telomere length also decreased with age [202].

The importance of these cardiac stem cells has been recently highlighted by new observations detailing their role as the origin of cycling and proliferating myocytes, more evident in the pathological failing and hypertrophic heart [203, 204], in particular in end-stage ischemic heart disease, in idiopathic DCM [205] and after myocardial infarction [206].

The role of these relatively new discovered CSCs has not yet been fully determined in either the normal or pathological heart. However, studies of human aortic stenosis have suggested that these cells play a role in maintaining cardiac cellular homeostasis and contribute to cardiac remodeling with intense new myocyte formation in the left ventricle outflow tract appearing to be the result of CSC differentiation, and resulting in an increased cardiac mass arising from a combination of myocyte hypertrophy and hyperplasia [204].

Stem cells derived from the adult heart are self-renewing, clonogenic and multipotent and show similar properties/markers in both rodent and human myocardium [207, 208], and can differentiate either *in vitro* or *in vivo*. After expansion *in vitro*, these human heart stem cells when injected into immunodeficient SCID beige mice could form the major specialized myocardial cell-types of the heart, including fully contractile myocytes and vascular cells (i.e., cells with endothelial or smooth muscle markers) and could repair myocardial injury forming functional myocardium. Recent studies of the architectural organization of the cardiac stem cell niches residing within the adult mouse heart have shown that CSCs contribute to myocyte turnover, which is heterogeneous across the heart, faster at the apex and atria, and slower at the base-midregion of the ventricle [209].

As previously noted, these cells may eventually be used for autologous cell transplantation to produce physiologically relevant myocardial regeneration to repair injury and cardiac dysfunction with the potential for longer-lasting improvement than with noncardiac cells. Gathered observations have suggested that the dominant beneficial effects are probably due to neoangiogenesis and arteriogenesis. However, there may be a synergism between the paracrine stimulation of arteriogenesis and myogenesis/myocyte differentiation. Recently, it has been found that stem cell engraftment and differentiation to cardiac myocytes (i.e., myogenesis) arising from transplantation of embryonic stem cells into injured myocardium is markedly enhanced with paracrine signaling [210–213]. This growth factor/paracrine stimulation can be supplemented by added factors (e.g., vascular endothelial growth factor, fibroblast growth factor [FGF]), and transforming growth factor β (TGF-β), generated from the transplanted cells or generated from endogenous cells. The cardiomyogenic potential of bone marrow-derived Oct3/4 stem cells was recently shown to be largely governed by age-dependent paracrine/platelet-derived growth factor (PDGF) pathways [214]. In bone marrow cell cultures from 3 month old mice, PDGF-AB induction was required for the generation of cardiomyogenesis, whereas in cells derived from (18 month) mice, diminished PDGF-B induction was associated with impaired cardiomyogenic potential, despite having Oct3/4 levels similar to those in the young cells. Importantly, the cardiac differentiation capacity of the old bone marrow cells could be restored with supplementation with PDGF-AB. Other reports have been less optimistic about the use of growth factors in the elderly. The therapeutic efficacy of granulocyte colony-stimulating factor (G-CSF) and stem cell factor (SCF) in old versus young adult rats has been evaluated in a model of experimental MI; G-CSF/SCF therapy in young animals reversed the cardiac dysfunction, attenuated LV dilation, decreased infarct size, and reduced cardiomyocyte hypertrophy, but had little effect in aging rats [215]. This effect was attributed to a lower reduction of apoptosis whose rate remained high in older rodents, despite cytokine treatment, and may be due to aging-mediated downregulation of myocardial cytokine receptors (or downstream signaling), which have been reported in conjunction with reduced tumor necrosis factor (TNF); aging impaired cardioprotection was attributable to downregulated TNF-α receptors [216].

Furthermore, despite the increased attention that these cells are receiving, high proliferation rates of pure CSCs have not been attained and complete differentiation of cardiac progenitor cells into adult cardiomyocytes either *in vitro* or *in vivo* remain poorly understood. More research is clearly needed to identify factors that influence their proliferation and differentiation [217].

Given that the development of a senescent phenotype in CSCs has been associated with a decline in function, cardiac stem cell transplantation may be less beneficial in the elderly due to their heightened susceptibility to apoptosis and senescence. Moreover, cardiac stem cells express IGF-1 receptors and synthesize and secrete the corresponding ligands, hepatocyte growth factor (HGF) and IGF-1, which mobilize the cardiac stem cells and promote their survival and proliferation respectively [218]. Resident CSCs might be activated by treatment with a novel cocktail of growth factors with the capacity to reverse the aged CSC phenotype and activate and mobilize these cells *in situ* in order to regenerate myocardium and microcirculation lost as a consequence of coronary obstruction. Such an approach would have the distinct advantage of being generally available for rapid administration of cells in the acute post-MI phase, without relying on highly invasive, difficult-to-obtain and often heterogenous cell preparations [219, 220]. Administration of combinations of growth factors in a porcine model of acute MI is being tested, since the importance of murine and canine data to human pathology is unclear. Preliminary findings showed that therapeutic *in situ* activation of CSCs can produce extensive formation of new myocardial tissue and significantly improve LV function in hearts similar in size and anatomy to human hearts [220, 221]. Future examination of the effect of aging in this model appears to be of critical significance.

In addition, to the effects of aging on cardiac stem cell number and function, there is a large body of evidence showing that vascular stem cells, in particular the endothelial progenitor cells (EPCs), are substantially affected by aging and by aging-associated diseases [222]. For instance, EPC mobilization following coronary artery bypass grafting is significantly impaired in older individuals compared with younger patients [223]. Other observations have documented an aging-associated decline in human EPC proliferation, migration and survival concomitant with a decline in endothelial-dependent dilation and overall dysfunction [224]. One study reported a significant decline in the levels of EPCs in a healthy elderly male cohort compared to a younger group, and circulating EPCs correlated this decline with a reduction in both small and large arterial elasticity [225]. Furthermore, gathered observations have demonstrated a pronounced depletion of circulating EPC cells in concert with the progression of age-associated vascular diseases, including coronary artery disease [223], diabetes [226, 227], and atherosclerosis [228]. Experimentally, bone marrow transplantation from young, but not old, nonatherosclerotic mice, prevented atherosclerosis progression in apolipoprotein E knockout recipients, suggesting that deficient vascular repair because of increased age is a critical determinant of disease initiation and progression [229]. It is important to note here that a wide range of environmental factors influence EPC generation and function. For example, decreased levels of estrogen at the onset of menopause are associated with reduced levels of circulating EPCs as well as with increased CVD incidence in postmenopausal women [222]. *In vitro* studies have shown that estrogen can attenuate human EPC senescence by augmenting telomerase activity and activating Akt [230]. Thus, the decrease in EPC levels at the time of menopause may be in part explained by the loss of estrogen's inhibitory effects on EPC senescence. Estrogen replacement can restore bone marrow-derived EPC levels in ovariectomized female mice, as well as diminishing the increased neointima formation that occurs after carotid artery injury [231]. Estrogen-mediated increase in EPCs was shown to involve a reduction in EPC apoptosis, in particular the caspase-8 pathway. Likely involved are also modulation of NO, and eNOS levels in EPCs since they are mediating factors in EPC mobilization, as well as downstream mediators in growth factor and estrogen signaling pathways [232–234].

Repair of tissues with EPC transplantation is complicated because the growth of atherosclerotic lesions, which involves increased vascularization of the neointimal tissue, will be enhanced by the presence of EPCs. Transplantation of bone marrow or spleen-derived EPCs into $ApoE^{-}/^{-}$ mice promoted atherosclerotic lesion development [235]. As previously discussed, future therapies might better utilize activation of resident EPCS using combined factors, which can enhance EPC function either at the site of mobilization from the bone marrow and/or at sites of homing to damaged blood vessels [236]. Moreover, the age-associated decline in factors such as VEGF and PDGF signaling and circulating estrogen levels, which contribute to decrease in EPC mobilization, might be targeted and reversed by restoration of these factors providing added protective benefit to the cardiovascular system and limiting the impact of CVD. Thum et al. [237] have used GH treatment to enhance IGF-1 levels and significantly restore EPC number and function (e.g., improved colony forming and migratory capacity, enhanced incorporation into tube-like structures, and augmented eNOS expression) in middle-aged men relative to young adults. Treatment of aged mice with IGF-1 or with GH (7 day) improved the number and function of EPC that significantly increases systemic IGF-1 levels, whereas a short term GH treatment did not increase IGF-1 or EPC levels. Additionally, interruption of IGF-1/IGF-1 receptor signaling completely prevented the GH-mediated increase in EPC number and function.

Targeting Specific Organelles in Aging: Mitochondria/Lysosome

Given the extreme importance of mitochondrial function and dysfunction in mechanisms and pathways of aging, it is no surprise that a considerable portion of the treatments intended to reverse or retard aging target the mitochondria. In rodent models the use of caloric and dietary restriction as well as specific fatty-acid regimens have shown promising results by reversing OS and oxidative damage, stemming from mitochondrial dysfunction in aging [238–240]. Similarly, the use of antioxidants as molecular supplements such as coenzyme Q10 and acetyl-L-carnitine and/or lipoic acid and melatonin appear to operate on the same targets [241–243]. Potent synthetic cell-permeable peptide antioxidants have been designed that concentrate at high levels in the inner mitochondrial membrane reducing mitochondrial-generated ROS, mitochondrial swelling, membrane damage and apoptosis [244], and appear to be promising in treatment of aging. Using gene transfer, overexpressed antioxidant proteins (e.g., metallotheinein and mitochondrial-targeted catalase) have shown modest but significant effects on life span and on cardiovascular health, particularly when introduced as cardiac-specific constructs [245–247]. However, at the present time there are many unknowns with the clinical application of gene therapy, an approach that also is highly invasive. Vectors will also have to be carefully and rigorously tested to ensure safety and efficacy. Some vectors don't appear to work in the elderly (e.g., adenoviral based constructs) and may have to be redesigned accordingly [248]. Gene therapy to treat mitochondrial mutations or defective mtDNA-encoded proteins is not yet available; re-engineering all 13 mtDNA-encoded proteins expressed as allotopic constructs from the nucleus has been recommended by de Grey [183], although this is a rather unlikely undertaking. The use of smaller specific agonists, co-factors and antagonists, which can be introduced systemically, the global transcriptional modulators (including PPAR, PGC-1), the sirtuin family and TOR, all of which either directly or indirectly impact mitochondrial metabolism including ROS generation, may be more easily adaptable to clinical use to modulate pathways involved in aging.

Another organelle targeted in aging is the lysosome and the over-accumulation of cell garbage. The limited data available (see Chapter 4) suggest that the intralysosomal degradative process, known as autophagy, is inefficient in the aging process [249]. Deposits of aggregated proteins and or organelles which are not effectively turned-over or removed have been implicated in a wide array of neurodegenerative disorders as well as in atherosclerosis [250]. Interestingly, according to de Grey, the degradation of these aggregates is helped by the addition of bacterial or fungal enzymes – "xeno-hydrolases" – that can degrade molecules that our natural machinery cannot [251, 252]. While this scenario is highly futuristic as envisioned, it is worth considering for potential adaptation (e.g., design of stem-cells that could be introduced with this capacity). Other less challenging venues include finding/designing drugs that can activate (in the short-term) autophagy. For instance, some forms are activated by chaperones [253].

It has been proposed that CR and disruption of insulin-like signals can modulate aging by prolonged stimulation of macroautophagy [254]. Recent studies reported that life-long weekly administration of an anti-lipolytic drug (3, 5-dimethylpyrazole, DMP), showed enhanced removal of mitochondria containing oxidatively damaged mtDNA, decreased glucose and insulin levels, stimulating autophagy and intensifying the anti-aging effects of submaximal CR [255, 256].

Techniques for targeting DNA damage and genomic instability, chromatin and telomeric remodeling and dysfunction are extremely complex issues that may prove extremely difficult to precisely target. The role of telomerase in some types of cell senescence has been demonstrated although its overall role in aging seems less clear.

Accelerating DNA repair may prove useful in reversing DNA damage, a frequent stimulus of senescent pathways. Targeting downstream signaling components and effectors in the senescent pathway with designer drugs appears promising; however, the balance between senescence and excessive proliferation (i.e., cancer) must be carefully considered before their use. Growth hormone, IGF-1 and components of their signaling pathways may stimulate/modulate survival pathways in cardioprotection; modulation of cardioprotective pathways needs further research, particularly in the elderly to assess whether there is a significant depression in cardioprotective responses and how this might be overcome [257, 258]. Again, reducing ROS and oxidative damage may obviate the need for treating DNA damage/telomere damage. Similarly, further investigation of the nexus between DNA transcription and damage, will help to identify targets that more precisely link particular transcriptional events, chromatin remodeling and aging phenotypes (e.g., senescence). Interestingly, resveratrol, a component of red wine and a putative ligand of the sirtuin deactylase family (involved in chromatin and metabolic remodeling) when fed to middle-aged mice, fed on a high-calorie diet, increased their survival and produced significant changes associated with longer life span, including increased insulin sensitivity, reduced IGF-1 levels, increased AMP-activated protein kinase (AMPK) and PGC-1α activity, increased mitochondrial number, and improved motor function [259]. This phytochemical compound has been implicated in increasing the longevity in multiple species (yeast, *C. elegans* and *Drosophila*), and in addition to its anti-aging properties has anti-inflammatory and multiple cardioprotective effects, including attenuation of myocardial ischemic reperfusion injury, atherosclerosis, and reduces ventricular dysrhythmias in both acute and chronic models [260, 261].

Several anti-aging approaches, which we should mention, are particularly important in targeting cardiac and vascular remodeling in aging and age-associated diseases. For example, one tact that has shown significant results in preclinical studies addresses cardiac fibrosis and the development of advanced glycation products that cause cross-linking, and is implicated in age-induced and diabetes-induced arterial stiffness and diastolic dysfunction. A variety of factors (including IGF-1, pitavastatin, aldosterone antagonists and long-term mineralocorticoid receptor blockade) can be used to reduce cardiac fibrosis and improve cardiac performance [262–265]. Current cross-linking breakers (e.g., alagebrium, of the thiazolium halide family) appear to be able to target a subset of the cross-linked protein structures enabling some reversal of the age- and disease-mediated damage to large arteries caused by AGE [266, 267]. In animal studies, alagebrium was effective in reducing large artery stiffness, slowing pulse-wave velocity, enhancing cardiac output, and improving left ventricular diastolic distensibility. In clinical trials alagebrium improved arterial compliance in elderly patients with vascular stiffening [268], and significantly improved peripheral artery endothelial function in older adults with isolated systolic hypertension [269]. Interestingly, the single most important collagen cross-link known to date in diabetes and aging is glucosepane, a lysyl-arginine cross-link that forms under nonoxidative conditions [270], and these are refractory to all current breakers. High-throughput screening and rational drug design might be well applied to glycation breaker discovery in order to find molecules that are able to break glucosepane cross-links of extracellular proteins.

Another important cardiovascular defect associated with aging, diastolic dysfunction, has been reversed in animal models with the introduction of genes involved in calcium cycling (SERCA, parvalbumin), antioxidant response (metallotheinein), ADH and signaling proteins (IGF-1). The overexpression of SERCA, a protein involved in sarcomeric calcium cycling, markedly improved rate-dependent contractility and diastolic function in senescent rat hearts [271]. Similarly, *in vivo* overexpression of parvalbumin, a calcium binding protein had no effect on systolic parameters but significantly improved diastolic dysfunction in two different rat models of senescence (i.e., the Fischer 344 [F344] and the Fischer 344 x Brown Norway F1 hybrid [F344 x BN]) [272]. Interestingly, SERCA content and activity was upregulated in mice overexpressing either IGF-1 [273], or alcohol dehydrogenase (ADH) [274]. Fang et al. have reported that the overexpression of metallotheinein in mice reversed aging-mediated insulin signaling changes (including restoring aging-reduced Akt and insulin receptor expression and phosphorylation) as well as attenuated aging-induced cardiac contractile dysfunction [275]. Unfortunately, SERCA levels were not assessed. The ways in which these preclinical findings may be translated and adapted to human clinical application remain to be determined.

Pharmacogenomics and Nutrigenomics

It would be injudicious to conclude this book concerning the molecular genetic aspects of aging and the outlook for future research without at least mentioning (actually reprising) the relatively nascent approaches of pharmacogenomics and nutrigenomics.

Nutrigenetics and pharmacogenetics probes how individual genetic make-up manifesting as single nucleotide polymorphisms, copy number polymorphisms and epigenetic factors affect susceptibility to diet and drugs respectively. In contrast, nutrigenomics (and pharmacogenomics) twists the relationship on its head to examine how diet (or drugs) influences gene transcription, protein expression and metabolism.

A long-term goal of nutrigenomics and pharmacogenomics is defining the right diet or drug treatment for the most effective way to maintain individual health and prevent disease. A prerequisite for "successful–omics" clearly involves the integration of genomics (gene analysis), transcriptomics (gene expression analysis), proteomics (protein expression analysis) and metabonomics (metabolite profiling or "the quantitative measurement of metabolic response of living systems to abnormal stimuli or genetic modification") to define an individualized "healthy" phenotype. Arguments for personalized or individually-tailored medicine promises several key benefits including better diagnosis and earlier interventions, more effective therapies, and more efficient drug development.

In regard to aging, several findings are worth mentioning. Ames et al. have noted that common micronutrient deficiencies including mineral and vitamin deficits can accelerate mitochondrial oxidative decay, thought to be a primary contributor of aging [276]. For instance, deficiencies in minerals including iron (25% of menstruating women ingest < 50% of the recommended daily allowance) can contribute to inhibition of the pathway of heme biosynthesis in mitochondria, leading to a heme-*a* deficit. Decline in heme-*a*, only found in respiratory complex IV, results in oxidant leakage and accelerates mitochondrial decay, leading to further DNA damage, neural decay, and aging. Several vitamin deficiencies, such as biotin or pantothenic acid also increase mitochondrial oxidants through a related mechanism. Furthermore, a folate deficiency can promote the formation of DNA double-strand breaks (DSBs), a serious DNA lesion caused by ionizing radiation. A comparative study of the effects of irradiation and folate deficiency on primary human lymphocytes, to assess cell proliferation, apoptosis, cell cycle, DSBs and changes in gene expression, revealed that both radiation and folate deficiency significantly decreased cell proliferation and induced DNA breaks, apoptosis, and cell cycle arrest [277]. Folate deficiency levels, commonly reported, produced similar levels of damage to those caused by a relatively high dose of radiation (1 Gy). While both radiation and folate deficiency caused DNA breaks, they affected the expression of different genes. Radiation treatment activates excision and DSB repair genes and represses mitochondrially-encoded genes. Folate deficiency activates base and nucleotide excision repair genes, represses folate-related genes and fails to induce DSB repair genes. This suggests that a diet poor in folate can pose a significant risk for DNA damage comparable to high doses of radiation.

An added feature to the potential for abnormalities is presented by genomic variants. Polymorphic variants in genes encoding enzyme subunits result in a lower affinity of the enzyme for coenzymes (i.e., vitamins). This poorer affinity (K_m) of the mutant enzyme for its coenzyme can be remedied by feeding high-dose of vitamin B, which raise levels of the corresponding coenzyme [278]. Therefore supplementation of micronutrients and metabolites, could provide an optimal level which varies with age and genetic constitution, would tune up metabolism and provide a marked improvement in health, particularly for the poor, obese, and elderly.

Polymorphic variations in the genes for the family of interleukin 1 (IL-1) proteins provide an example of the role of inflammatory genetics as a modifier of diseases of aging. IL-1 genetic variations are known to be associated with variation in both the inflammatory response and the clinical presentation of a number of age-associated diseases, including coronary artery disease and Alzheimer disease. Understanding how these genetic variants are linked to inflammation and chronic disease may allow the identification of healthy persons who are at increased risk of disease and the potential modification of the trajectory of disease to prolong healthy aging. Furthermore, an important application of nutritional modulation of chronic disease may be the identification of nutrients that regulate the expression of key inflammatory genes [279].

Previously, we discussed the multiple effects of resveratrol, a putative activator of the sirtuins that have been implicated in a broad series of highly conserved metabolic, signaling and chromatin remodeling changes in aging cells. Evaluation of environmental/nutritional factors that could impact on human sirtuin activity using a sensitive screen of a yeast heterochromatic derepression assay has been reported [280]. Unexpectedly, a common food/cosmetic additive was discovered to contain a potent sirtuin inhibitor activity. Dihydrocoumarin (DHC), a compound found in *Melilotus officinalis* (sweet clover), which is commonly added to food and cosmetics, disrupted heterochromatic silencing and inhibited yeast Sir2p as well as human SIRT1 deacetylase activity. In addition, when tested in human cells in culture, DHC increased p53 acetylation and apoptosis, a phenotype associated with senescence and aging.

Conclusion

Given the large range of potential therapeutic approaches – many which are novel, and others, more familiar – the possible reversal and/or retardation in aging and perhaps more importantly, more effective treatment of aging-associated diseases may become a reality within the next decade or two. Despite the fanciful claims of the SENS approach (that humans will live 100s if not 1000s of years if true aging pathway re-engineering was to take place) – the primary objective of many gerontologists and aging scientists remains to identify and eventually modulate genes, intracellular pathways and environmental factors – that will increasingly lead to what we term healthy aging. In this effort, the information from aging studies should contribute to identifying and targeting cellular dysfunction leading to a variety of degenerative diseases both at the cardiovascular and neurological levels. Further studies of the basic science of stem cells – including the isolation of factors involved in the acceleration of specific cell-type differentiation, mediating their migration, homing and proliferation *in vitro* as well as *in vivo* – and their responses to OS, apoptosis and injury – should contribute greatly to their potential use in clinical transplantation and as potential approaches to treatment of aging dysfunction and cardiovascular disease. Moreover, a number of the approaches discussed here such as CR, systems biology, gene profiling, proteomics, genetic analysis, the development of increasingly relevant animal and cellular models, nutrigenomics and pharmacogenomics, while promising at this time are really all relatively new approaches with a good deal still remaining to be learned. This increasingly armamentarium should contribute greatly to further understanding the role of basic cellular processes and adaptive capacities – including improving the understanding of organelle biology, metabolic modulation, DNA and protein damage and apoptosis, and their role as markers and causative factors in aging. In addition, findings from these basic studies as well as a larger multi-discipline based-perspective using integrative systems biology methods will likely increase our knowledge of critical interactions between multiple organ systems and their cross-talk through hormonal and inflammatory/immune signaling, which have only recently been found to play a significant role in human aging and aging-associated cardiovascular diseases. Finally, molecular-based tools of nutrigenomics and pharmacogenomics should provide further impetus to realize the development of a more effective highly individualized medicine. While there is a certainty that this research will be increasingly expensive, the alternative option of ignorance would be in the long run more costly.

Summary

- Studies of aging in a wide spectrum of model organisms from yeast to mice have identified a number of genes and highly conserved intracellular pathways that play a contributory role in aging and longevity.
- These models have proved useful in our understanding of human age-associated cardiovascular diseases, as well as in recapitulating many aspects of premature aging syndromes.
- While pathways involving oxidative DNA and telomeric damage have been shown to lead to replicative senescence in a variety of cell-type *in vitro* cells, their relevance to aging tissues *in vivo* remain unclear as underlined by the fact that there is no definitive evidence that cellular senescence *in vivo* limits animal life span. Nevertheless, the pathways identified in these studies have been increasingly implicated in aging-associated cardiovascular disease.
- Genetic analysis of centenarians, linkage analysis and case association studies have identified a number of genes, which modulate either frailty or susceptibility to disease or longevity, including inflammatory/immune genes, genes involved in lipid metabolism and mtDNA polymorphism.
- A number of the gene variants impact specific ethnic populations or are gender-specific suggesting the involvement of either environmental or other genetic factors, which modify the aging phenotypic expression.
- Search for aging biomarkers has shown a rather wide spectrum of potential candidates, many which remain to be validated. Identification of novel markers has been increasingly facilitated by gene profiling and proteomic analysis and nutrigenomic research.
- Post-translational oxidative modification of proteins, oxidative lesions of DNA and of cellular membranes and accumulation of glycation and lipofuscin aggregates also constitute informative aging biomarkers.
- The use of an integrative systems biology approach based on molecular, cellular, physiological and clinical data, and involving computational analysis and database availability, has been highly recommended. Such a multi-disciplinary approach may prove to be critical in our understanding of intraorgan cross-talk in aging, and in managing the enormous input and analysis of quantitative data furnished from diverse aging studies with heterogenous human populations and in developing testable (and/or *in silico*) models of aging.
- A number of methods for reversing and/or retarding aging and age-related diseases have shown significant promise in preclinical models. Targeting oxidative damage, enhanced cell death, DNA damage or inadequate DNA repair, replicative senescence, diminished "garbage" removal, altered intracellular signaling and metabolic inefficiency represent some of the primary foci attacked by these approaches.

- Other methods employed are pharmacological/hormonal supplementation, gene therapy, and lifestyle modification (including dietary restriction and exercise). Adapting these approaches with clinical studies is challenging, although some clinical trials are already underway.
- A variety of adult stem-cells including cardiac stem cells (CSCs) and endothelial progenitor cells (EPCs) which appear to play a regenerative role in injured and diseased tissues, including the heart and vasculature, are diminished either in number or are targeted with functional senescence with aging in either rodent or humans.
- Since transplantation or activation of resident stem cells with growth factors has proved to be a highly effective approach to repairing tissues including the heart, an understanding of how the limitations in stem cell efficacy can be overcome should be an important research priority.
- The development of nutrigenomics and pharmacogenomics might be effective methodologies to develop individualized medicine for the elderly potentially improving the management, diagnosis and treatment of age-associated diseases.

References

1. Jazwinski SM. New clues to old yeast. Mech Ageing Dev 2001;122:865–882
2. Johnson TE. A personal retrospective on the genetics of aging. Biogerontology 2002;3:7–12
3. Tower J. Transgenic methods for increasing Drosophila life span. Mech Ageing Dev 2000;118:1–14
4. Hasty P, Vijg J. Accelerating aging by mouse reverse genetics: a rational approach to understanding longevity. Aging Cell 2004;3:55–65
5. Liang H, Masoro EJ, Nelson JF, Strong R, McMahan CA, Richardson A. Genetic mouse models of extended life span. Exp Gerontol 2003;38:1353–1364
6. Miller RA. Genetic approaches to the study of aging. J Am Geriatr Soc 2005;53:S284–S286
7. Haigis MC, Guarente LP. Mammalian sirtuins – emerging roles in physiology, aging, and calorie restriction. Genes Dev 2006;20:2913–2921
8. Bordone L, Guarente L. Calorie restriction, SIRT1 and metabolism: understanding longevity. Nat Rev Mol Cell Biol 2005;6:298–305
9. Warner HR. Subfield history: use of model organisms in the search for human aging genes. Sci Aging Knowledge Environ 2003;2003(6):RE1
10. Butler RN, Austad SN, Barzilai N, Braun A, Helfand S, Larsen PL, McCormick AM, Perls TT, Shuldiner AR, Sprott RL, Warner HR. Longevity genes: from primitive organisms to humans. J Gerontol A Biol Sci Med Sci 2003;58:581–584
11. de Haan G, Williams RW. A genetic and genomic approach to identify longevity genes in mice. Mech Ageing Dev 2005;126:133–138
12. Ocorr K, Akasaka T, Bodmer R. Age-related cardiac disease model of Drosophila. Mech Ageing Dev 2007;128:112–116
13. Wessells RJ, Bodmer R. Age-related cardiac deterioration: insights from Drosophila. Front Biosci 2007;12: 39–48
14. Bienengraeber M, Olson TM, Selivanov VA, Kathmann EC, O'Cochlain F, Gao F, Karger AB, Ballew JD, Hodgson DM, Zingman LV, Pang YP, Alekseev AE, Terzic A. ABCC9 mutations identified in human dilated cardiomyopathy disrupt catalytic KATP channel gating. Nat Genet 2004;36:382–387
15. Hekimi S. How genetic analysis tests theories of animal aging. Nat Genet 2006;38:985–991
16. King MC, Marks JH, Mandell JB. New York breast cancer study group. Breast and ovarian cancer risks due to inherited mutations in BRCA1 and BRCA2. Science 2003;302:643–646
17. Barzilai N, Atzmon G, Schechter C, Schaefer EJ, Cupples AL, Lipton R, Cheng S, Shuldiner AR. Unique lipoprotein phenotype and genotype associated with exceptional longevity. JAMA 2003;290:2030–2040
18. Geesaman BJ, Benson E, Brewster SJ, Kunkel LM, Blanche H, Thomas G, Perls TT, Daly MJ, Puca AA. Haplotype-based identification of a microsomal transfer protein marker associated with the human life span. Proc Natl Acad Sci USA 2003;100:14115–14120
19. Gerdes LU, Jeune B, Ranberg KA, Nybo H, Vaupel JW. Estimation of apolipoprotein E genotype-specific relative mortality risks from the distribution of genotypes in centenarians and middle-aged men: apolipoprotein E gene is a "frailty gene", not a "longevity gene". Genet Epidemiol 2000;19:202–210
20. Atzmon G, Rincon M, Schechter CB, Shuldiner AR, Lipton RB, Bergman A, Barzilai N. Lipoprotein genotype and conserved pathway for exceptional longevity in humans. PLoS Biol 2006;4:e113

21. Ershler WB, Keller ET. Age-associated increased interleukin-6 gene expression, late-life diseases, and frailty. Annu Rev Med 2000;51:245–270
22. Pletcher SD, Khazaeli AA, Curtsinger JW. Why do life spans differ? Partitioning mean longevity differences in terms of age-specific mortality parameters. J Gerontol A Biol Sci Med Sci 2000;55:B381–B389
23. Terry DF, Wilcox M, McCormick MA, Lawler E, Perls TT. Cardiovascular advantages among the offspring of centenarians. J Gerontol A Biol Sci Med Sci 2003;58:M425–M431
24. Nebel A, Schreiber S. GEHA – the pan-European "Genetics of Healthy Aging" project. Sci Aging Knowledge Environ 2004;2004:pe23
25. Puca AA, Daly MJ, Brewster SJ, Matise TC, Barrett J, Shea-Drinkwater M, Kang S, Joyce E, Nicoli J, Benson E, Kunkel LM, Perls T. A genome-wide scan for linkage to human exceptional longevity identifies a locus on chromosome 4. Proc Natl Acad Sci USA 2001;98:10505–10508
26. Nebel A, Crouchr PJ, Stiegeler R, Nikolaus S, Krawczak M, Schreiber S. No association between microsomal triglyceride transfer protein (MTP) haplotype and longevity in humans. Proc Natl Acad Sci USA 2005;102:7906–7909
27. Candore G, Balistreri CR, Listi F, Grimaldi MP, Vasto S, Colonna-Romano G, Franceschi C, Lio D, Caselli G, Caruso C. Immunogenetics, gender, and longevity. Ann NY Acad Sci 2006;1089:516–537
28. De Benedictis G, Tan Q, Jeune B, Christensen K, Ukraintseva SV, Bonafe M, Franceschi C, Vaupel JW, Yashin AI. Recent advances in human gene-longevity association studies. Mech Ageing Dev 2001;122: 909–920
29. Melzer D, Hurst AJ, Frayling T. Genetic variation and human aging: progress and prospects. J Gerontol A Biol Sci Med Sci 2007;62:301–307
30. Tan Q, Kruse TA, Christensen K. Design and analysis in genetic studies of human ageing and longevity. Ageing Res Rev 2006;5:371–387
31. Tan Q, Christiansen L, Bathum L, Li S, Kruse TA, Christensen K. Genetic association analysis of human longevity in cohort studies of elderly subjects: an example of the PON1 gene in the Danish 1905 birth cohort. Genetics 2006;172:1821–1828
32. Singh R, Kolvraa S, Bross P, Christensen K, Gregersen N, Tan Q, Jensen UB, Eiberg H, Rattan SI. Heat-shock protein 70 genes and human longevity: a view from Denmark. Ann NY Acad Sci 2006;1067:301–308
33. Martin GM. Genetic modulation of senescent phenotypes in homo sapiens. Cell 2005;120:523–532
34. Zhang J, Asin-Cayuela J, Fish J, Michikawa Y, Bonafe M, Olivieri F, Passarino G, De Benedictis G, Franceschi C, Attardi G. Strikingly higher frequency in centenarians and twins of mtDNA mutation causing remodeling of replication origin in leukocytes. Proc Natl Acad Sci USA 2003;100:1116–1121
35. Niemi AK, Moilanen JS, Tanaka M, Hervonen A, Hurme M, Lehtimaki T, Arai Y, Hirose N, Majamaa K. A combination of three common inherited mitochondrial DNA polymorphisms promotes longevity in Finnish and Japanese subjects. Eur J Hum Genet 2005;13:166–170
36. Ross OA, McCormack R, Curran MD, Duguid RA, Barnett YA, Rea IM, Middleton D. Mitochondrial DNA polymorphism: its role in longevity of the Irish population. Exp Gerontol 2001;36:1161–1178
37. Santoro A, Salvioli S, Raule N, Capri M, Sevini F, Valensin S, Monti D, Bellizzi D, Passarino G, Rose G, De Benedictis G, Franceschi C. Mitochondrial DNA involvement in human longevity. Biochim Biophys Acta 2006;1757:1388–1399
38. Merriwether DA, Clark AG, Ballinger SW, Schurr TG, Soodyall H, Jenkins T, Sherry ST, Wallace DC. The structure of human mitochondrial DNA variation. J Mol Evol 1991;33:543–555
39. De Benedictis G, Rose G, Carrieri G, De Luca M, Falcone E, Passarino G, Bonafe M, Monti D, Baggio G, Bertolini S, Mari D, Mattace R, Franceschi C. Mitochondrial DNA inherited variants are associated with successful aging and longevity in humans. FASEB 1999;13:1532–1536
40. Niemi AK, Hervonen A, Hurme M, Karhunen PJ, Jylha M, Majamaa K. Mitochonrial DNA polymorphisms associated with longevity in a Finnish population. Hum Genet 2003;112:29–33
41. Dato S, Passarino G, Rose G, Altomare K, Bellizzi D, Mari V, Feraco E, Franceschi C, De Benedictis G. Association of the mitochondrial DNA haplogroup J with longevity is population specific. Eur J Hum Genet 2004;12:1080–1082
42. Brown MD, Starikovskaya E, Derbeneva O, Hosseini S, Allen JC, Mikhailovskaya IE, Sukernik RI, Wallace DC. The role of mtDNA background in disease expression: a new primary LHON mutation associated with Western Eurasian haplogroup. J Hum Genet 2002;110:130–138
43. Torroni A, Petrozzi M, D'Urbano L, Sellitto D, Zeviani M, Carrara F, Carducci C, Leuzzi V, Carelli V, Barboni P, De Negri A, Scozzari R. Haplotype and phylogenetic analyses suggest that one European-specific mtDNA background plays a role in the expression of leber hereditary optic neuropathy by increasing the penetrance of the primary mutations 11778 and 14484. Am J Hum Genet 1997;60:1107–1121
44. Reynier P, Penisson-Besnier I, Moreau C, Savagner F, Vielle B, Emile J, Dubas F, Malthiery Y. mtDNA haplogroup J: a contributing factor of optic neuritis. Eur J Hum Genet 1999;7:404–406

45. Rose G, Passarino G, Carrieri G, Altomare K, Greco V, Bertolini S, Bonafe M, Franceschi C, De Benedictis G. Paradoxes in longevity: sequence analysis of mtDNA haplogroup J in centenarians. Eur J Hum Genet 2001;9:701–707
46. Wallace DC. A mitochondrial paradigm of metabolic and degenerative diseases, aging, and cancer: a dawn for evolutionary medicine. Annu Rev Genet 2005;39:359–407
47. Tanaka M, Gong JS, Zhang J, Yoneda M, Yagi K. Mitochondrial genotype associated with longevity. Lancet 1998;351:185–186
48. Tanaka M, Gong J, Zhang J, Yamada Y, Borgeld HJ, Yagi K. Mitochondrial genotype associated with longevity and its inhibitory effect on mutagenesis. Mech Ageing Dev 2000;116:65–76
49. Yao YG, Kong QP, Zhang YP. Mitochondrial DNA 5178A polymorphism and longevity. Hum Genet 2002;111:462–463
50. Takagi K, Yamada Y, Gong JS, Sone T, Yokota M, Tanaka M. Association of a 5178C<001>A (Leu237Met) polymorphism in the mitochondrial DNA with a low prevalence of myocardial infarction in Japanese individuals. Atherosclerosis 2004;175:281–286
51. Mukae S, Aoki S, Itoh S, Sato R, Nishio K, Iwata T, Katagiri T. Mitochondrial 5178A/C genotype is associated with acute myocardial infarction. Circ J 2003;67:16–20
52. Wang D, Taniyama M, Suzuki Y, Katagiri T, Ban Y. Association of the mitochondrial DNA 5178A/C polymorphism with maternal inheritance and onset of type 2 diabetes in Japanese patients. Exp Clin Endocrinol Diabetes 2001;109:361–364
53. Matsunaga H, Tanaka Y, Tanaka M, Gong JS, Zhang J, Nomiyama T, Ogawa O, Ogihara T, Yamada Y, Yagi K, Kawamori R. Antiatherogenic mitochondrial genotype in patients with type 2 diabetes. Diabetes Care 2001;24:500–503
54. Kokaze A, Ishikawa M, Matsunaga N, Yoshida M, Sekine Y, Sekiguchi K, Harada M, Satoh M, Teruya K, Takeda N, Fukazawa S, Uchida Y, Takashima Y. Longevity-associated mitochondrial DNA 5178 A/C polymorphism and blood pressure in the Japanese population. J Hum Hypertens 2004;18:41–45
55. Kokaze A, Yoshida M, Ishikawa M, Matsunaga N, Makita R, Satoh M, Sekiguchi K, Masuda Y, Uchida Y, Takashima Y. Longevity-associated mitochondrial DNA 5178 A/C polymorphism is associated with intraocular pressure in Japanese men. Clin Experiment Ophthalmol 2004;32:131–136
56. Hayflick L. The longevity of cultured human cells. J Am Geriatr Soc 1974;22:1–12
57. Ben-Porath I, Weinberg RA. The signals and pathways activating cellular senescence. Int J Biochem Cell Biol 2005;37:961–976
58. Kregel KC, Zhang HJ. An integrated view of oxidative stress in aging: basic mechanisms, functional effects, and pathological considerations. Am J Physiol Regul Integr Comp Physiol 2007;292:R18–R36
59. Passos JF, von Zglinicki T. Mitochondria, telomeres and cell senescence. Exp Gerontol 2005;40:466–472
60. Chevanne M, Caldini R, Tombaccini D, Mocali A, Gori G, Paoletti F. Comparative levels of DNA breaks and sensitivity to oxidative stress in aged and senescent human fibroblasts: a distinctive pattern for centenarians. Biogerontology 2003;4:97–104
61. Foreman KE, Tang J. Molecular mechanisms of replicative senescence in endothelial cells. Exp Gerontol 2003;38:1251–1257
62. Bekaert S, De Meyer T, Van Oostveldt P. Telomere attrition as ageing biomarker. Anticancer Res 2005;25: 3011–3021
63. von Zglinicki T, Martin-Ruiz CM. Telomeres as biomarkers for ageing and age-related diseases. Curr Mol Med 2005;5:197–203
64. Lou Z, Chen J. Cellular senescence and DNA repair. Exp Cell Res 2006;312:2641–2646
65. de Magalhaes JP. From cells to ageing: a review of models and mechanisms of cellular senescence and their impact on human ageing. Exp Cell Res 2004;300:1–10
66. Erusalimsky JD, Kurz DJ. Cellular senescence in vivo: its relevance in ageing and cardiovascular disease. Exp Gerontol 2005;40:634–642
67. Cristofalo VJ, Lorenzini A, Allen RG, Torres C, Tresini M. Replicative senescence: a critical review. Mech Ageing Dev 2004;125:827–848
68. Hornsby PJ. Cellular senescence and tissue aging in vivo. J Gerontol A Biol Sci Med Sci 2002l;57:B251–B256
69. Minamino T, Komuro I. Vascular cell senescence: contribution to atherosclerosis. Circ Res 2007;100:15–26
70. Matthews C, Gorenne I, Scott S, Figg N, Kirkpatrick P, Ritchie A, Goddard M, Bennett M. Vascular smooth muscle cells undergo telomere-based senescence in human atherosclerosis: effects of telomerase and oxidative stress. Circ Res 2006;99:156–164
71. Carlson ME, Conboy IM. Loss of stem cell regenerative capacity within aged niches. Aging Cell 2007;6: 371–382
72. Geiger H, Rennebeck G, Van Zant G. Regulation of hematopoietic stem cell aging in vivo by a distinct genetic element. Proc Natl Acad Sci USA 2005;102:5102–5107

73. Torella D, Rota M, Nurzynska D, Musso E, Monsen A, Shiraishi I, Zias E, Walsh K, Rosenzweig A, Sussman MA, Urbanek K, Nadal-Ginard B, Kajstura J, Anversa P, Leri A. Cardiac stem cell and myocyte aging, heart failure, and insulin-like growth factor-1 overexpression. Circ Res 2004;94:514–524
74. Anversa P, Kajstura J, Leri A, Bolli R. Life and death of cardiac stem cells: a paradigm shift in cardiac biology. Circulation 2006;113:1451–1463
75. Butler RN, Sprott R, Warner H, Bland J, Feuers R, Forster M, Fillit H, Harman SM, Hewitt M, Hyman M, Johnson K, Kligman E, McClearn G, Nelson J, Richardson A, Sonntag W, Weindruch R, Wolf N. Biomarkers of aging: from primitive organisms to humans. J Gerontol A Biol Sci Med Sci 2004;59:B560–B567
76. Johnson TE. Recent results: biomarkers of aging. Exp Gerontol 2006;41:1243–1246
77. Voss P, Siems W. Clinical oxidation parameters of aging. Free Radic Res 2006;40:1339–1349
78. Ochi H, Cheng RZ, Kantha SS, Takeuchi M, Ramarathnam N. The JaICA-genox oxidative stress profile – an overview on the profiling technique in the oxidative stress assessment and management. Biofactors 2000;13:195–203
79. Chevion M, Berenshtein E, Stadtman ER. Human studies related to protein oxidation: protein carbonyl content as a marker of damage. Free Radic Res 2000;33:S99–S108
80. DiMarco T, Giulivi C. Current analytical methods for the detection of dityrosine, a biomarker of oxidative stress, in biological samples. Mass Spectrom Rev 2007;26:108–120
81. Kanski J, Behring A, Pelling J, Schoneich C. Proteomic identification of 3-nitrotyrosine-containing rat cardiac proteins: effects of biological aging. Am J Physiol Heart Circ Physiol 2005;288:H371–H381
82. Pero RW, Hoppe C, Sheng Y. Serum thiols as a surrogate estimate of DNA repair correlates to mammalian life span. J Anti-Aging Med 2000;3:241–249
83. Yan L-J, Levine RL, Sohal RS. Oxidative damage during aging targets mitochondrial aconitase. Proc Natl Acad Sci USA 1997;94:11168–11172
84. Yan L-J, Sohal RS. Mitochondrial adenine nucleotide translocase is modified oxidatively during aging. Proc Natl Acad Sci USA 1998;95:12896–12901
85. Navarro A. Mitochondrial enzyme activities as biochemical markers of aging. Mol Aspects Med 2004;25:37–48
86. Linton S, Davies MJ, Dean RT. Protein oxidation and ageing. Exp Gerontol 2001;36:1503–1518
87. Strehler BL, Mark DD, Mildvan AS, Gee MV. Rate of magnitude of age pigment accumulation in the human myocardium. J Gerontol 1959;14:430–439
88. Reichel E, Holander J, Clark HJ, Strehler BL. Lipofuscin pigment accumulation as a function of age and distribution in rodent brain. J Gerontol 1968;23:71–78
89. Kato Y, Maruyama W, Naoi M, Hashizume Y, Osawa T. Immunohistochemical detection of dityrosine in lipofuscin pigments in the aged human brain. FEBS Lett 1998;439:231–234
90. Sohal RS, Brunk UT. Lipofuscin as an indicator of oxidative stress and aging. Adv Exp Med Biol 1989;266: 17–26
91. Sitte N, Merker K, Von Zglinicki T, Davies KJ, Grune T. Protein oxidation and degradation during cellular senescence of human BJ fibroblasts: part II – aging of nondividing cells. FASEB J 2000;14:2503–2510
92. Baynes JW, Thorpe SR. Glycoxidation and lipoxidation in atherogenesis. Free Radic Biol Med 2000;28: 1708–1716
93. Schleicher ED, Wagner E, Nerlich AG. Increased accumulation of the glycoxidation product N(epsilon)-(carboxymethyl)lysine in human tissues in diabetes and aging. J Clin Invest 1997;99:457–468
94. Wautier JL, Schmidt AM. Protein glycation: a firm link to endothelial cell dysfunction. Circ Res 2004;95: 233–238
95. Ames BN, Shigenaga MK, Hagen TM. Oxidants, antioxidants, and the degenerative diseases of aging. Proc Natl Acad Sci USA 1993;90:7915–7922
96. Hudson EK, Hogue BA, Souza-Pinto NC, Croteau DL, Anson RM, Bohr VA, Hansford RG. Age-associated change in mitochondrial DNA damage. Free Radic Res 1998;29:573–579
97. Anson RM, Hudson E, Bohr VA. Mitochondrial endogenous oxidative damage has been overestimated. FASEB J 2000;14:355–360
98. Hamilton ML, Van Remmen H, Drake JA, Yang H, Guo ZM, Kewitt K, Walter CA, Richardson A. Does oxidative damage to DNA increase with age? Proc Natl Acad Sci USA 2001;98:10469–10474
99. Gianni P, Jan KJ, Douglas MJ, Stuart PM, Tarnopolsky MA. Oxidative stress and the mitochondrial theory of aging in human skeletal muscle. Exp Gerontol 2004;39:1391–1400
100. Dizdaroglu M, Jaruga P, Birincioglu M, Rodriguez H. Free radical-induced damage to DNA: mechanisms and measurement. Free Radic Biol Med 2002;32:1102–1115
101. Mohamed SA, Hanke T, Erasmi AW, Bechtel MJ, Scharfschwerdt M, Meissner C, Sievers HH, Gosslau A. Mitochondrial DNA deletions and the aging heart. Exp Gerontol 2006;41:508–517
102. Meissner C, Bruse P, Oehmichen M. Tissue-specific deletion patterns of the mitochondrial genome with advancing age. Exp Gerontol 2006;41:518–524

103. Brena RM, Huang TH, Plass C. Quantitative assessment of DNA methylation: potential applications for disease diagnosis, classification, and prognosis in clinical settings. J Mol Med 2006;84:365–377
104. Wojdacz TK, Hansen LL. Techniques used in studies of age-related DNA methylation changes. Ann NY Acad Sci 2006;1067:479–487
105. Bergamini E, Bizzarri R, Cavallini G, Cerbai B, Chiellini E, Donati A, Gori Z, Manfrini A, Parentini I, Signori F, Tamburini I. Ageing and oxidative stress: a role for dolichol in the antioxidant machinery of cell membranes? J Alzheimers Dis 2004;6:129–135
106. Parentini I, Cavallini G, Donati A, Gori Z, Bergamini E. Accumulation of dolichol in older tissues satisfies the proposed criteria to be qualified a biomarker of aging. J Gerontol A Biol Sci Med Sci 2005;60:39–43
107. Maggio M, Basaria S, Ble A, Lauretani F, Bandinelli S, Ceda GP, Valenti G, Ling SM, Ferrucci L. Correlation between testosterone and the inflammatory marker soluble interleukin-6 receptor in older men. J Clin Endocrinol Metab 2006;91:345–347
108. Bellido T, Jilka RL, Boyce BF, Girasole G, Broxmeyer H, Dalrymple SA, Murray R, Broxmeyer H, Dalrymple SA, Murray R, Manolagas SC. Regulation of interleukin-6, osteoclastogenesis, and bone mass by androgens. The role of the androgen receptor. J Clin Invest 1995;95:2886–2895
109. Khosla S, Atkinson EJ, Dunstan CR, O'Fallon WM. Effect of estrogen versus testosterone on circulating osteoprotegerin and other cytokine levels in normal elderly men. J Clin Endocrinol Metab 2002;87:1550–1554
110. Malkin CJ, Pugh PJ, Jones RD, Kapoor D, Channer KS, Jones TH. The effect of testosterone replacement on endogenous inflammatory cytokines and lipid profiles in hypogonadal men. J Clin Endocrinol Metab 2004;89:3313–3318
111. De Martinis M, Franceschi C, Monti D, Ginaldi L. Inflammation markers predicting frailty and mortality in the elderly. Exp Mol Pathol 2006;80:219–227
112. Cesari M, Penninx BW, Pahor M, Lauretani F, Corsi AM, Rhys Williams G, Guralnik JM, Ferrucci L. Inflammatory markers and physical performance in older persons: the InCHIANTI study. J Gerontol A Biol Sci Med Sci 2004;59:242–248
113. Kritchevsky SB, Cesari M, Pahor M. Inflammatory markers and cardiovascular health in older adults. Cardiovasc Res 2005;66:265–275
114. Cesari M, Penninx BW, Newman AB, Kritchevsky SB, Nicklas BJ, Sutton-Tyrrell K, Rubin SM, Ding J, Simonsick EM, Harris TB, Pahor M. Inflammatory markers and onset of cardiovascular events: results from the health ABC study. Circulation 2003;108:2317–2322
115. Lane MA, Ingram DK, Ball SS, Roth GS. Dehydroepiandrosterone sulfate: a biomarker of primate aging slowed by calorie restriction. J Clin Endocrinol Metab 1997;82:2093–2096
116. Perret M, Aujard F. Aging and season affect plasma dehydroepiandrosterone sulfate (DHEA-S) levels in a primate. Exp Gerontol 2005;40:582–587
117. Perrini S, Laviola L, Natalicchio A, Giorgino F. Associated hormonal declines in aging: DHEAS. J Endocrinol Invest 2005;28:85–93
118. Kontoleon PE, Anastasiou-Nana MI, Papapetrou PD, Alexopoulos G, Ktenas V, Rapti AC, Tsagalou EP, Nanas JN. Hormonal profile in patients with congestive heart failure. Int J Cardiol 2003;87:179–183
119. Jankowska EA, Biel B, Majda J, Szklarska A, Lopuszanska M, Medras M, Anker SD, Banasiak W, Poole-Wilson PA, Ponikowski P. Anabolic deficiency in men with chronic heart failure: prevalence and detrimental impact on survival. Circulation 2006;114:1829–1837
120. Moriyama Y, Yasue H, Yoshimura M, Mizuno Y, Nishiyama K, Tsunoda R, Kawano H, Kugiyama K, Ogawa H, Saito Y, Nakao K. The plasma levels of dehydroepiandrosterone sulfate are decreased in patients with chronic heart failure in proportion to the severity. J Clin Endocrinol Metab 2000;85:1834–1840
121. Feldman HA, Johannes CB, Araujo AB, Mohr BA, Longcope C, McKinlay JB. Low dehydroepiandrosterone and ischemic heart disease in middle-aged men: prospective results from the Massachusetts male aging study. Am J Epidemiol 2001;153:79–89
122. Wu FC, von Eckardstein A. Androgens and coronary artery disease. Endocr Rev 2003;24:183–217
123. von Muhlen D, Laughlin GA, Kritz-Silverstein D, Barrett-Connor E. The Dehydroepiandrosterone And WellNess (DAWN) study: research design and methods. Contemp Clin Trials 2007;28:153–168
124. Libby P, Ridker PM, Maseri A. Inflammation and atherosclerosis. Circulation 2002;105:1135–1143
125. Davis T, Kipling D. Werner Syndrome as an example of inflamm-aging: possible therapeutic opportunities for a progeroid syndrome? Rejuvenation Res 2006;9:402–407
126. Cadroy Y, Pierrejean D, Fontan B, Sie P, Boneu B. Influence of aging on the activity of the hemostatic system: prothrombin fragment 1+2, thrombin-antithrombin III complexes and D-dimers in 80 healthy subjects with age ranging from 20 to 94 years. Nouv Rev Fr Hematol 1992;34:43–46
127. Pieper CF, Rao KM, Currie MS, Harris TB, Chen HJ. Age, functional status, and racial differences in plasma D-dimer levels in community-dwelling elderly persons. J Gerontol A Biol Sci Med Sci 2000;55:M649–M657
128. Wilkerson WR, Sane DC. Aging and thrombosis. Semin Thromb Hemost 2002;28:555–568

129. Satyanarayana A, Rudolph KL. p16 and ARF: activation of teenage proteins in old age. J Clin Invest 2004;114:1237–1240
130. Shapiro GI, Edwards CD, Ewen M., Rollins BJ. p16INK4A participates in a G1 arrest checkpoint in response to DNA damage. Mol Cell Biol 1998;18:378–387
131. Krishnamurthy J, Torrice C, Ramsey MR, Kovalev GI, Al-Regaiey K, Su L, Sharpless NE. Ink4a/Arf expression is a biomarker of aging. J Clin Invest 2004;114:1299–1307
132. von Zglinicki T, Saretzki G, Ladhoff J, d'Adda di Fagagna F, Jackson SP. Human cell senescence as a DNA damage response. Mech Ageing Dev 2005;126:111–117
133. Gardner JP, Kimura M, Chai W, Durrani JF, Tchakmakjian L, Cao X, Lu X, Li G, Peppas AP, Skurnick J, Wright WE, Shay JW, Aviv A. Telomere dynamics in macaques and humans. J Gerontol A Biol Sci Med Sci 2007;62:367–374
134. Kittleson MM, Hare JM. Molecular signature analysis: using the myocardial transcriptome as a biomarker in cardiovascular disease. Trends Cardiovasc Med 2005;15:130–138
135. Lee CK, Klopp RG, Weindruch R, Prolla TA. Gene expression profile of aging and its retardation by caloric restriction. Science 1999;285:1390–1393
136. Park SK, Prolla TA. Gene expression profiling studies of aging in cardiac and skeletal muscles. Cardiovasc Res 2005;66:205–212
137. Anisimov SV, Boheler K. Aging-associated changes in cardiac gene expression: large scale transcriptome analysis. Adv Gerontol 2003;11:67–75
138. Ashton KJ, Willems L, Holmgren K, Ferreira L, Headrick JP. Age-associated shifts in cardiac gene transcription and transcriptional responses to ischemic stress. Exp Gerontol 2006;41:189–204
139. Edwards MG, Sarkar D, Klopp R, Morrow JD, Weindruch R, Prolla TA. Age-related impairment of the transcriptional responses to oxidative stress in the mouse heart. Physiol Genomics 2003;13:119–127
140. Spindler SR. Use of microarray biomarkers to identify longevity therapeutics. Aging Cell 2006;5:39–50
141. Fu C, Hickey M, Morrison M, McCarter R, Han ES. Tissue specific and non-specific changes in gene expression by aging and by early stage CR. Mech Ageing Dev 2006;127:905–916
142. Bender A, Beckers J, Schneider I, Holter SM, Haack T, Ruthsatz T, Vogt-Weisenhorn DM, Becker L, Genius J, Rujescu D, Irmler M, Mijalski T, Mader M, Quintanilla-Martinez L, Fuchs H, Gailus-Durner V, de Angelis MH, Wurst W, Schmidt J, Klopstock T. Creatine improves health and survival of mice. Neurobiol Aging 2007 Apr 6; [Epub ahead of print]
143. Gohil K. Functional genomics identifies novel and diverse molecular targets of nutrients in vivo. Biol Chem 2004;385:691–696
144. Mathers JC. Nutritional modulation of ageing: genomic and epigenetic approaches. Mech Ageing Dev 2006;127:584–589
145. Feil R. Environmental and nutritional effects on the epigenetic regulation of genes. Mutat Res 2006;600: 46–57
146. Welle S, Brooks AI, Delehanty JM, Needler N, Thornton CA. Gene expression profile of aging in human muscle. Physiol Genomics 2003;14:149–159
147. Volkova M, Garg R, Dick S, Boheler KR. Aging-associated changes in cardiac gene expression. Cardiovasc Res 2005;66:194–204
148. Zahn JM, Sonu R, Vogel H, Crane E, Mazan-Mamczarz K, Rabkin R, Davis RW, Becker KG, Owen AB, Kim SK. Transcriptional profiling of aging in human muscle reveals a common aging signature. PLoS Genet 2006;2:e115
149. Lu T, Pan Y, Kao SY, Li C, Kohane I, Chan J, Yankner BA. Gene regulation and DNA damage in the ageing human brain. Nature 2004;429:883–891
150. Kyng KJ, May A, Stevnsner T, Becker KG, Kolvra S, Bohr VA. Gene expression responses to DNA damage are altered in human aging and in werner syndrome. Oncogen 2005;24:5026–5042
151. Roy AK, Oh T, Rivera O, Mubiru J, Song CS, Chatterjee B. Impacts of transcriptional regulation on aging and senescence. Ageing Res Rev 2002;1:367–380
152. Kyng KJ, May A, Kolvraa S, Bohr VA. Gene expression profiling in werner syndrome closely resembles that of normal aging. Proc Natl Acad Sci USA 2003;100:12259–12264
153. Kyng KJ, Bohr VA. Gene expression and DNA repair in progeroid syndromes and human aging. Ageing Res Rev 2005;4:579–602
154. Csoka AB, English SB, Simkevich CP, Ginzinger DG, Butte AJ, Schatten GP, Rothman FG, Sedivy JM. Genome-scale expression profiling of Hutchinson-Gilford progeria syndrome reveals widespread transcriptional misregulation leading to mesodermal/mesenchymal defects and accelerated atherosclerosis. Aging Cell 2004;3:235–243
155. Anderson L. Candidate-based proteomics in the search for biomarkers of cardiovascular disease. J Physiol 2005;563:23–60

156. Ridker PM, Rifai N, Rose L, Buring JE, Cook NR. Comparison of C-reactive protein and low-density lipoprotein cholesterol levels in the prediction of first cardiovascular events. N Engl J Med 2002;347:1557–1565
157. Lopez MF, Melov S. Applied proteomics: mitochondrial proteins and effect on function. Circ Res 2002;90: 380–389
158. Gaucher SP, Taylor SW, Fahy E, Zhang B, Warnock DE, Ghosh SS, Gibson BW. Expanded coverage of the human heart mitochondrial proteome using multidimensional liquid chromatography coupled with tandem mass spectrometry. J Proteome Res 2004;3:495–505
159. McDonald TG, Van Eyk JE. Mitochondrial proteomics. Undercover in the lipid bilayer. Basic Res Cardiol 2003;98:219–227
160. Kiri AN, Tran HC, Drahos KL, Lan W, McRorie DK, Horn MJ. Proteomic changes in bovine heart mitochondria with age: using a novel technique for organelle separation and enrichment. J Biomol Tech 2005;16:371–379
161. Yan L, Ge H, Li H, Lieber SC, Natividad F, Resuello RR, Kim SJ, Akeju S, Sun A, Loo K, Peppas AP, Rossi F, Lewandowski ED, Thomas AP, Vatner SF, Vatner DE. Gender-specific proteomic alterations in glycolytic and mitochondrial pathways in aging monkey hearts. J Mol Cell Cardiol 2004;37:921–929
162. Dencher NA, Goto S, Reifschneider NH, Sugawa M, Krause F. Unraveling age-dependent variation of the mitochondrial proteome. Ann NY Acad Sci 2006;1067:116–119
163. Reifschneider NH, Goto S, Nakamoto H, Takahashi R, Sugawa M, Dencher NA, Krause F. Defining the mitochondrial proteomes from five rat organs in a physiologically significant context using 2D blue-native/SDS-PAGE. J Proteome Res 2006;5:1117–1132
164. Hunzinger C, Wozny W, Schwall GP, Poznanovic S, Stegmann W, Zengerling H, Schoepf R, Groebe K, Cahill MA, Osiewacz HD, Jagemann N, Bloch M, Dencher NA, Krause F, Schrattenholz A. Comparative profiling of the mammalian mitochondrial proteome: multiple aconitase-2 isoforms including N-formylkynurenine modifications as part of a protein biomarker signature for reactive oxidative species. J Proteome Res 2006;5: 625–633
165. Crampin EJ, Halstead M, Hunter P, Nielsen P, Noble D, Smith N, Tawhai M. Computational physiology and the Physiome Project. Exp Physiol 2004;89:1–26
166. Kirkwood TB, Proctor CJ. Somatic mutations and ageing in silico. Mech Ageing Dev 2003;124:85–92
167. Salvioli S, Capri M, Valensin S, Tieri P, Monti D, Ottaviani E, Franceschi C. Inflamm-aging, cytokines and aging: state of the art, new hypotheses on the role of mitochondria and new perspectives from systems biology. Curr Pharm Des 2006;12:3161–3171
168. Bassingthwaighte JB, Qian H, Li Z. The cardiome project: an integrated view of cardiac metabolism and regional mechanical function. Adv Exp Med Biol 1999;471:541–53
169. Kriete A, Sokhansanj BA, Coppock DL, West GB. Systems approaches to the networks of aging. Ageing Res Rev 2006;5:434–448
170. Kriete A. Biomarkers of aging: combinatorial or systems model? Sci Aging Knowledge Environ 2006;2006:pe1
171. Kirkwood TB, Kowald A. Network theory of aging. Exp Gerontol 1997;32:395–399
172. Kujoth GC, Hiona A, Pugh TD, Someya S, Panzer K, Wohlgemuth SE, Hofer T, Seo AY, Sullivan R, Jobling WA, Morrow JD, Van Remmen H, Sedivy JM, Yamasoba T, Tanokura M, Weindruch R, Leeuwenburgh C, Prolla TA. Mitochondrial DNA mutations, oxidative stress, and apoptosis in mammalian aging. Science 2005;309: 481–484
173. Kirkwood TB, Boys RJ, Gillespie CS, Proctor CJ, Shanley DP, Wilkinson DJ. Towards an e-biology of ageing: integrating theory and data. Nat Rev Mol Cell Biol 2003;4:243–249
174. de Magalhaes JP, Toussaint O. GenAge: a genomic and proteomic network map of human ageing. FEBS Lett 2004;571:243–247
175. de Magalhaes JP, Costa J, Toussaint O. HAGR: the human ageing genomic resources. Nucleic Acids Res 2005;33:D537–D543
176. Boyce K, Kriete A, Nagatomi S, Kelder B, Coschigano K, Kopchick JJ. Phenotypical enrichment strategies for microarray data analysis applied in a type II diabetes study. OMICS 2005;9:251–265
177. Noble D. Modelling the heart: insights, failures and progress. Bioessays 2002;24:1155–1163
178. Sastre J, Pallardo FV, Vina J. The role of mitochondrial oxidative stress in aging. Free Radic Biol Med 2003;35:1–8
179. Timiras PS, Yaghmaie F, Saeed O, Thung E, Chinn G. The ageing phenome: caloric restriction and hormones promote neural cell survival, growth, and de-differentiation. Mech Ageing Dev 2005;126:3–9
180. Lussier YA, Liu Y. Computational approaches to phenotyping: high-throughput phenomics. Proc Am Thorac Soc 2007;4:18–25
181. Butte AJ, Kohane IS. Creation and implications of a phenome-genome network. Nat Biotechnol 2006;24:55–62
182. Harris TB, Launer LJ, Eiriksdottir G, Kjartansson O, Jonsson PV, Sigurdsson G, Thorgeirsson G, Aspelund T, Garcia ME, Cotch MF, Hoffman HJ, Gudnason V. Age, gene/environment susceptibility-Reykjavik study: multidisciplinary applied phenomics. Am J Epidemiol 2007;165:1076–1087

183. de Grey AD, Ames BN, Andersen JK, Bartke A, Campisi J, Heward CB, McCarter RJ, Stock G. Time to talk SENS: critiquing the immutability of human aging. Ann NY Acad Sci 2002;959:452–62
184. de Grey AD, Baynes JW, Berd D, Heward CB, Pawelec G, Stock G. Is human aging still mysterious enough to be left only to scientists? Bioessays 2002;24:667–676
185. de Grey AD. Challenging but essential targets for genuine anti-ageing drugs. Expert Opin Ther Targets 2003;7:1–5
186. de Grey AD. Like it or not, life-extension research extends beyond biogerontology. EMBO Rep 2005;6:1000
187. Warner H, Anderson J, Austad S, Bergamini E, Bredesen D, Butler R, Carnes BA, Clark BF, Cristofalo V, Faulkner J, Guarente L, Harrison DE, Kirkwood T, Lithgow G, Martin G, Masoro E, Melov S, Miller RA, Olshansky SJ, Partridge L, Pereira-Smith O, Perls T, Richardson A, Smith J, von Zglinicki T, Wang E, Wei JY, Williams TF. Science fact and the SENS agenda. What can we reasonably expect from ageing research? EMBO Rep 2005;6:1006–1008
188. Yamamoto S, Yang G, Zablocki D, Liu J, Hong C, Kim SJ, Soler S, Odashima M, Thaisz J, Yehia G, Molina CA, Yatani A, Vatner DE, Vatner SF, Sadoshima J. Activation of Mst1 causes dilated cardiomyopathy by stimulating apoptosis without compensatory ventricular myocyte hypertrophy. J Clin Invest 2003;111:1463–1474
189. Wencker D, Chandra M, Nguyen K, Miao W, Garantziotis S, Factor SM, Shirani J, Armstrong RC, Kitsis RN. A mechanistic role for cardiac myocyte apoptosis in heart failure. J Clin Invest 2003;111:1497–1504
190. Holly TA, Drincic A, Byun Y, Nakamura S, Harris K, Klocke FJ, Cryns VL. Caspase inhibition reduces myocyte cell death induced by myocardial ischemia and reperfusion in vivo. J Mol Cell Cardiol 1999;31:1709–1715
191. Faubel S, Edelstein CL. Caspases as drug targets in ischemic organ injury. Curr Drug Targets Immune Endocr Metabol Disord 2005;5:269–287
191. Brocheriou V, Hagege AA, Oubenaissa A, Lambert M, Mallet VO, Duriez M, Wassef M, Kahn A, Menasche P, Gilgenkrantz H. Cardiac functional improvement by a human Bcl-2 transgene in a mouse model of ischemia/reperfusion injury. J Gene Med 2000;2:326–333
192. Jayasankar V, Woo YJ, Pirolli TJ, Bish LT, Berry MF, Burdick J, Gardner TJ, Sweeney HL. Induction of angiogenesis and inhibition of apoptosis by hepatocyte growth factor effectively treats postischemic heart failure. J Card Surg 2005;20:93–101
193. Haendeler J. Nitric oxide and endothelial cell aging. Eur J Clin Pharmacol 2006;62:137–140
194. Napoli C, Martin-Padura I, de Nigris F, Giorgio M, Mansueto G, Somma P, Condorelli M, Sica G, De Rosa G, Pelicci P. Deletion of the p66Shc longevity gene reduces systemic and tissue oxidative stress, vascular cell apoptosis, and early atherogenesis in mice fed a high-fat diet. Proc Natl Acad Sci USA 2003;100:2112–2116
195. Menini S, Amadio L, Oddi G, Ricci C, Pesce C, Pugliese F, Giorgio M, Migliaccio E, Pelicci P, Iacobini C, Pugliese G. Deletion of p66Shc longevity gene protects against experimental diabetic glomerulopathy by preventing diabetes-induced oxidative stress. Diabetes 2006;55:1642–1650
196. Rota M, LeCapitaine N, Hosoda T, Boni A, De Angelis A, Padin-Iruegas ME, Esposito G, Vitale S, Urbanek K, Casarsa C, Giorgio M, Luscher TF, Pelicci PG, Anversa P, Leri A, Kajstura J. Diabetes promotes cardiac stem cell aging and heart failure, which are prevented by deletion of the p66shc gene. Circ Res 2006;99:42–52
197. Pinton P, Rimessi A, Marchi S, Orsini F, Migliaccio E, Giorgio M, Contursi C, Minucci S, Mantovani F, Wieckowski MR, Del Sal G, Pelicci PG, Rizzuto R. Protein kinase C beta and prolyl isomerase 1 regulate mitochondrial effects of the life-span determinant p66Shc. Science 2007;315:659–663
198. Obreztchikova M, Elouardighi H, Ho M, Wilson BA, Gertsberg Z, Steinbeg SF. Distinct signaling functions for SHC isoforms in the heart. J Biol Chem 2006;281:20197–20204
199. Lee CK, Allison DB, Brand J, Weindruch R, Prolla TA. Transcriptional profiles associated with aging and middle age-onset caloric restriction in mouse hearts. Proc Natl Acad Sci USA 2002;99:14988–14993
200. Rohrbach S, Gruenler S, Teschner M, Holtz J. The thioredoxin system in aging muscle: key role of mitochondrial thioredoxin reductase in the protective effects of caloric restriction? Am J Physiol Regul Integr Comp Physiol 2006;291:R927–R935
201. Kwak HB, Song W, Lawler JM. Exercise training attenuates age-induced elevation in Bax/Bcl-2 ratio, apoptosis, and remodeling in the rat heart. FASEB J 2006;20:791–793
202. Anversa P, Rota M, Urbanek K, Hosoda T, Sonnenblick EH, Leri A, Kajstura J, Bolli R. Myocardial aging – a stem cell problem. Basic Res Cardiol 2005;100:482–493
203. Nadal-Ginard B, Kajstura J, Leri A, Anversa P. Myocyte death, growth, and regeneration in cardiac hypertrophy and failure. Circ Res 2003;92:139–150
204. Urbanek K, Quaini F, Tasca G, Torella D, Castaldo C, Nadal-Ginard B, Leri A, Kajstura J, Quaini E, Anversa P. Intense myocyte formation from cardiac stem cells in human cardiac hypertrophy. Proc Natl Acad Sci USA 2003;100:10440–10445
205. Kajstura J, Leri A, Finato N, Di Loreto C, Beltrami CA, Anversa P. Myocyte proliferation in end-stage cardiac failure in humans. Proc Natl Acad Sci USA 1998;95:8801–8805

206. Beltrami AP, Urbanek K, Kajstura J, Yan SM, Finato N, Bussani R, Nadal-Ginard B, Silvestri F, Leri A, Beltrami CA, Anversa P. Evidence that human cardiac myocytes divide after myocardial infarction. N Engl J Med 2001;344:1750–1757
207. Beltrami AP, Barlucchi L, Torella D, Baker M, Limana F, Chimenti S, Kasahara H, Rota M, Musso E, Urbanek K, Leri A, Kajstura J, Nadal-Ginard B, Anversa P. Adult cardiac stem cells are multipotent and support myocardial regeneration. Cell 2003;114:763–776
208. Messina E, De Angelis L, Frati G, Morrone S, Chimenti S, Fiordaliso F, Salio M, Battaglia M, Latronico MV, Coletta M, Vivarelli E, Frati L, Cossu G, Giacomello A. Isolation and expansion of adult cardiac stem cells from human and murine heart. Circ Res 2004;95:911–921
209. Urbanek K, Cesselli D, Rota M, Nascimbene A, De Angelis A, Hosoda T, Bearzi C, Boni A, Bolli R, Kajstura J, Anversa P, Leri A. Stem cell niches in the adult mouse heart. Proc Natl Acad Sci USA 2006;103: 9226–9231
210. Behfar A, Zingman LV, Hodgson DM, Rauzier JM, Kane GC, Terzic A, Puceat M. Stem cell differentiation requires a paracrine pathway in the heart. FASEB J 2002;16:1558–1566
211. Kofidis T, de Bruin JL, Yamane T, Tanaka M, Lebl DR, Swijnenburg RJ, Weissman IL, Robbins RC. Stimulation of paracrine pathways with growth factors enhances embryonic stem cell engraftment and host-specific differentiation in the heart after ischemic myocardial injury. Circulation 2005;111:2486–2493
212. Vandervelde S, van Luyn MJ, Tio RA, Harmsen MC. Signaling factors in stem cell-mediated repair of infarcted myocardium. J Mol Cell Cardiol 2005;39:363–376
213. Min JY, Chen Y, Malek S, Meissner A, Xiang M, Ke Q, Feng X, Nakayama M, Kaplan E, Morgan JP. Stem cell therapy in the aging hearts of Fisher 344 rats: synergistic effects on myogenesis and angiogenesis. J Thorac Cardiovasc Surg 2005;130:547–553
214. Pallante BA, Duignan I, Okin D, Chin A, Bressan MC, Mikawa T, Edelberg JM. Bone marrow Oct3/4+ cells differentiate into cardiac myocytes via age-dependent paracrine mechanisms. Circ Res 2007;100(1):e1–11
215. Lehrke S, Mazhari R, Durand DJ, Zheng M, Bedja D, Zimmet JM, Schuleri KH, Chi AS, Gabrielson KL, Hare JM. Aging impairs the beneficial effect of granulocyte colony-stimulating factor and stem cell factor on post-myocardial infarction remodeling. Circ Res 2006;99:553–560
216. Cai D, Xaymardan M, Holm JM, Zheng J, Kizer JR, Edelberg JM. Age-associated impairment in TNF-alpha cardioprotection from myocardial infarction. Am J Physiol Heart Circ Physiol 2003;285:H463–H469
217. van Vliet P, Sluijter JP, Doevendans PA, Goumans MJ. Isolation and expansion of resident cardiac progenitor cells. Expert Rev Cardiovasc Ther 2007;5:33–43
218. Urbanek K, Rota M, Cascapera S, Bearzi C, Nascimbene A, De Angelis A, Hosoda T, Chimenti S, Baker M, Limana F, Nurzynska D, Torella D, Rotatori F, Rastaldo R, Musso E, Quaini F, Leri A, Kajstura J, Anversa P. Cardiac stem cells possess growth factor-receptor systems that after activation regenerate the infarcted myocardium, improving ventricular function and long-term survival. Circ Res 2005;97:663–673
219. Torella D, Ellison GM, Mendez-Ferrer S, Ibanez B, Nadal-Ginard B. Resident human cardiac stem cells: role in cardiac cellular homeostasis and potential for myocardial regeneration. Nat Clin Pract Cardiovasc Med 2006;3:S8–S13
220. Torella D, Ellison GM, Karakikes I, Nadal-Ginard B. Growth-factor-mediated cardiac stem cell activation in myocardial regeneration. Nat Clin Pract Cardiovasc Med 2007;4:S46–S51
221. Ellison GM. The pig heart harbors cardiac stem-progenitor cells which respond to growth factor stimulation regenerating the infarcted myocardium [abstract]. Eur Heart J 2006;27:546
222. Ballard VL, Edelberg JM. Stem cells and the regeneration of the aging cardiovascular system. Circ Res 2007;100:1116–1127
223. Scheubel RJ, Zorn H, Silber RE, Kuss O, Morawietz H, Holtz J, Simm A. Age-dependent depression in circulating endothelial progenitor cells in patients undergoing coronary artery bypass grafting. J Am Coll Cardiol 2003;42:2073–2080
224. Heiss C, Keymel S, Niesler U, Ziemann J, Kelm M, Kalka C. Impaired progenitor cell activity in age-related endothelial dysfunction. J Am Coll Cardiol 2005;45:1441–1448
225. Tao J, Wang Y, Yang Z, Tu C, Xu MG, Wang JM. Circulating endothelial progenitor cell deficiency contributes to impaired arterial elasticity in persons of advancing age. J Hum Hypertens 2006;20:490–495
226. Hill JM, Zalos G, Halcox JP, Schenke WH, Waclawiw MA, Quyyumi AA, Finkel T. Circulating endothelial progenitor cells, vascular function, and cardiovascular risk. N Engl J Med 2003;348:593–600
227. Fadini GP, Sartore S, Albiero M, Baesso I, Murphy E, Menegolo M, Grego F, Vigili de Kreutzenberg S, Tiengo A, Agostini C, Avogaro A. Number and function of endothelial progenitor cells as a marker of severity for diabetic vasculopathy. Arterioscler Thromb Vasc Biol 2006;26:2140–2146
228. Fadini GP, Coracina A, Baesso I, Agostini C, Tiengo A, Avogaro A, de Kreutzenberg SV. Peripheral blood CD34+KDR+ endothelial progenitor cells are determinants of subclinical atherosclerosis in a middle-aged general population. Stroke 2006;37:2277–2282

229. Rauscher FM, Goldschmidt-Clermont PJ, Davis BH, Wang T, Gregg D, Ramaswami P, Pippen AM, Annex BH, Dong C, Taylor DA. Aging, progenitor cell exhaustion, and atherosclerosis. Circulation 2003;108:457–463
230. Imanishi T, Hano T, Nishio I. Estrogen reduces endothelial progenitor cell senescence through augmentation of telomerase activity. J Hypertens 2005;23:1699–1706
231. Strehlow K, Werner N, Berweiler J, Link A, Dirnagl U, Priller J, Laufs K, Ghaeni L, Milosevic M, Bohm M, Nickenig G. Estrogen increases bone marrow-derived endothelial progenitor cell production and diminishes neointima formation. Circulation 2003;107:3059–3065
232. Bernardini D, Ballabio E, Mariotti M, Maier JA. Differential expression of EDF-1 and endothelial nitric oxide synthase by proliferating, quiescent and senescent microvascular endothelial cells. Biochim Biophys Acta 2005;1745:265–272
233. Papapetropoulos A, Garcia-Cardena G, Madri JA, Sessa WC. Nitric oxide production contributes to the angiogenic properties of vascular endothelial growth factor in human endothelial cells. J Clin Invest 1997;100: 3131–3139
234. Lantin-Hermoso RL, Rosenfeld CR, Yuhanna IS, German Z, Chen Z, Shaul PW. Estrogen acutely stimulates nitric oxide synthase activity in fetal pulmonary artery endothelium. Am J Physiol 1997;273:L119–L126
235. George J, Afek A, Abashidze A, Shmilovich H, Deutsch V, Kopolovich J, Miller H, Keren G. Transfer of endothelial progenitor and bone marrow cells influences atherosclerotic plaque size and composition in apolipoprotein E knockout mice. Arterioscler Thromb Vasc Biol 2005;25:2636–2641
236. Ballard VL, Edelberg JM. Harnessing hormonal signaling for cardioprotection. Sci Aging Knowledge Environ 2005;2005:re6
237. Thum T, Hoeber S, Froese S, Klink I, Stichtenoth DO, Galuppo P, Jakob M, Tsikas D, Anker SD, Poole-Wilson PA, Borlak J, Ertl G, Bauersachs J. Age-dependent impairment of endothelial progenitor cells is corrected by growth-hormone-mediated increase of insulin-like growth-factor-1. Circ Res 2007;100:434–443
238. Navarro A, Boveris A. The mitochondrial energy transduction system and the aging process. Am J Physiol Cell Physiol 2007;292:C670–C686
239. Hunt ND, Hyun DH, Allard JS, Minor RK, Mattson MP, Ingram DK, de Cabo R. Bioenergetics of aging and calorie restriction. Ageing Res Rev 2006;5:125–143
240. Pepe S. Effect of dietary polyunsaturated fatty acids on age-related changes in cardiac mitochondrial membranes. Exp Gerontol 2005;40:751–758
241. Hagen TM, Moreau R, Suh JH, Visioli F. Mitochondrial decay in the aging rat heart: evidence for improvement by dietary supplementation with acetyl-L-carnitine and/or lipoic acid. Ann NY Acad Sci 2002;959: 491–507
242. Rodriguez MI, Carretero M, Escames G, Lopez LC, Maldonado MD, Tan DX, Reiter RJ, Acuna-Castroviejo D. Chronic melatonin treatment prevents age-dependent cardiac mitochondrial dysfunction in senescence-accelerated mice. Free Radic Res 2007;41:15–24
243. Kumaran S, Subathra M, Balu M, Panneerselvam C. Supplementation of L-carnitine improves mitochondrial enzymes in heart and skeletal muscle of aged rats. Exp Aging Res 2005;31:55–67
244. Zhao K, Zhao GM, Wu D, Soong Y, Birk AV, Schiller PW, Szeto HH. Cell-permeable peptide antioxidants targeted to inner mitochondrial membrane inhibit mitochondrial swelling, oxidative cell death, and reperfusion injury. J Biol Chem 2004;279:34682–34690
245. Schriner SE, Linford NJ, Martin GM, Treuting P, Ogburn CE, Emond M, Coskun PE, Ladiges W, Wolf N, Van Remmen H, Wallace DC, Rabinovitch PS. Extension of murine life span by overexpression of catalase targeted to mitochondria. Science 2005;308:1909–1911
246. Ren J, Li Q, Wu S, Li SY, Babcock SA. Cardiac overexpression of antioxidant catalase attenuates aging-induced cardiomyocyte relaxation dysfunction. Mech Ageing Dev 2007;128:276–285
247. Wu S, Li Q, Du M, Li SY, Ren J. Cardiac-specific overexpression of catalase prolongs life span and attenuates ageing-induced cardiomyocyte contractile dysfunction and protein damage. Clin Exp Pharmacol Physiol 2007;34:81–87
248. Communal C, Huq F, Lebeche D, Mestel C, Gwathmey JK, Hajjar RJ. Decreased efficiency of adenovirus-mediated gene transfer in aging cardiomyocytes. Circulation 2003;107:1170–1175
249. Terman A, Brunk UT. Autophagy in cardiac myocyte homeostasis, aging, and pathology. Cardiovasc Res 2005;68:355–365
250. Bergamini E. Autophagy: a cell repair mechanism that retards ageing and age-associated diseases and can be intensified pharmacologically. Mol Aspects Med 2006;27:403–410
251. de Grey AD, Alvarez PJ, Brady RO, Cuervo AM, Jerome WG, McCarty PL, Nixon RA, Rittmann BE, Sparrow JR. Medical bioremediation: prospects for the application of microbial catabolic diversity to aging and several major age-related diseases. Ageing Res Rev 2005;4:315–338
252. de Grey AD. Bioremediation meets biomedicine: therapeutic translation of microbial catabolism to the lysosome. Trends Biotechnol 2002;20:452–455

253. Massey AC, Zhang C, Cuervo AM. Chaperone-mediated autophagy in aging and disease. Curr Top Dev Biol 2006;73:205–235
254. Bergamini E, Cavallini G, Donati A, Gori Z. The anti-ageing effects of caloric restriction may involve stimulation of macroautophagy and lysosomal degradation, and can be intensified pharmacologically. Biomed Pharmacother 2003;57:203–208
255. Donati A. The involvement of macroautophagy in aging and anti-aging interventions. Mol Aspects Med 2006;27:455–470
256. Cavallini G, Donati A, Taddei M, Bergamini E. Evidence for selective mitochondrial autophagy and failure in aging. Autophagy 2007;3:26–27
257. Groban L, Pailes NA, Bennett CD, Carter CS, Chappell MC, Kitzman DW, Sonntag WE. Growth hormone replacement attenuates diastolic dysfunction and cardiac angiotensin II expression in senescent rats. J Gerontol A Biol Sci Med Sci 2006;61:28–35
258. Headrick JP, Willems L, Ashton KJ, Holmgren K, Peart J, Matherne GP. Ischaemic tolerance in aged mouse myocardium: the role of adenosine and effects of A1 adenosine receptor overexpression. J Physiol 2003;549:823–833
259. Baur JA, Pearson KJ, Price NL, Jamieson HA, Lerin C, Kalra A, Prabhu VV, Allard JS, Lopez-Lluch G, Lewis K, Pistell PJ, Poosala S, Becker KG, Boss O, Gwinn D, Wang M, Ramaswamy S, Fishbein KW, Spencer RG, Lakatta EG, Le Couteur D, Shaw RJ, Navas P, Puigserver P, Ingram DK, de Cabo R, Sinclair DA. Resveratrol improves health and survival of mice on a high-calorie diet. Nature 2006;444:337–342
260. de la Lastra CA, Villegas I. Resveratrol as an anti-inflammatory and anti-aging agent: mechanisms and clinical implications. Mol Nutr Food Res 2005;49:405–430
261. Das DK, Maulik N. Resveratrol in cardioprotection: a therapeutic promise of alternative medicine. Mol Interv 2006;6:36–47
262. Susic D, Varagic J, Ahn J, Matavelli L, Frohlich ED. Long-term mineralocorticoid receptor blockade reduces fibrosis and improves cardiac performance and coronary hemodynamics in elderly SHR. Am J Physiol Heart Circ Physiol 2007;292:H175–H179
263. Saka M, Obata K, Ichihara S, Cheng XW, Kimata H, Noda A, Izawa H, Nagata K, Yokota M. Attenuation of ventricular hypertrophy and fibrosis in rats by pitavastatin: potential role of the RhoA-extracellular signal-regulated kinase-serum response factor signalling pathway. Clin Exp Pharmacol Physiol 2006;33:1164–1171
264. Kumar A, Meyerrose G, Sood V, Roongsritong C. Diastolic heart failure in the elderly and the potential role of aldosterone antagonists. Drugs Aging 2006;23:299–308
265. Diaz-Araya G, Borg TK, Lavandero S, Loftis MJ, Carver W. IGF-1 modulation of rat cardiac fibroblast behavior and gene expression is age-dependent. Cell Commun Adhes 2003;10:155–165
266. Zieman S, Kass D. Advanced glycation end product cross-linking: pathophysiologic role and therapeutic target in cardiovascular disease. Congest Heart Fail 2004;10:144–149
267. Furber JD. Extracellular glycation crosslinks: prospects for removal. Rejuvenation Res 2006;9:274–278
268. Bakris GL, Bank AJ, Kass DA, Neutel JM, Preston RA, Oparil S. Advanced glycation end-product cross-link breakers. A novel approach to cardiovascular pathologies related to the aging process. Am J Hypertens 2004;17:23S–30S
269. Zieman SJ, Melenovsky V, Clattenburg L, Corretti MC, Capriotti A, Gerstenblith G, Kass DA. Advanced glycation endproduct crosslink breaker (alagebrium) improves endothelial function in patients with isolated systolic hypertension. J Hypertens 2007;25:577–583
270. Monnier VM, Mustata GT, Biemel KL, Reihl O, Lederer MO, Zhenyu D, Sell DR. Cross-linking of the extracellular matrix by the maillard reaction in aging and diabetes: an update on "a puzzle nearing resolution". Ann NY Acad Sci 2005;1043:533–544
271. Schmidt U, del Monte F, Miyamoto MI, Matsui T, Gwathmey JK, Rosenzweig A, Hajjar RJ. Restoration of diastolic function in senescent rat hearts through adenoviral gene transfer of sarcoplasmic reticulum Ca(2+)-ATPase. Circulation 2000;101:790–796
272. Schmidt U, Zhu X, Lebeche D, Huq F, Guerrero JL, Hajjar RJ. In vivo gene transfer of parvalbumin improves diastolic function in aged rat hearts. Cardiovasc Res 2005;66:318–323
273. Li Q, Wu S, Li SY, Lopez FL, Du M, Kajstura J, Anversa P, Ren J. Cardiac-specific overexpression of insulin-like growth factor 1 attenuates aging-associated cardiac diastolic contractil dysfunction and protein damage. Am J Physiol Heart Circ Physiol 2007;292:H1398–H1403
274. Guo KK, Ren J. Cardiac overexpression of alcohol dehydrogenase (ADH) alleviates aging-associated cardiomyocyte contractile dysfunction: role of intracellular Ca2+ cycling proteins. Aging Cell 2006;5:259–265
275. Fang CX, Doser TA, Yang X, Sreejayan N, Ren J. Metallothionein antagonizes aging-induced cardiac contractile dysfunction: role of PTP1B, insulin receptor tyrosine phosphorylation and Akt. Aging Cell 2006;5:177–185
276. Ames BN, Atamna H, Killilea DW. Mineral and vitamin deficiencies can accelerate the mitochondrial decay of aging. Mol Aspects Med 2005;26:363–378

277. Courtemanche C, Huang AC, Elson-Schwab I, Kerry N, Ng BY, Ames BN. Folate deficiency and ionizing radiation cause DNA breaks in primary human lymphocytes: a comparison. FASEB J 2004;18:209–211
278. Ames BN. A role for supplements in optimizing health: the metabolic tune-up. Arch Biochem Biophys 2004;423:227–234
279. Kornman KS. Interleukin 1 genetics, inflammatory mechanisms, and nutrigenetic opportunities to modulate diseases of aging. Am J Clin Nutr 2006;83:475S–483S
280. Olaharski AJ, Rine J, Marshall BL, Babiarz J, Zhang L, Verdin E, Smith MT. The flavoring agent dihydrocoumarin reverses epigenetic silencing and inhibits sirtuin deacetylases. PLoS Genet 2005;1:e77

Glossary

AAV Adeno-associated virus; vector useful for cardiomyocyte gene transfection.

ACH Acetylcholine.

ACS Acute coronary syndromes; a set of signs and symptoms suggestive of sudden cardiac ischemia, usually caused by disruption of atherosclerotic plaque in an epicardial coronary artery.

Adipokines Group of cytokines secreted by adipose tissue including leptin, resistin, adiponectin, TNF-α, interleukin-6 (IL-6) and plasminogen activator inhibitor-1 (PAI-1) which have critical roles in inflammation, modifying appetite, insulin resistance and atherosclerosis- some beneficial, others deleterious.

Adiponectin An adipokine exclusively secreted from adipose tissue into the bloodstream, whose plasma levels are inversely correlated with body mass index and which plays a role in suppression of metabolic derangements that may result in type 2 diabetes, obesity, and atherosclerosis.

AF Atrial fibrillation, the most common dysrhythmia seen in clinical cardiology, can be familial with both monogenic and more often heterogeneous genetic cases reported.

AGE Advanced glycation endproducts produced from glycation reactions have been implicated in aging-associated chronic diseases including type II diabetes and CVDs with particular damage to endothelium, collagen and fibrinogen.

AGT Angiotensinogin gene involved in the RAAS pathway

AIF Apoptosis-inducing factor. Released from mitochondrial intermembrane space in early apoptosis and subsequently involved in nuclear DNA fragmentation.

Akt Protein kinase B (PKB). Myocardial Akt phosphorylates a number of downstream targets, including cardioprotective factors involved in glucose and mitochondrial metabolism, apoptosis and regulators of protein synthesis

AL Ad libitum; in contrast to dietary restriction, free access to feed or water

ALCAR Acetyl-l-carnitine, supplementation with lipoic acid (LA) appears to improve myocardial bioenergetics and decrease oxidative stress associated with aging.

Allele An alternative form of a gene.

Allotopic expression Alternative method of mitochondrial gene therapy in which a mitochondrial gene is reengineered for expression from the nucleus and targeting its translation product to the mitochondria.

Angiogenesis Formation of new vessels from preexisting ones, and in particular the sprouting of new capillaries from postcapillary venules

J. Marín-García, *Aging and the Heart,*

Ang II Angiotensin II

ANT Adenine nucleotide translocator. A mitochondrial inner membrane carrier protein of ADP and ATP and constituent of the PT pore.

Antagonistic Pleiotropy Multiple gene effects in an organism, such that alleles which improve fitness early in life have detrimental effects later in life.

Antioxidants A nutrient, enzyme or chemical that reacts with and neutralizes oxidants, free radicals or chemicals that release free radicals; also called free radical scavengers.

APC Anesthetic preconditioning.

APOE Apolipoprotein E, a gene on chromosome 19 encoding a protein in lipoproteins of blood plasma, including HDL, LDL and VLDL. Among the common alleles of APOE gene E2, E3, and E4, E4 is associated with increased frailty and limited life span.

Apoptosis Programmed cell death.

Apoptosome Cytosolic complex involved in the activation of apoptotic caspases.

ARC protein Apoptosis repressor with a caspase recruitment domain (CARD), inhibitor of both the intrinsic and extrinsic apoptosis pathways.

ARVD Arrhythmogenic right ventricular dysplasia; the most common symptoms are ventricular dysrhythmias, palpitations, fainting or loss of consciousness (syncope), and sudden death.

ASO Allele specific oligonucleotides, useful in screening for specific mutations

ATM Ataxia-telangiectasia mutated gene product responsible for Ataxia telangiectasia, an immunodeficiency disorder; the ATM protein is a large serine-threonine kinase involved in regulating cell growth and cell cycle checkpoints in part by regulating p53, BRCA1 and CHEK2. ATM is involved in repair of double strand DNA and telomeres.

ATP Adenosine triphosphate.

Autophagy Digestion of the cell's organelles.

AV Atrioventricular.

AVC Atrioventricular canal.

AV node Atrioventricular node; a group of specialized cells located between the atria and ventricles that regulate electrical current passing to the ventricles.

AVNRT AV nodal reentrant tachycardia, the most common reentrant tachycardia. and most common regular supraventricular tachycardia in elderly patients.

Bacteriophage A virus that infects bacteria; useful as a vector for gene transfer.

β-AR Beta-adrenergic receptor, G-protein coupled receptors containing a seven transmembrane domain involved in signaling pathways of diverse cardiovascular functions including blood pressure control and cardiac contractility.

BER Base excision repair. DNA repair in which a missing or damaged base on a single strand is recognized, excised, and replaced by synthesizing a sequence complementary to the remaining strand.

BF Blood flow.

BH domains Features of proapoptotic proteins, (BH1-4) are essential for homo- and hetero-complex formation, as well as to induce cell death. Proapoptotic homologues can be subdivided into 2 major subtypes, the multidomain Bax subfamily (e.g., Bax and Bak) which possesses BH1-3 domains, and the BH3-only subfamily (e.g., Bad and Bid).

Bid A proapoptotic Bcl-2 related protein, which links the extrinsic and intrinsic apoptotic pathways.

Bilayer Arrangement of phospholipids in biological membranes.

Biomarker A measurable parameter of physiological age that is a more useful predictor of remaining life expectancy than chronological age.

BMC Bone-marrow-derived cells.

BN-PAGE Blue-native polyacrylamide gel electrophoresis allows the separation of large macromolecular complexes preserving protein-protein interactions.

BNP Brain natriuretic peptide, hemodynamic marker of neurohumoral and vascular stress.

bp Base pairs.

BrdU Bromodeoxyuridine, a DNA synthesis inhibitor.

CAC Coronary artery calcification, a marker of atherosclerosis

CAD Coronary artery disease. (See ischemic heart disease).

CAECs Endothelial cells from the coronary artery.

Calpain Calcium-dependent neutral proteases; non lysosomal.

CaM Calmodulin, an intracellular Ca^{2+} sensor that selectively activates downstream signaling pathways in response to local changes in Ca^{2+}.

CaMK Ca^{2+}/CaM dependent protein kinase.

Cameleons Fluorescent indicators for Ca^{2+} that can be targeted to specific intracellular locations.

cAMP Cyclic AMP; second messenger used extensively in cell signaling. Product of adenylyl cyclase (AC).

CAR Coxsackie adenovirus receptor; host protein involved in cellular penetration by adenoviruses and expression level of adenoviral-mediated transfected genes; levels/function may decline with aging impacting the efficacy of adenoviral-mediated gene therapy in the elderly.

Cardiomyocyte A single cell of a heart muscle.

Cardiolipin Anionic phospholipid located primarily in mitochondrial inner membrane.

Carnitine Carrier molecule involved in the transport of long-chain fatty acids into the mitochondria for β-FAO.

Caspases Intracellular cysteine proteases activated during apoptosis that cleave substrates at their aspartic acid residues.

Catalase Antioxidant enzyme which degrades H_2O_2; primarily localized in the peroxisome.

Caveolae Vesicular organelles which are specialized subdomains of the plasma membrane particularly abundant in cardiovascular cells which function both in protein trafficking and signal transduction.

Cell cycle The period between the release of a cell as one of the progeny of a division and its own subsequent division by mitosis into two daughter cells.

Cell fusion Fusion of two somatic cells creating a hybrid cell.

CETP Cholesteryl ester transfer protein plays role in reverse cholesterol transport with transfer of cholesteryl ester-rich HDL to triglyceride-rich lipoproteins (VLDL).

Channelopathy A disease involving dysfunction of an ion channel. Channelopathies involving potassium, sodium, chloride and calcium ion channels have been identified.

Chaperone Protein that assists in the proper folding and assembly into larger complexes of unfolded or misfolded proteins.

ChIP Chromatin immunoprecipitation, a procedure used to determine whether a given protein binds to a particular region of chromatin *in vivo*.

Chromatin The complex of DNA and histone and nonhistone proteins found in the nucleus of a eukaryotic cell that constitutes the chromosomes.

Chylomicron Large triglyceride-rich particles containing apoB48 packaged from dietary lipids in the intestinal enterocyte.

***Cis*-acting elements** Regulatory DNA sequences that affect the expression of genes only on the molecule of DNA where they reside; not protein encoding.

CK Creatine kinase. Both mitochondrial and cytosolic isoforms of this enzyme that catalyzes the reversible phosphorylation of creatine by ATP to form the high-energy compound phosphocreatine.

CML N (epsilon)-(Carboxymethyl)lysine, one of the better-characterized glycation elements (see AGE) which can be formed on proteins by both glycoxidation and lipid peroxidation pathways.

CS Cockayne syndrome: A rare autosomal recessive premature aging syndrome caused by mutations in the ERCC6 and ERCC8 genes involved in DNA repair (NER/TCR).

Comet assay A microgel electrophoresis technique that can measures DNA damage (i.e., single-strand or double strand breaks) at the level of single cells.

Connexins A group of transmembrane proteins that form gap junctions between cells.

CoQ Coenzyme Q (also ubiquinone). Electron carrier and antioxidant.

COX Cytochrome *c* oxidase (complex IV).

CP Cardioprotection.

CpG islands GC-rich regions of DNA often found in promoter regions; DNA methylation target.

CR Caloric restriction, a restricted dietary regimen that has been shown to increase the lifespan of a number of organisms including mammals and may have anti-aging effects in the heart.

CRC Calcium retention capacity, technique used to gauge mitochondrial permeability transition.

CRP C-reactive protein; a significant marker of inflammation and atherosclerotic progression; serum CRP levels are predictive of future cardiovascular events.

CRT Cardiac resynchronization therapy (also called biventricular pacing) is increasingly used to treat and/or prevent heart failure caused by DCM.

CsA Cyclosporin A. An inhibitor of PT pore opening.

CSC Cardiac stem cell.

cTnI Cardiac troponin I, widely used marker of myocardial ischemia and necrosis.

cTnT Cardiac troponin T, widely used marker of myocardial ischemia and necrosis.

Cu-Zn SOD Also SOD1; Copper-zinc superoxide dismutase; Cytosolic ROS scavenger.

CVD Cardiovascular disease.

Cyclin A family of proteins involved in the progression of cells through the cell cycle, and in activating the protein kinase function of its interacting partner, cyclin-dependent kinase (Cdk) and in modulating proliferative growth.

CyP-D Cyclophilin-D. CsA-binding mitochondrial matrix protein component of the PT pore.

Cytochrome A family of proteins that contain heme as a prosthetic group involved in electron transfer and identifiable by their absorption spectra.

Cytochrome c A mitochondrial protein involved in ETC at complex IV whose release from the mitochondrial into cytosol is a trigger of caspase activation and early myocardial apoptosis.

DAP kinase Death-associated protein kinase, a positive mediator of apoptotic cell death.

DCM Dilated cardiomyopathy.

DHEA Dehydroepiandrosterone, a steroid prohormone and precursor of testosterone and estrogen produced by adrenal glands, whose levels significantly decline in aging humans and monkeys, a potential aging biomarker.

DHEAS Dehydroepiandrosterone sulfate, common highly stable, sulfated form of DHEA found in blood.

DISC Death-inducing signaling complex, a multiprotein complex involved in the extrinsic apoptotic pathway triggered by the binding of specific ligands to the death receptor.

D-loop Noncoding regulatory region of mtDNA involved in controlling its replication and transcription.

DMD Duchenne muscular dystrophy caused by defects in the X-linked DMD gene encoding dystrophin.

Dolichol Long-chain unsaturated organic compounds primarily associated with membrane proteins and sugars which increase markedly with age.

DRVD Dysrhythmogenic right ventricular dysplasia (see ARVD).

DSB Double strand breaks, in which both strands in the DNA double helix are severed, are particularly deleterious DNA defects because they can lead to genome rearrangements.

DQAsomes Liposome-like vesicles formed in aqueous medium with a dicationic amphiphile dequalinium used as a mitochondrial-specific delivery system for gene therapy.

Dystrophin Cytoskeletal protein defective in Duchenne (DMD) and Becker (BMD) muscular dystrophy.

EB Embryoid bodies, aggregations of embryonic stem cells which can differentiate spontaneously in *vitro* to a variety of cell types including cardiomyocytes.

EC Endothelial cell.

ECM Extracellular matrix.

EcSOD Extracellular superoxide dismutase

Endocannabinoids Endogenous lipids capable of binding to two cannabinoid receptors, CB1 and CB2 involved in hunger-induced food intake and energy balance; in clinical trials, CB1 receptor blockade has shown effects in reducing abdominal obesity and directly improving lipid and glucose metabolism and insulin resistance in the metabolic syndrome.

eNOS Endothelial nitric oxide synthase.

EPC Endothelial progenitor cells.

Epigenetic Acquired and reversible modification of genetic material (e.g., methylation).

Epistasis Modification of the action of one gene by one or several genes that assort independently.

ER Endoplasmic reticulum. A membrane-bound cytosolic compartment where lipids and membrane-bound proteins are synthesized.

ERK Extracellular regulated kinase.

ERs Estrogen receptors.

ESC Embryonic stem cell.

ETC Electron transport chain. A series of complexes in the mitochondrial inner membrane to conduct electrons from the oxidation of NADH and succinate to oxygen.

Exon Segment of a gene that remains after the splicing of the primary RNA transcript and contains the coding sequences as well as 5' and 3 untranslated regions

FA Friedreich ataxia. An autosomal-dominant neuromuscular disorder with frequent HCM.

FADD Fas-associated via death domain, adaptor protein recruiting procaspase into the apoptotic-promoting complex DISC.

FAO Fatty acid oxidation.

FasL Fas ligand, death ligand in extrinsic apoptotic pathway.

FGF Fibroblast growth factor.

FH Familial hypercholesterolemia, relatively rare monogenic forms of dyslipidemia leading to atherosclerosis.

FIX Procoagulant factor IX.

Forkhead box proteins (FOX and FOXO proteins) play important roles in regulating the transcriptional expression of genes involved in cell growth, proliferation, differentiation, and longevity.

FPLD Familial partial lipodystrophy; a rare monogenic form of insulin resistance caused by mutations in LMNA or PPAR-γ which has used as a potential model of MetSyn.

FRDA Gene for frataxin, a mitochondrial-localized protein. Mutations in FRDA are responsible for Friedreich ataxia (FA).

FRTA Free radical theory of aging.

Functional genomics A branch of molecular biology that makes use of the enormous amount of data produced by genome sequencing to delineate genome function.

Gene transfection Introduction of DNA into eukaryotic cells.

Genotype Genetic constitution of a cell or an organism.

G-CSF Granulocyte colony-stimulating factor.

GH Growth hormone.

GIK Glucose, insulin and potassium. Applied as a metabolic "cocktail" to provide beneficial preconditioning effects to injured myocardium.

GLUT Glucose transporter.

Glycation A form of non-enzymatic glycosylation in which sugars such as fructose or glucose, bond to a protein or lipid molecule without the controlling action of an enzyme.

Glycolysis Cytosolic-located metabolic pathway present in all cells catalyzing the anaerobic conversion of glucose to pyruvate.

GPCR G-protein coupled receptors.

G-protein A heterotrimeric membrane-associated GTP-binding protein involved in cell-signaling pathways; activated by specific hormone or ligand binding to a 7-helix transmembrane receptor protein.

GPx Glutathione peroxidase. An antioxidant enzyme with both mitochondrial and cytosolic isoforms.

GSH Reduced glutathione.

GSK-3B Glycogen synthase kinase 3B, negative regulator of cardiac hypertrophy and of both normal and pathologic stress–induced growth.

GSSG Glutathione disulfide.

HAGR Human Aging Genomic Resources.

Haplotype A set of single nucleotide polymorphisms (SNPs) or multiple linked alleles, on a single chromatid whose genetic transmission is statistically associated.

Hayflick Limit The limit to the number of times a cell can divide during serial cell culture.

HbA1c Glycosylated (or glycated) hemoglobin; formed in a non-enzymatic pathway by hemoglobin's normal exposure to high plasma levels of glucose implicated in diabetes mellitus.

HCM Hypertrophic cardiomyopathy.

HDAC Histone deacetylases, enzymes that deacetylate lysine side chains in histones as well as in specific non-histone proteins leading to altered states of conformation and activity, resulting in chromatin remodeling, a major form of epigenetic modification.

HDL High-density lipoprotein.

HDOA High-density oligonucleotide array, technique for high-throughput mutation detection and genotyping.

Helicase Enzymes that separate the strands of DNA.

Heterochromatin Condensed regions of chromosomes containing less active genes.

Heteroplasmy Presence of more than 1 genotype in a cell.

5-HD 5-hydroxydecanoic acid, selective mitoK_{ATP} channel blocker.

HF Heart failure.

HF-NEF Heart failure with normal ejection fraction; more common in aging women than in men.

HGF Hepatocyte growth factor.

HGP Human Genome Project.

HGPS Hutchinson-Gilford Progeria Syndrome (see progeria).

Histones Chief proteins of chromatin acting as spools around which DNA winds. They play a role in regulation of gene expression.

HNE 4-hydroxynonenal. A major product of endogenous lipid peroxidation.

H_2O_2 Hydrogen peroxide; a form of ROS and marker of oxidative stress.

HO-1 Heme oxygenase, antioxidant enzyme with cardioprotective function.

Homocysteine A reactive amino acid intermediate in methionine metabolism whose adverse effects include endothelial dysfunction with associated platelet activation and thrombus formation and accumulation of vascular atheroslerotic lesions.

Homoplasmy Presence of a single genotype in a cell.

Hormesis The stimulating effect of a subinhibitory concentration of any toxic substance on an organism.

HR Homologous recombination; DNA repair pathway.

HRT Hormone replacement therapy.

HSC Hematopoietic stem cells.

HSP Heat-shock protein. A family of chaperones involved in protein folding.

HUVECs Human umbilical vein endothelial cells.

HPA Hybridization protection assay, rapid telomere analytical method.

Hydrophobic Lipophilic; insoluble in water.

ICAM-1 Intercellular adhesion molecule; along with integrins involved in the adhesion of inflammatory cells at the vascular surface, in the development of atherosclerotic plaques.

ICD Implantable cardioverter-defibrillator, implantation effective for treatment of short QT.

IEF Isolectric focusing, analytical technique useful to separate proteins on basis of charge; generally used in first dimension of 2D-PAGE.

IEG Immediate early response genes expressed early in response to stress

IFM Interfibrillar mitochondria.

IGF-1 Insulin-like growth factor, stimulates proliferative cardiomyocyte pathways and cell growth.

IMT Intima-media thickness; this measurement in carotid arteries are regarded as a valid index of atherosclerosis and have been associated with the incidence of myocardial infarction and stroke.

Integral membrane protein Protein with at least 1 transmembrane segment requiring detergent for solubilization.

Integrins Class of transmembrane, cell-surface receptor molecules that constitute part of the link between the extracellular matrix and the cardiomyocyte cytoskeleton and which act as signaling molecules and transducers of mechanical force.

Intermembrane space Space between inner and outer mitochondrial membranes.

Intron A segment of a nuclear gene that is transcribed into the primary RNA transcript but is excised during RNA splicing and not present in the mature transcript.

Ion channels Multisubunit transmembrane protein complexes that perform the task of mediating selective flow of millions of ions per second across cell membranes, and are the fundamental functional units of biological excitability

IP3 Inositol trisphosphate, second messenger produced by phospholipase C (see PLC).

IPC Ischemic preconditioning.

I/R Ischemia/reperfusion.

Ischemic heart disease – Also called coronary artery disease (CAD) and coronary heart disease (CHD), this condition is caused by narrowing of the coronary arteries, thereby causing a decreased blood supply to the heart.

Isoforms Related form of the same protein generated by alternative splicing, transcriptional starts or encoded by entirely different genes.

JC-1 Fluorometric dye used for measuring/imaging mitochondrial membrane potential.

KCOs Potassium channel openers (e.g., nicorandil, diazoxide, and pinacidil); can mediate cardioprotection.

KIR Potassium inward rectifier, key pore-forming subunit in sarcolemmal K_{ATP} channels.

Klotho A single-pass transmembrane protein that function in signaling pathways that suppress aging and which has β-glucuronidase activity.

Knock-out mutation A null mutation in a gene, abolishing its function (usually in transgenic mouse); allows evaluation of its phenotypic role.

Krebs cycle Central metabolic pathway of aerobic respiration occurring in the mitochondrial matrix; involves oxidation of acetyl groups derived from pyruvate to CO_2, NADH, and H_2O. The NADH from this cycle is a central substrate in the OXPHOS pathway. Also termed TCA or citric acid cycle.

KSS Kearns-Sayre syndrome. A mitochondrial neuropathy characterized by ptosis, ophthalmoplegia, and retinopathy frequently with cardiac conduction defects and cardiomyopathy

LA Lipoic acid, a potent thiol antioxidant and mitochondrial metabolite, appears to increase low molecular weight antioxidants, decreasing age-associated oxidative damage.

LBBB Left bundle branch block.

LCAD Long-chain acyl CoA dehydrogenase involved in FAO.

LCFA Long-chain fatty acid.

LCHAD Long-chain 3-hydroxylacyl-CoA dehydrogenase.

LDL Low-density lipoprotein, a cholesteryl ester-rich particle (containing only apoB100) whose plasma levels are elevated in several monogenic disorders of lipoprotein metabolism and lead to atherosclerosis.

LDLR Low-density lipoprotein receptor, cell-surface receptor in liver or peripheral tissues responsible for LDL removal from blood; defective LDLR results in FH.

Leptin An adipokine produced by adipose tissue that regulates energy intake and expenditure by decreasing appetite (e.g., downregulating endocannabinoids) and increasing metabolism. (e.g., increased oxygen consumption).

LHON Leber hereditary optical neuropathy, mitochondrial cytopathy.

LMNA Gene encoding Lamin A/C; mutations can cause a wide variety of disorders including DCM, FPLD or premature aging (HGPS).

Ligand Any molecule that binds to a specific site on a protein or a receptor molecule.

Lipofuscin Brown pigment granules composed of difficult-to-degrade lipid-containing residues of lysosomal digestion whose accumulation in several tissues/cells is associated with aging, hence the term age pigment.

Liposomes Lipid spheres with a fraction of aqueous fluid in the center used as vectors for gene transfection with plasmid DNA or oligonucleotides.

LPO Lipid peroxides

Lp-PLA2 Lipoprotein-associated phospholipase A2 (also known as platelet-activating factor acetylhydrolase); produced by inflammatory cells primarily of myeloid origin and highly expressed in vulnerable plaques and recognized as biomarker for predicting stroke risk associated with atherosclerosis.

LPO Lipid peroxidation, oxidative degradation of lipids most often attacking multiple double-bonds of polyunsaturated fatty acids after initiation by free radicals.

LQT Long QT syndrome; prolongation of the QT interval a significant cause of syncope and SCD in children; delayed or prolonged repolarization of the cardiac myocyte can be acquired (e.g., drugs) or congenital (e.g., mutations in specific ion channels).

LVAD Left-ventricular assist devices.

LVOTO Left ventricular outflow tract obstruction.

LVH Left ventricular hypertrophy.

LXR Liver X receptors; member of the nuclear receptor family of transcription factors closely related to PPARs. Regulator of cholesterol, fatty acid and glucose homeostasis. LXR is considered an orphan receptor since no endogenous activating ligand has been yet identified.

MAPCs Multipotent adult precursor cells.

MAPK Mitogen-activated protein kinases. A family of conserved serine/threonine protein kinases activated as a result of a wide range of signals involved in cell proliferation and differentiation; includes JNK and ERK.

Matrix Space enclosed by the mitochondrial inner membrane.

Membrane potential or cell potential. Combination of proton and ion gradients across the inner mitochondria membrane/or a cell's plasma membrane making the inside negative relative to the outside.

Metabonomics Quantitative assessment of multiple metabolic changes occurring in response to developmental, physiological or pathophysiological perturbations or genetic modification; also metabolomics.

MetR Methionine restriction; form of dietary restriction which promotes reduction of mtDNA oxidative damage, mitochondrial ROS production, and levels of markers of protein oxidation.

MetSyn Metabolic syndrome.

3-MA 3-methyladenine, inhibitor of autophagy.

MCFS Macrophage colony-stimulating factor; upregulated in response to oxLDLs binding and activation of macrophage enabling their survival and multiplication within atherosclerotic lesions.

MHC Myosin heavy chain.

MI Myocardial infarction.

Microarray A range of oligonucleotides immobilized onto a surface (chip) that can be hybridized to determine quantitative transcript expression or mutation detection.

Minisatellites Repetitive and variable DNA sequences, generally GC-rich, ranging in length from 10 to over 100 bp.

Missense mutation Mutation which causes substitution of one amino acid for another.

MitoK$_{ATP}$ channel Activation of the ATP-sensitive inner membrane mitoK$_{ATP}$ channel has been implicated as a central signaling event (both as trigger and end effector) in IPC and other cardioprotection pathways.

MitoQ Synthetic ubiquinone analog which can be selectively targeted to mitochondria used to provide antioxidant cardioprotection.

MitoPTP Mitochondrial permeability transition pore (see PT pore)

Mito VitE Synthetic analog of vitamin E which can reduce mitochondrial lipid peroxidation and protein damage and accumulate after oral administration at therapeutic concentrations within the cardiac tissue.

MLC Myosin light chain.

MLP Muscle LIM protein, localized in the cardiomyocyte cytoskeleton, a positive regulator of myogenic differentiation.

MMPs Metalloproteinases, enzymes involved in extracellular matrix remodeling.

MMR Mismatch repair, corrects errors of DNA replication and recombination that result in mispaired nucleotides following DNA replication.

MnSOD Also SOD2; manganese superoxide dismutase; mitochondrial ROS scavenger.

MODY Maturity onset diabetes of the young; rare monogenic form of diabetes due to dominantly inherited mutations impacting insulin production or secretion.

MOMP Mitochondrial outer-membrane permeabilization, channel formed as an apoptotic event in part mediated by binding of proapoptotic proteins (e.g., Bad, Bax, Bid) to mitochondria.

Modifier gene A gene that modifies a trait encoded by another gene.

MPTP See MitoPTP (also PT pore).

MR Mineralocorticoid receptor.

mRNA Messenger RNA. Specifies the amino acid sequence of a protein; translated into protein on ribosomes. Transcripts of RNA polymerase II

MSC Mesenchymal stem cells.

MT Metallothionein. An inducible antioxidant metal-binding protein with cardioprotective properties.

mtDNA Mitochondrial DNA.

mtTFA Mitochondrial transcription factor A (also called *TFAM*).

mTOR Mammalian target of rapamycin (also TOR).

MTP Microsomal triglyceride transfer protein; involved in both lipid metabolism and genetic variants have been associated with increased life span in several human populations.

Mutation Changes occurring in the genetic material (usually DNA or RNA).

Myocarditis An inflammatory disease of the myocardium associated with cardiac dysfunction and increased myocyte necrosis; can be a precursor to dilated cardiomyopathy (DCM).

NADH Nicotinamide adenine dinucleotide (reduced form).

NADPH oxidase (also NOX) Multicomponent enzyme which is a major source of endothelial superoxide; subject to specific regulation by diverse stimuli including oscillatory shear stress, hypoxia, angiotensin II, growth factors, cytokines and hyperlipidemia.

NCX Sodium-calcium exchanger, a mitochondrial form of NCX (also denoted mNCE) is primarily responsible for calcium efflux from the mitochondria.

Necrosis A form of cell death resulting from injury causing severe molecular and/or structural damage and leading to progressive, irreversible and catastrophic metabolic failure. This results in membrane disruption, cell swelling and eventual cell lysis and fragmentation with associated acute inflammatory response.

NHEJ Non-homologous end joining, a highly-conserved pathway present in humans requiring a number of proteins that can be used to repair DNA double-strand breaks

Nitrotyrosine The formation of 3-nitrotyrosine (3-NT) resulting from the nitration of tyrosine residues. Is a post-translational modification of selective proteins arising primarily from peroxynitrite reactions and is associated with aging.

NER Nucleotide excision repair.

NF-κB Nuclear Factor-Kappa B. Family of transcription factors involved in the control of a number of normal cellular and organismal processes, including immune and inflammatory responses, developmental processes, cellular growth, and apoptosis.

NO Nitric oxide; vasodilator.

Northern blot Molecular analytical technique by which RNA separated by electrophoresis is transferred and immobilized for the detection of specific transcripts by hybridization with labeled probe.

NOS Nitric oxide synthase

NRF-1 and NRF-2 Nuclear respiratory factors. Transcription factors that modulate expression of nuclear-DNA encoded mitochondrial proteins.

NSI-MS/MS Nano-electrospray ionization-tandem mass spectrometry, analytical technique used in proteomic analysis to assist in protein identification.

Nt nucleotide, the basic unit of DNA composed of a purine or pyrimidine base, a sugar (deoxyribose) and a phosphate group.

NT-proBNP N-terminal pro-brain natriuretic peptide, a marker for acute congestive HF.

NTG Nitroglycerin.

Null mutation Ablation or knock-out of a gene

Nutrigenomics Study of how different nutrients may interact with specific genes to increase the risk of common chronic diseases. Nutrigenomics also seeks to provide a molecular understanding of how common dietary factors affect health and aging by altering the expression of genes and the structure of an individual's genome.

OGGT Oral glucose tolerance test.

Oligonucleotide Short polymer of DNA or RNA that is usually synthetic in origin.

ORI Origin of replication. Unique DNA sequence at which DNA replication is initiated, from this point replication may proceed either bidirectionaly or unidirectionaly.

OS Oxidative stress.

OxLDL Oxidized LDL, a primary substrate for macrophage activation and involved in atherosclerosis progression.

8-oxodG 8-oxo-deoxyguanosine, major oxidative DNA lesion associated with aging, reparable by BER.

OXPHOS Oxidative phosphorylation. A process in mitochondria in which ATP formation is driven by electron transfer from NADH and $FADH_2$ to molecular oxygen and by the generation of a pH gradient and chemiosmotic coupling.

PAF Platelet-activating factor, potent inflammatory mediator binding to the PAF receptor found on platelets, monocytes and leukocytes which can lead to platelet aggregation; structure mimicked by oxidized LDL phospholipids.

PAGE Polyacrylamide gel electrophoresis.

PAI-1 Plasminogen activator inhibitor-1, a principal regulator of fibrinolysis.

PAR Protease-activated receptors; these G-coupled transmenbrane receptors are activated by extracellular proteolytic cleavage by serine proteases such as thrombin and trypsin.

Paraoxonase Antioxidant enzyme.

Parvalbumin Small, intracellular, calcium-binding protein found exclusively in fast-twitch muscle fibers; overexpression in senescent rats corrected myocardial diastolic dysfunction.

PARP Poly (ADP-ribose) polymerase; enzyme that plays diverse roles in many molecular processes, including DNA damage detection and repair, chromatin modification, transcription, and cell death pathways.

PC Anticoagulant factor protein C.

PCR Polymerase chain reaction. An amplification of DNA fragments using a thermostabile DNA polymerase and paired oligonucleotide primers subjected to repeated reactions with thermal cycling.

PDGF Platelet-derived growth factor.

PDH Pyruvate dehydrogenase, mitochondrial matrix enzyme producing acetyl-CoA from pyruvate linking glycolysis and Krebs cycle.

Penetrance The proportion of individuals with a specific genotype expressing the related phenotype.

Peptide Short polymer of amino acids that can be produced synthetically.

Peripheral membrane protein Protein associated with membrane via protein-protein interactions; solubilized by changes in pH or salt.

Peroxisome Small membrane-bounded organelle that uses oxygen to oxidize organic molecules, including fatty acids and contain enzymes that generate and degrade hydrogen peroxide (H_20_2) (e.g., catalase).

pFOX Partial fatty acid oxidation.

PGC-1α Peroxisome proliferator-activated receptor γ coactivator 1α. Transcriptional regulator of mitochondrial bioenergetic and biogenesis operative during physiological transitions.

Pharmaceutical preconditioning A large variety of drugs including the targeted use of volatile anesthetics, potassium channel openers, nitric oxide donors and modulators of downstream pathways including erythropoietin, statins, insulin and pyruvate have been shown to mimic ischemic preconditioning and provide cardioprotection when either substituted for the preconditioning period or applied at reperfusion.

Pharmacogenetics Study of the role of inheritance in interindividual variation in drug response.

Pharmacogenomics A branch of pharmaceutics dealing with the influence of genetic changes on drug response by correlating gene expression or SNPs with the drug's effect.

Phenome A set of all phenotypes expressed by a cell, tissue, organ, organism, or species including phenotypic traits due to either genetic or environmental influences.

Phenotype Observable physical characteristics of a cell or organism resulting from the interaction of its genetic constitution (genotype) with its environment.

Phospholamban Negative regulator of SERCA.

PI3-K Phosphatidylinositol 3-kinase; also PI3K.

PKA Protein kinase A. Activated by cAMP.

PKB Protein kinase B; also called Akt.

PKC Protein kinase C.

PKD Protein kinase D, a mitochondrial sensor of oxidative stress

Plasmid A relatively autonomous replicating non-chromosomal DNA molecule primarily found in bacteria that can be used as a vector for transferring recombinant genes to cells or tissues.

Pleiotropy The multiple phenotypic effects of a single gene.

PNA Peptide nucleic acids; an alternative delivery system for nucleic acids to mitochondria.

Polygenic A large number of genes, each contributing a small amount to the phenotype.

Polγ Nuclear-encoded catalytic subunit of mtDNA polymerase γ.

Porin Pore-forming protein in the outer mitochondrial membrane (see VDAC).

Postconditioning A series of brief interruptions of reperfusion applied at the very onset of reperfusion can reduce infarct size and apoptosis and provide cardioprotection.

Post-translational modification Postsynthetic modification of proteins by glycosylation, phosphorylation, proteolytic cleavage, or other covalent changes involving side chains or termini.

p66Shc Adaptor protein which controls oxidative stress; p66Shc-null mice have reduced systemic and tissue oxidative stress, vascular cell death and increased life span.

P70S6K 70-kDa ribosomal protein S6 kinase. It plays a key role in translational control of cell proliferation in response to growth factors in mammalian cells

PPARs Peroxisome proliferator-activated receptors. Nuclear receptor transcription factors that function as transcriptional regulators impacting cellular carbohydrate and lipid metabolism as well as cell differentiation in a variety of target tissues, including the heart.

PVBs Premature ventricular beats, often benign but can promote a more serious dysrhythmia.

Primer Short nucleotide sequence that is paired with 1 strand of DNA and provide a free 3'-OH end at which a DNA polymerase starts the synthesis of a nascent chain.

Progeria Human genetic disease resembling accelerated aging, typically affects children. Examples include Hutchinson-Gilford progeria syndrome (HGPS).

Progeroid A phenotype with features resembling accelerated aging.

Promoter Non-coding regulatory region of DNA sequence upstream of the gene coding sequences involved in the binding of RNA polymerase to initiate transcription.

Protein kinase Enzyme that transfers the terminal phosphate group of ATP to a specific amino acid of a target protein.

Proteome Entire complement of proteins contained within the eukaryotic cell.

Proteasome A cytosolic macromolecular complex of multicatalytic proteases that digest proteins that have been tagged with ubiquitin for destruction.

PT pore Permeability transition pore. A non-specific megachannel in the mitochondrial inner membrane. See also mitoPTP or MPTP.

PUFA Polyunsaturated fatty acids.

RAAS Renin-angiotensin-aldosterone system

RACKs Receptors for activated C kinase.

RAGE Receptors for AGE (advanced glycation endproducts); integral membrane proteins present in a wide array of cardiovascular cell-types that mediate production of pro-inflammatory cytokines and formation of free radicals.

Ras A small G protein (see G proteins).

RBBB Right bundle branch block.

RCM Restrictive cardiomyopathy, the rarest form of cardiomyopathy, involves impaired ventricular filling and reduced diastolic volume in the presence of normal systolic function and is most frequently caused by pathological conditions that stiffen the myocardium by promoting infiltration or fibrosis.

Real-Time PCR Quantitative PCR technique employs simultaneous DNA amplification and quantification often using fluorescent dyes that intercalate with double-strand DNA, and modified DNA oligonucleotide probes which fluoresce when hybridized with a complementary DNA.

Reactive fibrosis Occurs in the absence of cell loss as a maladaptive reaction to inflammation and is primarily perivascular and further extends into the neighboring interstitial space.

Redox reactions Oxidation-reduction reactions in which there is a transfer of electrons from an electron donor (the reducing agent) to an electron acceptor (oxidizing agent).

Replacement fibrosis Also called reparative fibrosis; occurs as a reaction to a loss of myocardium (due to necrosis or apoptosis, after myocardial ischemia or senescence), and it is mainly interstitial.

Replicative senescence Cessation of cell division, usually determined in a cell population that may or may not be accompanied by cell death.

RER Recombinational repair; overall class of DNA repair.

Resveratrol Plant-produced polyphenolic compound (found in red grapes and red wine) with anti-inflammatory and cardioprotective properties in rats and mice, as well as anti-aging effects (increasing lifespan) in yeast and mice; potential sirtuin (SIRT1) activator.

Ribosome A factory-like organelle that builds proteins from a set of genetic instructions. Composed of rRNA and ribosomal proteins, it translates mRNA into apolypeptide chain.

Rimonabant Specific CB1 receptor blocker stemming endocannabinoid action and tested in the RIO clinical trials to impact symptoms of the metabolic syndrome (see endocannabinoid).

RNAi RNA interference, use of a specific double-stranded RNA (dsRNA) construct to post-transcriptionally silence specific gene expression.

RNA polymerase Enzyme responsible for transcribing DNA as template into RNA

RNS Reactive nitrogen species (e.g., peroxynitrite)

ROS Reactive oxygen species, including superoxide, hydroxyl radicals, and hydrogen peroxide.

rRNA Ribosomal RNA. A central component of the ribosome.

RTK Receptor tyrosine kinase; this large family of proteins includes receptors for many growth factors and insulin; ligand binding results in dimerization and phosphorylation of downstream signaling targets as well as autophosphorylation.

RT-PCR Reverse transcription (RT) of RNA to DNA with the enzyme reverse transcriptase can be combined with traditional PCR to allow the amplification and determination of the abundance of specific RNA.

RXR Retinoid X receptor. On binding 9-cis retinoic acid, RXR acts as a heterodimer and as a repressor or activator of specific gene transcription, playing a key role in cardiac development and physiological gene expression.

Ryanodine receptor Major SR Ca^{2+} release channel in cardiac muscle; mutations in the cardiac isoform encoded by RyR2 result in ARVD and CVPT.

SAGE Serial analysis of gene expression. Quantitative analysis of RNA transcripts by using short sequence tags to generate a characteristic expression profile.

SAN Sinoatrial node (see SA node)

SA node The sinoatrial node is a group of specialized cells located in the right atrium which produces electrical impulses (a relatively simple action potential) that travel down to eventually reach the ventricular muscle causing the heart to contract and serving as the "natural" pacemaker of the heart.

Sarcopenia The degenerative loss of skeletal muscle mass and strength in senescence, reducing muscle performance in the elderly; an important independent predictor of disability, and linked to poor balance, gait speed, falls, and fractures.

SCD Sudden cardiac death.

SD Sudden death.

SDH Succinate dehydrogenase. A TCA cycle enzyme associated with respiratory complex II.

SDS Sodium dodecyl sulfate. An ionic detergent used for solubilization and denaturation of proteins, and their size separation in PAGE.

SENS Strategies for engineered negligible senescence, a proposal by A. de Grey that includes a detailed plan to reverse cellular and molecular age-related changes and cure human aging.

SERCA Sarcoplasmic reticulum Ca^{2+}-ATPase. There are 3 major isoforms which are variably expressed in different muscle types.

SERM Selective estrogen receptor modulators.

SHR Spontaneously hypertensive rats.

Sick sinus syndrome The failure of the sinus node to regulate the heart's rhythm.

SIPS Stress-induced premature senescence; stressful stimuli unrelated to telomere damage, including intracellular oxidative stress or persistent mitogenic stimulation cause cellular senescence.

siRNA Small interfering RNA. Sometimes known as short interfering RNA, they are a class of 20-25 nucleotide-long RNA molecules that interfere with the expression of genes.

Smac/Diablo Mitochondrial intermembrane protein released into the cytosol during early apoptosis stimulating caspase activation.

SMC Smooth muscle cell.

S-nitrosylation A ubiquitous post-translational modification involving the covalent attachment of NO to cysteine thiol moieties on targeted proteins.

SND Sinoatrial node dysfunction

SNP Single nucleotide polymorphism.

SOD Superoxide dismutase. An antioxidant ROS-scavenging enzyme with both cytosolic (Cu-Zn SOD)/SOD1 and mitochondrial (MnSOD)/SOD2 isoforms.

Southern blot Detection of separated restriction fragments after size separation on agarose gels, transfer to membranes and hybridization with labeled gene probes.

SP cells Side population cells; rare groups of multipotent progenitor cells capable of proliferation and differentiation.

SP-PCR Small pool PCR, a sensitive method for the detection and quantification of microsatellite instability (MSI) in somatic cells

Splicing Reaction in the nucleus in which introns are removed from primary nuclear RNA and exons joined to generate mRNA.

SR Sarcoplasmic reticulum. A network of internal membranes in muscle-cell cytosol that contains high Ca^{2+} concentration, which is released on excitation.

SSB Single-strand breaks; lesions in one of the two DNA strands often caused by oxidative damage and repàrable by NER or BER.

SSCP Single strand conformation polymorphism; technique for mutation detection.

SSM Subsarcolemmal mitochondria.

Statins HMG-CoA reductase inhibitors used to treat patients with elevated plasma LDL.

STELA Single telomere length analysis utilizing PCR analysis

STEMI ST-segment elevation myocardial infarction.

Supravalvular aortic stenosis Discrete narrowing of the ascending aorta resulting from mutations in the gene encoding a component of the extracellular matrix (i.e., elastin).

SUR Sulfonylurea receptor, components of potassium ion channels

SVECs Endothelial cells from the human saphenous vein

SVT Superventricular tachycardia.

T1D Type 1 diabetes; Also juvenile diabetes. Primarily autoimmune-mediated disease associated with the destruction of insulin-producing pancreatic B cells; has multiple genetic and environmental risk factors.

T2D Type 2 diabetes; also known as non insulin-dependent or adult-onset diabetes; a polygenic metabolic disorder that is primarily characterized by insulin resistance, relative insulin deficiency, and hyperglycemia. most common form of diabetes and particularly prevalent in the elderly.

TAG Intracellular triacylglycerols.

Taq polymerase Thermostable DNA polymerase isolated from the bacterium *Thermus aquaticus* used extensively in PCR.

TCA cycle Tricarboxylic acid cycle (see Krebs cycle).

TCR Transcription-coupled repair, form of NER (see NER) which deploys high-priority NER repair enzymes to genes that are being actively transcribed.

TD Tangier disease; a rare autosomal-recessively inherited atherosclerotic disease characterized by severe reduction in plasma HDL levels due to defective ABCA1 transporters.

TdP *Torsade de pointes*, a polymorphic ventricular tachycardia which can be followed by syncope and SD; this can be acquired by exercise (swimming) or congenital (any of the LQTs).

Telomere Special structure containing tandem repeats of a short G-rich sequence present at the end of a chromosome.

Telomerase An enzyme that recognizes the G-rich strand, and elongates it using an RNA template that is a component of the enzyme itself.

TEA Tetraethylammonium chloride, a specific inhibitor of some types of K^+ currents including the calcium-activated K^+ (K_{Ca}) channel

TERC Telomerase RNA component.

TERT Telomerase reverse transcriptase catalytic subunit.

TF Tissue factor.

TGF Transforming growth factor.

TH Thyroid hormone (also thyroxin), a stimulus for cardiac hypertrophic growth and myocardial mitochondrial biogenesis.

Titin Large polypeptide, anchored in the Z-disc spanning the sarcomere contributes to sarcomere organization, myofibrillar elasticity and myofibrillar cell signaling.

TLR Toll-like receptors involved in the innate-immunity signaling response of the macrophage, including pattern-recognition of pathogens and oxidized LDL, leukocyte recruitment and production of local inflammation and downstream signaling in atherosclerotic progression.

TNF-α Tumor necrosis factor α

tPA Tissue-type plasminogen activator, a primary regulator of fibrinolysis.

TR Thyroid hormone receptor, mediates both nuclear genomic effects of TH (largely as a transcription factor) as well as non-genomic effects of TH.

Transgenic animal Animal that has stably incorporated one or more genes from another cell or organism.

Transcript Specific RNA product of DNA transcription.

Transcription factor Protein required for the initiation of transcription by RNA polymerase at specific sites and functioning as a regulatory factor in gene expression.

Transcriptome Comprehensive transcript analysis for expression profiling.

Translation Synthesis of protein from the mRNA template at the ribosome.

TRF2 Telomere repeat- binding factor, telomere-associated protein critical for the control of telomere structure and function.

tRNA Transfer RNA. A small RNA molecule used in protein synthesis as an adaptor between mRNA and amino acids.

TTD Trichothiodystrophy; premature aging disorder caused by mutations in XPD, a DNA helicase, involved in both DNA repair and transcription

TTT Tilt table test, diagnostic test to detect cause of syncope or near-syncope

TUNEL Terminal deoxynucleotidyl transferase mediated dUTP Nick End Labeling assay; a fluorescence method for detecting DNA fragmentation associated with apoptotic cell death.

2-dimensional electrophoresis Technique for separating proteins based on their size and charge differences; also 2DE.

TZD Thiazolidinediones; PPAR-γ agonist used in treating type 2 diabetes and potentially MetSyn.

UCP Uncoupling protein.

Uncoupler Protein or other molecule capable of uncoupling electron transport from oxidative phosphorylation.

VDAC Voltage-dependent anion channel in mitochondrial outer membrane (see porin).

VEGF Vascular endothelial growth factor.

VF Ventricular fibrillation, the most serious dysrhythmia resulting in little blood pumped from the heart, fainting and if not treated, heart attack; higher risk groups include the elderly with history of CAD, or myocardial ischemia.

VGCC Voltage-gated calcium channels.

VLCAD Very long-chain acyl CoA-dehydrogenase; enzyme involved in mitochondrial β-oxidation of fatty acids.

VLDL Very low density lipoprotein, a triglyceride-rich lipoprotein containing apoB100 which progressively become enriched in cholesteryl ester (CE) as a result of CE transfer from HDL and is converted by lipolysis to LDL and/or taken up as VLDL remnants by the liver.

VT Ventricular tachycardia, a potentially life threatening cardiac dysrhythmia. VT may degrade to the more serious ventricular fibrillation, and is a common and often lethal complication of myocardial infarction.

Western blot Immunochemical detection of proteins immobilized on a filter after size separation by PAGE.

Wild-type The common genotype or phenotype of a given organism occurring in nature.

WPW Wolff-Parkinson-White syndrome may present with hypertrophic cardiomyopathy, conduction defects and accumulation of cardiac glycogen.

WS Werner syndrome, a very rare autosomal recessive genetic disorder resembling accelerated aging. Typically has an adult onset. The defect is in the WRN gene localized on the short arm of chromosome 8 encoding a DNA helicase protein involved in DNA repair.

XIAP X-linked inhibitor of apoptosis; Member of the family of inhibitor of apoptosis proteins (IAPs) which binds to and inhibits already activated caspases-9, -3, and -7, and interferes with procaspase-9 dimerization and activation.

XO Xanthine oxidase, cytosolic enzyme involved in purine metabolism. XO is involved in myocardial ROS production (e.g., superoxide radicals) particularly after I/R injury.

Z-discs Cardiomyocyte component positioned at the junction between the cytoskeleton and the myofilaments, providing a physical connection between the sarcomere, nucleus, membrane and sarcoplasmic reticulum (SR) with role in cardiac contraction and signaling.

Index

ABCA1 gene expression, 249
ACAD, enzyme, 399
ACC/AHA/NASPE guidelines, 351
Actin cytoskeleton and aging neutrophils, 185
Acute coronary syndrome (ACS), 256–258, 324
Adaptive immune system, age-associated changes in, 182
Adenine nucleotide translocase, 40, 116, 400
Adiponectin, 327
β-Adrenergic receptor (β-AR), 328, 487
β-Adrenergic stimulation on LV filling, 46
Adult cardiomyocyte proliferative growth and IGF/IGFR pathway, 73
Adult-onset X-linked DCM, 219
Advanced glycation end-products (AGEs), 19, 117, 229, 426
Advanced heart failure, 351–352
Adverse drug events (ADE), 211
Age-associated
  changes in adaptive immune system, 182
  CVDs and gender, 309–320
  diseases, reversing aging/dysfunction, 516–517
  diseases and SNP analysis in, 430–432
Age-independent mortality component, 20
Age-mediated damage in elements of angiogenic response, 169
Aging
  angiogenesis/neovascularization in, 168–169
  antidysrhythmic therapy in, 355
  antioxidant metallothionein (MT) role in, 451
  arterial remodeling and, 149–154
  AV conduction in, 345–346
  biomarkers in, 506–513
  and blood-brain barrier, 196–198
  Ca^{2+} transporter in, 361–364
  caloric restriction (CR) dietary regimen effects on, 79
  cardiac function in, 52
  cardiomyopathy and heart failure in, 209
  and cardiovascular function, 213
  cell culture study in, 72
  cell proteomics in, 427–428
  and cellular components of innate immune system, 184
  CR mimetics effect on, 483
  definition of, 3
  dietary and lifestyle change, 58
  DNA damage and mutations in, 82–84
  DNA repair enzymes in, 85–87
  electrophysiological studies in animal models of, 341–342
  free radical theory of, 118
  gender issues in, 21–22
  gene overexpression and cardiovascular phenotype in, 77
  gene profiling studies in, 79
  genes mapping, 429
  genetics, 429–431
  genomic instability and, 132
  hemostatic changes during, 167
  hormesis and, 21
  and hypothalamic hormone, 193
  immune system, 182–190
  inflammatory pathway induction and, 168
  lysosome in, 457
  macrophage TLR expression in, 185
  mediated cardiac pathology, 229
  microarray gene profiling analysis of murine and monkey skeletal muscle transcripts, 80
  mitochondrial ion channels in, 365
  mitochondrial K-ATP channel in, 365–367
  mitochondrial PTP in, 367–369
  modulation of mitochondrial ion function, 371
  mouse models, 401–404
  mtDNA polymorphisms and, 6
  myocardial remodeling and, 213–229
  and neurohormonal regulation, 191–198
  pharmacogenetics/pharmacogeneomics in dysrhythmias/channelopathies of, 370–371
  proteomic analysis for, 81–82
  related downregulation of MHC and SERCA expression, 487
  role of altered immunity in atherosclerosis in, 255–256
  sarcolemmal K_{ATP} channels in, 356–357
  sarcopenia and, 197
  and skeletal muscle, 194–196
  SNP analysis in, 430–432
  stem cells and, 518–521
  studies of aging skeletal muscle transcriptome and, 80
  sympathetic nerve system in, 340

targeting cellular atrophy and depletion in, 517–518
targeting specific organelles in, 521–523
theories of, 12–20
thrombosis, fibrinolysis and inflammation in, 166–168
transgenic mouse, specific gene knock-outs as models of, 78
vascular function and structure in, 194
and vascular smooth muscle cells (SMCs), 162–168
Aging-associated diseases
and cross-talk of immune cells, 188
immune gene variants, 189
Aging heart
adrenergic (and muscarinic) receptors, 46–47
structural and functional changes, 104
thyroid hormone/SERCA, 48–49
Akt phosphorylation in myocytes, 41
Akt/PI3K/PKB signaling pathway, 446
ALA-fed cardiomyopathic hearts, 229
Alkyltransferase protein O6-methylguanine DNA methyltransferase (MGMT), 124
Allele of apo E4 frequency and nonagenarians, 7
Alpha-lipoic acid (ALA)-enriched diet, 229
Amadori product, 117
American Academy of Clinical Endocrinologists (AACE) definition, 278
Aminoguanidine (AG), protein crosslinking inhibitor, 485, 489
AMP-activated protein kinase (AMPK), 483
cAMP-dependent signaling pathway, 105
cAMP response element-binding protein, 446
Amyloidosis, 221
Androgen receptor (AR), 316
Androgen replacement therapy (ART), 308
Angiogenesis, 168
See also Aging
Angiotensin-aldosterone system, 310
Angiotensin-converting enzyme (ACE) inhibitor (perindopril) therapy, 161, 261
Angiotensin I-converting enzyme (ACE), 431
Angiotensin II (Ang II), 447
Angiotensin II-mediated EPC senescence, 162
Angiotensin II type 1A receptor gene (AT1A), 316–317
Angiotensinogen gene (AGT), 263
Animal models of cardiomyopathy and HF, 222–229
ANT, *see* Adenine nucleotide translocase
Antagonistic Pleiotropy Theory, 12
Anticoagulation and risk factors in AF, 314
Antihypertensive and Lipid-Lowering Treatment to Prevent Heart Attack Trial (ALLHAT), 260
Antinitrotyrosine antibody, 115
Aortic aneurysm, 165
Aortic vascular SMC polyploidy, 166
AP endonuclease (APE), 477
ApoE-deficient animals, 256
Apolipoprotein (apo), 430
Apolipoprotein D (ApoD), 401
Apoptosis, 106–110
inducing Factor (AIF), 109, 445
intrinsic and extrinsic pathways, 109
repressor with a caspase recruitment domain (CARD [ARC]), 110
APT, *see* Antagonistic Pleiotropy Theory
Arginine vasopressin (AVP) basal release, 192
Aromatase (CYP19A1), 319
Arrhythmogenic right ventricular dysplasia/cardiomyopathy (ARVD/ARVC), 216
Atg proteins (Atg 12 and Atg8), 113
Atherosclerotic lesion's fibrous cap, 250
ATM-mediated p53 activation, 133
ATP binding cassette transporter (ABCA1) gene, 241
ATRIA, *see* Anticoagulation and Risk factors in AF
Atrial dysrhythmias, 342–345
Atrial Fibrillation (AF), 313, 331, 344–345, 352
Atrioventricular (AV), 313
Atrioventricular Nodal Reentrant Tachycardia (AVNRT), 343–344
Attenuating cell-death and remodeling, 444–446
Atypical Werner Syndrome, 220
Autophagocytosis and mitochondria, 114
Autophagy
associated cell death, 115
steps, 113

Base excision repair (BER), 124, 476
BCL2-associated athanogene 3 (Bag3), 421
Becker (BMD) muscular dystrophies, 219
BER/DNA-metabolizing enzymes, 124
Beta-Blocker Evaluation of Survival Trial (BEST), 310
4E binding protein (4EBP1), 310
Bioavailable Testosterone (BT), 283
Biological CV aging, 34
β-Blocker nebivolol and HF, 211
Bloom's syndrome, 23
Blue-native PAGE electrophoresis (BN-PAGE), 425
Bone morphogenetic protein (BMP), 421
B-type natriuretic peptide in diagnosis of HF, 211
Bulky photodimer single-strand lesions, 124

C5178A polymorphism and anti-atherosclerotic effects in diabetes, 6
CAC, *see* Coronary artery calcification
Calcium/calmodulin-dependent protein kinase II (CamKII) pathways, 240
Calcium channels, 357–358
Calcium-dependent neutral proteases (calpains), 113
Caloric restriction (CR), 396, 417, 422–424, 434, 452, 471–472, 489
in heart and skeletal muscle, 472–473
mediated reduction in mtDNA damage, 474
mimetics development, 482–483
process dissection, 481–482
role in mitochondrial biogenesis, 475
Cannabinoid receptors (CB), 280
β Cardiac-adrenergic receptor (β-AR), 46
Cardiac E-C coupling cycle, 34
Cardiac excitation–contraction (E-C) coupling, 34
Cardiac G protein-coupled receptors, 47–48
Cardiac hypertrophy, 316–318

Cardiac K_{ATP} channel, 219
Cardiac PKC-ERK1/2 signaling modules, 47
Cardiac proteins
  and HCM-causing genes, 216
  proteomic analysis in aging rat, 82
Cardiac remodeling and insulin resistance in elderly, 285–286
Cardiac resynchronization therapy, 212
Cardiac sarcoplasmic reticular Ca^{2+}-adenosine triphosphatase (SERCA2a) pump, 219
Cardiac-specific HO-1 transgene expression, 451
Cardiac stem cells
  differentiation, 214
  mediated myocyte regeneration, 41
Cardiac-targeted adenoviral-mediated gene transfer of SOD, 450
Cardiac targeted-overexpression of antioxidant, 229
Cardiac Troponin (cTn), 317, 324, 331
Cardiometabolic risk factors
  and cardiovascular disease in elderly, 286
  in elderly, 282
Cardiomyocyte loss (replacement fibrosis), 105
Cardiomyopathy, 216
Cardioprotection pathways, 447–450
Cardiovascular (CV) aging, 33
  apoptosis role in, 38
  autophagy and, 51–52
  cellular damage/cell loss, mitochondria and, 37–41
  cellular mechanisms and, 34
  epigenetic and environmental factors in, 53–55
  genetic make-up in, 52–53
  inflammation and, 45
  modifying/delaying, 57
  neuroendocrine mechanisms in, 45–46
  and oxidative phosphorylation (OXPHOS) deficiency, 38
  ROS generation and, 41–45
  somatic mutations in mtDNA, 43
  stem cells and, 58
  targeted therapies in, 444
  telomeres and, 35–37
  transcriptome profiling in, 424–425
Cardiovascular genes analysis in aging, 417–440
Carnitine Palmitoyl Transferase-I (CPT1), 418, 419
Carotid sinus syndrome, 348
Cathepsin B, 252
CB1 blockade on cardiometabolic risk, 280–281
CD94-NKG2A inhibitory signaling pathway, 187
C. elegans, metabolic pathways involved in longevity, 392–395
Cell-based therapy, 58
Cell-engineering and transplantation, 89–91
Cell senescence
  mechanisms of, 157–158
  role of, 155–157
  telomere/telomerase theory of aging, 15
  theory, 19
Cellular Garbage theory, 19
Cellular hypertrophy, 72
Cellular mechanisms and cardiac aging, 34
Cellular retinol-binding protein, 428
Centimorgan (cM), 429
CETP, *see* Cholesteryl ester transfer protein
CETP deficiency, 243
Channelopathies, calcium and potassium currents, 355–356
Charcot-Marie-Tooth-disease, 220
Chemotaxis, 247
Cholesterol acyltransferase, 242
Cholesteryl ester transfer protein, 430
Chromatin immunoprecipitation (ChIP), 86
Cockayne's syndrome (CSA and CSB), 125, 460
Cockayne syndrome protein, 85
Coding polymorphism (Met235Thr), 263
Coenzyme Q_{10} (CoQ_{10}), 394, 484
Cognitive impairment and HF, 211
Comet assay and DNA damage, 84
Complete heart block (CHB), 315
Connexins, 358
Copenhagen City Study, AF prevalence, 313
Coronary artery calcification, 326
Coronary artery disease (CAD), 209, 308, 320–324
Coronary artery spasm (CAS), 322
Corticotropin-releasing factor (CRF), 191
Corticotropin-releasing hormone (CRH)-induced ACTH release in aged rats, 192
Cortisol/DHEA ratio, 193
Coxsackie adenovirus receptor (CAR), 75
CREB, *see* cAMP response element-binding protein
CRF binding protein (CRF-BP) synthesis, 192
CRH-R1 receptor mRNA expression, 192
Cross-linkage theory, 19
CRPB, *see* Cellular retinol-binding protein
CRP-mediated regulation of GADD153 mRNA expression in vascular SMCs, 253
CRT, *see* Cardiac resynchronization therapy
CSB, *see* Cockayne syndrome protein
Cultured neonatal cardiomyocyte, 72
CXC chemokine receptor 2 (CXCR2), 255
Cyclic guanosine monophosphate (cGMP), 427, 475
Cyclin B1-CDC2 genes overexpression in adult cardiomyocytes, 73
Cyclophilin-D (CyP-D), 445
Cyclosporin A (CsA), 445, 448
Cysteine protease (caspase) activation cascade, 107
Cytochrome P450 (CYP), 309
Cytomegalovirus (CMV), 182
Cytosolic Ca^{2+} overload-induced dysregulation, 34

Damaged DNA in aging tissues, 118
Death-associated protein (DAP) kinase, 253
Death-inducing signaling complex (DISC), 108
Dehydroepiandrosterone (DHEA), 321
Dehydroepiandrosterone sulfate (DHEAS), 472, 509
Demethoxyubiquinone (DMK), 393
Depression and HF, 211
Diabetes and genes, 291
7,8-Dihydro-8-oxoguanine (8-oxoG), 453

Dilated cardiomyopathy (DCM), 216, 218–222
3,5-dimethylpyrazole (DMP), 456
2,4-dinitrophenol (DNP), 400
Direct reversal pathway, 123, 124
Disposable Soma Theory, 12
DNA
damage and mutations, 117–123
See also Aging
damage types, 83
dependent Protein Kinase (DNA-PK), 477
dependent Protein Kinase complex (DNA-PKcs), 126
genetic theory, 15
methyltransferases (Dnmts), 432
repair, 19, 123–128
repair and human diseases of aging, 129–131
and telomere damage in aging and DNA repair pathways, 126
Dolichol, 508
Double-strand break (DSB), 125, 477
Drosophila melanogaster
aging, genetic factors in, 398–401
aging process study, 9
Sir2 (dSir2), 396
DST, *see* Disposable Soma Theory
Duchenne (DMD) muscular dystrophies, 219
Dysrhythmias, 313–316
Dysrhythmogenic Right Ventricular Dysplasia in Elderly (DRVD), 354–355

E2F transcriptional activity, 164
Electron-transfer flavoprotein (ETF), 426
Electron transport chain (ETC), 323, 392, 418
Embryonic stem (ES), 393
Emery-Dreifuss muscular dystrophy (EDMD), 220
Endogenous sex hormones and metabolic syndrome in elderly, 283–284
Endonuclease G (Endo G), 445
Endothelial cell (EC), 308, 420, 427, 444, 462
aging and oxidative stress, 160–162
centrality of dysfunction in vascular aging phenotype, 163
dysfunction, effect of glycation and age on, 152
function and remodeling, 155–162
senescence functional effects, 158–160
Endothelial-leukocyte adhesion molecule 1 (E-selectin), 325
Endothelial nitric oxide synthase (eNOS), 37, 475
Endothelial progenitor cells (EPCs), 263, 321–322, 458
Endothelin-1 (ET-1), 316
Endothelium-dependent vasodilation, 263
Enoxaparin and Thrombolysis Reperfusion for Acute Myocardial Infarction Treatment (ExTRACT), 257
Epigenetics, 432–433
Erythropoietin (EPO), 448
Estradiol (E2), 316, 318
Estrogen
genomic and post-genomic effects on vascular cells, 319
non-genomic effects, 22
Estrogen receptors (ER), 307, 310, 318–319
Eukaryotic initiation factor (eIF4G), 310
Evolutionary theories for aging, 12–14
Excision repair, 123
Exercise clinical applications, 488–489
Exertional dyspnea and HF, 210
Extracellular matrix (ECM), 418
Extracellular signal regulated kinase (ERK), 157, 449
Extracellular superoxide dismutase (ECSOD), 450
ExTRACT-TIMI 25, 257
Extrinsic cardiac aging, 34

Factor IX (FIX), 166
Familial amyloidosis, 221
Familial partial lipodystrophy (FPLD), 289
Farnesyl transferase Inhibitors (FTIs), 459
Fas-associated via death domain (FADD), 108
Fatty acid chain-length-specific dehydrogenase enzyme (VLCAD and LCAD), 228
Fatty acid metabolism mutations, 217
Fatty acid oxidation (FAO), 418, 423, 484
FGF receptors (FGFRs), 392
Fibrinolysis, 166
Fibroblast growth factor23 (Fgf23), 391
Fibrosis, 105–106
Finkel-Biskis-Jenkins osteosarcoma gene, 254
Fischer 344 (F344) rat, 419, 424, 426, 447, 461, 485–487
Fischer 344 × Brown Norway hybrid (F344 × BN) rat, 449
Fish eye disease, 242
FLICE-like (Fas-associated death domain protein-like-interleukin-1-converting enzyme- like) inhibitory protein (FLIP), 109
Fluorescein-labeled peptide nucleic acid (PNA), 89
Forkhead box O1 (Foxo1), 478
Forkhead transcription factor (FOXO), 9
Forkhead/winged helix box (FOX) gene family and DCM, 219
Formyl methionyl leucyl peptide (FMLP), 182
Frailty and aging, 210
Framingham Heart Study, stroke, 314
Frataxin homologue (frh-1), 394–395
Free radical theory of aging (FRTA), 16–18, 42

Gamma-H2AX-positive cells, 84
gata2 gene, 252
Gender
cardiovascular diseases in aging, 307–338
and pharmacogenomics, 328–329
specific CV markers, 324–329
specific effects of gene variants in aging-associated CVD, 328
Gene-longevity association studies, 4–8
Gene polymorphisms, 5
and diabetes, 293
in gender-specific age-related CVDs, 327–328
See also Gene-longevity association studies

Genes
in clinical HCM, 217
in DCM, 218
expression profiling and atherosclerosis, 251–254
Genetics of life span, 387–415
Genomic instability, 459–460
Genomics and cardiomyopathy, 216
4G/5G polymorphism and PAI-1 gene transcription, 6
GH-releasing hormone (GHRH), 50
Gi-coupled signaling pathways in heart, 47–48
Glucocorticoid action in aging, 192
Glucose-insulin-potassium (GIK), 448
Glucose transporter (GLUT) 1 protein, 324
Glutamine to histidine at amino acid 95 (Q95H), 429
Glutathione Peroxidase (GPx), 403, 421
Glycated Hemoglobin A1c (HbA1c), 325
Glycation, 117
post-transcriptional protein modification, 426–427, 482, 485, 489
See also Aging
Glycogen synthase kinase-3β (GSK-3β), 397–398
Glycosylation theory of aging, *see* Cross-linkage theory
GM-CSF receptor, 185
gm2 ganglioside activator protein, 252
Gompertz law of mortality, 20
Gompertz-Makeham law, 20
Goto-Kakizaki (GK), rat, 324
GPCR, *see* Cardiac G protein-coupled receptors
G-protein G_aq overexpression, 226
Granulocyte colony-stimulating factor (G-CSF), 456
Granulocyte colony-stimulating factor (G-CSF) therapeutic efficacy, 90
Granulocyte macrophage colony stimulating factor (GM-CSF), 182–183
Growth-factor-dependent signaling, 104
Growth factor signaling pathways, 40
Growth hormone (GH), 390, 447, 477–478
Growth hormone receptor knockout (GHR-KO), 478

Hamster model of cardiomyopathy, 114
Hamsters cardiomyopathic-prone strains, 229
Hayflick limit theories, 19
Hayflick theory, 19
Heart and Estrogen/Progestin Replacement Study (HERS), 308
Heart failure (HF), 309–313, 349, 351–352, 424, 462
atypical clinical features of, 211
clinical considerations and, 209–213
cognitive impairment and, 211
device and replacement therapy in, 212–213
disease management programs for, 212
etiologies in aged population, 210
model of triggers and cellular pathways in, 214
with normal ejection fraction (HF-NEF), 312
pathophysiologic of, 213
pharmacotherapy of, 211–212
with preserved ejection fraction (HfnlEF), 312
Heart fatty-acid binding protein (HFABP), 418
Heart muscle/cardiomyocyte-specific gene transcription studies, 80
Heart transplantation, 212–213
Heat-shock proteins (HSPs), 40, 388
Heat shock-transcription factor (HSF-1), 388
Helix-distorting DNA lesions, 125
Heme oxygenase (HO-1), 419, 450–451
Hemostatic genes, age-sensitive regulatory elements in, 168
Heparin-binding domain (HBD), 450
Hepatocyte growth factor (HGF), 447
Hereditary amyloidosis, 221
HERG potassium channel gene (LQT2), 315, 346
HFE mutations, 222
High-density lipoprotein (HDL), 430
High-density oligonucleotide arrays (HDOA), 87–88
Histone deacetylase (HDAC), 396, 432–433, 459
HMG-CoA inhibition, 255
Homeostasis model assessment of insulin resistance (HOMA), 284
Honolulu-Asia Aging Study (HAAS), 287
Hormesis and aging, 21
Hormone-IGF-1 Axis Hypothesis, 21
Hormone Replacement Therapy (HRT), 307
Human aging and aging-related diseases, molecular genetic studies, 500
Human cholinergic receptors, age-dependent alterations, 46
Human dilated cardiomyopathy (DCM), 310
Human ECs from umbilical vein (HUVECs), 72
Human extracellular superoxide dismutase (ECSOD), 76
Human genes
for nicotinamide phosphoribosyltransferase (Nampt/Visfatin), 76
polymorphisms and aortic stiffness, 153
polymorphisms and longevity, 6
Human Genome Project (HGP), 24
Human genotyping and gene analysis, advances in, 501–506
Human growth hormone (hGH), 326
Human haplotype maps (HAPMAP) databases, 503
Human hRad50-hMre11-p95 complex, 23
Human hypertension loci, 264
Human *KCNQ* genes mutations, 501
Human *PON1* and *PON2* gene polymorphisms, 245
Human segmental progeroid disorders, 130
Human umbilical vein endothelial cells (HUVECs), 254, 427
Human uncoupling protein UCP2 (hUCP2), 400
Human X-linked FIX gene, 166
Hutchinson-Gilford Progeria Syndrome (HGPS), 220, 459
3-hydroxyacyl CoA dehydrogenase *(HAD),* 419
8-hydroxydeoxy-guanosine (8OHdG), 476
4-hydroxy-2-nonenal (HNE), 115–116
Hypertension, 317–320
in elderly, 259–261
genes and candidate genes, 262–264
genetics and environmental factors in, 261–262
in Very Elderly Trial (HYVET), 261
Hypertrophic cardiomyopathy (HCM), 216, 310, 349

Hypothalamic paraventricular nucleus (PVN), 192
Hypothalamo-neurohypophysial system (HNS), 191
Hypothalamo-pituitary-adrenocortical (HPA), 191

Idiopathic DCM and gender-based differences in cardiac remodeling, 311
Idiopathic dilated cardiomyopathy (IDC), 215
Idiopathic right ventricular tachycardia (VT), 313
IGF/IGFR pathway, 72
IGF binding protein (IGFBP1), 428, 460
IIS pathway activity, 11
Immediate early response genes (IEGs), 421
Immunoglobin amyloidosis (AL), 221
I'm Not Dead Yet (INDY) gene, 400
Impaired exercise tolerance and HF, 210
Implantable cardioverter defibrillator (ICD), 212
Inactive 4E binding protein (4EBP1)/eIF4E complex, 310
Inactive X chromosome (Xi), 459
InCHIANTI study, 509
INdividual Data ANalysis of Antihypertensive (INDANA) meta-analysis, 261
Inflammation and atherosclerosis, 246–250
Inflammatory signaling, 45
Initiating pro-survival pathways, 446–447
Insertion/deletion loops (IDLs), 125
Insulin/IGF-1
  like growth factor I (IGF-I) signal response pathway, 49
  pathway in *C. elegans,* 388–390
  signaling (IIS) pathway and aging regulation, 9, 10
  signaling in eucaryotes, 390–392
  signaling tissue-specific roles, 392
Insulin-like growth factor 1 (IGF-1), 477
Insulin-like receptor (InR), 390, 392
Insulin resistance syndrome, 278
Insulin response element (IRS)-driven genes (IGFBP1), 480
Insulin signaling pathway, 22
Intercellular adhesion molecule 1 (ICAM-1), 481
Interleukin-1b (IL1b), 424
Interleukin-8 (IL-8) receptors, 183
Intermyofibrilar (IFM), 487
International Diabetes Federation (IDF), 278
Interventricular septum (IVS), 317
Intima-media thickness (IMT), 327
Invecchiare in Chianti (InCHIANTI) study, 284
I/R-Induced myocardial apoptosis, 486
Ischemia-mediated nuclear DNA degradation in postnatal cardiomyocytes, 38
Ischemia-reperfusion (I/R), 311, 331, 421
Ischemic preconditioning (IPC), 447, 462
Isoproterenol (ISO), 317, 343, 355

Janus tyrosine kinase (Jak)2-signal transducer, 184
Jun N-terminal kinase (JNK), 399

KCNQ1 potassium channel gene (LQT1), 315, 346
KCNQ potassium channel, 358–359
Kearns-Sayre (KSS) and Pearson syndromes, 128
Killer cell immunoglobulin-like receptor (KIR) expression, 187
Klotho, aging suppressor gene, 391–392, 431
Klotho protein, 51
Knock-out transgenic animal models, 77–78
Kruppel-like transcription factors (Klf), 421
Ku autoantigen (Ku), 477
Ku80 null cells, 131

lacZ reporter gene, 87, 122
Lamin A (LMNA), 459
Langendorff perfusion, 323
Late-onset HCM, 217
LCAT, *see* Cholesterol acyltransferase
Leber hereditary optic neuropathy (LHON), 504
Left ventricle ejection fraction (LVEF), 310
Left ventricular hypertrophy (LVH), 285
Left ventricular outflow tract obstruction (LVOTO) in patients with HCM, 310
Left ventricular peak developed pressure (LVPDP), 446
Left Ventricular Systolic Function (LVSF), 312
Leptin and metabolic syndrome in elderly, 284
Leucine-rich receptors RXFP1/ RXFP2, 48
Life span definition, 4
Limb girdlemuscular dystrophy (LGMD), 220
Lipid peroxides (LPO), 326, 331
Lipofuscin-like autofluorescent material, 72
Lipoprotein-associated Phospholipase A2 (Lp-PLA2), 325
Lipoprotein oxidation and modification, 244–246
Liver X receptors (LXRs), 249
LMNA
  mediated myopathies, 220
  mutations, 221
Lmna$^{N195K/N195K}$ mice, 224
Logarithm of odds (LOD), 429
Longevity, 4
LongQT Syndrome (LQTS), 315
Losartan For Endpoint reduction (LIFE), 260
Lowdensity lipoprotein (LDL), 430
Lower extremities edema and HF, 210
LV mass (LVM), 317
LV wall thickness (LVWT), 310, 317
Lysosomal rupture, 115

Macrophage colony-stimulating factor (MCSF), 247
MacrophageMAPK activation with IFN and ROS production, 185
Macrophage MHC gene expression, 185
Maillard glycation reaction, 118
Maillard reaction, *see* Glycation
Malate dehydrogenase (MDH), 426
Mammalian Sir2 homologue (SIRT1) and gluconeogenic/glycolytic pathways in liver, 478–489
Mammalian target of rapamycin (mTOR), 113
Manganese superoxide dismutase (MnSOD), 391
MAPK and NFkB signaling pathways, 22
Matrix-assisted laser desorption ionization peptide mass fingerprinting (MALD1-PMF), 425

Matrix-associated Lon protease, 113
Matrix metalloproteinase (MMP), 311
Matrix metalloproteinase-9 (MMP-9), 252
Matrix proteins rat glypican 3 (OCI-5), 166
Membrane-bound AAA proteases, 113
Membrane theory of aging, 19
Metabolic syndrome (MetSyn), 277–279
 clinical management and trials in, 281–282
 and diabetes, 294–295
 genes and, 289–291
 and oxidative stress in elderly, 284–285
 rimonabant effect on, 282
Metallothionein 1L (Mt1l), 424
Metallothionein (MT), 451
Methionine restriction (MetR), 452, 481
Methyl-methane sulphonate (MMS), 124
Methyltetrahydrofolate-reductase (MTFHR), 430
α-MHC Arg403Gln missense mutation (α-MHC403/+), 317
Microsatellite instability, 83
Microsomal triglyceride transfer protein (MTTP), 429
Mismatch repair, 123
Mitochondria
 apoptosis induced channels (MAC) activation, 40
 autophagy, 113
 calcium homeostasis and AGE/RAGE, 117
 channels, 359–360
 DNA repair, 128–129
 electron transport chain (ETC) flux, 323
 and extracellular matrix remodeling in HF, 311
 fatty acid oxidation (FAO) pathways, 228
 free matrix calcium ([Ca^{2+}]Mito), 323
 function and biogenesis, 474–475
 mediated intrinsic apoptotic pathway, 38–39
 mtDNA damage and repair, 476
 outer membrane permeabilization (MOMP), 445
 8-oxodG incision activity, 124
 related apoptosis, 41
 ROS generation, 42
 ROS production and telomere-dependent replicative senescence, 38
 trifunctional protein (MTP), 228
Mitochondrial Ca^{2+}
 channels/transporter, 360
 cycling, 361
Mitochondrial Creatine Kinase (Mi-CK), 419, 424
Mitochondrial DNA (mtDNA), 419, 452–453, 476, 481
Mitochondrial intermembrane space (IMS), 445
Mitochondrial transcription factor A gene (TFAM), 128–129, 402
Mitogen-activated protein (MAP), 449
Mitogen-activated protein kinase kinase (MAPKK), 421
Mitoquinone (MitoQ), 400
MnSOD protein expression, 452
Modern evolutionary synthesis (MES), 12
Molecular/genome mutations/deletions theory, 14–16
Monocyte chemotactic protein (MCP), 247
Mouse embryo fibroblasts (MEFs), 405, 460
Mouse models
 cardiomyopathy and HF-signaling genes, 225
 metabolic genes involved in CM and HF, 227
 premature aging model, 123
Mre11/RAD50/Nbs1 (MRN) protein complex, 127
MST-FOXO signaling pathway, 11
mtDNA deletions, 118–119
mtDNA mutations in heart, 41
mtDNA polymorphisms and aging, 6
Murine myocardial genes, 423
Muscarinic M(2)-receptors, 48
Mutant LDL receptor gene and plasma cholesterol concentrations, 7
Mutation analysis, 87–88
MYBPC3 encoding cardiac myosin binding protein-C mutations, 217
Myeloperoxidase (MPO), 480
Myocardial gene therapy, 451
Myocardial infarction (MI), 309, 349, 446, 486
Myocardial transplant/cell-type specific advantages and limitations, 91
Myocarditis, 258
Myocarditis/endocarditis in elderly, 258–259
a-Myosin heavy chain (a-MHC), 316
Myosin heavy chain (MHC) isoform expression, 34

Na^{+} /Ca^{2+} exchanger (NCX), 229
Naïve CD4^{+} T cells, 182
Nanoelectrospray ionization-tandemmass spectrometry (NSI-MS/MS), 426
National Cholesterol Education Program Adult Treatment Panel III (NCEP ATP III), 278
Nε-carboxymethyl lysine (CML), 485
Necrosis cell death, 107
Neointimal formation, aging, 425
NER pathway, 125
Neural apoptosis-regulated convertase 1 (NARC-1), 240
Neurocardiogenic syncope, 348
Neuro endocrine changes in aging, 191
Neuro-endocrine/immunological theory, 20
Neurohormonal regulation, 191
Neutrophil NADPH oxidase, 161
Neutrophil receptor signaling, 184
N(G)-Nitro-L-arginine methyl ester (L-NAME), 309
NHANES data, 259
Nitric oxide synthase (NOS), 449
NK cell activity, 185
Nonhelix-distorting DNA lesions, 124
Nonsarcomeric/non-cytoskeletal proteins and HCM-causing genes, 216
Non-ST-segment elevation myocardial infarction (NSTEMI), 256, 321
 ACS clinical trials, 257
Novel cardiac troponin T mutation (A171S), 317
NOX inhibitors diphenyleneiodonium (DPI), 161
NOX-mediated OS, 162
Nuclear corepressor (N-CoR), 249–250
Nuclear receptor co-repressor (NCoR), 319, 478
Nuclear respiratory factors (NRF), 419

Nucleophosmin (NPM), 428
Nucleotide excision repair (NER), 124
Null mutation in frataxin (FRDA), 228
Nutrition and exercise in cardiovascular aging, 471–490

Orthopnea and HF, 210
OS aging hypothesis, 118
Ovariectomized (OVX), 309, 311, 316, 318
Oxidative Damage Attenuation hypothesis, 21
Oxidative phosphorylation (OXPHOS), 111, 323
Oxidative stress (OS), 326, 390, 473–474
  induced senescence and aging, molecular and subcellular events, 18
  and ROS, 473
Oxidative Stress Profiles (JaICA-Genox OSP), 507
Oxidized LDL (oxLDL) infiltration, 244
Oxidized LDL receptor 1 *(olr1)* gene, 252
OxLDL-induced ROS formation, 246
8-oxo-2-deoxyguanosine (8oxodG), 402
oxo8dG levels in nuclear DNA, 118
Oxoguanine DNA glycosylase (OGG1), 403
Oxygen-dependent degradation (ODD), 451

Pace maker therapy, 352
Pacer therapy in elderly, 351
Parvalbumin, adenoviral construct, 461, 463
p53-dependent pathway, 158
PDGF-B induction pathway, 155–156
Peak and end of T wave (Tpe), 315
Peptide nucleic acids (PNAs), 453
Peripheral-type benzodiazepine receptors (PBRs), 445
Permeability transition (PT), 397
Peroxisomal proliferating activating receptor (PPAR), 419
Peroxisome Proliferator activated receptor g (PPARg), 396
Peroxisome Proliferator activated receptor g coactivator 1a (PGC-1a), 396
PGC-1a signaling pathway, 474
Phagocyte-type NADPH oxidase (NOX), 161
Pharmacogenomics
  and gender, 328–329
  nutrigenomics, 523–524
  supplements, new directions, 484–485
Phenyl-4,5-dimethylthazolium chloride (ALT-711), 117
Phenylephrine (PE), 317, 340
Phosphatidylinositol 3-kinase-I (PI3K-I)/PKB, 113
Phosphatidylinositol 3-OH kinase (PI3-K), 388
Phosphatidylinositol 3, 4, 5-trisphosphate (PIP3), 388
Phosphofructokinase (PFK), 418, 423
Phospholipase A(2), 325
PI3K/Akt pathway in mediating TERT induction by estrogen, 37
p16INK4a expression, 41
Pituitary proopiomelanocortin (POMC), 192
PKC-ε translocation inhibitor peptide (PKC-ε-TIP), 449
Plaque rupture and acute coronary syndromes (ACS) and MI, 250
Plasminogen activator inhibitor-1 (PAI-1), 159, 166, 321
Platelet-activating factor (PAF), 244
Platelet-derived growth factor-AB (PDGF-AB), 449
Podospora anserine, aging process study, 8
Poly(ADP-ribose) polymerase 1 (PARP-1), 406
Polycystic ovarian syndrome (PCOS), 321
Polymorphonuclear neutrophilic leukocytes (PMN), 182
PON-1 gene, 190
Population aging, 24–25
Porcine model of chronically instrumented pigs, 113–114
Potassium channel opener (KCO), 448
Pravastatin in elderly at risk (PROSPER), 325
Premature aging syndromes and progeria models, 404–406
Progeria cells and G608G LMNA mutation, 459
Proliferating cell nuclear antigen (PCNA), 404
Prolonged heart rate corrected QT and sudden death, 346–350
Prostaglandin E2 (PGE2), 480
G-protein coupled receptor (GPCR), 399
Protein C receptor *(procr)* gene, 252
Protein kinase C (PKC), 318, 449
Protein kinase D (PKD), 451
GProtein mediated signal transduction, 46
Protein restricted (PR), 481
Protein sulfhydryls oxidation in aged tissues, 116–117
p66Shc gene, 41, 401–402, 407, 431
Pyruvate dehydrogenase kinase4 (pdk4), 420

RAAS, *see* Angiotensin-aldosterone system
Rate control versus electrical cardioversion (RACE), 314
Rb and p53 tumor suppressor proteins, 24
Reactive fibrosis, 105
Reactive oxygen species (ROS), 462
C-reactive protein (hs-CRP), 321, 324–325
Receptor for AGE (RAGE), 117
Receptors for activated C kinase (RACKs), 46
Recombinant adeno-associated virus (rAAV), 450
Recombinational repair (RER), 123
Regulatory sulfonylurea receptors (SUR), 364
Relaxin family peptide (RXFP) receptors, 48
Reliability theory, 19–20
Renin-angiotensin-aldosterone system (RAAS), 310
Replication Protein A (RPA), 404
Resistin, 327
Restrictive cardiomyopathy (RCM), 216, 221–222
Reversing cardiovascular and cardiac aging damage, primary targets in, 444–459
RIO programme, 281
RNA-mediated interference (RNAi), 387
RNA polymerase II (RNAP II) complex, 129
ROS generation, antioxidant response and signaling, 112
ROS-mediated oxidative damage lipids and proteins in aging heart, 111

Sarcoplasmic reticulum (SR) function, 34
Sarcoplasmic reticulum Ca^{2+}-ATPase (SERCA2), 419
SCN5A sodium channel gene (LQT3), 315, 346
Segmental progeroid syndromes, 129

E-selectin/atherosclerosis, 325–326
Selective Estrogen Receptor Modulators (SERMs), 307
Senescence-associated
gene products, 41
nuclear protein, p16ink4a expression, 215
Senescence signaling pathways, 158
Senescent heart, nitration in, 116
SERCA protein, 49, 75
Sex Hormone Binding Globulin (SHBG), 283, 316
Signal transducer and activator of transcription 3 (STAT3), 226
Silencing mediator of retinoid and thyroid hormone receptors (SMRT), 478
Silent information regulator (SIR), 395
Single nucleotide polymorphism (SNP), 315, 339, 349
Single-strand (SSBs) and double-strand breaks (DSBs) in DNA analysis, 83
Single telomere length analysis (STELA), 89
Sinoatrial Node Dysfunction (SND), 342–343
Sinus node dysfunction, 348
SIRT1 overexpression, 480
Sirtuins, 395–396, 433, 475, 478
Skeletal muscle aging, 194–196
Skeletal muscle protein degradation and synthesis in aging, 197
Small ubiquitin-like modifiers (SUMO), 249–250
SMC markers of in aging and aging-related diseases, 165–166
Smooth muscle cell (SMC), 308, 319, 425
Sodium-hydrogen exchanger (NHE), 449
Specific molecular mechanism (s), 307
Spontaneously hypertensive rats (SHR), 309, 316
SR Ca^{2+-}ATPase (SERCA), 312
STAT5 signaling pathway, 184
Sterol regulatory element binding protein (SREBPs), 289, 478
Stress-induced premature senescence (SIPS), 157
Stress-responsive Jun-N-terminal kinase (JNK) pathway, 11
ST-segment elevation myocardial infarction (STEMI) in, 21, 256
Subsarcolemmal (SSM), 487
Superoxide dismutase (Sod) overexpression, 17, 421
Syncope/Tilt test, 350–351
Syndrome X, 278
System biology, 513–516
Systemic hypertension, 209
Systolic Blood Pressure (SBP), 431
Systolic shortening (SS), 446

Tachycardia, 348
Tangier disease (TD), 241
Taq1B polymorphism, 243
Targeted therapies in cardiac aging, 444
Targeting sarcomere and SR, 461
Target of Rapamycin (TOR), 113, 397–398
Target of Rapamycin (TOR) pathway, 21
Telomerase (TERC), 405, 428, 446, 457–459
and cell proliferation, 36
dependent/telomerase-independent DNA repair pathways, 23
Telomerase reverse transcriptase (TERT), 15, 36
Telomerase RNA component (Terc), 36
Telomeres
analysis, 88–89
and CV aging, 35–37
independent pathway, 157
length and cardiovascular disease (CVD), 36
repeat-binding factor (TRF2), 36–37
structure with associated proteins, 133
and telomerase in human and animal's models with cardiovascular disease (CVD), 39
and telomere-related proteins, 131–134
Testosterone (T), 308, 316, 321
Thrombolysis in Myocardial Infarction (TIMI) 25 study, 257
Thrombosis and acute coronary syndromes (ACS) and MI, 250
Thromboxane A2 (TXA2), 480
Thromboxane A2 and endothelin-1, 159
Thyroid hormone (TH), 420, 487
Thyroid hormone response element (TRE), 487
Thyroid receptor (TR), 487
Tissue engineering, 91–92
Tissue inhibitor of metalloproteinases (TIMPs) in aged cells, 163, 421
Tissue-specific and cardiovascular-specific transcriptional and proteomic profiling of CR, 472–473
Tissue-type plasminogen activator (tPA), 488
TNFa-converting enzyme (TACE), 425
Toll-like receptors (TLRs), 184
Torsades de pointes (TdP), 315
Transcriptional gene profiling, 418–428
Transcription-coupled repair pathway (TCR), 125
Transferase-mediated dUTP nick end labeling (TUNEL), 107
Transferrin (TRFE), 428
Translational targets, 443–470
Transmural dispersion of ventricular repolarization (TDR), 315
Tricarboxylic acid (TCA), 426
Trichothiodystrophy (TTD), 131, 460
3,3'-Triiodothyronine (T3), 488
Truncated allele of troponin T (TnT-trunc), 317
TTR mutation, 222
Tuberous sclerosis complex genes 1 and 2 (dTsc1, dTsc2), 397
TUNEL-positive cardiomyocytes, 109

Ubiquitin-like proteins, 113
Uncoupling protein (UCP3), 418, 420
Unstable angina (UA), 321, 325
Upstream activating sequence (UAS), 400
UracilDNA glycosylase (UNG), 453
USA's National Institute of Aging (NIA), 34

Vascular (Ea), 312
Vascular adhesion molecule-1 (VCAM-1), 481

Vascular SMC senescence mechanisms and significance, 164–165
Vectors for gene transfer and expression comparison, 75
Ventricular diastolic (Ed), 312
Ventricular fibrillation (VF), 354
Ventricular systolic (Ees), 312
Ventricular tachycardia (VT), 353
Voltage-dependent anion channel (VDAC), 426
Voltage-gated Ca^{2+} channel structure, 358

Warfarin, anticoagulant, 314
Wear-and Tear-theories, 16–19
Werner and Hutchinson-Gilford Progeria syndromes, 159–160
Werner syndrome (WS), 23, 129, 404–406
Werner syndrome protein (WRN), 85
Women's Health Initiative (WHI), 308
Women's Ischemia Syndrome Evaluation (WISE), 320–321
WRN helicase protein, 126

Xenohydrolases, hydrolytic microbial enzymes, 456
Xeroderma pigmentosum human disease, 125, 460
X-linked defect GLA gene, 217
X-linked inhibitor of apoptosis (XIAP), 110

Yeast mother cells life span and *SIR* genes, 9, 10